W9-BRD-296

DIAGNOSIS OF BONE AND JOINT DISORDERS

VOLUME 1

Donald Resnick, M.D.

Chief,
Department of Radiology
Veterans Administration Medical Center
San Diego, California
and
Professor of Radiology
Department of Radiology
University of California, San Diego
San Diego, California

Gen Niwayama, M.D., D.Med.Sc.

Director, Autopsy Division
Department of Pathology
Brotman Medical Center
Culver City, California
and
Associate Clinical Professor
Department of Pathology
School of Medicine
University of California, Los Angeles

With Emphasis on Articular Abnormalities

1981

W.B. SAUNDERS COMPANY Philadelphia • London • Toronto

W. B. Saunders Company: West Washington Square
Philadelphia, PA 19105

1 St. Anne's Road
Eastbourne, East Sussex BN21 3UN, England

1 Goldthorne Avenue
Toronto, Ontario M8Z 5T9, Canada

Library of Congress Cataloging in Publication Data

Resnick, Donald.

Diagnosis of bone and joint disorders.

1. Joints — Diseases — Diagnosis. 2. Joints — Radiography. 3. Bones — Radiography. 4. Bones — Diseases — Diagnosis. I. Niwayama, Gen, joint author. II. Title. [DNLM: 1. Bone diseases — Diagnosis. 2. Joint diseases — Diagnosis. 3. Joints — Abnormalities. R43d] RC932.R46 616.7′1′075
79-3791 ISBN 0-7216-7561-1

Diagnosis of Bone and Joint Disorders

ISBN 0-7216-7561-1 Volume 1
ISBN 0-7216-7562-X Volume 2
ISBN 0-7216-7563-8 Volume 3
ISBN 0-7216-7564-6 Set

Last digit is the print number: 9 8 7 6 5 4 3 2 1

To my father, Benjamin Resnick, M.D., who illuminated my first viewbox and with it, my mind, and to my mother.

D.R.

and

To my parents, teachers, Sumiko, Eriko, and Akira.

G.N.

CONTRIBUTORS

ROGER J. ADAMS, D.M.D., M.S.
Formerly Assistant Professor of Radiology and Pathology, Schools of Medicine and Dental Medicine, Washington University, St. Louis, Missouri; Resident in Oral Surgery, Mayo Graduate School of Medicine, Rochester, Minnesota
The Temporomandibular Joint

WAYNE H. AKESON, M.D.
Professor and Chief, Division of Orthopaedics and Rehabilitation, University of California Medical Center, San Diego, California
Articular Cartilage Physiology and Metabolism

NAOMI ALAZRAKI, M.D.
Associate Professor of Radiology, University of California Medical School, San Diego; Chief, Nuclear Medicine Service, Veterans Administration Medical Center, San Diego, California
Bone Imaging by Radionuclide Techniques

RODNEY BLUESTONE, M.B., F.R.C.P.
Clinical Professor of Medicine, University of California, Los Angeles, School of Medicine; Associate Attending Physician, Cedars-Sinai Medical Center, Los Angeles, California
Symptoms and Signs of Articular Disease; Laboratory Signs of Articular Disease

JOHN A. BONAVITA, M.D.
Assistant Professor of Radiology, University of Pennsylvania School of Medicine, Philadelphia; Director of Emergency Radiology, Section of Orthopedic Radiology, Hospital of the University of Pennsylvania, Philadelphia, Pennsylvania
Radiation Changes

JOSEPH J. BOOKSTEIN, M.D.
Professor of Radiology, University of California Medical School, San Diego; Chief of Vascular Radiology, University of California Medical Center and Veterans Administration Hospital; Consulting Angiographer, Naval Regional Medical Center, San Diego, California
Angiography of Articular and Para-Articular Disease

MARC N. COEL, M.D.
Formerly Associate Professor, University of California Medical School, San Diego, California; Staff Physician, The Queen's Medical Center, Honolulu, Hawaii
Imaging Modalities in Intraspinal Disorders

MURRAY K. DALINKA, M.D.
Professor of Radiology and Orthopedics, University of Pennsylvania School of Medicine, Philadelphia; Section Chief, Orthopedic Radiology, Hospital of the University of Pennsylvania, Philadelphia, Pennsylvania
Radiation Changes

DAVID S. FEIGIN, M.D.
Assistant Professor of Radiology, University of California Medical School, San Diego; Chief, Chest Radiology, Veterans Administration Medical Center; Attending Radiologist, University of California Medical Center, San Diego, California
General Organ Systems

FRIEDA FELDMAN, M.D., F.A.C.R.
Professor of Radiology, Columbia University College of Physicians and Surgeons, New York; Attending Radiologist, Columbia-Presbyterian Medical Center, New York, New York
Tuberous Sclerosis, Neurofibromatosis, and Fibrous Dysplasia

ERICH FISCHER, M.D.
Professor of Radiology, University of Tübingen; Department of Radiology, Robert-Bosch-Krankenhaus, Stuttgart, Federal Republic of Germany
Low Kilovolt Radiography

HARRY K. GENANT, M.D.
Professor of Radiology and Chief of Skeletal Section, Department of Radiology, University of California, San Francisco; Consultant Radiologist, Letterman General Hospital, Veterans Administration Medical Center, San Francisco; Veterans Administration Hospital, Martinez; Oakland Naval Hospital, Oakland, California
Magnification Radiography; Xeroradiography; Computed Tomography; Quantitative Bone Mineral Analyses

DAVID H. GERSHUNI, M.D., F.R.C.S.
Assistant Professor of Orthopaedics, University of California Medical Center, San Diego; Chief of Orthopaedics, Veterans Administration Medical Center, San Diego, California
Articular Cartilage Physiology and Metabolism

THOMAS GOERGEN, M.D.
Assistant Clinical Professor of Radiology, University of California Medical School, San Diego; Attending Radiologist, Pomerado Hospital, Poway, California
Radiographic Evaluation of the Postoperative Patient

AMY BETH GOLDMAN, M.D.
Associate Professor, Cornell University Medical College, New York; Attending Radiologist, Hospital for Special Surgery and New York Hospital, New York, New York
Collagen Disease, Epiphyseal Dysplasias, and Related Conditions

THEODORE E. KEATS, M.D.
Professor of Radiology and Chairman, Department of Radiology, University of Virginia School of Medicine, Charlottesville; Attending Radiologist, University of Virginia Hospital, Charlottesville, Virginia
Normal Variants and Artifacts

JOEL E. LICHTENSTEIN, M.D.
Assistant Professor of Radiology, Uniformed Services University of the Health Sciences, Bethesda, Maryland; Chief, Division of Diagnostic Radiologic Pathology, Armed Forces Institute of Pathology, Washington, D.C.
General Organ Systems

JOHN E. MADEWELL, M.D.
Associate Professor, Department of Radiology and Nuclear Medicine, Uniformed Services University of the Health Sciences, Bethesda, Maryland; Chairman and Registrar, Department of Radiologic Pathology, Armed Forces Institute of Pathology, Washington, D.C.
Tumors and Tumor-like Lesions in or About Joints; Pathogenesis of Osteonecrosis

WILLIAM A. MURPHY, M.D.
Associate Professor of Radiology, Washington University School of Medicine, St. Louis; Co-director, Musculoskeletal Section, Edward Mallinckrodt Institute of Radiology; Associate Radiologist, Barnes Hospital and Saint Louis Children's Hospital, St. Louis, Missouri
The Temporomandibular Joint

TIMOTHY R. O'BRIEN, D.V.M., Ph.D.
Professor of Radiological Sciences, School of Veterinary Medicine, University of California, Davis; Radiologist, Veterinary Medical Teaching Hospital, University of California, Davis, California
Naturally Occurring Arthropathies of Animals

JOHN A. OGDEN, M.D.
Professor of Orthopedic Surgery and Pediatrics and Director, Skeletal Growth and Development Study Unit, Yale University School of Medicine, New Haven; Chief of Orthopedics, Yale-New Haven Hospital, New Haven; Attending Physician, Newington Children's Hospital, Newington, Connecticut
Congenital Dysplasia of the Hip

NIELS C. PEDERSEN, D.V.M., Ph.D.
Associate Professor of Medicine, School of Veterinary Medicine, University of California, Davis; Clinician, Small Animal Internal Medicine, Veterinary Medical Teaching Hospital, University of California, Davis, California
Naturally Occurring Arthropathies of Animals

MICHAEL J. PITT, M.D.
Associate Professor of Radiology and Associate Professor of Orthopedic Surgery, University of Arizona College of Medicine, Arizona Health Sciences Center, Tucson, Arizona
Rickets and Osteomalacia

ROY R. POOL, D.V.M., Ph.D.
Associate Professor of Pathology, School of Veterinary Medicine, University of California, Davis; Pathologist, Veterinary Medical Teaching Hospital, University of California, Davis, California
Naturally Occurring Arthropathies of Animals

WILLIAM SCHEIBLE, M.D.
Assistant Professor of Radiology, University of California Medical School, San Diego, California
Diagnostic Ultrasound

CLEMENT B. SLEDGE, M.D.
John B. and Buckminster Brown Professor of Orthopedic Surgery, Harvard Medical School, Cambridge; Orthopedist-in-Chief, Peter Bent Brigham and Robert B. Brigham Hospitals, Boston, Massachusetts
Developmental Anatomy of Joints; Orthopedic Intervention in Articular Disease

DONALD E. SWEET, M.D.
Clinical Associate Professor of Pathology, Uniformed Services University of the Health Sciences, Bethesda, Maryland; Chairman and Registrar, Department of Orthopedic Pathology, Armed Forces Institute of Pathology, Washington, D.C.
Tumors and Tumor-like Lesions in or About Joints; Pathogenesis of Osteonecrosis

PETER S. WALKER, Ph.D.
Lecturer in Orthopedic Surgery, Harvard Medical School, Boston, Massachusetts; Director of Product Development, Howmedica, Inc., Rutherford, New Jersey
Biomechanics of Joints

PREFACE

> I profess both to learn and to teach anatomy, not from books but from dissection; not from positions of philosophers but from the fabric of nature.
>
> William Harvey (1587-1657)
> De Motu Cordis et Sanguinis (1628)
>
> An Anatomical Disquisition on the Motion of the Heart and Blood in Animals, translated from the Latin by Robert Willis (1847)

The roentgenographic features of many common and some not so common musculoskeletal disorders, particularly those that affect articulations, can be explained by closely correlating the radiographic, gross pathologic, and histologic abnormalities. Although this technique is not new, it is seldom applied to the evaluation of skeletal diseases. When radiographic and pathologic correlation was utilized in the past to analyze these diseases, the discussion generally centered upon primary bone neoplasms, which, although important, are rare occurrences indeed. The common "everyday" disorders have, in large part, been neglected, requiring the student of radiology to memorize lists of roentgenographic signs and differential diagnoses without regard to disease mechanisms and pathogeneses. Yet, the radiograph is but a mirror, and its image a reflection of the underlying anatomy and pathology. When the student is armed with an understanding of the basic pathologic aberrations of disease, perception of the "image" takes on new meaning.

There are several reasons why correlation of radiology and pathology is infrequently encountered in descriptions of many musculoskeletal diseases. Such studies require the close cooperation of two interested parties, a radiologist and a pathologist. For the radiologist, the development and the refinement of newer and more sophisticated diagnostic modalities, such as ultrasonography and computed tomography, have led to some degree of complacency and disinterest in the older and more established techniques of plain film radiography and standard tomography. The radiographic information presented by routine examination of the skeleton no longer evokes the excitement it once did, particularly when compared to the enthusiasm that accompanies an unusual sectional display on ultrasound or computed tomographic examination. For the pathologist, skillful and meticulous postmortem and surgical pathologic examinations have been neglected, in many institutions, in favor of histologic studies and complicated chemical analyses. Some regard anatomic pathology as "descriptive" in nature, static, and of little importance. Nothing is farther from the truth.

The difficulty in obtaining adequate pathologic material is another reason for the infrequency of close radiographic and pathologic correlation in musculoskeletal disorders. The energetic investigator, however, can find several sources of such material. First, tissues can be obtained at postmortem examination. Although there is a general reluctance to remove large samples of bones and joints during autopsy, portions of the spine, sacroiliac articulations, symphysis pubis, sternum, sternoclavicular and acromioclavicular joints, and ribs can be examined in detail without deforming the body in any fashion. In certain situations, special permission to allow more extensive skeletal examination can be obtained, although this may require knowledge of the presence in a hospital of patients who are seriously ill and personal interviews with these individuals or their immediate family members. A second source of material is derived from surgical specimens. In many institutions, osseous and articular specimens are examined superficially, yet material obtained from total joint replacements, biopsy procedures, and amputations can shed light on many common and important disorders. A third source of pathologic material is the anatomy department of nearby medical centers. Body donation programs exist in many such departments, and careful analysis of donated cadavers can uncover various musculoskeletal diseases. Body donation programs may also be associated with local chapters of organizations such as the Arthritis Foundation.

Once the material has been collected, meticulous radiographic and pathologic study is mandatory. We have routinely obtained radiographs and photographs of all intact specimens. Subsequently, tissue freezing with sectioning followed by radiographic and pathologic evaluation, or tissue maceration followed by similar evaluation, is useful. Histologic material can then be obtained from appropriate tissue sections.

This textbook utilizes such radiographic and pathologic correlation, wherever possible, in a variety of musculoskeletal disorders. Although the original intent of the authors was to discuss only "articular" problems, it soon became apparent that any discussion of joint diseases that did not encompass alterations of neighboring bones and soft tissue was incomplete. Thus, the scope of the textbook has been expanded to cover additional local and systemic disease processes, although in all cases articular findings are emphasized. The major portion of the discussion is directed toward radiographic and pathologic features that aid in accurate diagnosis, although some attention is focused upon major clinical and laboratory alterations. The methods and goals of therapy of the various diseases are not included, as these are given in other available sources.

The organization of the material appears quite logical. Initially, developmental and comparative anatomy, physiology, biochemistry, and biomechanics of articulations are studied. This discussion of the basic sciences is followed by an evaluation of the role of available radiographic and related modalities in the diagnosis of musculoskeletal diseases, of normal anatomic variants and artifacts that simulate disease, and of methods of classification of articular disorders. Subsequently, four chapters summarize the principles of medical and surgical examination in patients with articular diseases and of radiographic evaluation of the postoperative patient. In the remaining portions of the text, individual musculoskeletal disorders are evaluated. These are grouped into specific categories, although we recognize that some disagreement might exist regarding the manner in which the diseases are divided. In the final chapters, additional sites of abnormality are discussed, including the temporomandibular joint, soft tissues, and other organ systems. A summary of the patterns of distribution of articular abnormalities is included. Four appendixes consider additional diagnostic and investigative modalities. By design, some degree of overlap in discussion appears in certain segments of the book to provide emphasis.

The choice of contributing authors was made carefully and deliberately. Each is a recognized authority in the field of musculoskeletal disease and most are well known for their interest in the area of radiographic-pathologic correlation. Although the writing style of one author might differ from that of another, these differences are minimal, and the terminology that is utilized is remarkably consistent throughout the textbook. Furthermore, great care has been exercised in the choice and in the preparation of the illustrations. When necessary, color photographs are used, and the orientation of the radiographic and pathologic material is such to facilitate correlation of the findings. A conscious effort has also been made to arrange many of the radiographs and photographs throughout the textbook in such a fashion that it appears that the same side of the body has been examined. This technique will enable comparison of disease processes discussed in different sections of the book. An extensive and up-to-date bibliography is included for those who might wish to consult pertinent references for additional information. Each reference has been carefully verified in the final stages of preparation to assure accuracy.

In conclusion, creation of this text has indeed been a labor of love. We sincerely hope that it will bring an equal amount of enjoyment to those who read it.

D. Resnick, M.D.
G. Niwayama, M.D.

ACKNOWLEDGMENTS

Without the help of many people, this book would have remained an idea and nothing more. We would like to take this opportunity to thank some of these people. To each of the contributors to this text, we are indeed indebted. They approached their task not in a perfunctory fashion but with a genuine interest in organizing and teaching a specific subject, and the first-rate manuscripts that they produced testify to this fact. Numerous other individuals contributed illustrations. We would especially like to thank the following physicians who were kind enough to let us use some of their case material: Kaneyoshi Akazaki, Alan Altman, Akbar Bonakdarpour, Jack Bowerman, E. G. L. Bywaters, Clifford W. Colwell, Jr., W. Peter Cockshott, F. Richard Convery, Larry Danzig, David Edwards, George Ehrlich, Robert Freiberger, Richard Gelberman, Richard Gold, Guerdon Greenway, John Joyce III, Jeremy Kaye, Sidney Madden, Jerrold Mink, Alex Norman, Mike Ozonoff, Victor Rosen, Ronald Saldino, H. Ralph Schumacher, Jr., Robert Shapiro, Frederick Silverman, Richard Smith, Kornel Terplan, Alvin Turken, James Usselman, Vinton Vint, John Weston, and Nathan Zvaifler. To two individuals we are particularly indebted for innumerable illustrations: Drs. Anne Brower and Murray Dalinka. Whatever the disease, no matter how exotic or rare, we could almost be certain that one or both of these people would have an example and would share it with us. We should also like to express our appreciation to Thomas E. Callear and Alice R. Russell of Eastman Kodak Company for providing us with exquisite material from previous issues of Medical Radiography and Photography, and to the late Dr. Henry Jaffe and to Lea & Febiger, Publishers, for supplying many original illustrations from Dr. Jaffe's inspiring work, *Metabolic, Degenerative, and Inflammatory Diseases of Bones and Joints*. This work, more than any other, provided the foundation upon which our ideas took shape.

A text of this length requires an extraordinary amount of typing, yet in large part, two individuals, Elizabeth O'Brien and Sallie Rostad, managed to avoid backache and boredom in struggling through more than 15,000 pages of manuscript. To these two people, we can offer only our admiration and our thanks, although this hardly seems sufficient.

To Kurt Smolen and Janet Julien, who contributed the excellent art work, to Sydney Sandoz, David Sandoz, Sue Brown, and Robert Turner, for the photography, and to Debbie Trudell, Peggy Gorball, Mary Gonsalves, John Sykes, and Clark Neal for providing specimens for gross pathology and histology, we again offer our sincere appreciation. We would also like to thank Judith Dodson for checking the accuracy of each of the references in an extensive bibliography; Rose Tyson and Liz Alcauskas and the San Diego Museum of Man for allowing us to photograph and radiograph a portion of the museum's remarkable skeletal collection; and the Picker and Pfizer Corporations for their assistance during the last five years.

Finally we would like to express great appreciation to those individuals at the W. B. Saunders Company who guided and even cajoled us during the preparation of this text: to Lisette Bralow, the tireless editor, to Catherine Fix, the talented copyeditor, and to Herbert Powell, the meticulous production manager, we are indeed indebted.

CONTENTS

Section VIII DEGENERATIVE DISEASE

Section IX CRYSTAL-INDUCED AND RELATED DISEASES

Section X METABOLIC DISEASES

Section XI ENDOCRINE DISEASES

PROLOGUE

BONE AS A HISTORIC MARKER OF DISEASE

by Donald Resnick, M.D.

Paleopathology represents the study of pathologic conditions in fossil organisms. When this study is directed at the skeletal remains from ancient human populations, the results of the investigation provide documentation of the antiquity of a certain disorder and information regarding its natural course.

The paleopathologic specimens illustrated in the following pages belong to the San Diego Museum of Man and, in large part, were collected in the mountains and coastal regions of Peru in 1913 by Dr. Ales Hrdlicka for exhibition at the Panama-California Exposition of 1915.* Dr. Hrdlicka visited more than 20 Peruvian burial sites and was quickly able to obtain an enormous collection because local grave robbers, in searching for pottery and precious metals, had exposed and scattered the bones, leaving the ground littered with skeletal remains. As Hrdlicka remarked, "The place looked like a veritable Golgotha, or some great barbaric battlefield, with skulls and bones whitening the ground and ruins in every direction." He gathered all the well-preserved crania and other bones and, with the permission of the Peruvian government, transferred them to Lima and, from there, to the United States.

The results of Hrdlicka's expedition(s) to Peru represent one of the most important anthropology collections in the United States despite the fact that the exploration was limited to those specimens that lay exposed on the ground. Although it was difficult to determine the age of many of the burial grounds and thus precisely place the recovered material in a historical timetable, a large majority of the specimens are almost certainly pre-Columbian. The pathologic conditions evident in the collection appeared diverse in nature and variable in severity and, as Hrdlicka noted, included "symmetrical osteoporosis of the skull, in infancy and early childhood; a strange progressive arthritic process affecting the head of the femur and the cotyloid cavity in the adult or rarely the adolescent called here from its most characteristic feature the 'mushroom head' femur (arthritis deformans); and characteristic exostoses in the distal part of the auditory meatus, tending towards its occlusion. There was a great scarcity of fractures, but on the other hand there were everywhere numerous traumatic lesions of the skull, showing fighting and perhaps executions."

The illustrations on the following pages (Figs. 1 to 25) serve to emphasize man's chronic battle against the ravages of skeletal disease. Although it is not possible to verify specific diagnoses, disease states suggested by the gross pathologic and radiologic findings are indicated, and, in many cases, similarities of the ancient and modern responses of bones and joints to insult are apparent.

*Additional material in the museum's collection was recovered during the excavation of Paa-Ko (also known locally as San Pedro), an Indian village in north central New Mexico during the years 1935 to 1937.

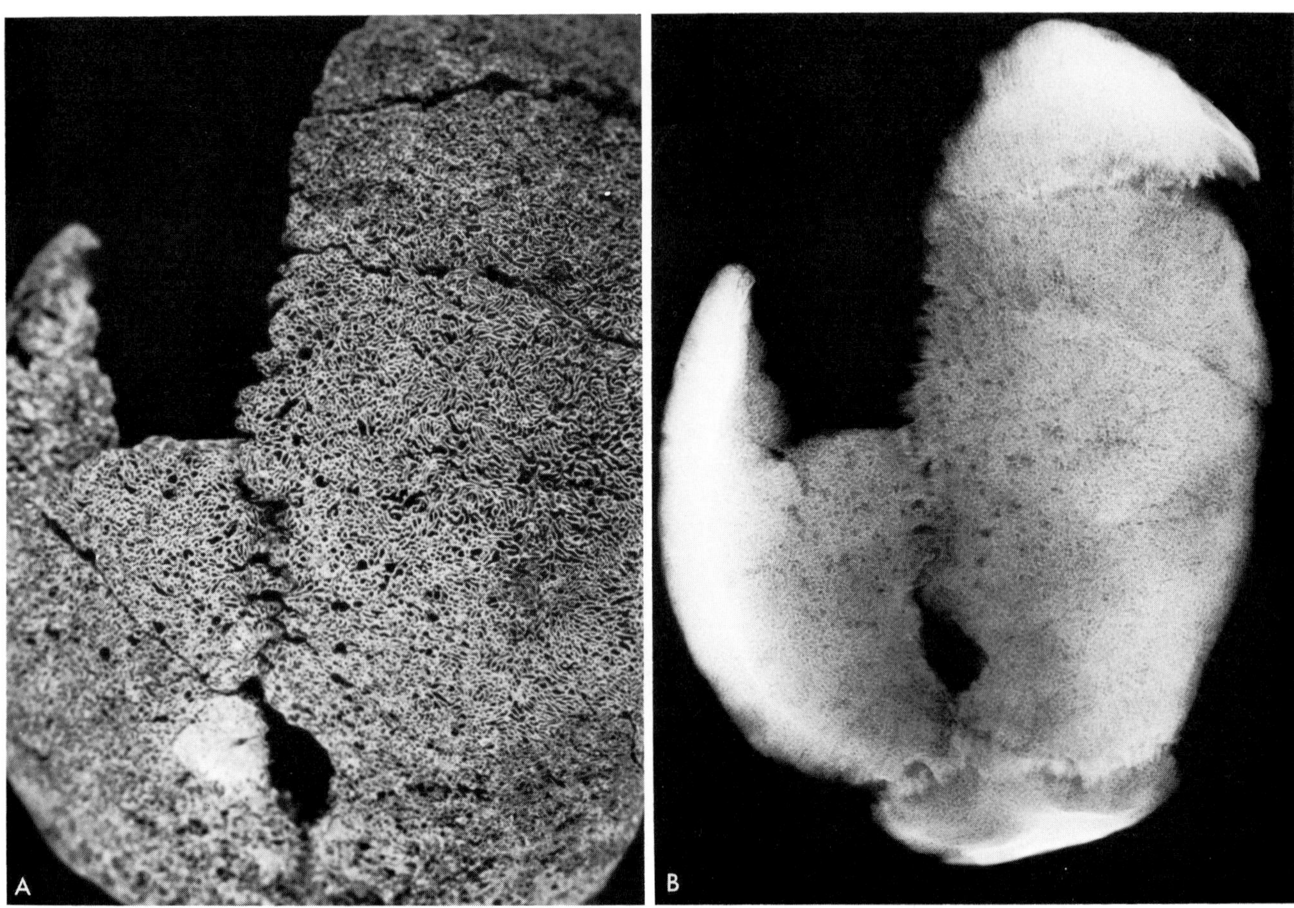

Figure 1.

Object: Partial calvarium.

Source: Panama-California Exposition.

Date of Receipt: 1915.

Date or Period of Specimen: Prehistoric.

Diagnosis: Porotic hyperostosis — related to anemia.

Remarks: Findings include widening of the diploic space due to overgrowth of the bone marrow, coarsening of the trabecular pattern, and a "hair-on-end" appearance.

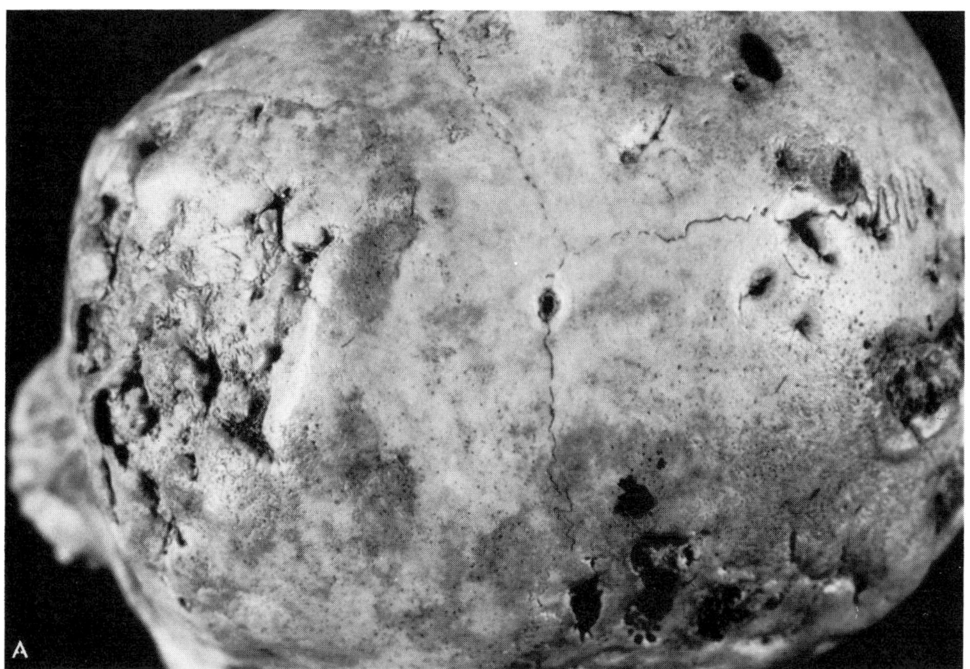

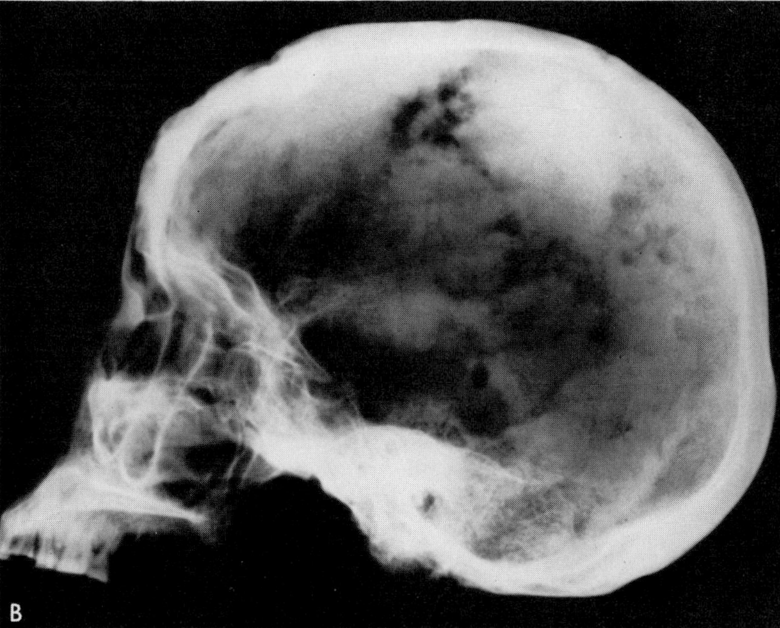

Figure 2.
Object: *Calvarium.*
Source: *Panama-California Exposition.*
Date of Receipt: *1915.*
Date or Period of Specimen: *Modern.*
Diagnosis: Osteomyelitis, possibly syphilis.
Remarks: *Bony destruction is evident throughout the skull but is most prominent in the frontal region.*

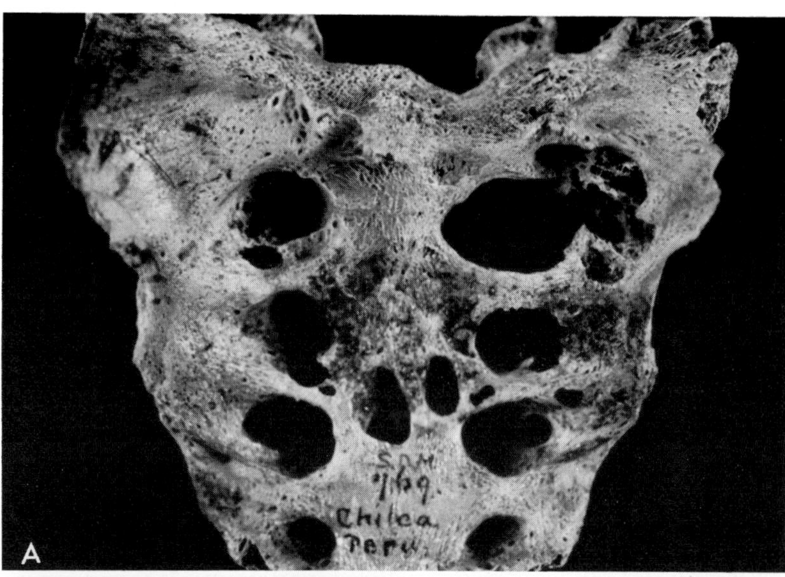

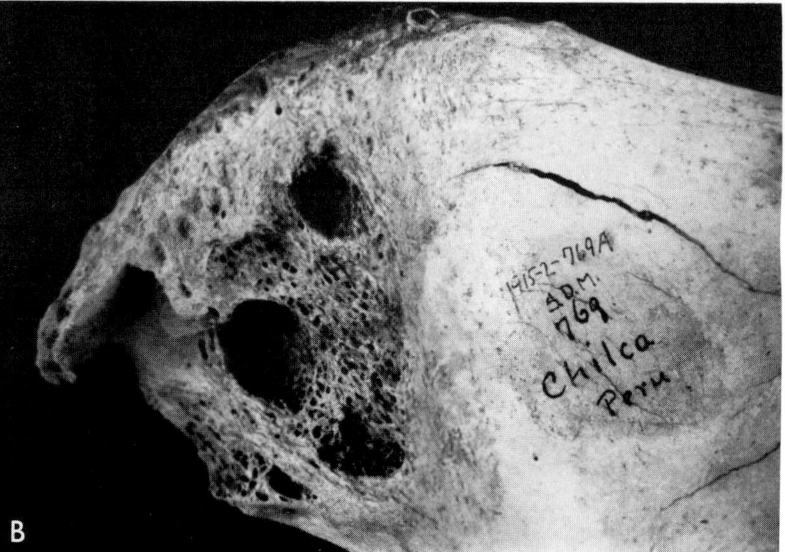

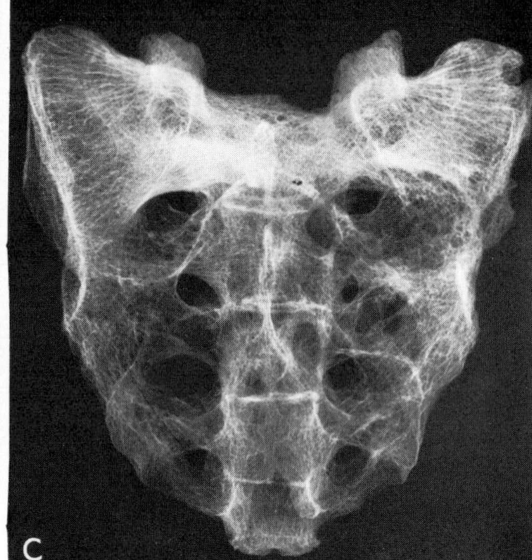

Figure 3.

Object: Sacrum and left ilium.

Source: Panama-California Exposition.

Date of Receipt: 1915.

Date or Period of Specimen: Post-Columbian (?).

Diagnosis: Osteomyelitis and septic arthritis, possibly tuberculosis.

Remarks: osseous destruction involves the central sacrum and para-articular region about the left sacroiliac joint.

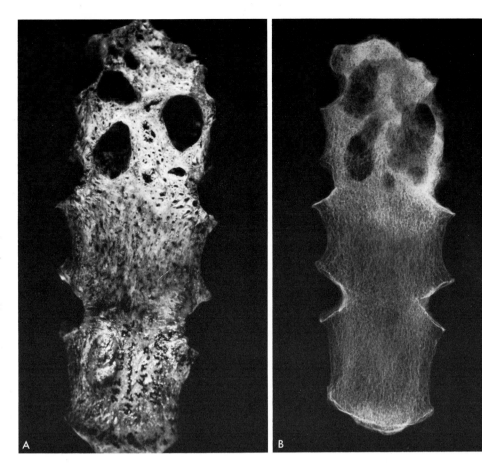

Figure 4.

Object: Sternum.

Source: Panama-California Exposition.

Date of Receipt: 1915.

Date or Period of Specimen: Historic.

Diagnosis: Osteomyelitis, possibly tuberculosis.

Remarks: Several circular lytic lesions of the sternum are surrounded by reactive sclerosis. Infection is the most likely diagnosis, although the exact agent responsible for the changes cannot be determined.

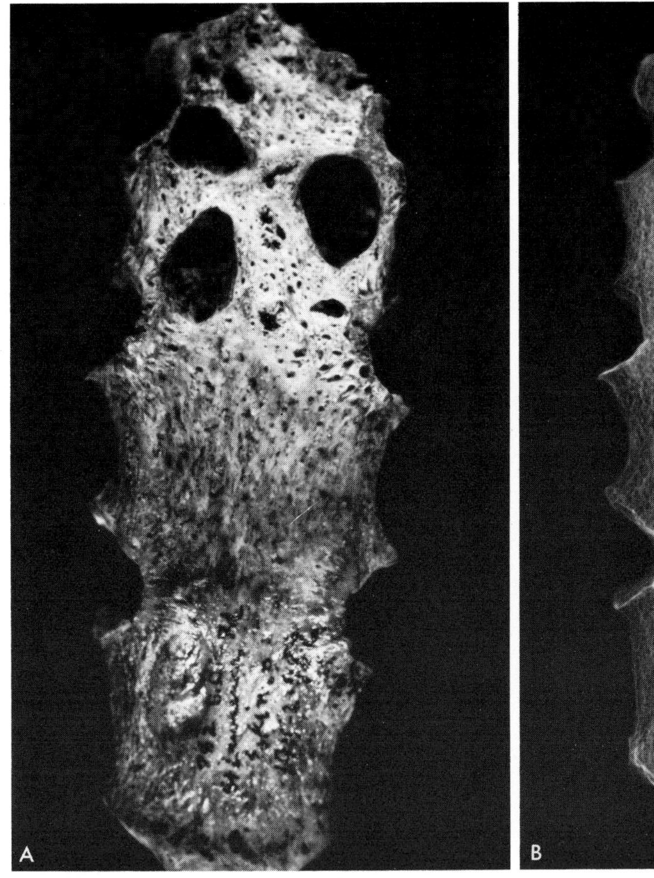

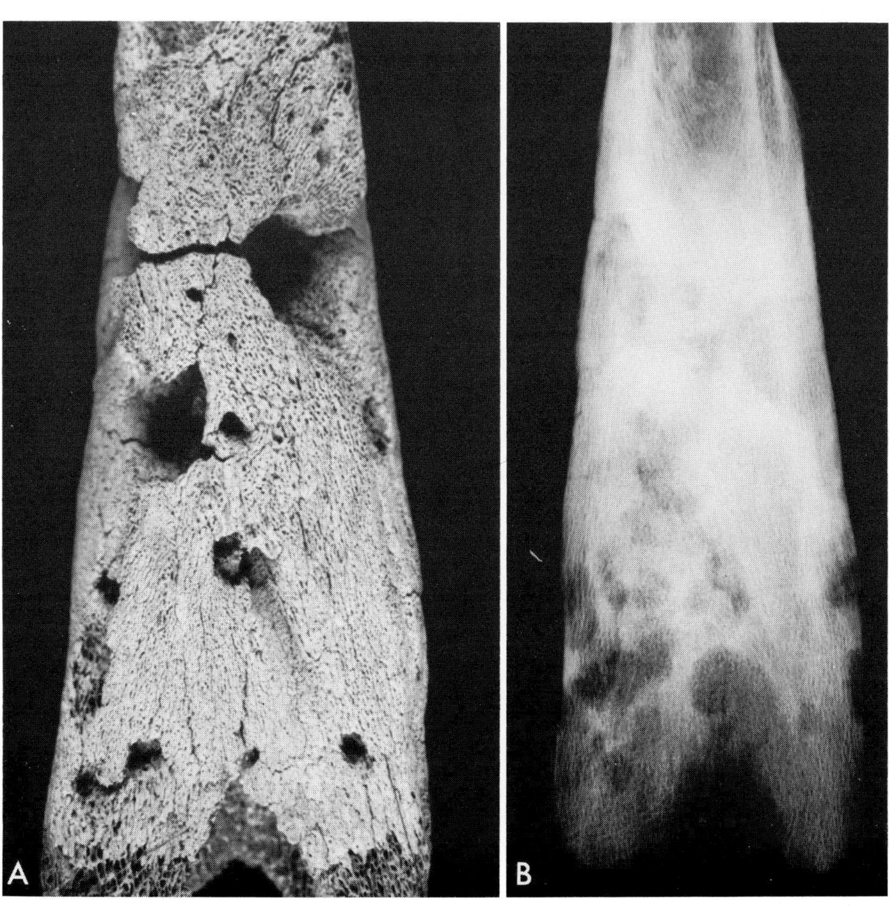

Figure 5.

Object: Femur.

Source: Panama-California Exposition.

Date of Receipt: 1915.

Date or Period of Specimen: Prehistoric.

Diagnosis: Osteomyelitis.

Remarks: Findings include bone destruction with reactive sclerosis, involucrum formation, and possible sequestra.

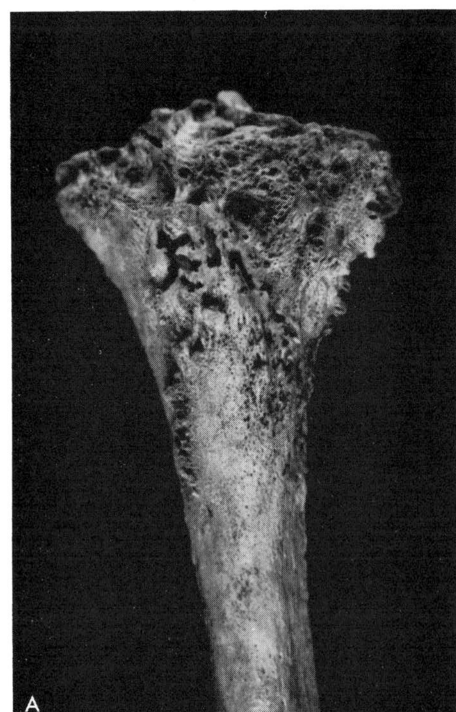

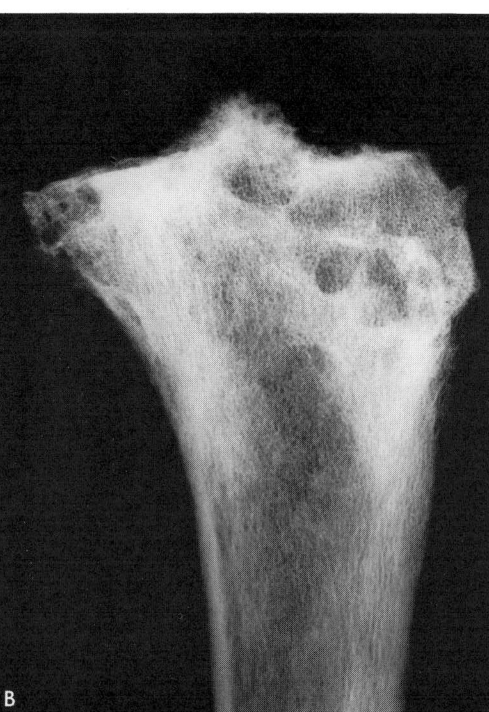

Figure 6.

Object: Tibia.

Source: Panama-California Exposition.

Date of Receipt: 1915.

Date or Period of Specimen: Historic.

Diagnosis: Osteomyelitis and septic arthritis.

Remarks: Observe the destruction of the proximal tibia with irregularity of articular bone.

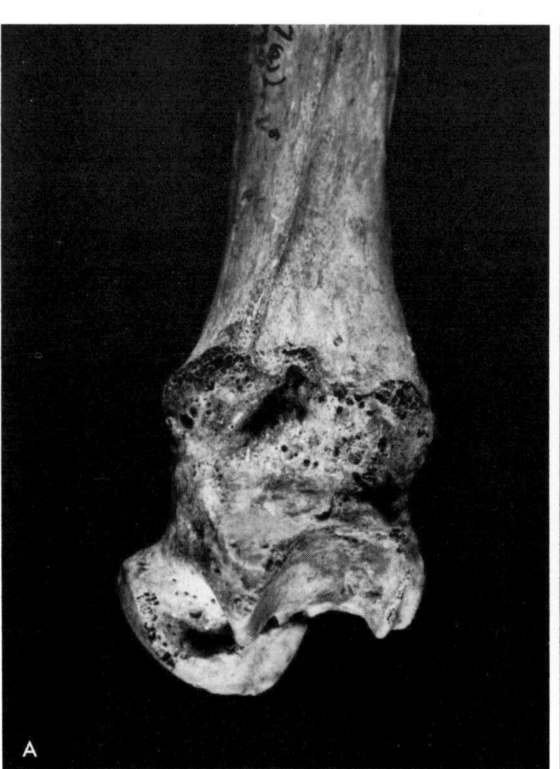

Figure 7.

Object: Tibia and talus.

Source: Panama-California Exposition.

Date of Receipt: 1915.

Date or Period of Specimen: Prehistoric.

Diagnosis: Osteomyelitis and septic arthritis.

Remarks: Complete intra-articular bony ankylosis between distal tibia and talus has apparently resulted from a previous infection.

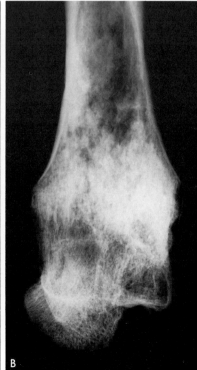

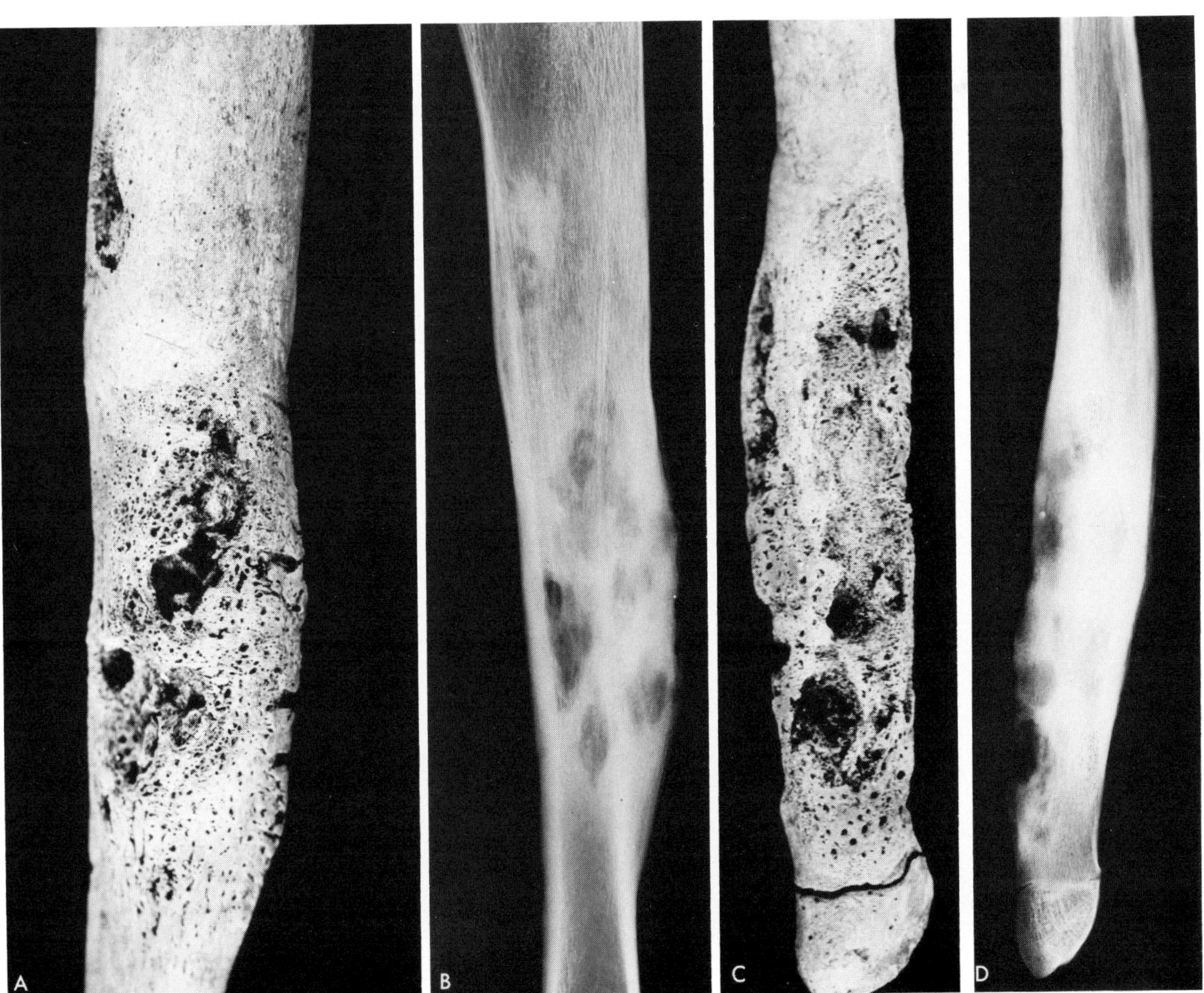

Figure 8.

Object: Tibia and fibula.

Source: Panama-California Exposition.

Date of Receipt: 1915.

Date or Period of Specimen: Historic.

Diagnosis: Osteomyelitis.

Remarks: Pronounced osteomyelitis involves the middle third of the tibia and the distal third of the fibula in this young patient with an open distal fibular growth plate. Observe the extensive osseous destruction with associated sclerosis and periostitis. Possible sequestra are identified.

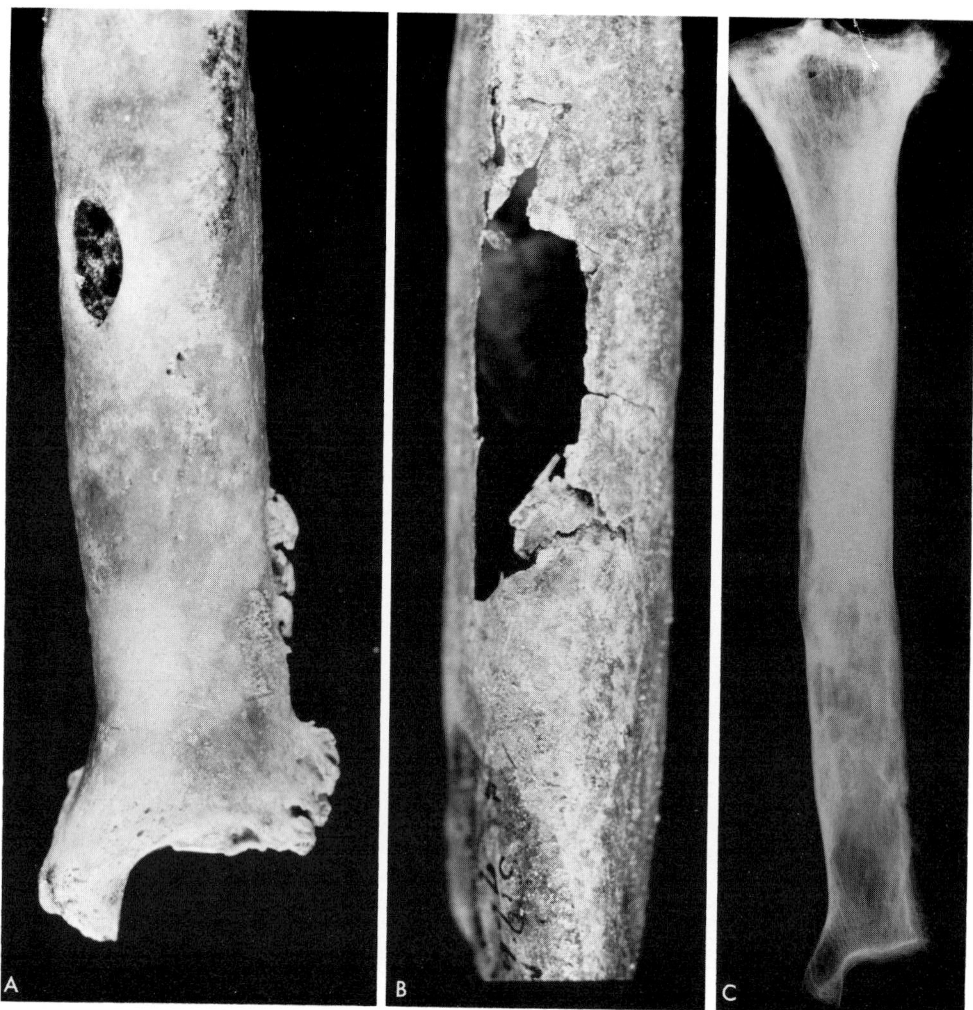

Figure 9.

Object: Tibia and overlying skin.

Source: Panama-California Exposition.

Date of Receipt: 1915.

Date or Period of Specimen: Prehistoric.

Diagnosis: Osteomyelitis.

Remarks: The changes of osteomyelitis are apparent in the distal tibia and extend into the tibiotalar joint. Similarly, there is involvement of the lateral aspect of the proximal tibia. In the lower tibia, note the focal area of destruction containing a sequestrum. This sequestrum had led to a fistulous tract with breakdown of the overlying skin, which is well shown in the accompanying specimen photograph of the mummified skin that was overlying this portion of the tibia.

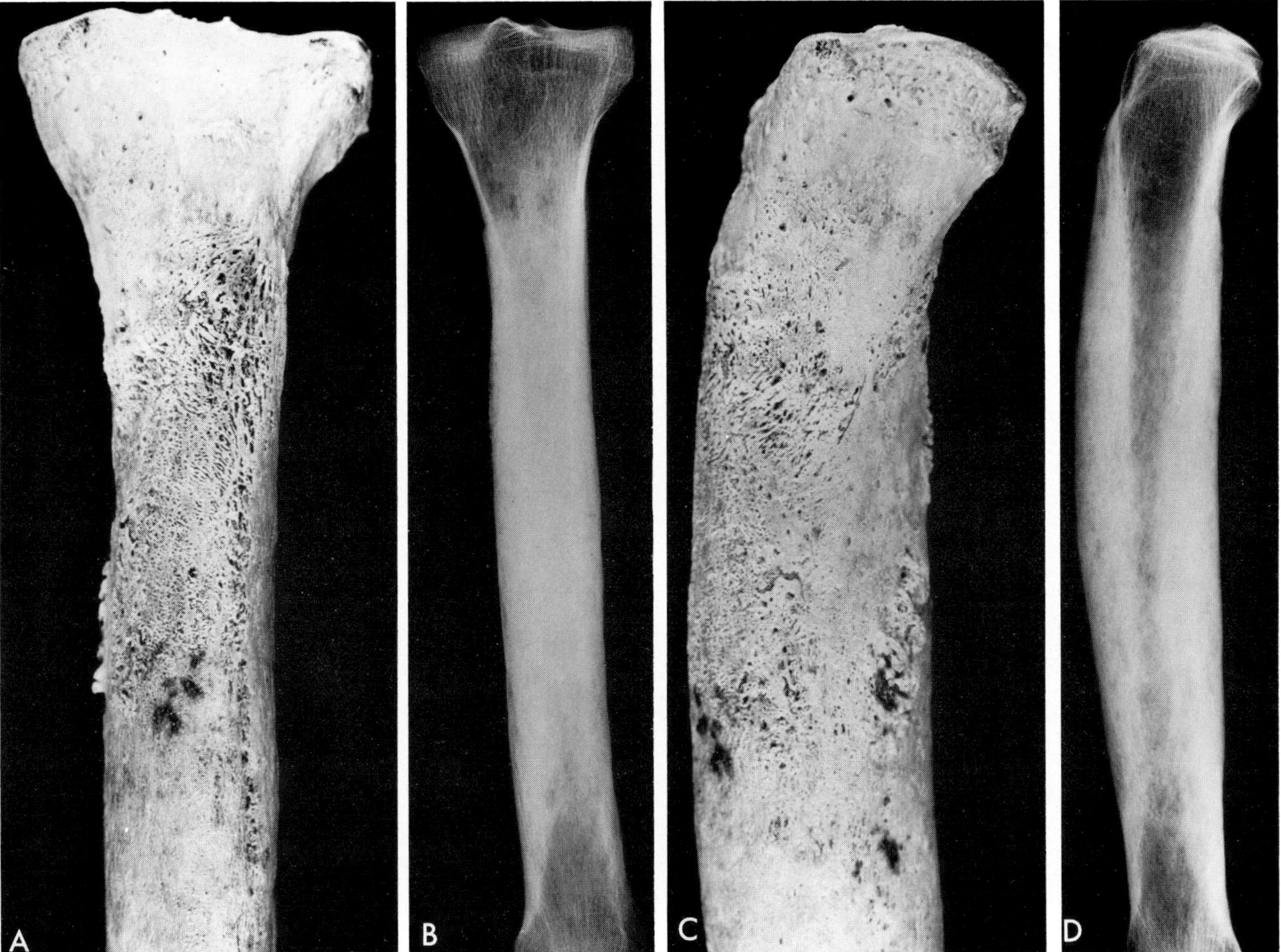

Figure 10.

Object: Tibia.

Source: Panama-California Exposition.

Date of Receipt: 1915.

Date or Period of Specimen: Prehistoric.

Diagnosis: Osteomyelitis.

Remarks: Frontal and lateral views of the proximal tibia indicate the osseous changes of chronic infection. Considerable bony eburnation is seen. The cortex is thickened owing to periosteal and endosteal proliferation. The anterior surface of the tibia appears bowed.

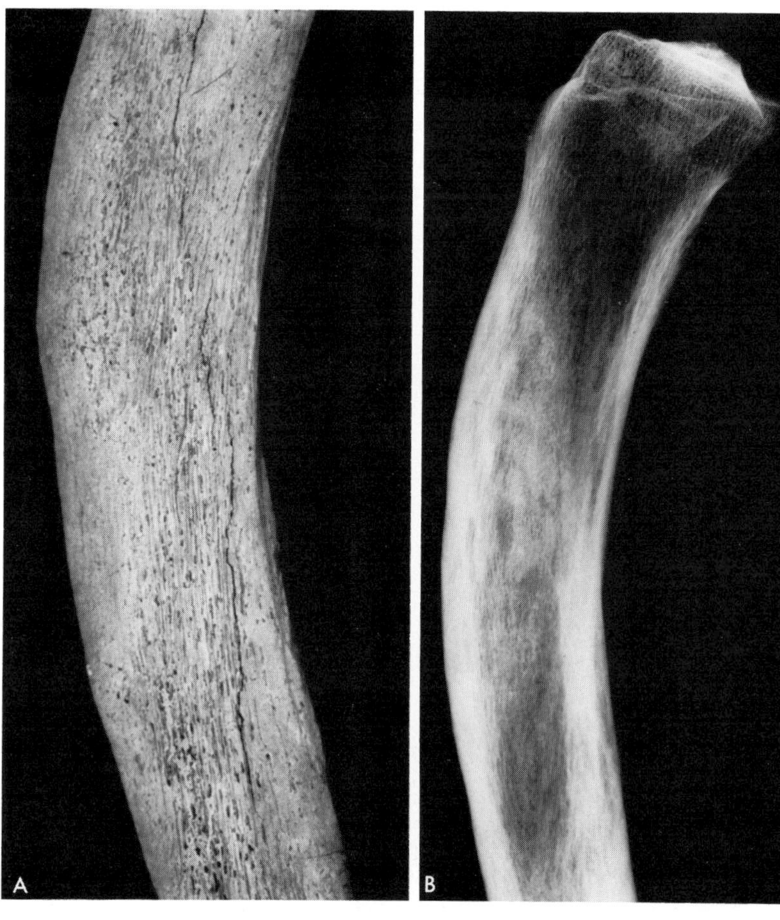

Figure 11.
Object: Tibia.
Source: Panama-California Exposition.
Date of Receipt: 1915.
Date or Period of Specimen: Possibly post-Columbian.
Diagnosis: Probable syphilis.
Remarks: Bony expansion and deformity have resulted in a typical saber-shin appearance.

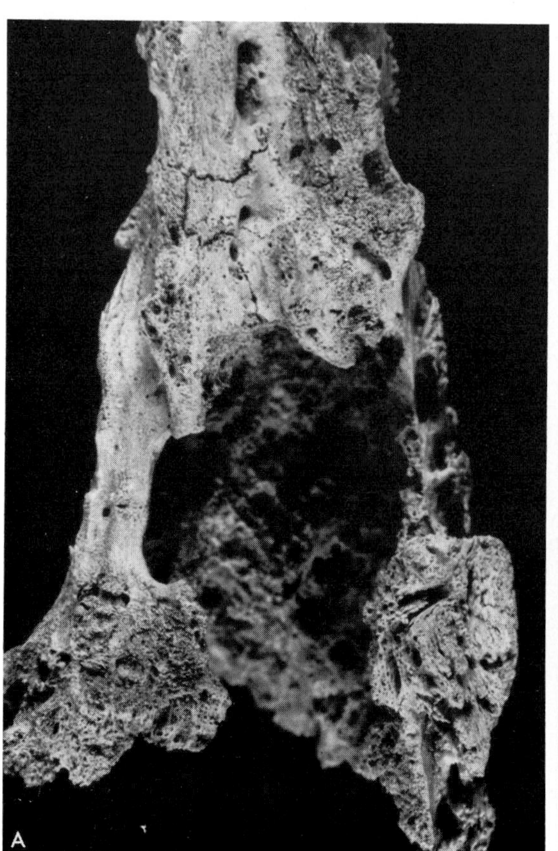

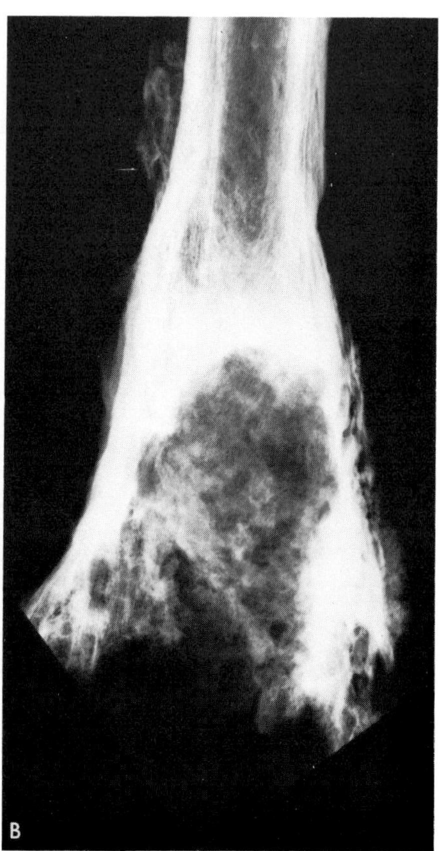

Figure 12.
Object: Femur.
Source: Panama-California Exposition.
Date of Receipt: 1915.
Date or Period of Specimen: Prehistoric.
Diagnosis: Tumor, possibly chondrosarcoma.
Remarks: Extensive bone destruction is associated with reactive sclerosis and periostitis. A radiograph of the proximal end of this bone indicated an enchondroma, suggesting the possibility that a similar lesion in the distal femur had undergone malignant transformation.

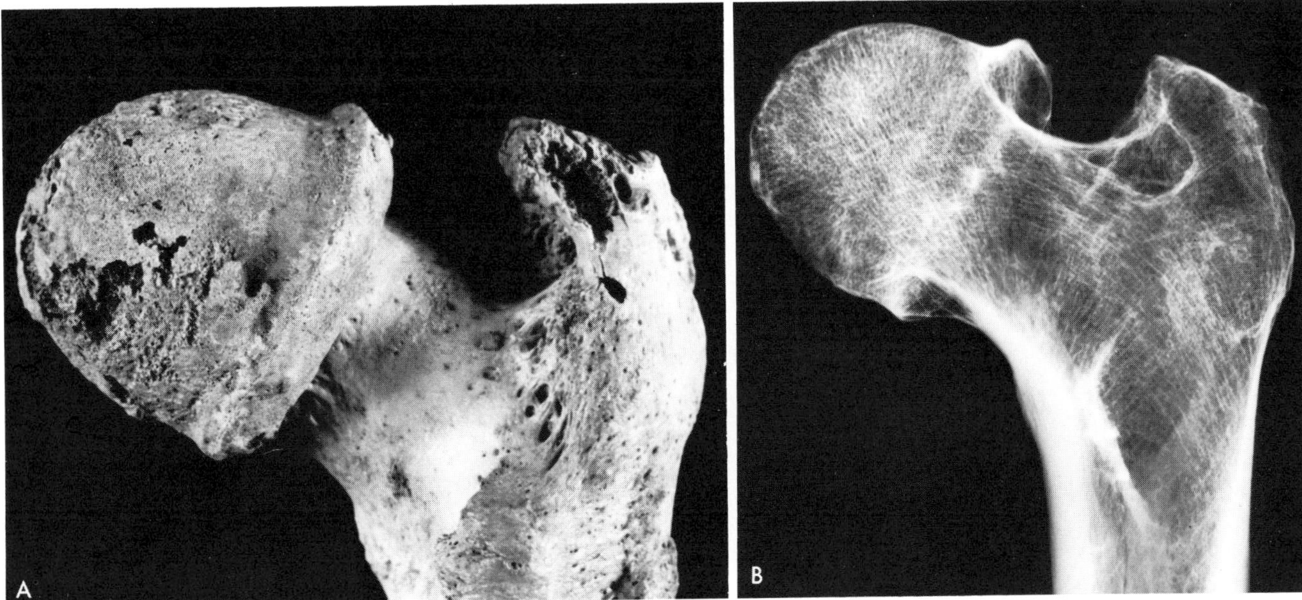

Figure 13.
Object: Femur.
Source: Panama-California Exposition.
Date of Receipt: 1915.
Date or Period of Specimen: Prehistoric.
Diagnosis: Osteoarthritis.
Remarks: Findings include flattening of the superior aspect of the femoral head and prominent osteophytosis at the femoral head–femoral neck junction. Buttressing along the medial aspect of the femoral neck is seen.

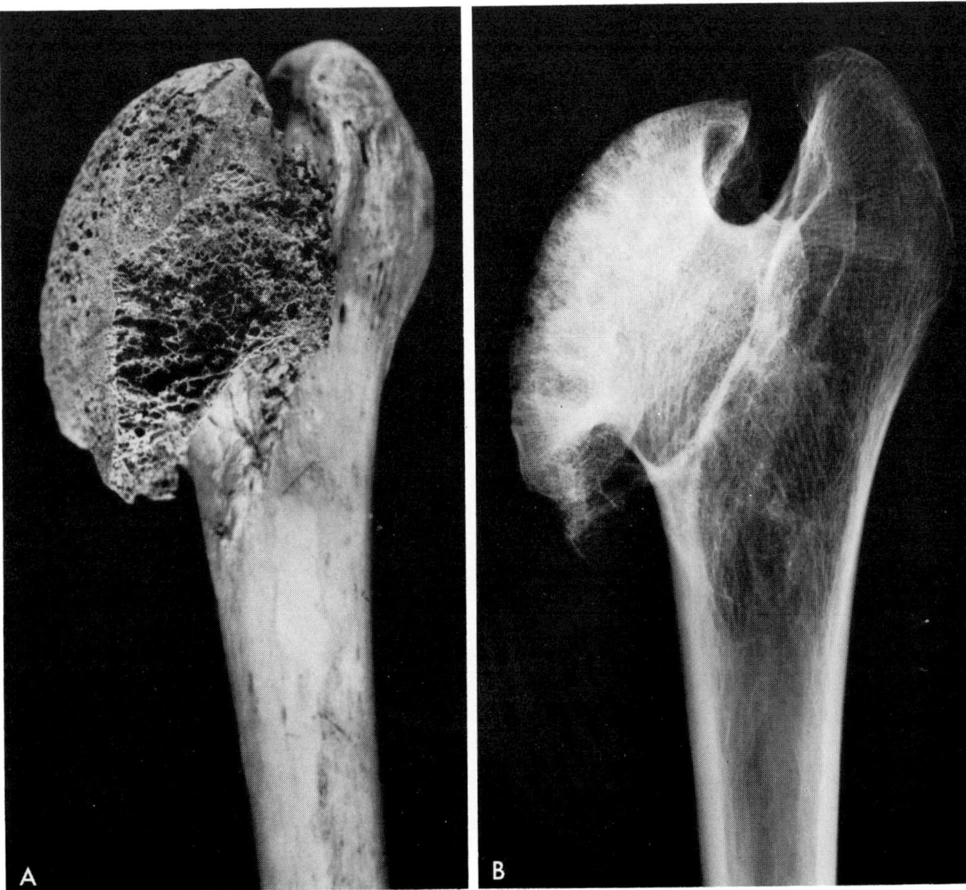

Figure 14.
Object: Femur.
Source: Panama-California Exposition.
Date of Receipt: 1915.
Date or Period of Specimen: Prehistoric.
Diagnosis: Possibly Legg-Calvé-Perthes disease.
Remarks: The flattening and deformity of the femoral head, osteophytosis, and widening of the femoral neck could be the result of previous Legg-Calvé-Perthes disease, although other diagnoses could certainly be considered.

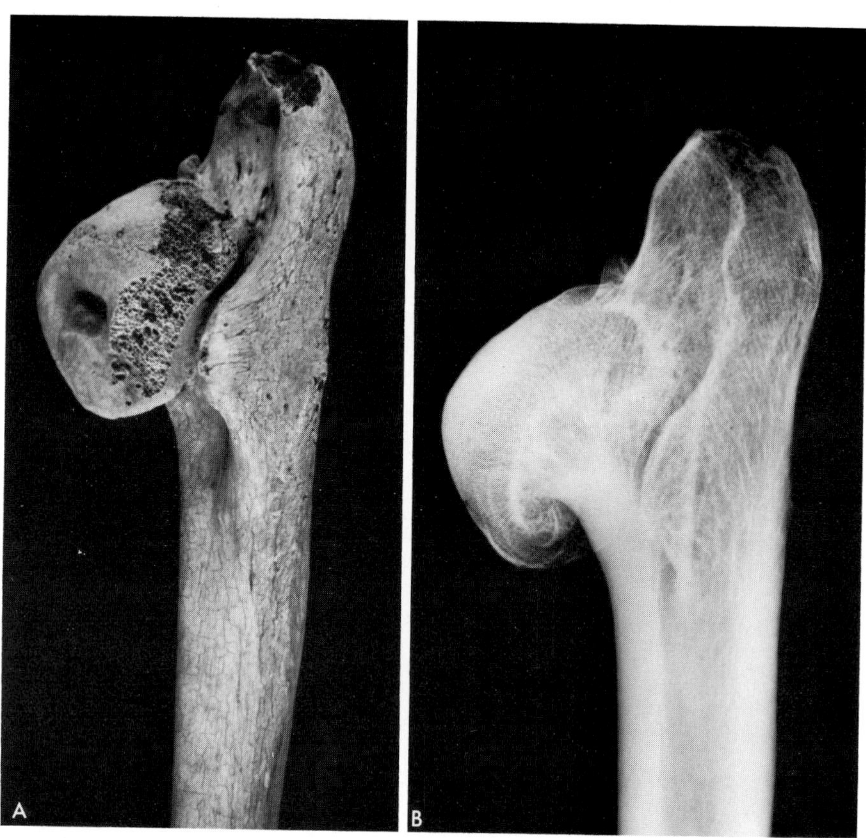

Figure 15.

Object: Femur.

Source: Panama-California Exposition.

Date of Receipt: 1915.

Date or Period of Specimen: Prehistoric.

Diagnosis: Coxa vara.

Remarks: Findings include varus deformity of the proximal femur, shortening of the femoral neck, prominence of the greater trochanter, and osteophytosis at the femoral head–femoral neck junction.

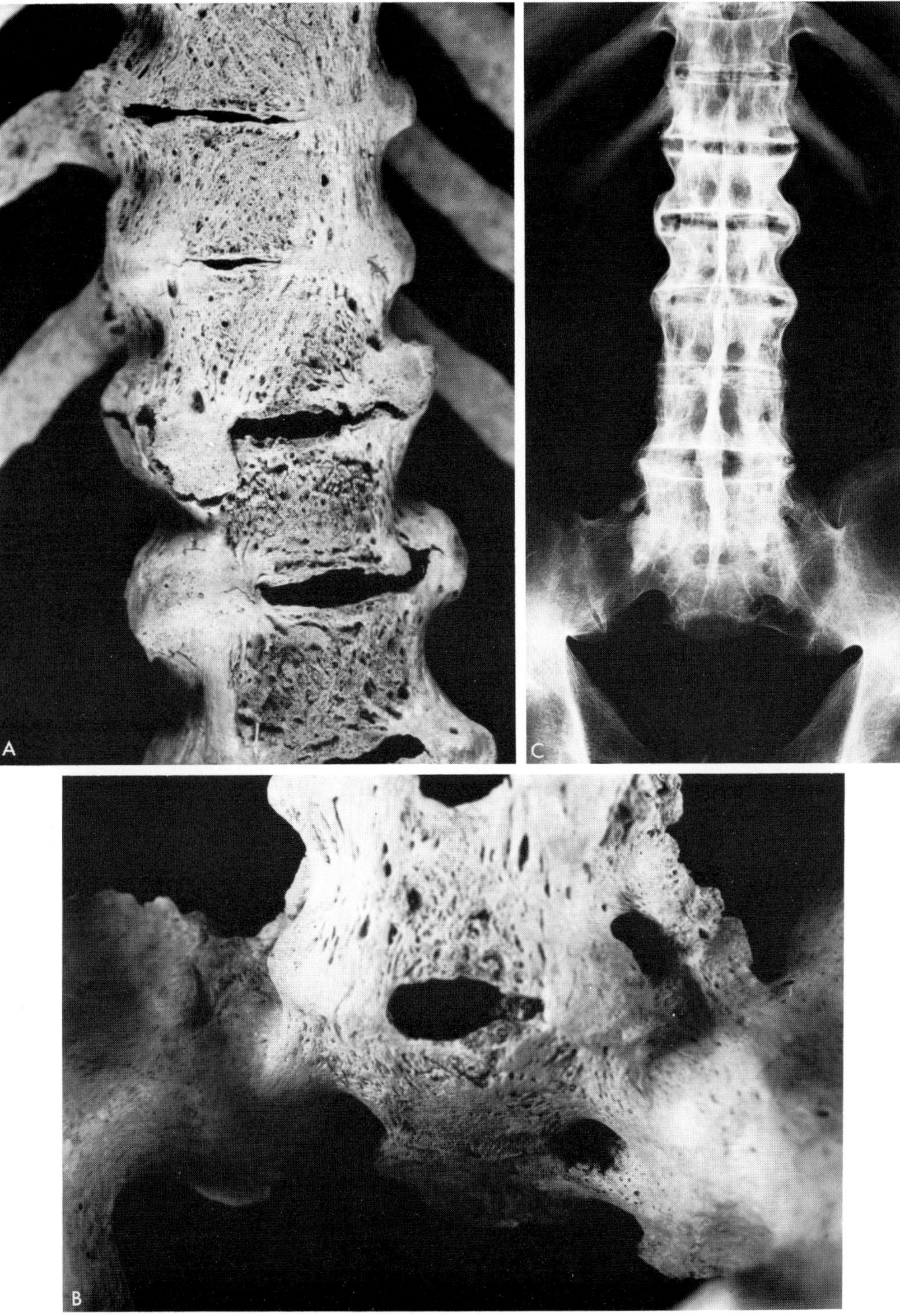

Figure 16.

Object: Thoracolumbar spine and pelvis.

Source: Panama-California Exposition.

Date of Receipt: 1915.

Date or Period of Specimen: Historic.

Diagnosis: Ankylosing spondylitis.

Remarks: Changes include widespread syndesmophytosis and costovertebral and sacroiliac joint bony ankylosis. In some locations, the outgrowths resemble the changes in diffuse idiopathic skeletal hyperostosis.

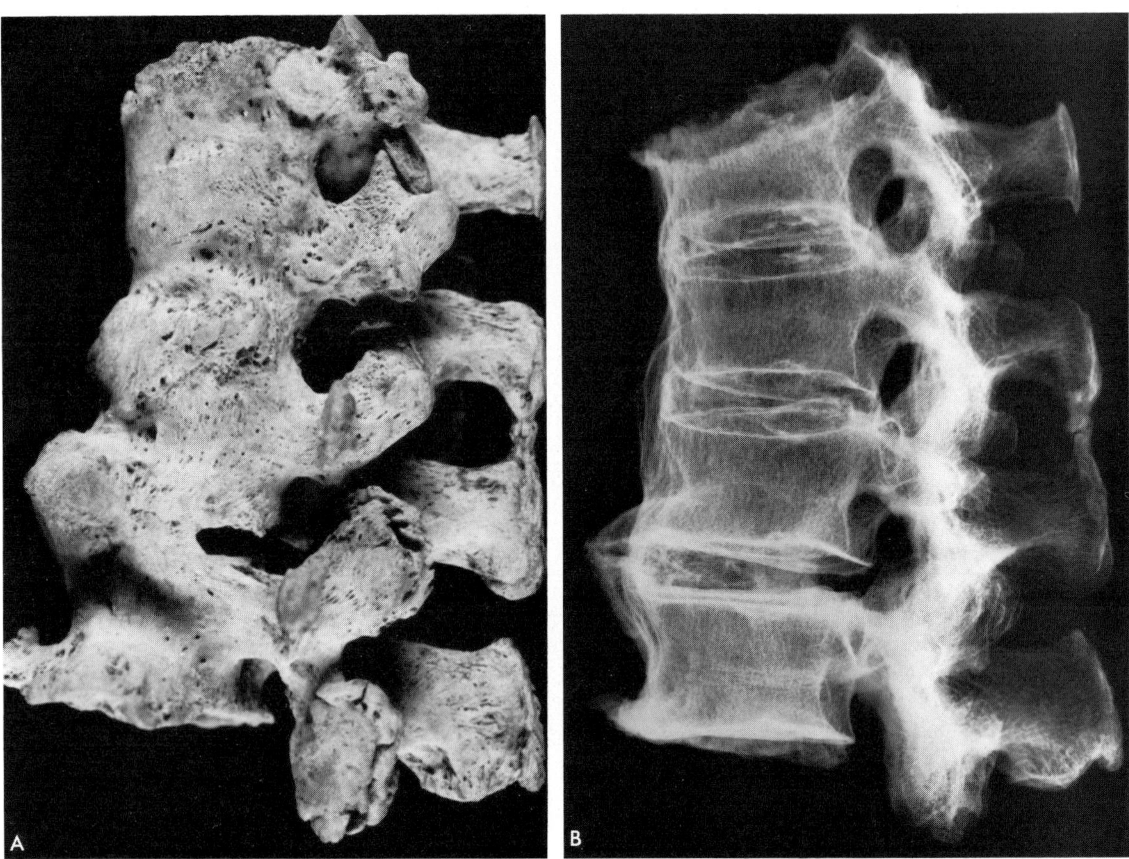

Figure 17.

Object: Spine, pelvis, calcaneus, ulna.

Source: Sheriff's Department, San Diego, California.

Date of Receipt: Early 1930s.

Date or Period of Specimen: Early 1930s.

Diagnosis: Diffuse idiopathic skeletal hyperostosis.

Remarks: The widespread nature of this ossifying diathesis is well shown in these specimens. The findings include typical spinal excrescences with ligament ossification, "whiskering" about the bony pelvis, para-articular bridging osteophytes at the sacroiliac joints, and ulnar and calcaneal bony proliferation at sites of tendon and ligament attachment.

Illustration continued on the opposite page

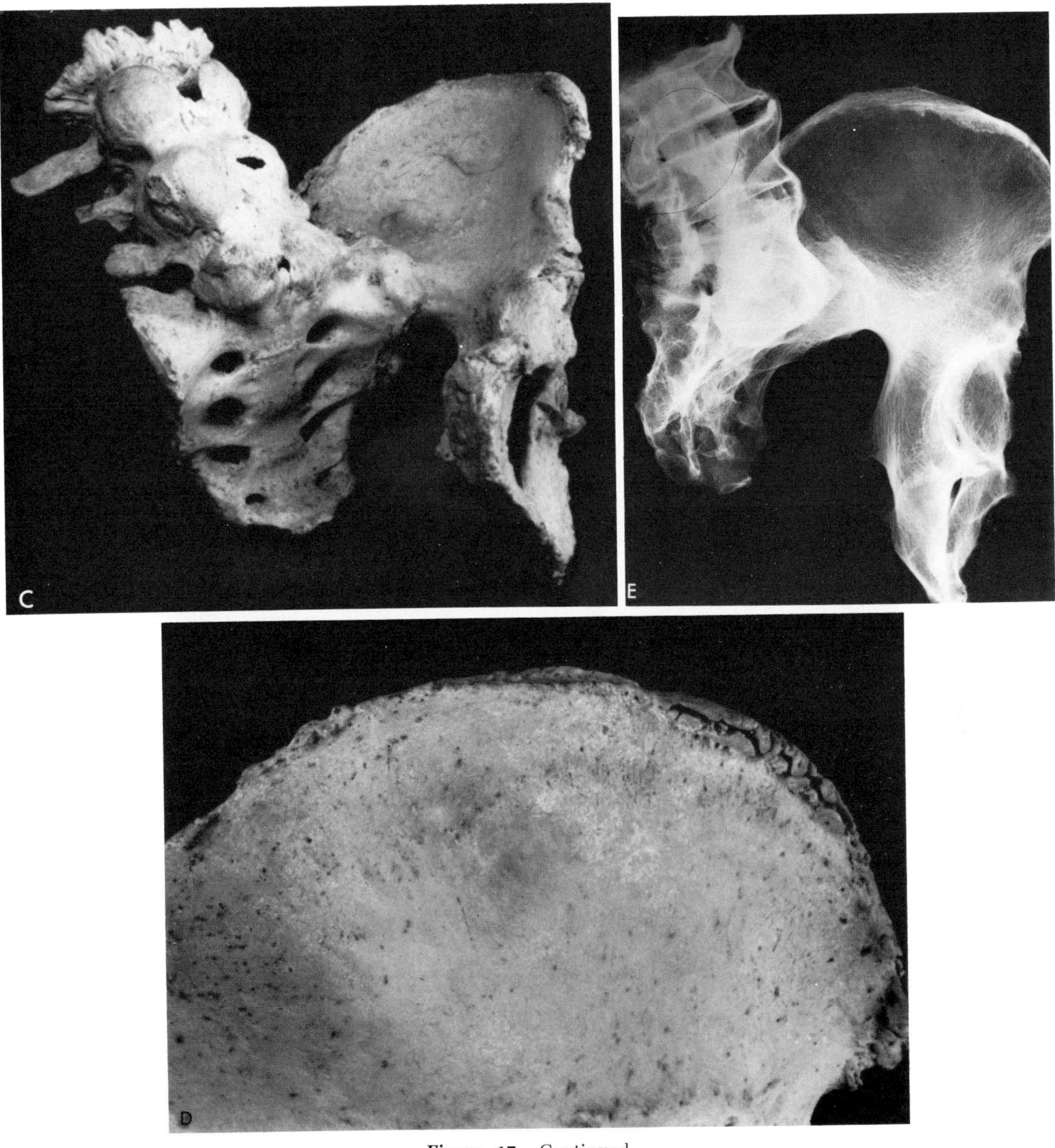

Figure 17. Continued
Illustration continued on the following page

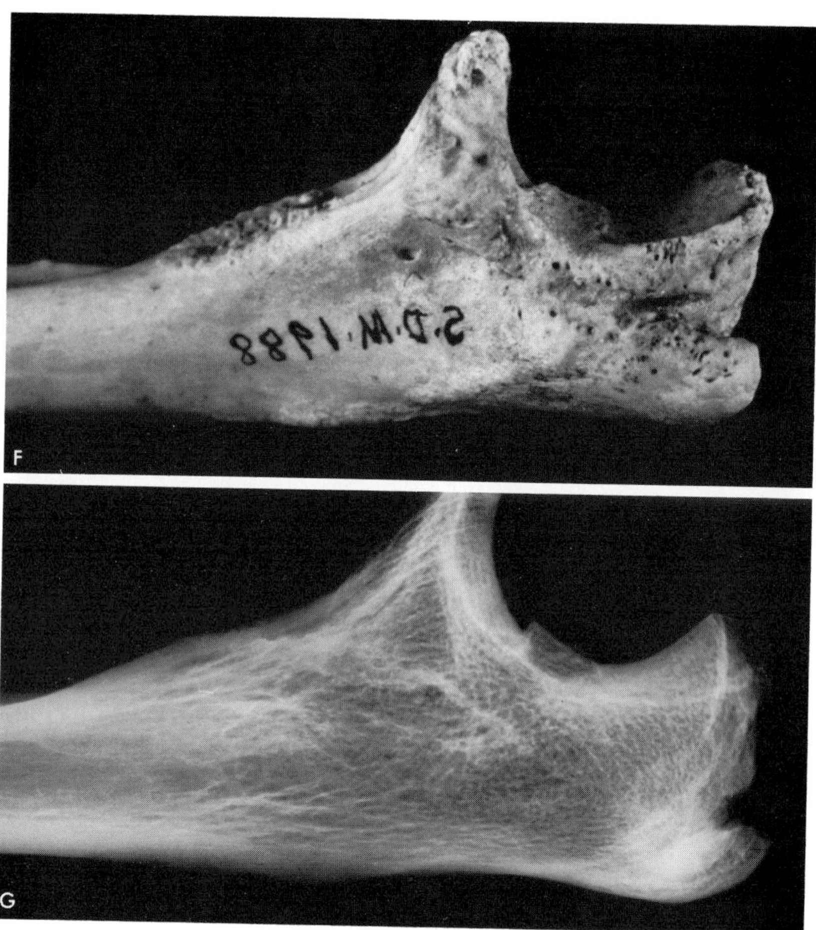

Figure 17. Continued

Illustration continued on the opposite page

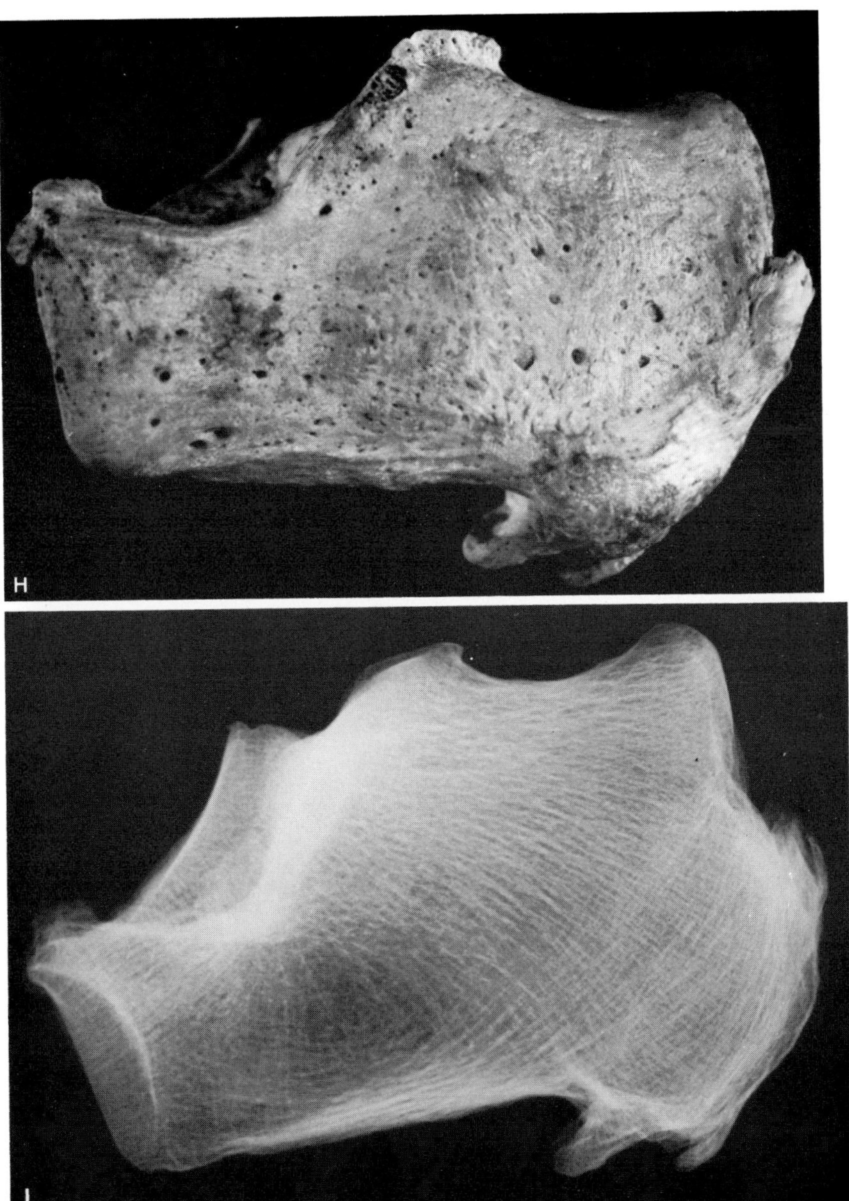

Figure 17. Continued

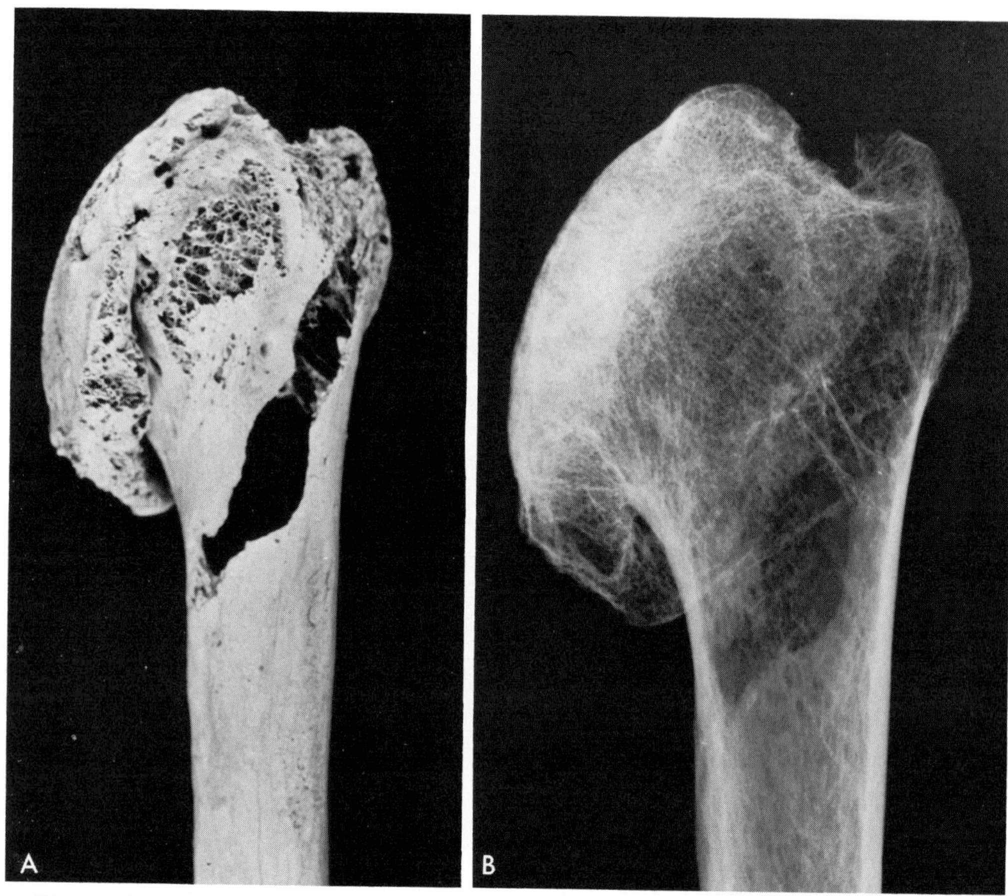

Figure 18.

Object: Humerus.

Source: Panama-California Exposition.

Date of Receipt: 1915.

Date or Period of Specimen: Prehistoric.

Diagnosis: Osteoarthritis.

Remarks: The sclerosis and osteophytosis of the humeral head are consistent with osteoarthritis. The cause of these changes in the glenohumeral joint, which is infrequently involved with degenerative disease, is unknown. The degree of flattening of the head of the humerus suggests that osteonecrosis may have been a primary or secondary abnormality.

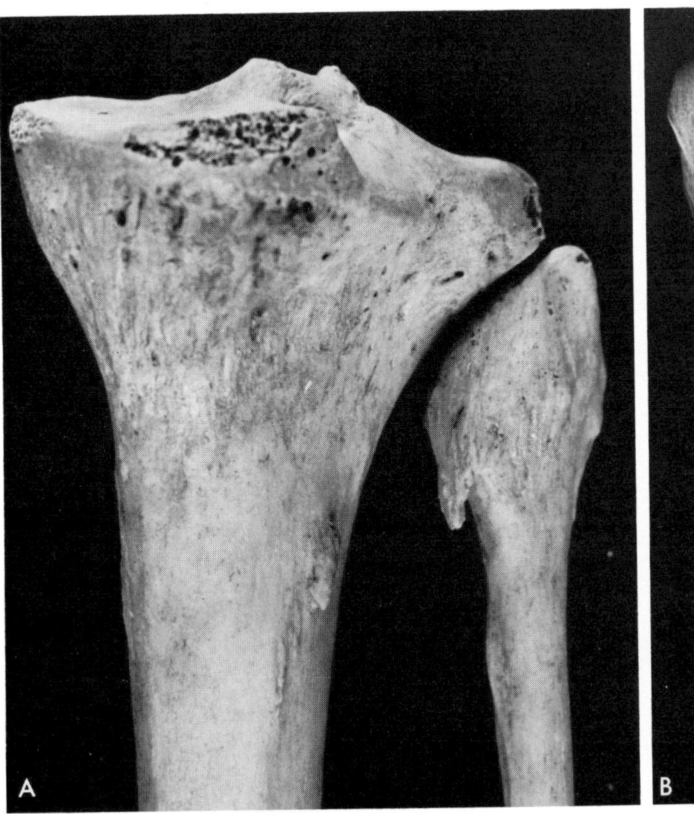

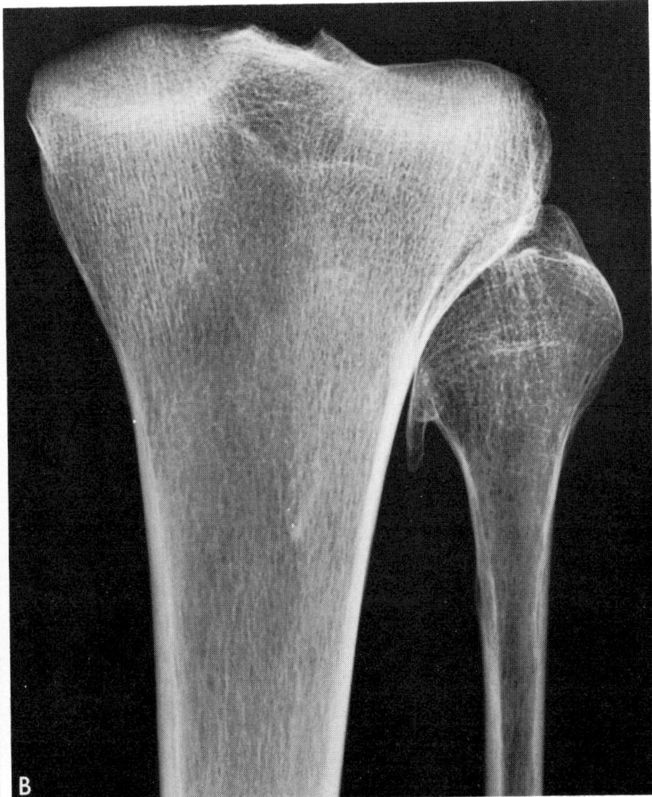

Figure 19.
Object: Tibia and Fibula.
Source: Panama-California Exposition.
Date of Receipt: 1915.
Date or Period of Specimen: Prehistoric.
Diagnosis: Healed fractures of the distal tibia and fibula with secondary osteoarthritis of the proximal tibiofibular joint.
Remarks: The well-healed fractures of the distal tibia and fibula are associated with osseous deformity. An inferior fibular osteophyte at the proximal tibiofibular joint is noted. The possibility of mild lateral subluxation of the fibular head is raised.

Illustration continued on the following page

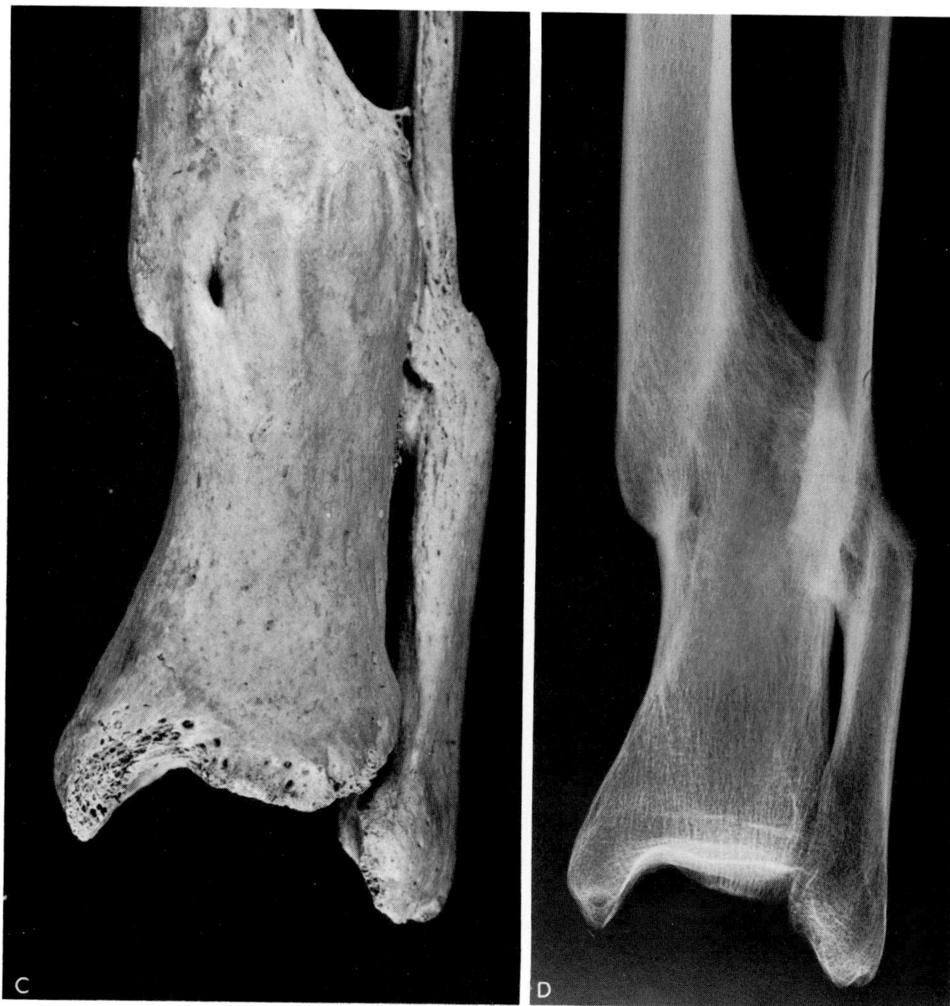

Figure 19. Continued

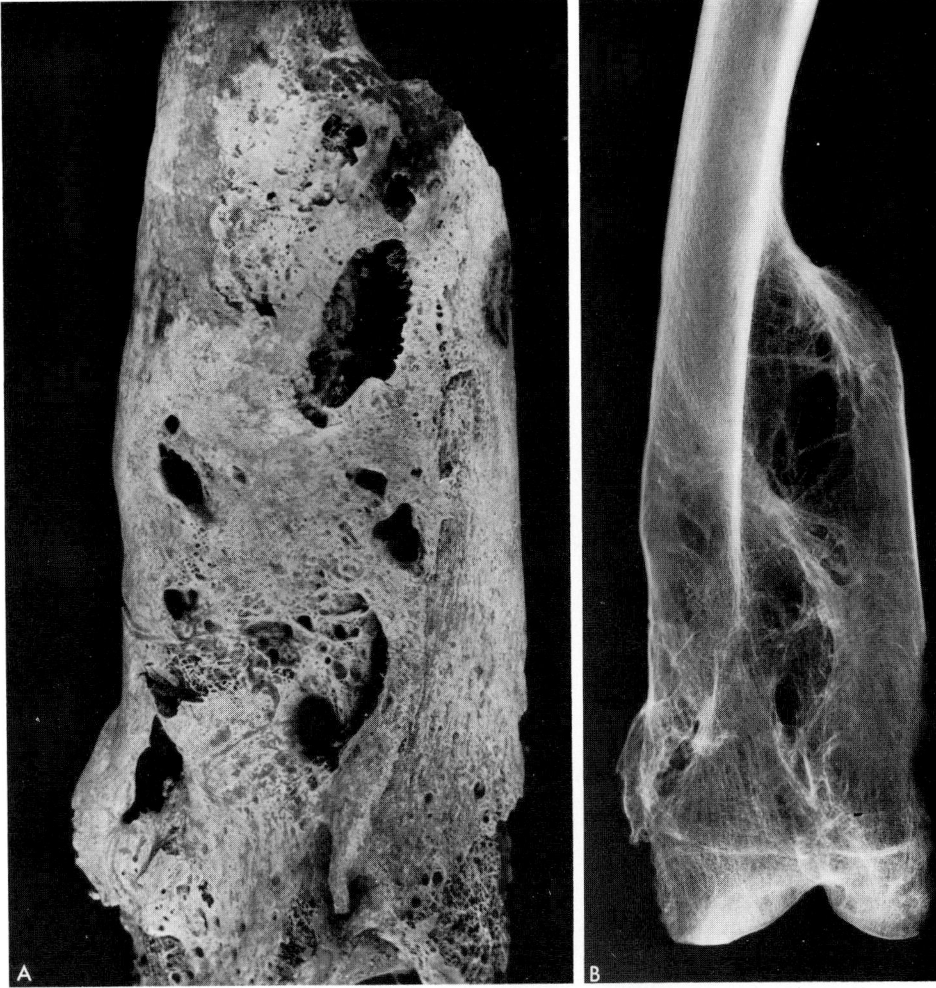

Figure 20.
Object: Femur.
Source: Panama-California Exposition.
Date of Receipt: 1915.
Date or Period of Specimen: Prehistoric.
Diagnosis: Healed fracture of the distal femur.
Remarks: extensive deformity of the distal femur has accompanied healing of this oblique fracture. The absence of significant bony sclerosis would suggest that osteomyelitis had not been present. Note the eburnation of subchondral bone in the distal femur.

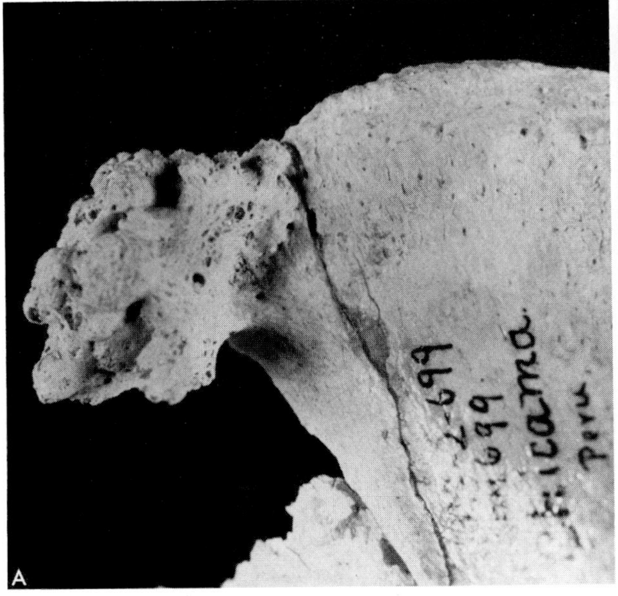

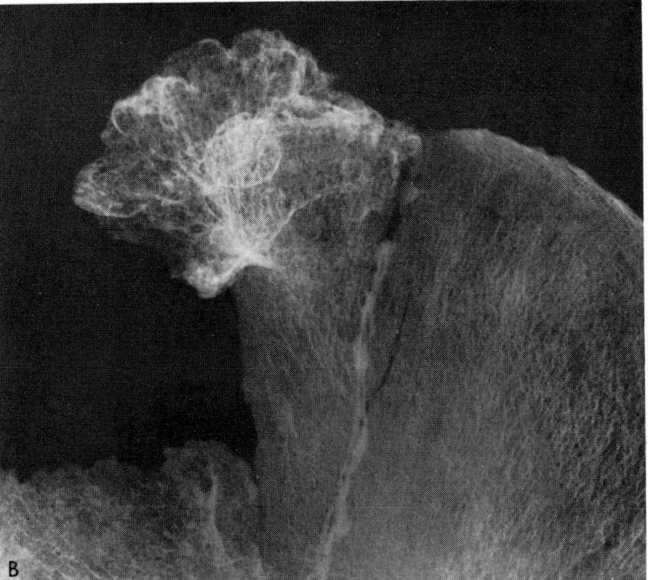

Figure 21.
Object: Ilium.
Source: Panama-California Exposition.
Date of Receipt: 1915.
Date or Period of Specimen: Prehistoric.
Diagnosis: Osteochondroma.
Remarks: A proliferating tumor is arising from the posterior aspect of the iliac bone. No features suggesting malignancy can be detected.

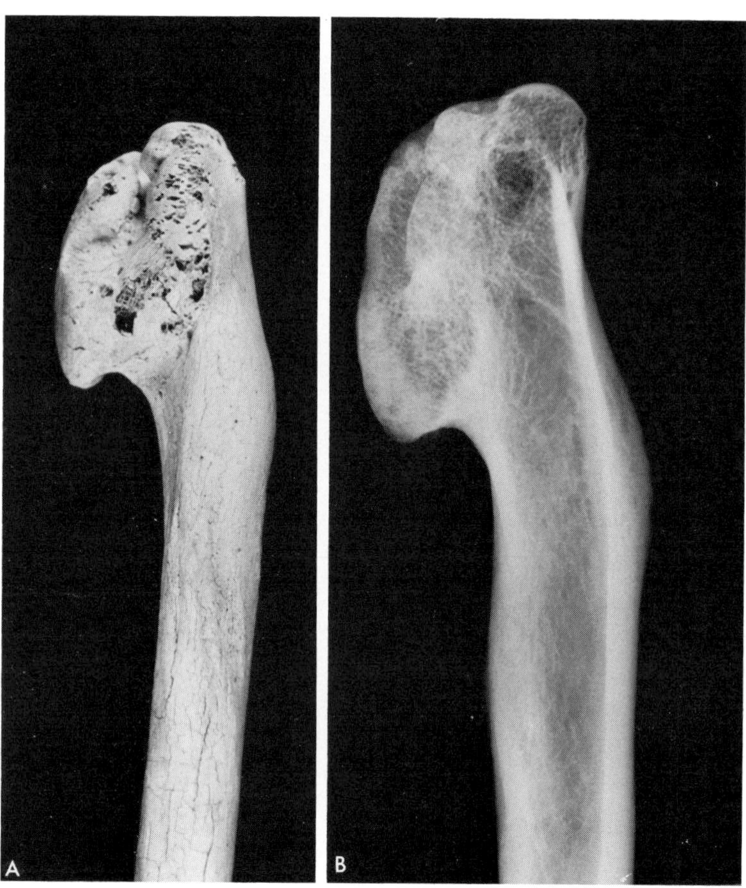

Figure 22.

Object: Humerus.

Source: Panama-California Exposition.

Date of Receipt: 1915.

Date or Period of Specimen: Prehistoric.

Diagnosis: Possible achondroplasia.

Remarks: The entire humerus was significantly shortened. Observe the varus deformity of the proximal humerus with irregularity of the humeral head and neck.

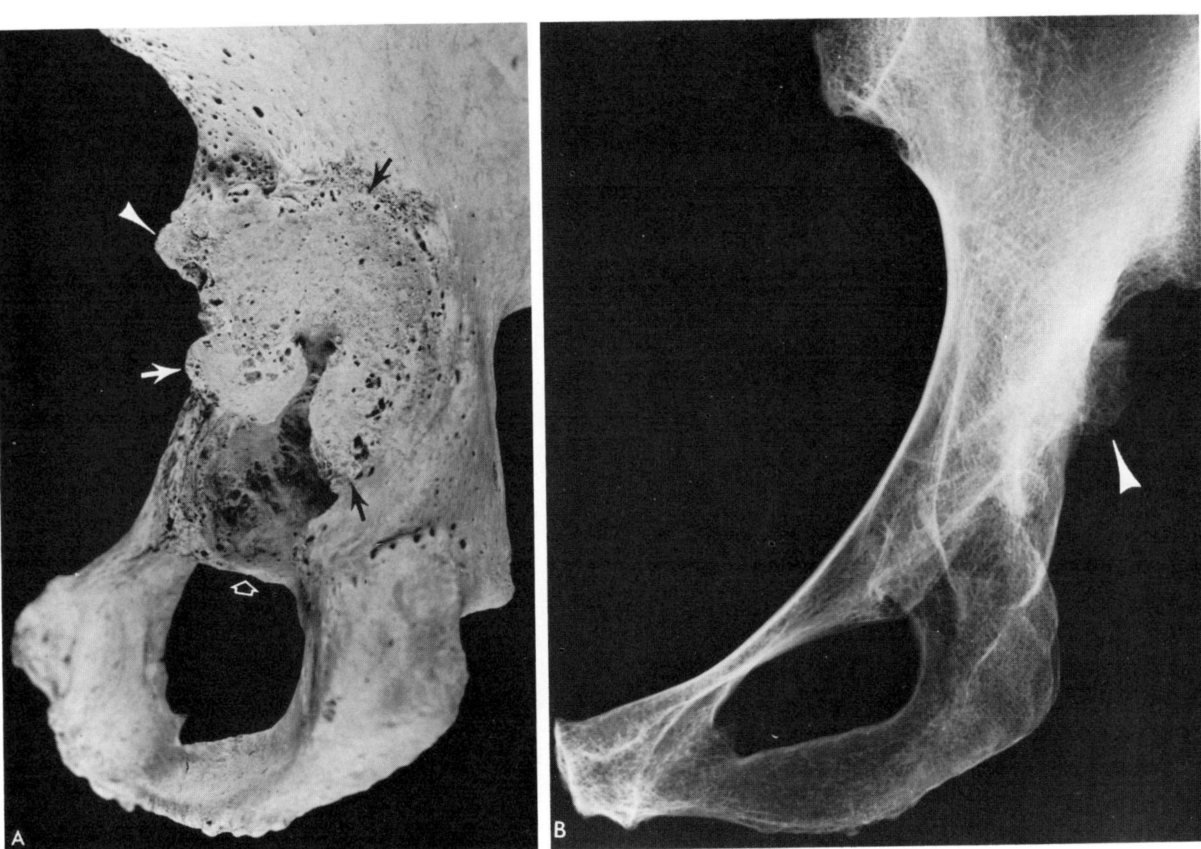

Figure 23.
Object: Pelvis.
Source: Panama-California Exposition.
Date of Receipt: 1915.
Date or Period of Specimen: Prehistoric.
Diagnosis: Congenital dislocation of the hip.
Remarks: Acetabular deformity is evident. The original acetabulum (open arrow) is shallow, and a pseudoacetabulum (arrows) has been created by a dislocated femoral head. Note the osseous excrescence (arrowhead).

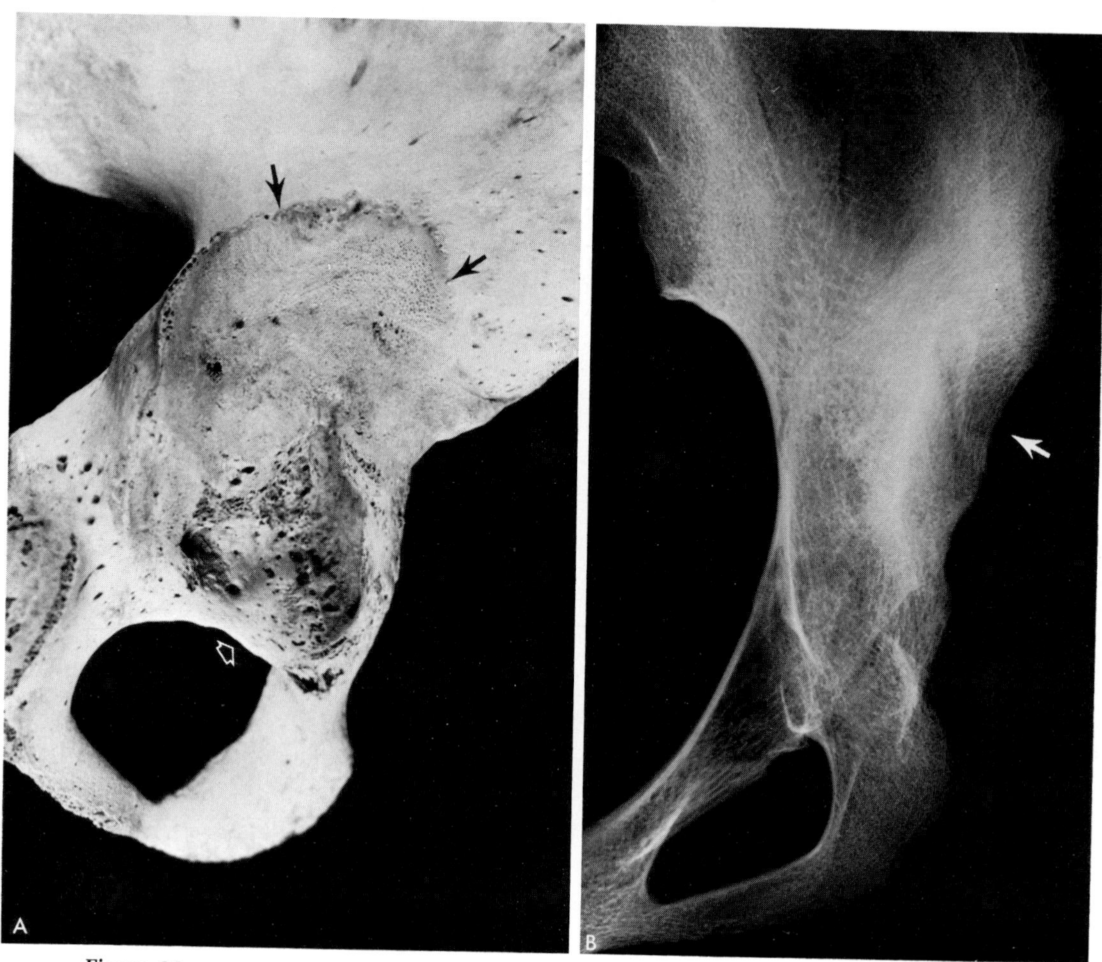

Figure 24.

Object: Pelvis.

Source: Panama-California Exposition.

Date of Receipt: 1915.

Date or Period of Specimen: Prehistoric.

Diagnosis: Congenital dislocation of the hip.

Remarks: Observe the shallow and deformed acetabulum (open arrow) and a pseudoacetabulum (solid arrows) created by a dislocated femoral head.

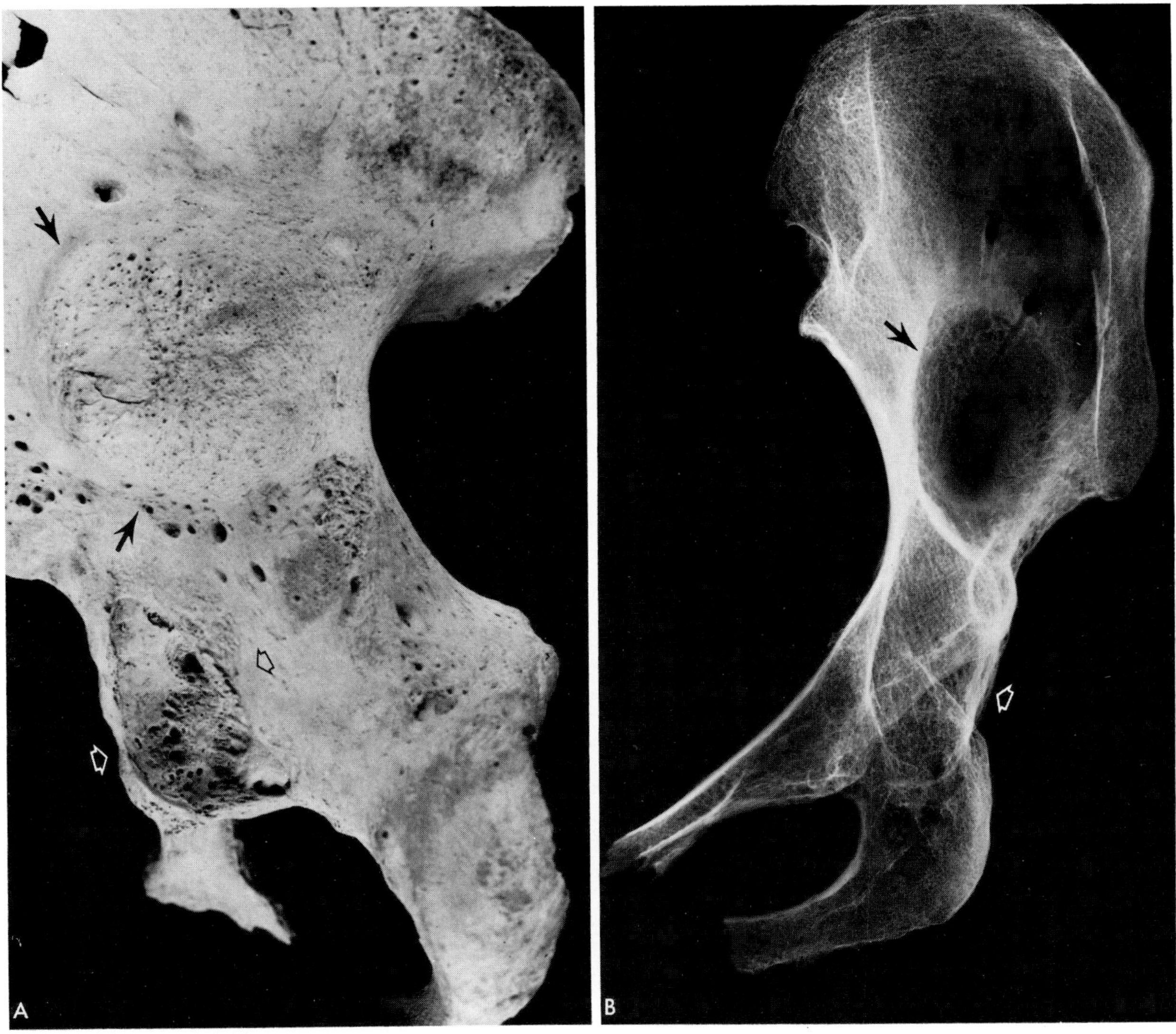

Figure 25.
Object: Pelvis.
Source: Panama-California Exposition.
Date of Receipt: 1915.
Date or Period of Specimen: Prehistoric.
Diagnosis: Congenital dislocation of the hip.
Remarks: A flattened, shallow, and deformed acetabulum (open arrows) is identified. Above this, a pseudoacetabulum (solid arrows) is seen.

REFERENCES

1. Hrdlicka A: Anthropological work in Peru in 1913, with notes on the pathology of the ancient Peruvians. Smithsonian Misc Collections *61*(18), 1914.
2. Moodie RL: Studies in paleopathology XXI. Injuries to the head among the pre-Columbian Peruvians. Ann Med History *9*:277, 1927.
3. Hrdlicka A: Disease, medicine and surgery among the American aborigines. JAMA *99*:1661, 1932.
4. Burton FA: Aural exostosis. Ann Otol Rhinol Laryngol *32*:97, 1923–1924.
5. Moodie RA: Archeological evidences of the antiquity of disease in South America. Scientific Monthly *29*:193, 1929.
6. Hrdlicka A: Some results of recent anthropological exploration in Peru. Smithsonian Misc Collections *56*:(16):1, 1911.
7. Lambert M: Paa-Ko: Archaeological chronicle of an Indian village in North Central New Mexico. Monograph 19, Parts I–V. Santa Fe, NM, School of American Research, page 1.
8. Steinbock RT: Paleopathological Diagnosis and Interpretation. Bone Diseases in Ancient Human Populations. Springfield, Ill, Charles C Thomas, 1976.

INTRODUCTION

BONE AS A LIVING TISSUE: AN OVERVIEW

by Donald Resnick, M.D., and Gen Niwayama, M.D.

Bone is a remarkable tissue. Although its appearance on the radiograph might be misinterpreted as indicating inactivity, bone is constantly undergoing change, not only in the immature skeleton, in which growth and development are readily apparent, but in the mature skeleton as well, through the constant and balanced processes of bone formation and resorption. It is when these processes are modified such that one or the other dominates that a pathologic state may be created. In some instances, the resulting imbalance between bone formation and destruction is easily detectable on the radiograph. In others, a more subtle imbalance exists that may only be identified on the histologic level. In order to clarify some of the concepts that are discussed in this book, the following comments are offered as an overview of the development and structure of the living tissue bone. This overview represents a synthesis of the detailed descriptions that are provided by Jaffe and others,[1,2] and the interested reader should consult these excellent reference sources.

THE DEVELOPING BONE

A bone develops by the process of intramembranous bone formation or endochondral bone formation, or both. At some locations, such as the bones of the cranial vault, intramembranous (mesenchymal) ossification is detected; in other locations, such as the tubular bones of the extremities, both endochondral and intramembranous ossification can be identified.

Intramembranous ossification is initiated by the proliferation of mesenchymal cells about a network of capillaries. At this site, a transformation of mesenchymal cells is accompanied by the appearance of a meshwork of collagen fibers and amorphous ground substance. The primitive cells change in number, shape, and size. They proliferate, enlarge, and become arranged in groups, which extend in a strand-like configuration into the surrounding tissue. The cells have now become osteoblasts and are intimately associated with the development of an eosinophilic matrix that appears within the collagenous tissue. This sequence represents the initial stage of the ossification process, which becomes more prominent and more widespread as the osteoid matrix undergoes calcification with the deposition of calcium phosphate. Some of the osteoblasts on

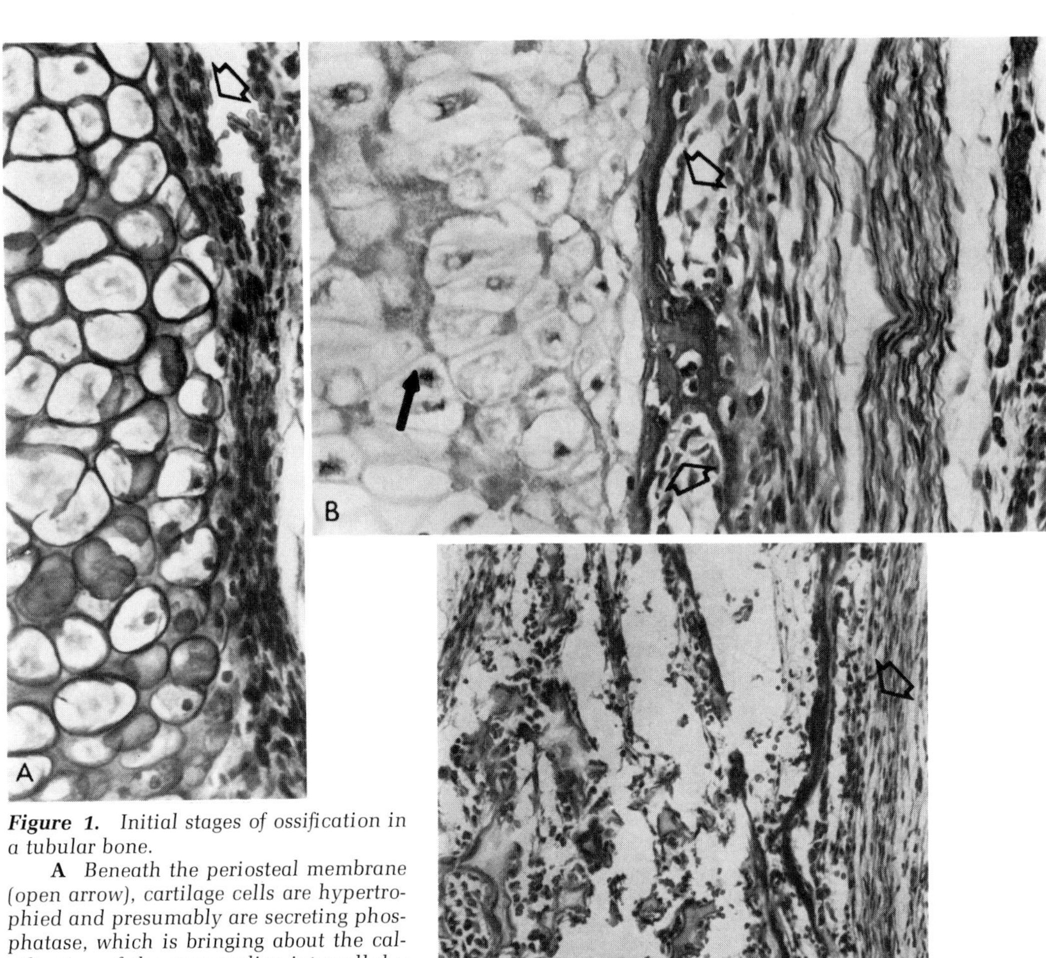

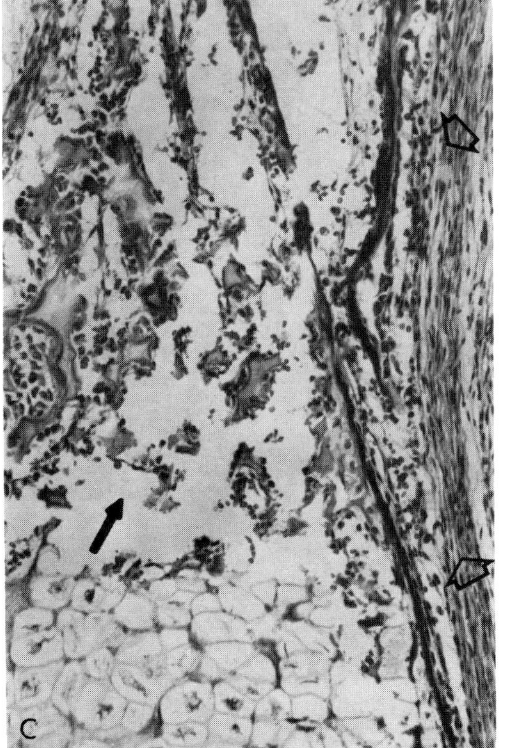

Figure 1. *Initial stages of ossification in a tubular bone.*

A *Beneath the periosteal membrane (open arrow), cartilage cells are hypertrophied and presumably are secreting phosphatase, which is bringing about the calcification of the surrounding intercellular substance. (Phalanx of fetus, 100×.)*

B *Observe subperiosteal bone formation (open arrows) and partly calcified hypertrophied cartilage (solid arrow). (Femur of fetus, 200×.)*

C *The osteogenic cells and vascular channels from the periosteum (open arrows) have grown into the spaces in the degenerating cartilage, and the osteogenic cells in this area are beginning to differentiate into osteoblasts and to lay down bone on what is left of the calcified cartilage matrix (solid arrow). (Radius of fetus, 100×.)*

the surface of the osteoid and woven-fibered bone become entrapped within the substance of the matrix in a space called a lacuna. Here, the osteoblast becomes an osteocyte, and although it is isolated in some respects from the neighboring proliferating mesenchymal tissue, it maintains some contact with the precursor cells by developing elongated processes or projections, termed canaliculi, that are surrounded by condensed matrix. The embedded osteocyte will now be devoted primarily to maintaining the integrity of the surrounding matrix rather than be directly involved in the future ossification process. Through the continued transformation of mesenchymal cells to osteoblasts, the elaboration of an osteoid matrix, and the entrapment of osteoblasts within the matrix, the primitive mesenchyme is converted into osseous tissue. The ultimate characteristics of the tissue depend upon its location within the bone: In the cancellous areas of the bone, the meshwork of osseous tissue contains intervening vascular connective tissue representing the embryonic precursor of the bone marrow; in the compact areas of the bone, the osseous tissue becomes more condensed, forming cylindrical masses containing a central vascular channel, the haversian system. On the external and internal surfaces of the compact bone, fibrovascular layers develop (periosteum and endosteum) that contain cells which remain osteogenic, giving bone its ever-changing quality. In the process of further development, coarse-fibered nonlamellar primitive bone is eventually converted to fine-fibered lamellar mature bone.

Endochondral (intracartilaginous) ossification is prominent in the bones of the appendicular skeleton, the axial skeleton, and the base of the skull. In this process, cartilaginous tissue derived from mesenchyme is destroyed and subsequently replaced with bone (Figs. 1 and 2). The initial sites of bone formation are called centers of ossification (primary and secondary), and their precise location within the bone is very much dependent upon the specific bone that is being analyzed. In the tubular bones, the primary center of ossification is located in the central portion of the cartilaginous model, whereas later-appearing centers of ossification (secondary centers) are located at the ends of the models within epiphyses and apophyses. About the cartilaginous model exists vascular mesenchymal tissue or perichondrium, whose deeper layers contain cells with osteogenic potential.

The initial change in the primary center that indicates the inception of endochondral ossification is hypertrophy of cartilage cells, glycogen accumulation, and reduction of intervening matrix. Subsequently, these cells degenerate, die, and become calcified. Simultaneously, the deeper or subperichondrial cells undergo transformation to osteoblasts and, through a process identical to intramembranous ossification, these osteoblasts produce a subperiosteal collar or cuff of bone, which encloses

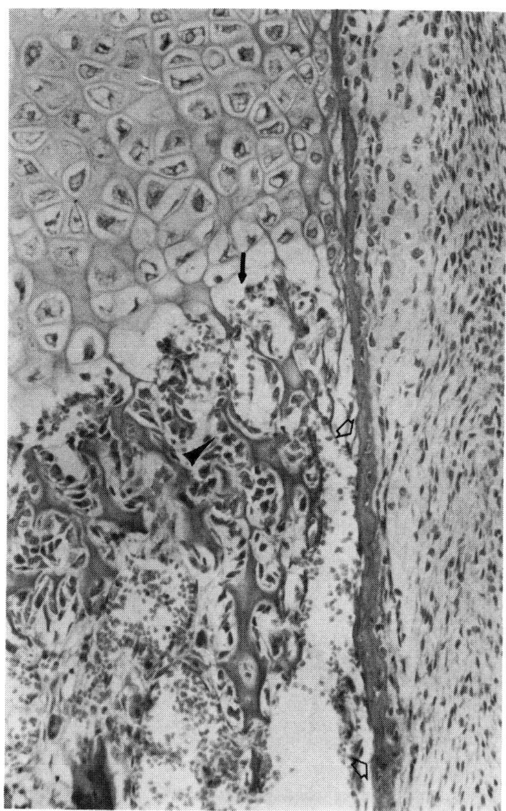

Figure 2. *Endochondral and intramembranous ossification in a tubular bone: the radius of a 4½-month old fetus. The large and confluent cartilage cell lacunae are being penetrated by vascular channels (solid arrow), thus exposing intervening cores of calcified cartilage matrix. The osteoblasts are depositing osseous tissue on these cartilage matrix cores (arrowhead). Observe subperiosteal bone formation (open arrows).*

the central portions of the cartilaginous tissue. Periosteal tissue is converted into vascular channels, and these channels perforate the shell of bone, entering the degenerating cartilaginous foci. The aggressive vascular tissue disrupts the lacunae of the cartilage cells, creating spaces that fill with embryonic bone marrow. Osteoblasts appear, which transform the sites of degenerating and dying cartilage cells into foci of ossification by laying down osteoid tissue in the cartilage matrix. Osteoblasts become trapped within the developing bone as osteocytes in a fashion similar to that occurring in the process of intramembranous ossification. The entire area is alive with activity as the cartilaginous model is gradually replaced with bone. From the center of the tubular bone, ossification proceeds toward the ends of the bone as cells in adjoining cartilaginous areas undergo hypertrophy, death, calcification in association with vascular invasion, osteoblast transformation, and conversion to bone. Similarly, the periosteal collar, which is actively participating in intramembranous ossification, spreads towards the end of the bone, slightly ahead of the band of endochondral ossification. Through a process of resorption of some of the initially formed trabeculae, a marrow space is created, and through a process of subperiosteal deposition of bone, a cortex becomes evident, grows thicker, and is converted into a system with longitudinally arranged compact bone surrounding vascular channels (haversian system). The frontier of endochondral ossification that is advancing toward the end of the bone becomes better delineated, appearing as a plate of cellular activity. It is this plate that ultimately becomes located between the epiphysis and diaphysis of a tubular bone, forming the growth plate (cartilaginous plate) that is the predominant site of longitudinal growth of the bone. The plate contains clearly demarcated zones: a resting zone of flattened and

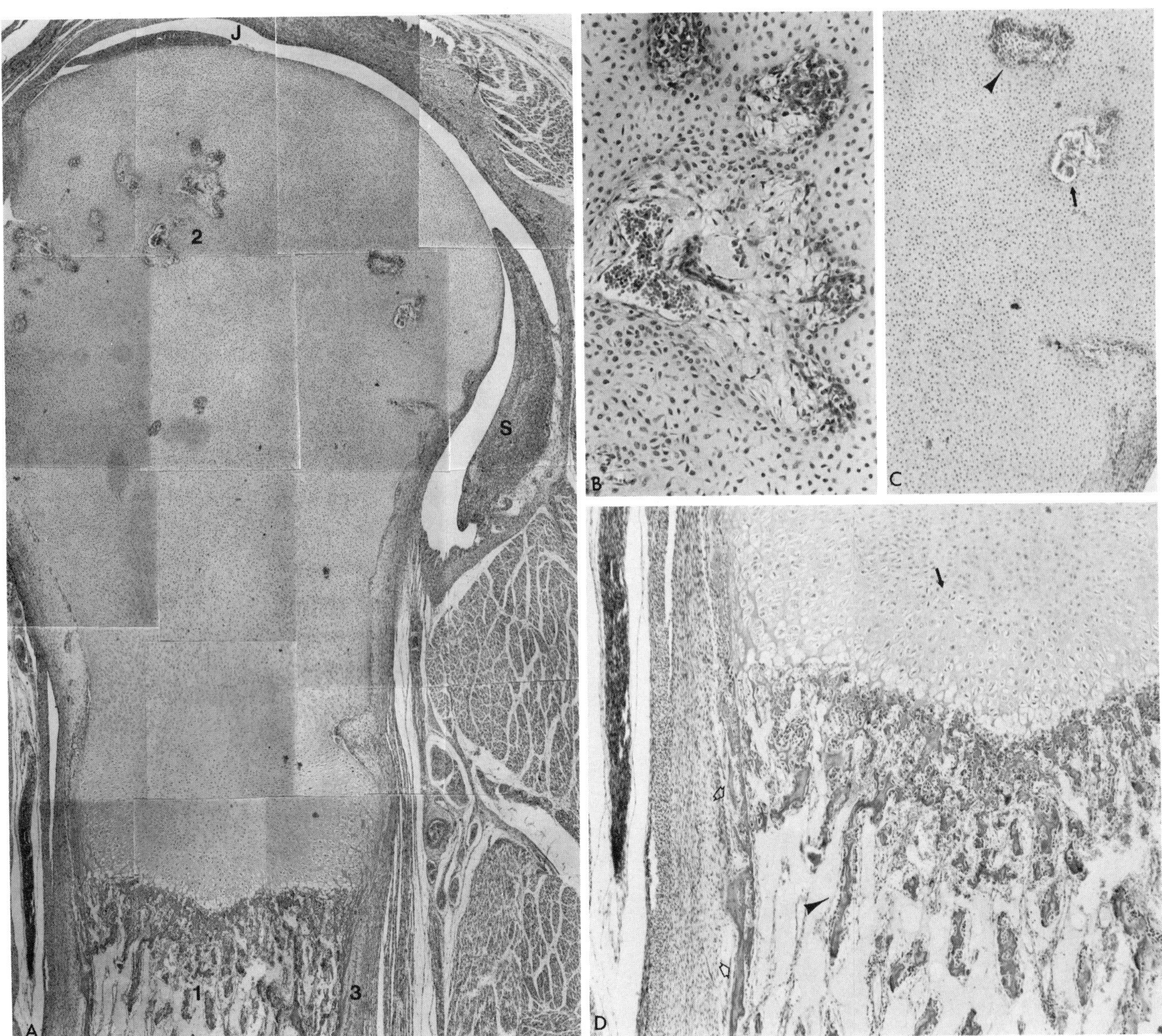

Figure 3. *Endochondral and intramembranous ossification in a tubular bone: The proximal humerus of a 4½-month old fetus.*

A *A composite photomicrograph (25×). Observe sites of endochondral ossification in the diaphysis (1) and several foci in the epiphysis (2) and of intramembranous ossification related to the periosteal membrane (3). J, glenohumeral joint space; S, synovial membrane.*

B *A high power photomicrograph (215×) shows a developing ossification center of the epiphysis with a vessel-rich focus of developing osteoblasts.*

C *A high power photomicrograph (86×) of a portion of the proximal humeral epiphysis demonstrates blood vessels (arrow) about a small ossifying focus (arrowhead).*

D *A high power photomicrograph (86×) demonstrates the features of the band of endochondral ossification that exists between the cartilage (solid arrow) and diaphyseal bone (arrowhead). Observe a layer of bone (open arrows) beneath the periosteal membrane related to intramembranous ossification.*

immature cells on the epiphyseal aspect of the plate, and zones of cell growth and hypertrophy and of transformation with provisional calcification and ossification on the metaphyseal or diaphyseal aspect of the plate.

In this setting of progressive ossification of the diaphysis with longitudinal spread toward the ends of the bone, characteristic changes appear within the epiphysis (Fig. 3). Epiphyseal invasion by vascular channels is later followed by the initiation of endochondral bone formation, creating secondary centers of ossification. The process is again characterized by cartilage cell hypertrophy and death, followed by calcification. Vascular mesenchyme invades these epiphyseal foci, and osteoblasts appear, which deposit osseous tissue on the calcified matrix. In this fashion, an enlarging ossification nucleus is created whose peripheral margins contain zones of cell hypertrophy, degeneration, calcification, and ossification. The epiphyseal ossification center at first develops rapidly, although later the process slows. The epiphyseal cartilage is thus converted to bone, although a layer on its articular aspect persists, destined to become the articular cartilage of the neighboring joint. With continued maturation of both the epiphysis and diaphysis, the growth plate is thinned still further (Fig. 4). Gradually, cellular activity within the plate diminishes and a layer of bone is applied to its diaphyseal surface. Soon, vascular invasion of the plate's remaining cartilage cells is associated with ossification via the process of creeping substitution. In this fashion, the growth plate disappears, allowing fusion of epiphyseal and diaphyseal ossification centers, followed by cessation of endochondral bone formation deep to the articular cartilage of the epiphysis, with formation of a subchondral bone plate. Although the growth plate has now ceased to function, a band of horizontally oriented trabeculae may persist, marking the previous location of the plate as a transverse radiopaque fusion line.

This process of endochondral ossification has its counterpart in bones other than the tubular ones of the extremities. Enlarging ossification nuclei are recognized in the developing carpus and tarsus, while in the vertebral column, multiple centers of ossification appear in the vertebral body and the neural arches and, through a process of enlargement and fusion, create the vertebral structure that characterizes the mature skeleton (Fig. 5).

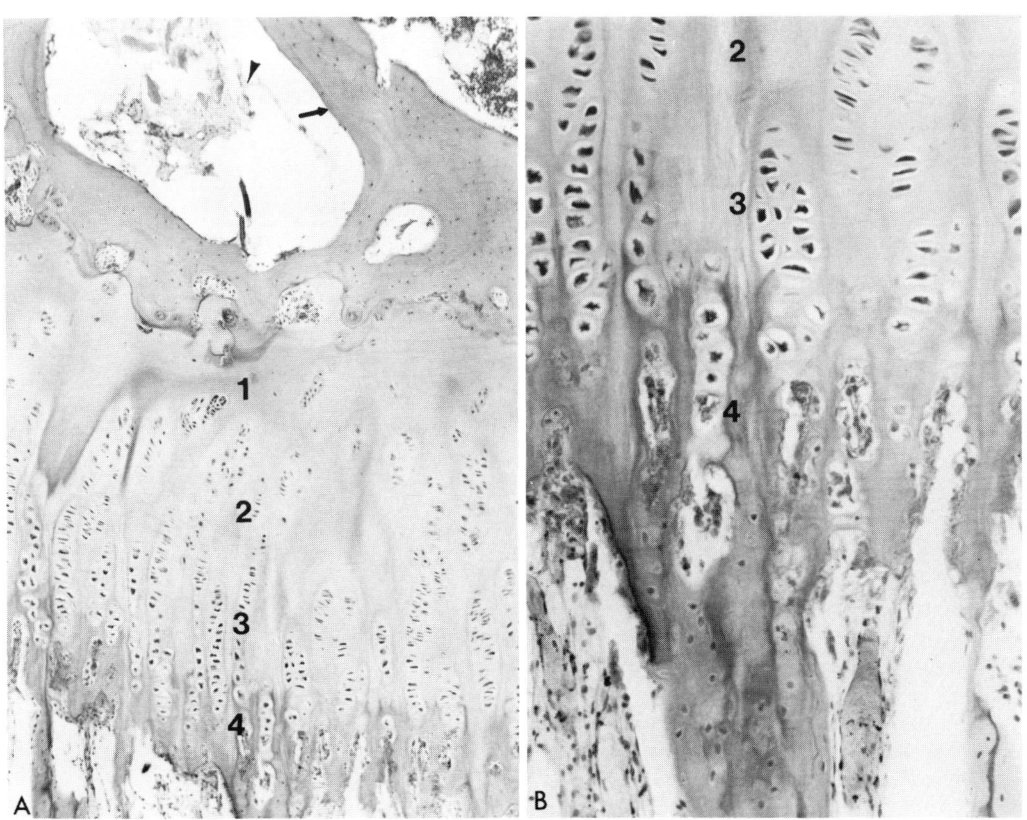

Figure 4. *Cartilaginous growth plate in a 16 year old patient. Observe the bone (arrow) and marrow (arrowhead) of the epiphysis. The areas of the growth plate include a zone of resting cartilage (1), proliferating cartilage (2), maturing cartilage (3), and calcifying cartilage (4). (**A**, 86 ×; **B**, 215×.)*

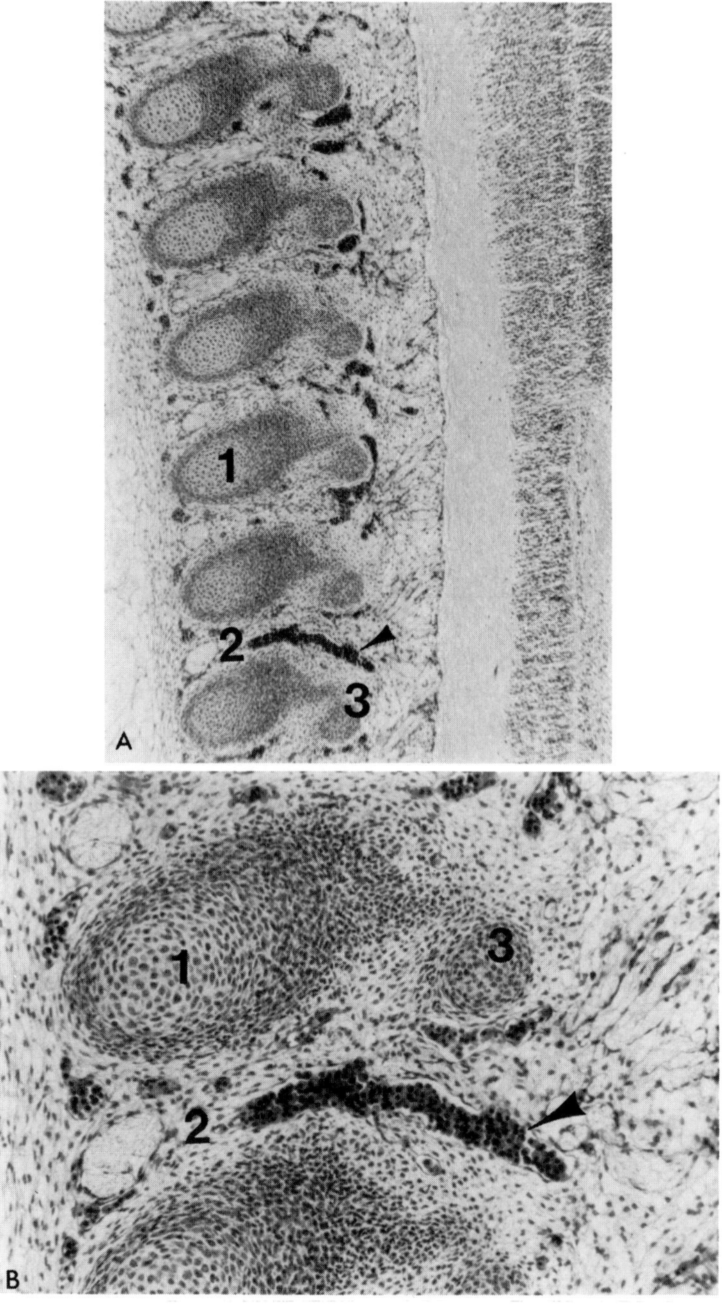

Figure 5. *Development of vertebra and intervertebral disc.*

A, B *Photomicrographs of a sagittal section of a young embryo. Observe sites of the primitive vertebral body (1), intervertebral disc (2), and posterior elements (3). Blood vessels are evident (arrowhead). (**A**, 20×; **B**, 56×.)*

Illustration continued on the opposite page

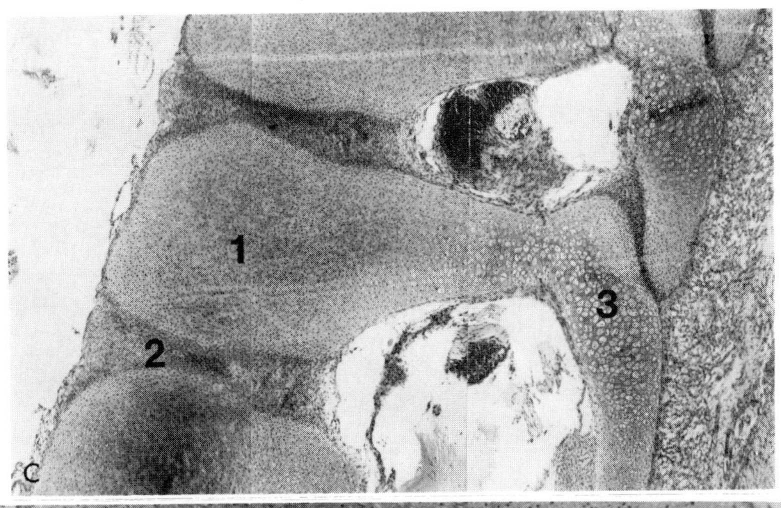

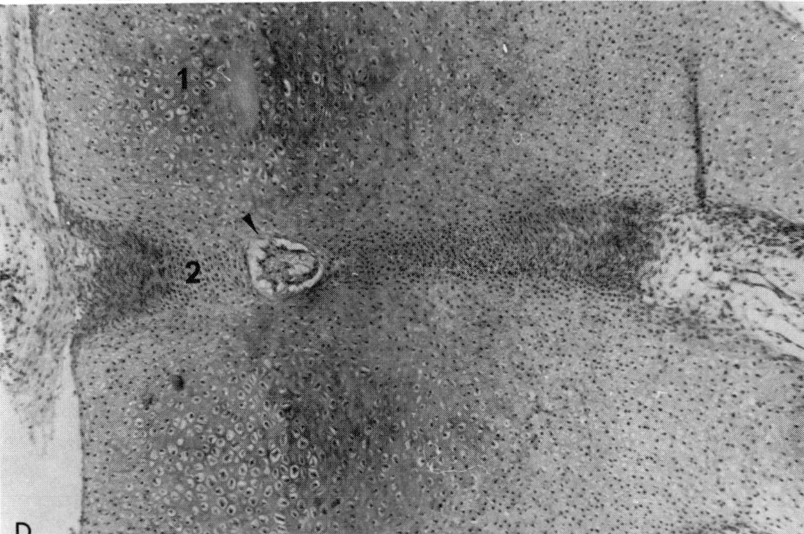

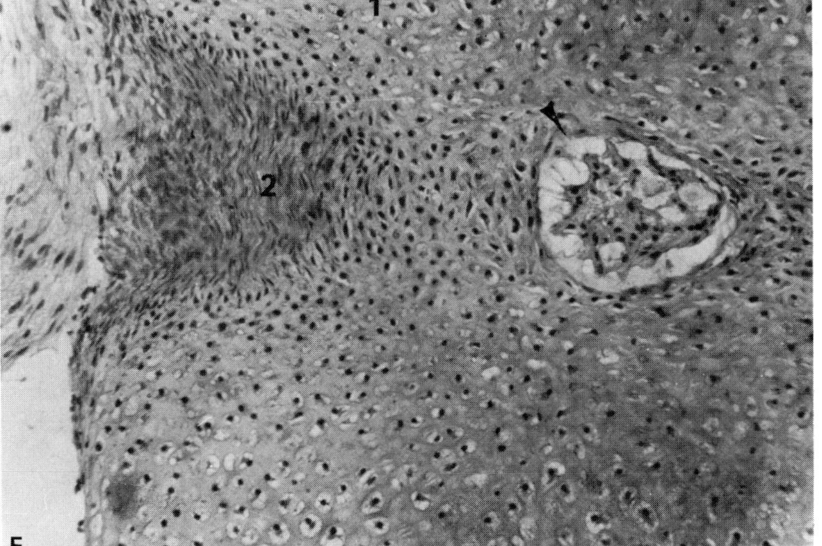

Figure 5. Continued

C *At this stage of chondrification of the mesenchyme of the primitive vertebral column, proliferation of cartilage cells is most evident in the posterior elements (3). 1, Vertebral body; 2, intervertebral disc.) (56×.)*

D, E *Within the intervertebral disc, an aggregate of notocord cells (arrowhead) can be identified. The cells form a syncytial mass separated by clefts in which mucoid material is found. 1, Vertebral body; 2, intervertebral disc. (**D**, 100×; **E**, 250×.)*

Illustration continued on the following page

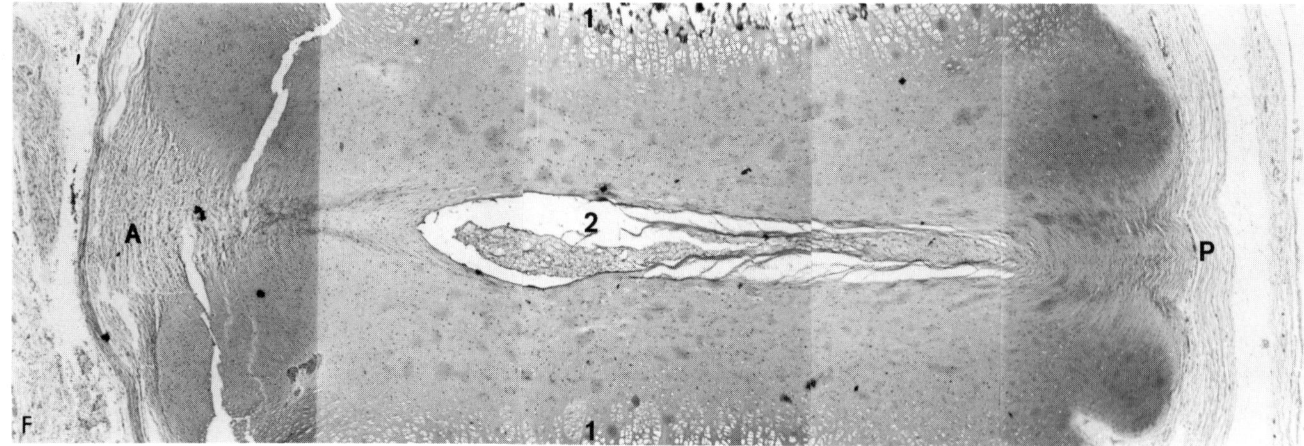

Figure 5. Continued
F *At this stage, observe the ossifying vertebral bodies (1), the primitive nucleus pulposus of the intervertebral disc (2), and the sites of the anterior (A) and posterior (P) longitudinal ligaments. (56×.)*

THE DEVELOPING JOINT

Although a description of the embryology of articular structures is contained in Chapter 1, a few comments regarding the development of articulations are appropriate here. An articulation appears in the mesenchyme that is placed between the developing ends of the bones. In this interzone, mesenchyme is not converted to cartilage or bone but rather undergoes change that is influenced by the type of articulation destined to be formed. In a fibrous joint, the interzonal mesenchyme is modified to form the fibrous tissue that will connect the adjacent bones; in a synchondrosis it is converted into hyaline cartilage; and in a symphysis it is changed into fibrocartilage. At the site of a synovial joint, the central portion of the mesenchyme becomes loose-meshed in nature and is continuous in its periphery with adjacent mesenchyme that is undergoing vascularization (Figs. 6 and 7). The synovial mesenchyme that is created will later form the synovial membrane as well as some additional intra-articular structures, whereas the central aspect of the mesenchyme undergoes liquefaction and

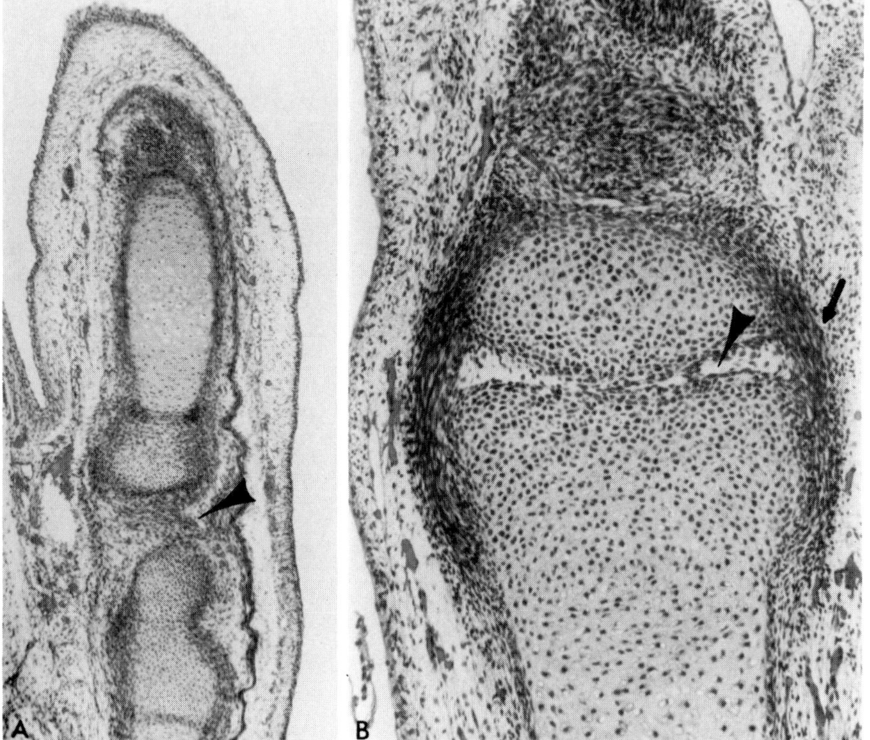

Figure 6. *Development of a synovial joint.*
A *The site of the primitive joint (arrowhead) can be identified as an interspace between the phalanges of a finger. (56×.)*
B *At this stage, cavitation (arrowhead) within the interzone has created the primitive joint cavity. (140×.) Condensation at the periphery of the joint (arrow) will lead to capsule formation.*
Illustration continued on the opposite page

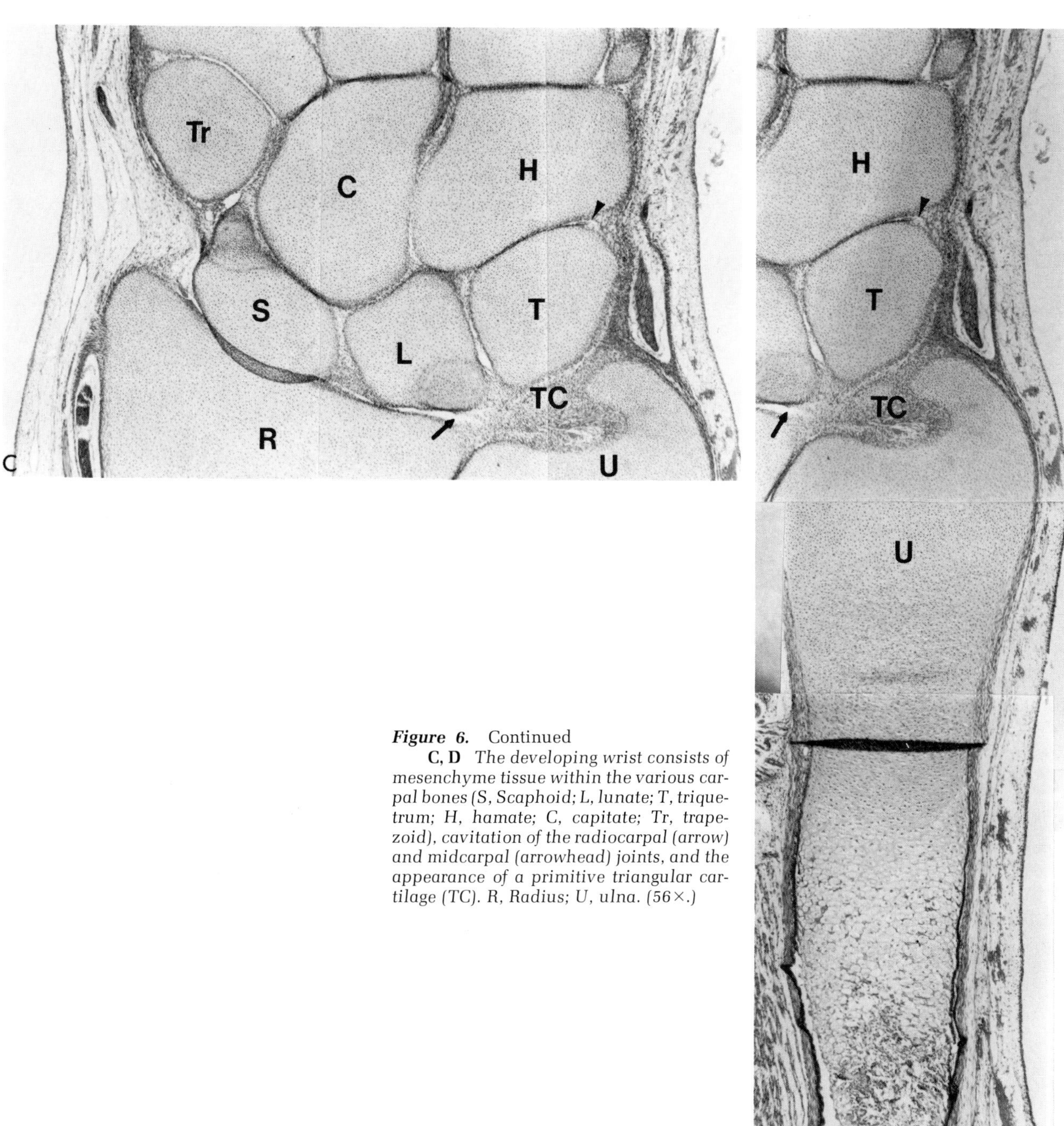

Figure 6. Continued

C, D *The developing wrist consists of mesenchyme tissue within the various carpal bones (S, Scaphoid; L, lunate; T, triquetrum; H, hamate; C, capitate; Tr, trapezoid), cavitation of the radiocarpal (arrow) and midcarpal (arrowhead) joints, and the appearance of a primitive triangular cartilage (TC). R, Radius; U, ulna. (56×.)*

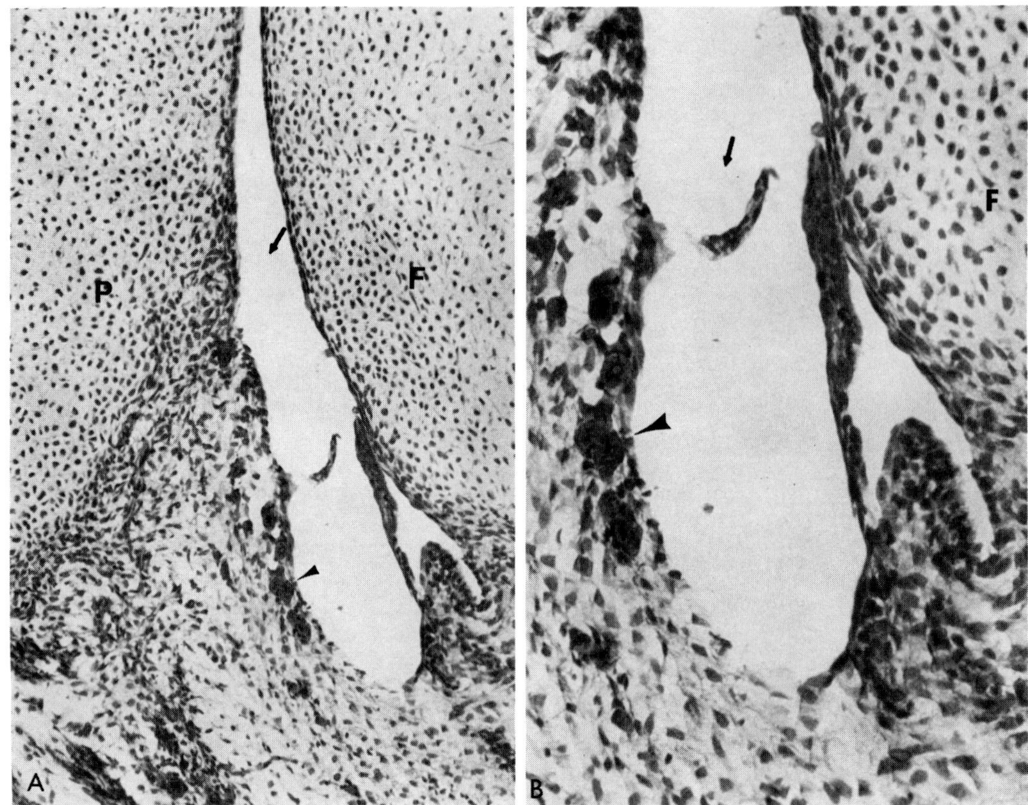

Figure 7. *Development of the synovial membrane. In the knee joint, a space between the femur* (F) *and patella* (P) *can be identified (arrow), which is lined by a synovial membrane. The synovial membrane consists of flat synovial cells and well-formed vascular channels (arrowhead). (**A**, 215×; **B**, 430×.)*

cavitation, creating the joint space. Condensation of the peripheral mesenchyme leads to joint capsule formation.

THE STRUCTURE OF MATURE BONE

The prime ingredients of the mature bone are an outer shell of compact bone termed the cortex, which encloses a more loosely appearing meshwork of trabeculae, the cancellous or spongy bone, with its anastomosing spaces containing myeloid or fatty marrow, or both. The cortical bone is clothed by a periosteal membrane, which contains arterioles and capillaries that pierce the cortex, entering the medullary canal (Fig. 8). These vessels, along with larger structures that enter one or more nutrient canals, provide the blood supply to the bone. The periosteum is continuous about the bone except for that portion that is intra-articular and covered with synovial membrane or cartilage. At sites of attachment to bone, the fibers of tendons and ligaments blend with the periosteum (entheses) (Fig. 9). The structure of the periosteal membrane varies with the age of the individual, being thicker, vascular, active, and loosely attached in the infant and child, and thinner, inactive, and more firmly adherent in the adult. For this reason, the periosteal membrane in the immature skeleton contains two relatively well defined layers, an outer fibrous and an inner osteogenic layer, whereas that in the mature skeleton is characterized by a single layer, which has resulted from fusion of the fibrous and osteogenic layers. These structural characteristics underscore the augmented ability of the infant's and child's periosteum to be lifted from the parent bone and to be stimulated to form osseous tissue. Although a layer that may be identified on the inner surface of the cortex is sometimes called an endosteum to emphasize its similarities with the periosteum, this layer is less well defined than the periosteum, may be involved with significant normal bone formation only in the fetus, and may be absent in the adult.

A closer look at the cortex identifies its remarkable structure (Figs. 10 and 11). Cylindrical units, called haversian systems or osteons, consist of a central haversian canal containing neurovascular ingredients, which is surrounded by concentric lamellae of osseous tissue. The haversian canals run in a more or less longitudinal direction, with branches connecting each system to neighboring haversian canals. These branching vessels are normal findings and should not be confused with Volkmann's canals, which represent abnormal channels

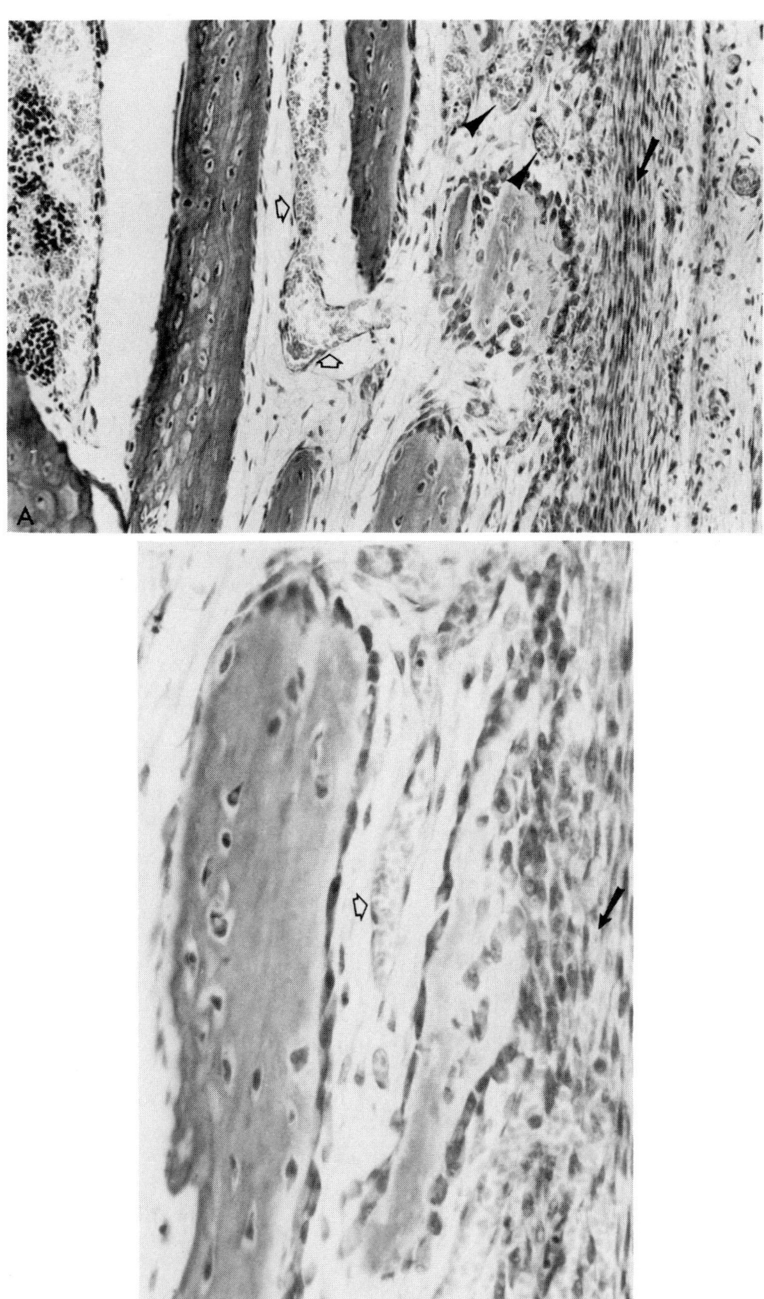

Figure 8. *Development of the periosteum and the process of intramembranous ossification (tibia in a 4½-month old fetus). The periosteum (solid arrow) is a vascular tissue. Its capillaries (arrowheads) enter the vascular channels of the underlying cortex (open arrows). The developing bone is lined by numerous osteoblasts and contains osteocytes. (***A***, 420×;* **B**, *840×.)*

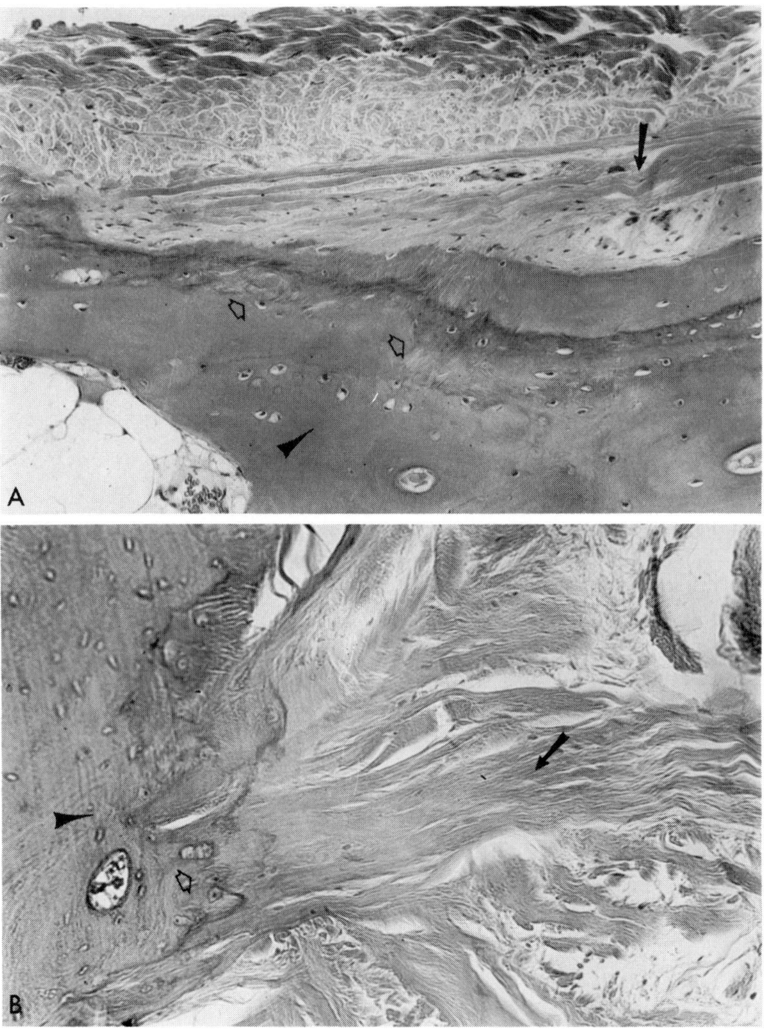

Figure 9. *Sites of ligament attachment to bone (entheses). The ligament (solid arrow) and the bone (arrowhead) can be identified. Note that the fibers of the ligament are incorporated into the osseous tissue (open arrows).* (**A,** *210×;* **B,** *420×.*)

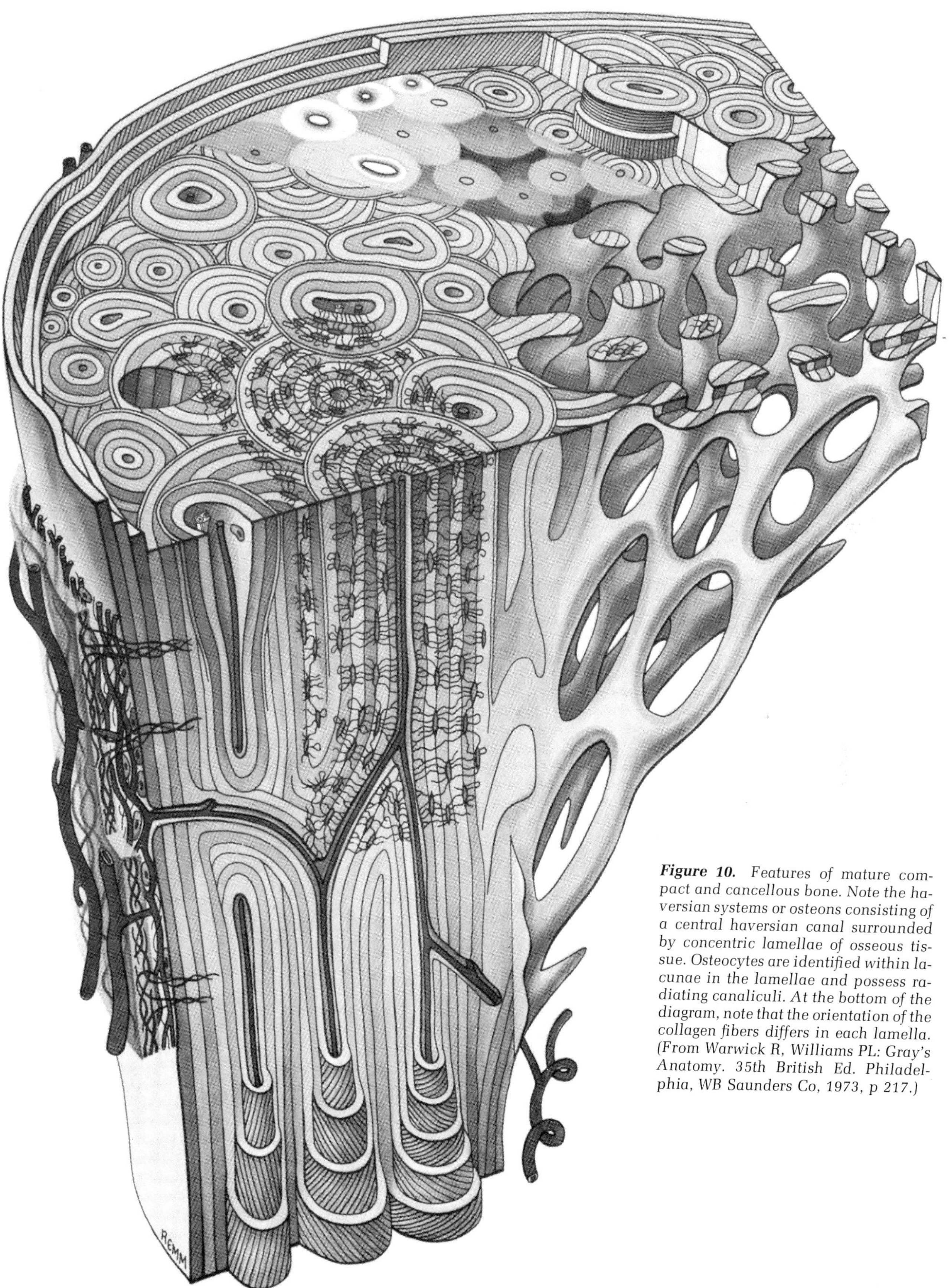

Figure 10. Features of mature compact and cancellous bone. Note the haversian systems or osteons consisting of a central haversian canal surrounded by concentric lamellae of osseous tissue. Osteocytes are identified within lacunae in the lamellae and possess radiating canaliculi. At the bottom of the diagram, note that the orientation of the collagen fibers differs in each lamella. (From Warwick R, Williams PL: Gray's Anatomy. 35th British Ed. Philadelphia, WB Saunders Co, 1973, p 217.)

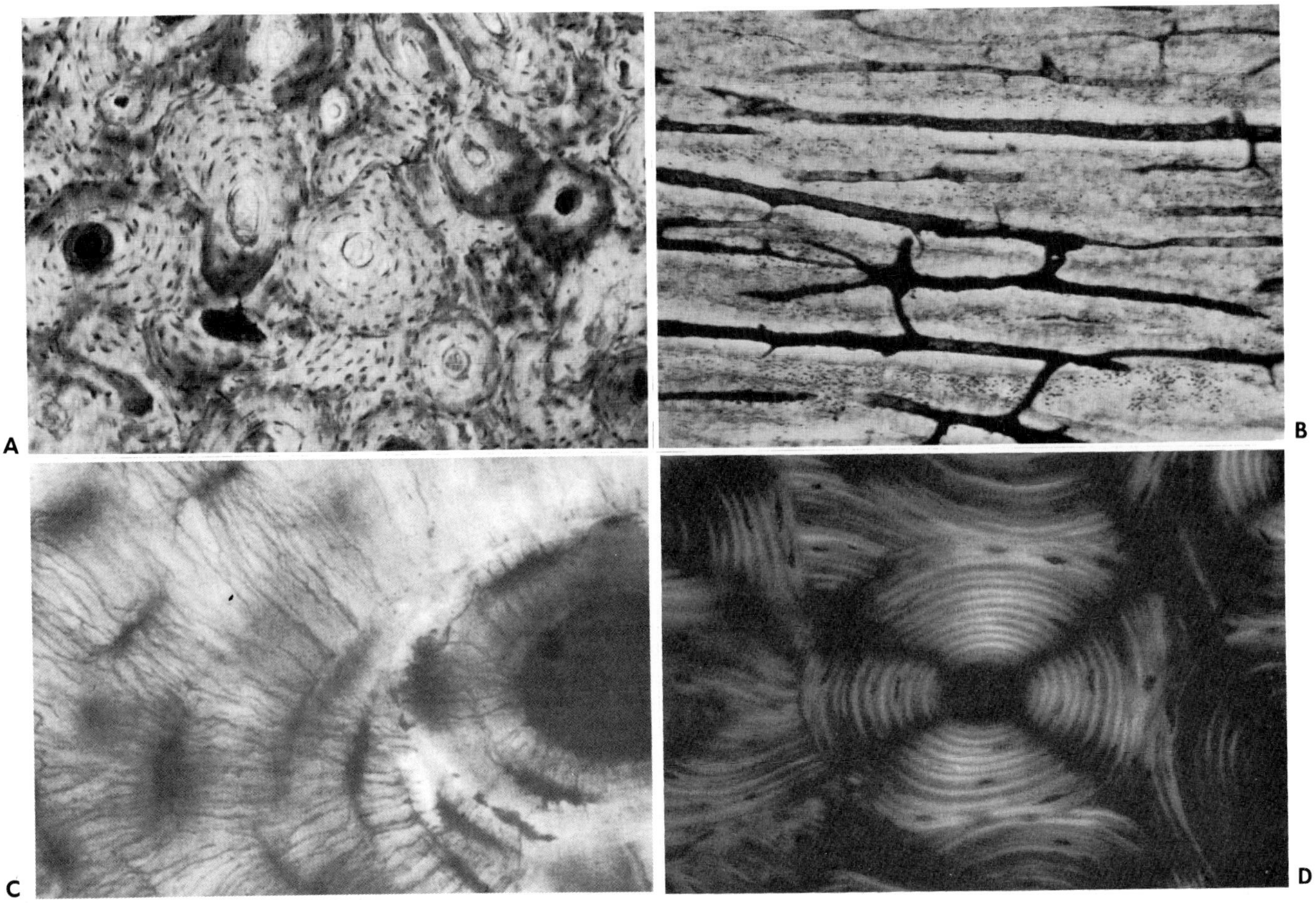

A B C D

Figure 11. *Features of mature compact bone.*

A, B *Transverse* **(A)** *and longitudinal* **(B)** *ground sections of compact bone from a human femoral shaft. Note the variation in shape and size of the osteons and their canals and in the distribution of lacunae in* **A.**

C *A high power view of part of an osteon in transverse section as seen with transmitted light. Note the relation of the osteocyte lacunae and their canaliculi to each other and to the central haversian canal.*

D *A single secondary osteon viewed with high power polarization optics to illustrate its lamellar architecture.*

(From Warwick R, Williams PL: Gray's Anatomy, 35th British Ed. Philadelphia, WB Saunders Co, 1973, pp 218, 219.)

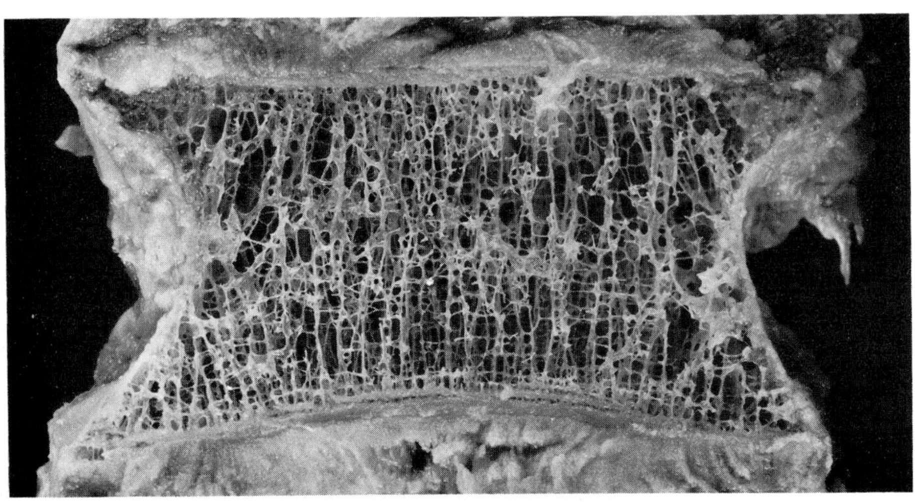

Figure 12. *Features of mature spongy bone. The macerated coronal section of a vertebral body reveals the honeycomb appearance of the trabeculae. Some accentuation of vertical trabeculae can be seen as they align themselves according to physiologic stress.*

whose formation is provoked by a pathologic state associated with neovascularity and bone resorption. Interstitial lamellae exist in spaces between the haversian systems. The haversian systems and most of the interstitial systems are separated from their neighbors by basophilic smoothly curved or indented lines, called cement lines. Surrounding each haversian canal and contained within the individual lamellae are the osteocytes, each in its own lacuna, which are connected to other osteocytes and to the central canal by radiating canaliculi. Within a single lamella, collagen fiber bundles and hydroxyapatite crystals are oriented in a specific and complex fashion, which differs from the orientation of these substances in adjacent lamellae.

The spongiosa bone differs in structure from the cortical bone. A cross-hatched or honeycomb distribution of individual trabeculae can be identified, which divide the marrow space into communicating compartments (Fig. 12). The precise distribution, orientation, and size of the individual trabeculae differ from one skeletal site to another, although the trabeculae often appear most numerous and prominent in areas of normal stress, at which site they align themselves in the direction of physiologic strain. The major difference, then, between spongy and cortical bone is in the porosity of the osseous tissue. In the compact bone of the cortex, porosity is less striking than in the spongiosa, in which large spaces and a paucity of bone are characteristic.

CELLULAR CONSTITUENTS OF BONE

The osteoblast is intimately involved in the processes of intramembranous and endochondral bone formation (Fig. 13). It is a mononuclear cell whose shape is dependent upon its level of activity: When actively involved in the production of bone matrix, the osteoblast is cuboidal or columnar in configuration, whereas in its quiescent phase, the osteoblast is flat and elongated. Although numerous and large in the developing skeleton, osteoblasts decrease in number and size as the skeleton reaches maturity. Despite this decrease in size and number, a dormant osteoblast is capable of responding to the stimulus produced by a pathologic process by demonstrating the same degree of cellular activity that characterizes the osteoblast in the fetus. Osteoblasts are fundamental to the process of collagen and mucopolysaccharide production in bone. Their life span as osteoblasts may cease rather abruptly with their incorporation into the osseous tissue in the form of a new cell, the osteocyte.

The osteocytes arise from the gradual evolution of preosteoblasts and osteoblasts. The osteoblasts, after spending some time at the surface of the bone, become entrapped within the osseous tissue as an osteocyte (Fig. 13). Here, the osteocyte lies in a lacuna and sends out branching canaliculi into the surrounding tissue. Three phases in the life of an osteocyte have been described: formative phase, resorptive phase, and degenerative phase.[3] In the formative phase, the osteocyte acts as an active secretory cell and reveals many of the structural characteristics of an osteoblast, with a sizable nucleus, an extensive endoplasmic reticulum, a large Golgi complex, and numerous mitochondria. In the resorptive phase, the endoplastic reticulum and mitochondria are less prominent, whereas in the degenerative phase, vacuolization of the cytoplasm, mitochondria, and Golgi apparatus is observed. The osteocyte is concerned with proper maintenance of the bone matrix, a process that is facilitated by the transport of material and fluid via the canaliculi. This exchange is usually confined to that space outlined by the cement lines in the bone. The osteocyte has the ability to synthesize bone matrix, although this ability is less pronounced than that of the osteoblast. The osteocyte may also be

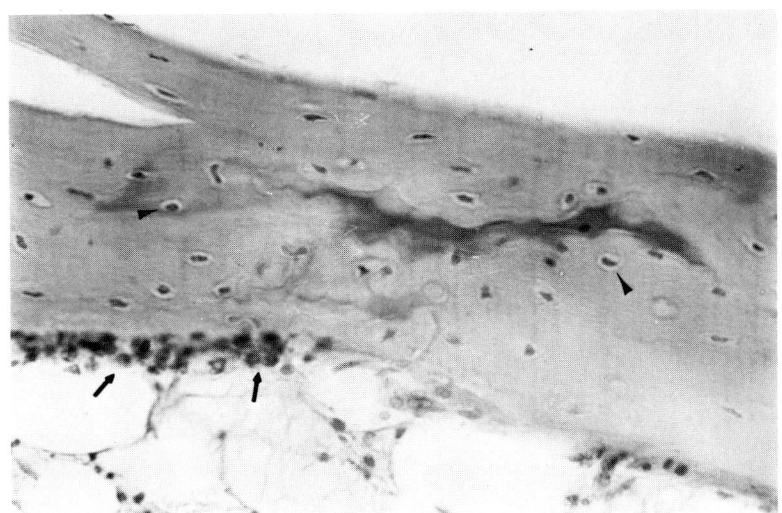

Figure 13. *Cellular constituents of bone: Osteoblasts and osteocytes. The osteoblasts (arrows) can be identified along the surface of the trabeculae, whereas the osteocytes (arrowheads) are found within the osseous tissue, enclosed in lacunae. An occasional osteoclast is identified. (210×.)*

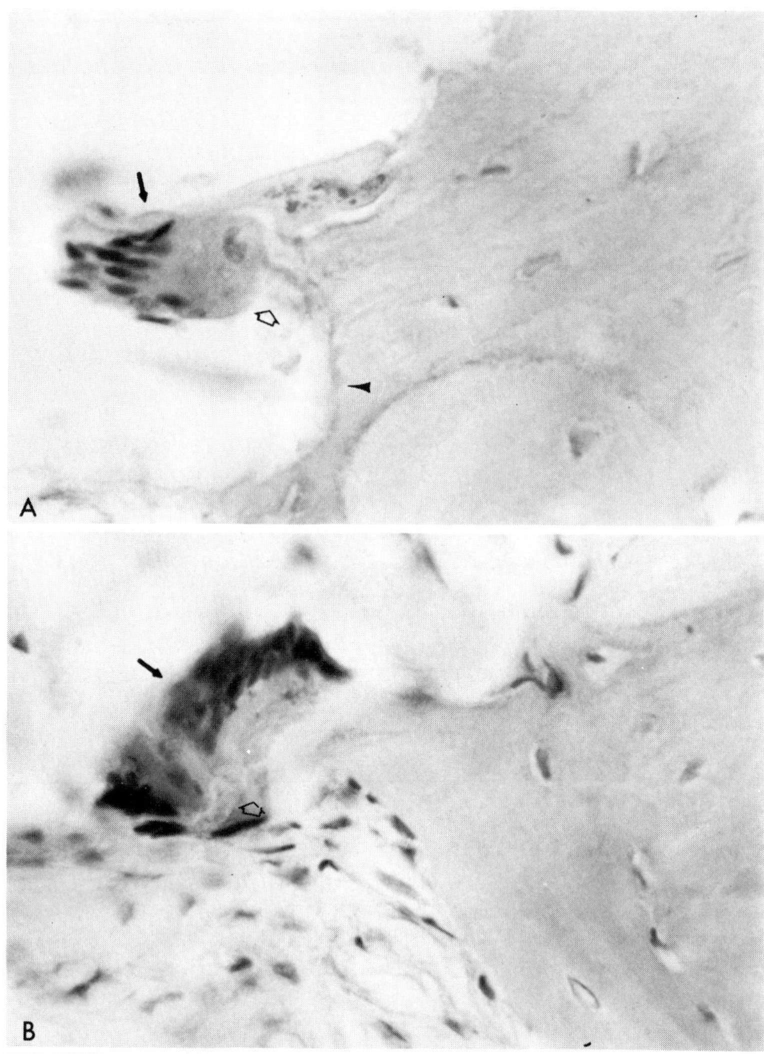

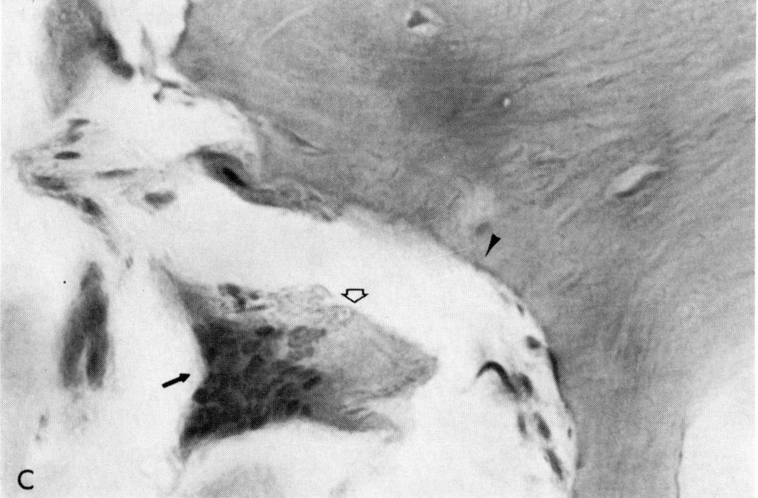

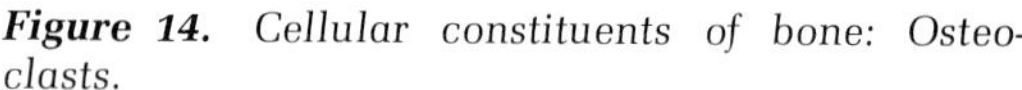

Figure 14. *Cellular constituents of bone: Osteoclasts.*

A–C *Observe the osteoclasts (solid arrow) containing multiple nuclei located within Howship's lacunae (arrowhead). A brush-like cellular border is perceptible (open arrow). (840 ×.)*

Illustration continued on the opposite page

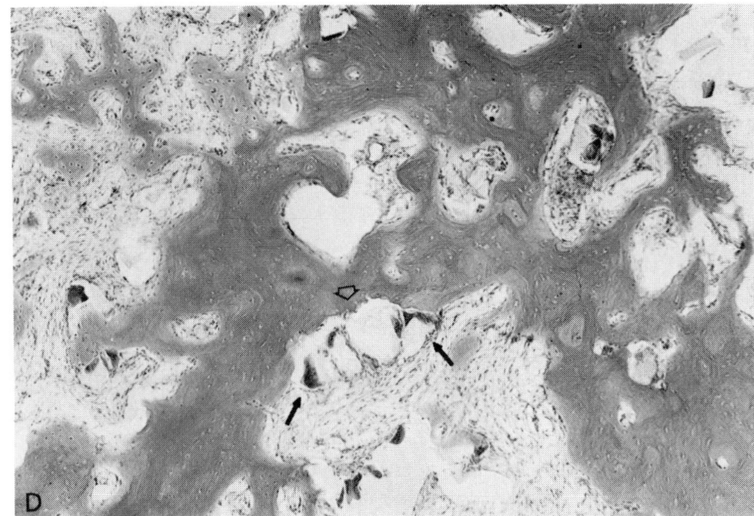

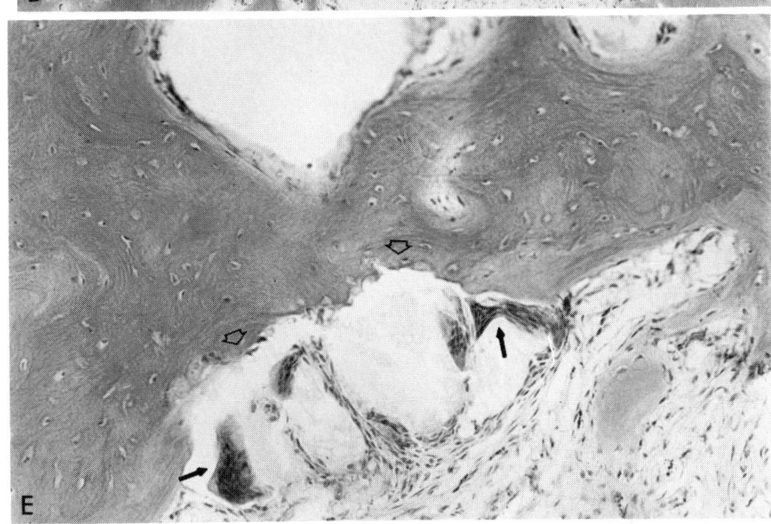

Figure 14. Continued

D, E *In a patient with chronic renal disease and secondary hyperparathyroidism, numerous osteoclasts (solid arrows) are evident in Howship's lacunae (open arrows). New bone formation and periosseous fibrosis are seen. (**D**, 84×; **E**, 420×.)*

involved in bone resorption, a process called osteocytic osteolysis. This process involves the active participation of the cells, in which surrounding matrix is modified by the extraction of specific ions. Parathyroid hormones stimulate this resorptive function and thus shorten the life span of the osteocyte.

A third cell, the osteoclast, has been the subject of much interest and investigation.[4,5] It is a multinucleated cell with a short life span which appears to be intimately related to the process of bone resorption (Fig. 14). Although it is generally believed that osteoclasts arise from fusion of mononucleated precursor cells, the nature of the precursor cell is debated. Some investigators have suggested that osteoclasts have a skeletal origin, arising from the fusion of osteoblasts or osteocytes, or both. Other investigators support the concept that osteoclasts have an extraskeletal origin, being derived from blood-borne cells. In this latter process, osteoclasts might originate from mononuclear phagocytic cells, although their further development might depend upon the incorporation of osteoblastic and other osteoclastic cells by the preosteoclast. Whatever their precise origin, osteoclasts are actively engaged in bone resorption. The exact manner in which bone resorption takes place about the osteoclast is not known, although two different mechanisms may be important: the secretion of lytic enzymes that result in modifications of the structure of the collagen and mucopolysaccharide; and the incorporation and digestion of the liberated matrix and mineral components. It is generally agreed upon that a modification in the ground substance of bone must occur prior to the resorption of the osseous tissue by the osteoclasts. This process is associated with the appearance of resorption pits or Howship's lacunae. The osteoclasts within the lacunae have prominent nuclei and cytoplasmic granules, as well as vacuoles that may contain degenerating osteocytes. The active osteoclast may reveal a finely striated or brush border where it is in contact with the bone. When the erosive process is terminated, osteoclasts become less numerous and may even disappear entirely.

NONCELLULAR CONSTITUENTS OF BONE

The cellular components—the osteoblasts, osteocytes, and osteoclasts—account for a very small fraction of the total weight of bone. The other constituents of bone include the remaining organic matrix (collagen and mucopolysaccharides), accounting for approximately 35 per cent of osseous tissue by weight, and the inorganic material, accounting for approximately 65 per cent of osseous tissue by weight. It is these constituents, in physiologic amounts, that create osseous tissue that is both dynamic and uniquely capable in providing the support which the body requires.

Collagen is the major ingredient of the organic matrix of bone; the collagen is embedded in a gelatinous mucopolysaccharide substance (ground substance). The mucopolysaccharides of bone include chondroitin sulfate A, keratosulfate, and other sulfated and nonsulfated substances. Although these ingredients represent a minor quantitative part of the structure of osseous tissue, they appear to be very important in the process of bone matrix maturation and mineralization. The collagen fiber consists of an aggregate of rod-shaped tropocollagen subunits, each unit being composed of three coiled polypeptide chains wound about each other.[6] The collagen of bone is characterized by the presence of two identical coils and a third coil with a different amino acid composition; important amino acid constituents are hydroxylysine and hydroxyproline. Linked to the amino acid components of collagen are carbohydrates, the principal one being galactosylhydroxylysine.

The inorganic mineral of bone exists in a crystalline form that resembles hydroxyapatite—$Ca_{10}(PO_4)_6 OH_2$—although the precise nature and structure of bone mineral is not known and it appears that structural characteristics of the mineral change somewhat during the processes of bone formation and dissolution, reflected by changing molar ratios of calcium and phosphate.[7] In terms of its ionic composition, the inorganic matter of bone consists principally of calcium, magnesium, sodium, potassium, and strontium as cations, and phosphorus, carbon dioxide, citric acid, chlorine, and fluorine as anions.[2] It is the calcium, phosphates, and carbonates that represent the major inorganic constituents of bone.

PROCESS AND CONTROL OF BONE CALCIFICATION

The complicated factors that constitute the process of bone calcification have been well described by Glimcher and Krane[6] and Jaffe[2] and summarized by Potts and Deftos[7] as well as others.[8] Some aspects of these analyses are included here. The initial nucleation or deposition of inorganic calcium and phosphate is associated with changes occurring at regular intervals along the longitudinal axis of the collagen fibril. Although the specific site of nucleation in bone is debated, the majority of the inorganic crystals appear to form within the collagen fibrils; it has been suggested that these crystals gain access to the substance of the fibril by normal gaps or holes resulting from overlap of linear polymers of collagen. In fact, it is likely that the precise structure of the collagen is of fundamental importance in calcium deposition and must be maintained if nucleation is to be initiated, as chemical modifications of collagen in vitro interfere with this process. If proper nucleating sites exist, structural components in the organic matrix of bone are able to induce calcification. Collagen seems to be the most important constituent of the organic matrix of bone that is required for calcium deposition, although it is not clear whether specific amino acid residues or the side-chain functional groups of these amino acids represent the most important factor in calcification. The possibility that phosphorylation of collagen or other matrix component is an essential step in the calcification of bone has also been suggested.

Although the basic role of collagen in initiating calcification is generally accepted, it is also possible that other components within the matrix of bone are essential in controlling the calcifying process. These components include the mucopolysaccharides, which may serve to alter the precipitability of calcium and phosphorus, specific enzymes, which might degrade substances that normally inhibit calcification, and phosphorylated glycoproteins, which might promote crystal formation in bone and inhibit such formation in other tissues.[7]

After nucleation has been initiated, further precipitation of calcium and phosphate ions leads to growth of the hydroxyapatite crystal, which becomes oriented with its long axis parallel to the long axis of the collagen fibrils. Eventually, the further growth of the crystal is terminated, although the mechanisms controlling the termination of the process have not been elucidated.[2]

BONE REMODELING AND RESORPTION

Although the histologic characteristics of each of the cellular constituents of bone—the osteoblast, osteocyte, and osteoclast—are well known, the function of each cell is not so precisely defined. Classic descriptions of bone physiology have emphasized the predominant role of the osteoblast in the formation of bone and a similar role of the osteoclast in the resorption of bone. The osteocyte was regarded as a relatively inactive cellular component of bone, which was held prisoner in its lacuna within the osseous tissue. More recent evidence obtained through use of a variety of sophisticated techniques has indicated that osteoclastic resorption of bone (osteoclasia) is not the only process that can lead to loss of osseous tissue. A second process, apparently related to the metabolic activity of the osteocyte, has been defined (osteocytic osteolysis).[9] The process of osteocytic osteolysis is associated with alterations in the histologic characteristics of the osteocyte and its neighboring tissue, characterized by enlargement of the osteocyte and its lacuna and metachromasia and basophilia of the surrounding matrix. Increased accumulation of certain enzymes, such as proteases, hydrolases, and alkaline phosphatase, relates to release of these substances by the osteocyte, which is being modified in response to certain stimuli, such as an increase in parathyroid gland activity. Thus, osteocytic osteolysis appears to be important in certain physiologic and pathologic states in humans, such as pregnancy, hyperparathyroidism, and hyperthyroidism. The cellular response of the osteocyte is quite rapid when compared with that of the osteoclast,[10] suggesting that osteocytic osteolysis represents the primary mechanism of bone resorption and that osteoclasia is a secondary phenomenon that allows removal of bone that has already been altered. Osteocytic osteolysis is an important mechanism of bone resorption not only in pathologic states but also under normal circumstances, such as those related to metaphyseal remodeling in the immature skeleton.[11,12]

The renewed interest in the function of the osteocyte as a cell active in bone lysis should not be misinterpreted as suggesting that the osteoclast is not also important in this activity.[13] The increased numbers of osteoclasts in disease states associated with accelerated osteolysis and the intimate relationship of these cells with resorption pits or Howship's lacunae in the abnormal bone underscore the osteoclast's role in bone resorption, a role that may be more operative in conditions associated with chronic osteolysis.

The processes of resorption and deposition are continuously occurring in normal bone (Fig. 15). In the immature skeleton, major modifications in the

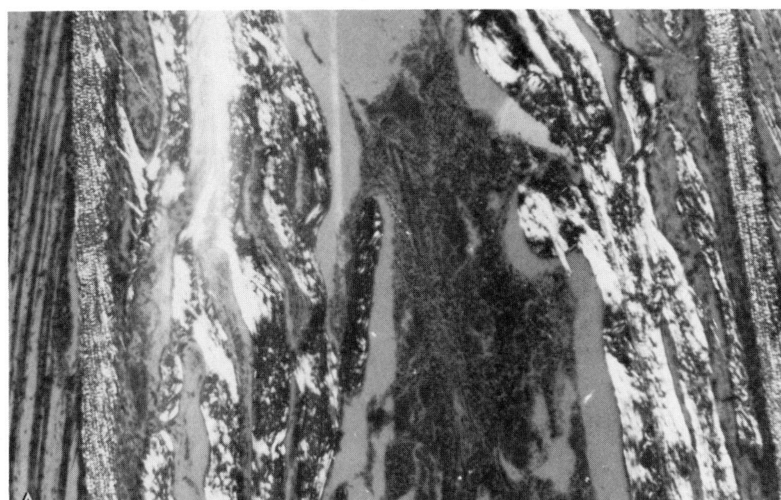

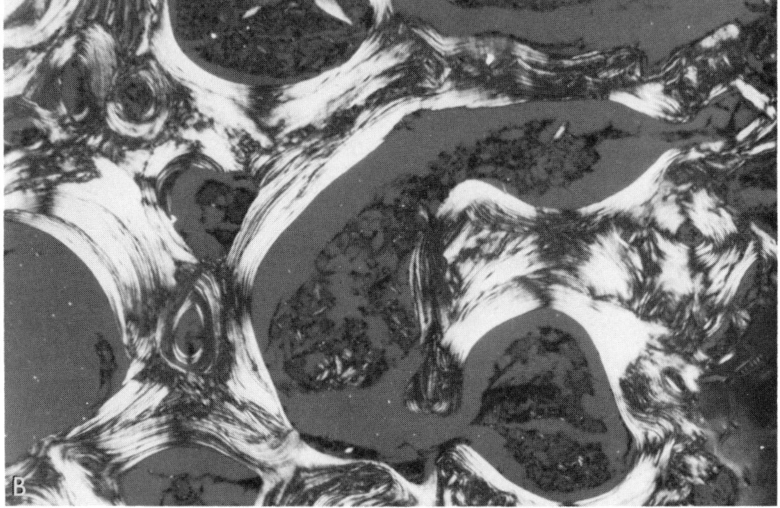

Figure 15. *Changing structure of osseous tissue.*

A *In a 4½ month old fetus, a polarized photomicrograph (84×) of the femoral shaft indicates the absence of a lamellated cortical structure.*

B *In the adult skeleton, a polarized photomicrograph (210×) indicates the organized structure of the cortex.*

size and shape of the osseous tissue that characterize the normal remodeling process are accomplished by deposition of osseous tissue on some surfaces and by resorption of osseous tissue on others. In the normal mature skeleton, a similar but less dramatic interaction of bone formation and resorption is constantly occurring. The normal carefully balanced interaction of these two processes is significantly disrupted in the presence of a variety of disease states, which results in skeletal alterations that may be readily detected on radiographic examination. It is these radiographic changes and their pathologic counterparts that are illustrated throughout the pages of this textbook.

REFERENCES

1. Warwick R, Williams PL: Gray's Anatomy. 35th British Ed. Philadelphia, WB Saunders Co, 1973, p 207.
2. Jaffe HL: Metabolic, Degenerative, and Inflammatory Diseases of Bones and Joints. Philadelphia, Lea & Febiger, 1972, p 1.
3. Jande SS, Bélanger LF: The life cycle of the osteocyte. Clin Orthop Rel Res *94*:281, 1973.
4. Hanaoka H: The origin of the osteoclast. Clin Orthop Rel Res *145*:252, 1979.
5. Göthlin G, Ericsson JLE: The osteoclast. Review of ultrastructure, origin and structure-function relationship. Clin Orthop Rel Res *120*:201, 1976.
6. Glimcher MK, Krane SM: Organization and structure of bone and the mechanism of calcification. *In* BS Gould, GN Ramachandran (Eds): Treatise on Collagen. New York, Academic Press, 1965, p 68.
7. Potts JT Jr, Deftos LJ: Parathyroid hormone, calcitonin, vitamin D, bone and bone mineral metabolism. *In* PK Bondy, LE Rosenberg (Eds): Duncan's Diseases of Metabolism. 7th Ed. Vol II. Endocrinology. Philadelphia, WB Saunders Co, 1974, p 1225.
8. Irving JT: Theories of mineralization of bone. Clin Orthop Rel Res *97*:225, 1973.
9. Belanger LF: Osteolyses: Outlook on its mechanisms and etiology. *In* PJ Gaillard, et al (Eds): The Parathyroid Glands; Ultrastructure, Secretion, and Function. Chicago, University of Chicago Press, 1965, p 137.
10. Talmage RV: A study of the effect of parathyroid hormone on bone remodeling and on calcium homeostasis. Clin Orthop Rel Res *54*:163, 1967.
11. Whalen JP, Winchester P, Krook L, Dische R, Nunez E: Mechanisms of bone resorption in human metaphyseal remodeling. A roentgenographic and histologic study. Am J Roentgenol *112*:526, 1971.
12. Whalen JP: The resorption of bone and its control: Its roentgen significance. Radiology *113*:257, 1974.
13. Chambers TJ: The cellular basis of bone resorption. Clin Orthop Rel Res *151*:283, 1980.

SECTION I

BASIC SCIENCES

1
DEVELOPMENTAL ANATOMY OF JOINTS

by Clement B. Sledge, M.D.

In the course of evolution each joint has developed a unique size and shape so that motion required of it can be achieved while maintaining a uniform mechanical environment. Articular cartilage, which has little capability of repair, functions for the lifetime of the organism only if the physical demands placed upon it are kept within a narrow range. The most important physical parameter is unit load — the force applied divided by the area over which the load is spread. Assuming constancy of load, three mechanisms are available to protect joints: compliance of the cartilage-cancellous bone unit; joint incongruency, which allows increasing contact area with increasing load; and transfer of forces into surrounding soft tissue ligaments and muscles.

The demands placed upon each joint dictate the precise relationships among the three mechanisms of force dissipation. The shoulder, having an enormous range of motion, must have a small area of contact and minimal constraint. Stress overload is prevented by two mechanisms: (1) dissipation of forces into the soft tissues supporting the mechanically unstable articulation, and (2) high compliance conferred by virtue of having one side of the articulation (the scapula) "floating" in a highly compliant mass of muscle. The ankle, which provides limited and essentially uniaxial motion, experiences enormous forces but must remain small, with limited contact areas, because of its distance from the fulcrum (the hip) and the inertia that would prevent the acceleration of a large, heavy body segment through a distance. Here the solution is by significant dissipation of forces to the fibula and, to a lesser extent, by incongruency and expansion of the articulation with increasing force.

Each joint has achieved optimal configuration, suiting its form to its function, through a different balance of protective mechanisms. A meaningful discussion of the developmental anatomy of joints, therefore, must keep mechanical features clearly in mind while dealing with the articulation as a functional entity consisting of cartilage, underlying bone, synovium, and surrounding soft tissues. Since the ultimate and unrenewable bearing surface is articular cartilage, and its mechanical function is closely linked to its chemical composition, the "chemical embryology" of this tissue must be considered. Implicit also is the need to consider limb development as well as joint development.

The skeletal system is beautifully suited to its function. It is composed of hollow cylinders of bone with the strength of oak, and the articular ends of these cylinders are flared to provide the largest articular surface for joint contact and thereby to minimize the unit load on articular cartilage. The flared end is composed of trabecular bone aligned along stress lines, minimizing weight while providing optimal strength and resilience to absorb joint impact forces. The basic structural features of the skeleton, including the articulations, are self-differentiating; the developing limb carries the genetic information to complete its differentiation from primitive mesenchyme to a normally formed structure composed of bone, cartilage, synovium, and so forth. As will be seen, it is the primary form of the cartilaginous model that is entirely self-differentiating; the bony replacement of this model is highly responsive to physical forces.

LIMB DEVELOPMENT

Staging

Although human embryonic material has been studied for generations, most of our detailed knowledge of limb and joint development comes from the study of lower vertebrate forms. Such experimental tissues may be more readily obtained, more perfectly fixed and prepared for chemical and histologic evaluation, and subjected to experimental manipulation in vivo or in vitro. Since the processes of determination and differentiation of bones and joints are basically similar in all animal forms, much of the experimental work has been done in the chick limb.

To compare embryologic events from one specimen to another within the same species, it is necessary to have a reference point for this comparison. Because of the difficulties and uncertainties associated with the accurate determination of embryonic age or length, it is preferable to refer to stages of development. For human embryologic material, Streeter formulated a scheme of developmental stages or horizons and divided the period from the single cell stage to the end of the embryonic period at 8 weeks into 23 stages (Table 1–1).

By the end of Stage 23, the chief aspects of differentiation are completed, and the remainder of the gestational period, called the fetal period, is concerned primarily with growth. As will be seen in

Table 1–1

CHRONOLOGY OF HUMAN LIMB DEVELOPMENT

Age (days)	C-R (Crown-Rump) Length (mm)	Stage	Morphologic Events
		1	One-celled egg.
		2	Segmenting egg.
		3	Free blastocyst.
6		4	Implanting ovum.
9–10		5	Implanted but avillous ovum.
11–15		6	Primitive villi, distinct yolk sac.
16–20		7	Branching villi, axis of germinal disk defined.
20–21		8	Hensen's node, primitive groove evident.
21–22		9	Neural folds, elongated notochord.
23		10	Early somite stage.
24		11	13–20 somites.
26	3–5	12	21–29 somites. Arm bud appears.
28	4–6	13	Leg bud appears.
31	5–7	14	Arm bud curving slightly. Marginal vessel appears.
33	7–9	15	Hand segment appears. Blood supply established.
36	8–11	16	Nerve trunks enter brachial muscles.
41	11–14	17	Finger rays evident. Musculoskeletal condensation extends from scapula to forearm.
44	12–17	18	Individual muscle groups surrounding early cartilage.
47+	16–19	19	Joint areas evident as opaque zones.
50+	18–23	20	Arm bent at elbow.
51	22–24	21	Toes well formed.
54	23–28	22	Periosteal bone appears in humerus.
56+	27–31	23	Nutrient vessel penetrates humerus. End of embryonic period.
60	37	Fetus	Marrow cavity forming in humerus.
90	55		Endochondral trabeculae forming in marrow cavity.
120	100		Growth zone nearing level of capsular attachment.
150	150		Active remodeling—osteoclasts seen on periosteal surface.

Table 1–2
FORMATION OF THE SHOULDER JOINT*

Stage	C-R (Crown-Rump) Length	Event
	11 mm	Chondrification centers present in scapula and humerus.
17	12 mm	Form of joint evident at junction of intersecting arcs from adjacent chondrification centers.
	13 mm	External features, such as condyles, tuberosities, etc., visible. Interzone appears as single condensed layer.
18	16 mm	Fibrous capsule appears as condensation in mesenchyme surrounding joint area.
	19 mm	Capsule well formed. Synovial mesenchyme evident.
19	20 mm	Intra-articular tendon of biceps appears.
21	23 mm	Glenoid labra evident.
23	30 mm	Beginning liquefaction of interzone.
	34 mm	Joint cavity forming by coalescence of smaller clefts.
	40 mm	Adjacent articular surfaces well separated.
	55 mm	Synovial villi seen.

*Data from Haines RW: The development of joints. J Anat *81*:33, 1947.

the section on histologic aspects of limb development, the most constant and reliable index marking the end of the embryonic period is vascular penetration of the humerus and formation of a primitive marrow cavity[1] (Table 1–2).

In the discussion of the events of limb development, two terms that are widely utilized by embryologists but which have only loose definitions will be used. A *blastema* is a growing mass of embryonic mesenchymal tissue before definitive tissues or organs can be distinguished. The term is usually used in conjunction with a condensation of cells destined to give rise to a particular structure; for example, the blastemal condensation of the femur. An *anlage* is the first visible and identifiable precursor of a specific organ; for example, the cartilaginous anlage of the humerus refers to the cartilaginous model from the time it first becomes identifiable until it reaches the conclusion of the embryonic period.

As the developmental stages described by Streeter end with the formation of the first primitive marrow cavity in the humerus, many of the critical events in formation of the skeleton and joints occur during the fetal period, for which no adequate staging has been devised.[1] For this reason, most investigators rely on the crown-rump (C-R) length for a rough approximation of gestational age. There is, however, no fixed relationship between crown-rump length and age, and comparisons based upon this criterion are merely approximations.

Limb Development

Two time gradients exist in the development of the appendicular skeleton; the first is proximodistal, by which is implied the fact that proximal structures develop in advance of more distal structures. Thus the glenohumeral articulation develops before the wrist and hand. The second gradient is from craniad

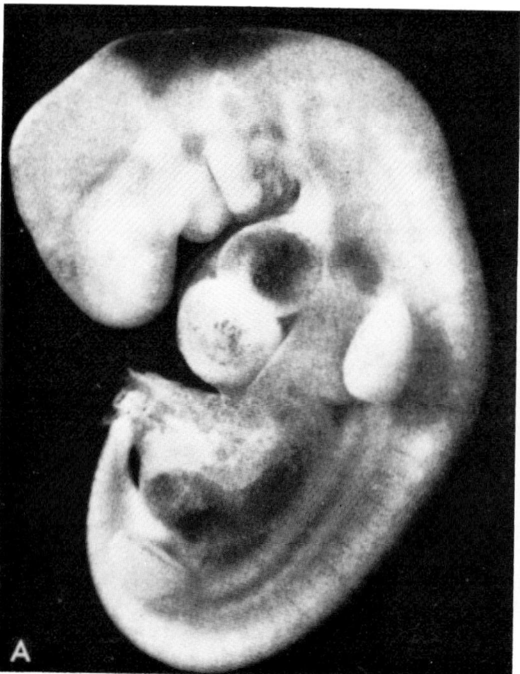

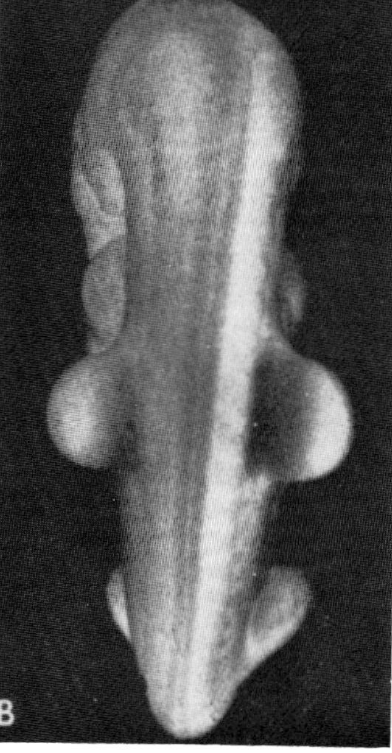

Figure 1–1. *Stage 13 embryo, lateral* **(A)** *and posterior* **(B)** *views, showing the elongating limb bud for the upper extremity and the sessile swelling marking the more primitive lower extremity limb bud. (From Streeter, G. L.: Contrib Embryol Carnegie Institution of Washington, 31:48, 1945.)*

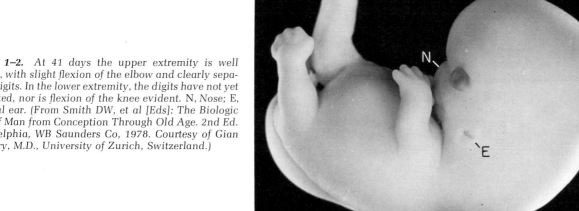

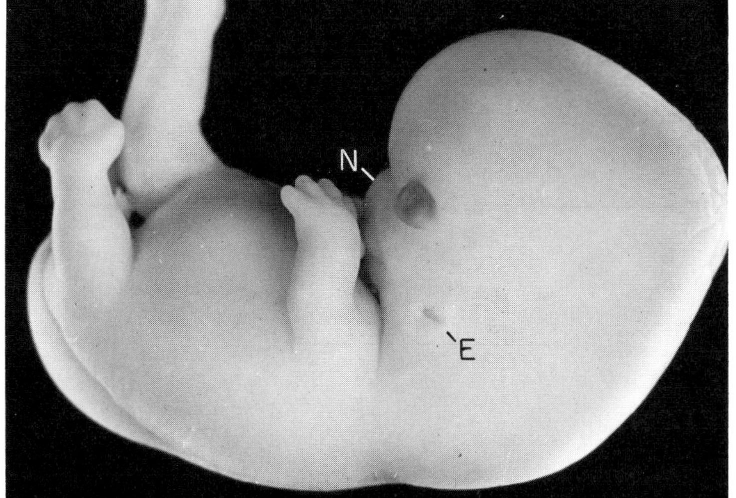

Figure 1–2. At 41 days the upper extremity is well formed, with slight flexion of the elbow and clearly separated digits. In the lower extremity, the digits have not yet separated, nor is flexion of the knee evident. N, Nose; E, external ear. (From Smith DW, et al [Eds]: The Biologic Ages of Man from Conception Through Old Age. 2nd Ed. Philadelphia, WB Saunders Co, 1978. Courtesy of Gian Töndury, M.D., University of Zurich, Switzerland.)

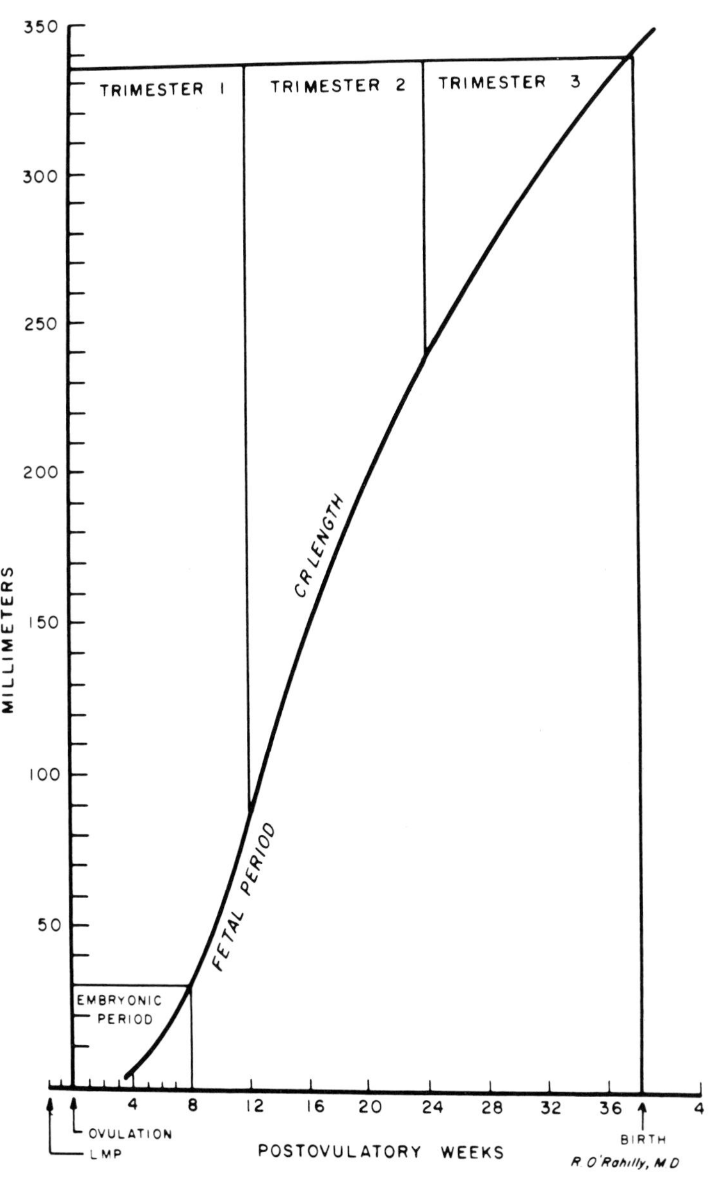

Figure 1–3. Graphic representation of the embryonic and fetal periods demonstrating the relatively short period of time during which the musculoskeletal system (as well as other organ systems) are formed. During the fetal period, enormous growth occurs and some increased complexity in organs is seen, but the full features of each organ have been developed during the embryonic period. (From O'Rahilly R: In CH Frantz [Ed]: Normal and Abnormal Embryological Development. Washington, DC, National Research Council, 1947, p 5.)

to caudad; this refers to the fact that the upper extremity develops approximately 24 hours earlier than analogous portions of the lower limb. The importance of this lies in trying to understand the influence of environmental factors on congenital anomalies; insults to embryologic development during the period of limb formation will affect a more distal portion of the upper extremity than of the lower extremity.

The arm bud appears at the end of Stage 12, when the crown-rump length of the embryo is 3 to 5 mm, the estimated age is 26 days, and 21 to 29 somites are present. The first visible evidence of the future upper limb is a sessile swelling of the lateral body wall at the level of the fifth to seventh cervical somites. This swelling occurs along a small cylindric zone that extends down the lateral aspect of the developing embryo and is known as Wolff's crest. Intense mitotic activity along Wolff's crest at the location of the future upper and lower limbs produces swellings that are readily visible in Stages 12 and 13 embryos. By Stage 13, the arm bud is easily visible, and the leg bud is just appearing (Fig. 1–1). In the next 24 hours the arm bud elongates considerably; by Stage 14 it has assumed a slight forward curvature and caudal angulation, and the distal portion is flattened in the region of the future hand. By Stage 15, the hand segment is easily visible, whereas the leg bud, about one stage behind in development, does not as yet display a definite foot segment. By Stage 17, finger rays are visible as rounded cylindric areas separated by thin, flattened web spaces. The fingers have separated into individual rays by Stage 18, while the foot is still a paddle with the individual rays linked by web spaces (Fig. 1–2). By Stage 21, well-formed toes are visible, and all the external characteristics of the adult limb are identifiable. During Stage 22 (approximately 54 days of gestation), periosteal bone is laid down around the humerus, and 2 days later a nutrient vessel penetrates the humerus, signaling the start of Stage 23 and the end of the embryonic period; thus, approximately 4 weeks have elapsed since the first swelling heralded the beginning of the arm bud (Fig. 1–3).

Histologic Features and Tissue Interactions

The first proliferative activity in the lateral nonsegmented body wall (somatopleure) extends along the entire length of that layer from the cardiac to the cloacal level and produces a small cylindric zone known as "Wolff's crest."[2, 3] Subsequent proliferation is greatest at the two extremes of this region, giving rise to the limb buds themselves. There is good evidence that the limb buds are largely the result of local proliferation, and ingrowth or migration of somitic or neural crest cells is limited in humans.[4-6] Intense mitotic activity leads to an accumulation of somewhat more closely packed cells just under the outgrowing ectoderm covering the developing limb bud. The apex of the ectodermal pouch becomes thickened and by Stage 14 has formed a well-defined ridge-like structure called the apical ectodermal ridge (AER).[7] It is generally agreed that the presence of the AER is necessary for the orderly, sequential elaboration of limb elements. Under its influence, the mesoderm is stimulated to elaborate limb elements in a proximodistal sequence. These mesodermal structures are self-differentiating and when isolated from the limb they will continue to develop into a recognizable skeletal element in the absence of ectoderm, whether they are implanted in other animals[8-10] or grown as grafts[11, 12] or in tissue culture.[13] If the AER is removed, mesodermal proliferation ceases, and only the proximal structures develop; in other words, only those structures laid down under the influence of the AER will continue to differentiate. Some regulation, however, is possible. By regulation is meant the ability of the embryo to form a complete organ following the elimination of part of its tissue at an earlier stage. The classic work of Saunders and co-workers[10, 14-19] and Zwilling and associates[20-24] has established that the induction and maintenance of the AER is a function of the subjacent limb mesoderm through the elaboration of an apical ectoderm maintenance factor (AEMF). Thus, there is a mutual interdependence of the developing mesoderm and the overlying ectoderm in the developing limb. In chick embryos it has been shown that it is the mesoderm that determines limb type; when mesoderm from the leg bud is placed in an ectodermal jacket from the wing and grown as a graft, a typical leg is formed instead of a wing.[15-17] If mesoderm derived from the duck is placed in a jacket of chick ectoderm, a web-footed limb develops.[22] If nonlimb mesoderm is placed in a limb ectoderm jacket, the AER degenerates and no limb structures are formed; if limb mesoderm is covered by nonlimb ectoderm, again no limb elements develop. Limb mesoderm that has been completely dissociated into its component cells will form an essentially normal limb when placed inside an ectodermal jacket derived from a limb and containing a viable AER.[22] There are two possible explanations of this result: The cells may migrate back to their previous position, axial or peripheral, or cells that now find themselves in an axial position may be induced by the local environment to differentiate into cartilage. Further discussion of the organization of the mesenchymal cells is given below.

Some of the characteristics of the AEMF have been determined by a series of elegant experiments by Saunders and Gasseling.[16, 25] They have shown that the AEMF is a transmissible factor, manufactured by the mesoderm and responsible for viability of the AER. Interposition of a thin piece of mica between the mesoderm and the ectoderm of the limb for only 1 or 1.5 hours leads to flattening and eventual disappearance of the ectodermal ridge. Furthermore, by interposing cellulose acetate filters of varying pore size, these investigators have demonstrated that the AEMF can exert its influence through filters as small as 0.05 mμm in pore size but not through a thin Mylar film. These experiments strongly suggest that the AEMF is a large molecule. Certain anomalous limb patterns in animals result from faulty distribution or absence of the AEMF and others from genetically inactive ectoderm. Thus, in chicks, polydactyly is found to be associated with an abnormally extensive AER and amelia and ectromelia with deficiencies of the ridge.[26-29]

Although the mesenchymal cells composing the early blastemal condensation in the limb bud appear to be homogeneous, it is known that the ability of these cells to differentiate into muscle or cartilage is determined from the earliest stage of limb formation.[30] It has been shown that the myogenic and chondrogenic precursors have separate embryonic origins and remain distinct cell types that do not mix to any great extent in the blastema. The chondrogenic cells are confined to a central core while the myogenic cells are located peripherally around this core. When small fragments of tissue were isolated from 4 day old chick limb buds and grown in tissue culture, some fragments produced cartilage, whereas others produced primitive muscle and fibrous tissue, suggesting that some cells had already been "determined" to form cartilage and others to form noncartilaginous limb structures.[13] Skeletogenic, myogenic, and chondrogenic areas of the histologically undifferentiated mandible of the chick embryo develop according to their normal histogenetic patterns when exposed to the same conditions in culture, and produce bone, muscle, or cartilage according to their site of origin.[31] This early determination has been termed mosaicism. Mosaicism suggests that the mesenchyme is composed of at least two cell types — premyoblasts and prechondroblasts — that are intermixed but not yet recognizable since they have not formed matrix. The central question is "how do prechondrocytes end up in the center of the developing extremity to form the cartilage model?" Currently two theories are held with equal fervor by their proponents. The first suggests that a massive process of cell sorting occurs early in the course of limb development; prechondrogenic cells migrate to the central portion, whereas premyogenic cells attain a peripheral location. Support for this concept of cell migration has come largely from experiments with disaggregated limb mesenchyme in tissue culture.[32] Steinberg has shown, both experimentally and theoretically, that the more adhesive chondrocytes will seek a central position while the less adhesive myoblasts seek a peripheral position.[33, 34] This sorting is dictated by the greater adhesion of the chondrocytes and the increased thermodynamic stability conferred by their central location. Contrary evidence has been provided by Searls, who grafted labeled prechondrogenic chick limb bud tissue into unlabeled embryos.[35] He was not able to demonstrate any migration of labeled cells and concluded that, until late in development, "every cell in the limb bud mesenchyme is equally capable of mucopolysaccharide synthesis." He further concluded that an environmental process, superimposed upon the cells, forces chondrogenic expression upon the central cells, whereas peripheral cells find themselves in an environment that favors muscle phenotypic expression (Fig. 1–4).

The consensus at the present time "indicates that the limb mesoderm, like the somite, contains a heterogeneous distribution of chondrogenic and myogenic cells . . . ." The "common precursor 'mesenchyme' cell ancestral to myoblasts and chondroblasts must have divided into cells in the myogenic and chondrogenic lineages at least two generations prior to the appearance of terminally differentiated

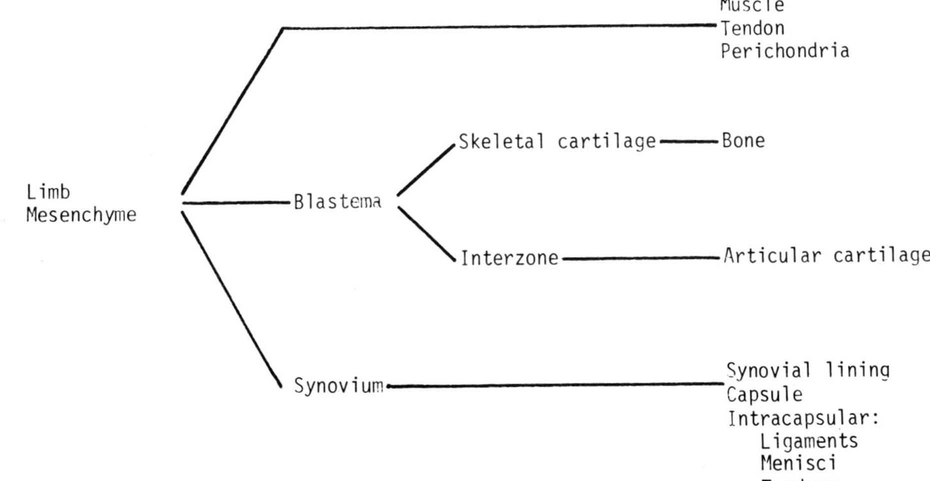

Figure 1–4. *Diagram of differentiation of primitive limb mesenchyme into the various cell types constituting the musculoskeletal system.*

muscle and cartilage cells."[36] What, then, determines that cartilage will form centrally and muscle peripherally? Caplan has suggested that it is the pattern of vascularization of the early limb bud that provides the environment in which either premyogenic or prechondrogenic cells will thrive.[37,38] He and others have proposed a regulatory role for intracellular nicotinamide adenine dinucleotide (NAD) and have shown a direct relationship between intracellular NAD concentrations and extracellular nicotinamide levels.[39] Myoblasts are rich in NAD, whereas chondroblasts lack this energy intermediary. As nicotinamide is brought into the limb by the circulation, vascularized areas will have a high level and avascular central zones a low level. This theory suggests that centrally placed cells in the mosaic of limb bud mesenchyme will be "directed" into chondrogenic expression, whereas peripheral cells will be "directed" into myogenic expression. In addition, many investigators have shown that low tissue pO_2 favors chondrogenic expression,[38,40] whereas high pO_2 levels lead to cartilage destruction.[41] This vascular theory suggests that "prospective myogenic and chondrogenic areas become differentially vascularized before the onset of molecular differentiation, thus indicating that the vascular pattern is capable of establishing metabolic gradients across the limb."[37]

Perhaps the most exciting and plausible theory of tissue organization in the developing limb bud arises from attempts to produce mathematical models that explain the biochemical and histologic events.[42-44] Except for the interrelationship of the apical ectodermal ridge and its underlying mesoderm, little biochemical information has been available to explain the sequence of pattern formation in the developing limb. Newman and Frisch have recently proposed an ingenious and plausible theory to explain the pattern of skeletal development in the limb.[44] They address the problem "how a field of cells that are competent to diversify along more than one pathway do so in a patterned fashion such that appropriate structures appear in the correct positions." The model they propose assumes that two distinct cell populations are found in the blastema — myogenic and chondrogenic — and that these cell types, although indistinguishable microscopically, are geographically separate. The more central cells are chondrogenic and are surrounded by myogenic cells. This arrangement can be predicted on thermodynamic grounds by differences in cell-to-cell adhesion, as discussed earlier. The chondrogenic cells have three options: cartilage formation, differentiation into fibroblasts, or cell death. Newman and Frisch propose that a molecule that promotes cell-to-cell contact produces chondrification in competent cells. A further postulate is that there must also be an inhibitor of chondrification. On the basis of analysis of the size of various compartments in the developing chick embryo and the diffusion rates of various sized molecules through the dilute hyaluronate gel of the developing limb, they have proposed that the chondrogenic molecule is fibronectin and that the inhibitor is hyaluronidase. These molecules meet the size requirements dictated by the mathematical model. Furthermore, both can be demonstrated in precartilage mesenchyme at the tip of the developing limb bud[45,46]; hyaluronate has been shown to inhibit chondrogenesis,[47] and the presence of hyaluronidase in the base of the limb bud[48] provides a mechanism to remove the inhibitory hyaluronate and allow chondrogenesis to proceed from the proximal to the distal end of the limb. Further physicochemical considerations allow the model to predict the arithmetic progression in the number of skeletal elements found from the proximal to the distal sites: one humerus, one radius plus one ulna, three to four carpal bones, and five digits. Furthermore, subtle changes in concentration of any of the three critical molecules or changes in the size of the compartments can produce congenital anomalies such as polydactyly or intercalary defects. The mathematical model awaits experimental confirmation but provides a rational explanation for the sequence of events observed in the developing limb bud.

The early skeletal anlage is self-differentiating at the gross anatomic as well as the histologic level. Much of our knowledge of the anatomic differentiation of skeletal structures has been obtained from the organ cultures of Fell[13,49] and the transplant studies of Murray and co-workers,[11,12,50] Felts,[8,9] and Chalmers.[51] These workers have demonstrated that isolated limb buds, obtained at a stage prior to any histologic differentiation (Stage 13 in the human), continued to differentiate at the anatomic level and formed jointed cartilaginous structures when grafted onto the chorioallantoic membrane, implanted subcutaneously or into the spleen, or cultivated on a plasma embryo-extract clot. Thus, the typical shape of the shaft of the femur develops even when the precartilaginous mesenchyme is isolated in culture; condyles, trochanters, and the head and neck maintain their structural characteristics during culture while undergoing extensive growth and enlargement. The salient features of the cartilaginous rudiment, therefore, develop in response to intrinsic, genetic factors. However, external factors may override these intrinsic capabilities and distort the normal form. If normal functional relationships do not become established, dedifferentiation and loss of specificity occur.

The first histochemical change seen in the limb bud is an accumulation of RNA in the outer layers of the mesoderm; this accumulation is most marked initially just under the area destined to form the AER.[2,52] Immediately before the apical thickening appears, the ectoderm in this area also shows an increase of both RNA and alkaline and acid phosphatases. As development proceeds, an axial condensation within the spongy core of the limb bud outlines the future skeletal anlage. This condensed core, or blastema, fades gradually into the looser surrounding mesoderm, and no definite boundary is yet visible. The central cells begin to accumulate glycogen and lose the alkaline phosphatase activity characteristic of their precursors. At first oval, the prechondral cells soon elongate at right angles to the limb axis, continue to accumulate glycogen, and enlarge slightly. By Stage 16, the skeletal blastema is distinguished from the surrounding muscular blastema by the ingrowth of blood vessels and nerve fibers into the latter (Fig. 1–5). At this stage, when precartilage is evident in the proximal humerus, the hand is visible externally as a paddle-shaped structure filled with undifferentiated mesoderm. During Stages 16 and 17, the most central precartilage cells begin to lose glycogen and become enclosed by a metachromatic capsule, constituting the first cartilage matrix. The first center of chondrification occurs in the middle of the humeral blastema and shortly thereafter additional centers are formed in the middle of the radial and ulnar blastemas. From each chondrification center, hypertrophy spreads centrifugally, proximally, and distally. The less differentiated chondroblasts in these proximal and distal locations thereby become somewhat flattened as hypertrophy in the center progresses. Separating adjacent chondrification centers, dense cellular areas known as interzones appear and mark the location of the future joint. By Stage 17, there exists a continuous core of cartilage from the forearm to the scapula; the outline of the humerus is now complete, and this structure is surrounded by a cellular condensation recognizable as a perichondrium and enveloped by innervated and vascularized muscular tissue. The AER, which appeared at Stage 14, has now become separated into five localized areas over the digits and finally disappears during Stage 18, before the carpal elements begin to chondrify. Thus, in spite of its critical relationship to limb development, the ridge is present only during the fifth week of embryonic development.[7]

After its development from precartilage, cartilage goes through an orderly sequence of maturational changes. The sequence is basically identical in many species, from chick to human.[53, 54] Streeter described five phases of cartilage maturation in human material,[1] whereas Fell[53] distinguished proliferating, flattened, hypertrophic, and necrotic cells.

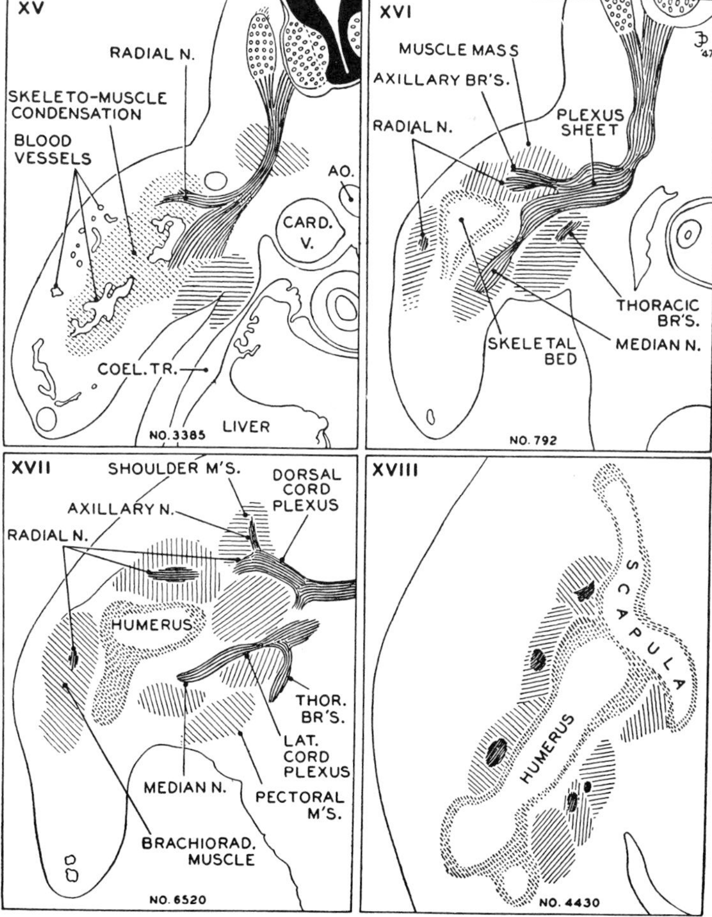

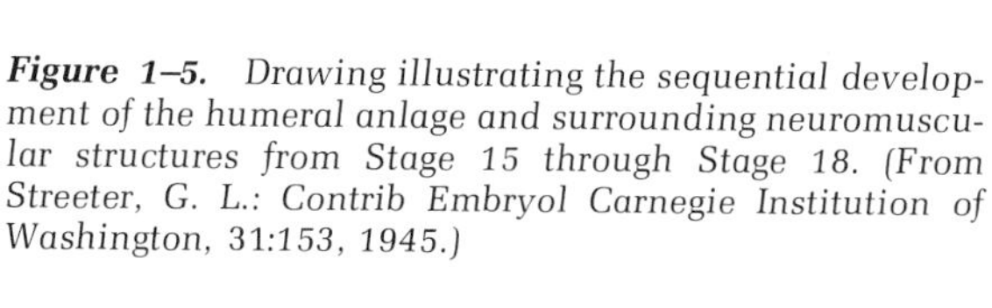
Figure 1–5. *Drawing illustrating the sequential development of the humeral anlage and surrounding neuromuscular structures from Stage 15 through Stage 18. (From Streeter, G. L.: Contrib Embryol Carnegie Institution of Washington, 31:153, 1945.)*

The sequence of maturation at first occupies the entire rudiment, with the older, hypertrophic cells occurring in the midshaft and the youngest, proliferative cells at either end. Later, after a marrow cavity is formed, all the zones are telescoped into a small area at either end of the rudiment and persist as the epiphysis and growth plate.

The compressed, longitudinally oriented cells surrounding the cartilaginous rudiment continue to proliferate and form a two-layered perichondrium that is thickest in the midshaft over the hypertrophic cells. By Stage 22 a thin collar of periosteal bone is seen (Fig. 1–6). Stage 23 is characterized by the penetration of the periosteal sleeve by the ingrowing nutrient vessel, followed by excavation of the hypertrophic cartilage cells and formation of the primitive marrow cavity (Fig. 1–7). As the vascular bud invades the calcified hypertrophic cartilage in the center of the rudiment, the cartilaginous model is replaced by bone. The process is visible externally in the embryo when reviewed by transillumination, and it is also visible radiographically; it constitutes the *primary center of ossification.*[55] An identical process occurs later in the epiphyseal cartilage and forms a secondary center of ossification, which will be described in the discussion of joint development.

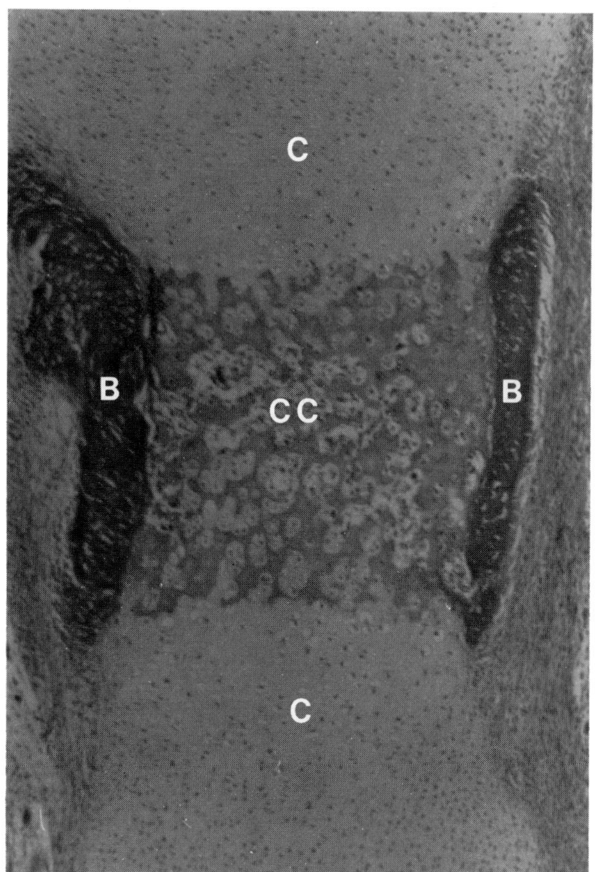

Figure 1–6. *The centrally placed hypertrophic cells in this cartilage model have altered the surrounding matrix to induce calcification. Concomitant with calcification in the cartilage matrix, periosteal cells lay down a "napkin ring" of more darkly stained bone, reinforcing this area so that when vascular invasion and excavation of the cartilage model occur, structural integrity will be maintained by the bony collar. C, Cartilage; B, periosteal bone; CC, calcified cartilage.*

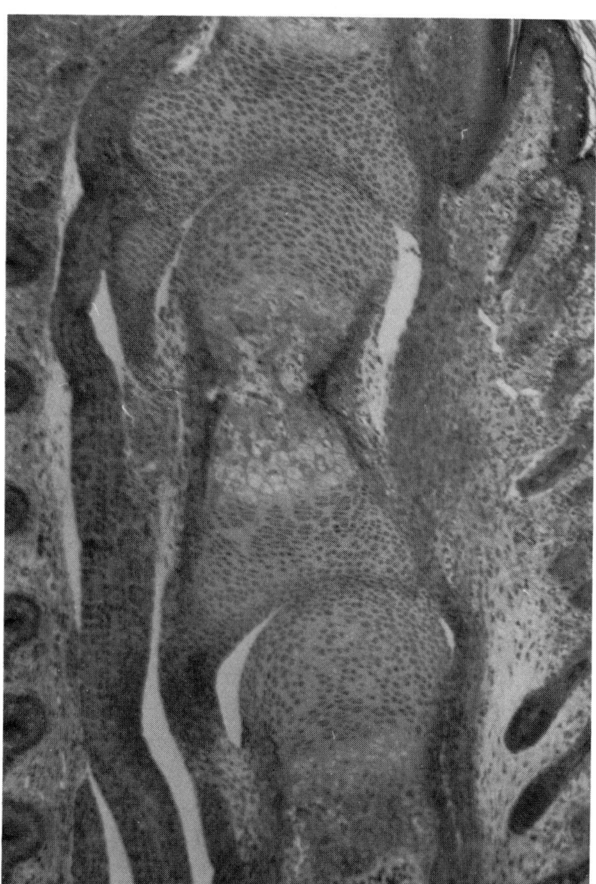

Figure 1–7. *In the middle phalanx of this guinea pig embryo, the periosteal collar of bone has been perforated by the nutrient vessel, and excavation of the marrow cavity is beginning. As the cartilage model is removed, the remaining cores of cartilage are encased in primitive woven bone, constituting the primary center of ossification. The zones of proliferating and hypertrophic cartilage can readily be distinguished, as can the primitive articular surface separating adjacent rudiments.*

The Role of Cell Death in Morphogenesis

Saunders and associates have described the mechanism by which areas of unwanted tissue are removed during limb development.[18] The process, termed "programed cell death," results in removal of tissue from the antecubital area to form a flexion crease and removal of tissue between the chondrification center of the developing radius and ulna, as well as removal of interdigital tissue to convert the paddle-shaped hand into a structure with five independent digits[56, 57] (Fig. 1–8). When tissue from such a zone, destined to degenerate, is transplanted at an early stage, the cells survive; if tissue is transplanted at a slightly later stage, but still well before any

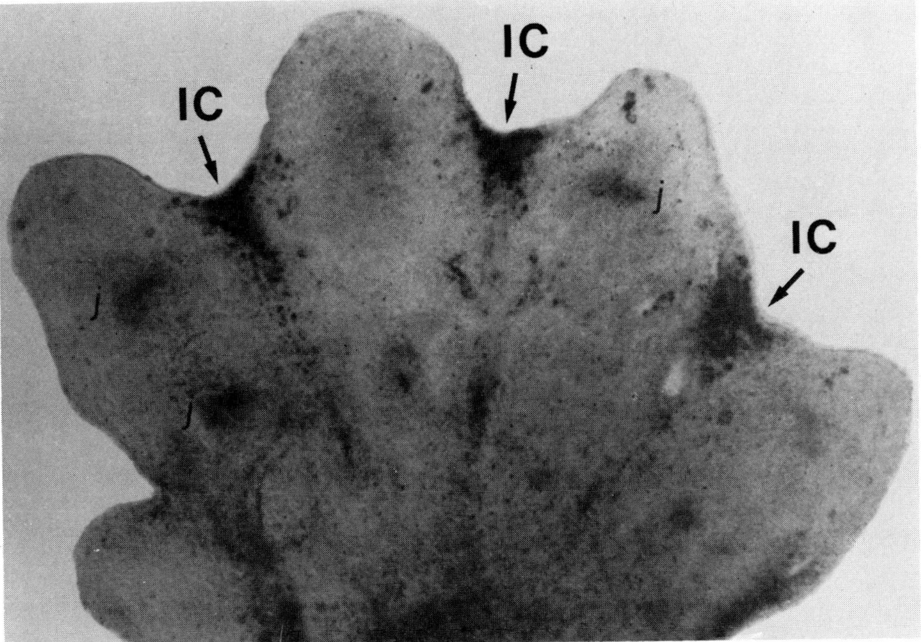

Figure 1–8. Acid phosphatase stain demonstrating intense lysosomal activity both in the interdigital area (IC) and the zone of future joint development (j). (From Ballard KJ, Holt SJ: J Cell Sci 3:245, 1968.)

histologic evidence of abnormality can be seen, the cells die in their new site at precisely the time when they would have degenerated in their original position. The necrosis of these cells, and the concomitant removal of unwanted intercellular material, is brought about through the release of lysosomal enzymes. Cortisone is capable of stabilizing the lysosome and preventing release of its degradative enzymes; it is interesting to note that the congenital malformations associated with cortisone exposure during embryologic development are syndactyly and cleft palate.[58, 59] In both of these situations, unwanted tissue (either between the two developing palatal structures or between the digits) is "stabilized" by the steroid and the predicted anomaly results.

The differentiation of the bones and joints of the limbs from a generalized cellular blastema to structures possessing a form and arrangement similar to those in the adult occurs during the period from 4½ to 7 weeks of development. This extremely rapid process of differentiation occurs in a precise sequence that has captured the interest of embryologists for generations. A knowledge of the sequence of events and their timing in organogenesis is important also in determining the relationship between intrauterine insults (trauma, anoxia, toxic medications, febrile episodes, and so forth) and the development of congenital malformations of the limb.[60, 61]

JOINT DEVELOPMENT

Joint development can be thought of in three separate but interrelated stages: segmentation of the chondrogenic limb core with formation of the articular surface of each anlage, joint cavity formation, and development of intra-articular structures such as synovium. Each stage merges into the others, influences subsequent stages, and must occur in the proper sequence and in proper temporal relationship with other aspects of development, such as that of the neuromuscular system.

Segmentation and Formation of the Articular Surfaces

Centers of chondrification first appear in the interior of each presumptive skeletal element. By the time chondrocytes have reached the hypertrophic stage, they have become surrounded by concentric rings of flattened cells extending toward either end of the cartilaginous anlage. Where these arches of flattened cells in adjacent anlagen meet, the intervening undifferentiated tissue forms what is known as the *interzone*. The interzone is the blastemal condensation that gives rise to the joint cavity and articular ends of the bone. In the human embryo the interzone is formed in the shoulder joint by Stage 16 and in the knee joint by Stage 17 or 18.[62, 63] At first the cells of the interzone are identical to those of the undifferentiated mesenchyme and differ from the chondrogenic cells in that they do not form matrix. Somewhat later, three distinct zones can be identified: a central loose layer of randomly arranged cells lying between two denser zones in which the cells are aligned parallel to the surface of the subjacent proliferating epiphyseal region.[64-66] The inter-

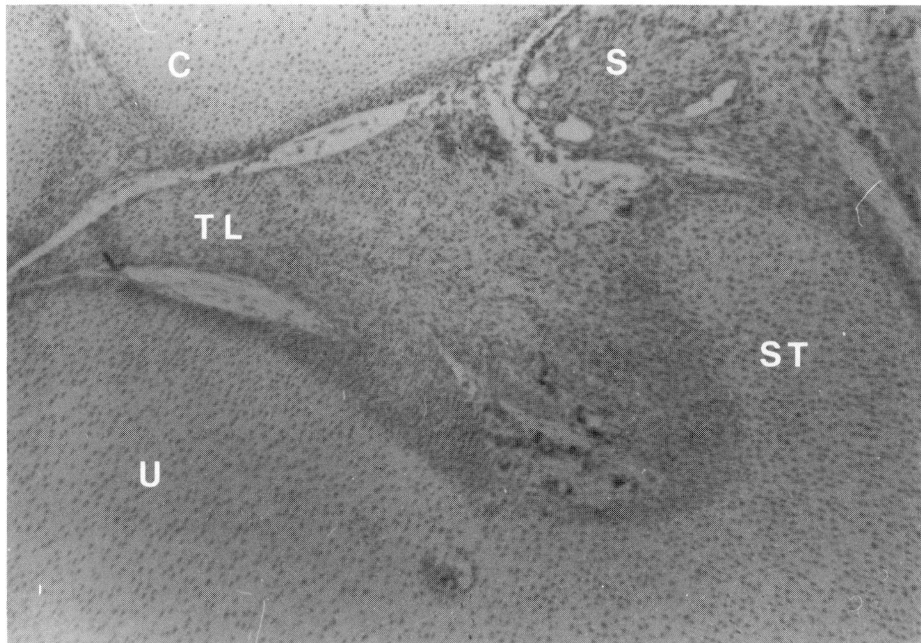

Figure 1–9. Distal ulna in a human fetus demonstrating the in situ development of the triangular fibrocartilage (TL) separating the ulna from the proximal carpal row. U, Ulna; ST, styloid process; C, carpal bone; S, synovium.

mediate zone, which merges laterally into the surrounding mesenchyme, produces a scant metachromatic matrix, presumably hyaluronate. The denser zones form parallel bundles of collagen and resemble the perichondrium, with which they are continuous; they later give rise to the articular cartilage. The fibrous joint capsule rises as a condensed layer of mesenchyme surrounding the future joint and first becomes evident before the three layers of the interzone are well formed. The general mesenchymal tissue included within the future joint space by this peripheral capsular condensation is distinguished from the axial skeletal blastema in that the latter is avascular, whereas the entrapped mesenchyme is well vascularized. It is from this entrapped vascularized tissue (synovial mesenchyme) that the synovium and other intracapsular structures such as tendons, ligaments, and menisci arise[66] (Fig. 1–9). Intra-articular structures such as the long head of the biceps arise in situ in the joint and do not migrate in from a developmentally more primitive extra-articular position. Thus, ontogeny does not recapitulate phylogeny in this instance.

Cavitation

For a true joint to appear in the solid cartilaginous core of the limb bud, the various cartilaginous anlagen must be separated by a joint cavity. The process of cavitation begins in the loose central portion of the interzone, separating the dense chondrogenic layers.[67] The process of cavitation has been described in a number of species and appears to occur initially either centrally or peripherally, with

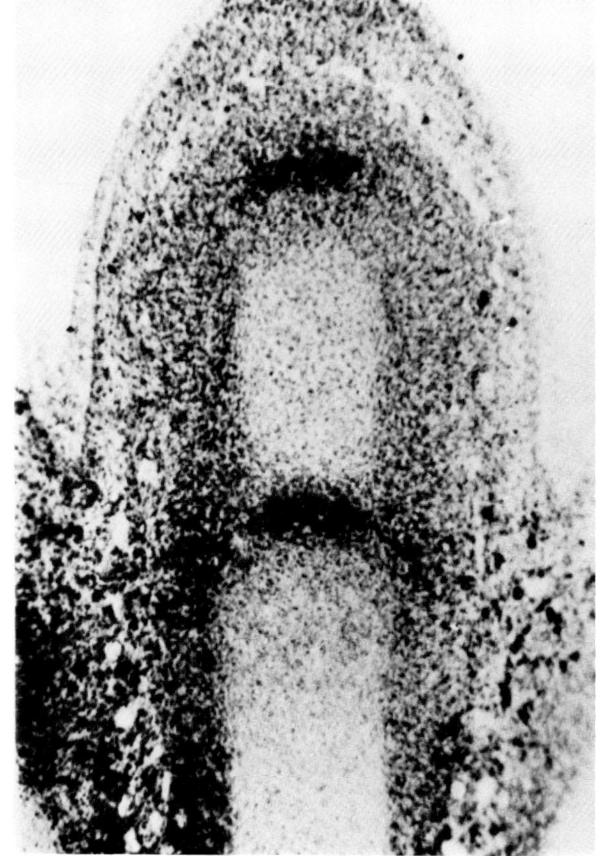

Figure 1–10. Histochemical preparation demonstrating intense localization of acid phosphatase (representing lysosomal activity) in the zone of presumptive joint formation in a mouse embryo. This enzymatic removal of matrix allows cavitation to occur, separating the limb elements. (From Milaire J: In CH Frantz [Ed]: Normal and Abnormal Embryological Development. Washington, DC, National Research Council, 1947, p 61.)

later coalescence of many small cavities into a single joint cavity. Whether the process is enzymatic in nature or whether it is an example of programed cell death remains to be determined. Several features of the process suggest that it is enzymatic (Fig. 1–10). Cavitation is preceded by vascular invasion; hyaluronate can be demonstrated histochemically in the areas of cavitation; and necrotic cells are not seen in the synovial lining immediately after cavitation.[67, 68] The process of vascular invasion to produce a cavity has been discussed earlier with regard to marrow cavity formation. The enzymatic events surrounding that process have been described[69] and appear to be related to the release of lysosomal enzymes from the chondrocytes as they are approached by a capillary, with an attendant increase in tissue oxygenation. Studies on the formation of joint fluid have indicated that the molecular sieve effect of hyaluronate will determine the characteristics of joint fluid.[70, 71] Thus, early secretion of hyaluronate by synovial cells would lead to an accumulation of "joint fluid" within the earliest areas of cavitation. Regardless of the precise molecular events in the formation of the joint cavity, it appears to be a self-differentiating process and occurs even in vitro after removal of a presumptive joint area. Fell and Canti demonstrated that chondrifying skeletal elements were necessary for joint formation in vitro.[72] When a whole limb was explanted, the joint developed; when presumptive knee joint tissue was explanted without adjacent cartilaginous tissue, only a single piece of cartilage without a joint appeared.

Drachman and co-workers, in an elegant series of experiments, demonstrated that the process of ultimate joint formation depends upon mechanical factors, especially joint motion.[73-75] If motion does not occur shortly after the stage of initial cavitation, regressive changes occur, and the joint becomes fused by fibrous tissue. By infusing the chick embryo with curare and other neuromuscular blocking agents, these workers demonstrated that even transient paralysis of 24 to 48 hours occurring at the crucial stage of cavitation produces joint ankylosis. In humans, muscular activity begins during the second month of gestation, just as the first synovial joints have reached the cavitation stage. It is probable that failure of movement at this time, whether due to neuromuscular failure or mechanical abnormalities, may produce congenital joint disease, such as arthrogryposis, clubfoot, and so forth, in which regressive changes in the joint are seen.[76]

A recent series of experiments carried out by Holder has shed some light on the relationship between development of the cartilaginous anlage and development of the joint.[77] By excising the presumptive joint area prior to its histologic differentiation, Holder was able to demonstrate that the absence of distal structures does not influence formation of the articular surface of proximal structures. That is, the specific cells that develop into the articular surface resemble cells that form the perichondrium, arise in situ, and are determined very early in limb development to form articular cartilage. Removal of these cells removes the capability to form the joint. Furthermore, after excision of the presumptive joint area, fusion of the proximal and distal cartilaginous foci occurred, suggesting that differentiation of remaining cells into a new joint was not possible in this situation. This work also suggested that the matrix secreted by the joint cells was different from the matrix secreted by the cartilage anlage cells in the underlying epiphysis (see discussion later in this chapter).

To summarize the work of Fell and Canti, Hampe, Drachman and Holder, the cells forming the articular end of the cartilage anlage are a distinct cell type differentiating according to information acquired at an early stage. They differ from the underlying epiphyseal chondrocytes, and this difference remains fixed well into adolescence. The mechanical stresses brought about by development of adjacent centers of chondrification are necessary for the formation of the interzone, and excision of part or all of a more distal chondrification center results in abnormality of joint formation. Finally, although the formation of interzone clefts is genetically programed, a true joint cavity will not form or persist in the absence of motion.

Although formation of a number of synovial joints differs from the general process described previously, the similarities outweigh the differences. Some small joints show a considerable delay between differentiation and cavitation. The acromioclavicular joint does not display the homogeneous three-layered interzone and the temporomandibular joint develops where a continuous blastema never existed.[78, 79]

Development of the Synovial Lining

As soon as the multiple cavities within the interzone begin to coalesce, the first synovial lining cells can be distinguished.[67] At this stage only one type of synovial cell can be recognized. Somewhat later, there is an invasion of synovial mesenchyme by blood vessels, with macrophages and other cell types accompanying this vascular invasion. After the primitive joint cavity is formed, expansion takes place rapidly. In all large joints in the human, complete joint cavities are seen at the beginning of the fetal period. The synovial lining cells form a smooth surface one or two cells thick overlying a richly vascularized subjacent mesenchyme (Fig. 1–11). The synovial lining cells demonstrate acid phosphatase, beta glucuronidase, and

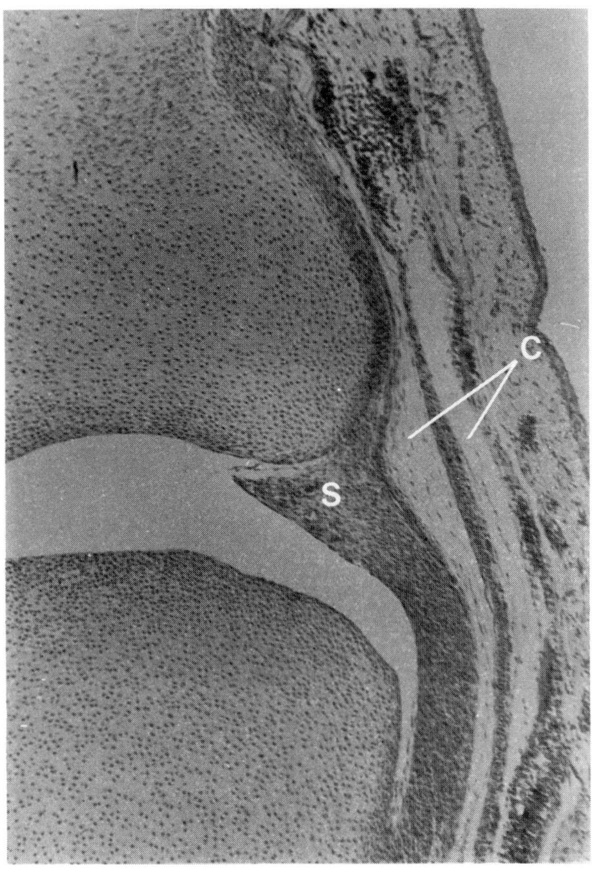

Figure 1–11. Adjacent phalanges in a human embryo hand are separated by a clearly demarcated joint space containing early synovial tissue. The densely collagenous joint capsule lying exterior to the synovium is clearly demonstrated. S, Synovium; C, capsule.

ATPase activity at this stage.[80] As the joint cavity increases in size, significant proliferation of synovial lining cells must occur to maintain a continuous lining. With continued enlargement of the joint, the synovial cavity develops its characteristic recesses and bursae, and it acquires its lining of several layers of rounded synovial cells interspersed with the lymphocytes, plasma cells, mast cells, and macrophages that accompanied vascular invasion (Fig. 1–12). The individual synovial lining cells are not connected by means of desmosomes or tight junctions but rather lie loosely in a bed of hyaluronate interspersed with collagen fibrils (Figs. 1–13 and 1–14). This meshwork of synovial cells, hyaluronate, and collagen overlies a vascular stroma surrounded by the joint capsule. In common usage, the term synovium refers both to the true synovial lining and to the subjacent vascular and areolar tissue, up to but excluding the capsule. Since tight junctions are not found in normal human synovium, the use of the term "synovial membrane" is not entirely correct. The semipermeable nature of the synovium is imparted not by cell-to-cell junctions but by the macromolecular sieve effect of the hyaluronate surrounding the synovial lining cells.[70, 71]

The histochemical aspects of limb and joint development have been reviewed by Kelley,[81] Milaire,[3] and Pinner and Swinyard,[82] as well as Andersen[83-86] and Andersen and Bro-Rasmussen.[87] All investigators have demonstrated metachromatic intercellular substance in the interzone prior to cavitation. The precise nature of the metachromatic material is debatable. Some investigators have reported chondroitin-6-sulfate and chondroitin-4-

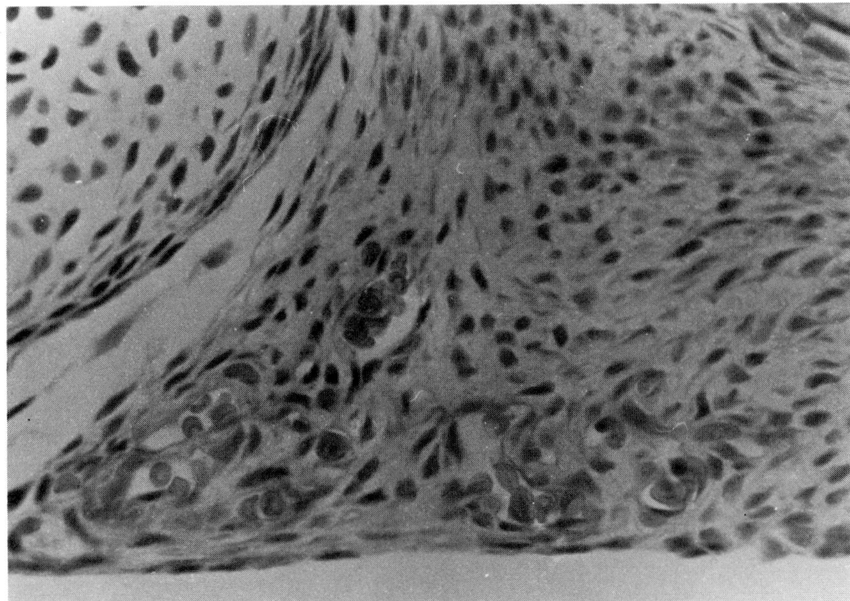

Figure 1–12. Higher magnification demonstrates the richly vascular nature of the primitive synovium with thin-walled capillaries lying immediately beneath the joint cavity.

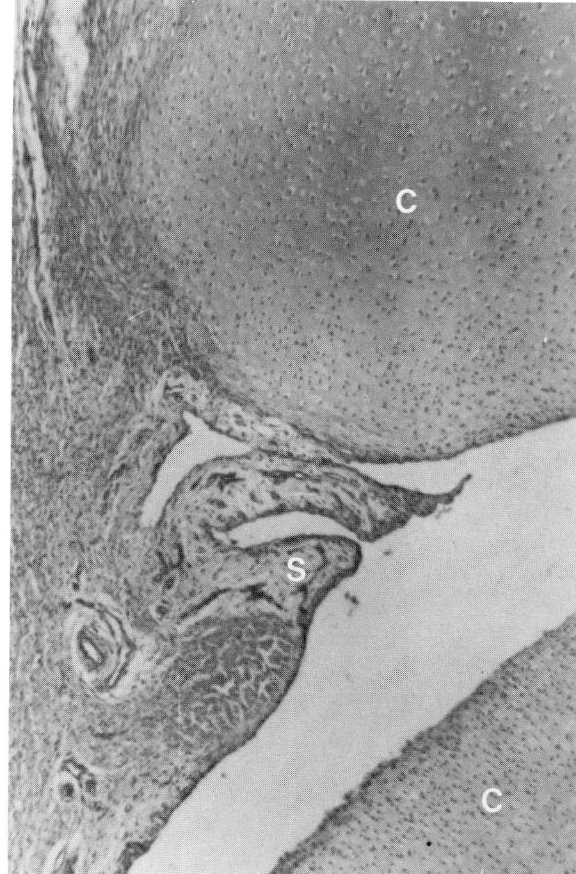

Figure 1–13. With further development of the synovial lining, the surface is thrown up into multiple folds or villi, which greatly increase the surface area available for diffusion from the subsynovial vessels into the joint space and vice versa. S, Synovium; C, cartilage.

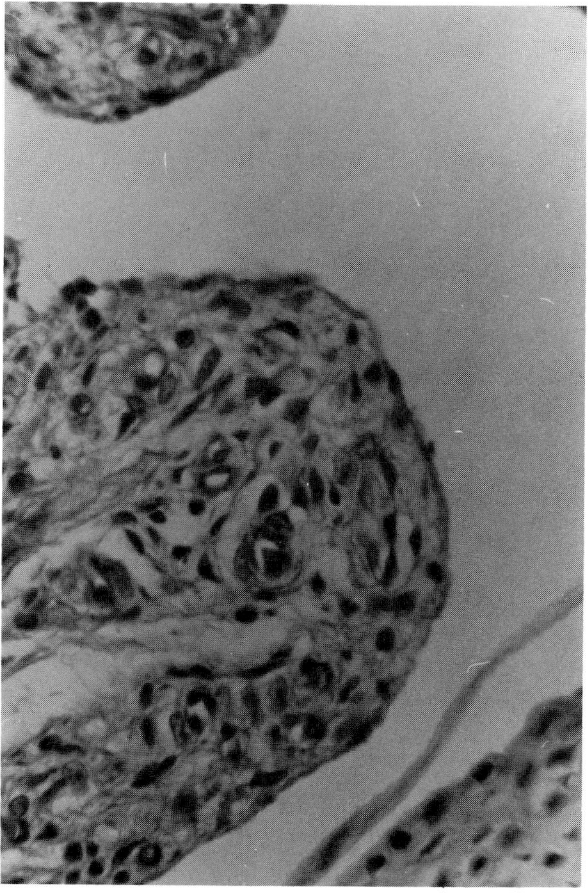

Figure 1–14. A single synovial villus is illustrated, covered by a single cell layer overlying numerous capillaries and an admixture of fibroblasts, lymphocytes, and macrophages.

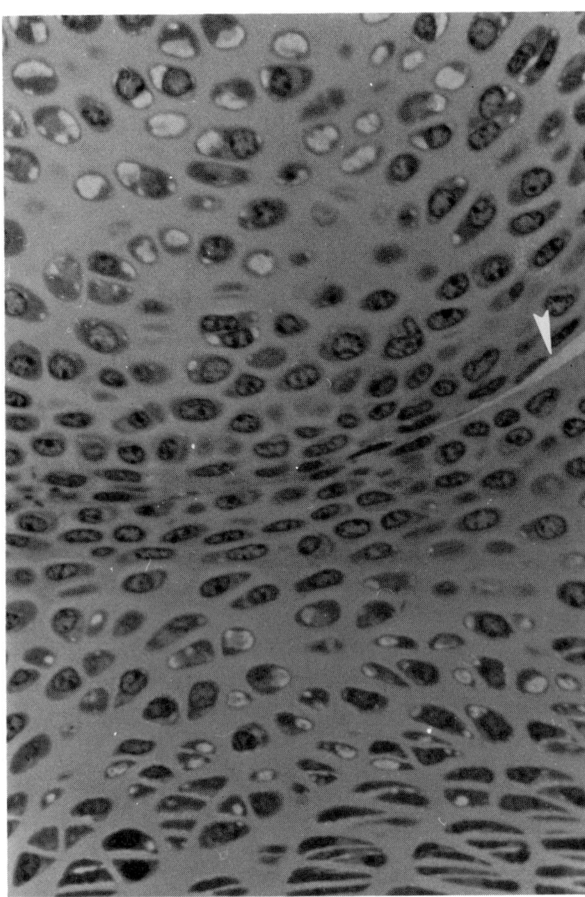

Figure 1–15. Two adjacent articular surfaces in the developing guinea pig interphalangeal joint. The early joint cleft is seen on the right (arrowhead) and cytologic differences between the articular surface cells and the more deeply placed chondroblasts can be distinguished.

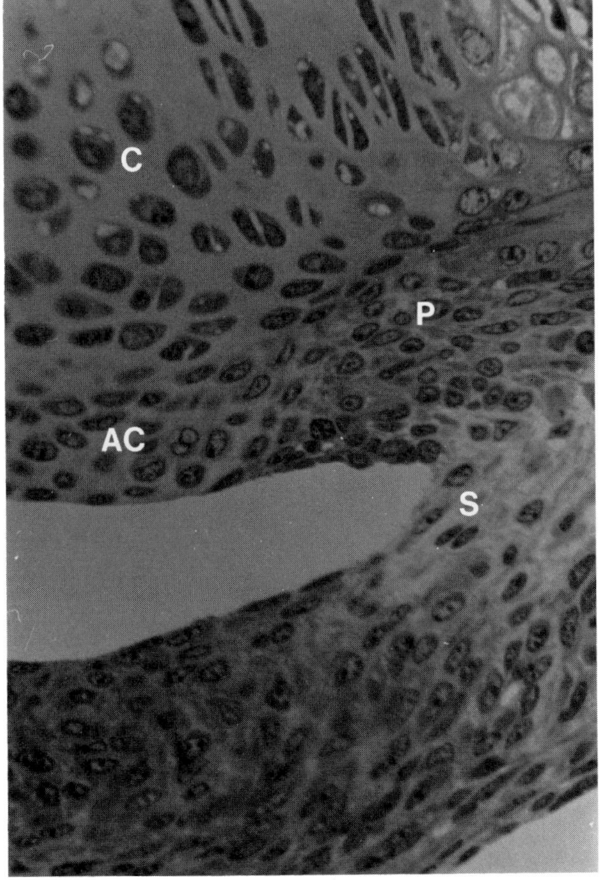

Figure 1–16. At the periphery of the developing joint, a zone can be seen where synovium (S), periosteum (P), and true articular lining cells merge gradually into one another. Subtle differences help distinguish the true articular chondrocytes (AC) from the subjacent blastemal chondrocytes (C). The common origin of the periosteal, perichondrial, and synovial cells from the interzone structure is suggested.

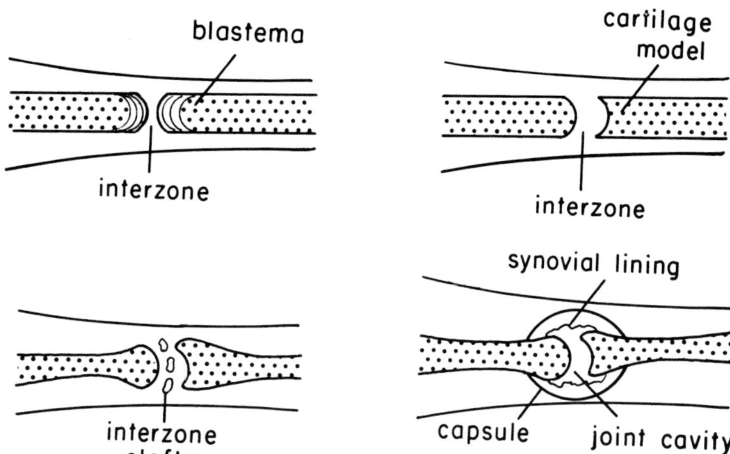

Figure 1–17. Diagrammatic representation of the stages of joint development.

sulfate without hyaluronic acid, and others have reported finding hyaluronic acid. The synovial mesenchyme that forms in the peripheral portion of the interzone becomes looser in appearance than the dense, articular portions of the interzone, and it is distinguished by early metachromasia. This metachromasia also clearly distinguishes it from the surrounding general mesenchyme.

Articular cartilage develops from the dense layers of the interzone and the continuous intracapsular portion of the perichondrium (Fig. 1–15). At birth, this articular cartilage is still only slightly more fibrous than the subjacent epiphyseal cartilage, which it resembles (Fig. 1–16). Although not much biochemical information is available, it appears that the earliest articular cartilage is much richer in chondroitin-4-sulfate and poorer in keratan sulfate than its adult counterpart.[88]

Synovial villi do not appear until the end of the second month, early in the fetal period. They greatly increase the surface area available for exchange between the joint cavity and the vascular space.

The salient features of joint formation are diagrammed in Figure 1–17.

Postfetal Development

After formation of the periosteal collar of bone around the cartilaginous anlage and its penetration by a blood vessel to form the primary center of ossification, the endochondral process spreads rapidly toward either end of the rudiment.[89] During this process, the rate of cartilage removal greatly exceeds the rate of formation of new cartilage, and the marrow cavity extends proximally and distally. By a process that is not understood, this extension slows when it reaches a certain level, where it forms the epiphyseal growth plate that separates the cartilaginous epiphysis from the flared metaphysis containing the primitive cancellous bone and marrow. Thereafter, the rate of cartilage proliferation on the epiphyseal side of the plate is equalled by the rate of resorption on the metaphyseal side, and longitudinal growth proceeds. At the same time, the epiphysis (above the physis or growth plate) enlarges in a hemispheric fashion by interstitial growth. As the blastemal chondrocytes of the epiphysis replicate and the structure enlarges, proliferation of the articular chondrocytes covering the end of the bone keeps pace so that the enlarging epiphysis is covered by a uniform thickness of articular cartilage. As the epiphysis enlarges, it is traversed by cartilage canals containing blood vessels. The role of these vessels in cartilage nutrition seems obvious, but the precise relationship remains unknown. In most instances (such as formation of the primary center of ossification and vascular invasion of the growth plate), vascular invasion of cartilage is destructive. Indeed, at a slightly later stage of development the same process will result in formation of the secondary center of ossification. The character of the vessels in the cartilage canals may be different from other vessels, or the fibrous lining of the canal and its large size relative to the small caliber of the vessel may protect the cartilage from invasion. Nonetheless, the cartilaginous epiphysis continues to expand by interstitial growth until a critical size is reached, whereupon the most central and oldest cells undergo hypertrophy and chemically alter the matrix, which then calcifies and institutes true vascular invasion, with replacement of calcified cartilage by bone. In this manner, the secondary center of ossification is formed and expands centrifugally, to occupy most of the cartilaginous epiphysis; the secondary center is visible radiographically and is often incorrectly referred to on radiographs as the "epiphysis," of which it is only a part. The mechanisms that control the time of onset of development of the secondary center are complex; hypothyroidism and hypogonadism delay the onset, and physical forces are necessary for its timely appearance. Thus, "skeletal age," determined radiographically by counting secondary centers, is delayed in hypothyroidism and hypogonadism, and the appearance of the secondary center is delayed in the proximal femoral epiphysis of a dislocated hip.

The secondary center expands rapidly until it reaches the top of the growth plate on the one side and the articular cartilage on the other side. In the latter location, a miniature growth plate is formed deep to the articular cartilage. This growth plate is actually hemispheric in shape and allows growth of the articular end of the bone, whereas the true growth plate produces growth in length. Utilizing tritiated thymidine in growing rabbits, Mankin has demonstrated two zones of cell replication in the articular end.[90] One is located within the articular cartilage and represents offspring of the interzone cells, now contributing new articular cartilage to cover the expanding joint. The second zone of proliferation is deep to the first and is in every way analogous to the zone of replication in the growth plate; that is, it contributes new cells for continued centrifugal expansion of the secondary center. McKibbin and Holdsworth demonstrated the unique nature of these two layers of the developing joint surface by removing full-thickness plugs from the rabbit joint and replacing them in an inverted position.[91] Each layer remained distinct and continued its previous function, demonstrating that the dual origin of the two-layered structure, not location, nutrition, or other extraneous factors, was responsible for its different form and function.

As mentioned earlier, joint structures develop during the embryonic period. Fetal development of joint structures is characterized by increase in size and complexity. Thus, synovial villi appear during the third month, as do various bursae, some of which develop communications with adjacent joints. Intra-articular fat cells and fat pads appear at 4 to 5 months, and nerve fibers, present at the end of the embryonic period, develop specific nerve endings.[79]

Following the adolescent growth spurt, mitotic activity ceases in the growth plate, the secondary center, and the articular cartilage. The growth plate is remodeled to the point where only a thin horizontal plate of trabecular bone marks its previous location. The miniature growth plate in the deep portion of the articular surface produces a thicker bony layer known as the subchondral bone plate. Mitotic activity in the articular cartilage itself ceases and is not seen again except in advanced stages of degenerative arthritis. Although subtle changes in size and shape of the articular ends of bone have been demonstrated in adults, the mechanisms are unknown.[92] In addition, reinstitution of endochondral proliferation with the formation of osteophytes covered by articular cartilage is seen in late stages of degenerative arthritis, but the mechanism by which the growth process is reinstated remains unknown. In acromegaly, continued stimulation of chondrocyte replication by somatomedin produces continued growth in the depths of articular cartilage, most evident in the mandible and in the hand.

These examples of regeneration and growth capacity by adult articular cartilage provide enticing shreds of evidence that, given the proper biochemical signal, it should be possible to bring about cartilage healing and to reverse the process of degenerative joint disease.

SUMMARY

The development of the musculoskeletal system requires remarkable organization of cells and tissues and a precise sequence of events in order to form the osseous and articular structures. Disturbances in any of these sensitive events of development can lead to a variety of congenital anomalies.

The author of this chapter would like to thank Sonya Shortkroff and Phyllis White for their preparative assistance and Marcia Chapin for her photographic assistance.

REFERENCES

1. Streeter GL: Developmental horizons in human embryos. IV. A review of the histogenesis of cartilage and bone. Contrib Embryol *33*:149, 1949.
2. Milaire J: Histochemical aspects of limb morphogenesis in vertebrates. Adv Morphog *2*:183, 1962.
3. Milaire J: Some histochemical considerations of limb development. *In* CA Swinyard (Ed): Limb Development and Deformity: Problems of Evaluation and Rehabilitation. Springfield, Ill, Charles C Thomas, 1969, p 70.
4. Raynaud A: Somites and early morphogenesis in reptile limbs. *In* DA Ede, et al (Eds): Vertebrate Limb and Somite Morphogenesis. Cambridge, Cambridge University Press, 1977, p 373.
5. Chevallier A, Kieny M, Mauger A, Sengel P: Developmental fate of the somitic mesoderm in the chick embryo. *In* DA Ede, et al (Eds): Vertebrate Limb and Somite Morphogenesis. Cambridge, Cambridge University Press, 1977, p 421.
6. Chevallier A, Kieny M, Mauger A: Limb-somite relationship: Origin of the limb musculature. J Embryol Exp Morphol *41*:245, 1977.
7. O'Rahilly R, Gardner E, Gray DJ: The ectodermal thickening and ridge in the limbs of staged human embryos. J Embryol Exp Morphol *4*:254, 1956.
8. Felts WJ: Transplantation studies of factors in skeletal organogenesis. I. The subcutaneously implanted immature long-bone of the rat and mouse. Am J Phys Anthropol *17*:201, 1959.
9. Felts WJ: In vivo implantation as a technique in skeletal biology. Int Rev Cytol *12*:243, 1961.
10. Saunders JW Jr: The experimental analysis of chick limb bud development. *In* DA Ede, et al (Eds): Vertebrate Limb and Somite Morphogenesis. Cambridge, Cambridge University Press, 1977, p 1.
11. Murray PDF, Huxley JS: Self-differentiation of the grafted limb-bud of the chick. J Anat (Lond) *59*:379, 1925.

12. Murray PDF, Selby D: Intrinsic and extrinsic factors in the primary development of the skeleton. Wilhelm Roux' Arch Entwicklungsmech Org *122*:629, 1930.
13. Fell HB: Experiments on the differentiation in vitro of cartilage and bone. Part I. Arch Exp Zell *7*:390, 1928.
14. Saunders JW Jr: The proximo-distal sequence of origin of the parts of the chick wing and the role of the ectoderm. J Exp Zool *108*:363, 1948.
15. Saunders JW Jr, Cairns JM, Gasseling MT: The role of the apical ridge of ectoderm in the differentiation of the morphological structure and inductive specificity of limb parts in the chick. J Morphol *101*:57, 1957.
16. Saunders JW Jr, Gasseling MT: Transfilter propagation of apical ectoderm maintenance factor in the chick embryo wing bud. Dev Biol *7*:64, 1963.
17. Saunders JW Jr, Gasseling MT, Cairns JM: The differentiation of prospective thigh mesoderm grafted beneath the apical ectodermal ridge of the wing bud in the chick embryo. Dev Biol *1*:281, 1959.
18. Saunders JW Jr, Gasseling MT, Saunders LC: Cellular death in morphogenesis of the avian wing. Dev Biol *5*:147, 1962.
19. Saunders JW Jr, Gasseling MT, Gfeller MD: Interaction of ectoderm and mesoderm in the origin of axial relationships in the wing of the fowl. J Exp Zool *137*:39, 1958.
20. Zwilling E: Ectoderm-mesoderm relationship in the development of the chick embryo limb bud. J Exp Zool *128*:423, 1955.
21. Zwilling E: Limb morphogenesis. Adv Morphog *1*:301, 1961.
22. Zwilling E: Development of fragmented and of dissociated limb bud mesoderm. Dev Biol *9*:20, 1964.
23. Zwilling E: Interaction between limb bud ectoderm and mesoderm in the chick embryo. III. Experiments with polydactylous limbs. J Exp Zool *132*:219, 1956.
24. Zwilling E, Saunders JW Jr, Gasseling MT: Involvement of the apical ectodermal ridge in chick limb development. Anat Rec *136*:307, 1960.
25. Gasseling MT, Saunders JW Jr: Duplication of foot parts after reorientation of the leg-bud apex in the chick embryo. Anat Rec *136*:195, 1960.
26. Goetinck PF, Abbott U: Tissue interaction in scaleless mutant and the use of scaleless as an ectodermal marker in studies of normal limb differentiation. J Exp Zool *154*:7, 1963.
27. Goetinck PF, Abbott U: Studies on limb morphogenesis. I. Experiments with the polydactylous mutant, talpid. J Exp Zool *155*:161, 1964.
28. Goetinck PF: Studies on limb morphogenesis. II. Experiments with polydactylous mutant eudiplopodia. Dev Biol *10*:71, 1964.
29. Goetinck PF, Pennypacker JP: Controls in the acquisition and maintenance of chondrogenic expression. *In* DA Ede, et al (Eds): Vertebrate Limb and Somite Morphogenesis. Cambridge, Cambridge University Press, 1977, p 139.
30. Ahrens PB, Solursh M, Reiter RS, Singley CT: Position-related capacity for differentiation of limb mesenchyme in cell culture. Dev Biol *69*:436, 1979.
31. Jacobson W, Fell HB: The developmental mechanics and potencies of the undifferentiated mesenchyme of the mandible. Quart J Micr Sci *82*:563, 1941.
32. Moscona A: Patterns and mechanisms of tissue reconstruction from dissociated cells. *In* D Rudnick (Ed): Developing Cell Systems and Their Control. 18th Symposium of the Society for the Study of Development and Growth. New York, The Ronald Press, 1960, p. 45.
33. Steinberg MS: Mechanism of tissue reconstruction by dissociated cells. II. Time-course of events. Science *137*:762, 1962.
34. Steinberg MS: Does differential adhesion govern self-assembly processes in histogenesis? Equilibrium configurations and the emergence of a hierarchy among populations of embryonic cells. J Exp Zool *173*:395, 1970.
35. Searls RL: The role of cell migration in the development of the embryonic chick limb bud. J Exp Zool *166*:39, 1967.
36. Dienstman SR, Biehl J, Holtzer S, Holtzer H: Myogenic and chondrogenic lineages in developing limb buds grown in vitro. Dev Biol *39*:83, 1974.
37. Caplan AI, Koutroupas S: The control of muscle and cartilage development in the chick limb: the role of differential vascularization. J Embryol Exp Morphol *29*:571, 1973.
38. Caplan AI: Muscle, cartilage and bone development and differentiation from chick limb mesenchymal cells. *In* DA Ede, et al (Eds): Vertebrate Limb and Somite Morphogenesis. Cambridge, Cambridge University Press, 1977, p 199.
39. Landauer W: Niacin antagonists and chick development. J Exp Zool *136*:509, 1957.
40. Bassett CAL, Herrmann I: Influence of oxygen concentration and mechanical factors on differentiation of connective tissues in vitro. Nature *190*:460, 1961.
41. Sledge CB, Dingle JT: Activation of lysosomes by oxygen: Oxygen induced resorption of cartilage in organ culture. Nature *205*:140, 1965.
42. Wilby OK: A model for the control of limb growth and development. *In* DA Ede, et al (Eds): Vertebrate Limb and Somite Morphogenesis. Cambridge, Cambridge University Press, 1977, p 299.
43. Bryant SV: Pattern regulation in amphibian limbs. *In* DA Ede, et al (eds): Vertebrate Limb and Somite Morphogenesis. Cambridge, Cambridge University Press, 1977, p 311.
44. Newman SA, Frisch HL: Dynamics of skeletal pattern formation in developing chick limb. Science *205*:662, 1979.
45. Lewis CA, Pratt RM, Pennypacker JP, Hassell JR: Inhibition of limb chondrogenesis in vitro by vitamin A: Alterations in cell surface characteristics. Dev Biol *64*:31, 1978.
46. Baheri A, Ruoslahti E, Mosher D (Eds): Fibroblast Surface Protein. New York, New York Academy of Sciences, 1978.
47. Toole BP, Jackson G, Gross J: Hyaluronate in morphogenesis: Inhibition of chondrogenesis in vitro. Proc Natl Acad Sci *69*:1384, 1972.
48. Toole BP: Hyaluronate turnover during chondrogenesis in the developing chick limb and axial skeleton. Dev Biol *29*:321, 1972.
49. Fell HB: Skeletal development in tissue culture. *In* GH Bourne (Ed): Biochemistry and Physiology of Bone. New York, Academic Press, 1956 p 401.
50. Murray PDF: Bones. A study of the development and structure of the vertebrate skeleton. Cambridge, Cambridge University Press, 1936.
51. Chalmers J: A study of some of the factors controlling growth of transplanted skeletal tissue. *In* LJ Richelle, MJ Dallemagne (Eds): Calcified Tissues. Liège, Belgium, University of Liège, 1965, p. 177.
52. Sledge CB: Some morphologic and experimental aspects of limb development. Clin Orthop *44*:241, 1966.
53. Fell HB: The histogenesis of cartilage and bone in the long bones of the embryonic fowl. J Morphol Physiol *40*:417, 1925.
54. Godman GC, Porter KR: Chondrogenesis, studied with the electron microscope. J Biophys Biochem Cytol *8*:719, 1960.
55. Gardner E: Osteogenesis in the human embryo and fetus. *In* GH Bourne (Ed): The Biochemistry and Physiology of Bone. 2nd Ed. Vol III. New York, Academic Press, 1971, p 77.
56. Dawd DS, Hinchliffe JR: Cell death in the "opaque patch" in the central mesenchyme of the developing chick limb: A cytological, cytochemical and electron microscopic analysis. J Embryol Exp Morphol *26*:401, 1971.
57. Ballard KJ, Holt SJ: Cytological and cytochemical studies on cell death and digestion in foetal rat foot; the role of macrophages and hydrolytic enzymes. J Cell Sci *3*:245, 1968.
58. Fraser FC, Fainstat TD: Production of congenital defects in the offspring of pregnant mice treated with cortisone. Pediatrics *8*:527, 1951.
59. Fainstat T: Cortisone-induced congenital cleft palate in rabbits. Endocrinology *55*:502, 1954.
60. Millen JW, Woollam DHM: Influence of cortisone on teratogenic effect of hypervitaminosis-A. Br Med J *2*:196, 1957.
61. O'Rahilly R, Gardner E: The timing and sequence of events in the development of the limbs in the human embryo. Anat Embryol *148*:1, 1975.
62. Gardner E, Gray DJ: Prenatal development of the human shoulder and acromioclavicular joints. Am J Anat *92*:219, 1953.
63. Gardner E, O'Rahilly R: The early development of the knee joint in staged human embryos. J Anat *102*:289, 1968.
64. Sledge CB: Structure, development, and function of joints. Orthop Clin North Am *6*:619, 1975.
65. Drachman DB: Normal development and congenital malformation of joints. Bull Rheum Dis *19*:536, 1969.
66. Haines RW: The development of joints. J Anat *81*:33, 1947.
67. Henrickson RC, Cohen AS: Light and electron microscopic observations of the developing chick interphalangeal joint. J Ultrastruct Res *13*:129, 1965.
68. Andersen H: Development, morphology and histochemistry of the early synovial tissue in human foetuses. Acta Anat *58*:90, 1964.
69. Sledge CB: Biochemical events in the epiphyseal plate and their physiologic control. Clin Orthop *61*:37, 1968.
70. Nettelbladt E, Sundblad L: On the significance of hyaluronic acid changes in the pathogenesis of joint effusion. Opusc Med *12*:224, 1964.
71. Simkin PA, Pizzorno JE: Transynovial exchange of small molecules in normal human subjects. J Appl Physiol *36*:581, 1974.
72. Fell HB, Canti RG: Experiments on the development in vitro of the avian knee-joint. Proc Soc Lond [Biol] *116*:316, 1934.
73. Drachman DB, Coulombre AJ: Experimental clubfoot and arthrogryposis multiplex congenita. Lancet *2*:523, 1962.
74. Drachman DB, Sokoloff L: The role of movement in embryonic joint development. Dev Biol *14*:401, 1966.
75. Drachman DB, Weiner LP, Price DL, Chase J: Experimental arthrogryposis caused by viral myopathy. Arch Neurol *33*:362, 1976.
76. Yasuda Y: Differentiation of human limb buds in vitro. Anat Rec *175*:561, 1973.
77. Holder N: An experimental investigation into the early development of the chick elbow joint. J Embryol Exp Morphol *39*:115, 1977.

78. O'Rahilly R, Gardner E: The embryology of bone and bones. *In* LV Ackerman, et al (Eds): Bones and Joints. Baltimore, Williams & Wilkins Co, 1976, p 1.
79. O'Rahilly R, Gardner E: The embryology of movable joints. *In* L Sokoloff (Ed): The Joints and Synovial Fluid. New York, Academic Press, 1978, p 49.
80. Wassilev W: Elektronenmikroskopische und histochemische Untersuchungen zur Entwicklung des Kniegelenkes der Ratte. Z Anat Entwicklungsgesch *137*:221, 1972.
81. Kelley RO: An electron microscopic study of mesenchyme during development of interdigital spaces in man. Anat Rec *168*:43, 1970.
82. Pinner B, Swinyard CA: Histochemical studies of limb development. *In* CA Swinyard (Ed): Limb Development and Deformity: Problems of Evaluation and Rehabilitation. Springfield, Ill, Charles C Thomas, 1969, p 56.
83. Andersen H: Histochemical studies on the histogenesis of the knee joint and superior tibio-fibular joint in human fetuses. Acta Anat *46*:279, 1961.
84. Andersen H: Histochemical studies of the development of the human hip joint. Acta Anat *48*:258, 1962.
85. Andersen H: Histochemical studies of the histogenesis of the human elbow joint. Acta Anat *51*:50, 1962.
86. Andersen H: Histochemistry and development of the human shoulder and acromioclavicular joints with particular reference to the early development of the clavicle. Acta Anat *55*:124, 1963.
87. Andersen H, Bro-Rasmussen F: Histochemical studies on the histogenesis of the joints in human fetuses with special reference to the development of the joint cavities in the hand and foot. Am J Anat *108*:111, 1961.
88. Simunek Z, Muir H: Changes in the protein-polysaccharides of pig articular cartilage during prenatal life, development and old age. Biochem J *126*:515, 1971.
89. O'Rahilly R, Gardner E: The initial appearance of ossification in staged human embryos. Am J Anat *134*:291, 1972.
90. Mankin HJ: Localization of tritiated thymidine in articular cartilage of rabbits. I. Growth in immature cartilage. J Bone Joint Surg *44A*:682, 1962.
91. McKibbin B, Holdsworth FW: The dual nature of epiphyseal cartilage. J Bone Joint Surg *49B*:351, 1967.
92. Johnson LC: Morphologic analysis in pathology: The kinetics of disease and general biology of bone. *In* HM Frost (Ed): Bone Biodynamics. Boston, Little, Brown and Co, 1964, p 543.

2

ARTICULAR ANATOMY AND HISTOLOGY

by Donald Resnick, M.D. and Gen Niwayama, M.D.

Skeletal structures are connected to each other in a variety of ways; these junctions have been termed articulations, arthroses, juncturae, and joints. Methods used to classify articulations have included divisions based upon (a) extent of joint motion, and (b) type of articular histology. Neither of these two systems is ideal.

The classification of articulations based upon the extent of joint motion is as follows:

Synarthroses: Fixed or rigid articulations.

Amphiarthroses: Slightly movable articulations.

Diarthroses: Freely movable articulations.

This classification fails to disclose the fact that motion between rigid skeletal structures may result from either apposition of two sliding surfaces, as occurs in synovial joints, or changes and deformity of intervening tissue, which may be noted in fibrous or cartilaginous joints. Thus, any classification based solely upon the extent of joint motion will group together articulations whose histologic components are very dissimilar.

The classification of articulations based upon histology emphasizes the type of tissue that characterizes the junctional area.[1,2] The following categories are recognized:

Table 2–1
TYPES OF ARTICULATIONS

Fibrous	
Suture	Skull
Syndesmosis	Distal tibiofibular interosseous membrane Radioulnar interosseous membrane Sacroiliac interosseous ligament
Gomphosis	Teeth
Cartilaginous	
Symphysis	Symphysis pubis Intervertebral disc Sternomanubrial joint Central mandible
Synchondrosis	Epiphyseal plate (growth plate) Neurocentral joint Spheno-occipital joint
Synovial	
	Large, small joints of extremities Sacroiliac joint Apophyseal joint Costovertebral joint Sternoclavicular joint

Fibrous articulations: Apposed bony surfaces are fastened together by fibrous connective tissue.

Cartilaginous articulations: Apposed bony surfaces are initially or eventually connected by cartilaginous tissue.

Synovial articulations: Apposed bony surfaces are separated by an articular cavity that is lined by synovial membrane.

This second method of classification leads to difficulty because joints that are similar histologically may differ considerably in function. Furthermore, some articulations contain admixtures of a variety of tissues, such as fibrous and cartilaginous tissues, whereas others change their constituency as they develop.

Despite these obvious weaknesses in current classification systems, the following discussion will utilize one of these methods of classification — that based upon joint histology — rather than introduce new problems by deviating from these customary schemes (Table 2–1).

FIBROUS ARTICULATIONS

In this type of articulation, apposed bony surfaces are fastened together by intervening fibrous tissue. Fibrous articulations can be further subdivided into three types.

Suture

Limited to the skull, sutures (Fig. 2–1) allow no active motion and exist where broad osseous surfaces are separated only by a zone of connective tissue. This connective tissue, along with two layers of periosteum on the outer and inner surfaces of the articulating bone, is termed the sutural membrane or ligament. The precise structure of a suture has been outlined by Pritchard and associates.[3] There are five layers that intervene between the ends of the bone: cambial, capsular, middle, capsular, and cambial. The cambial layer, a zone of flattened osteogenic cells, is covered by a capsular layer. The middle

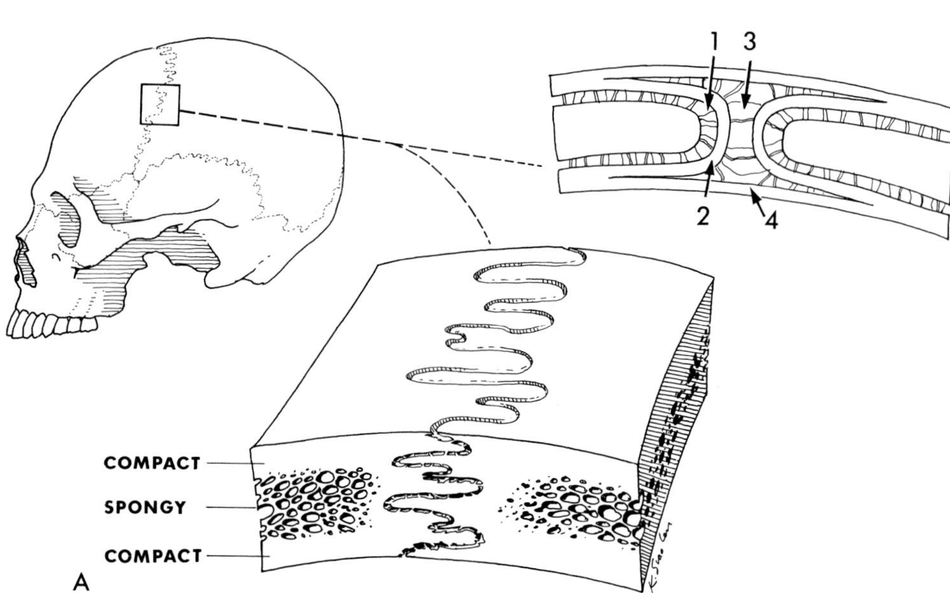

Figure 2–1. *Fibrous articulation: Suture.*

A *Schematic drawings indicating structure of typical suture in the skull. Note the interdigitations of the osseous surfaces. The specific layers that intervene between the ends of the bones are indicated at the upper right. These include the cambial (1), capsular (2), and middle (3) layers. A uniting (4) layer is also indicated. (Reproduced in part from Pritchard JJ, Scott JH, Girgis FG: The structure and development of cranial and fascial sutures. J Anat 90:73, 1956. Courtesy of Cambridge University Press.)*

Illustration continued on the opposite page

layer consists of loose fibrous connective tissue of varying thickness, containing blood vessels that communicate with the diploic vessels of the cranial vault.

Although classically a suture is considered to be a fibrous articulation, areas of secondary cartilage formation may be observed during the growth period, and in later life, sutures may undergo bony union or synostosis. Bony obliteration of the sutures is somewhat variable in its time of onset and cranial distribution.[4-8] It commences on the inner or deep surface of the suture between the ages of 30 and 40 years and on the outer or superficial surface approximately 10 years later. This obliteration usually occurs at the bregma and subsequently extends into the sagittal, coronal and lambdoid sutures, in that order. There are also minor variations in the way in which the two osseous surfaces approach each other and are fitted together. The bony surfaces are rarely smooth. When they possess minimal roughness or irregularities, the articulation is termed a plane suture. Serrated sutures contain irregular projections of bone that interdigitate with similar outgrowths on the adjacent bone, whereas denticulate sutures con-

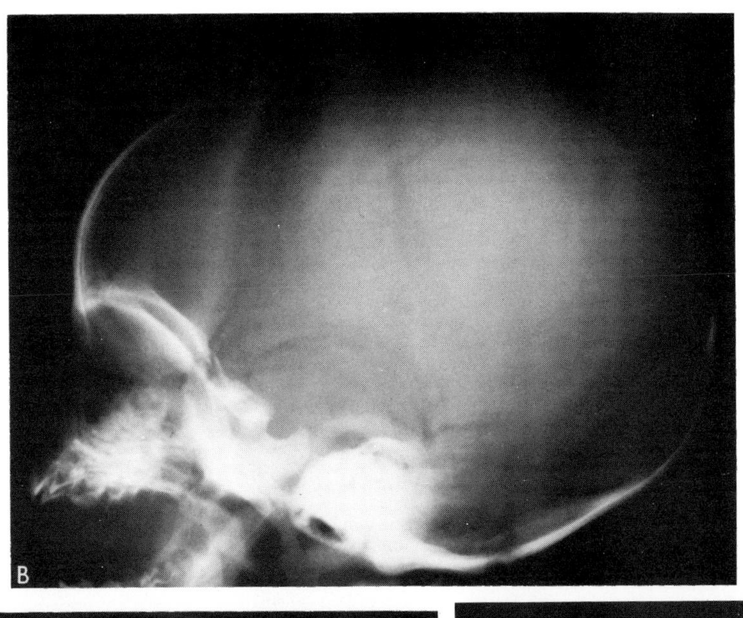

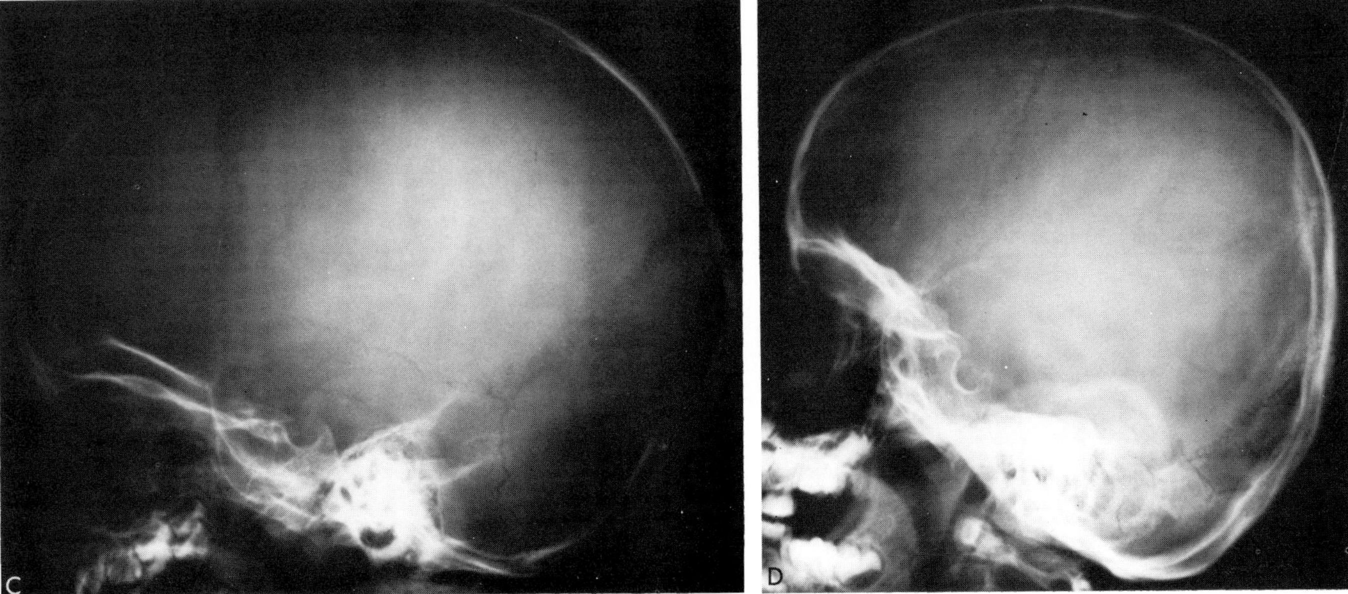

Figure 2–1. Continued
B–D *Appearance of skull sutures in a 4 week old child (B), the somewhat more narrowed sutures of a child aged 14 months (C), and further narrowing of the sutures in a child of 7 years (D).*

tain similar bony excrescences that are finer in nature. A squamous suture occurs when the margin of one bone overlaps its neighbor to some degree.

Syndesmosis

A syndesmosis (Fig. 2–2) is a fibrous articulation in which adjacent bony surfaces are united by an interosseous ligament, as in the distal tibiofibular joint, or an interosseous membrane, as at the diaphyses of radius and ulna and tibia and fibula. An additional example of a syndesmosis is the interosseous ligament between the superior aspect of sacrum and ilium. In fact, one could utilize the term syndesmosis for almost all ligaments in the body, as such ligaments are "interosseous" in nature. A syndesmosis may demonstrate minor degrees of motion related to stretching of the interosseous ligament or flexibility of the interosseous membrane.

Gomphosis

This special type of fibrous articulation (Fig. 2–3) is located between the teeth and maxilla or mandible. At these sites, the articulation resembles a peg which fits into a fossa or socket. The intervening membrane between tooth and bone is termed the periodontal ligament. This ligament varies in width from 0.1 to 0.3 mm and decreases in thickness with advancing age. The ligament has no elastic fibers, although its structure does allow slight movement of the tooth.

CARTILAGINOUS ARTICULATIONS

There are two types of cartilaginous joints, symphysis and synchondrosis.

Symphysis

In symphyses (Figs. 2–4, 2–5), adjacent bony surfaces are connected by a cartilaginous disc, which arises from chondrification of intervening mesenchymal tissue. This tissue is composed eventually of fibrocartilaginous or fibrous connective tissue, although a thin layer of hyaline cartilage usually persists, covering the articular surface of

Text continued on page 28

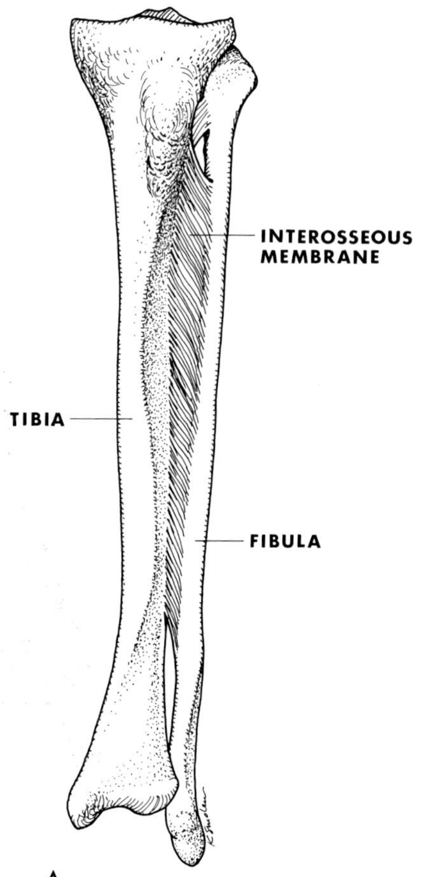

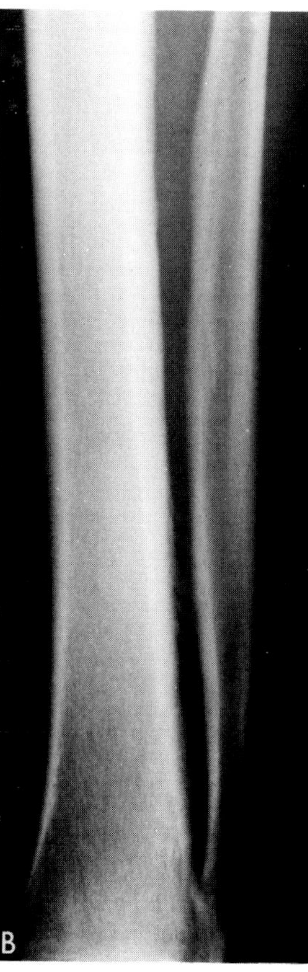

Figure 2–2. *Fibrous articulation: Syndesmosis.*

A, B *An interosseous membrane exists between the lateral border of the tibia and the medial border of the fibula. Note the orientation of its fibers and observe the slight irregularity of the apposing osseous surfaces on the radiograph.*

Illustration continued on the opposite page

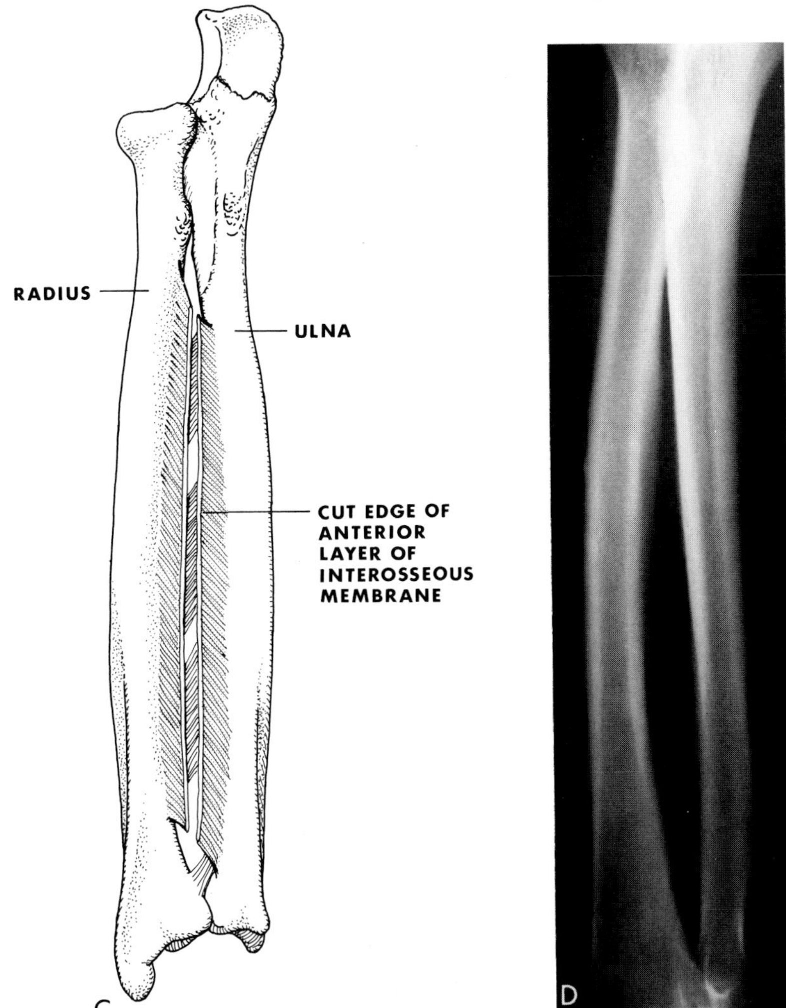

Figure 2–2. Continued

C, D *The interosseous membrane between the medial aspect of the radius and the lateral aspect of the ulna originates approximately 3 cm below the radial tuberosity and extends to the wrist, containing apertures for various interosseous vessels. The radiograph reveals an osseous crest on apposing surfaces of bone.*

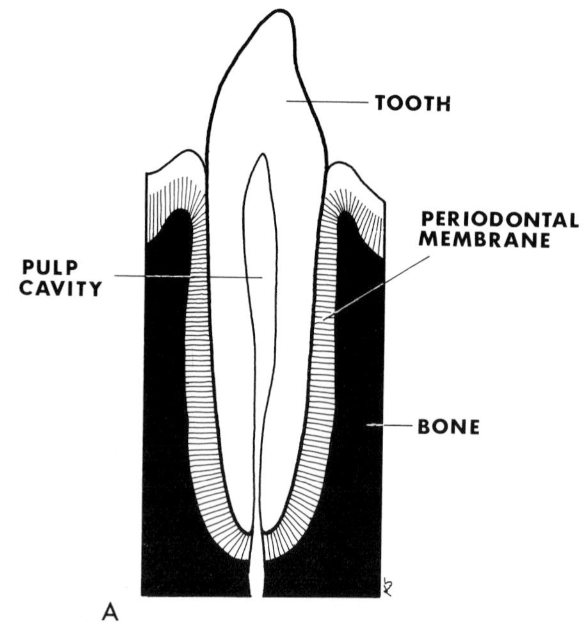

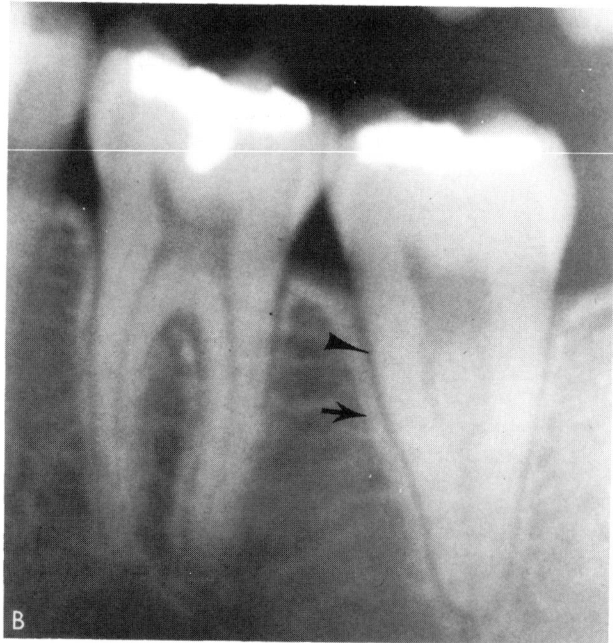

Figure 2–3. *Fibrous articulation: Gomphosis.*

A *A diagrammatic representation of this special type of articulation located between the teeth and the maxilla or mandible. Note the location of the periodontal membrane.*

B *A radiograph reveals the radiolucent periodontal membrane (arrowhead) and the radiopaque lamina dura (arrow).*

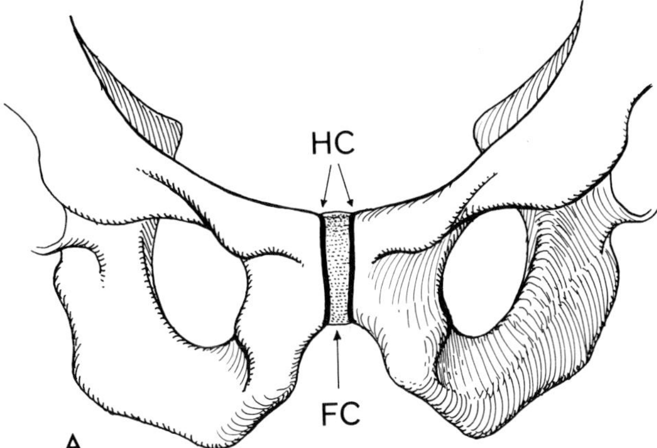

Figure 2–4. *Cartilaginous articulation: Symphysis (symphysis pubis).*

A *On the diagram, note the central fibrocartilage (FC), with a thin layer of hyaline cartilage (HC) adjacent to the osseous surfaces of the pubis.*

B *A photograph of a partially macerated symphysis pubis better delineates the structure of the central fibrocartilage (FC), peripheral hyaline cartilage (HC), and subchondral bone (arrowhead).*

C *A photomicrograph (8×) of a symphysis pubis outlines central fibrocartilage, surrounding hyaline cartilage, and subchondral trabeculae.*

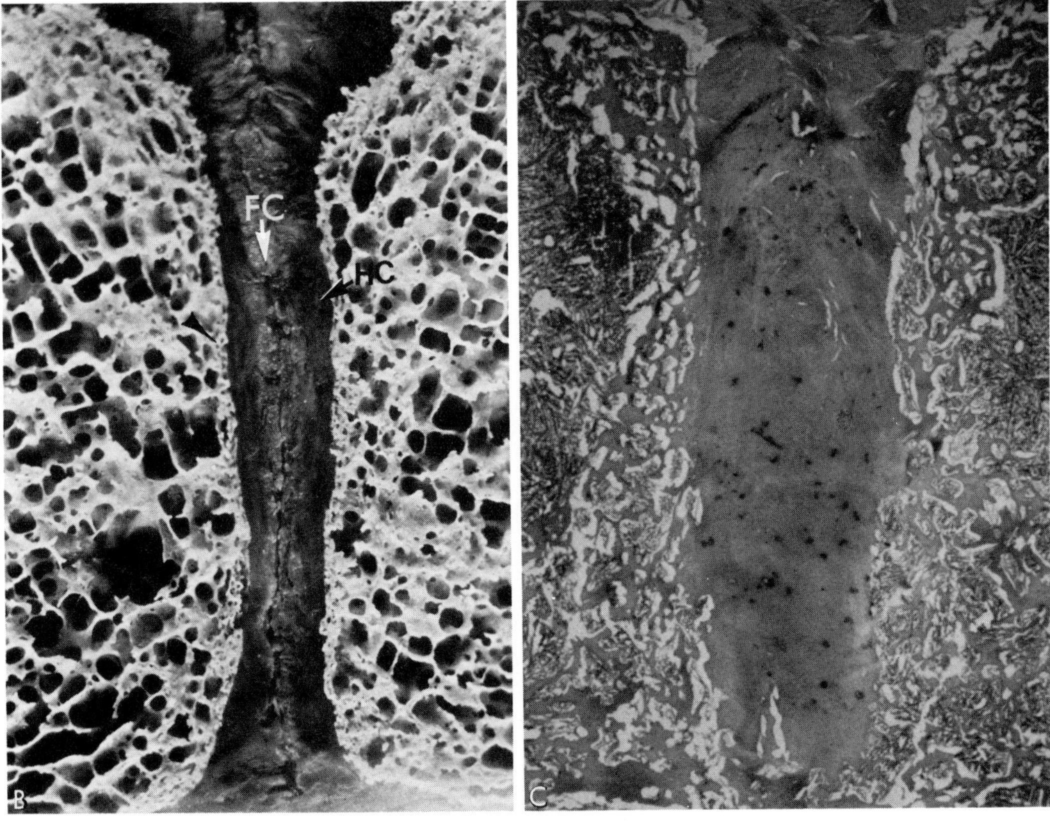

the adjacent bone. The hyaline cartilage contributes to the growth of the neighboring osseous tissue. Symphyses, of which typical examples are the symphysis pubis and the intervertebral disc, allow a small amount of motion, which occurs through compression or deformation of the intervening connective tissue.

Some symphyses, such as the symphysis pubis and sternomanubrial joint, reveal a small cleft-like central cavity that contains fluid and which may enlarge with advancing age. This feature is reminiscent of cavities within synovial articulations, perhaps indicating an intermediate phase of joint evolution. Furthermore, fibrous ligaments at the peripheral area of a symphysis bear some resemblance to joint capsules about synovial articulations.

Symphyses are located within the midsagittal plane of the human body and are permanent structures, unlike synchondroses, which are temporary articulations. Rarely, intra-articular ankylosis or synostosis may obliterate a symphysis, such as occurs at the sternomanubrial joint.

Synchondrosis

Synchondroses (Fig. 2–6) are temporary joints that exist during the growing phase of the skeleton

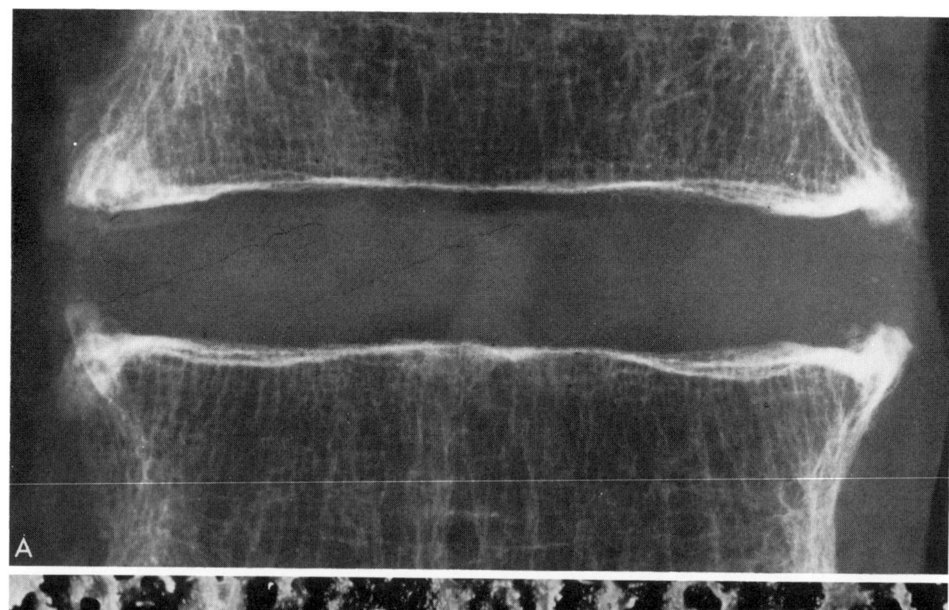

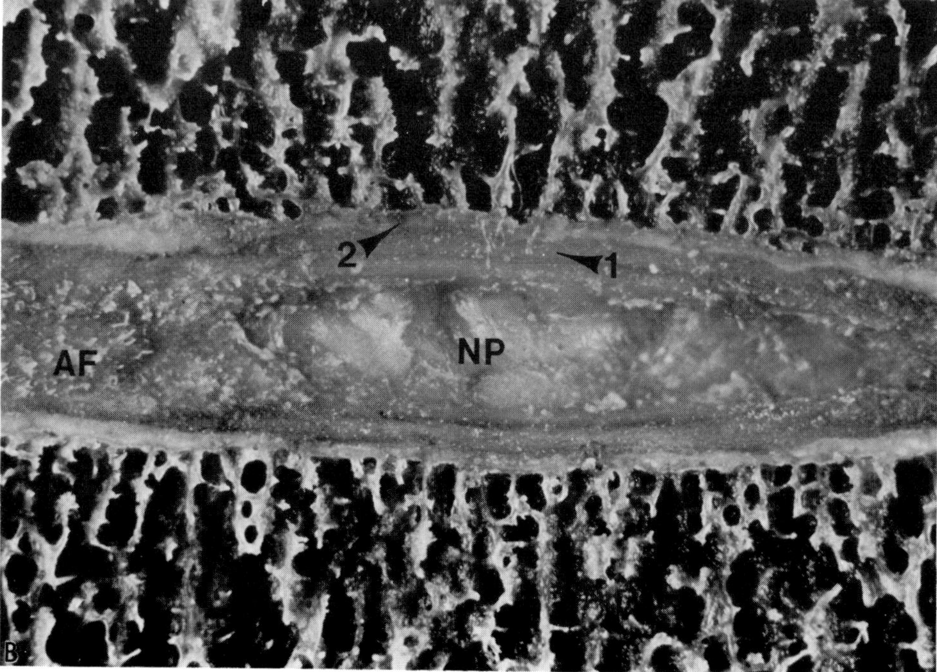

Figure 2–5. *Cartilaginous articulation: Symphysis (intervertebral disc).*

A *A magnification radiograph of the discovertebral junction reveals the radiolucent intervertebral disc surrounded by two vertebral bodies. Note the well-defined subchondral bone plate of each vertebra.*

B *A photograph of the discovertebral junction reveals the nucleus pulposus (NP), anulus fibrosus (AF), cartilaginous endplate (1), and subchondral bone plate (2).*

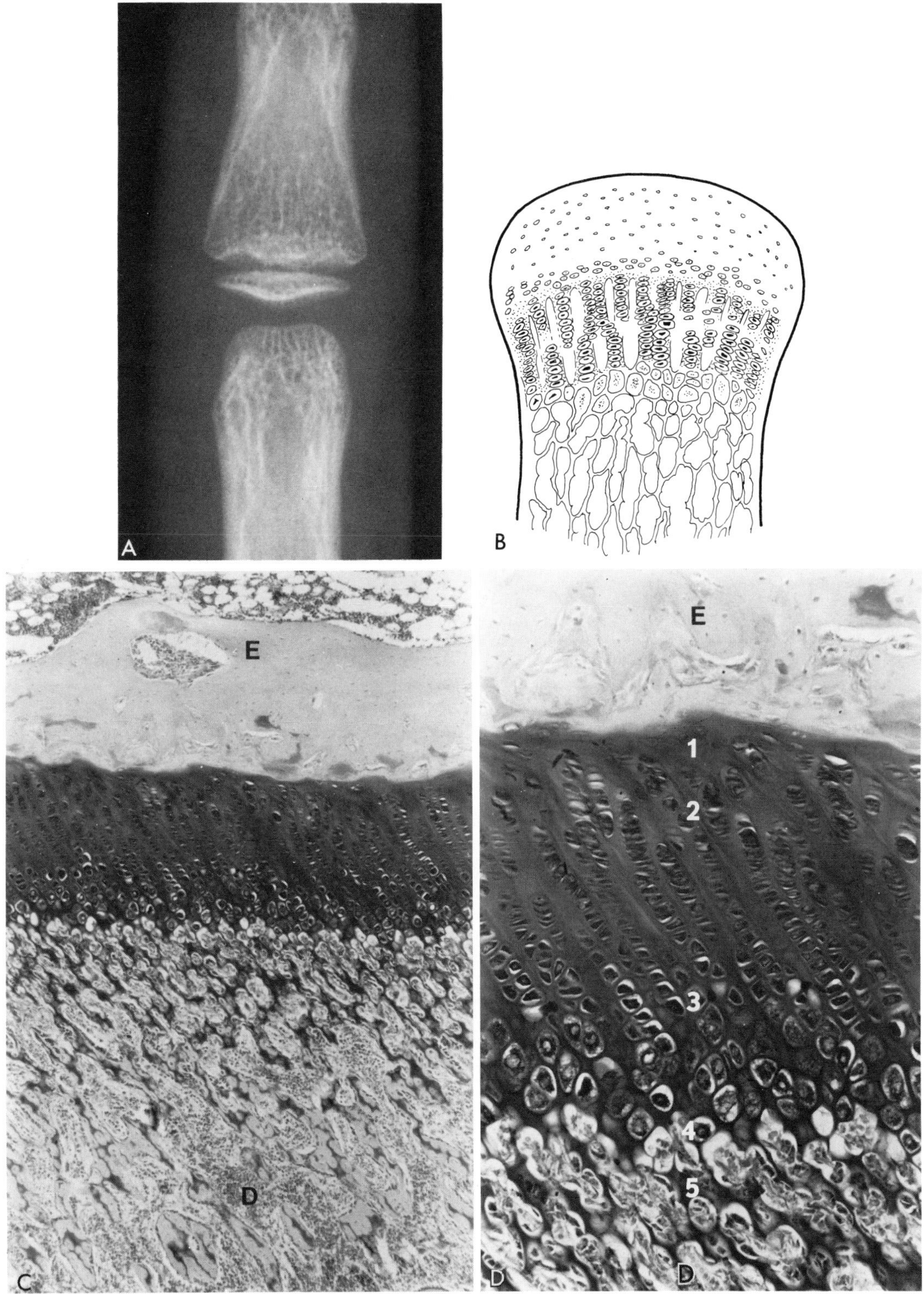

Figure 2–6. *Cartilaginous articulation: Synchondrosis.*

A *A radiograph of the phalanges in a growing child demonstrates a typical epiphysis separated from the metaphysis and diaphysis by the radiolucent growth plate.*

B *A schematic drawing of a growth plate between the cartilaginous epiphysis and the ossified diaphysis of a long bone. Note the transition from hyaline cartilage through various cartilaginous zones, including resting cartilage, cell proliferation, cell hypertrophy, cell calcification, and bone formation.*

C, D *Photomicrographs of an epiphyseal (growth) plate in a rabbit femur. The lower power (20×) and higher power (50×) photomicrographs reveal the various zones of cartilage in the epiphyseal plate separating the epiphysis (E) and diaphysis (D). These zones include resting cartilage (1), cell proliferation (2), cell hypertrophy (3), cell calcification (4), and ossification (5).*

Illustration continued on the following page

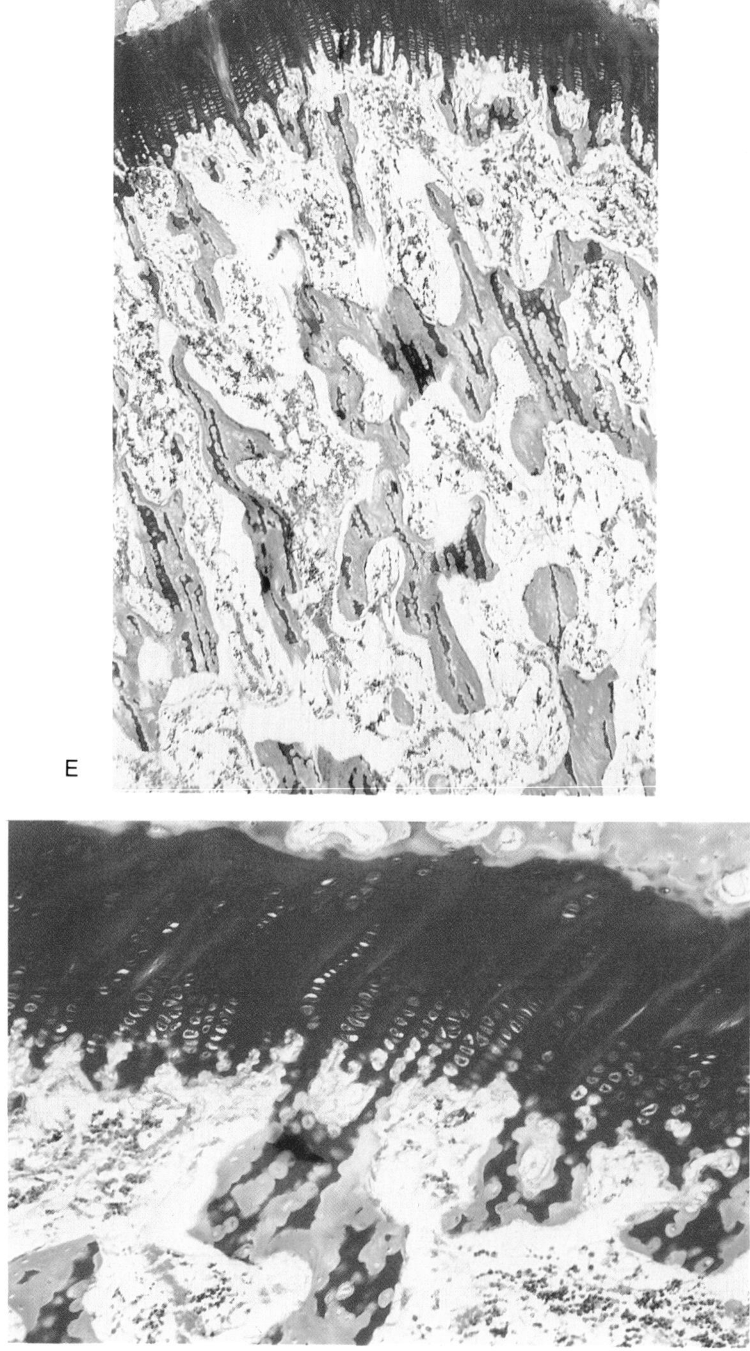

Figure 2–6. Continued
E, F *Color photomicrographs (10×, 20×) demonstrate these same cartilaginous zones.*

and are composed of hyaline cartilage. Typical synchondroses are the cartilaginous growth plate between the epiphysis and diaphysis of a tubular bone, the neurocentral vertebral articulations, and the unossified cartilage in the chondrocranium, the spheno-occipital synchondrosis. With skeletal maturation, synchondroses become thinner and are eventually obliterated by bony union or synostosis. Two synchondroses that persist into adult life are the first sternocostal and the petrobasilar articulations.

SYNOVIAL ARTICULATIONS

A synovial articulation is a specialized type of joint that is located primarily in the appendicular skeleton (Fig. 2–7). Synovial articulations generally allow unrestricted motion.[9] The structure of a synovial joint differs fundamentally from that of fibrous and cartilaginous joints; osseous surfaces are bound together by a fibrous capsule, which may be reinforced by accessory ligaments. The inner portion of the articulating surface of the apposing bones is separated by a space, the articular or joint cavity. Articular cartilage covers the ends of both bones; motion between these cartilaginous surfaces is characterized by a low coefficient of friction. The inner aspect of the joint capsule is formed by the synovial membrane, which secretes synovial fluid into the articular cavity. This synovial fluid acts both as a lubricant, encouraging motion, and as a nutritive substance, providing nourishment to the adjacent articular cartilage. In some synovial joints, an intra-articular disc of fibrocartilage partially or completely divides the joint cavity. Additional intra-articular structures, including fat pads and labra, may be noted.

The important constituents of a synovial joint are articular cartilage, subchondral bone plate, articular capsule (fibrous capsule and synovial membrane), intra-articular disc, fat pad and labrum, and synovial fluid. Surrounding structures include tendon sheaths, bursae, and small accessory bones or sesamoids.

Articular Cartilage

The articulating surfaces of the bone are covered by a layer of glistening connective tissue, the articular cartilage (Fig. 2–8). In most synovial joints, the cartilage is hyaline in type. The deep layers of the articular cartilage are involved in the growth of the underlying bone via endochondral ossification. At the cessation of growth, a narrow zone of calcification, the calcified zone of articular cartilage, appears and merges with the subjacent subchondral bone plate. At its periphery, articular cartilage merges with joint capsule and periosteum.

Articular cartilage is devoid of lymphatics, blood vessels, and nerves. A large portion of the cartilage derives its nutrition through diffusion of fluid from the synovial cavity. This cartilage–synovial fluid interface is indeed a dynamic area; synovial fluid may be expressed into the joint cavity from articular cartilage during movement and reabsorbed by cartilage when movement ceases.[10] A second source of cartilage nourishment is vascular in nature.[11] Small blood vessels pass from the subchondral bone plate into the deepest stratum of cartilage, providing nutrients to this area of articular cartilage. Additionally, a vascular ring is located within the synovial membrane at the periphery of the cartilage. At this site, larger vessels of the synovium form a vascular circle. The terminal branches of this circle overlie the margin of the cartilage.[12] This latter source of vascularity at the peripheral aspect of the cartilage may explain marginal new bone formation or osteophytes, which are characteristic of such diseases as osteoarthritis.

Articular cartilage is variable in thickness. It may be thicker on one articulating bone than on another. Furthermore, articular cartilage is not necessarily of uniform thickness over the entire osseous surface. In general, it varies from 1 to 7 mm in thickness, averaging 2 or 3 mm in thickness. Jaffe[13] noted other principles governing the thickness of articular cartilage; such cartilage is thicker (a) in large joints than in small joints; (b) in joints or areas of joints in which there is considerable functional pressure or stress, such as those in the lower extremity; (c) at sites of extensive frictional or shearing force; (d) in poorly fitted articulations as compared to smoothly fitted ones; and (e) in young and middle-aged individuals; it is thinner in older people. Non-use of a joint may lead to cartilage thinning, whereas excessive use during exercise may lead to temporary cartilage swelling related to imbibition of fluid by cartilage cells and matrix.

The color of articular cartilage varies with age; it is white or bluish-white in children, white and glossy in young adults, yellowish-white in middle-aged individuals and yellowish-brown in elderly persons.[13] Although cartilage appears perfectly smooth when viewed by the naked eye, microscopic examination, particularly utilizing electron microscopy, demonstrates minor surface irregularities produced by wear and tear of normal life.[1] These surface undulations may vary between 76.2×10^{-6} cm and 508×10^{-6} cm. With advancing age, the undulating cartilaginous surface may become even more irregular. Synovial fluid may pool between the surface irregularities, accounting for the low coefficient of friction that is characteristic of articular cartilage.

Histologic examination of articular cartilage demonstrates a cellular component (chondrocytes) embedded within an intercellular matrix consisting of collagenous fibrils in a homogeneous ground substance. The ground substance contains water and

Text continued on page 35

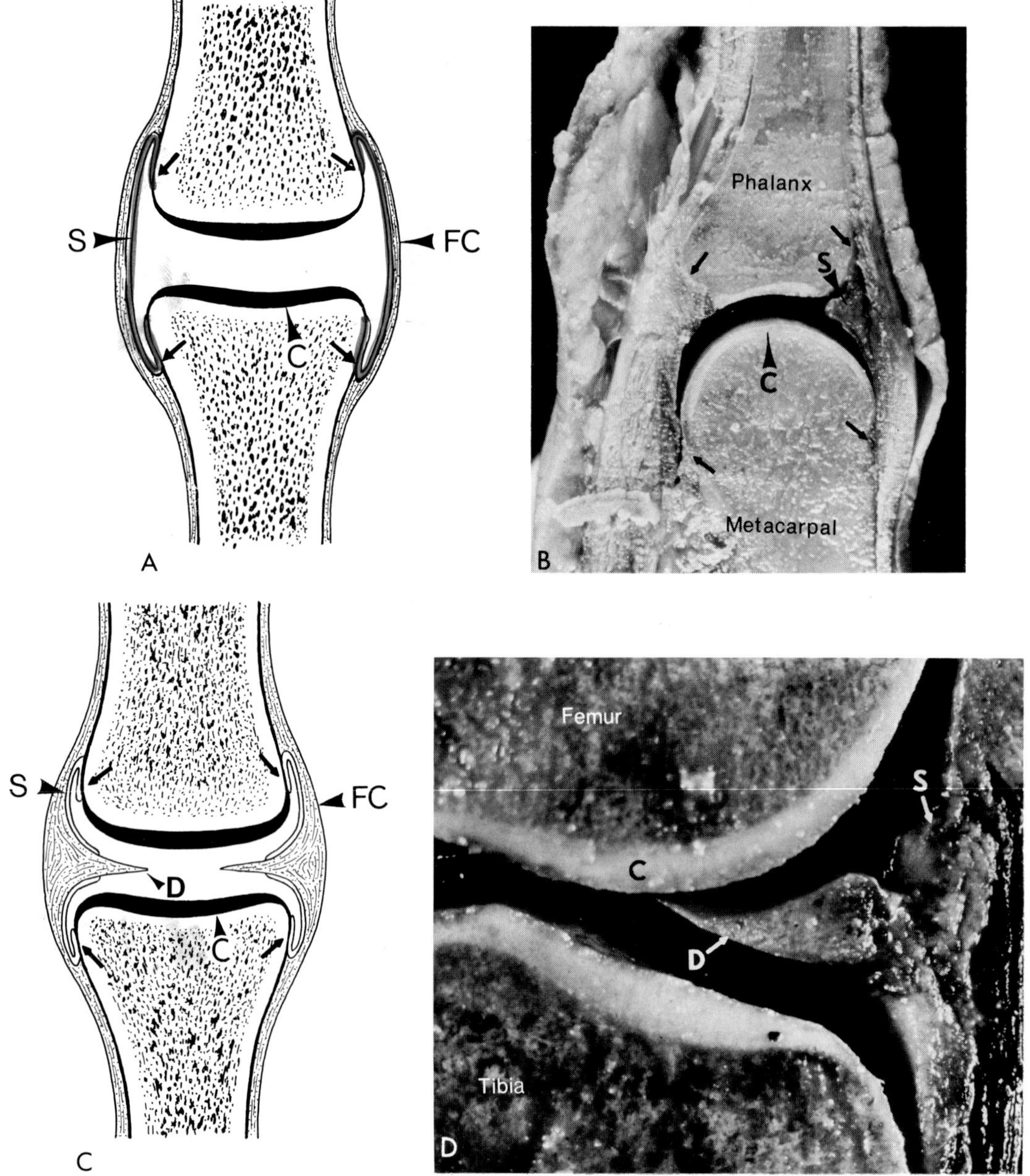

Figure 2–7. *Synovial articulation: General features.*

A, B *Typical synovial joint without an intra-articular disc. A diagram and photograph of a section through a metacarpophalangeal joint outline important structures, including fibrous capsule (FC), synovial membrane (S), and articular cartilage (C). Note that there are marginal areas of the articulation where synovial membrane abuts bone without protective cartilage (arrows).*

C, D *Typical synovial joint containing an articular disc that partially divides the joint cavity. Diagram and photograph of a section through the knee joint reveal fibrous capsule (FC), synovial membrane (S), articular cartilage (C), and articular disc (D). The marginal areas of the joint are again indicated by arrows.*

Illustration continued on the opposite page

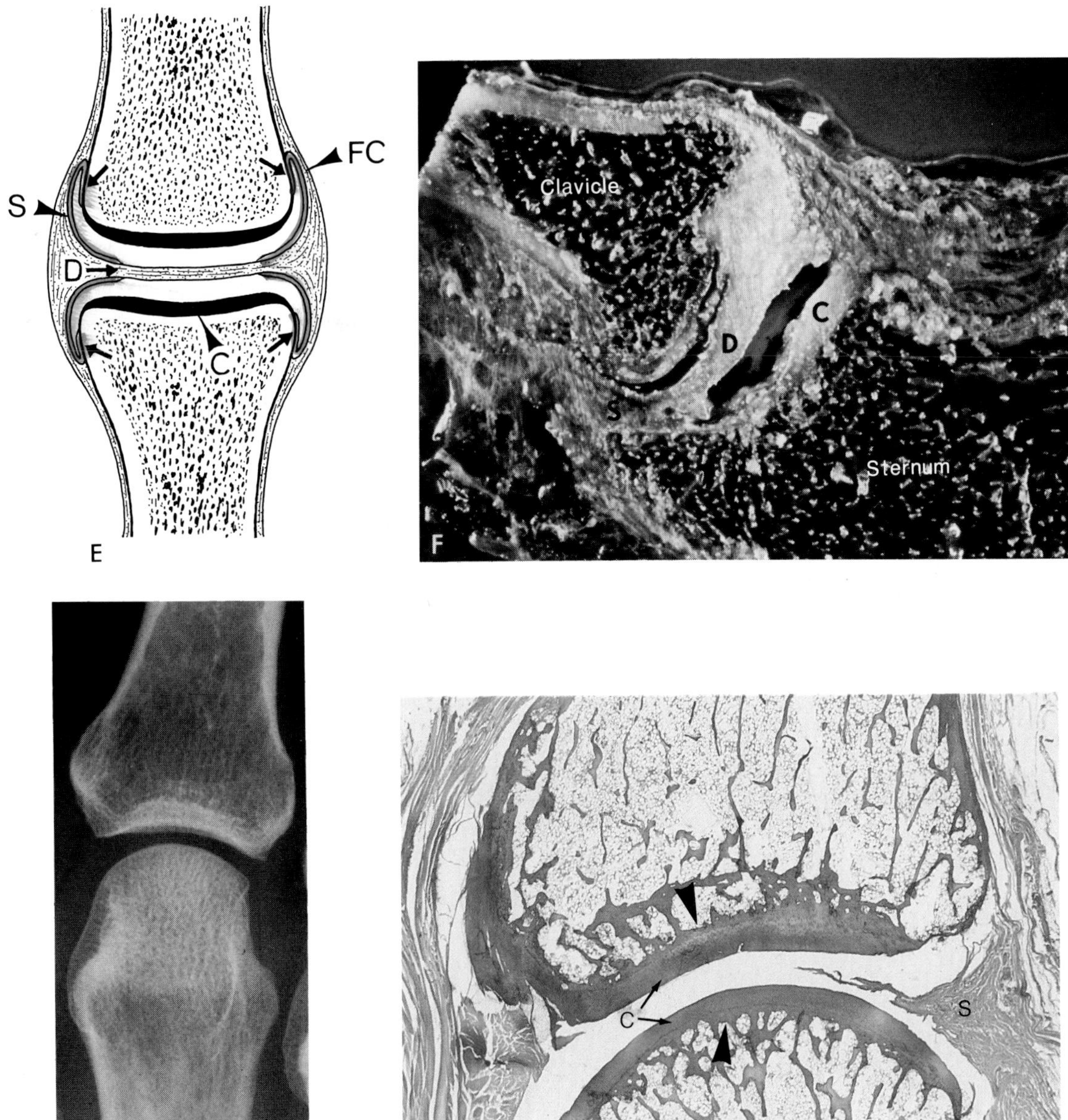

Figure 2–7. Continued

E, F *Typical synovial joint with an articular disc that completely divides the joint cavity. Diagram and photograph of a section through the sternoclavicular joint reveal fibrous capsule (FC), articular cartilage (C), synovial membrane (S), and intra-articular disc (D). The marginal areas are indicated by arrows.*

G *A radiograph of a metacarpophalangeal joint, indicating smooth articular surfaces of the metacarpal head and proximal phalanx separated by a joint cavity.*

H *A photomicrograph (10×) of a metacarpophalangeal joint. Observe synovium (S), articular cartilage (C), and subchondral bone plate (arrowheads).*

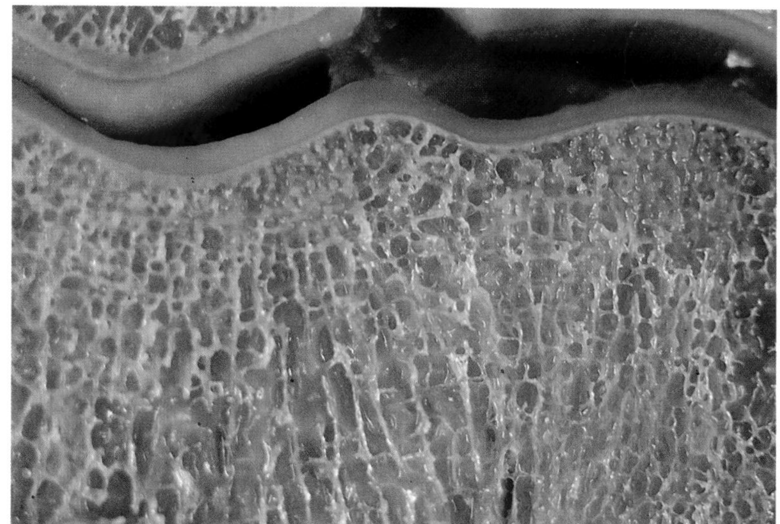

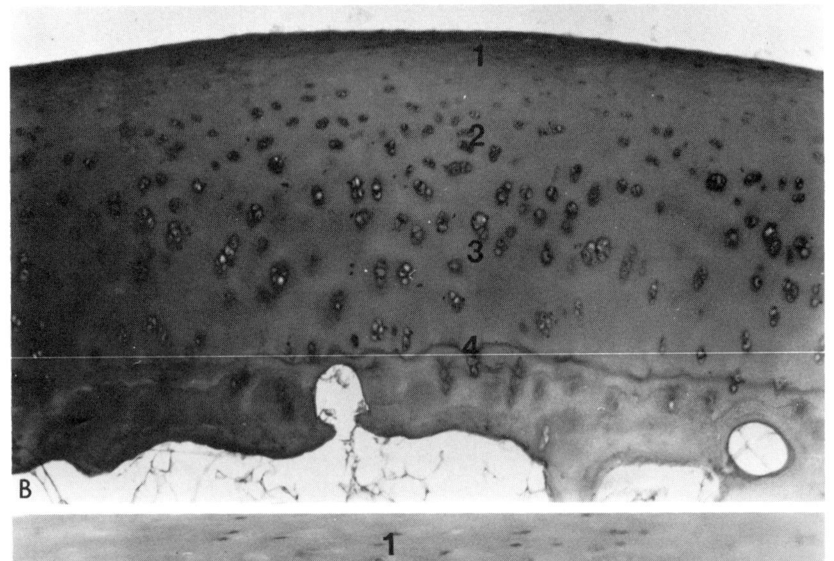

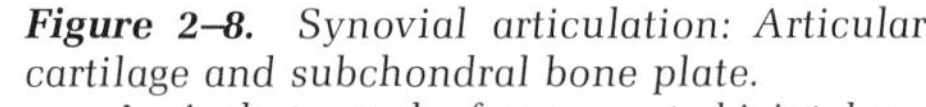

Figure 2–8. *Synovial articulation: Articular cartilage and subchondral bone plate.*

A *A photograph of a macerated joint demonstrates the articular cartilage, subchondral bone plate, and adjacent trabeculae.*

B, C *Photomicrographs at low power (80×) and high power (200×). Observe the tangential zone (1) with flattened cartilage cells, the transitional zone (2) with numerous irregularly distributed cells, the radial zone (3) with columnar arrangement of cells, and the calcified zone (4) adjacent to the osseous surface.*

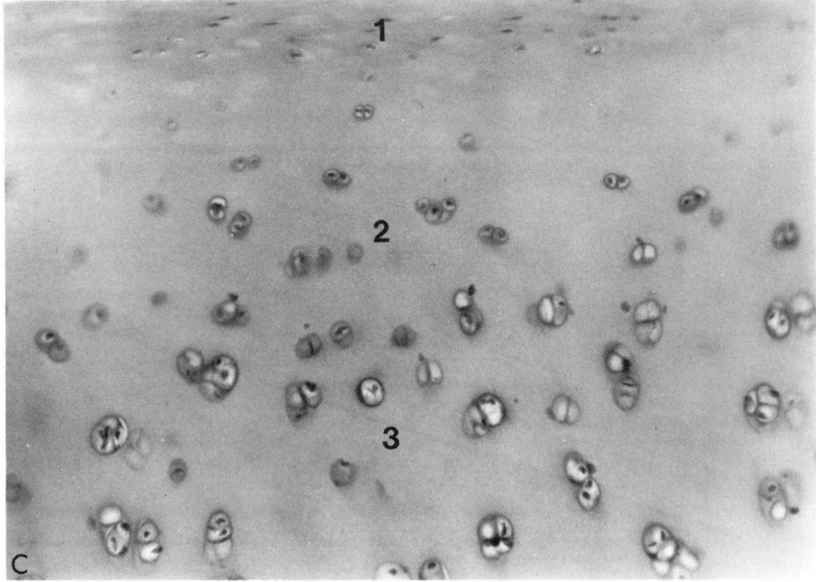

mucopolysaccharides, particularly chondroitin sulfate. The superficial tangential zone of cartilage consists of densely packed collagen fiber bundles, 20 to 32 nm in diameter.[14] Many of these fibers parallel the articular surface. Beneath the superficial zone, collagen fiber bundles have a more random orientation, and individual collagen fibers have a diameter of approximately 80 nm. A cross-linked latticework of fine fibrils can be noted.

There are differences in the appearance of cells in these various zones of articular cartilage. Cells in the superficial layer are generally smaller in size, flattened in shape, and arranged parallel to the articular surface. In the more deeply situated transitional and radial zones of cartilage, cells appear less flattened and may be arranged in groups or columns.[13] The radial zone is the largest layer, beneath which is the calcified zone of articular cartilage, which connects the hyaline cartilage to the subarticular bone.

Cartilage has a high water content, being approximately 70 to 75 per cent water by weight. The water is distributed within the cells in the matrix.[15, 16] The dry weight composition of hyaline cartilage is approximately one half collagen and one half chondroitin sulfate bound to protein.[9] Chondroitin sulfate occurs in two forms — the A and C types — and is important in regulating the consistency and elasticity of the cartilage matrix.[15, 17, 18] In elderly patients, small amounts of kerato-sulfate may also be noted.

Subchondral Bone Plate and "Tidemark"

The bony or subchondral end-plate is a layer of osseous tissue of variable thickness that is located beneath the cartilage (Fig. 2–8). Its features have been well delineated by Jaffe.[13] In most articulations the subchondral bone plate consists of trabeculae, which curve around the inferior aspect of the cartilage. Occasionally the plate consists of thick trabeculae resembling a subchondral cortex, which is perforated in certain areas by vessels extending from subchondral bone into overlying cartilage.

Immediately superficial to the subchondral bone plate is the calcified zone of articular cartilage, termed the "tidemark."[19-21] Projections from this zone interdigitate with indentations on the osseous surface and firmly anchor the calcified cartilage to the subchondral bone. Furthermore, fibrils within the deepest part of the noncalcified cartilage are attached to the calcified zone of cartilage. Thus, the tidemark serves a mechanical function; it anchors the collagen fibers of the noncalcified portion of cartilage and, in turn, is anchored to the subchondral bone plate. These strong connections resist disruption by shearing force.

The calcified layer of cartilage may have additional functions. Some investigators believe that this layer limits harmful diffusion of water and solutes between bone and cartilage.[22, 23] In addition, the calcified layer forms an integral part of the enlarging epiphysis[24] and is therefore important in endochondral ossification during growth and remodeling.

Articular Capsule

The articular capsule is connective tissue that envelops the joint cavity. It is composed of a thick, tough outer layer, the fibrous capsule, and a more delicate thin inner layer, the synovial membrane.

Fibrous Capsule. The fibrous capsule consists of parallel and interlacing bundles of dense white fibrous tissue. At each end of the articulation, the fibrous capsule is firmly adherent to the periosteum of the articulating bones. The site of attachment of the capsule to the periosteum is variable; in some articulations, a large segment of bone may be intracapsular whereas in other articulations, a short segment of bone is present within the capsule.

The fibrous capsule is not of uniform thickness. Ligaments and tendons may attach to it, producing focal areas of increased thickness. In fact, at some sites the fibrous capsules are replaced by tendons or tendinous expansions from neighboring muscles. Extracapsular accessory ligaments, such as those about the sternoclavicular joint, and intracapsular ligaments, such as the cruciate ligaments of the knee, may also be found. These ligaments are tough strands of connective tissue that resist excessive or abnormal motion. They are generally inelastic, although they may demonstrate small degrees of elasticity.[25]

The fibrous capsule is richly supplied with blood and lymphatic vessels and nerves, which may penetrate the capsule and extend down to the synovial membrane. Capsular blood vessels are particularly prominent and numerous at the margin of the articular cartilage. Additional openings in the capsule may be found that allow the synovial membrane to protrude in the form of a pouch or sac.

Microscopic evaluation of the fibrous capsule reveals tissue of varying cellularity.[13] Areas exist that appear tendinous in quality, being poorly supplied with cells, whereas other areas consist of richly cellular connective tissue.

Synovial Membrane. The synovial membrane is a delicate, highly vascular inner membrane of the articular capsule (Fig. 2–9). It lines the non-

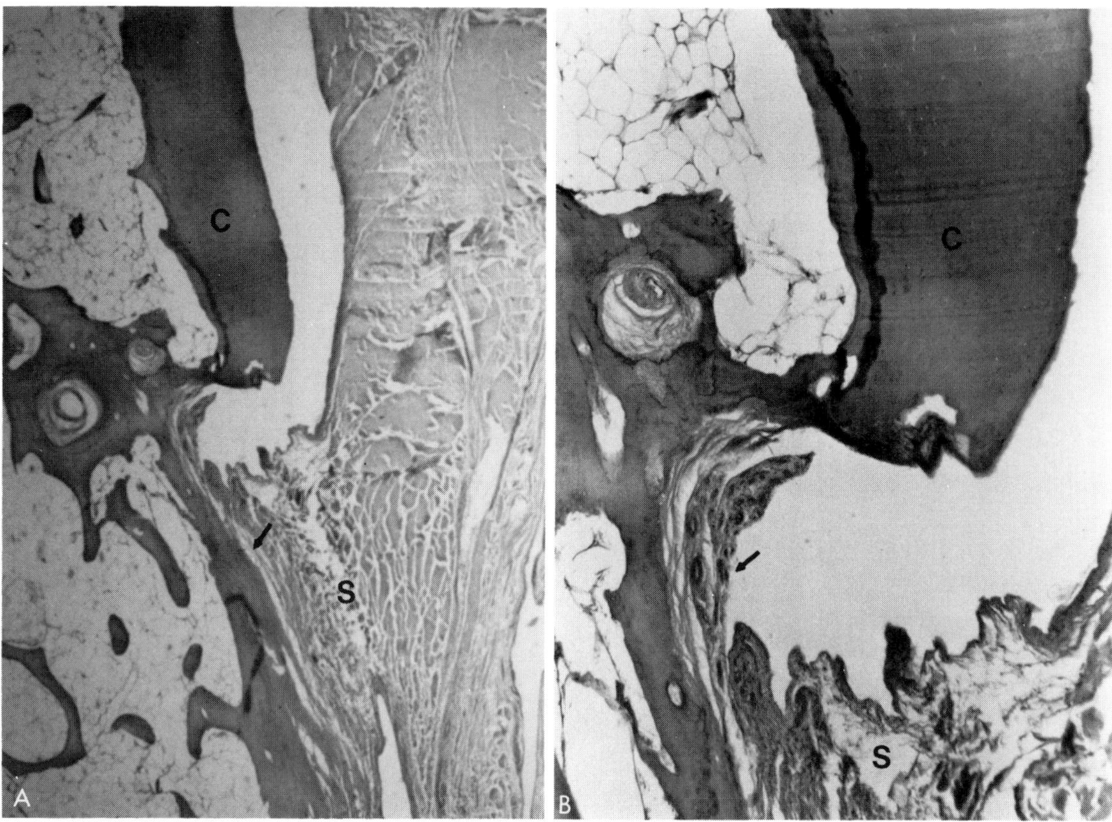

Figure 2–9. *Synovial articulation: Synovial membrane. Low power (80×) and high power (200×) photomicrographs of the chondro-osseous junction about a metacarpophalangeal joint delineate the synovial membrane (S) and articular cartilage (C). The marginal area of the joint at which synovial membrane abuts bone is well demonstrated (arrow).*

articular portion of the synovial joint and any intra-articular ligaments or tendons. The synovial membrane also covers the intracapsular osseous surfaces which are clothed by periosteum or perichondrium, but which are without cartilaginous surfaces. These latter areas frequently occur at the peripheral portion of the articulation and are termed "marginal" or "bare" areas of the joint. Sleeve-like extensions of synovial tissue may extend for short distances between the cartilage-covered bones,[26] but the central cartilaginous tissue and intra-articular discs are free of synovial tissue. Synovial tissue also lines bursae and tendon sheaths.

The synovial membrane is generally pink, moist, and smooth, although small finger-like projections, synovial villi, may be apparent on its inner surface.[27, 28] These villi, which are visible microscopically, are vascular, variable in size and shape, and composed of collagenous fibrils. They are found in special areas of the joint — for example, in sites at which the synovial membrane covers loose areolar tissue. Synovial membrane inflammation or irritation causes excessive villi formation, and in pathologic situations, villous projections may cover the entire inner surface of the synovial membrane.

In addition to synovial villi, the synovial membrane may also reveal thickened folds that extend into the articular cavity (e.g., alar folds and ligamentum mucosum of knee). Furthermore, adipose tissue may accumulate within the synovial membrane, forming articular fat pads. These latter collections act as flexible, compressible cushions extending into irregular areas of the joint cavity. In some joints, such as the elbow, the fat pads occupy a depression on the osseous surface and are displaced during articular motion.

The synovial membrane demonstrates variable structural characteristics in different segments of the articulation. In general, there are two synovial layers, a thin cellular surface layer (intima) and a deeper vascular underlying layer (subintima). The subintimal layer merges on its deep surface with the fibrous capsule. In certain locations, the synovial membrane is attenuated and fails to demonstrate two distinct layers. Sites at which the synovial membrane lines intra-articular ligaments or tendons, such as the cruciates and quadriceps, may not possess a distinct subintima, as the fibrous tissue merges imperceptibly with the adjacent capsule or tendon.

Synovial Intima. This layer consists of one to four rows of synovial cells embedded in a granular, fiber-free intercellular matrix.[2] The cells are of variable shape and may appear flattened and elongated or polyhedral in configuration.[29] The cells may be closely packed in some areas of the articular cavity and poorly apposed elsewhere, allowing subintimal tissue to be interspersed among the surface cells and to be in direct contact with the synovial cavity. Recently, two types of synovial lining cells have been identified: Type A cells resemble macrophages and appear important in phagocytic functions, whereas Type B cells, which are less numerous, have a somewhat different appearance and may be responsible for hyaluronate secretion.[9]

Synovial Subintima. This layer usually contains areolar tissue. Occasionally it is composed of either loose or more fibrous connective tissue.[30] Cellular constituents include fat cells, fibroblasts, macrophages, and mast cells. An elastic component consisting of elastin fibers paralleling the surface of the membrane prevents the formation of redundant synovial folds, which might be compromised during articular motion.

The synovial membrane has several functions (Table 2–2). It is involved in the secretion of sticky mucoid substance into the synovial fluid. In addition, the synovial membrane aids the removal of substances from the articular cavity. The route of egress of these intra-articular substances depends upon the size of the particles; small particles may traverse the synovial membrane and enter subintimal capillaries and venules directly, whereas larger particles may be removed via lymphatic channels.

Intra-articular Disc (Meniscus), Labrum, and Fat Pad

A fibrocartilaginous disc or meniscus may be found in some articulations, such as the knee, wrist, temporomandibular, acromioclavicular, sternoclavicular, and costovertebral joints (Fig. 2–10). The peripheral portion of the disc attaches to the fibrous capsule. Blood vessels and afferent nerves may be noted within this peripheral zone of the disc. Most of the articular disc, however, is avascular. The disc may partially or completely divide the joint cavity; complete discs are found in the sternoclavicular and wrist joints, whereas partial discs are noted in the knee and acromioclavicular articulations. In the temporomandibular joint, the disc may be partial or complete. Even the complete disc may reveal small perforations. Although the tissue of the intra-articular disc is generally referred to as fibrocartilage, it may more accurately represent fibroelastic connective tissue.[13] Collagenous connective tissue is interspersed with elastic fibers. The elastic tissue is particularly prominent in the central portion of a disc. Cellular components are also evident.

Table 2–2
SYNOVIAL MEMBRANE

Function	Site
Mucin component of synovial fluid	?Type B cells
Dialysate component of synovial fluid	Capillaries
Phagocytosis	Type A cells
Drainage of wastes from cavity	Lymphatics Capillaries
Regulation of entry of nutrients	Entire synovial membrane

The exact function of intra-articular discs is unknown. Suggested functions include shock absorption, distribution of weight over a large surface, facilitation of various motions (such as rotation) and limitation of others (such as translation), and protection of the articular surface.[31] It has been suggested that intra-articular discs play an important role in the effective lubrication of a joint.[32] For example, in the knee joint, interposed menisci separate the synovial fluid into two wedge-shaped collections of lubricant. These collections provide efficient lubrication, which allows one surface to roll over an adjacent one. Further evidence that articular discs play an important role in joint motion is the presence of these structures in articulations that display translation movements.[2] In these articulations, such as the temporomandibular joint, intra-articular cartilaginous discs may provide increased congruity of joint surface and even distribution of intervening synovial fluid.

Some joints, such as the hip and glenohumeral articulations, contain circumferential cartilaginous folds termed labra (Fig. 2–10). These lips of cartilage are usually triangular in cross section and are attached to the peripheral portion of an articular surface, thereby acting to enlarge or deepen the joint cavity. They may also serve to increase contact and congruity of adjacent articular surfaces, particularly at the extremes of joint motion.

Fat pads represent additional structures that may be present within a joint (Fig. 2–10). These structures possess a generous vascular and nerve supply, contain few lymphatic vessels, and are covered by a flattened layer of synovial cells. Fat pads may act as cushions, absorbing forces generated across a joint, thus protecting adjacent bony processes. They may also distribute lubricants in the joint cavity.

Synovial Fluid

Minute amounts of clear, colorless to pale yellow, highly viscous fluid of slightly alkaline pH are present in healthy joints. The exact composition, viscosity, volume, and color vary somewhat from joint to joint. This fluid represents a dialysate of

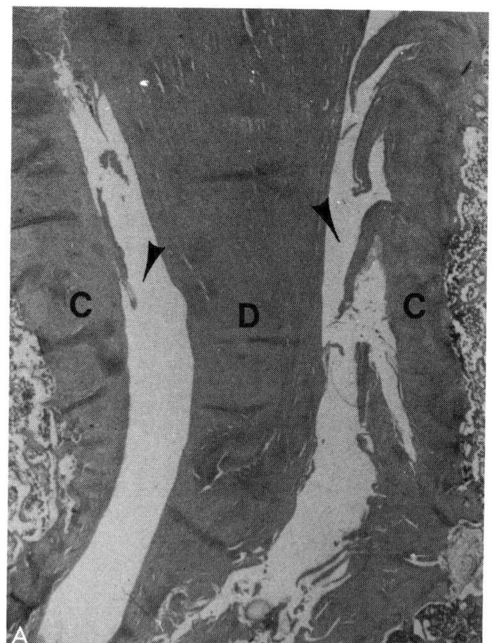

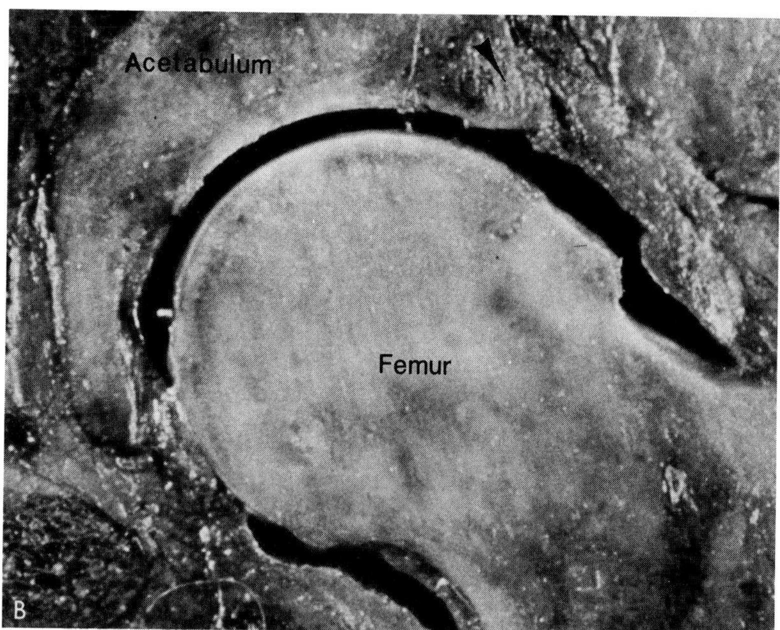

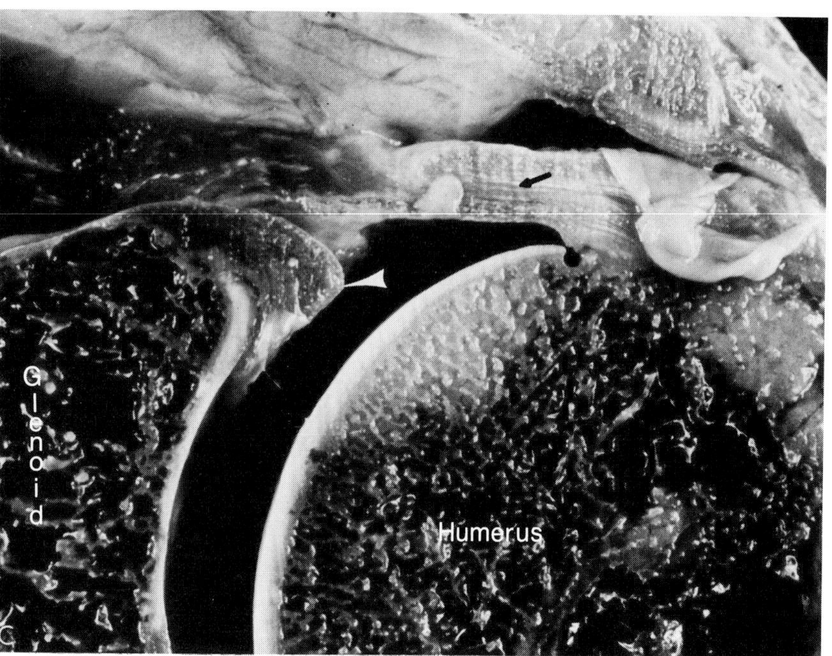

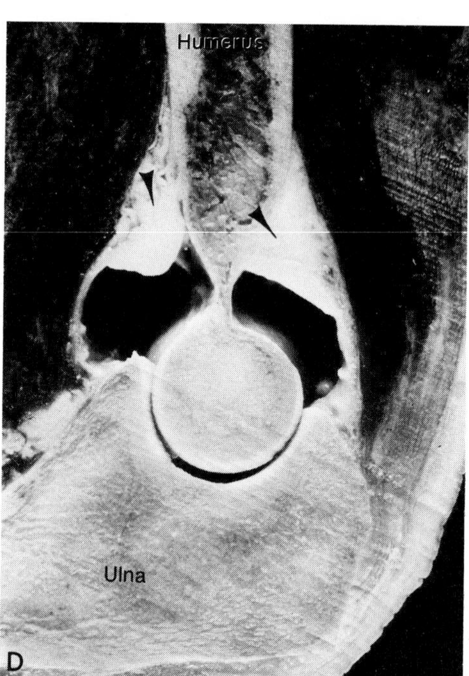

Figure 2–10. *Synovial articulation: Intra-articular disc, labrum, and fat pad.*

A *A photomicrograph (10×) reveals the structure of the intra-articular disc (D) of the sternoclavicular joint. Note the two joint cavities (arrowheads) and articular cartilage (C) of sternum and clavicle.*

B *A photograph of a coronal section through the hip joint outlines the labrum (arrowhead) along the outer aspect of the acetabulum.*

C *A photograph of a coronal section through the superior aspect of the glenohumeral joint demonstrates a cartilaginous labrum (arrowhead) along the superior aspect of the glenoid. Note the adjacent rotator cuff tendons (arrow).*

D *In a photograph of a sagittal section through the humeroulnar aspect of the elbow joint, note the intra-articular anterior and posterior fat pads (arrowheads) which are elevated by a large amount of intra-articular air.*

blood plasma to which has been added a mucoid substance secreted by the synovial cells. A small number of cells present within the synovial fluid consists of monocytes, lymphocytes, macrophages, polymorphonuclear leukocytes, and free synovial cells.[33] Erythrocytes are occasionally noted in normal synovial fluid, most likely representing contamination of the fluid due to the trauma of joint aspiration. Particles, cell fragments, and fibrous tissue may also be seen in the synovial fluid as a result of wear and tear of the articular surface. Various enzymes, such as alkaline phosphatase, are found in synovial fluid.

Functions of the synovial fluid are nutrition of the adjacent articular cartilage and disc and lubrication of joint surfaces, which decreases friction and increases joint efficiency. The cells within the synovial fluid are important in phagocytosis, removing microorganisms and joint debris.

Synovial Sheaths and Bursae

Synovial tissue is also found about various tendon sheaths and bursae (Fig. 2–11). This tissue is located at sites where closely apposed structures move in relationship to each other. Typical examples include tendons that are reflected or angulated about bony surfaces, and bursae that separate skin from subjacent bony protuberances.

Tendon sheaths completely or partially cover a portion of the tendon where it passes through fascial slings, osseofibrous tunnels, and ligamentous bands. Tendon sheaths are composed of two coats separated by a thin film of synovial fluid. The inner coat or visceral layer is attached to the surface of the tendon by loose areolar tissue. The outer coat or parietal layer is attached to adjacent connective tissue or periosteum. The invaginated tendon allows apposition of visceral and parietal layers in the form of a mesotendon. This latter structure carries blood vessels and is attached to a longitudinal line or hilus along the nonfrictional surface of the tendon. The tendon sheath also contains nerves and lymphatics. The microscopic structure of the tendon sheath resembles that of a synovial membrane.[13] Some areas are cellular, whereas others are poorly cellular. Small amounts of areolar tissue are focally interposed between the two coats of the tendon sheath.

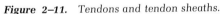

Bursae represent enclosed flattened sacs consist-

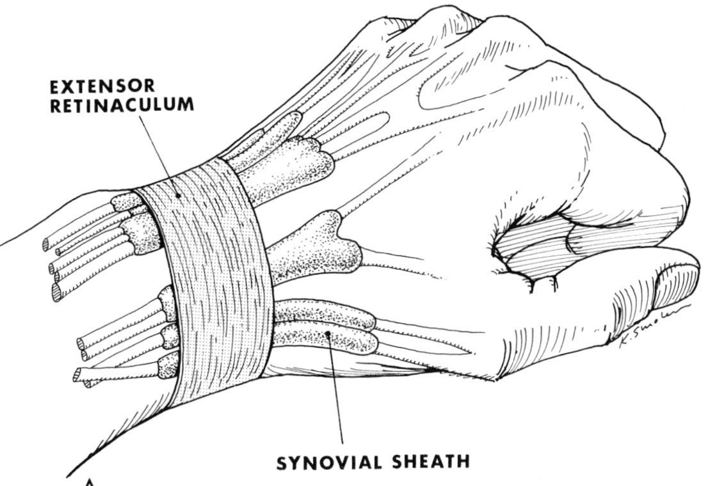

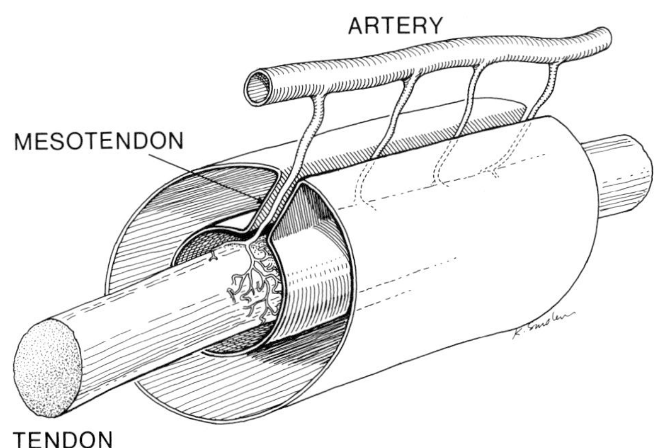

Figure 2–11. *Tendons and tendon sheaths.*

A *Extensor tendons with surrounding synovial sheaths pass beneath the extensor retinaculum on the dorsum of the wrist.*

B *A drawing of the fine structure of a tendon and tendon sheath reveals an inner coat or visceral layer adjacent to the tendon surface and an outer coat or parietal layer. Note that the invaginated tendon allows apposition of visceral and parietal layers in the form of a mesotendon. This latter structure provides a passageway for adjacent blood vessels.*

ing of synovial lining and a thin film of synovial fluid, which provides both lubrication and nourishment for the cells of the synovial membrane. Intervening bursae facilitate motion between apposing tissues. Subcutaneous bursae are found between skin and underlying bony prominences, such as the olecranon and patella; subfascial bursae are placed between deep fascia and bone; subtendinous bursae exist where one tendon overlies another tendon; submucosal bursae are located between muscle and bone, tendon, or ligament; interligamentous bursae separate ligaments. When bursae are located near articulations, the synovial membrane of the bursa may be continuous with that of the joint cavity, producing communicating bursae. At certain sites where skin is subject to pressure and lateral displacement, adventitious bursae may appear, allowing increased freedom of motion.

Sesamoid Bones

Sesamoids are generally ovoid nodules of small size which are embedded in tendons (Fig. 2–12). They are found in two specific situations in the skeleton.

Type A. The sesamoid is located adjacent to an articulation, and its tendon is incorporated into the joint capsule. The sesamoid nodule and adjacent bone form an extension of the articulation. Examples of this type are the patella and the hallucis and pollicis sesamoids.

Type B. The sesamoid is located at sites where tendons are angled about bony surfaces. They are separated from the underlying bone by a synovium-lined bursa. An example of this type of sesamoid is the sesamoid of the peroneus longus.

In both Type A and Type B situations, the arrangement of the sesamoid nodule and surrounding tissue resembles a synovial joint. Osseous surfaces are covered by cartilage and are intimate with the synovium-lined cavity. This type of arrangement has led many investigators to consider sesamoids as primarily articular in nature, their association with tendons representing a secondary phenomenon. In the hand, sesamoid nodules adjacent to joints (Type A) are most frequently present on the palmar aspect of the metacarpophalangeal joints, particularly the first. In this location, two sesamoids are found in the tendons of the adductor pollicis and flexor pollicis brevis, articulating with facets on the palmar surface of the metacarpal head. Additional sesamoids are most frequent in the second and fifth metacarpophalangeal joints and adjacent to the interphalangeal joint of the thumb.[34] This distribution of sesamoids in the hand is not constant. Examples of decreased and increased numbers of sesamoids have been described.[35]

Sesamoid distribution in the foot parallels that

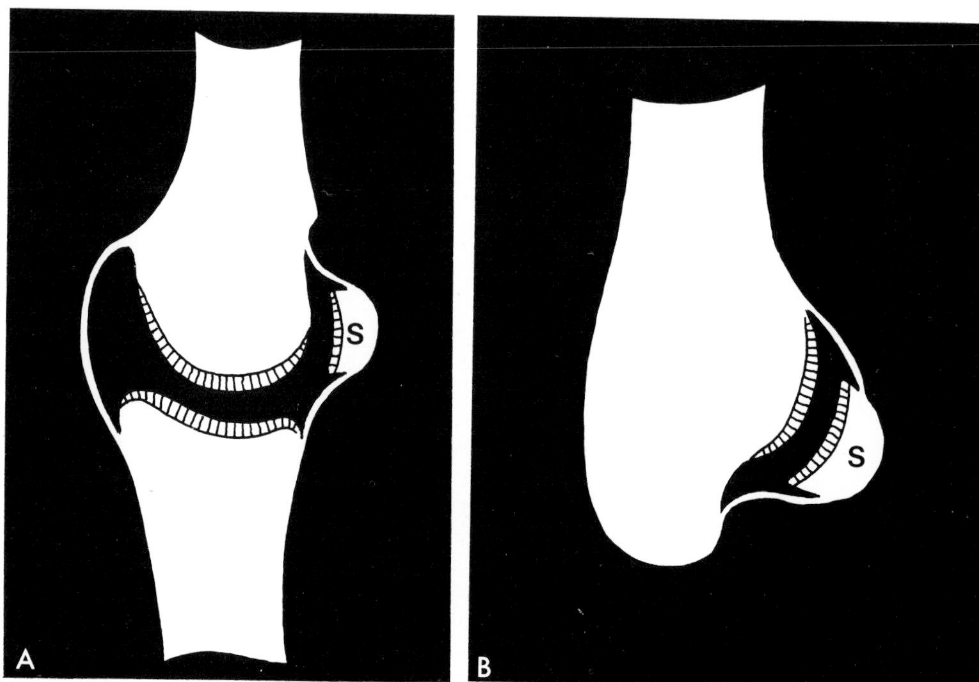

Figure 2–12. *Sesamoid bones.*

A, B *There are two types of sesamoids[2]: Type A* **(A),** *in which the sesamoid is located adjacent to an articulation, and Type B* **(B),** *in which the sesamoid is separated from the underlying bone by a bursa. In both types, the sesamoid is intimately associated with a synovial lining and articular cartilage (hatched areas).*

Illustration continued on the opposite page

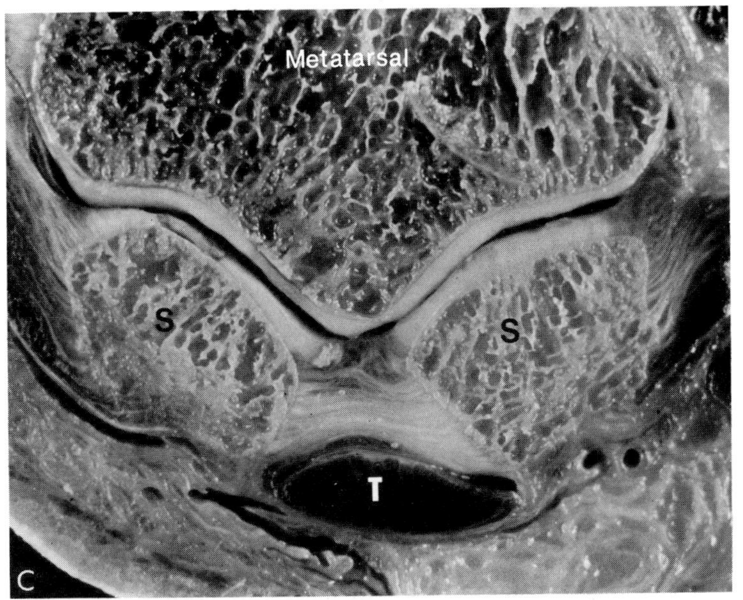

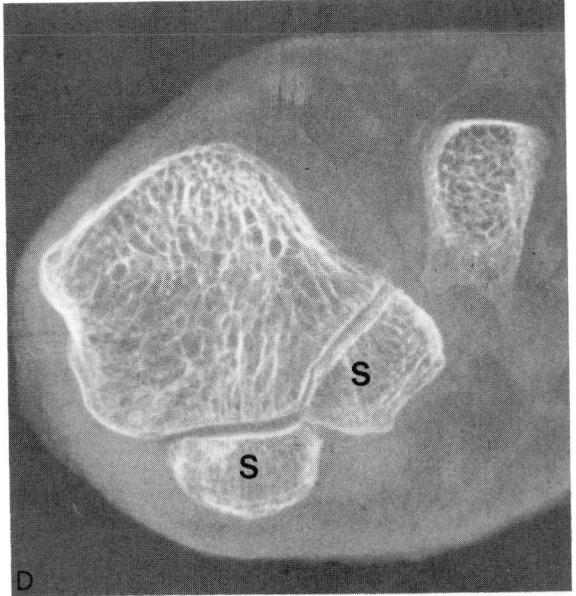

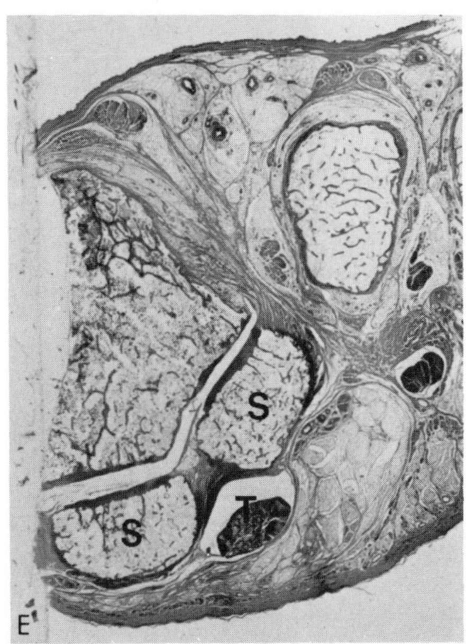

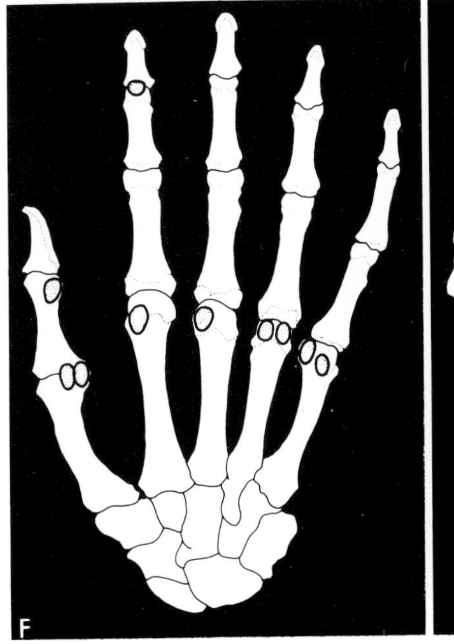

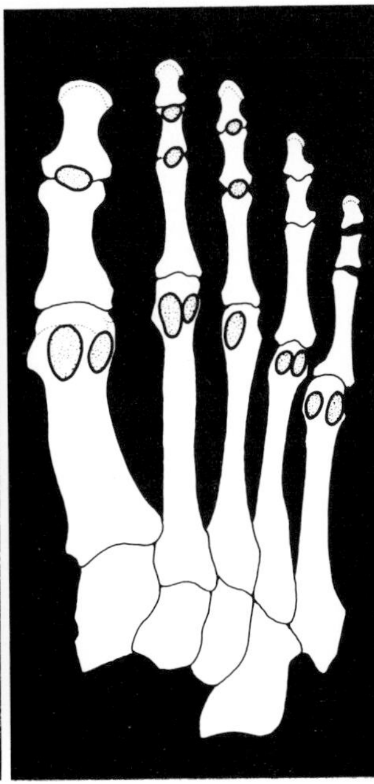

Figure 2–12. Continued

C–E *A photograph, radiograph, and photomicrograph (2×) of the sesamoids* (S) *of the first metatarsophalangeal joint. At this articulation, there are medial and lateral sesamoid bones* (S) *embedded in the plantar part of the capsule of the joint within the tendon of the flexor hallucis brevis* (T). *Note the articular cartilage on the sesamoids and adjacent metatarsal.*

F *The sesamoid distribution in the hand and foot is revealed. Type A sesamoids are most constantly present about the metacarpophalangeal joint and interphalangeal joint of the first digit of the hand and the metatarsophalangeal joint and interphalangeal joint of the first digit of the foot. Inconstant sesamoids may be located about any metacarpophalangeal, metatarsophalangeal, or interphalangeal joint.*

*(***A–C** *and* **F,** *From Resnick D, Niwayama G, Feingold ML: Radiology 123:57, 1977.)*

in the hand. Two sesamoids are located on the plantar aspect of the first metatarsophalangeal joint in the tendons of the flexor hallucis brevis. Sesamoid nodules may also be present at other metatarsophalangeal joints and the interphalangeal joint of the great toe. Sesamoid bones unassociated with synovial joints (Type B) are more frequent in the lower extremity than in the upper extremity. In the foot, sesamoids of this type are noted in the tendon of the peroneus longus adjacent to a facet on the tuberosity of the cuboid bone, in the tendon of the tibialis anterior muscle in contact with the medial surface of the medial cuneiform bone, and in the tendon of the tibialis posterior muscle adjacent to the medial aspect of the talus.

SUPPORTING STRUCTURES

A variety of supporting structures exist in periarticular locations or in a more general distribution; these structures influence articular disorders. In some disorders, the supporting structures are themselves involved. Rather than review in depth all of these structures, several important ones are identified below.

Tendons

Tendons represent a portion of a muscle of unvarying length, consisting of collagen fibers. They are flexible cords, white in color, smooth in texture, that can be angulated about bony protuberances, changing the direction of pull of the muscle. On the surface of the tendon, areolar connective tissue, the epitendineum, allows passage of vessels and nerves. Synovial sheaths may surround portions of the tendon.

Aponeuroses

Aponeuroses consist of several flat layers or sheets of dense collagen fibers associated with the attachment of a muscle. The fasciculae within one layer of an aponeurosis are parallel and different in direction from fasciculae of an adjacent layer.

Fasciae

Fascia is a general term used to describe a focal collection of connective tissue. Superficial fascia consists of a layer of loose areolar tissue of variable thickness beneath the dermis. It is most distinct over the lower abdomen, perineum, and limbs. Deep fascia resembles an aponeurosis, consisting of regularly arranged compact collagen fibers. Parallel fibers of one layer are angled with respect to the fibers of an adjacent layer. Deep fascia is particularly prominent in the extremities, and in these sites, muscle may arise from the inner aspect of the deep fascia. At sites where deep fascia contacts bone, the fascia fuses with the periosteum. It is well suited to transmit the pull of adjacent musculature. Intermuscular septae extend from deep fascia between groups of muscles, producing functional compartments. Retinaculae are transverse thickenings in the deep fascia that are attached to bony protuberances, creating tunnels through which tendons can pass. An example is the dorsal retinaculum of the wrist, under which extend the extensor tendons and their synovial sheaths.

VASCULAR, LYMPHATIC, AND NERVE SUPPLY

The blood supply of joints arises from periarticular arterial plexuses that pierce the capsule, break up in the synovial membrane, and form a rich and intricate network of capillaries. Many of the vessels are superficially located in the synovium, perhaps explaining the frequency of hemorrhage following even relatively insignificant trauma to the joint.[36] A circle of vessels (circulus articuli vasculosus) within the synovial membrane is adjacent to the peripheral margin of articular cartilage.

The lymphatics form a plexus in the subintima of the synovial membrane. Efferent vessels pass toward the flexor aspect of the joint and then along blood vessels to regional deep lymph nodes.

The nerve supply of movable joints generally arises from the same nerves that supply the adjacent musculature. The fibrous capsule and to a lesser extent the synovial membrane are both supplied by nerves. Each nerve supplies a specific segment of the capsule, but a good deal of overlap in innervation exists. Some of the nerves in the fibrous capsule have encapsulated nerve endings; others have free nerve endings. The encapsulated endings are thought to be proprioceptive in nature,[37, 38] whereas the free nerve endings, numerous at the attachments of fibrous capsule and ligaments, are believed to mediate pain sensation.[39] This would explain the extreme pain that is common following injury to joint ligaments. The synovial membrane itself is relatively insensitive to pain.[40]

REFERENCES

1. Walmsley R.: Joints. *In* GJ Romanes (Ed): Cunningham's Textbook of Anatomy. 11th Ed. London, Oxford University Press, 1972, p 207.
2. Warwick R, Williams PL: Arthrology. *In* Gray's Anatomy. 35th British Ed. Philadelphia, WB Saunders Co, 1973, p 388.
3. Pritchard JJ, Scott JH, Girgis FG: The structure and development of cranial and facial sutures. J Anat *90*:73, 1956.
4. Todd TW, Lyon DW Jr: Endocranial suture closure. Its progress and age relationship. Part I. Adult males of white stock. Am J Phys Anthropol *7*:325, 1924.
5. Todd TW, Lyon DW Jr: Cranial suture closure. Part II. Ectocranial closure in adult males of white stock. Am J Phys Anthropol *8*:23, 1925.
6. Todd TW, Lyon DW Jr: Suture closure. Part III. Endocranial closure in adult males of negro stock. Am J Phys Anthropol *8*:47, 1925.
7. Todd TW, Lyon DW Jr: Suture closure. Its progress and age relationship. Part IV. Ectocranial closure in adult males of negro stock. Am J Phys Anthropol 8:149, 1925.
8. Abbie AA: Closure of cranial articulations in the skull of the Australian aborigine. J Anat *84*:1, 1950.
9. Hamerman D, Rosenberg LC, Schubert M: Diarthrodial joints revisited. J Bone Joint Surg *52B*:725, 1970.
10. Barnett CH, Cobbold AF: Lubrication within living joints. J Bone Joint Surg *44B*:662, 1962.
11. Ingelmark BE: The nutritive supply and nutritional value of synovial fluid. Acta Orthop Scand 20:144, 1951.
12. Hunter W: On the structure and diseases of articular cartilage. Phil Trans B *42*:514, 1743.
13. Jaffe HL: Metabolic, Degenerative and Inflammatory Diseases of Bones and Joints. Philadelphia, Lea & Febiger, 1972, p 80.
14. Weiss C, Rosenberg L, Helfet AJ: An ultrastructural study of normal young adult human articular cartilage. J Bone Joint Surg *50A*:663, 1968.
15. Linn FC, Sokoloff L: Movement and composition of interstitial fluid of cartilage. Arthritis Rheum *8*:481, 1965.
16. Eichelberger L, Akeson WH, Roma M: Biochemical studies of articular cartilage. I. Normal values. J Bone Joint Surg *40A*:142, 1958.
17. Linn FC, Radin EL: Lubrication of animal joints. III. The effect of certain chemical alterations of the cartilage and lubricant. Arthritis Rheum *11*:674, 1968.
18. Sokoloff L: Elasticity of articular cartilage: effect of ions and viscous solutions. Science *141*:1055, 1963.
19. Redler I, Mow VC, Zimny ML, Mansell J: The ultrastructure and biomechanical significance of the tidemark of articular cartilage. Clin Orthop Rel Res *112*:357, 1975.
20. Green WT Jr, Martin GN, Eanes ED, Sokoloff L: Microradiographic study of the calcified layer of articular cartilage. Arch Pathol *90*:151, 1970.
21. Fawns HT, Landells JW: Histochemical studies of rheumatic conditions; observations on the fine structures of the matrix of normal bone and cartilage. Ann Rheum Dis *12*:105, 1953.
22. Maroudas A, Bullough P, Swanson SAV, Freeman MAR: The permeability of articular cartilage. J Bone Joint Surg *50B*:166, 1968.
23. Ishido B: Gelenkuntersuchungen. Virchows Arch Pathol Anat *244*:424, 1923.
24. Mankin HJ: The calcified zone (basal layer) of articular cartilage of rabbits. Anat Rec *145*:73, 1963.
25. Smith JW: The elastic properties of the anterior cruciate ligament of the rabbit. J Anat *88*:369, 1954.
26. Grant JCB: Interarticular synovial folds. Br J Surg *18*:636, 1931.
27. Palmer DG: Synovial villi: an examination of these structures within the anterior compartment of the knee and metacarpo-phalangeal joints. Arthritis Rheum *10*:451, 1967.
28. Sigurdson LA: The structure and function of articular synovial membranes. J Bone Joint Surg *12*:603, 1930.
29. Barland P, Novikoff AB, Hamerman D: Electron microscopy of the human synovial membrane. J Cell Biol *14*:207, 1962.
30. Davies DV: The structure and functions of the synovial membrane. Br Med J *1*:92, 1950.
31. Barnett CH, Davies DV, MacConaill MA: Synovial Joints; Their Structure and Mechanics. Springfield, Ill, Charles C Thomas, 1961.
32. MacConaill MA: The function of intra-articular fibrocartilages, with special reference to the knee and inferior radio-ulnar joints. J Anat *66*:210, 1932.
33. Bauer W, Ropes MW, Waine H: The physiology of articular structures. Physiol Rev *20*:272, 1940.
34. Gray DJ, Gardner E, O'Rahilly R: The prenatal development of the skeleton and joints of the human hand. Am J Anat *101*:169, 1957.
35. Jacobs P: Multiple sesamoid bones of the hand and foot. Clin Radiol *25*:267, 1974.
36. Davies DV: Anatomy and physiology of diarthrodial joints. Ann Rheum Dis *5*:29, 1945.
37. Stopford JSB: The nerve supply of the interphalangeal and metacarpo-phalangeal joints. J Anat *56*:1, 1921.
38. Mountcastle VB, Powell TPS: Central nervous mechanisms subserving position sense and kinesthesis. Bull Johns Hopkins Hosp *105*:173, 1959.
39. Gardner ED: Physiology of movable joints. Physiol Rev *30*:127, 1950.
40. Kellgren JH, Samuel EP: The sensitivity and innervation of the articular capsule. J Bone Joint Surg *32B*:84, 1950.

ANATOMY OF INDIVIDUAL JOINTS

by Donald Resnick, M.D.,
and Gen Niwayama, M.D.

WRIST
- Radiocarpal Compartment
- Inferior Radioulnar Compartment
- Midcarpal Compartment
- Pisiform-triquetral Compartment
- Common Carpometacarpal Compartment
- First Carpometacarpal Compartment
- Intermetacarpal Compartments

METACARPOPHALANGEAL JOINTS

INTERPHALANGEAL JOINTS OF THE HAND

RADIOULNAR SYNDESMOSIS (MIDDLE RADIOULNAR JOINT)

ELBOW

GLENOHUMERAL JOINT

ACROMIOCLAVICULAR JOINT

STERNOCLAVICULAR JOINT

STERNAL JOINTS
- Manubriosternal Joint
- Xiphisternal Joint

STERNOCOSTAL AND INTERCOSTAL JOINTS
- Sternocostal (Sternochondral) Joints
- Intercostal (Interchondral) Joints

COSTOVERTEBRAL JOINTS
- Joints of the Heads of Ribs
- Costotransverse Joints

JOINTS OF THE VERTEBRAL BODIES
- Intervertebral Disc
- Anterior and Posterior Longitudinal Ligaments

JOINTS OF THE VERTEBRAL ARCHES
- Articular Processes (Synovial Joints)
- Ligamentous Articulations (Syndesmoses)

MOVEMENTS OF THE VERTEBRAL COLUMN

ATLANTO-AXIAL JOINTS
- Lateral Atlanto-axial Joints
- Median Atlanto-axial Joints

ATLANTO-OCCIPITAL JOINTS
- Atlanto-occipital Synovial Joints
- Atlanto-occipital Membranes

OCCIPITAL-AXIAL SYNDESMOSES

OSSEOUS RELATIONSHIPS OF CERVICOBASILAR JUNCTION

JOINTS OF THE SACRUM AND COCCYX
- Lumbosacral Joints
- Sacrococcygeal Joint
- Intercoccygeal Joints

SACROILIAC JOINTS

PELVIC-VERTEBRAL LIGAMENTS

SYMPHYSIS PUBIS

HIP

KNEE

TIBIOFIBULAR JOINTS
- Proximal Tibiofibular Joint
- Crural Interosseous Membrane
- Distal Tibiofibular Joint

ANKLE (TALOCRURAL JOINT)

TENDON SHEATHS AND BURSAE ABOUT THE ANKLE AND CALCANEUS

INTERTARSAL JOINTS
- Talocalcaneal Joints
- Calcaneocuboid Joint
- Cuneonavicular, Intercuneiform, Cuneocuboid, and Cuboideonavicular Joints

TARSOMETATARSAL AND INTERMETATARSAL JOINTS

METATARSOPHALANGEAL JOINTS

INTERPHALANGEAL JOINTS OF THE FOOT

3

Anatomic features related to articular and periarticular soft tissue and osseous structures govern the manner in which disease processes become evident on roentgenograms. This chapter summarizes important osseous and soft tissue anatomy about individual articulations in the body.

WRIST

Osseous Anatomy

The bony structures about the wrist are the distal radius and ulna, the proximal and distal rows of carpal bones, and the metacarpals[1,2] (Figs. 3–1 and 3–2).

The distal aspects of the radius and ulna articulate with the proximal row of carpal bones. On the lateral surface of the radius is the radial styloid process, which extends more distally than the remainder of the bone, and from which arises the radial collateral ligament of the wrist joint. The articular surface of the radius is divided into an ulnar and a radial portion by a faint central ridge of bone. The ulnar portion articulates with the lunate and the radial portion with the scaphoid. The articular surface is continuous medially with that of the triangular fibrocartilage. The medial surface of the distal radius contains the concave ulnar notch, which articulates with the distal ulna. The posterior surface of the distal radius is convex and grooved or irregular in outline to allow passage of tendons and tendon sheaths. A prominent ridge in the middle of this surface is the dorsal tubercle of the radius. The anterior surface of the distal radius allows attachment of the palmar radiocarpal ligament.

The distal end of the ulna contains a small round head and a styloid process. The lateral aspect contains an articular surface for contact with the ulnar notch of the radius. The ulna also has a distal articular surface, which is intimate with the triangular fibrocartilage. The ulnar styloid process, which extends distally from the posteromedial aspect of the bone, gives rise to the ulnar collateral ligament. Between the styloid process and inferior articular surface, the ulna has an area for attachment of the triangular fibrocartilage and a dorsal groove for the extensor carpi ulnaris tendon and sheath.

The proximal row of carpal bones consists of the scaphoid, lunate, and triquetrum, as well as the pisiform bone within the tendon of the flexor carpi ulnaris. The distal row of carpal bones contains the trapezium, trapezoid, capitate, and hamate bones. The dorsal surface of the carpus is convex from side to side, and the palmar surface presents a deep concavity, termed the carpal groove or canal. The medial border of this palmar carpal groove contains the pisiform and hook of the hamate. The lateral border of the carpal groove contains the tubercles of the scaphoid and the trapezium. A strong fibrous retinaculum attaches to the palmar surface of the carpus, converting the groove into a carpal tunnel, through which pass the median nerve and flexor tendons.

The distal row of carpal bones articulates with the bases of the metacarpals. The trapezium has a saddle-shaped articular surface for the first metacarpal. The trapezoid fits into a deep notch in the second metacarpal. The capitate articulates mainly with the third metacarpal, but also with the second and fourth metacarpals. The hamate articulates with the fourth and fifth metacarpals. The bases of the metacarpals articulate not only with the distal row of carpal bones but also with each other.

Text continued on page 49

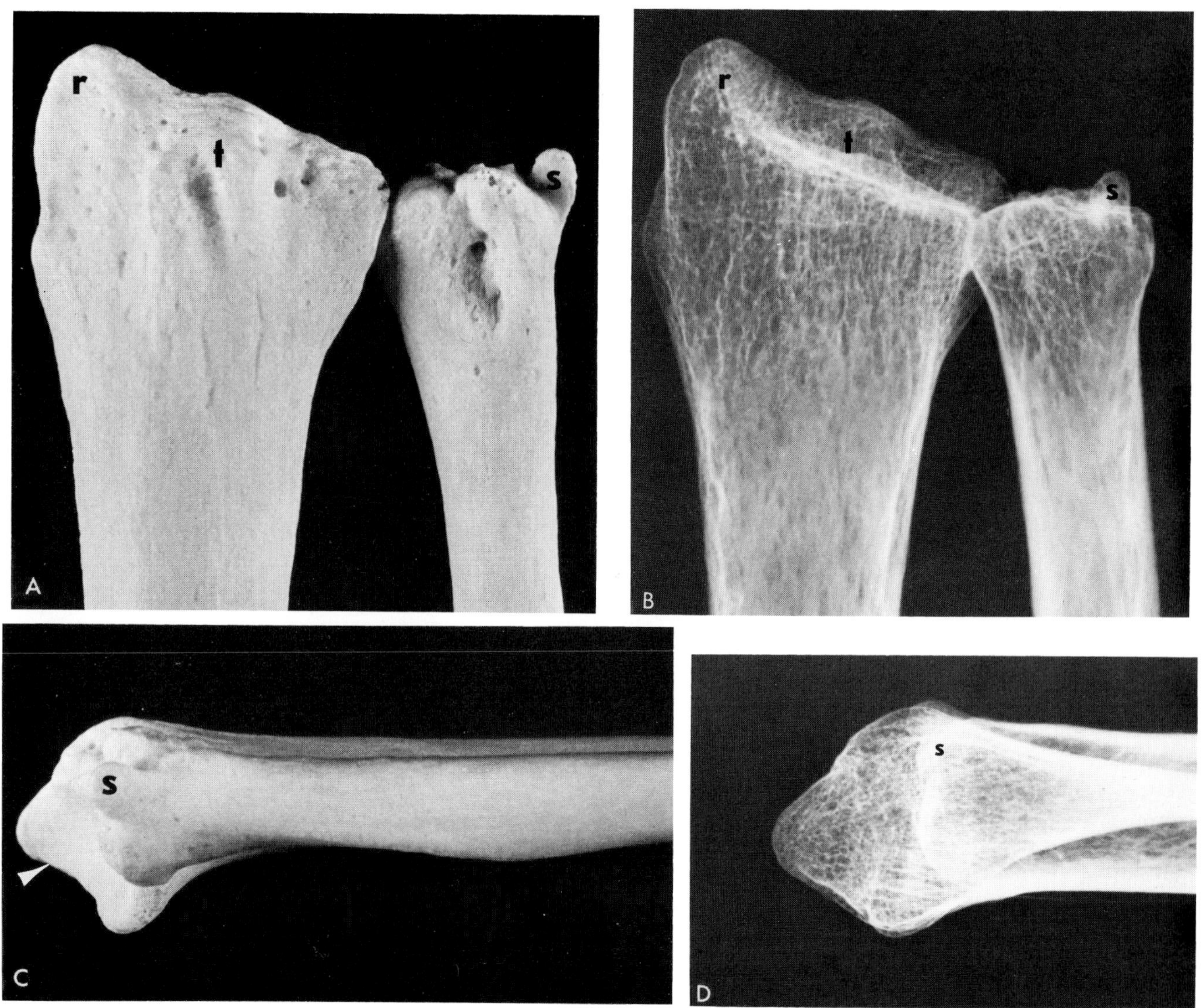

Figure 3–1. *Distal radius and ulna: Osseous anatomy.*

A, B *Posterior aspect. Note convex surface of the distal radius with radial styloid process* (r), *dorsal tubercle* (t) *and grooves for passage of various tendons and tendon sheaths, and the surface of the distal ulna with styloid process* (s) *and groove for the extensor carpi ulnaris tendon and tendon sheath.*

C, D *Ulnar aspect. Observe ulnar styloid* (s) *and articular surface of distal radius (arrowhead).*

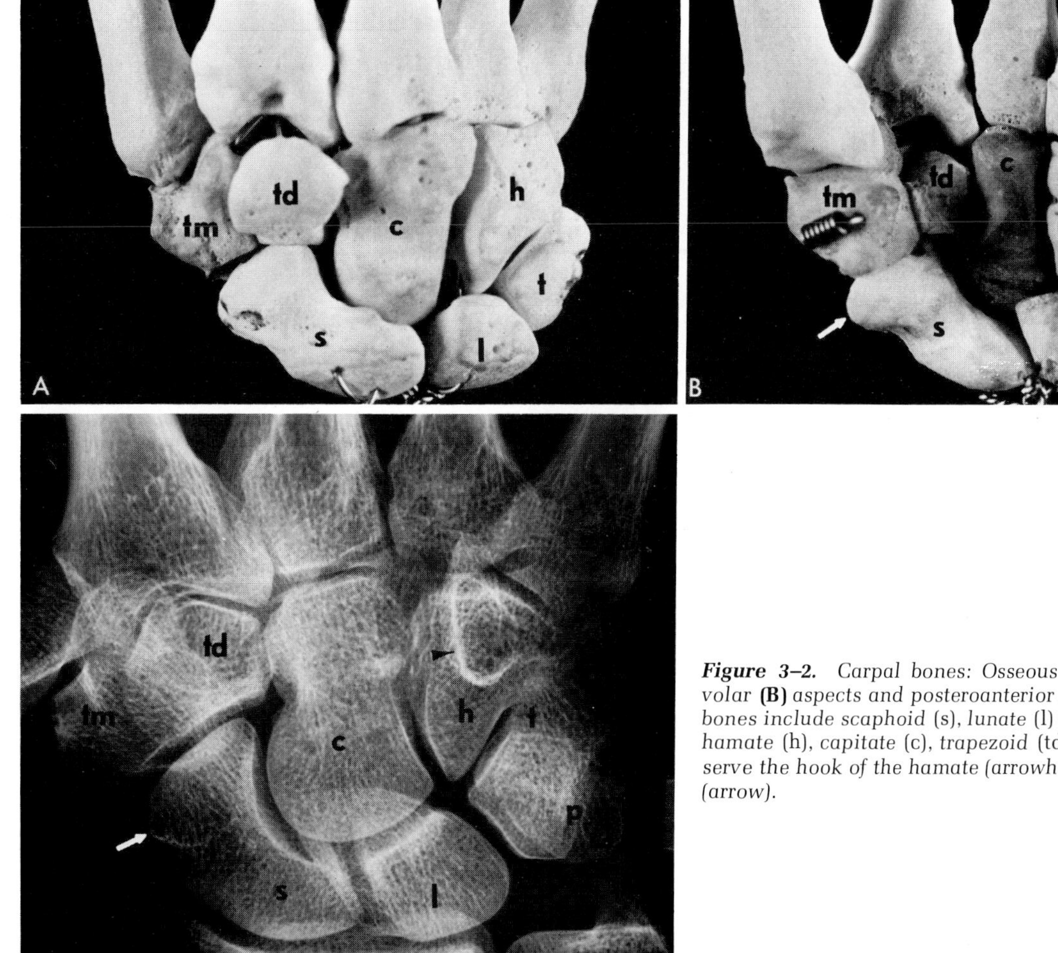

Figure 3–2. *Carpal bones: Osseous anatomy. Dorsal* **(A)** *and volar* **(B)** *aspects and posteroanterior radiograph* **(C).** *The carpal bones include scaphoid (s), lunate (l) triquetrum (t), pisiform (p), hamate (h), capitate (c), trapezoid (td), and trapezium (tm). Observe the hook of the hamate (arrowhead) and scaphoid tubercle (arrow).*

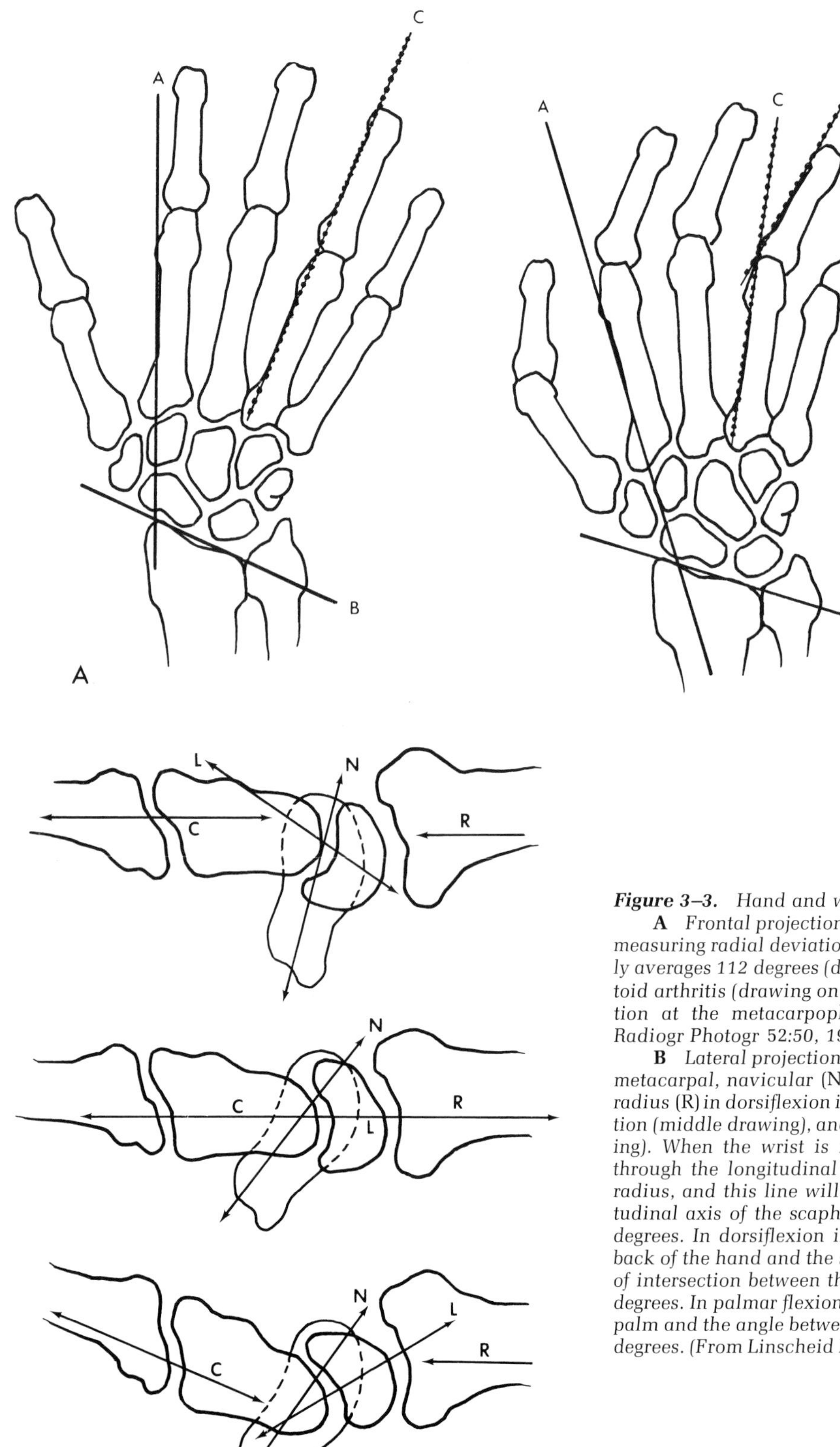

Figure 3–3. *Hand and wrist: Normal and abnormal alignment.*

A *Frontal projection. The angle of intersection of lines A and B, measuring radial deviation of the radiocarpal compartment, normally averages 112 degrees (drawing on left) and is increased in rheumatoid arthritis (drawing on right). Lines C and D measure ulnar deviation at the metacarpophalangeal joints. (From Resnick D: Med Radiogr Photogr 52:50, 1976.)*

B *Lateral projection. Line drawings of longitudinal axes of third metacarpal, navicular (N) or scaphoid, lunate (L), capitate (C), and radius (R) in dorsiflexion instability (upper drawing), in normal situation (middle drawing), and in palmar flexion instability (lower drawing). When the wrist is normal, a continuous line can be drawn through the longitudinal axes of the capitate, the lunate, and the radius, and this line will intersect a second line through the longitudinal axis of the scaphoid, creating an angle of 30 degrees to 60 degrees. In dorsiflexion instability, the lunate is flexed toward the back of the hand and the scaphoid is displaced vertically. The angle of intersection between the two longitudinal axes is greater than 60 degrees. In palmar flexion instability, the lunate is flexed toward the palm and the angle between the two longitudinal axes is less than 30 degrees. (From Linscheid RL, et al: J Bone Joint Surg 54A:1612, 1972.)*

The alignment of the bones of the wrist articulations varies with wrist position (Fig. 3–3). When the wrist is in neutral position without dorsal or palmar flexion, the distal end of the radius articulates with the scaphoid and approximately 50 per cent of the lunate. The degree of radial deviation of the radiocarpal compartment can be measured on a posteroanterior radiograph with the wrist in this neutral attitude. A line is drawn through the longitudinal axis of the second metacarpal at its radial cortex.[3] A second line is constructed from the ulnar limit of the distal radius to the tip of the radial styloid process. The second line intersects the first, creating an obtuse angle, which normally averages 112 degrees (range, 92 to 127 degrees).[4] In the neutral position, the space between carpal bones is approximately equal in the normal wrist. An abnormal widening of the scaphoid-lunate space is termed scaphoid-lunate dissociation. On a posteroanterior radiograph of a normal wrist, a line drawn tangentially from the distal tip of the radial styloid through the base of the ulnar styloid process intersects a second line drawn along the midshaft of the radius with an average angle of 83 degrees (72 to 95 degrees).[5]

On a lateral radiograph of a normal wrist in neutral position without palmar flexion or dorsiflexion, a continuous line can be drawn through the longitudinal axes of the radius, lunate, capitate, and third metacarpal.[6] A second line through the longitudinal axis of the scaphoid intersects this first line, creating a scaphoid-lunate angle of 30 to 60 degrees. A scaphoid-lunate angle of less than 30 degrees or more than 60 degrees suggests carpal instability which can be classified as (a) dorsiflexion instability, in which the lunate is dorsiflexed and displaced in a palmar direction and the scaphoid is vertically displaced, or (b) palmar flexion instability, in which the lunate is flexed in a palmar direction. On the lateral view, a line drawn tangentially along the distal articular surface of the radius intersects a second line through the midshaft of the radius with an average angle of 86 degrees (79 to 94 degrees).[5]

Radial and ulnar deviation and flexion and extension of the wrist cause changes in the alignment of the carpal bones.[7, 216] In radial deviation, palmar flexion of the proximal carpal bones is noted as the distal end of the scaphoid rotates into the palm. In ulnar deviation, the scaphoid is seen in full profile, the lunate and triquetrum become more closely apposed, and the pisiform becomes intimate with the tip of the ulnar styloid. Dorsiflexion of the wrist is particularly prominent at the capitate-lunate space, and palmar flexion is pronounced at the lunate-radial space.[7] During wrist flexion, the pisiform tilts on the triquetrum and moves in a volar direction for 2 to 3 mm.[8] During wrist extension, the pisiform slides distally and undergoes some rotation.

Soft Tissue Anatomy

The wrist is not a single joint. Rather it consists of a series of articulations or compartments[1, 2, 9-12] (Figs. 3–4, 3–5):

1. Radiocarpal compartment.
2. Inferior radioulnar compartment.
3. Midcarpal compartment.
4. Pisiform-triquetral compartment.
5. Common carpometacarpal compartment.
6. First carpometacarpal compartment.
7. Intermetacarpal compartments.

Radiocarpal Compartment. The radiocarpal compartment (Fig. 3–6*A*, *B*) is formed proximally by the distal surface of the radius and the triangular cartilage and distally by the proximal row of carpal bones exclusive of the pisiform. In the coronal plane, the radiocarpal compartment is a C-shaped cavity with a smooth shallow curve, which is concave distally. In the sagittal plane, this compartment is also C-shaped, but the curve is more acute. Interosseous ligaments extend between the carpal bones of the proximal row and prevent communication of this compartment with the midcarpal compartment. A triangular fibrocartilage prevents communication of the radiocarpal and inferior radioulnar compartments, whereas a meniscus may attach to the triquetrum, preventing communication of the radiocarpal and pisiform-triquetral compartments.

The radial collateral ligament is located at the radial limit of the radiocarpal compartment, whereas the ulnar limit of this compartment is the point at which the meniscus is firmly attached to the triquetrum. This ulnar area is Y-shaped; a proximal limb or diverticulum, termed the prestyloid recess, approaches the ulnar styloid[10] and a distal limb is intimate with two thirds of the proximal aspect of the triquetrum.

Palmar radial recesses extend proximally from the radiocarpal compartment beneath the distal articulating surface of the radius.[13] These recesses vary in number and size.

The meniscus occasionally contains ossification, termed the lunula,[10] which produces a circular radiodensity of variable size adjacent to the ulnar styloid.

Inferior Radioulnar Compartment. The inferior radioulnar compartment (Fig. 3–6C) is an L-shaped articulation whose proximal border is the cartilage-covered head of the ulna and

Text continued on page 53

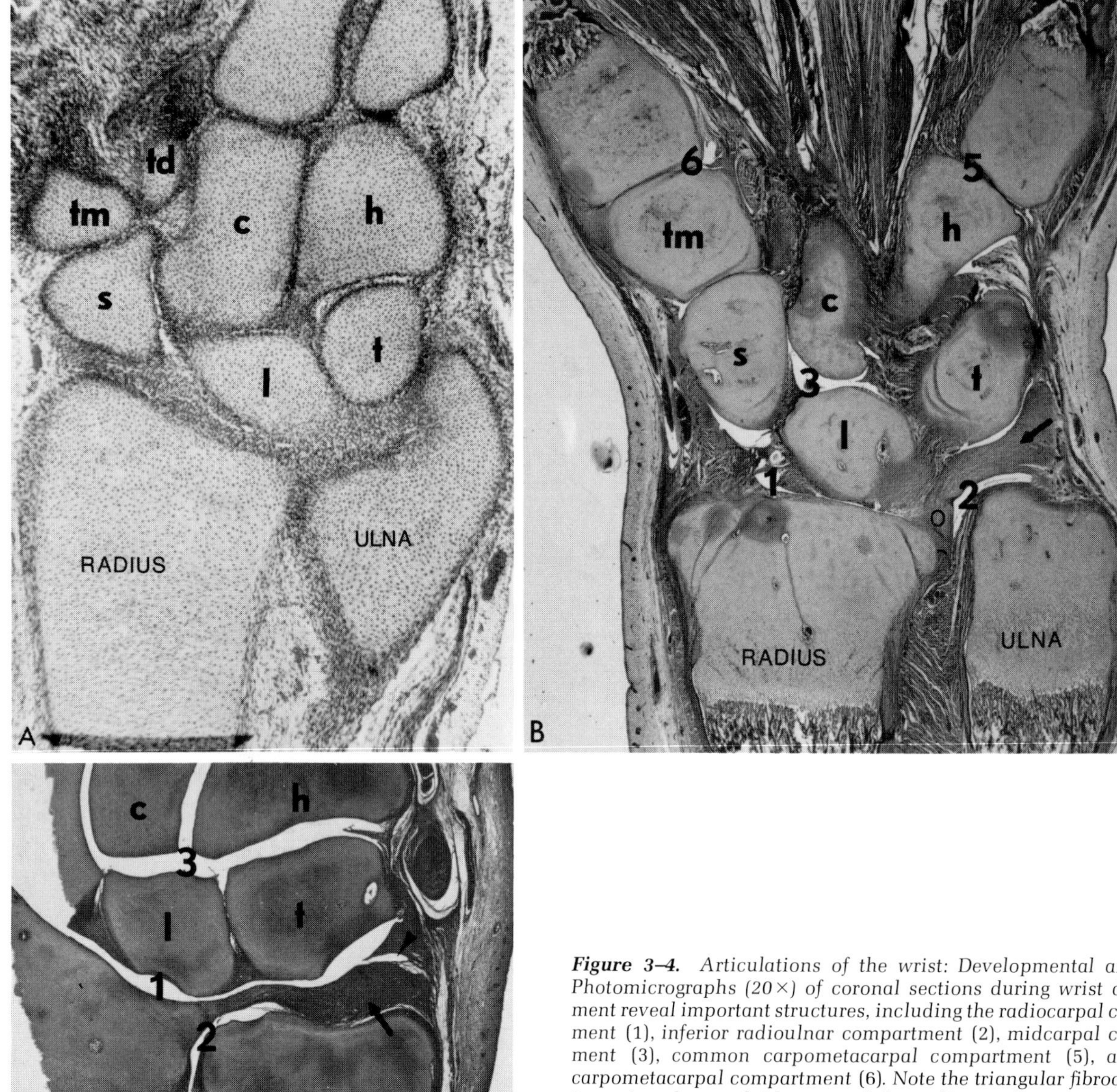

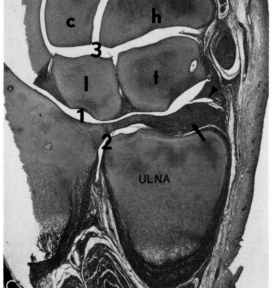

Figure 3–4. *Articulations of the wrist: Developmental anatomy. Photomicrographs (20×) of coronal sections during wrist development reveal important structures, including the radiocarpal compartment (1), inferior radioulnar compartment (2), midcarpal compartment (3), common carpometacarpal compartment (5), and first carpometacarpal compartment (6). Note the triangular fibrocartilage (arrow) and prestyloid recess of the radiocarpal compartment (arrowhead). s, Scaphoid; l, lunate; t, triquetrum; h, hamate; c, capitate; td, trapezoid; tm, trapezium.*

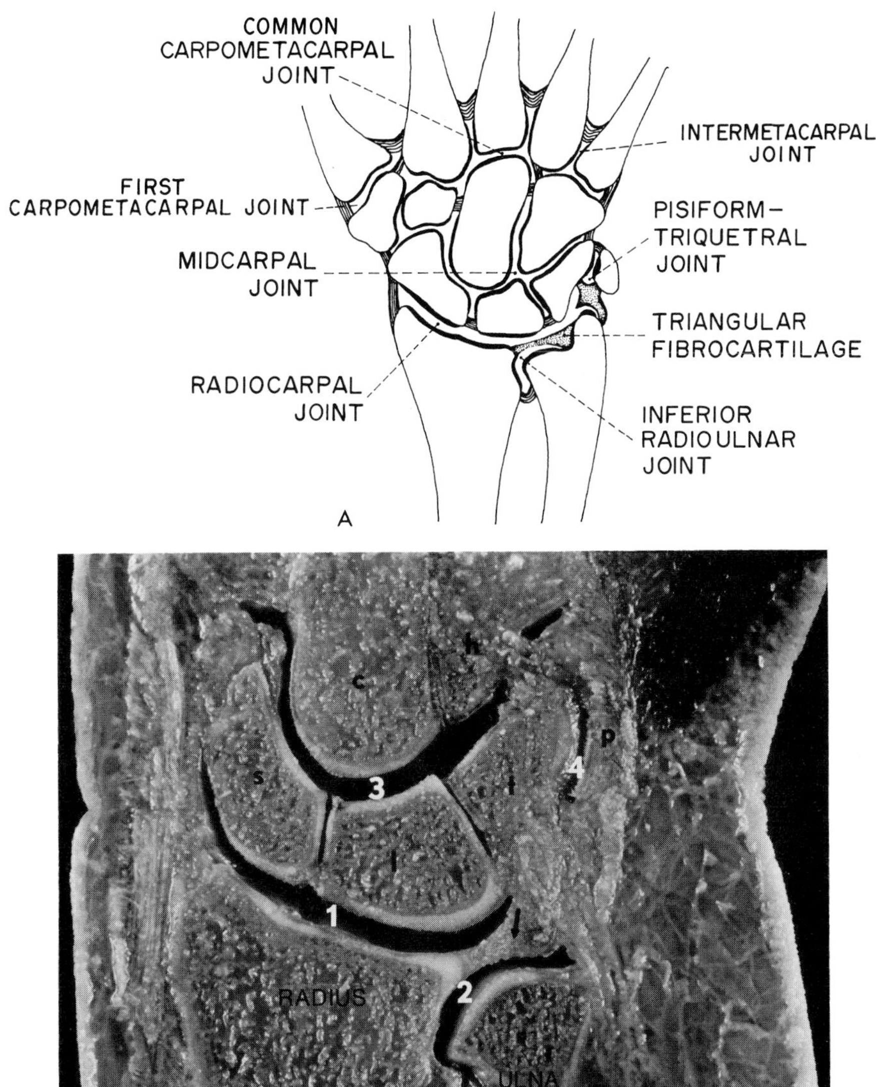

Figure 3–5. *Articulations of the wrist: General anatomy. Observe the various wrist compartments on a schematic drawing and photograph of a coronal section. These include the radiocarpal* (1), *inferior radioulnar* (2), *midcarpal* (3), *and pisiform-triquetral* (4) *compartments. Note the triangular fibrocartilage (arrow).* s, Scaphoid; l, *lunate;* t, *triquetrum;* p, *pisiform;* h, *hamate;* c, *capitate.*

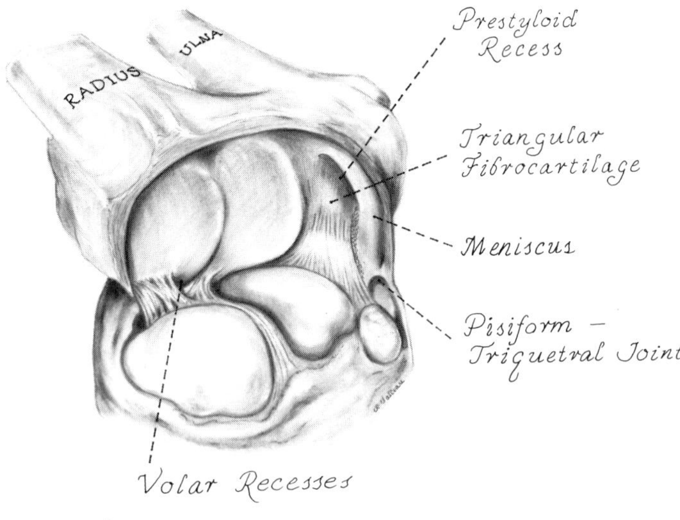

Figure 3–6. *Articulations of the wrist: Specific compartments.*

A *Radiocarpal compartment, open and flexed. The prestyloid recess approaches the ulnar styloid process. Observe the palmar (volar) radial recesses and the pisiform-triquetral joint, which communicates with the radiocarpal compartment in this drawing. (From Lewis OJ, et al: The anatomy of the wrist joint. J Anat 106:539, 1970. Courtesy of Cambridge University Press.)*

B *Ulnar limit of radiocarpal compartment (coronal section). Note the extent of this compartment (1), its relationship to the inferior radioulnar compartment (2), the intervening triangular fibrocartilage (arrow), and the prestyloid recess (arrowhead), which is intimate with the ulnar styloid (s).*

C *Inferior radioulnar compartment (coronal section). This L-shaped compartment (2) extends between the distal radius and ulna and is separated from the radiocarpal compartment (1) by the triangular fibrocartilage (arrow). Note the sac-like proximal contour of the inferior radioulnar compartment.*

Illustration continued on the opposite page

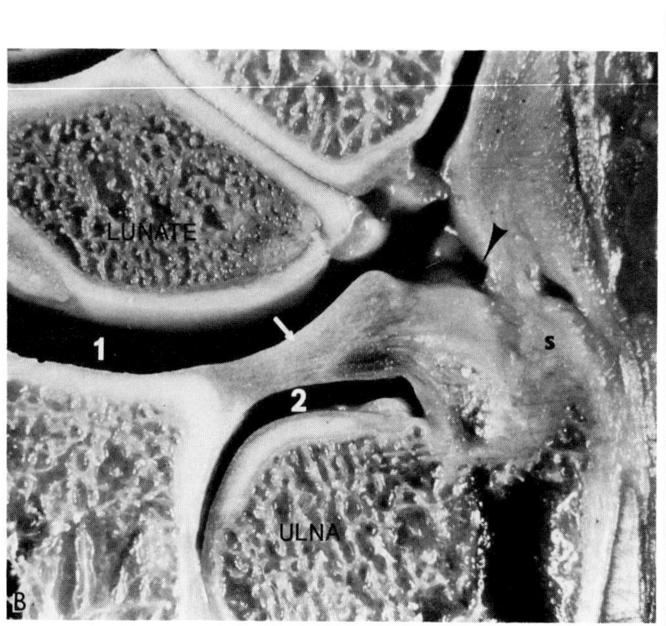

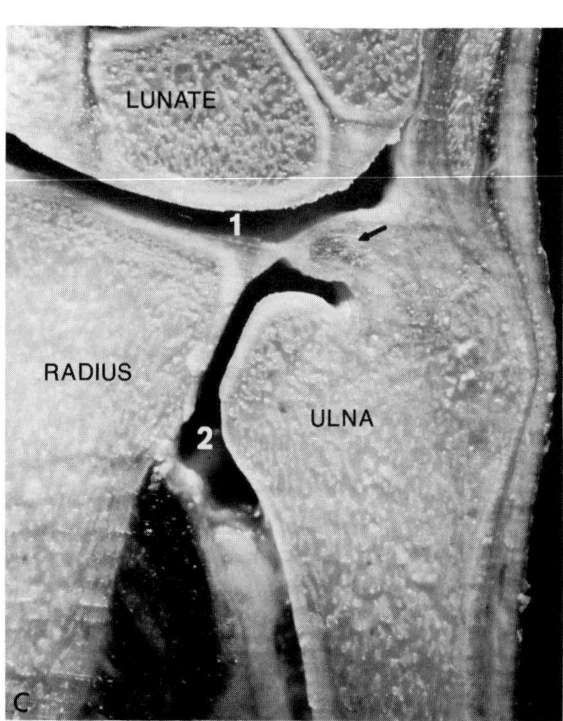

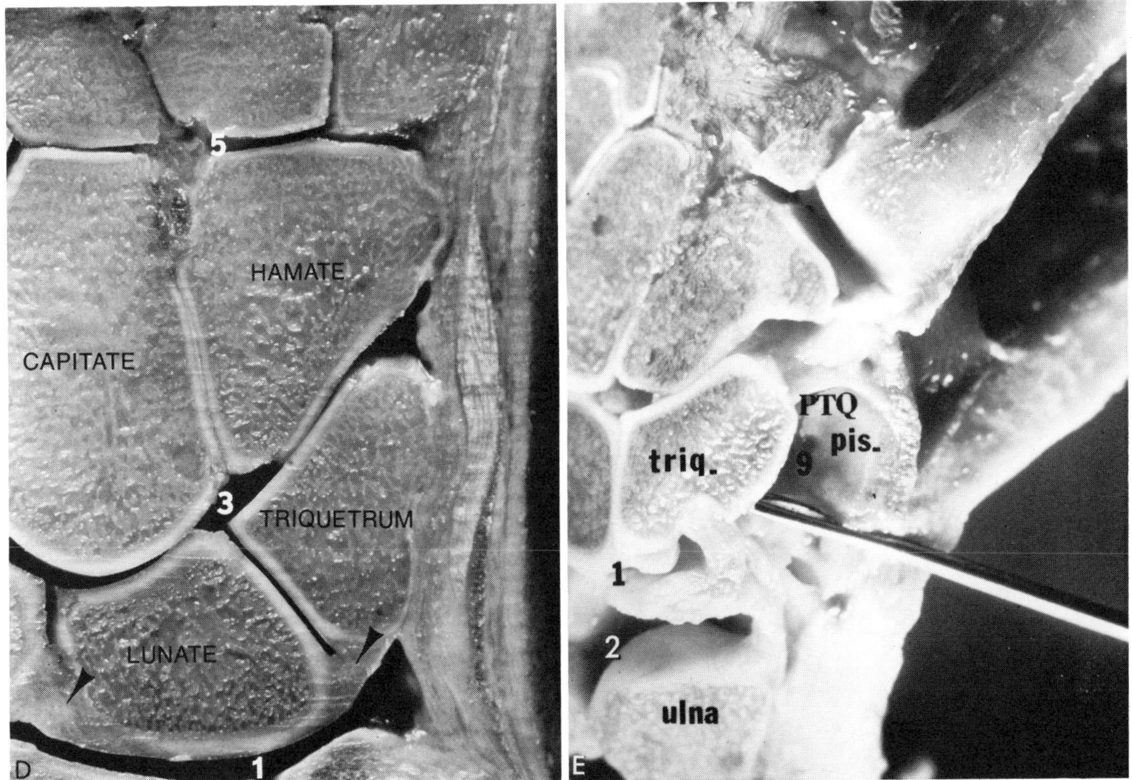

Figure 3–6. Continued

D *Midcarpal compartment (coronal section). The ulnar side of the midcarpal compartment* (3) *is well shown. This compartment is separated from the radiocarpal compartment* (1) *by interosseous ligaments (arrowheads) extending between bones of the proximal carpal row. Observe the common carpometacarpal compartment* (5) *between the distal carpal row and the bases of the four ulnar metacarpals.*

E *Pisiform-triquetral compartment (coronal section). This compartment (PTQ-9) exists between the triquetrum* (triq.) *and pisiform* (pis.)*. The radiocarpal* (1) *and inferior radioulnar* (2) *compartments are also indicated.*

ulnar notch of the radius. Its distal limit is the triangular fibrocartilage. This latter ligament is a band of tough fibrous tissue that extends from the ulnar aspect of the distal radius to the base of the ulnar styloid.

Midcarpal Compartment. The midcarpal compartment (Fig. 3–6*D*) extends between the proximal and distal carpal rows. On the ulnar aspect of this compartment, the head of the capitate and the hamate articulate with a concavity produced by the scaphoid, lunate, and triquetrum. This ulnar side widens between the triquetrum and hamate. On the radial aspect of the midcarpal compartment, the trapezium and trapezoid articulate with the distal aspect of the scaphoid. The radial side of this compartment is termed the trapezioscaphoid space.

Pisiform-Triquetral Compartment. The pisiform-triquetral compartment (Fig. 3–6*E*) exists between the palmar surface of the triquetrum and the dorsal surface of the pisiform. A large proximal synovial recess can be noted. The pisiform-triquetral compartment is surrounded by a loose fibrous articular capsule.

Common Carpometacarpal Compartment. The common carpometacarpal compartment exists between the base of each of the four medial metacarpals and the distal row of carpal bones. This synovial cavity extends proximally between the distal portion of the carpal bones, and distally between the bases of the metacarpals, to form three small intermetacarpal joints. Occasionally, the articulation between the hamate and the fourth and fifth metacarpals is a separate synovial cavity, produced by a ligamentous attachment between the hamate and fourth metacarpal (Fig. 3–5*A*).

First Carpometacarpal Compartment. The carpometacarpal compartment of the thumb is a separate saddle-shaped cavity between the trapezium and base of the first metacarpal.[14] It possesses a loose, thick fibrous capsule, which is thickest laterally and dorsally.

INTERMETACARPAL COMPARTMENTS. Three intermetacarpal compartments extend between the bases of the second and third, the third and fourth, and the fourth and fifth metacarpals. These compartments usually communicate with each other and the common carpometacarpal compartment.

Although the compartments of the wrist are distinct structures, communication among these compartments has been demonstrated anatomically[10, 15] and arthrographically[13, 16, 17] (Fig. 3–7) (Table 3–1).

Communication Between Radiocarpal and Inferior Radioulnar Compartments. Direct communication between these compartments has been noted in radiocarpal compartment arthrograms in 7 per cent[16] and in 16 per cent[17] of cadavers. Dissection of anatomic specimens has outlined similar connections in 30 per cent[15] and 60 per cent[10] of cadavers. This communication results from perforation of the triangular cartilage, a finding seen more frequently in elderly individuals which relates to cartilaginous degeneration. Small defects within this structure may not be revealed during arthrographic examination of the wrist.

Communication Between Radiocarpal and Midcarpal Compartments. Communication between these two compartments results from disruption of the interosseous ligaments which extend between the bones of the proximal carpal row. Anatomic study of elderly cadaveric wrists has revealed disruption of the scaphoid-lunate ligament in 40 per cent of cadavers and of the lunate-triquetral ligament in 36 per cent of cadavers.[10] Arthrography has demonstrated communication between the radiocarpal and midcarpal compartments in 13 per cent of cadavers.[17]

Communication Between Radiocarpal and Pisiform-Triquetral Compartments. Dissection of cadaveric wrists has outlined communication between these two compartments in 34 per cent of cadavers.[10] This communication may be demonstrated during arthrography.[8, 13, 18, 19]

Communication Among Midcarpal, Carpometacarpal, and Intermetacarpal Compartments. Arthrographic demonstration of communication among the midcarpal, common carpometacarpal, and intermetacarpal compartments is frequent. Such communication with the first carpometacarpal joint is unusual.

Movement of the wrist is complex, related to the associated changes in many of these compartments[1, 2, 11-14, 20-26] Wrist flexion occurs at both the radiocarpal and midcarpal joints, particularly the latter. In wrist extension, movement again occurs at both of these compartments but is greater at the radiocarpal joint. Adduction or ulnar deviation of the hand occurs mainly at the radiocarpal compartment, whereas abduction or radial deviation occurs predominantly at the midcarpal compartment. The movements at the common carpometacar-

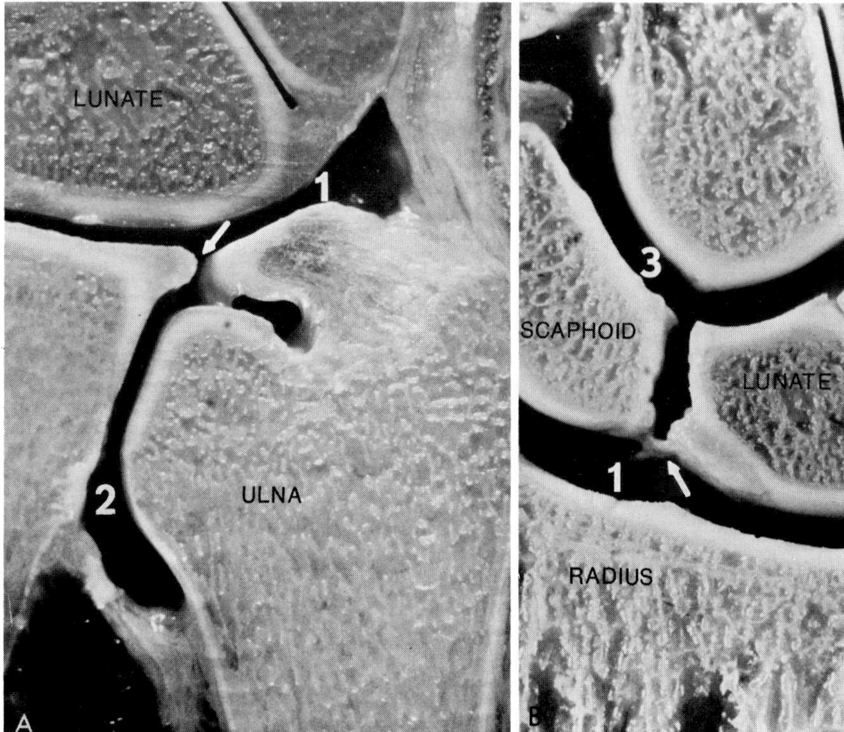

Figure 3–7. Compartmental communications.

A *In elderly patients, perforation of the triangular fibrocartilage (arrow) may allow communication between the radiocarpal (1) and inferior radioulnar (2) compartments (coronal section).*

B *In elderly patients, perforation of the interosseous ligaments (arrow) between bones of the proximal carpal row allows communication between radiocarpal (1) and midcarpal (3) compartments (coronal section).*

Table 3–1
COMMUNICATIONS WITH RADIOCARPAL COMPARTMENT IN CONTROL SUBJECTS

	Anatomic Dissections (Per Cent)	Arthrograms (Per Cent)
Radiocarpal compartment with inferior radioulnar compartment	30,[15] 60[10]	7,[16] 16[17]
Radiocarpal compartment with midcarpal compartment	36 to 40[10]	13[17]
Radiocarpal compartment with pisiform-triquetral compartment	34[10]	–

pal and intermetacarpal compartments are almost limited to mild gliding of one articular surface on an adjacent one. This movement is most pronounced in the fourth and fifth digits. Movement at the first carpometacarpal joint includes flexion, extension, abduction, adduction, rotation, and circumduction of the thumb.[14, 22, 23] Pronation and supination of the hand result from movement at the inferior and superior radioulnar joints.

The joint capsule of the wrist compartment is strengthened by various ligaments that extend from the radius and ulna toward the carpal bones. The dorsal radiocarpal ligament passes downward and medially from the posterior edge of the distal radius to the proximal row of carpal bones, particularly the triquetrum. The stronger palmar radiocarpal ligament is attached to the anterior edge of the distal radius and radial styloid and extends downward and medially to the scaphoid, lunate, and triquetrum. In its intracapsular course, the palmar radiocarpal ligament is incorporated into a groove near the tubercle of the scaphoid as the radial collateral ligament. On the ulnar aspect of the wrist, the palmar radiocarpal ligament extends from the distal ulna and triangular fibrocartilage to the capitate. The ulnar collateral ligament extends from the ulnar styloid to the triquetrum and pisiform. The tip of the ulnar styloid is devoid of ligamentous attachment. Pisohamate and pisometacarpal ligaments connect the pisiform, the hook of the hamate, and the base of the fifth metacarpal.

Extensor tendons traverse the dorsum of the wrist, surrounded by synovial sheaths (Fig. 3–8). The attachment of the dorsal carpal ligament to the adjacent radius and ulna creates six separate compartments or bundles of tendons. Flexor tendons

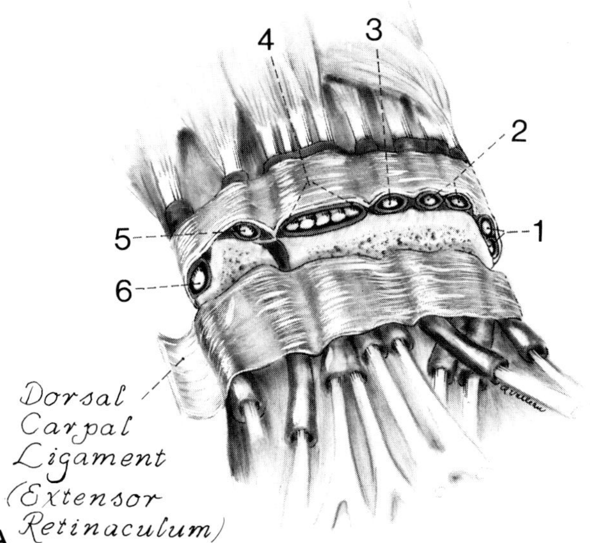

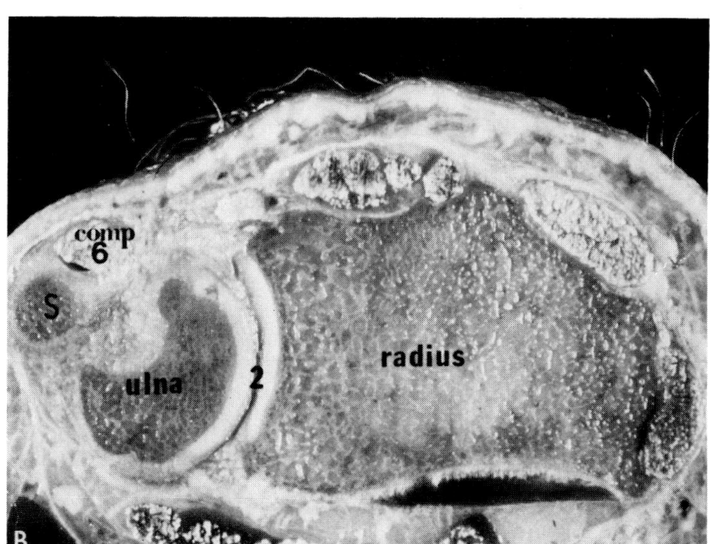

Figure 3–8. *Extensor tendons and tendon sheaths.*

A *Drawing showing dorsal carpal ligament and extensor tendons surrounded by synovial sheaths traversing dorsum of wrist within six separate compartments. These compartments are created by the insular attachment of the dorsal carpal ligament on the posterior and lateral surfaces of the radius and ulna. The extensor carpi ulnaris tendon and its sheath are in the medial compartment (6) and are closely applied to the posterior surface of the ulna.*

B *Cross section through distal end of radius and distal ulna reveals relationship of the extensor carpi ulnaris tendon and tendon sheath (comp 6) and ulnar styloid (S). The inferior radioulnar compartment (2) is also shown.*

(From Resnick D: Med Radiogr Photogr 52:50, 1976.)

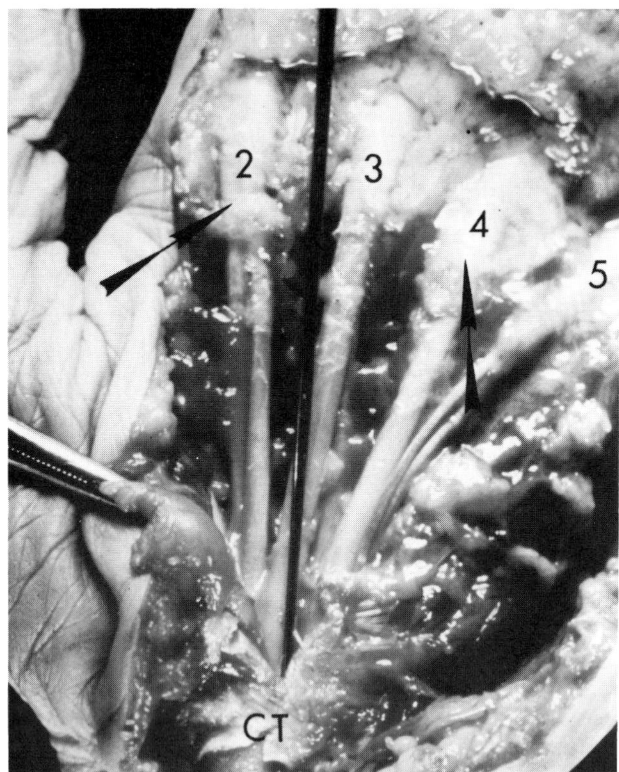

Figure 3–9. *Flexor tendons and tendon sheaths. Photograph of dissected palmar surface of wrist reveals the flexor tendons as they pass beneath the flexor retinaculum within the carpal tunnel (CT). As they approach the metacarpophalangeal joints (2–5), the tendons are surrounded by synovial sheaths (arrows.) (From Resnick D: Med Radiogr Photogr 52:50, 1976.)*

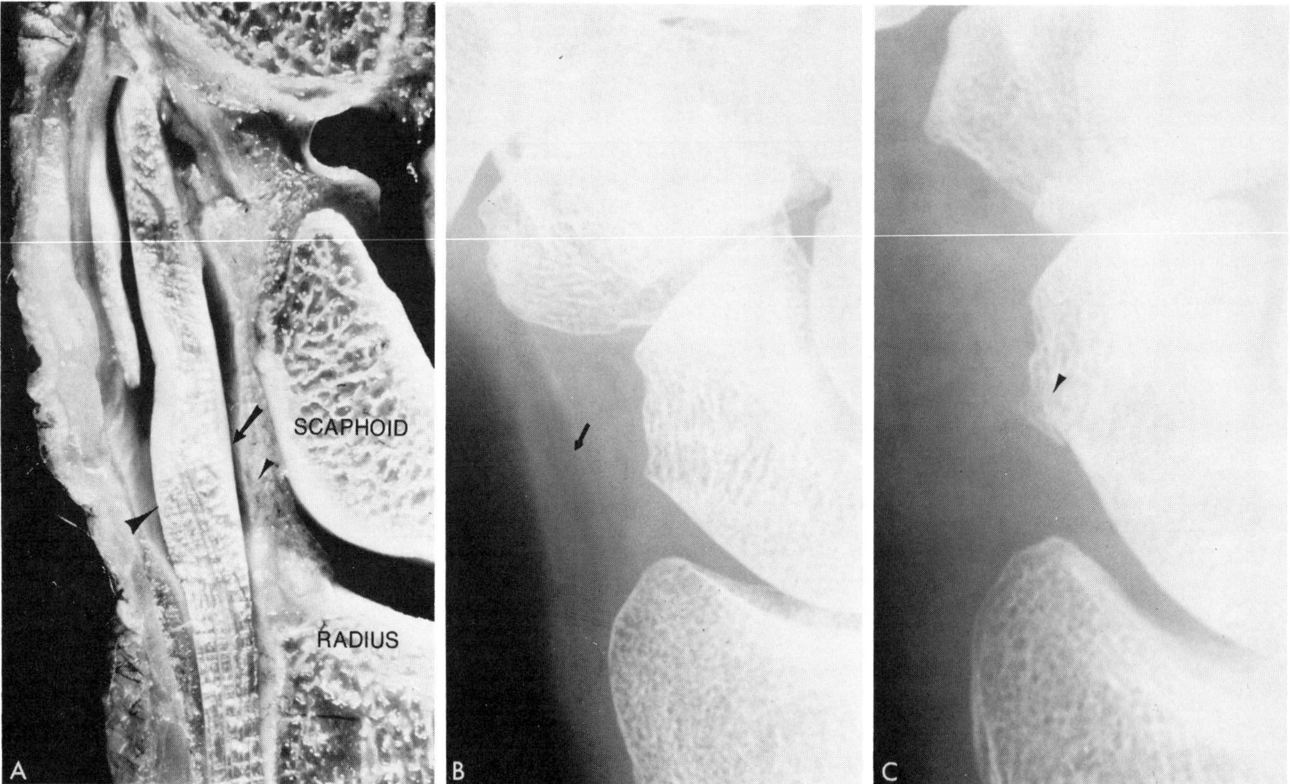

Figure 3–10. *Navicular (scaphoid) fat pad.*

A *A coronal section demonstrates the radial aspect of the wrist. Note the location of the fat plane (arrow) between the radial collateral ligament (small arrowhead) and the synovial sheath and tendons of the abductor pollicis longus and extensor pollicis brevis (large arrowhead).*

B *On a normal radiograph, the navicular fat pad (arrow) produces a triangular or linear radiolucent shadow paralleling the lateral surface of the scaphoid.*

C *This fat plane may be obscured with acute fractures of the neighboring bones. In this patient, a subtle scaphoid fracture (arrowhead) has resulted in obliteration of the navicular fat pad.*

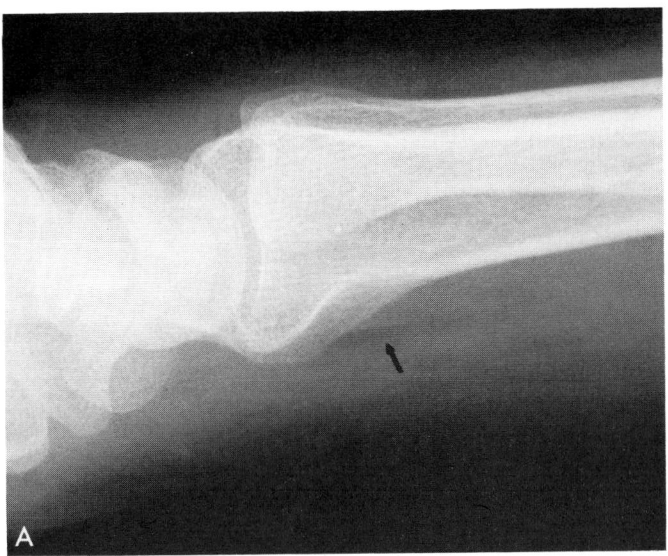

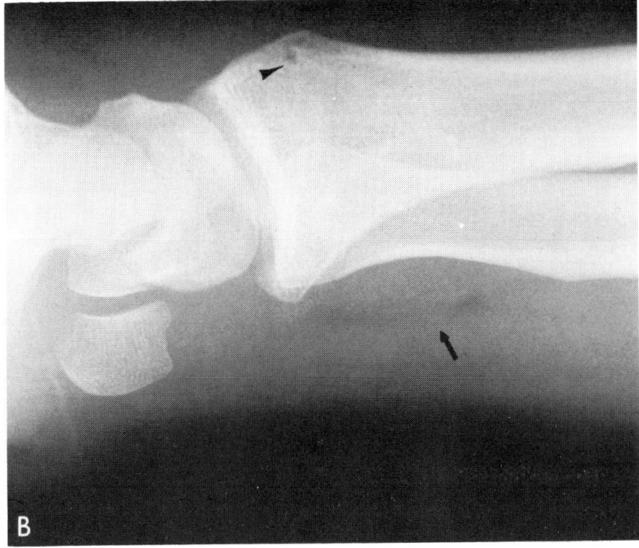

Figure 3–11. *Pronator fat pad.*

A *In normal situations, a fat plane between the pronator quadratus and tendons of the flexor digitorum profundus creates a radiolucent area (arrow) on the volar aspect of the wrist.*

B *With fractures, such as a subtle fracture of the distal radius (arrowhead), this fat plane may be obscured or displaced (arrow).*

with surrounding synovial sheaths pass through the carpal tunnel on the palmar aspect of the wrist (Fig. 3–9).

Certain tissue planes about the wrist have received attention in the literature. The navicular fat pad[27] is a triangular or linear collection of fat between the radial collateral ligament and the synovial sheath of the abductor pollicis longus and extensor pollicis brevis (Fig. 3–10). On radiographs, this fat pad may produce a thin radiolucent line or triangle paralleling the lateral surface of the scaphoid. It is more difficult to discern in children less than 11 to 12 years of age. Obliteration, obscuration, or displacement of this fat plane is reported to be common in acute fractures of the scaphoid, the radial styloid process, and the proximal first metacarpal bone.

A second important soft tissue landmark is the fat plane that exists between the pronator quadratus muscle and the tendons of the flexor digitorum profundus[28] (Fig. 3–11). On a lateral radiograph, the fat pad produces a radiolucency on the volar aspect of the wrist, which appears as a gentle convex curve beneath the distal aspect of the radius and ulna in almost all individuals from infancy to advanced age. Displacement, distortion, or obliteration of the pronator quadratus fat pad has been reported in fractures of the distal radius and ulna, osteomyelitis, and septic arthritis of the wrist.[28, 29]

METACARPOPHALANGEAL JOINTS

Osseous Anatomy

At the metacarpophalangeal articulations, the metacarpal heads articulate with the proximal phalanges (Fig. 3–12). The medial four metacarpal bones lie side by side; the first metacarpal lies in a more anterior plane and is rotated medially along its long axis through an angle of 90 degrees.[1] In this fashion, the dorsal surface of the thumb is aligned in a radial direction, whereas its ulnar surface is oriented superiorly. This position allows the thumb to oppose the other four metacarpals during flexion and rotation.[22, 23]

The metacarpal heads are smooth and round, extending further on the palmar than on the dorsal aspect of the bone.[30] On the palmar aspect, the articular surface of the metacarpal head is divided in such a fashion that it resembles condyles. The head of the first metacarpal is less convex than those of the other metacarpals and has two palmar articular eminences, which relate to sesamoid bones. Tubercles are found on the heads of all metacarpals; these tubercles occur at the sides of the metacarpal heads where the dorsal surface of the body of the bone extends onto the head. Collateral ligaments attach to the metacarpal tubercles. The bases of the phalanges contain concave oval surfaces that articulate with the metacarpal heads.

Soft Tissue Anatomy

Articular cartilage covers the osseous surfaces of metacarpals and phalanges,[30] and the synovial membrane is attached to the articular margin of the metacarpal head[31] (Fig. 3–13). This membrane is particularly prominent on the volar aspect of the metacarpal head and neck. The capsule about the metacarpophalangeal joint is somewhat loose, al-

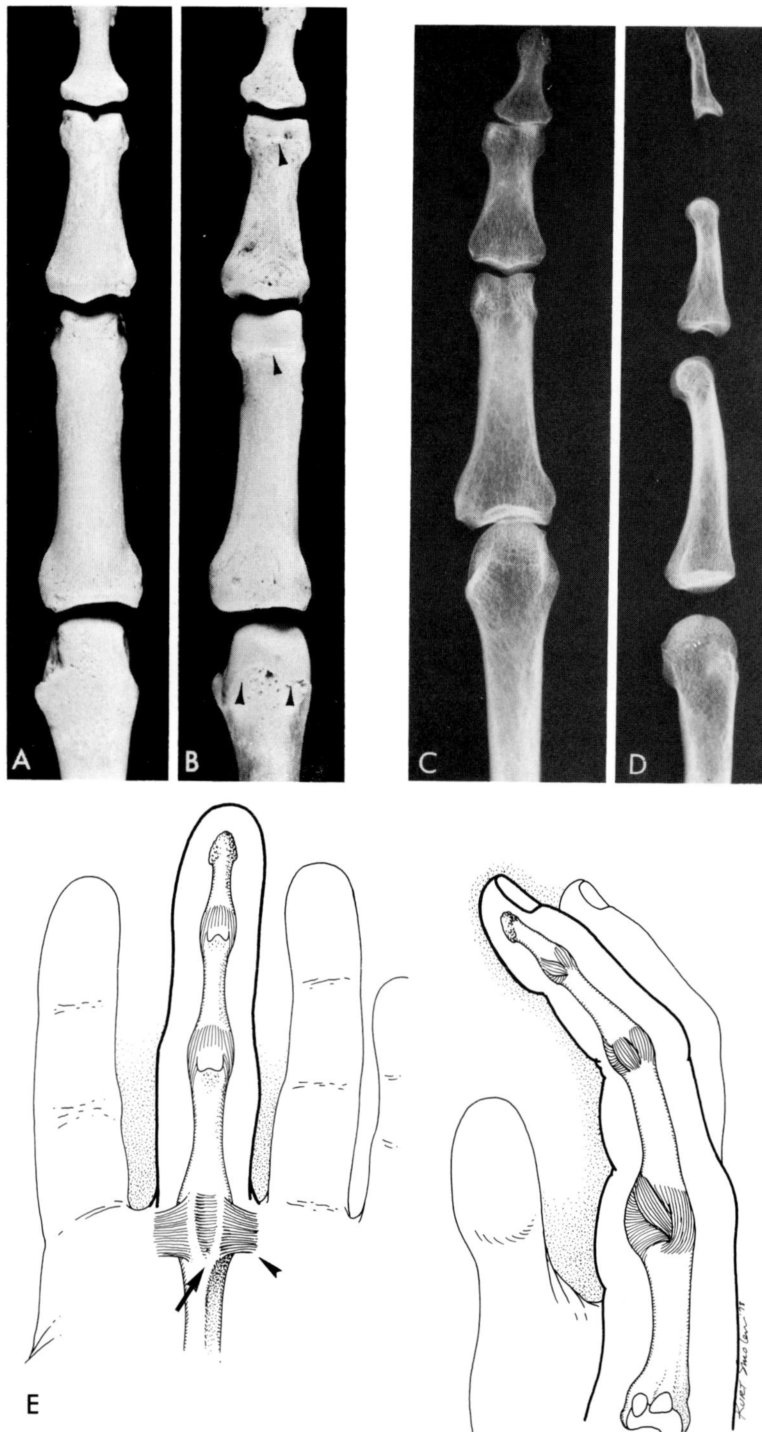

Figure 3–12. Metacarpals and phalanges: Osseous anatomy.

A, B Dorsal **(A)** and ventral **(B)** aspects of third metacarpal and phalanges. Note the more extensive articular surface on the volar aspect of the metacarpal heads and phalanges (arrowheads).

C, D Anteroposterior **(C)** and lateral **(D)** radiographs of second digit, demonstrating smooth osseous surfaces.

E Drawings of the palmar and medial aspects of the metacarpophalangeal and interphalangeal joints of the fourth digit reveal the deep transverse metacarpal ligament (arrowhead) with its central groove for the flexor tendons (arrow) and the capsule of the interphalangeal articulations.

lowing motion of the proximal phalanx. It attaches to the elevated bony crest surrounding the smooth articular surface of the metacarpal head and to the bony ridge about the articular surface of the base of the phalanx. On the dorsal surface of the metacarpophalangeal joints, the fibrous capsule is thin; in this location, a bursa separates the capsule from the extensor tendon.

Each metacarpophalangeal joint has a palmar ligament and two collateral ligaments.[1, 2, 12] The palmar ligament is located on the volar aspect of the articulation and is firmly attached to the base of the proximal phalanx and loosely united to the metacarpal neck. Laterally the palmar ligament blends with the collateral ligaments, and volarly the palmar ligament blends with the deep transverse metacarpal ligaments, which connect the palmar ligaments of the second through fifth metacarpophalangeal joints. The palmar ligament is also grooved for the passage of the flexor tendons, whose fibrous sheaths are attached to the sides of the groove. The collateral ligaments reinforce the fibrous capsule laterally.

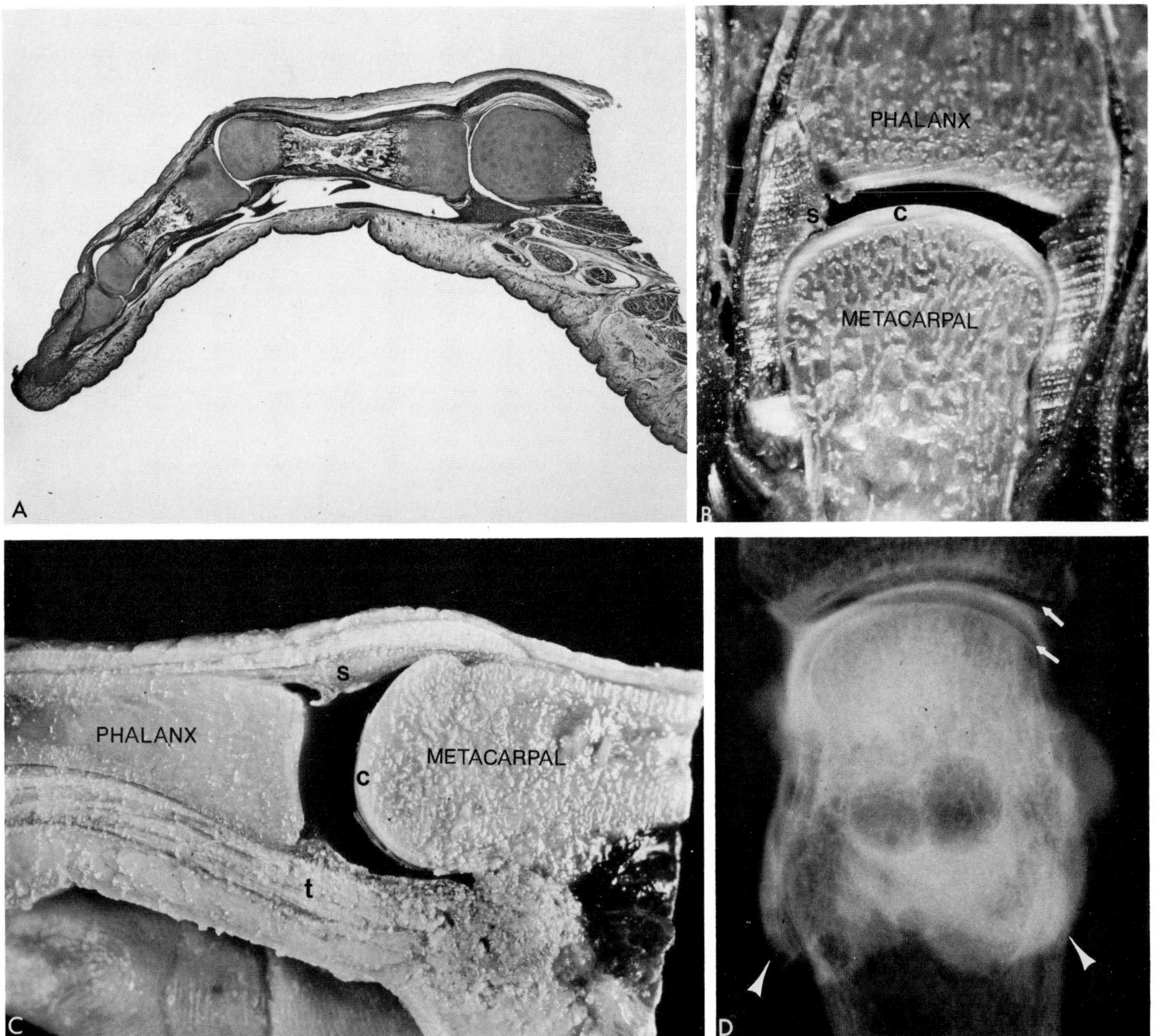

Figure 3–13. *Metacarpophalangeal and interphalangeal joints: Normal development and anatomy.*

A *During a stage of development, these articulations are well demonstrated between the unossified epiphyses of the metacarpal and phalanges on this sagittal section of a finger (20×).*

B, C *Metacarpophalangeal joint. Coronal* **(B)** *and sagittal* **(C)** *sections. Observe the articular cavity, cartilage (c), synovial membrane (s), and flexor tendon (t).*

D *On an arthrogram of a metacarpophalangeal joint, the proximal extent of the contrast-filled articular cavity is well seen (arrowheads). Observe the radiolucent cartilage of the metacarpal head and proximal phalanx (arrows).*

These ligaments pass obliquely from the posterior tubercles and depressions on the radial and ulnar aspect of the metacarpal to attach to the base of the proximal phalanx.

Active movements of the metacarpophalangeal articulations include flexion, extension, adduction, abduction, circumduction, and limited rotation. Accessory movements comprise rotation, gliding, and distraction. The metacarpophalangeal joint of the thumb, in general, has less extensive movement than the others; movement of the thumb occurs in two planes, that parallel to the remainder of the hand and that at right angles to this first plane.[22, 23]

INTERPHALANGEAL JOINTS OF THE HAND

Osseous Anatomy

The interphalangeal joints of the hand consist of four distal interphalangeal articulations, four proximal interphalangeal articulations, and an interphalangeal joint of the first digit.

At the proximal interphalangeal joints, the head of the proximal phalanx articulates with the base of the adjacent middle phalanx. The articular surface of the phalangeal head is wide (from side to side), with a central groove and ridges on either side for attachment of the collateral ligaments. The base of the middle phalanx contains a ridge that fits into the groove on the head of the proximal phalanx.

At the distal interphalangeal joints, the head of the middle phalanx articulates with the base of the distal phalanx. This phalangeal head, like that of the proximal phalanx, is pulley-like in configuration and conforms to the base of the adjacent phalanx. This latter structure is relatively large.

The interphalangeal joint of the thumb separates the proximal and distal phalanges of that digit. These phalanges are similar in structure to those of the other digits but are in general shorter and broader.

Soft Tissue Anatomy

Apposing surfaces of bone are covered by articular cartilage. A fibrous capsule surrounds the articulation and on its inner aspect, the capsule is covered by synovial membrane, which extends over intracapsular bone not covered by articular cartilage.[31, 32] At the interphalangeal joints, synovial pouches exist proximally on both dorsal and palmar aspects of the articulation.[32, 33] The interphalangeal articulations have a palmar and two collateral ligaments whose anatomy is similar to those about the metacarpophalangeal joints. Active movements at these joints include flexion and extension, both of which may be accompanied by a small amount of rotation; accessory movements are rotation, abduction, adduction and gliding.[1, 2, 12, 32, 34]

RADIOULNAR SYNDESMOSIS (MIDDLE RADIOULNAR JOINT)

The diaphyses of radius and ulna are united by an interosseous membrane whose fibers run in an inferior and medial direction from radius to ulna. This membrane originates approximately 3 cm below the radial tuberosity, extends to the wrist, and contains an aperture for various interosseous vessels.[229] A crest can be noted on both bones at the interosseous border.

ELBOW

The articulation about the elbow has three constituents: (a) humeroradial — the area between the capitulum of the humerus and the facet on the radial head; (b) humeroulnar — the area between the trochlea of the humerus and the trochlear notch of the ulna; and (c) superior (proximal) radioulnar — the area between the head of the radius and radial notch of the ulna and the annular ligament.

Although the superior or proximal radioulnar area is generally considered a separate articulation, it is convenient to discuss all three areas of the elbow region together.

Osseous Anatomy

The osseous structures about the elbow include the proximal end of the ulna and radius and the distal end of the humerus[1, 2] (Fig. 3–14).

The proximal end of the ulna contains two processes, the olecranon and the coronoid. The olecranon process is smooth posteriorly at the site of attachment of the triceps tendon. Its anterior surface provides the site of attachment of the capsule of the elbow joint. The coronoid process contains the radial notch, below which is the ulnar tuberosity.

The proximal end of the radius consists of head, neck, and tuberosity. The radial head is disc-shaped, containing a shallow, cupped articular surface, which is intimate with the capitulum of the humerus. The articular circumference of the head is largest medially, where it articulates with the radial notch of the ulna. The radial neck is the smooth, constricted part of the bone below the radial head. The radial tuberosity is located beneath the medial aspect of the neck.

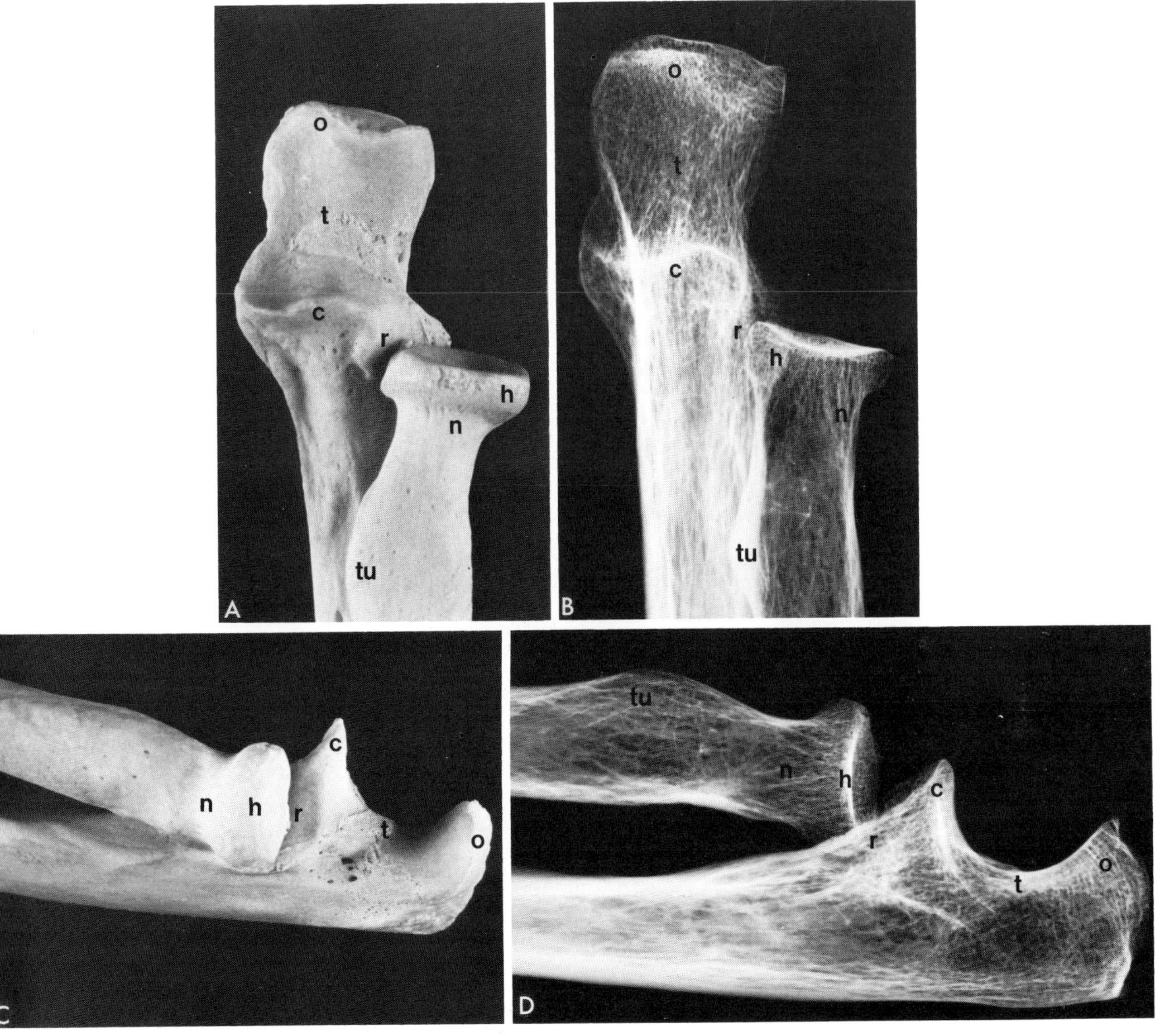

Figure 3–14. *Elbow joint: Osseous anatomy.*

A, B *Radius and ulna, anterior aspect. Note the olecranon* (o), *coronoid process* (c), *trochlear notch* (t), *radial notch* (r), *radial head* (h), *radial neck* (n) *and radial tuberosity* (tu).

C, D *Radius and ulna, lateral aspect.*

Illustration continued on the following page

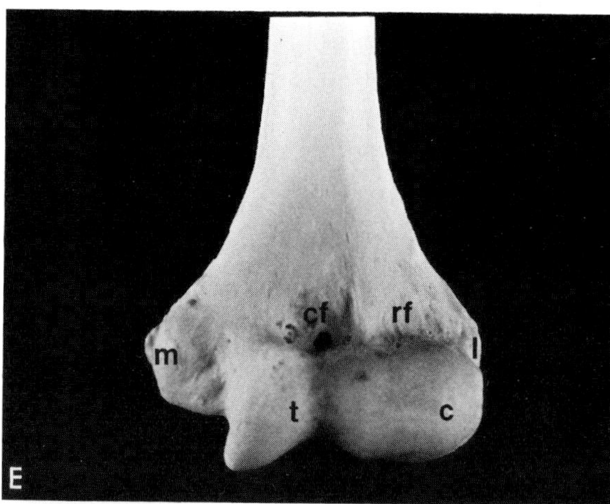

Figure 3–14. Continued

E–G *Distal humerus, anterior and posterior aspects. An anterior view* **(E)** *reveals the trochlea* (t), *capitulum* (c), *medial epicondyle* (m), *lateral epicondyle* (l), *coronoid fossa* (cf), *and radial fossa* (rf). *A posterior view* **(F)**, *oriented in the same fashion, outlines some of the same structures and, in addition, the olecranon fossa* (of). *An anteroposterior radiograph* **(G)** *demonstrates pertinent osseous anatomy.*

H, I *Distal humerus, lateral aspect. Observe the capitulum* (c), *lateral epicondyle* (l), *and lateral supracondylar ridge* (r). *Although there is superimposition of structures on the lateral radiograph, the areas of the coronoid fossa* (cf) *and olecranon fossa* (of) *are indicated.*

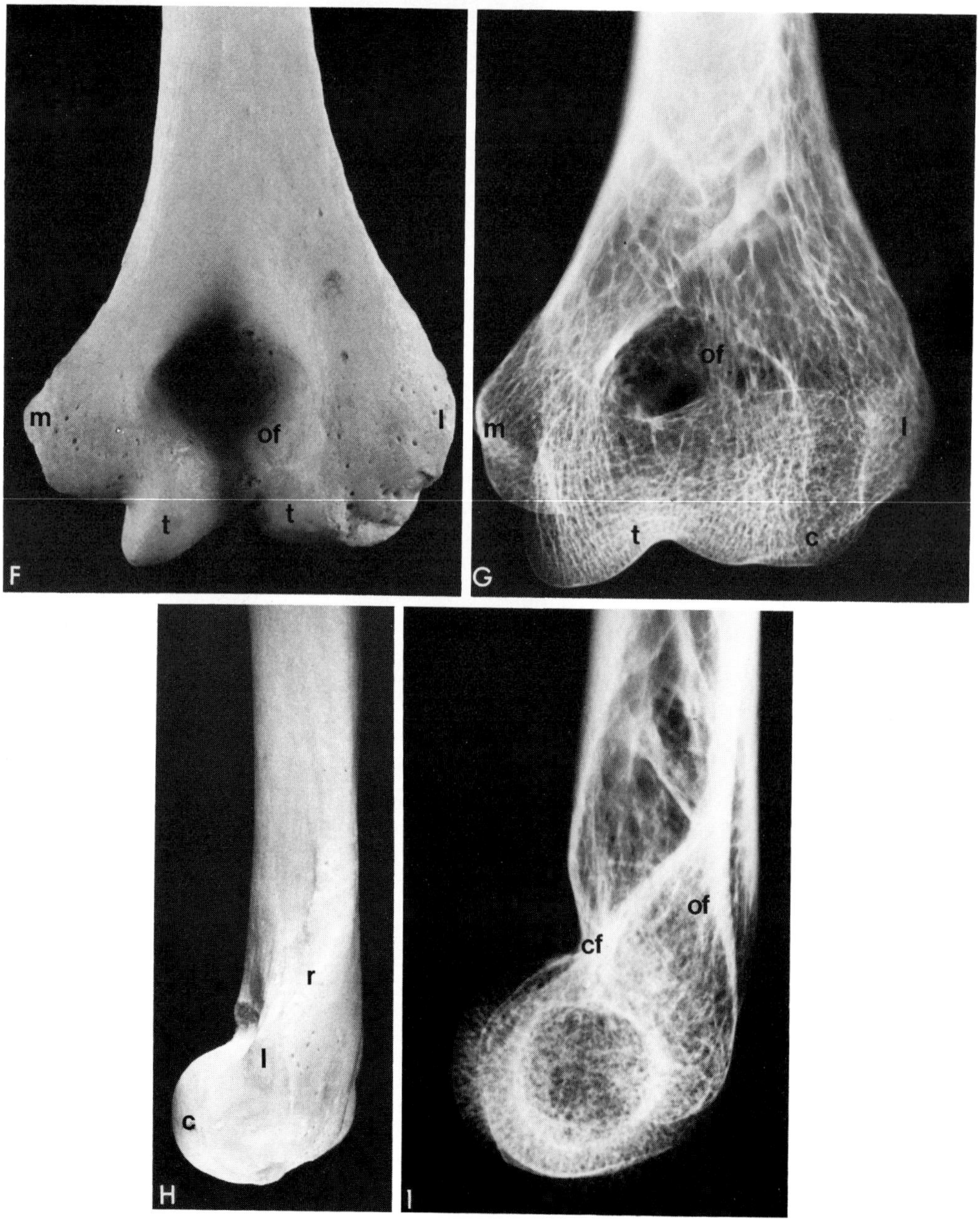

The distal aspect of the humerus is a wide, flattened structure. The medial third of its articular surface, termed the trochlea, is intimate with the ulna. Lateral to the trochlea is the capitulum, which articulates with the radius. The sulcus is between the trochlea and the capitulum. A hollow area is found on the posterior surface of the humerus above the trochlea, termed the olecranon fossa; the posterior capsular attachment of the humerus is located above this fossa. A smaller fossa, the coronoid fossa, lies above the trochlea on the anterior surface of the humerus, and a radial fossa lies adjacent to it, above the capitulum. The anterior capsular attachment to the humerus is located above these fossae. When the elbow is fully extended, the tip of the olecranon process is located in the olecranon fossa, and when the elbow is flexed, the coronoid process of the ulna is found in the coronoid fossa and the margin of the radial head is located in the radial fossa.

The medial epicondyle is a blunt osseous projection of the distal humerus. The posterior smooth surface of this epicondyle is crossed by the ulnar nerve. The anterior surface of the medial epicondyle is the site of attachment of superficial flexor muscles of the forearm. The lateral epicondyle is located on the lateral surface of the distal humerus. Its lateral and anterior surface represents the site of origin of the superficial group of extensor muscles of the forearm.

The degree of congruity of apposing articulating surfaces of radius, ulna, and humerus varies in different positions of the elbow joint; the greatest congruity exists when the forearm is in a position midway between full supination and full pronation and the elbow is flexed to a right angle.[2] When the elbow is extended, the inferior and posterior aspects of the trochlea contact the ulna; when the elbow is flexed, the trochlear notch slides forward on the anterior aspect of the ulna, exposing the posterior aspect of that bone. The capitulum and the radial head are reciprocally curved; in a midprone position, extensive contact occurs between radius and capitulum.

Roentgenographic anatomy of the axial relationships at the elbow has been described.[5] The carrying angle of the elbow is described as the obtuse angle created by the intersection of the longitudinal axes of the shafts of the humerus and ulna measured on the radial side. In men this angle averages 169 degrees (154 to 178 degrees), and in women it averages 167 degrees (158 to 178 degrees). The humeral angle is formed by the intersection of a line through the longitudinal axis of the humerus with a second line drawn tangentially to the articular surface of the trochlea and capitulum. In men this angle averages 85 degrees (77 to 95 degrees) and in women it averages 83 degrees (72 to 91 degrees). The ulnar angle is formed by the intersection of a line through the longitudinal axis of the ulna with a second line drawn tangentially to the articular surfaces of the trochlea and capitulum. The ulnar angle averages 84 degrees (74 to 99 degrees) in men and 84 degrees (72 to 93 degrees) in women.

Soft Tissue Anatomy

The articular surface of the humerus consists of a grooved trochlea, the spheroidal capitulum, and a sulcus between them[1, 2] (Fig. 3–15). It is covered with a continuous layer of articular cartilage. The ulnar articulating surface is the trochlear notch. This notch is covered with cartilage which is interrupted in a transverse fashion across its deepest aspect. The trochlear notch of the ulna and the trochlea of the humerus articulate. The radial articulating area is the radial head, which is covered with articular cartilage. This cartilage is continuous with that along the sides of the radial head including an area in the superior radioulnar articulation. The radial head articulates with the capitulum and the capitulotrochlear groove.

A fibrous capsule completely invests the elbow. The attachments of its broad, thin, and weak anterior part are the anterior humerus along the medial epicondyle and above the coronoid and radial fossae, the anterior surface of the ulnar coronoid process, and the annular ligament. The superior attachments of its thin, weak posterior part are the posterior surface of the humerus behind the capitulum, the olecranon fossa, and the medial epicondyle. Inferomedially the capsule is attached to the upper and lateral margins of the olecranon. Laterally the capsule is continuous with that about the superior radioulnar joint. The fibrous capsule is strengthened at the sides of the articulation by the radial and ulnar collateral ligaments.

The synovial membrane of the elbow lines the deep surface of the fibrous capsule and annular ligament. It extends from the articular surface of the humerus and contacts the olecranon, radial, and coronoid fossae and the medial surface of the trochlea. A synovial fold projects into the joint between the radius and ulna, partially dividing the articulation into humeroulnar and humeroradial portions.[1]

There are several fat pads located between fibrous capsule and synovial membrane (Fig. 3–16). Fat pads are located near the synovial fold between the radius and ulna, and over the olecranon, coronoid, and radial fossae. These fat pads, which are extrasynovial but intracapsular, are of radiographic significance.[35-40] On lateral roentgenograms, an anterior radiolucency represents the summation of radial and coronoid fossae fat pads. These fat pads are pressed into their respective fossae by the brachialis muscle during extension of the elbow. A posterior radiolucency represents the olecranon fossa fat pad. It is pressed into this fossa by the triceps muscle during flexion of the elbow. The

Text continued on page 68

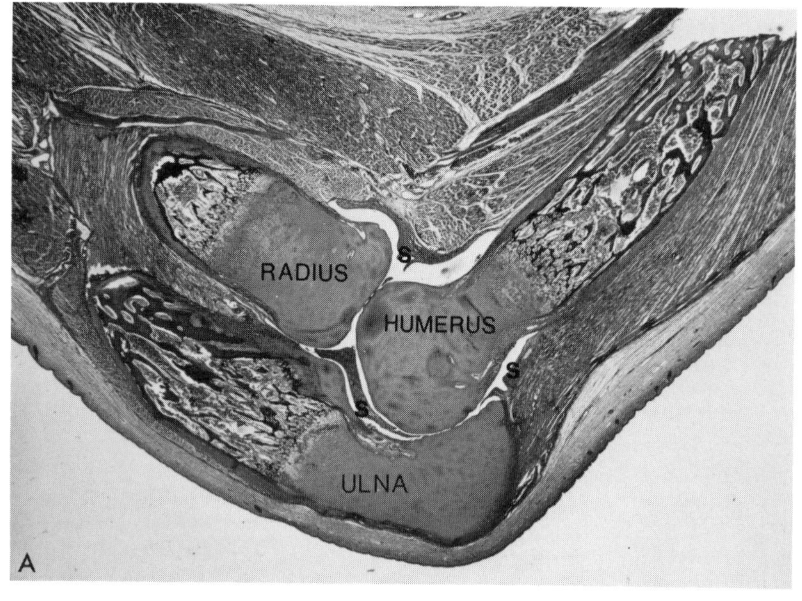

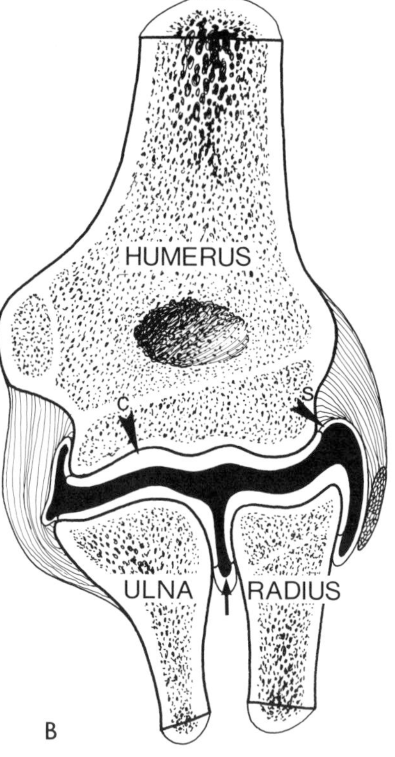

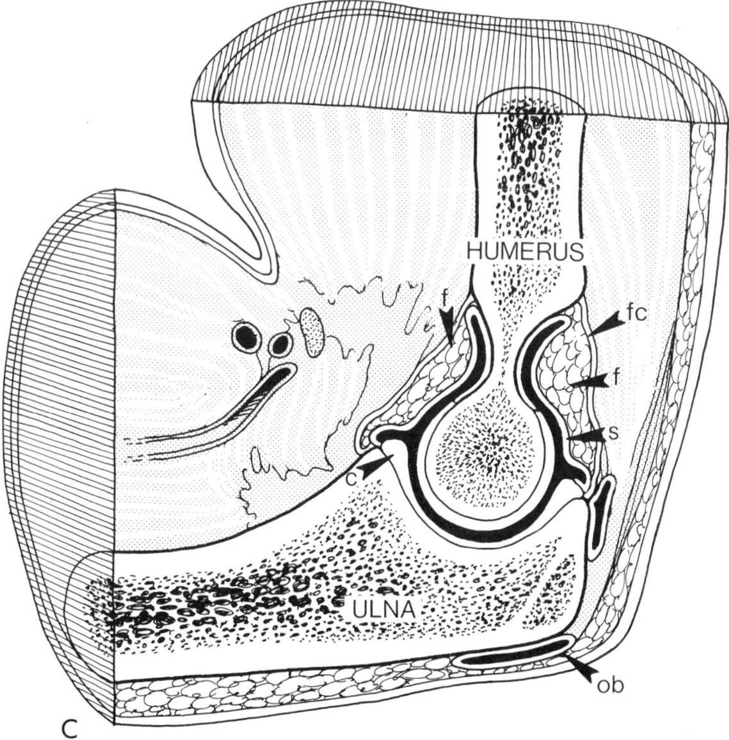

Figure 3–15. Elbow joint: Normal development and anatomy.

A *A sagittal section of the developing elbow outlines the articular cavity between unossified epiphyses of radius, ulna, and humerus. Synovial tissue (s) can be seen (20×).*

B, C *Drawings of coronal* **(B)** *and sagittal* **(C)** *sections. Observe synovium (s), articular cartilage (c), fibrous capsule (fc), anterior and posterior fat pads (f), and olecranon bursa (ob). Note the extension of the elbow joint between radius and ulna as the superior radioulnar joint (arrow).*

Illustration continued on the opposite page

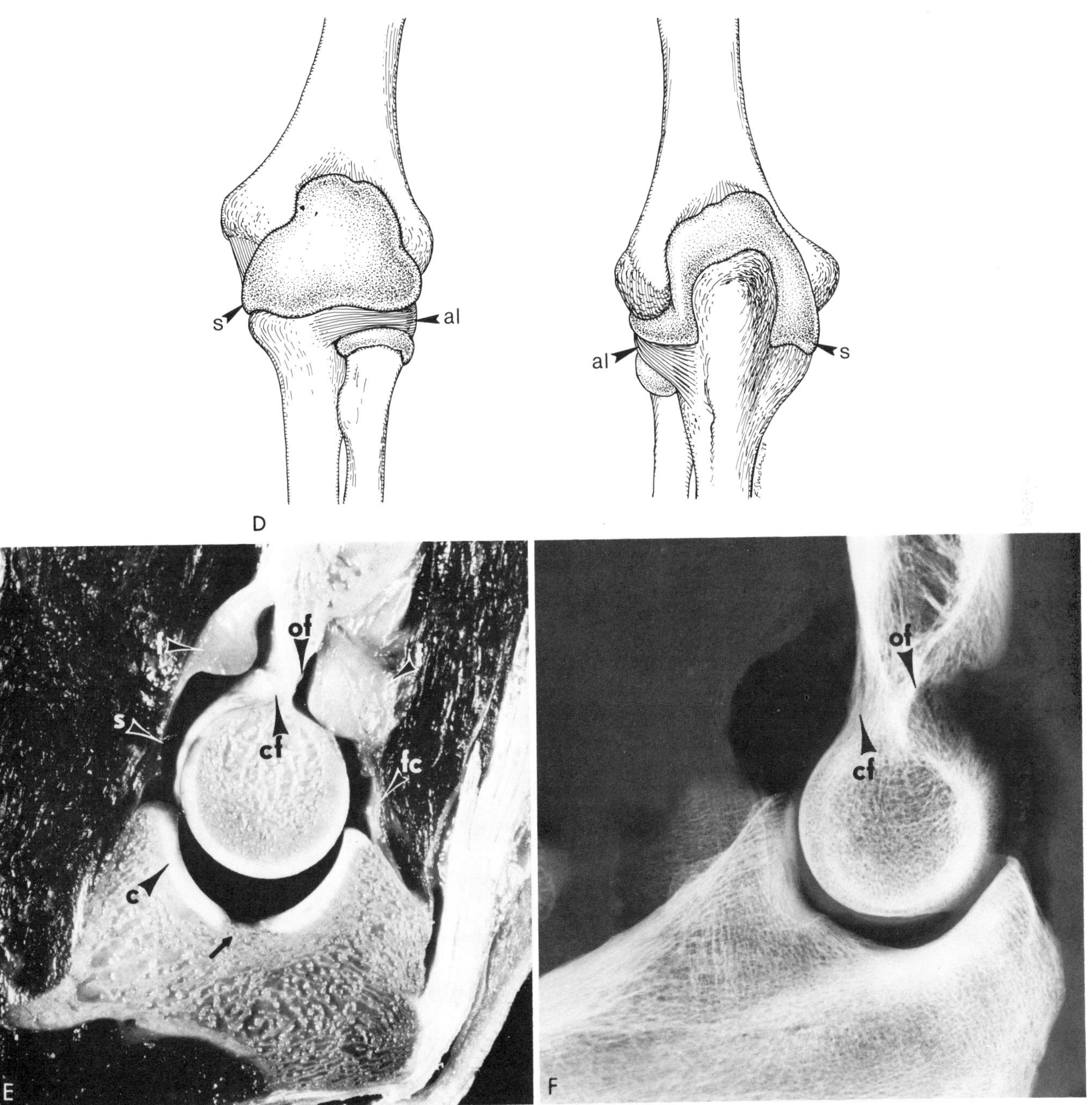

Figure 3–15. Continued

D *A drawing of the anterior (left) and posterior (right) aspects of the distended elbow joint with the fibrous capsule removed. Observe the synovial membrane (s) and the annular ligament (al) extending around the proximal radius, constricting the joint cavity. (From Warwick R, Williams P: Gray's Anatomy. 15th British Ed. Philadelphia, WB Saunders Co, 1973.)*

E, F *Photograph and radiograph of a sagittal section through the ulnar aspect of the elbow joint following air arthrography, showing distended articular cavity, fat pads (f), synovium (s), articular cartilage (c), fibrous capsule (fc), olecranon fossa (of), and coronoid fossa (cf). Note the area of the trochlear notch, which is normally devoid of cartilage (arrow).*

Illustration continued on the following page

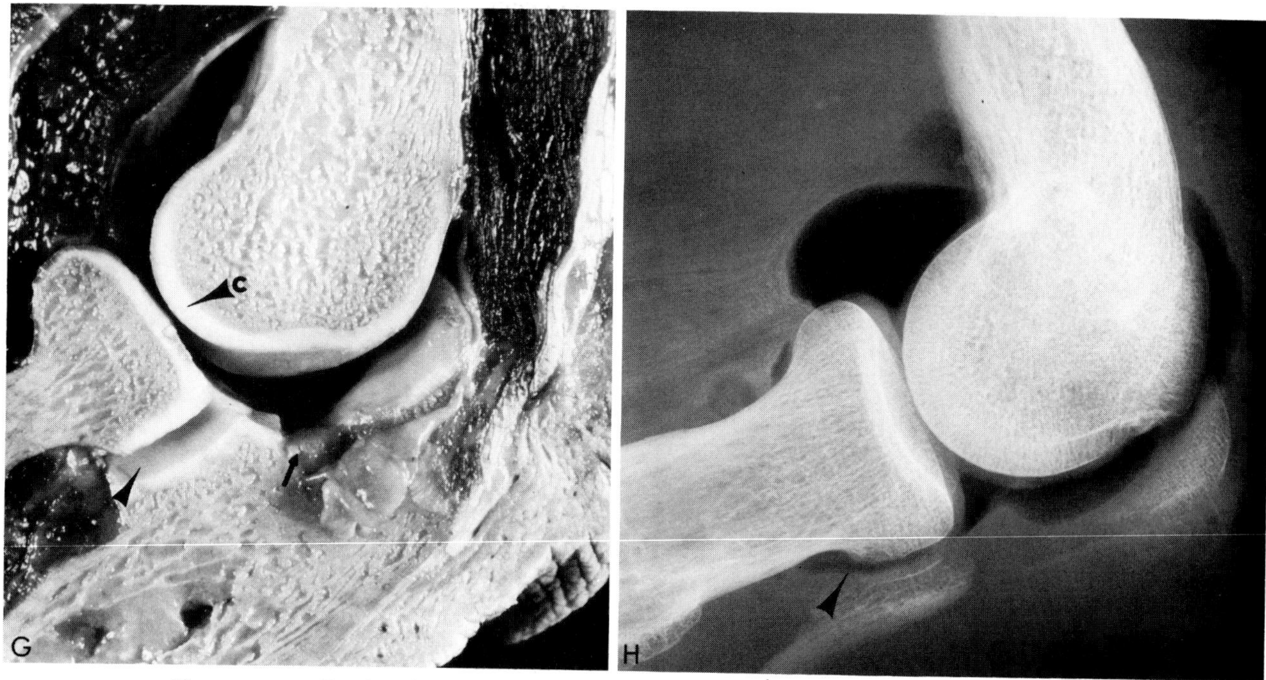

Figure 3–15. Continued

G, H *Photograph and radiograph of a more lateral sagittal section through humerus, radius, and ulna outlining air-filled distended joint cavity extending between radius and ulna as superior radioulnar joint (arrowheads). Again observe the cartilage-covered bones (c) with a normal cartilaginous defect on the trochlear notch (arrow).*

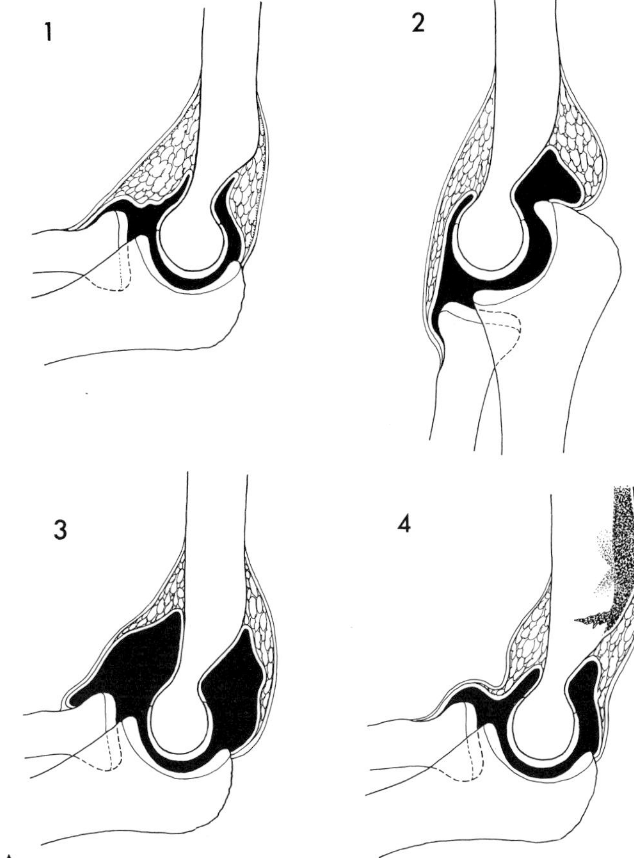

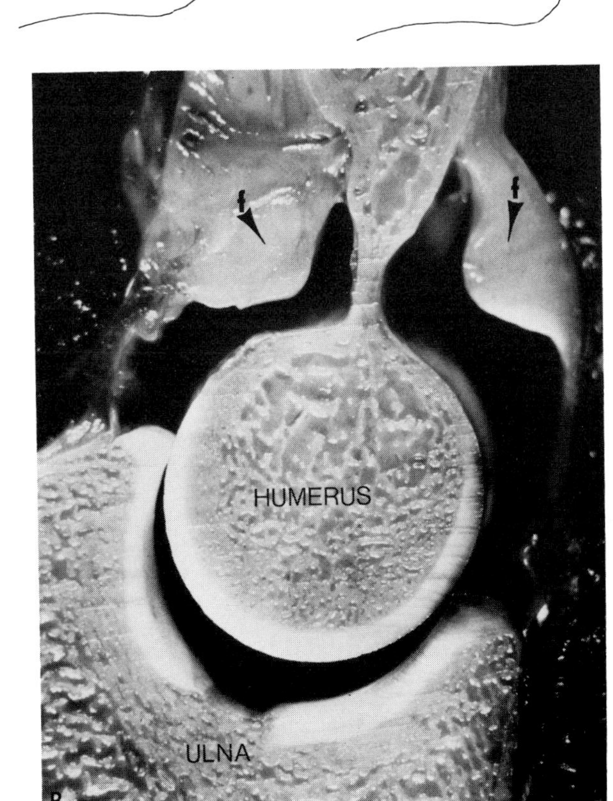

Figure 3–16. *Elbow joint: Normal and abnormal appearance of fat pads.*

A *Schematic drawings of anterior and posterior fat pads in normal and abnormal situations. Normally (1), the extrasynovial anterior and posterior fat pads are closely applied to the distal humerus. In extension (2), the anterior fat pad is pressed tightly against the humerus, whereas the posterior fat pad may be elevated by contact between the olecranon and humerus. With a joint effusion (3), both anterior and posterior fat pads may be elevated by intra-articular fluid. With distal humeral fractures (4), a paradoxic elevation of the posterior fat pad may occur. (From Murphy, WA, Siegel MJ: Radiology 124:659, 1977.)*

B *A sagittal section of the elbow following marked distention of the joint with air reveals the elevated anterior and posterior fat pads (f).*

Illustration continued on the following page

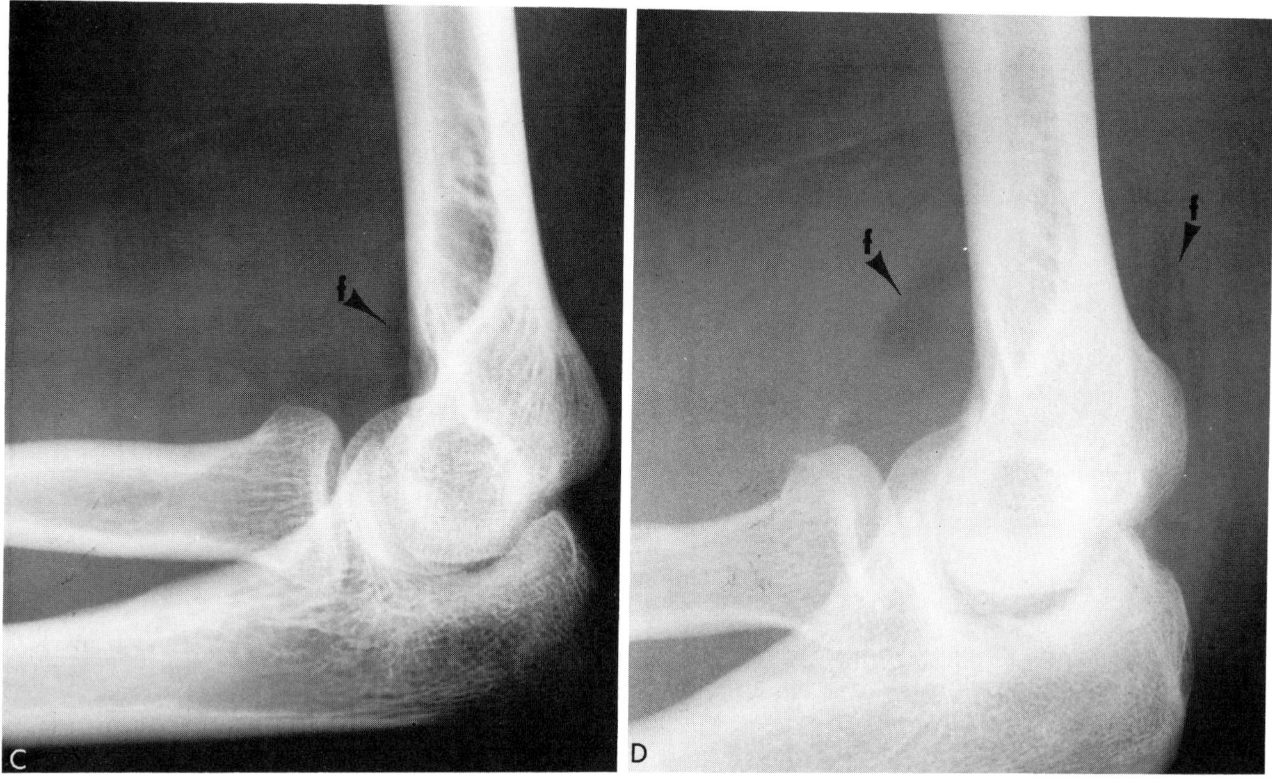

Figure 3–16. Continued
C *On a radiograph of the normal elbow flexed to approximately 90 degrees, the anterior fat pad (f) assumes a teardrop configuration and the posterior fat pad is not visible.*
D *With a joint effusion, both fat pads (f) are elevated. The anterior fat pad assumes a "sail" configuration, whereas the posterior fat pad becomes visible.*

anterior fat pad normally assumes a teardrop configuration anterior to the distal humerus on lateral radiographs of the elbow exposed in approximately 90 degrees of joint flexion. The posterior fat pad is normally not visible in radiographs of the elbow exposed in flexion. Its occasional appearance on such roentgenograms may reflect unusually large fat pads or slightly oblique projections.[37] Any intra-articular process that is associated with a mass or fluid may produce a "positive fat-pad sign" characterized by elevation and displacement of anterior and posterior fat pads. A variety of disease processes can present in this fashion.[40]

Radial and ulnar collateral ligaments reinforce the fibrous capsule. The radial collateral ligament attaches superiorly to the lateral epicondyle of the humerus and inferiorly to the radial notch of the ulna and the annular ligament. The ulnar collateral ligament is composed of three distinct bands that are continuous with each other. The anterior band extends from the anterior aspect of the medial epicondyle of the humerus to the medial edge of the coronoid process; a posterior band passes from the posterior aspect of the medial epicondyle to the medial edge of the olecranon; a thin intermediate band extends from the medial epicondyle to merge via a transverse or oblique band with the anterior and posterior bands on the coronoid process and the olecranon.

The superior radioulnar joint exists between the radial head and the osseous-fibrous ring formed by the annular ligament and the radial notch of the ulna. This notch is lined with articular cartilage that is continuous with that on the lower part of the trochlear notch. The radial head is also covered with cartilage. The annular ligament is attached anteriorly to the anterior margin of the radial notch. It encircles the head of the radius, and posteriorly it contains several bands that attach to the ulna near the posterior margin of the radial notch. The superior portion of the annular ligament is lined with fibrocartilage where it apposes the circumference of the radial head. The inferior portion of the annular ligament is covered with synovial membrane, which extends downward onto the radial neck. The quadrate ligament, a thin, fibrous layer, covers the synovial membrane.[41]

Various extracapsular fat planes can be observed on roentgenograms of the elbow. Extracapsular fat may be apparent on an anteroposterior projection as a radiolucent line closely applied to the lateral aspect of the capitulum, continuing downward over the lateral aspect of the radial head and neck.[42] Lateral to this fat, a second fat plane may be seen

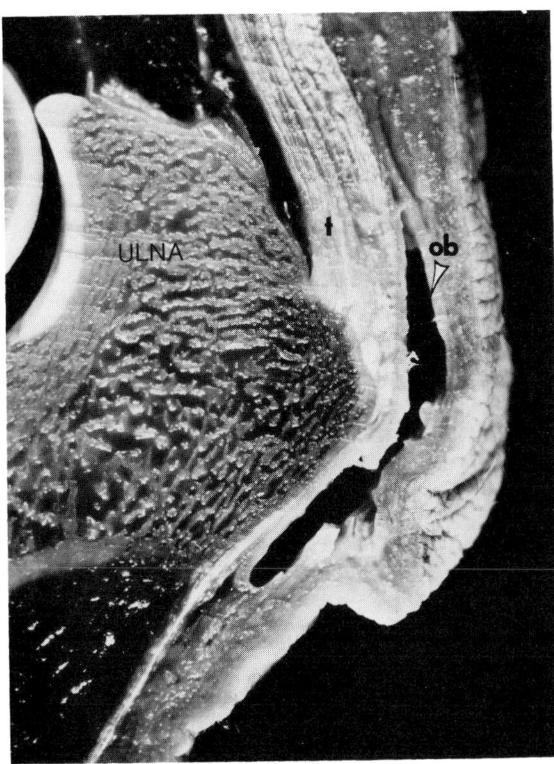

Figure 3–17. Olecranon bursa. A sagittal section through the ulna demonstrates the synovium-lined olecranon bursa (ob) between the skin and ulnar olecranon. Note the triceps tendon (t).

over the supinator muscle in this projection. On a lateral radiograph, the normal fat plane over the supinator muscle can appear as a radiolucent line, 4 to 5 cm in length, paralleling the radial head, neck, and upper shaft.[43] Changes in this latter fat plane have been reported in various elbow disorders.

Along the posterior aspect of the elbow, a subcutaneous bursa, the olecranon bursa, separates the skin from the ulnar olecranon (Fig. 3–17). This synovium-lined sac can be outlined by contrast material, revealing that it is situated like a cap on the olecranon process.[44]

Active movements of the elbow include flexion and extension. Accessory movements are slight screw action, abduction and adduction of the ulna, and forward and backward movement of the radial head on the capitulum. Supination and pronation result, in part, from movement at the superior radioulnar joint.

GLENOHUMERAL JOINT

The glenohumeral joint lies between the roughly hemispheric head of the humerus and the shallow cavity of the glenoid region of the scapula. Stability of this articulation is limited, for two reasons: the scapular "socket" is small compared to the size of the adjacent humeral head, so that apposing osseous surfaces provide little inherent stability; the joint capsule is quite redundant, providing little additional support. Stability of the glenohumeral joint is supplied by surrounding musculature.[45, 46]

Osseous Anatomy

The upper end of the humerus consists of the head and the greater and lesser tuberosities (tubercles) (Fig. 3–18). With the arm at the side of the body, the humeral head is directed medially, upward and slightly backward to contact the glenoid cavity of the scapula. Beneath the head is the anatomic neck of the humerus, a slightly constricted area that encircles the bone, separating the head from the tuberosities. The anatomic neck is the site of attachment of the capsular ligament of the glenohumeral joint. The greater tuberosity is located on the lateral aspect of the proximal humerus. The tendons of the supraspinatus and infraspinatus muscles insert on its superior portion, whereas the tendon of the teres minor muscle inserts on its posterior aspect. The lesser tuberosity is located on the anterior portion of the proximal humerus, immediately below the anatomic neck. The subscapularis tendon attaches to the medial aspect of this structure. Between the greater and lesser tuberosities is located the intertubercular sulcus or groove (bicipital groove) through which passes the tendon of the long head of the biceps brachii, surrounded by a synovial sheath, fixed by a transverse ligament extending between the tuberosities. The rough lateral lip of the groove is the site of attachment of the tendon of the pectoralis major; the floor of the groove gives rise to the attachment of the tendon of the latissimus dorsi; the medial lip of the groove is the site of attachment of the tendon of the teres major.

The shallow glenoid cavity is located on the lateral margin of the scapula (Fig. 3–19). Although there is variation in the osseous depth of the glenoid region,[45] a fibrocartilaginous labrum encircles and deepens the glenoid cavity. The glenoid contour may be almost flat or slightly curved, or it may possess a deep socket-like appearance. A supraglenoid tubercle is located above the glenoid cavity, to which is attached the long head of the biceps tendon. Below the cavity is a thickened ridge of bone, the infraglenoid tubercle, which is a site of attachment for the long head of the triceps.

Radiographic landmarks about the glenohumeral joint have been described.[47] With the arm in external rotation, the angle of intersection of two lines is calculated. The first line is drawn along the longitudinal axis of the humerus. The second line is drawn between the apex of the greater tuberosity and the junction of the shaft with the distal articular surface of the head. The average angle of intersection of these lines is 60 degrees (52 to 70 degrees) in men

Text continued on page 74

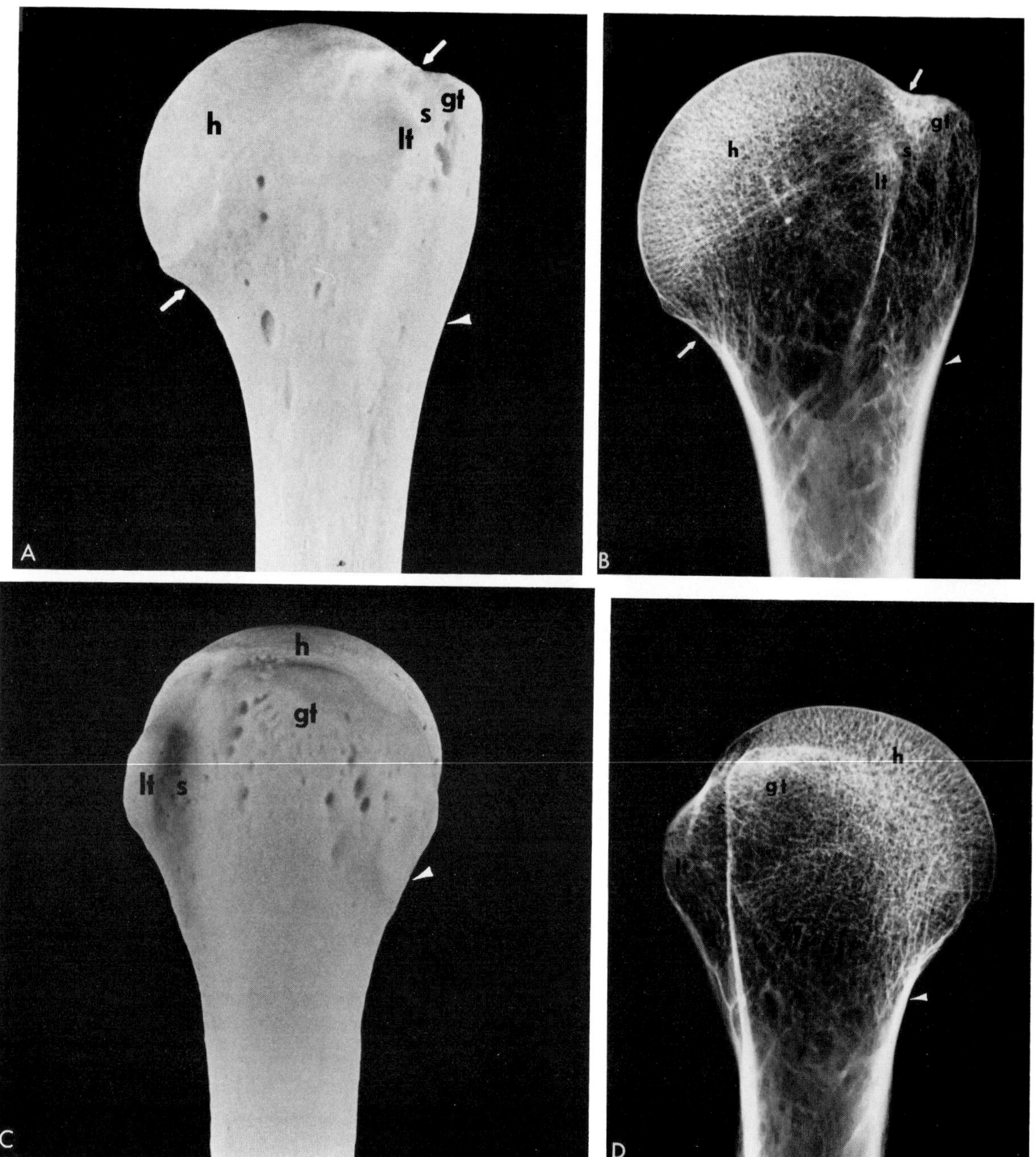

Figure 3–18. *Proximal humerus: Osseous anatomy.*

A, B *Anterior aspect, external rotation. Observe the articular surface of the humeral head (h), greater tuberosity (gt), lesser tuberosity (lt), intertubercular sulcus (s), anatomic neck (arrows), and surgical neck (arrowhead).*

C, D *Anterior aspect, internal rotation. The same structures as in* **A** *and* **B** *are indicated. The lesser tuberosity is seen in profile on the medial aspect of the humeral head and the greater tuberosity is seen en face.*

Illustration continued on the opposite page

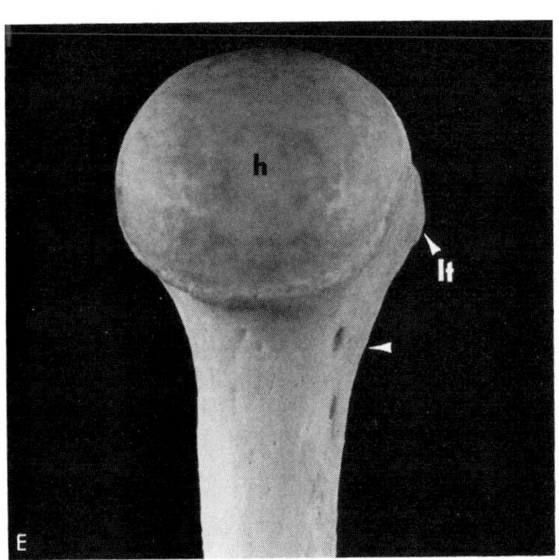

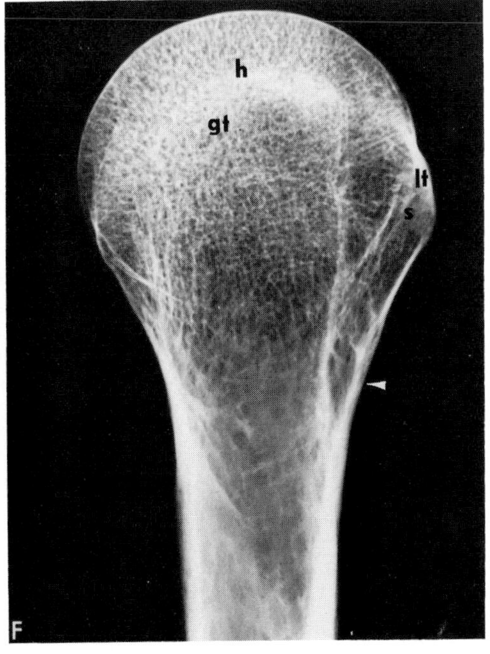

Figure 3–18. Continued
E, F *Medial aspect with same structures as in* **C** *and* **D** *identified.*

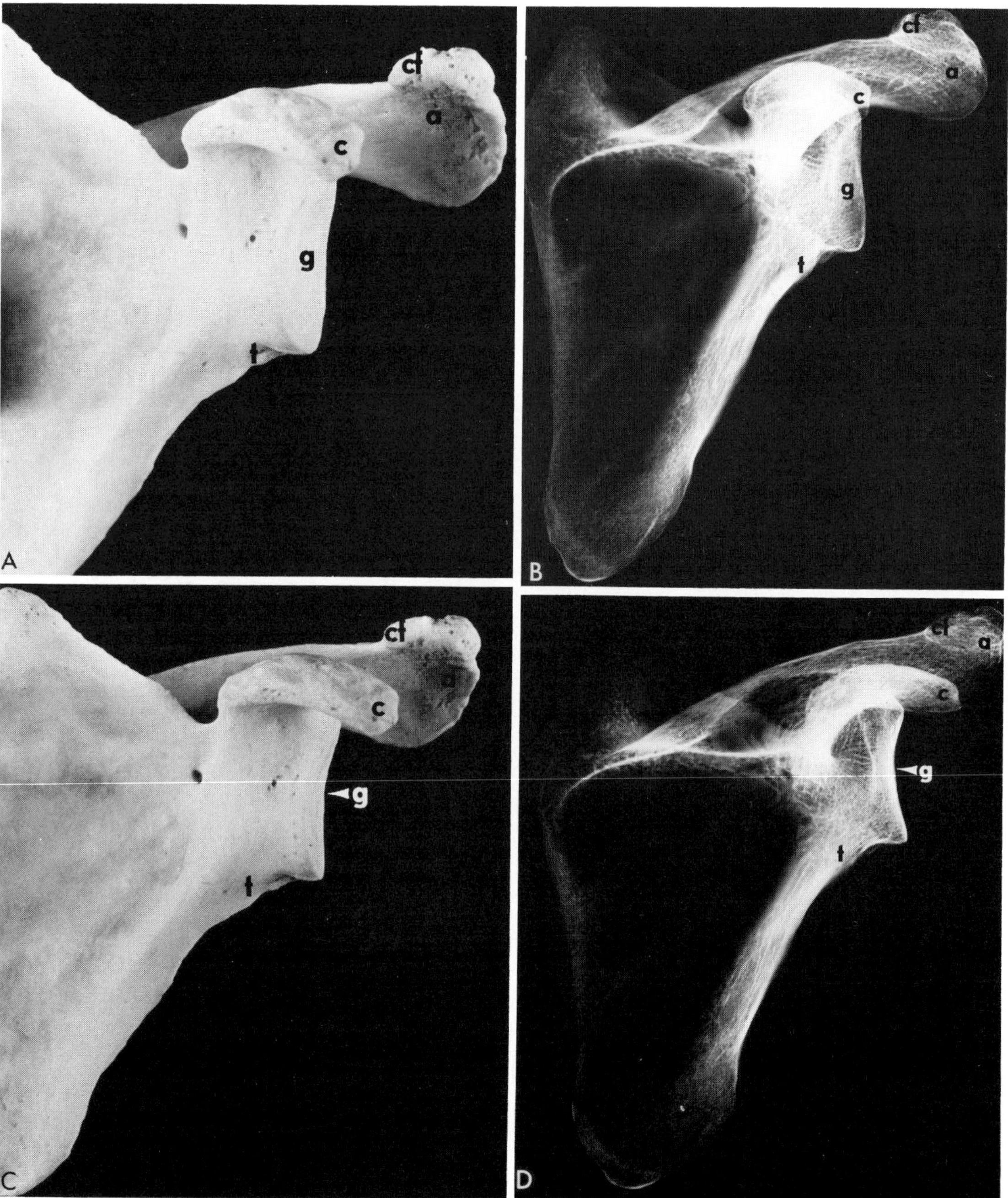

Figure 3–19. *Scapula: Osseous anatomy.*

A, B *Anterior (costal) aspect. The scapula is viewed in the position it maintains when an anteroposterior radiograph of the shoulder is obtained. Observe the acromion (a), clavicular facet (cf), coracoid process (c), glenoid cavity (g), and infraglenoid tubercle (t). Note that the glenoid cavity is not seen tangentially.*

C, D *Anterior (costal) aspect. The scapula is now positioned in a true anterior projection. The same structures are identified as in* **A** *and* **B**. *Observe that the glenoid cavity is now seen tangentially.*

Illustration continued on the opposite page

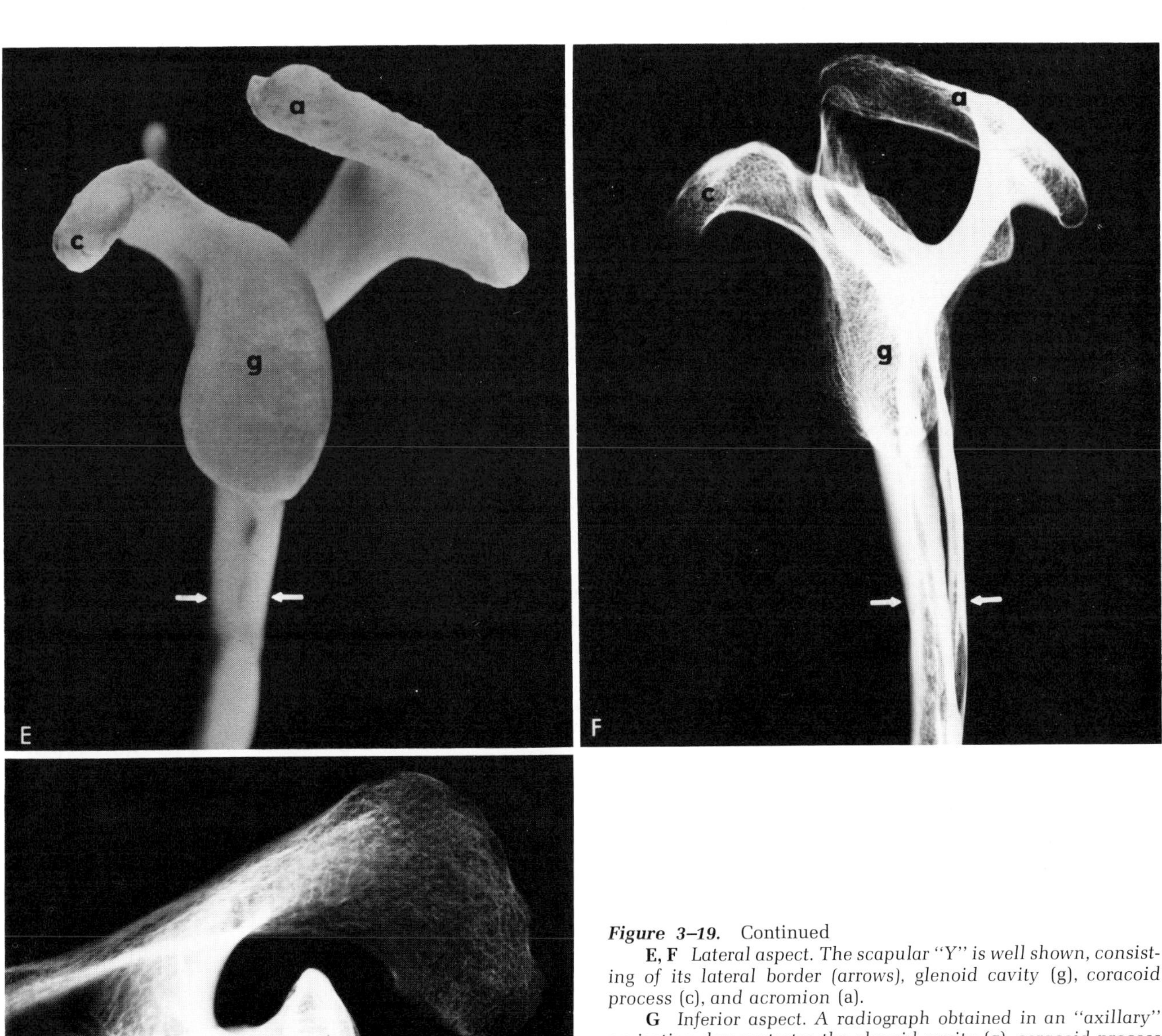

Figure 3–19. Continued

E, F *Lateral aspect. The scapular "Y" is well shown, consisting of its lateral border (arrows), glenoid cavity (g), coracoid process (c), and acromion (a).*

G *Inferior aspect. A radiograph obtained in an "axillary" projection demonstrates the glenoid cavity (g), coracoid process (c), and acromion (a).*

and 62 degrees (50 to 70 degrees) in women. The value for the width of the glenohumeral joint surface at the central portion of the glenoid is generally less than 6 mm.[48] The angle of "humeral torsion" is defined as the angle between the upper and lower articulating surfaces of the humerus.[1] This angle equals approximately 164 degrees, being greater in men than in women, and in adults than in children.

Soft Tissue Anatomy

The articular surfaces of the glenoid and the humerus are covered with hyaline cartilage (Fig. 3–20). The cartilage on the humeral head is thickest at its center and thinner peripherally, whereas the reverse is true on the glenoid portion of the joint.[1] A fibrocartilaginous structure, the labrum, attaches to the glenoid rim and adds an element of stability to the glenohumeral articulation.[49]

A loose fibrous capsule arises medially from the circumference of the glenoid labrum. It inserts distally into the anatomic neck of the humerus and periosteum of the humeral diaphysis. In certain areas the fibrous capsule is strengthened by its intimate association with surrounding ligaments; it is reinforced above by the supraspinatus, below by the long head of the triceps, anteriorly by the subscapularis, and posteriorly by the infraspinatus and teres minor. The tendons of the supraspinatus, infraspinatus, teres minor, and subscapularis form a cuff — the rotator cuff — which blends with and reinforces the fibrous capsule. The coracohumeral ligament strengthens the upper part of the capsule. It arises from the lateral edge of the coracoid process, extends over the humeral head, and attaches to the greater tuberosity. Anteriorly, the capsule may thicken to form the superior, middle, and inferior glenohumeral ligaments.[1, 46] These ligaments and the recesses formed between them are variable in configuration. The fibrous capsule is strengthened additionally by extensions from the tendons of the pectoralis major and teres major.

Three openings may be found in the fibrous capsule.[1] An anterior perforation below the coracoid process establishes joint communication with the bursa behind the subscapularis tendon, the subscapularis "recess." A second opening between the greater and lesser tuberosities allows passage of the tendon and synovial sheath of the long head of the biceps. A third, inconstant perforation may exist posteriorly, allowing communication of the articular cavity and a bursa under the infraspinatus tendon.

A synovial membrane lines the inner aspect of the fibrous capsule. It covers the anatomic neck of the humerus and extends to the articular cartilage on the humeral head. The synovium passes distally to line the bicipital groove and is reflected over the biceps tendon.

There are several bursae about the glenohumeral joint:

Subscapular "Recess." This bursa lies between the subscapularis tendon and the scapula, communicating with the joint via an opening between the superior and middle glenohumeral ligaments. This bursa is readily apparent on shoulder arthrograms as a tongue-shaped collection of contrast material extending medially from the glenohumeral space underneath the coracoid process.[50] It is prominent in internal rotation but is less obvious in external rotation, as the taut subscapularis muscle compresses the bursa.

Bursa About the Infraspinatus Tendon. This inconstant bursa separates the infraspinatus tendon and joint capsule and may communicate with the joint cavity.

Subacromial (Subdeltoid) Bursa. This important bursa lies between the deltoid muscle and joint capsule.[51] It extends underneath the acromion and the coraco-acromial ligament. The subacromial bursa is separated from the articular cavity by the rotator cuff and does not communicate with the joint unless there has been a perforation of the cuff. Layers of fat tissue about this bursa have been identified on radiographs of the normal shoulder[52]; a thin, crescentic radiolucency passes from the inferior aspect of the acromion process and distal clavicle along the outer margin of the upper humerus.

Bursa Above the Acromion. This bursa is located on the superior surface of the acromion process of the scapula.

Miscellaneous Bursae. Additional bursae[1] may be found between the coracoid process and the capsule, behind the coracobrachialis, between the teres major and the long head of the triceps, and about the latissimus dorsi.

The glenohumeral joint is active in a variety of movements, including flexion, extension, abduction, adduction, circumduction, and medial and lateral rotation. Accessory movements of this articulation include upward, downward, forward, and backward motions.[1, 46, 53-55]

ACROMIOCLAVICULAR JOINT

The acromioclavicular joint is a synovial articulation between the lateral aspect of the clavicle and the medial aspect of the acromion.[1, 2, 56]

Osseous Anatomy

The lateral or acromial end of the clavicle is a flattened structure with a small, oval articular facet that faces laterally and slightly downward (Fig. 3–21). This facet articulates with the acromial facet of the scapula and is the site of attachment of the

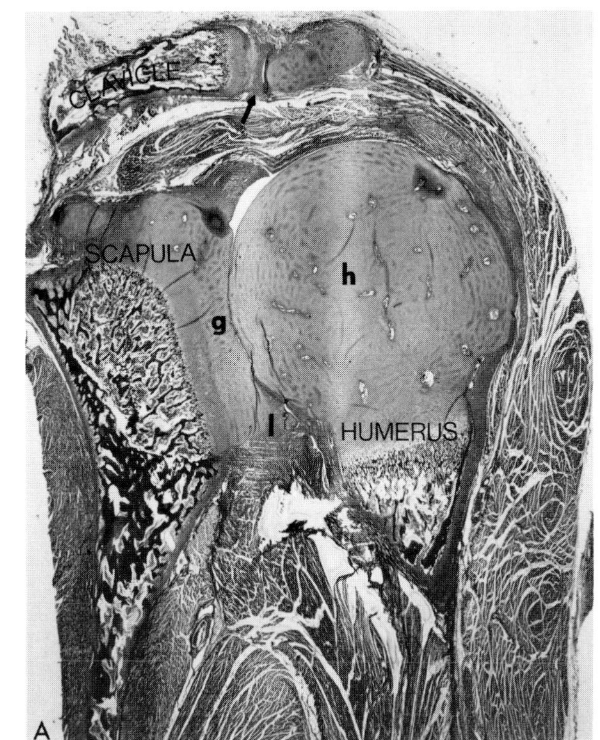

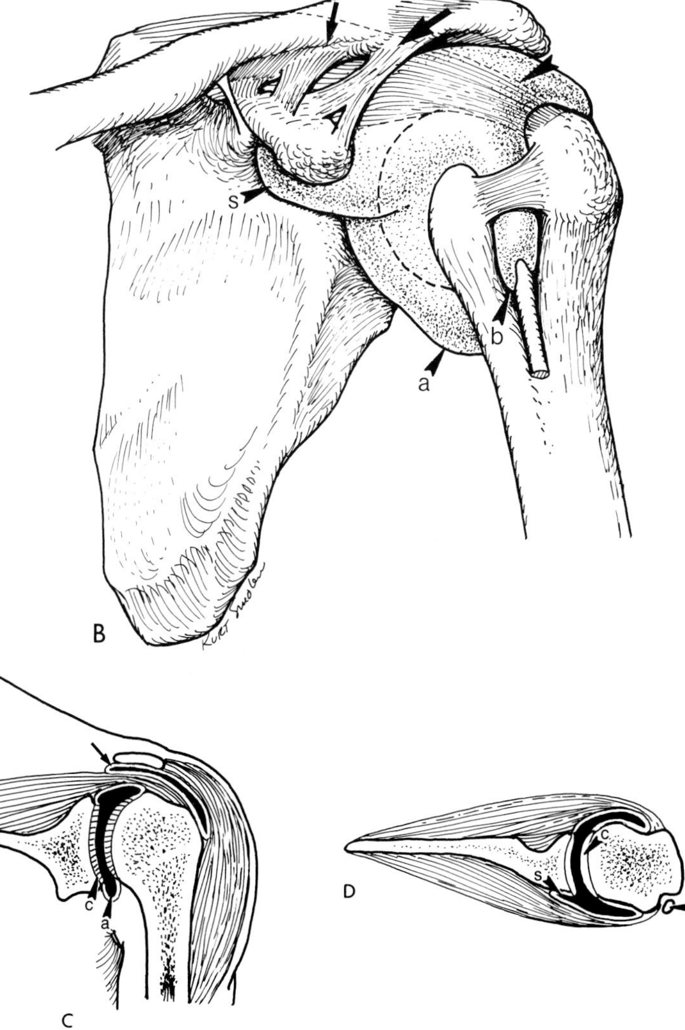

Figure 3–20. *Glenohumeral joint: Normal development and anatomy.*

A *A coronal section of the developing glenohumeral joint (20×) reveals the articulation between unossified humeral head* (h) *and glenoid cavity* (g). *Additional structures are the acromioclavicular joint (arrow) between acromion and distal clavicle, and the glenoid labrum* (l).

B *A drawing of the anterior aspect of the distended glenohumeral joint depicts axillary pouch* (a), *subscapular recess* (s), *and synovial extension over the bicipital tendon* (b). *Note the rotator cuff (arrowhead), coracoacromial ligament (heavy arrow) and coracoclavicular ligament (light arrow).*

C, D *Drawings of coronal* **(C)** *and transverse* **(D)** *sections of glenohumeral joint outline extent of the synovial cavity, articular cartilage* (c), *axillary pouch* (a), *subscapular recess* (s), *subacromial (subdeltoid) bursa (arrow), and bicipital tendon* (b).

Illustration continued on the following page

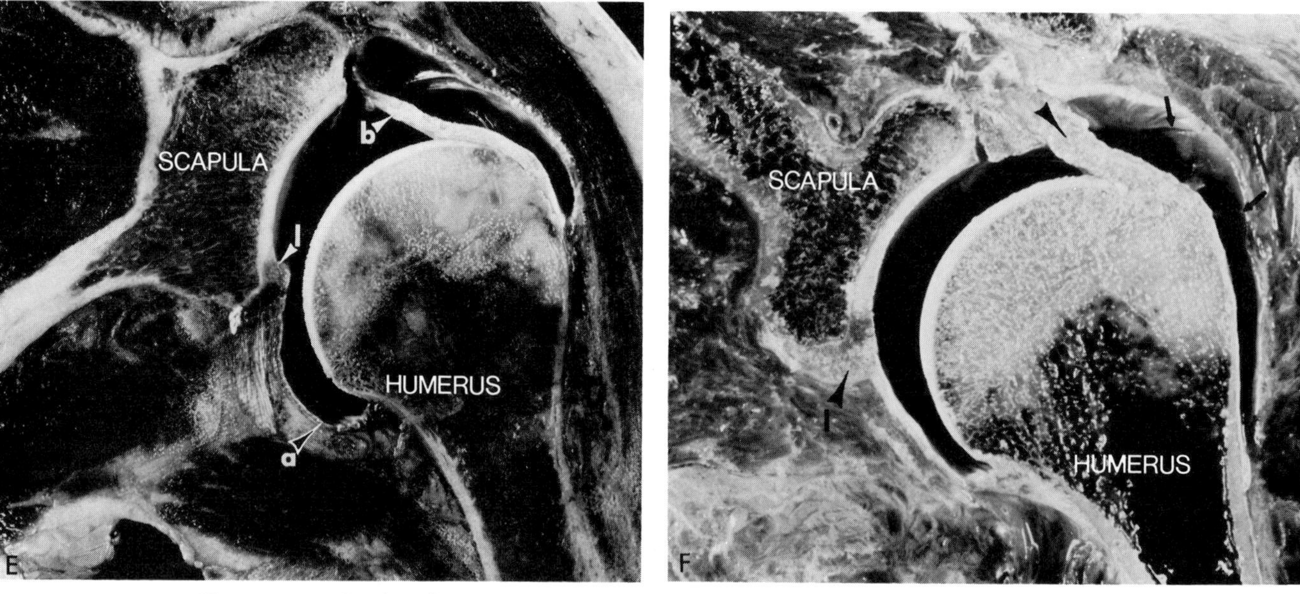

Figure 3–20. Continued

E, F *Two coronal sections through different portions of the air-distended glenohumeral joint outline articular cavity, axillary pouch* (a), *tendon of the long head of biceps* (b), *glenoid labrum* (l), *rotator cuff (arrowhead), and subacromial (subdeltoid) bursa (arrows).*

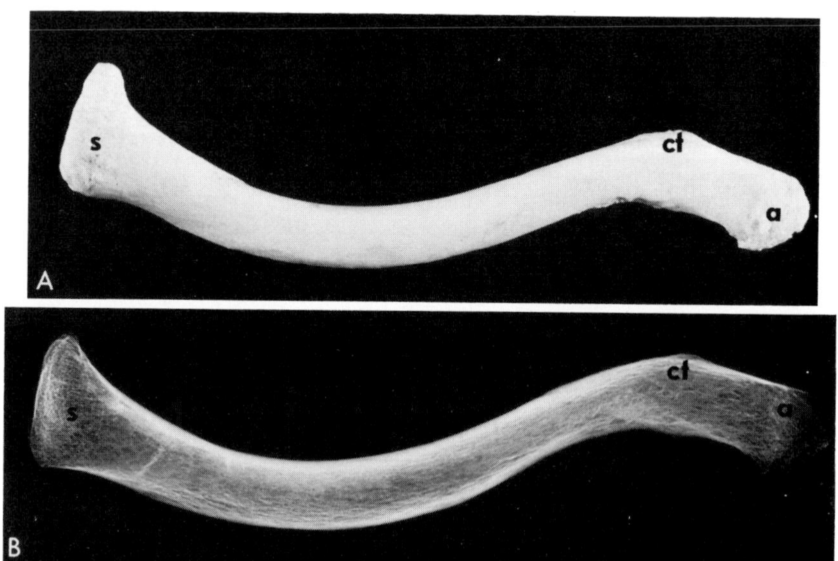

Figure 3–21. *Clavicle: Osseous anatomy.*

A, B *Superior aspect. Photograph and radiograph delineate sternal* (s) *and acromial* (a) *ends of clavicle. Note the conoid tubercle* (ct) *on the posterior surface of the distal clavicle.*

joint capsule of the acromioclavicular joint. The inferior surface of the acromial end of the clavicle possesses a rough osseous ridge, termed the trapezoid line. A conoid tubercle is located at the posterior aspect of the lateral clavicle. The trapezoid line and conoid tubercle are the sites of attachment of the trapezoid and conoid parts of the coracoclavicular ligament.

The acromion is a forward protuberance of the lateral aspect of the scapula. An articular facet, the acromial facet, is located on the medial border of the acromion and is small and oval in size and configuration, directed medially and superiorly.

Soft Tissue Anatomy

The articular surfaces about the acromioclavicular joint are covered with fibrocartilage (Fig. 3–22). In the central portion of the articulation is an articular disc[56, 57] that partially or, more rarely, completely divides the joint cavity. The fibrous capsule surrounds the articular margin and is reinforced on its superior and inferior surfaces. Surrounding ligaments include the acromioclavicular and coracoclavicular ligaments. The former ligament, which is located at the superior portion of the joint, extends between the clavicle and acromion. The coracoclavicular ligament, which attaches to the coracoid process of the scapula and clavicle, is composed of a trapezoid part and a conoid part. The trapezoid portion extends from the upper surface of the coracoid process to the trapezoid line on the inferior aspect of the clavicle; the conoid portion extends from the coracoid process to the conoid tubercle on the inferior clavicular surface. The trapezoid and conoid parts of the coracoclavicular ligament may be separated by fat or a bursa.

A joint may be noted between the clavicle and coracoid process in 0.1 to 1.2 per cent of people.[220-223] In these cases, a triangular outgrowth from the undersurface of the clavicle approaches the dorsomedial surface of the coracoid process. On dissection, the articulation may contain a capsule and synovial membrane as well as a cartilaginous disk.[218]

Normal anteroposterior radiographs of the acromioclavicular joint may reveal a soft tissue plane about the articulation related to the aponeurosis associated with the trapezius and deltoid muscles.[58, 59] Contrast opacification of the joint reveals an L-shaped articular cavity with a horizontal limb extending under the inferior surface of the distal clavicle.[59]

The acromioclavicular joint allows the acromion to glide in a forward and backward direction and to rotate on the clavicle. These movements depend upon additional movements at the sternoclavicular joint.[1]

STERNOCLAVICULAR JOINT

At the sternoclavicular articulation, the medial end of the clavicle articulates with the clavicular notch of the manubrium sterni and with the cartilage of the first rib[1, 56] (Fig. 3–23 to 3–25).

Osseous Anatomy

The enlarged medial or sternal end of the clavicle projects above the upper margin of the manubrium and is directed medially, inferiorly, and anteriorly (Fig. 3–21). The articular surface is smooth except on its superior portion, where a roughened area allows attachment of an articular disc. The inferior portion of the articular surface is extended to allow articulation with the first costal cartilage. The medial portion of the inferior surface of the clavicle has a rough impression for attachment of the costoclavicular ligament.

The superolateral portions of the manubrium

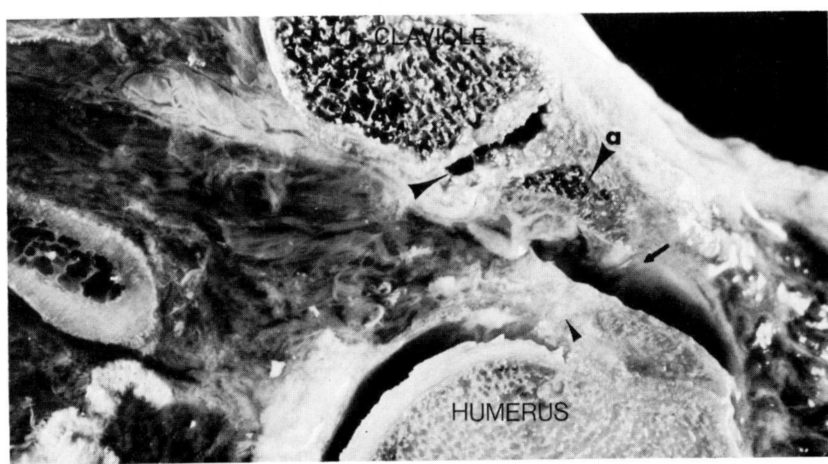

Figure 3–22. *Acromioclavicular joint: Normal anatomy. Visualized structures on this coronal section are the articular space (large arrowhead) between distal clavicle and acromion (a) (an articular disc is not visible), rotator cuff (small arrowhead), and subacromial (subdeltoid) bursa (arrow).*

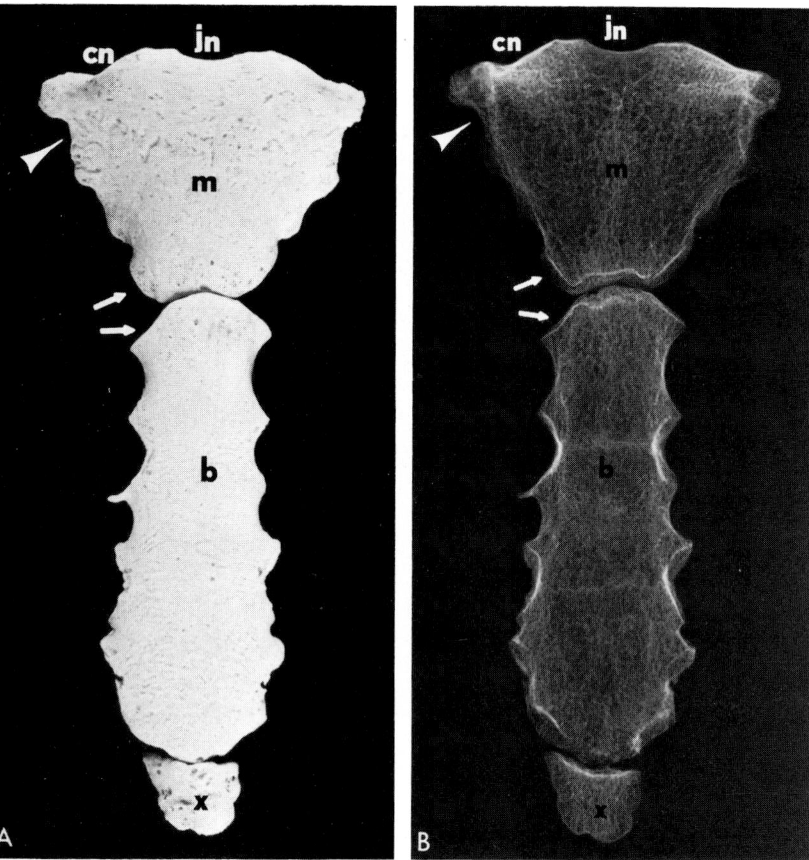

Figure 3–23. Sternum: Osseous anatomy. Anterior aspect. The three segments of the sternum are the manubrium (m), body (b), and xiphoid process (x). Additional landmarks are the clavicular notch (cn) and jugular notch (jn). A sternal facet for articulation with the first costal cartilage (arrowhead) and hemifacets for articulation with the second costal cartilage (arrows) are indicated. Other articular facets are also apparent on the body of the sternum.

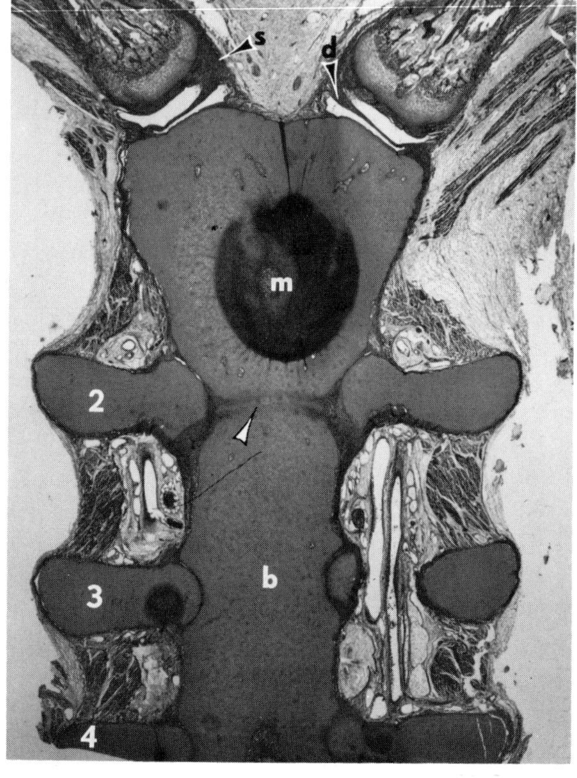

Figure 3–24. Sternum and clavicle: Developmental anatomy. A photomicrograph (20×) of a coronal section through the sternum and clavicle outlines the unossified manubrium (m) and body (b) of the sternum, partially ossified medial clavicle, and costal cartilage of the second (2), third (3), and fourth (4) ribs. Observe the sternoclavicular joints with synovium (s) and articular disc (d), and manubriosternal joint (arrowhead).

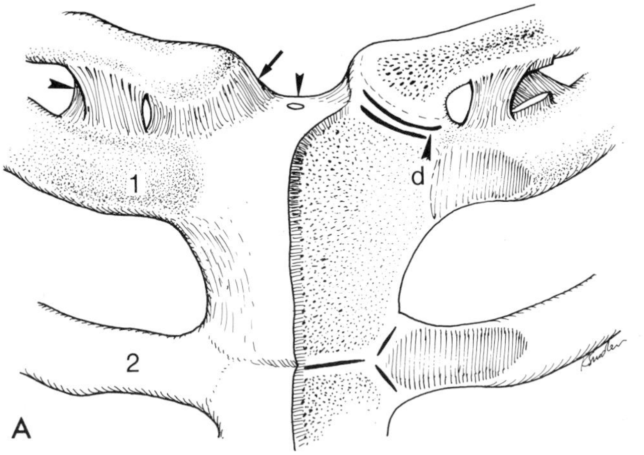

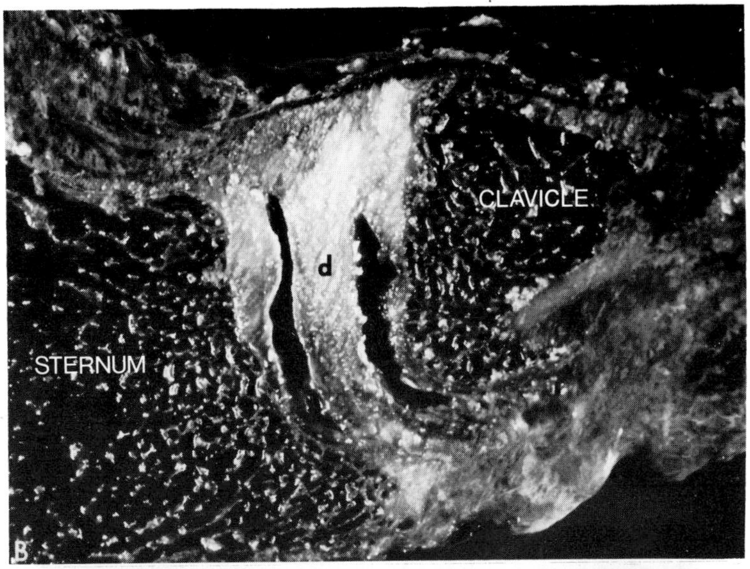

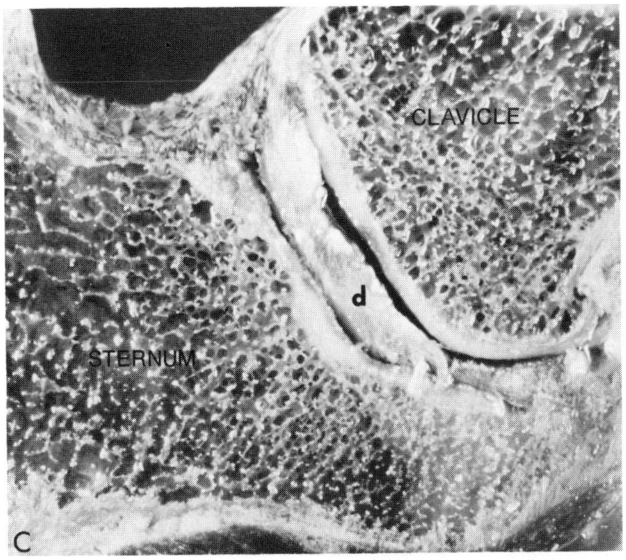

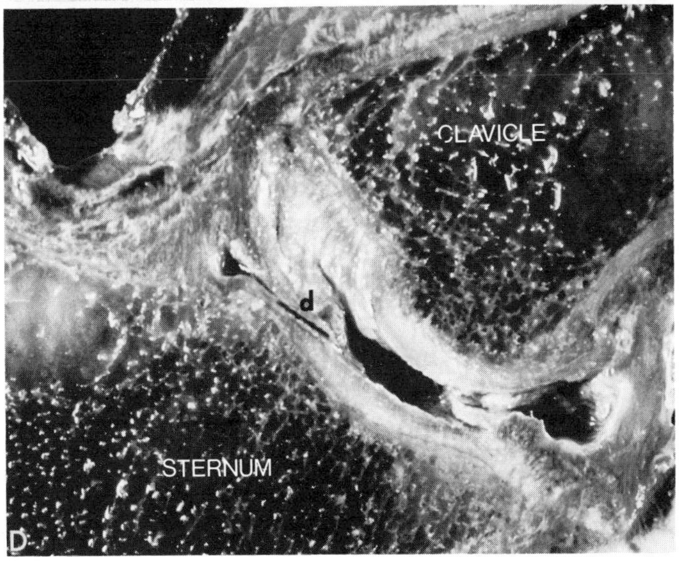

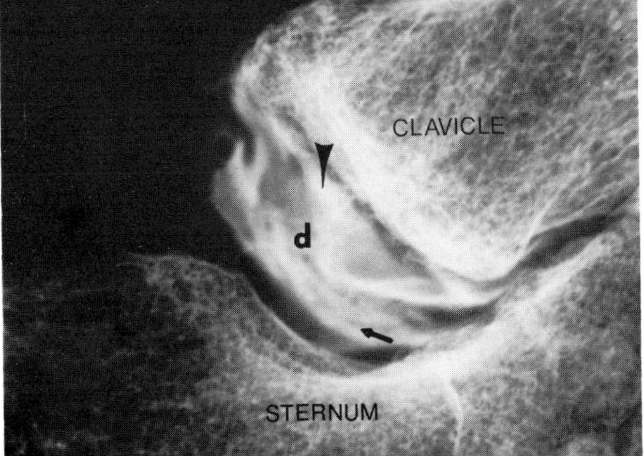

Figure 3–25. *Sternoclavicular joint: Normal anatomy.*

A *A diagrammatic depiction of the anterior aspect of the upper sternum and medial clavicles. On the right-hand side, the superficial bone has been removed, exposing the sternoclavicular, manubriosternal, and second sternocostal articulations. Identified structures are the anterior sternoclavicular ligament (arrow), costoclavicular ligament (large arrowhead), interclavicular ligament (small arrowhead) and articular disc (d). Note the first (1) and second (2) costal cartilages. (From Warwick R, Williams P: Gray's Anatomy. 35th British Ed. Philadelphia, WB Saunders Co, 1973.)*

B–D *Photographs of coronal sections through the sternoclavicular articulation in three different cadavers reveal characteristics of the intra-articular disc (d). Observe a relatively normal articular disc* **(B)**, *a slightly irregular disc* **(C)**, *and a perforated disc* **(D)**. *In the latter instance, the two articular cavities communicate.*

E *An arthrogram with injection of contrast material into the lateral articular space (arrowhead) results in opacification of the medial joint space (arrow) via defects in the intra-articular disc (d).*

contain oval articular surfaces, the clavicular facets or notches, which are directed superiorly, posteriorly, and laterally. Below each clavicular notch is a rough projection which receives the first costal cartilage.

Soft Tissue Anatomy

The articular end of the clavicle is covered with a layer of fibrocartilage that is thicker than the cartilage on the sternum. A flat circular disc is located between the articulating surfaces of the clavicle and sternum; it is attached superiorly to the posterior border of the clavicle, inferiorly to the cartilage of the first rib, and (elsewhere) to the fibrous capsule, and divides the joint into two articular cavities.[227] The disc acts as a checkrein against medial displacement of the inner clavicle. Perforations in the disc are frequent in older patients. A fibrous capsule surrounds the articulation[60] and is attached to the clavicular and sternomanubrial articular surfaces. The inferior portion of the capsule is weak as it passes between the clavicle and superior surface of the first costal cartilage. Elsewhere the capsule is strong, reinforced by the anterior and posterior sternoclavicular ligaments and the interclavicular ligament. Nearby, the costoclavicular ligament attaches below to the upper surface of the first rib and adjacent cartilage and above to the inferior surface of the medial end of the clavicle. This ligament consists of anterior and posterior portions, between which is located a bursa.[61] It resists forces that attempt to displace the medial clavicle anteriorly, posteriorly, upward, or laterally.

The sternoclavicular joint is freely mobile. It participates in movements of the upper extremity, including elevation, depression, protraction, retraction, and circumduction.[54, 62]

STERNAL JOINTS

Osseous Anatomy

The sternum consists of three portions, a proximal portion termed the manubrium, a middle portion, the body, and a distal portion, the xiphoid process (Fig. 3–23). The pattern of ossification during the development of the sternum is variable.[63-65, 226] The sternomanubrial junction usually remains unossified in the adult. Ossification between segments in the lower portion of the sternal body occurs soon after puberty; ossification between segments in the upper portion of the body occurs between puberty and the twenty-fifth year of life. Ossification between the body and xiphoid process occurs at approximately 40 years of age.

The manubrium is the widest portion of the sternum and is quadrilateral in shape. The jugular (suprasternal) notch is located at the midportion of the superior border of the manubrium. The body of the sternum is approximately twice as long as the manubrium. Its anterior surface contains three transverse ridges of bone, representing the sites of union between osseous sternal segments. The posterior surface has similar but less marked ridges. The xiphoid process is the smallest part of the sternum and is quite variable in appearance. It may be perforated in its central portion.

Soft Tissue Anatomy

Two articulations exist between segments of the sternum: the manubriosternal joint, and xiphisternal joint (Fig. 3–26).

Manubriosternal Joint. This articulation between manubrium and body of the sternum is a symphysis; the apposing osseous surfaces are covered with hyaline cartilage and separated by a fibrocartilaginous disc. In approximately 25 to 30 per cent of individuals, the central portion of the disc undergoes cavitation; in approximately 10 to 15 per cent of individuals over the age of 30 years, complete ossification produces a synostosis between these two segments of the sternum, a process which increases with advancing age.[66, 67, 217] Synostosis may be related to persistence of a synchondrosis rather than a symphysis at this junction.[68]

Xiphisternal Joint. This articulation is a symphysis that exists between the sternal body and xiphoid. Although it may remain unossified even in elderly persons, it usually becomes a synostosis by the fortieth year of life.[1]

STERNOCOSTAL AND INTERCOSTAL JOINTS

The anterior aspect of each rib is firmly attached to a column of hyaline cartilage, termed the costal cartilage at the costochondral junction.[69] The first costal cartilage is united with the sternum, the second through seventh costal cartilages articulate with sternal facets, and the lower costal cartilages, except for the eleventh and twelfth, articulate with each other. Costal cartilage calcification proceeds with advancing age, and the pattern of ossification appears different in men and women.[70-74]

Osseous Anatomy

On the manubrium is a rough facet below each clavicular notch, which articulates with the first

Text continued on page 84

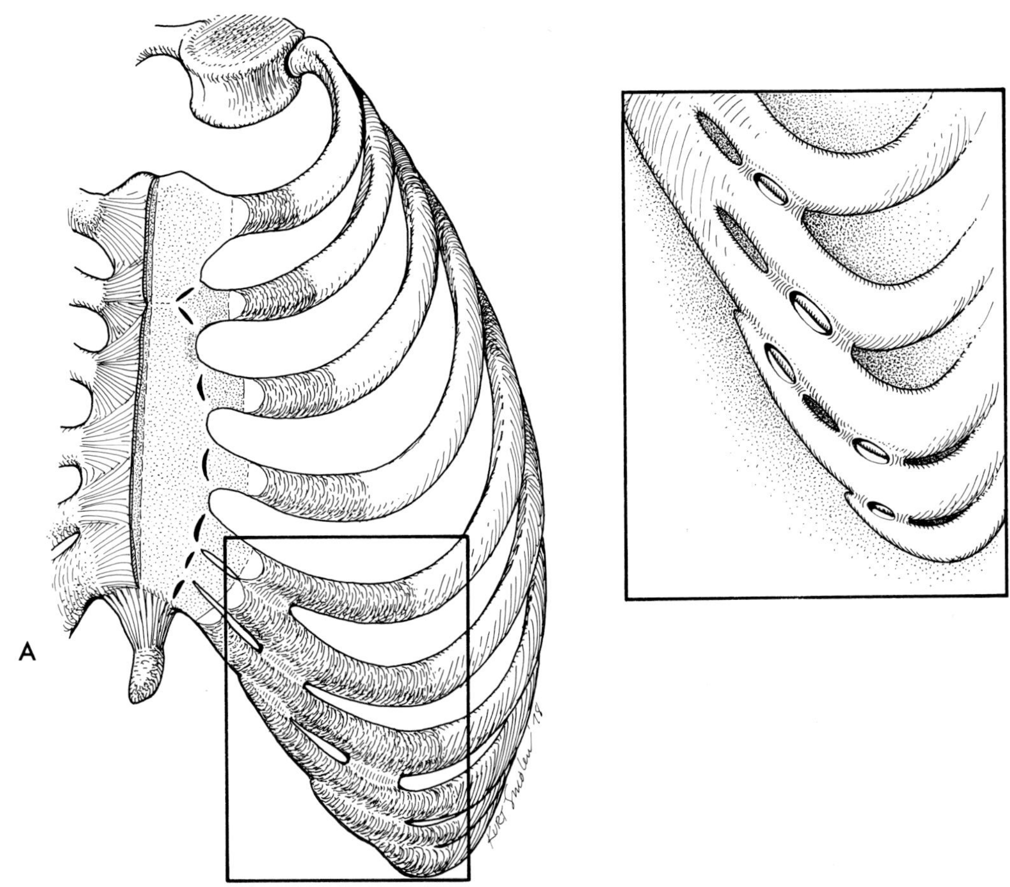

Figure 3–26. Sternal, sternocostal, and intercostal joints: Normal anatomy.

A *A schematic drawing of the anterior aspect of the chest wall depicts the manubriosternal and sternocostal articulations. At the manubriosternal joint, hemifacets on the sternum articulate with the second costal cartilage. A synchondrosis exists at the articulation between the first costal cartilage and the sternum. The third through seventh costal cartilages also articulate with the sternum. A close-up of the intercostal joints (inset) demonstrates facets separated by synovial cavities. (From Warwick R, Williams P: Gray's Anatomy. 35th British Ed. Philadelphia, WB Saunders Co, 1973.)*

Illustration continued on the following page

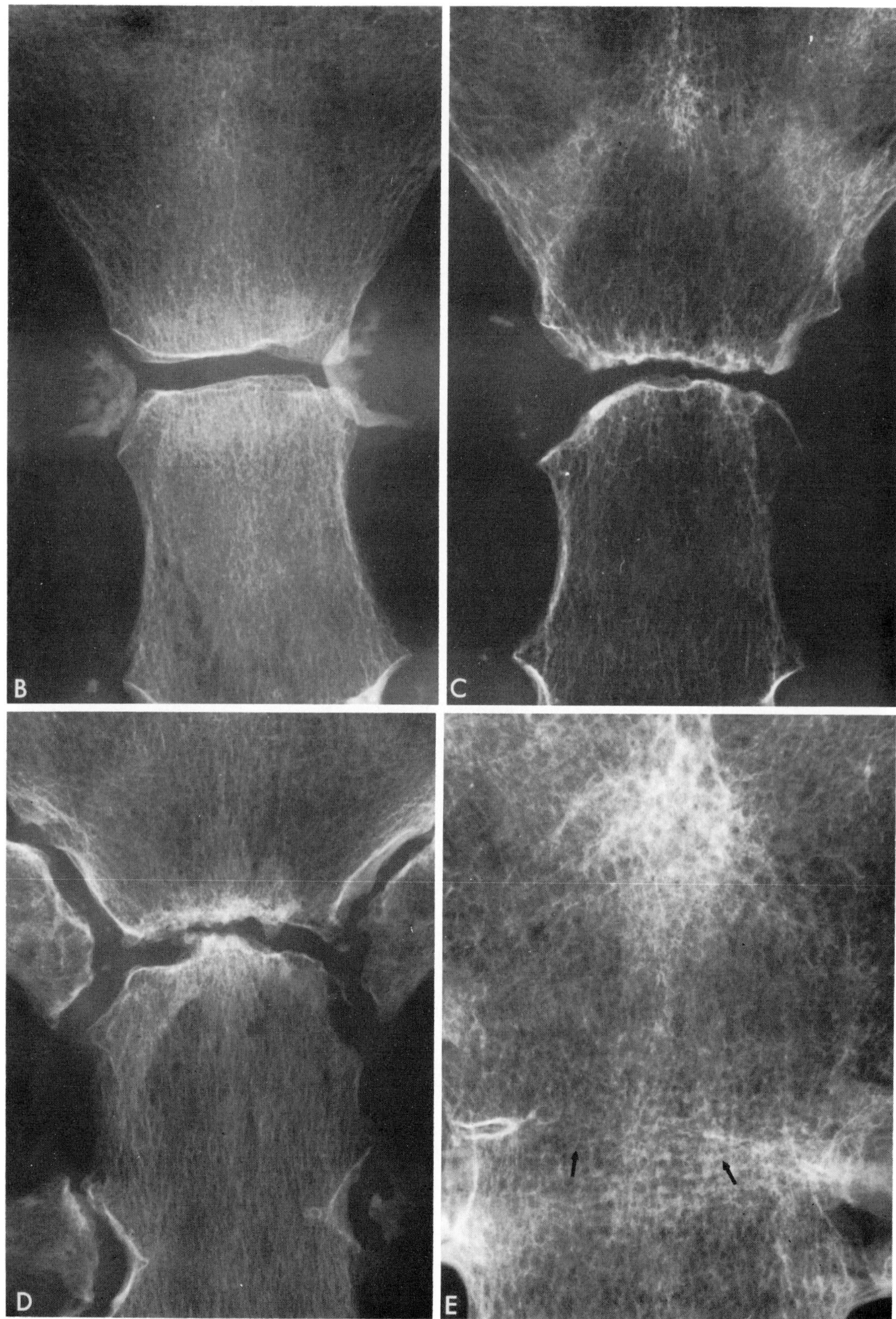

Figure 3–26. Continued

B–E *Frontal radiographs of the manubriosternal joint in four different cadavers outline sequential stages of ossification resulting in a synostosis (arrows) between manubrium and body of the sternum.*

Illustration continued on the opposite page

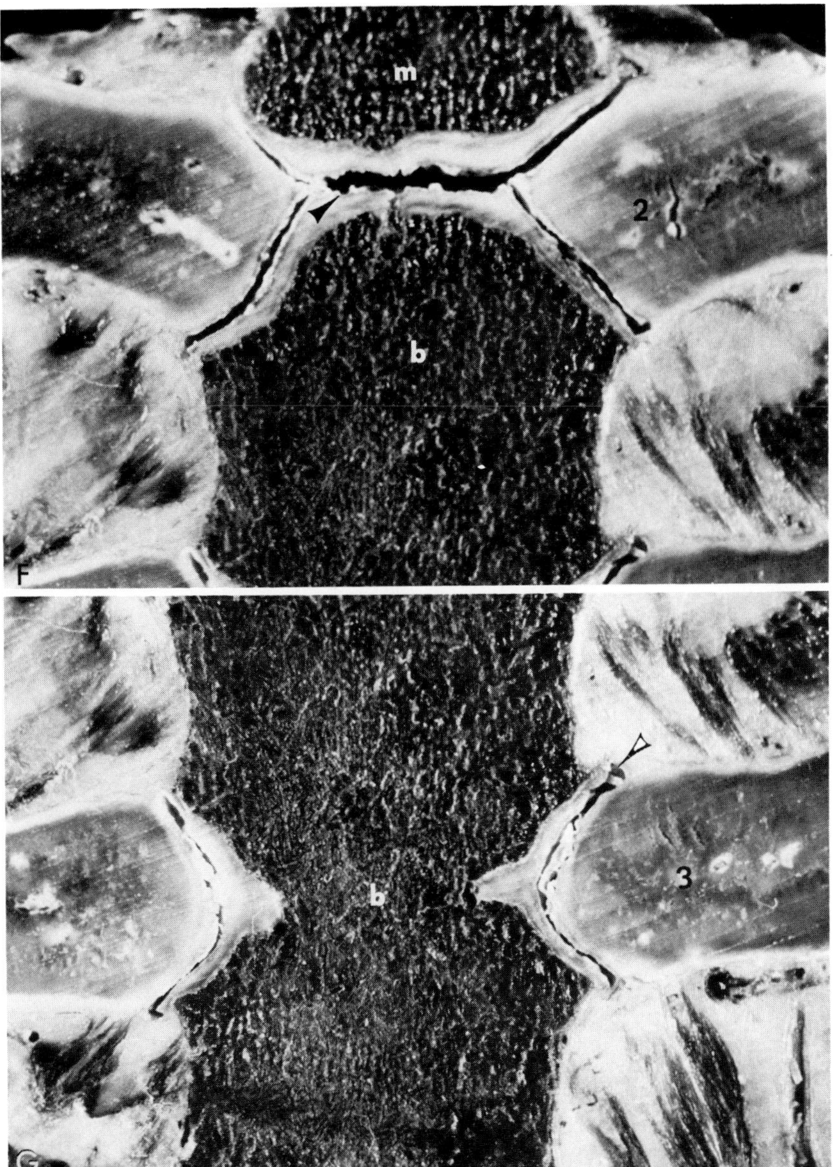

Figure 3–26. Continued

F *Manubriosternal and second sternocostal articulations (coronal section). In this cadaver, the manubriosternal joint has undergone cavitation (arrowhead). This articulation is communicating with the sternocostal joint (*m, *manubrium;* b, *body;* 2, *second costal cartilage).*

G *Third sternocostal articulation (coronal section). Observe sternal body* (b), *third costal cartilage* (3), *and intervening synovial articulation (arrowhead).*

Illustration continued on the following page

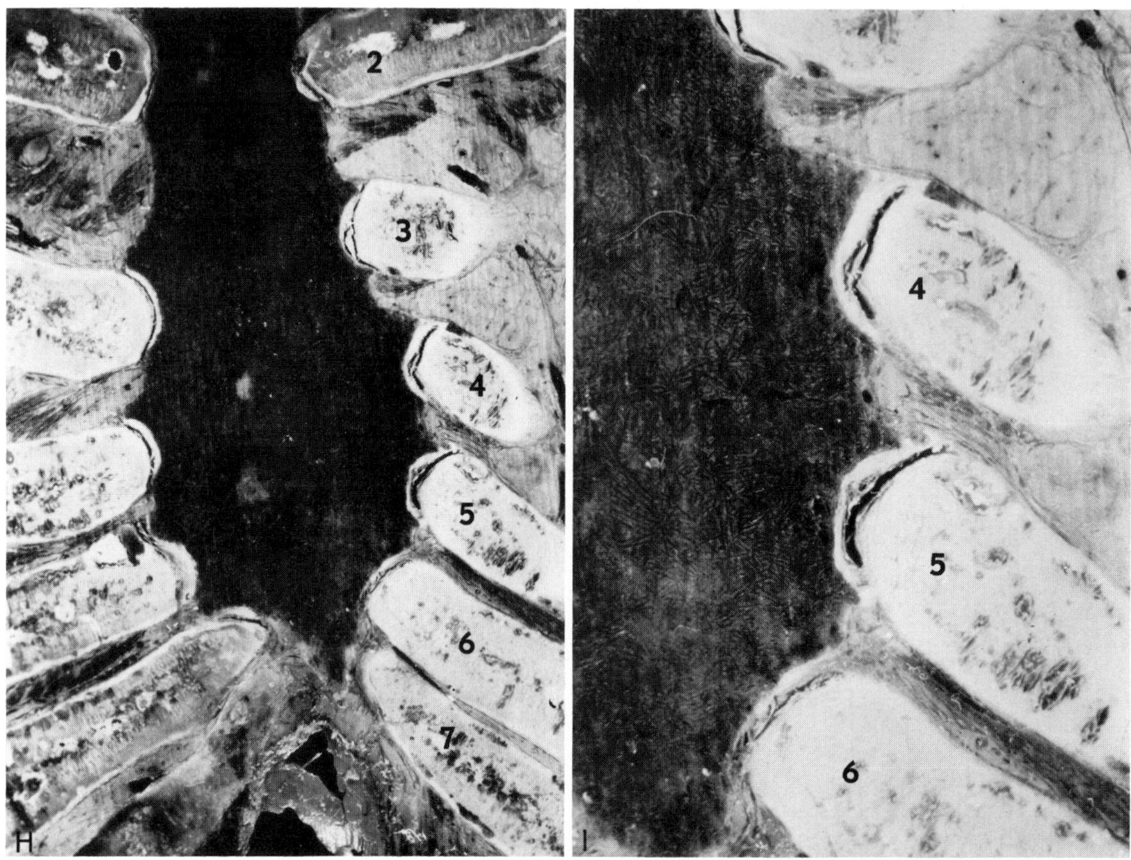

Figure 3–26. Continued
H, I *Sternocostal articulations. A coronal section of a cadaveric sternum, demonstrating second through seventh (2–7) sternocostal joints.*

costal cartilage (Fig. 3–23). At the manubrium-body junction, hemifacets are present, which articulate with the second costal cartilage. Additional articular facets occur between the segments of the body for articulation with the third to fifth costal cartilages, on the fourth segment of the body for articulation with the sixth costal cartilage, and at the xiphisternal junction for articulation with the seventh costal cartilage.

Soft Tissue Anatomy

The costal cartilages are involved in two types of articulations (Fig. 3–26).

STERNOCOSTAL (STERNOCHONDRAL) JOINTS. The articulation between the first costal cartilage and the sternum is a synchondrosis.[228] Elsewhere synovial articulations exist at the sternocostal junctions. The synovial cavity in each of these junctions is divided into two by an intra-articular ligament. This cavity persists at the second costal cartilage-sternal junction, but the other synovial cavities usually become obliterated with advancing age as ossification in the fibrocartilage-clothed articular surfaces unites costal cartilage and sternum.[75] Fibrous capsules about the articulations are strengthened in front and back by radiating fibers, termed the anterior and posterior radiate ligaments. Slight gliding motions, important in respiration, occur at the sternocostal joints.[1, 76]

INTERCOSTAL (INTERCHONDRAL) JOINTS. Contiguous borders of certain costal cartilages articulate with each other via facets separated by a synovial cavity, surrounded by a fibrous capsule, and strengthened laterally and medially by interchondral ligaments. This situation most frequently occurs between the sixth and seventh, seventh and eighth, and eighth and ninth costal cartilages. Occasionally a similar situation exists between the fifth and sixth, and between the ninth and tenth, costal cartilages, although at the latter site, a syndesmosis is more common.

COSTOVERTEBRAL JOINTS

The ribs and vertebral column articulate at two areas: between the heads of the ribs and vertebral

Table 3–2

ARTICULATIONS OF THE SPINE

Synovial Joints
Apophyseal (facet) joints
Atlas-odontoid process
Odontoid process-transverse ligament
Costovertebral joints
Joints of the heads of the ribs
Costotransverse joints
Joints of Luschka*
Symphyses
Intervertebral discs
Syndesmoses
Ligamentous connections of vertebral bodies
Ligamentous connections of vertebral arches

*Resemble synovial joints.

bodies; and between the necks and tubercles of the ribs and transverse processes of the vertebrae[77-82] (Table 3–2).

Osseous Anatomy

The posterior end of a typical rib contains an enlarged head with two sloping articular facets and an intervening osseous ridge or crest (Fig. 3–27). The neck of a rib is a flattened structure adjacent to the head, which lies anteriorly to the transverse process of the corresponding vertebra. The obliquely oriented neck contains an anterior surface that faces forward and upward. The upper border is the sharp crest of the neck of the rib. The lower border of the neck is round. The tubercle of the rib occurs at its

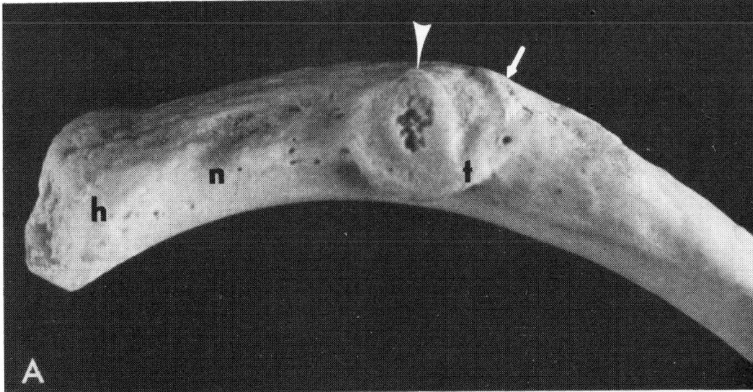

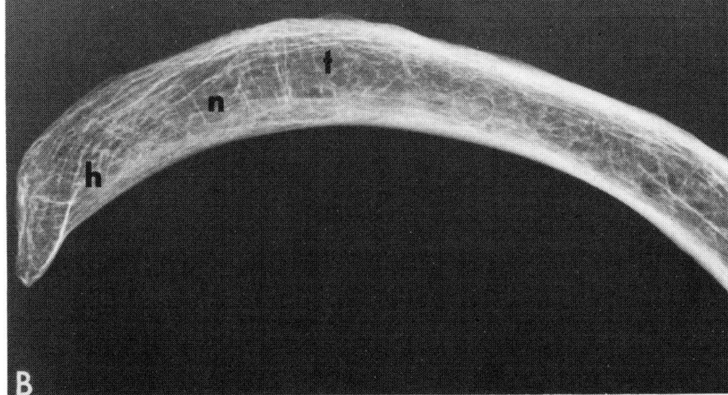

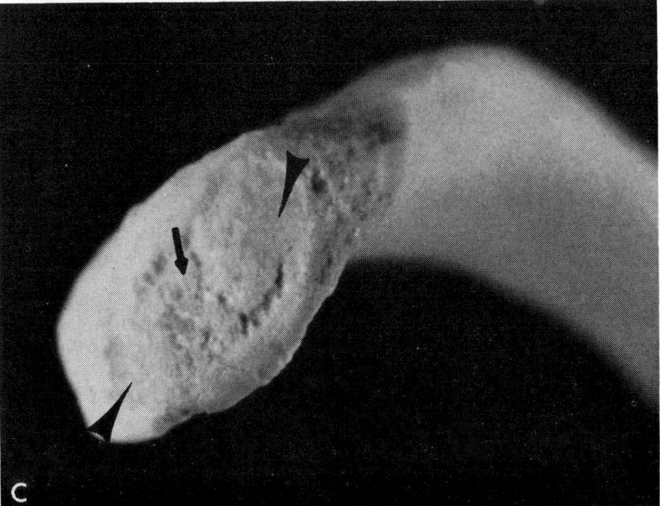

Figure 3–27. *Posterior rib: Osseous anatomy.*

A, B *Inferior aspect of typical rib. Note the head (h), neck (n), and tubercle (t). The latter consists of an articular (arrowhead) and nonarticular (arrow) portion.*

C *Medial aspect. A photograph of the head of a typical rib outlining two articular facets (arrowheads) with intervening osseous crest (arrow).*

posterior surface at the junction of the neck and body. The tubercle has an articular and a nonarticular portion. The former area contains a small, oval facet that articulates with the transverse process of the vertebra, and the latter area, which is roughened, represents the site of attachment of the lateral costotransverse ligament.

The first rib contains a small head with a single articular facet. It also possesses a long narrow neck and a large tubercle, which has a medial oval facet for articulation with the transverse process of the first thoracic vertebra. The tenth rib has a single articular facet on its head. The eleventh and twelfth ribs also have articular facets on their heads but have no necks or tubercles.

A typical thoracic vertebra contains two costal facets on each side of the body. The larger upper facet is located at the superior margin of the vertebral body in front of the pedicle. The smaller inferior facet is apparent at the inferior margin of the vertebral body, anterior to the vertebral notch. Additionally, an oval facet is located at the tip of the transverse process. This facet articulates with the tubercle of the numerically corresponding rib.

The upper costal facets on the body of the first thoracic vertebra are circular in appearance, as they articulate with the entire facet of the first pair of ribs. The ninth thoracic vertebral body may not articulate with the joints of the tenth rib; in these cases, inferior facets are absent on this vertebra. Similarly, its transverse process may or may not have an articular facet. The transverse processes of the eleventh and twelfth ribs also do not have articular facets.

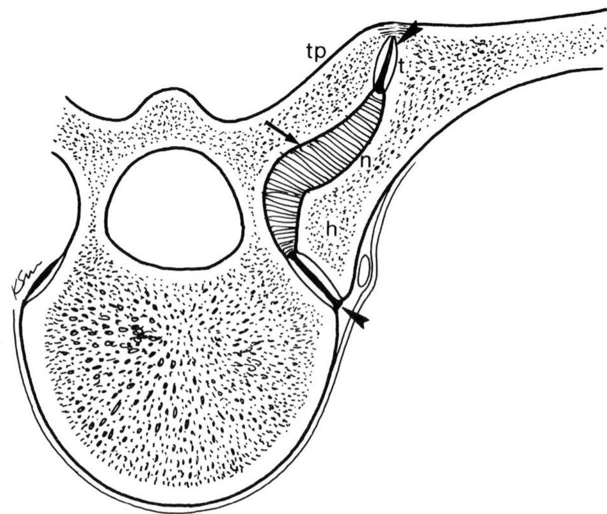

Figure 3–28. *Costovertebral joints: Normal anatomy (transverse section). There are two synovial cavities (arrowheads) separated by costotransverse ligaments (arrow). The head* (h), *neck* (n), *and tubercle* (t) *of the rib are indicated. The head articulates with the vertebral body and the tubercle articulates with the transverse process* (tp) *of the vertebra.*

Soft Tissue Anatomy

Joints of the Heads of Ribs (Fig. 3–28). A short, thick intra-articular ligament extends from the bony crest of the second through ninth ribs to the adjacent intervertebral disc, separating the articular cavity into two parts, each containing synovial membrane. The first, tenth, eleventh, and twelfth ribs articulate with a single vertebral body and hence create a single synovial joint. The articulations are surrounded by a fibrous capsule whose thickened anterior portion is termed the radiate ligament of the head of the rib.

Costotransverse Joints (Fig. 3–28). The costotransverse joint is a synovial articulation surrounded by a fibrous capsule. The lateral costotransverse ligament strengthens the posterolateral aspect of the articulation. The costotransverse ligament also binds the rib and adjacent transverse process, whereas the superior costotransverse ligament attaches the rib to the transverse process of the vertebra above. The costotransverse ligaments of the lowest two ribs are poorly defined or absent, and synovial joints between tubercles of rib and transverse processes of these vertebrae are not present.

At the costotransverse and rib head articulations, minimal gliding movements between articular surfaces are possible. Movements at these two sets of articulations occur simultaneously. The direction of movement varies between upper and lower ribs as the shape of the tubercle facets on these ribs is different.[1] The facets on the upper six ribs are oval in shape and convex from above downward; they fit into concavities on the anterior portion of the transverse processes, allowing upward and downward movement of the tubercle and rotation of the neck of the rib on its longitudinal axis. The facets on the tubercles of the seventh through tenth ribs are relatively flat, facing downward, backward, and medially. They articulate with the superior aspects of the transverse processes. In these articulations, the rib and neck move upward, backward and medially, or downward, forward, and laterally.

JOINTS OF THE VERTEBRAL BODIES

Osseous and Soft Tissue Anatomy

Articulations separating vertebral bodies are two in type: articulations between vertebral bodies that consist of intervertebral discs are symphyses; those between vertebral bodies that consist of anterior and posterior longitudinal ligaments are syndesmoses[1, 2, 83, 84] (Fig. 3–29).

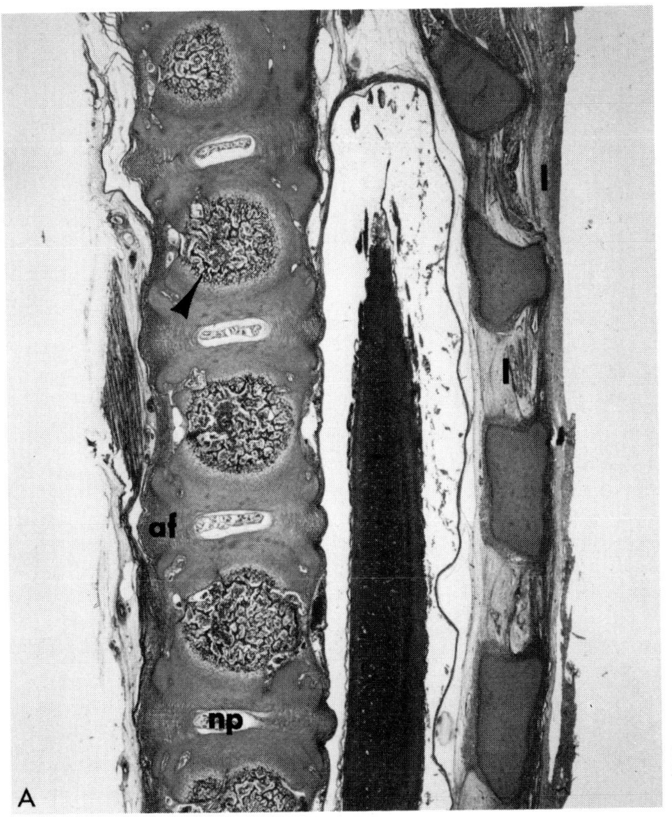

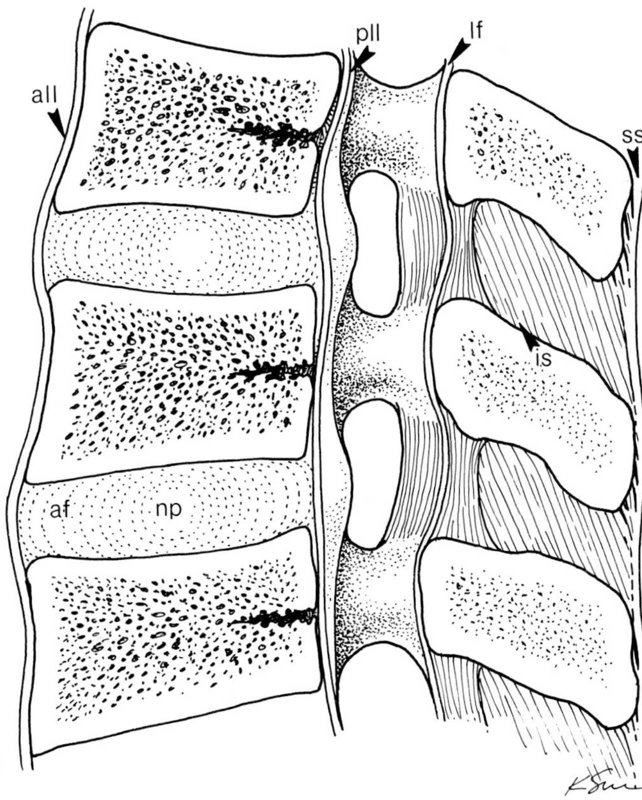

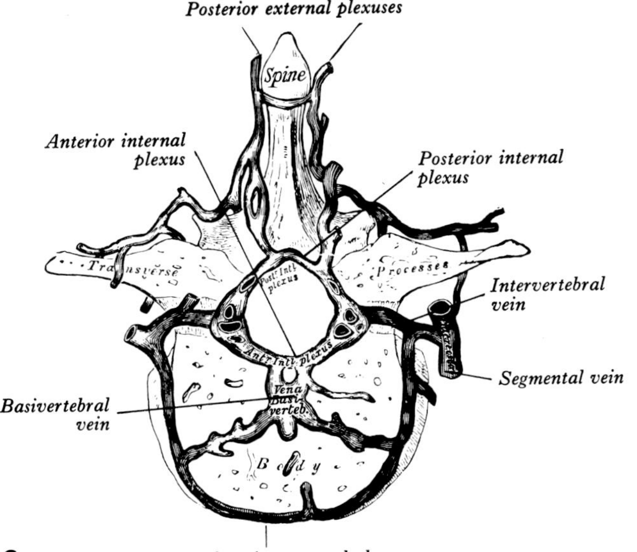

Figure 3–29. Vertebral column. Normal development and anatomy.

A Sagittal section (20×) of fetal spine. Ossification (arrowhead) within the vertebral bodies can be identified. Observe the developing intervertebral disc, consisting of anulus fibrosus (af) and nucleus pulposus (np), spinal cord, and interspinous and supraspinous ligaments (l).

B Drawing of a sagittal section of adult spine depicts vertebral bodies separated by intervertebral discs, consisting of anulus fibrosus (af) and nucleus pulposus (np). The anterior longitudinal ligament (all), posterior longitudinal ligament (pll), ligamentum flavum (lf), and interspinous (is) and supraspinous (ss) ligaments are indicated.

C A transverse section through the body of a thoracic vertebra, showing the vertebral venous plexuses and basivertebral veins. (**C**, From Warwick R, Williams P: Gray's Anatomy. 35th British Edition. Philadelphia, WB Saunders Co, 1973.)

Intervertebral Discs (Fig. 3–29). Intervertebral discs separate the vertebral bodies from the axis to the sacrum. The attachments of the discs include the anterior and posterior longitudinal ligaments and the intra-articular ligaments, which extend to some of the heads of the ribs. The intervertebral discs change in shape and thickness at various levels of the vertebral column. Discs are thickest in the lumbar region and thinnest in the upper thoracic area. In the cervical and lumbar regions, they are thicker anteriorly than posteriorly, whereas in the thoracic region, they are of uniform thickness.

The intervertebral discs between the cervical vertebrae do not extend to the lateral edges of the vertebral bodies (Fig. 3–30). In this area, articular modifications are found on both sides of the intervertebral discs as cleft-like cavities between the superior surface of the uncinate process of one vertebra and

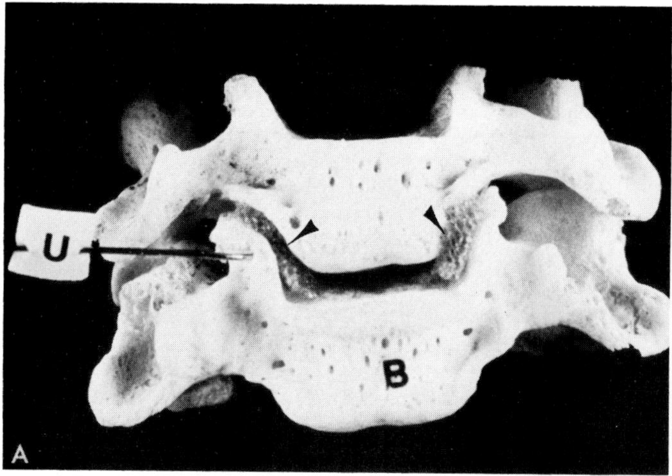

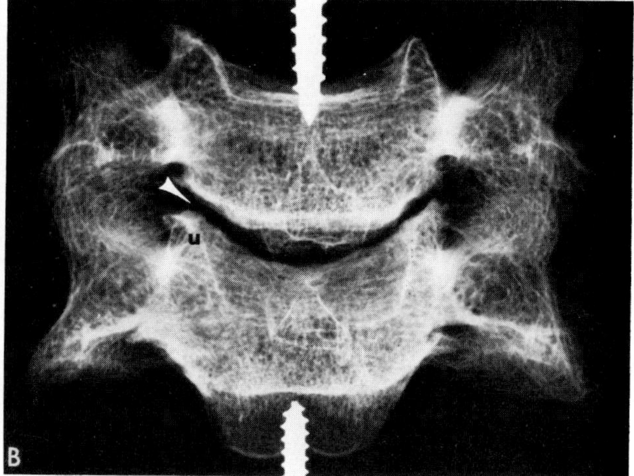

Figure 3–30. *Cervical spine: Joints of Luschka.*

A *On a photograph of the anterior aspect of the cervical spine, the joints of Luschka (arrowheads) are seen between the superior surface of the uncinate process* (U) *of one vertebra* (B) *and the lateral lips of the inferior articulating surface of the vertebra above.*

B *A radiograph of the specimen in* **A** *indicates the structure of the joints of Luschka (arrowhead) and the uncinate processes* (u).

the lateral lips of the inferior articulating surface of the vertebra above. These modifications, called the joints of Luschka, are a source of controversy.[2, 83-86] In the fetus, there are no joints of Luschka. These joints, which form postnatally by fibrillation and fissuring in the marginal fibers of the anulus fibrosus, are usually apparent by 4 years of age and well established by 14 years of age.[85] They may not be present in all individuals or at all cervical spine levels. The lining of the Luschka joint is provided by the cartilaginous end-plate of the vertebral body. A serum transudate is usually present within the cleft, and the arrangement simulates that of a synovial joint. However, a true synovial lining is not apparent.

The individual discs are adherent to hyaline cartilaginous end-plates which cover the central depressions of the upper and lower aspects of the vertebrae (Fig. 3–31). The deep surface of the cartilaginous end-plate contains calcified cartilage. The subchondral bone of the vertebral body is variable in appearance. In some areas, a thick layer of subchondral bone and calcified cartilage can be identified; elsewhere, the bony surface may be thin, with numerous perforations allowing direct contact of bone marrow and nonmineralized cartilage.[87] Complete perforations of the chondro-osseous junction by blood vessels may be noted at the discovertebral junction.[87] Vascular channels embedded within the cartilaginous end-plates are particularly prominent in very young children. They allow diffusion of fluid from bone marrow to intervertebral disc.[88]

Each disc consists of an inner portion, the nucleus pulposus, surrounded by a peripheral portion, the anulus fibrosus. The nucleus pulposus is particularly well developed in the cervical and lumbar segments of the spine. It is eccentrically located, more closely related to the posterior surface of the disc. The nucleus pulposus is soft and gelatinous in young individuals, but it gradually becomes replaced by fibrocartilage with increasing age. In older patients, the nucleus pulposus becomes amorphous, discolored, and dehydrated, and it is difficult to differentiate it from the remainder of the intervertebral disc.[89-92]

The anulus fibrosus encircles the nucleus pulposus and firmly unites the vertebral bodies. This structure consists of a peripheral zone of collagenous fibers and an inner zone of fibrocartilage. The lamellae of the anulus fibrosus are thinner and more closely packed between the nucleus and dorsal aspect of the intervertebral disc. Anteriorly, the lamellae are stronger and more distinct. The direction in which they are oriented varies with their relative position in the intervertebral disc.[83] In central areas, lamellae of the anulus fibrosus curve inward with their convexity facing the nuclear substance. More peripherally, the bands of fibers are vertical. At the extreme periphery of the intervertebral disc, the lamellae may again become curved, with their convexity facing the periphery of the intervertebral disc.

The anulus fibrosus is attached to the adjacent vertebral bodies. This attachment consists essentially of fibers that penetrate the cartilaginous end-plate and subchondral bony trabeculae. A stronger attachment between anulus fibrosus and vertebral body is apparent at the periphery of the intervertebral disc. Here, the fibers of the stoutest external lamellar bands pierce the elevated rim of compact bone on the vertebral body. These fibers, termed Sharpey's fibers, enter the bone at different angles and extend beyond the confines of the intervertebral disc, blending with the periosteum of the vertebral body and longitudinal ligaments.

The two components of the intervertebral disc,

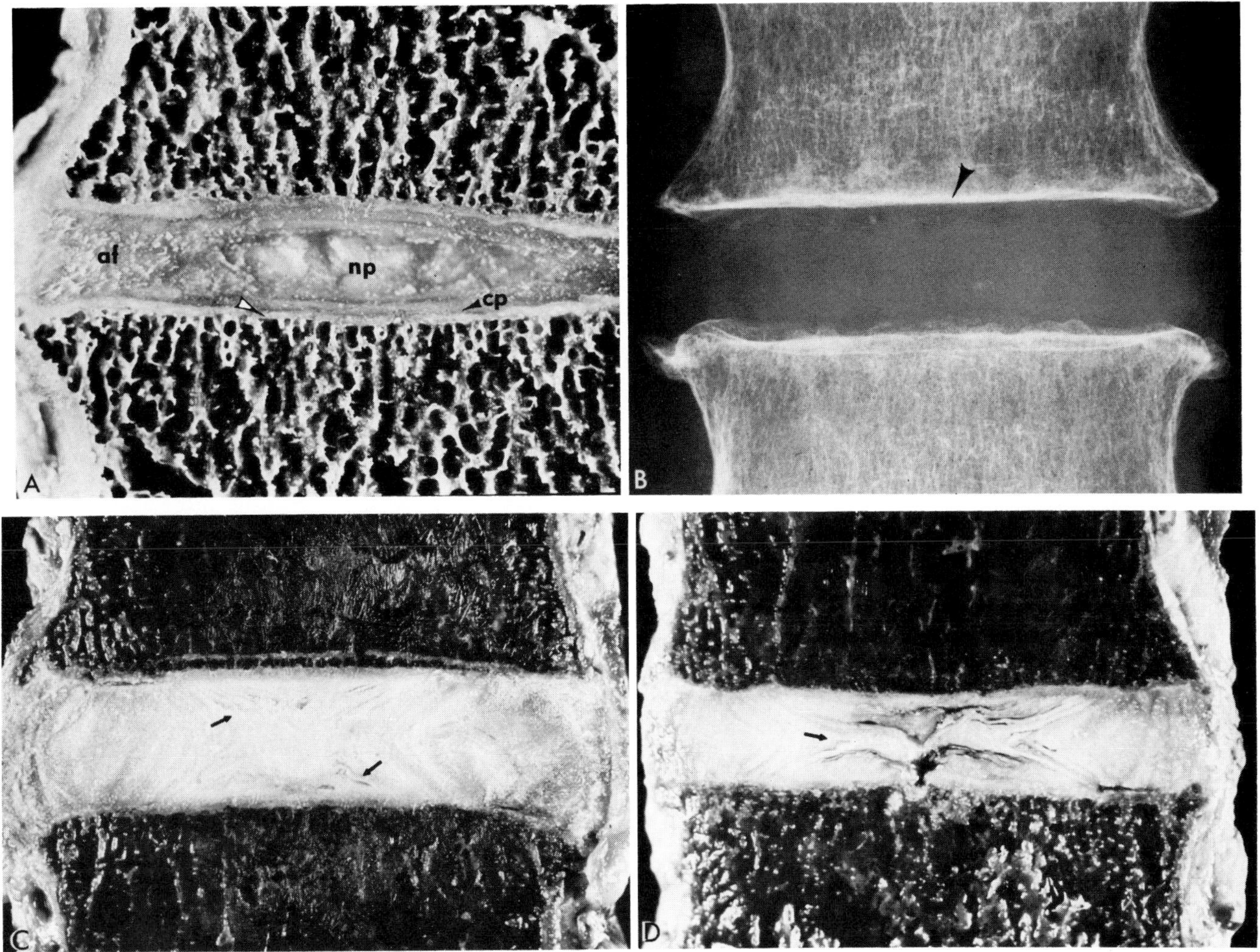

Figure 3–31. *Discovertebral junction: Normal anatomy (coronal section).*

A, B *Labeled structures are the nucleus pulposus (np), anulus fibrosus (af), cartilaginous end-plate (cp), and subchondral bone (arrowhead).*

C, D *Nucleus pulposus. Progressive changes of dehydration and degeneration in two cadavers (coronal sections). Discoloration and fragmentation (arrows) are apparent.*

the anulus fibrosus and nucleus pulposus, are avascular except for the most peripheral fibers of the anulus, which receive a blood supply from adjacent vessels.[93] These penetrating vessels are more prominent in children than in adults,[87] although a secondary ingrowth of vessels may be associated with disc degeneration in older patients.[87, 94] The nutrition of the intervertebral disc is dependent upon (a) diffusion of fluid from the marrow of the vertebral bodies through the porous upper and lower vertebral end-plates in the central portion of the plate, and (b) diffusion of fluid through the anulus fibrosus from the surrounding vessels.[95]

Both external and internal venous plexuses are associated with the vertebral column[95] (Fig. 3–29). The external plexus consists of an anterior and a posterior set of veins. The internal plexus is a series of irregular valveless epidural sinuses that extend from coccyx to foramen magnum. The internal plexus consists of anterior and posterior cross-connected collecting vessels. The anterior channels extend along the posterior surface of the vertebral body just medial to the pedicles and connect to a large unpaired basivertebral sinus that arises within the spongiosa and drains the intraosseous labyrinth of sinusoids. As the internal plexus is valveless, blood can pass in any direction according to shifts in intra-abdominal and intrathoracic pressure. Batson[96] has emphasized that retrograde flow from venous connections to pelvic organs provides an important route for metastasis to both the spine and the trunk areas.

Anterior and Posterior Longitudinal Ligaments. The anterior longitudinal ligament is a strong band of fibers that descends along the anterior surface of the vertebral column. It is relatively narrow in the cervical region and expands in width in the thoracic and lumbar regions, and in the latter area, it covers most of the anterolateral surface of the vertebral bodies and discs. The anterior longitudinal ligament consists of three sets of fibers: deep fibers span only one intervertebral articulation; intermediate fibers unite two or three vertebrae; the superficial layer connects four or five vertebrae.[83] The anterior longitudinal ligament is fixed to the intervertebral discs and vertebral bodies. It is particularly adherent to the articular lip at the edge of each vertebral body but loosely attached at intermediate levels of the bodies. The anterior longitudinal ligament is most readily separated or elevated at the midportion of the intervertebral disc, at which site it is loosely attached to the anulus.

The posterior longitudinal ligament extends along the posterior surface of the vertebral bodies and discs from skull to sacrum, within the vertebral canal. Its fibers are attached only to the intervertebral discs and margins of the vertebral bodies and not to the mid-posterior surface of the bone. In this latter area, the ligament is strung like a bow across the concavity of the posterior osseous surface, allowing venous structures to enter and leave the medullary sinus beneath its fibers. In the cervical and upper thoracic regions, the posterior longitudinal ligament is broad and uniform in width; in the lower thoracic and lumbar regions, it is narrow at the level of the vertebral bodies and broad at the level of the intervertebral discs.

Normal osseous and soft tissue radiography of the anterior vertebral column has received considerable attention. Normal values for the vertical and sagittal diameters of thoracic and lumbar vertebrae and intervertebral discs have been established.[97, 98] Additionally, a cervical prevertebral fat stripe has been described as a linear radiolucency that parallels the anterior surface of the cervical vertebral bodies,[99] which may be a more reliable indicator of disease than other cervical prevertebral soft tissue changes.[100] This lucency, which corresponds to areolar tissue in retropharyngeal and retroesophageal spaces, slants anteriorly at the level of the sixth cervical vertebral body, becoming continuous with areolar tissue behind the scalenus muscles. It is more readily identifiable in adult than in pediatric roentgenograms. Displacement or blurring of this fat plane may be associated with fracture, inflammation, or neoplasm.

JOINTS OF THE VERTEBRAL ARCHES

Articulations between vertebral arches consist of synovial joints (between articular processes of vertebrae) and syndesmoses (ligamentum flavum, interspinous, supraspinous, and intertransverse ligaments, and ligamentum nuchae).

Osseous Anatomy

The vertebral arch contains two pedicles and two laminae, the latter joining posteriorly to become the spinous process. The transverse process and two articular facets originate from a mass of bone at the junction of lamina and pedicle. One articular facet passes superiorly and a second one inferiorly, to articulate with a facet from the vertebrae above and below, respectively.

The orientation and appearance of the articular processes of the vertebrae vary, depending upon the region of the vertebral column. In the cervical spine (C3–C7) the articular processes are large, forming part of a pillar of bone termed the articular mass (Fig. 3–32). The flat, oval facets on these articular processes lie in an oblique coronal plane. The inferior articular facets of the axis (C2) have the same general orientation. In the thoracic spine, the superior articular processes, which face backward, slightly upward, and laterally, appose inferior articular processes, which face in the opposite direction (Fig. 3–33). In the lumbar spine, superior processes face medially and posteriorly, while inferior processes face laterally and anteriorly (Fig. 3–34). These regional differences in the orientation of articular processes require that different projections be utilized for their demonstration on radiographs.[101-104] The articulations of the cervical and thoracic portions of the spine are best demonstrated on lateral roentgenograms, whereas oblique projections are necessary for the lumbar spine. Tomography may be required.

The transverse processes of the vertebrae also demonstrate regional differences. In a typical cervical vertebra, the transverse processes have an anterior and a posterior tubercle, connected by a costotransverse lamella. The adjacent foramen transversarium transmits the vertebral artery, veins, and nerves. The transverse process of the axis (C2) is small and contains no anterior tubercle; that of the atlas (C1) closely resembles that of the axis. In the seventh cervical vertebra, the transverse process may extend anteriorly as a cervical rib. The transverse processes of the thoracic vertebrae have a tubercle for articulation with the corresponding rib tubercle. Transverse processes in the lumbar spine are flat, and the processes of the third lumbar vertebra may be the longest.

In the cervical spine, the spinous processes of the second to fifth vertebrae are frequently bifid. The atlas has no spinous process. In the thoracic spine, spinous processes are long and sloping, whereas in the lumbar spine, these processes are broad and horizontal.

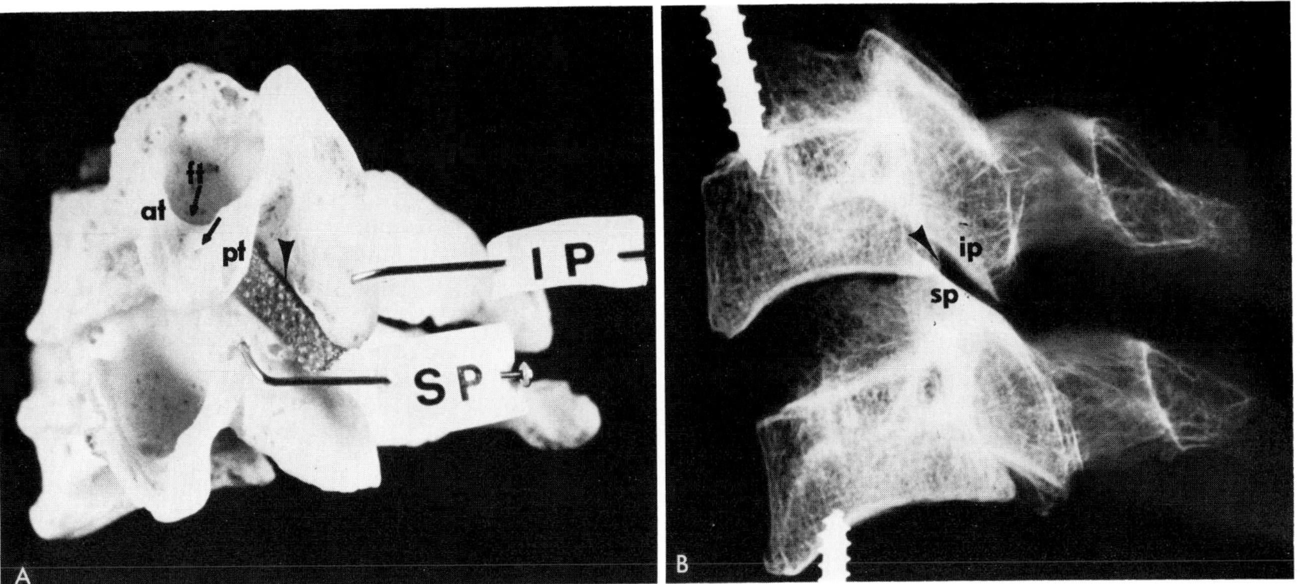

Figure 3–32. Articular processes: Cervical spine. A photograph and radiograph of the lateral aspect of two cervical vertebrae reveal the inferior articular process (ip) and superior articular process (sp), separated by a synovial joint (arrowhead). Observe the anterior tubercle (at) and posterior tubercle (pt) of the transverse process, sulcus for the ventral ramus of spinal nerve (arrow) and foramen transversarium (ft).

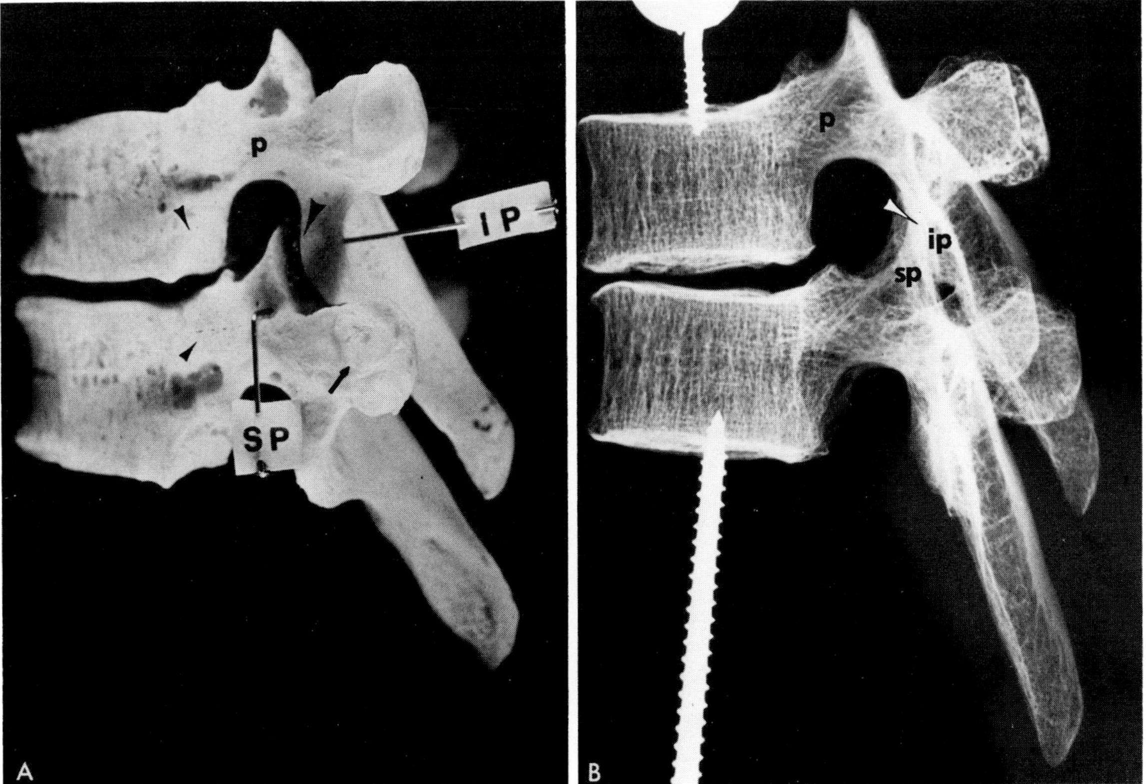

Figure 3–33. Articular processes: Thoracic spine. A photograph and radiograph of the lateral aspect of two thoracic vertebrae demonstrate the inferior articular process (ip) and superior articular process (sp), separated by a synovial joint (large arrowhead). Note the pedicle (p), hemifacets for the head of the rib (small arrowheads), and facet for the rib tubercle (arrow).

Soft Tissue Anatomy

Synovial joints and syndesmoses exist at the joints of the vertebral arches.

Articular Processes (Synovial Joints). The superior articulating process of one vertebra is separated from the inferior articulating process of the vertebra above by a synovial articulation, termed the apophyseal joint. This articulation is surrounded by a loose, thin articular capsule, which is attached to the bones of the adjacent articulating processes. The fibers of the articular capsule are longer and looser in the cervical region and are most taut as one proceeds downward in the vertebral column.

Ligamentous Articulations (Syndesmoses). The syndesmoses between the vertebral arches are formed by the paired sets of ligamenta flava, intertransverse ligaments, and interspinous ligaments, and the unpaired supraspinous ligament.[1, 2, 83]

The ligamenta flava connect the laminae of adjacent vertebrae from the second cervical to the lumbosacral levels. The attachment of the ligamenta flava extends from the articular capsule of the apophyseal joint to the area where the laminae fuse to form the spinous process. A small space or cleft between the two ligaments at this site allows passage of veins from the internal to the external venous plexuses. The ligamentum flavum, which consists predominantly of yellow elastic fibers extending in a perpendicular fashion, is thin and broad in the cervical region, and thicker in the thoracic and lumbar areas. It is the most marked elastic ligament in the human body; it permits separation of the

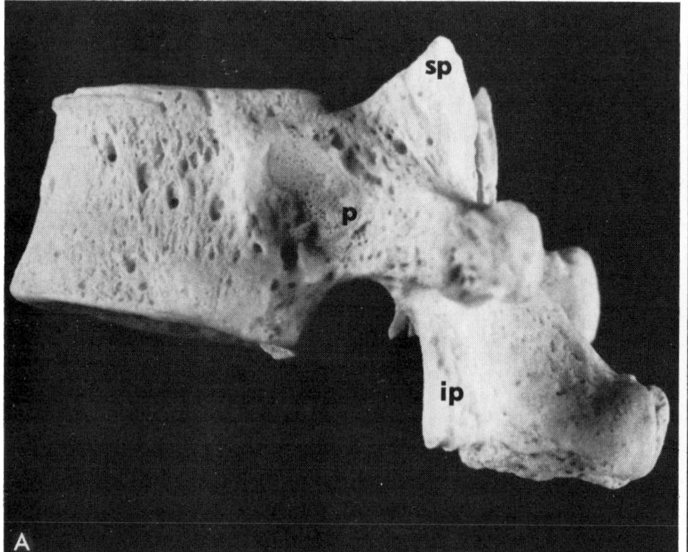

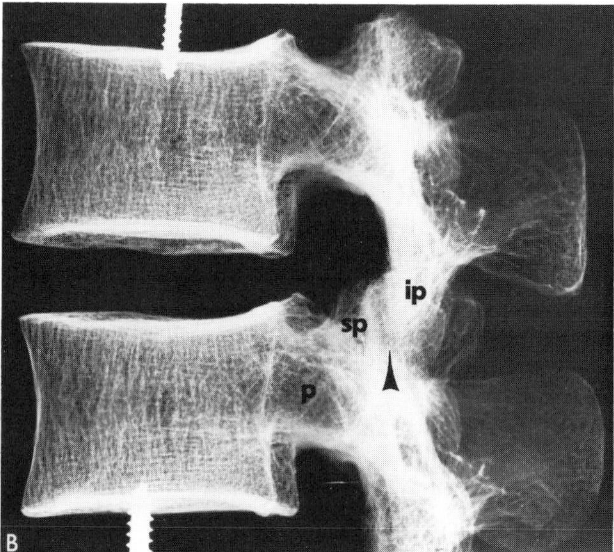

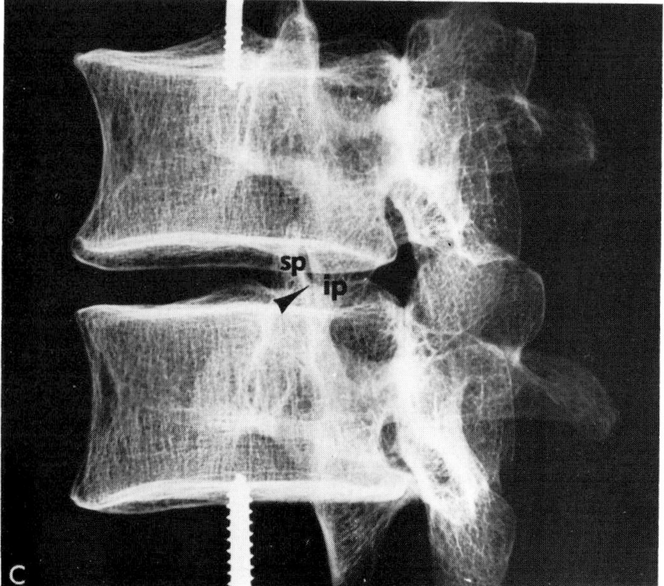

Figure 3–34. *Articular processes: Lumbar spine.*

A, B *A photograph and radiograph of the lateral aspect of the lumbar vertebrae outline the superior articular process (sp) and inferior articular process (ip), separated by a synovial joint (arrowhead). Also observe the pedicles (p).*

C *On a radiograph of the lumbar vertebrae in an oblique projection, the synovial articulation (arrowhead) between superior articular process (sp) and inferior articular process (ip) is better shown.*

laminae with flexion of the vertebral column and does not form redundant folds, which might otherwise compromise adjacent nervous tissue when the spine resumes an erect posture.

Intertransverse ligaments extend between transverse processes. Their appearance varies at different levels of the spine: in the cervical spine, they are absent or consist of a few irregular, scattered fibers; in the thoracic spine they are cords of tissue associated with the deep musculature of the back; and in the lumbar spine, they are thin and membranous.

Interspinous ligaments connect adjoining spinous processes where their attachment extends from the root to apex of the process. These ligaments, which are placed between the ligamentum flavum in front and the supraspinous ligament behind, are longest and strongest in the lumbar spine. Contrast examination of these ligaments has been described.[105]

The supraspinous ligament extends along the tips of the spinous processes from the seventh cervical vertebra to the sacrum. It is fused with the posterior edges of the interspinous ligaments. The most superficial fibers of the supraspinous ligament extend over three to four vertebrae. More deeply situated fibers extend over two to three vertebrae. The supraspinous ligament is broader and thicker in the lumbar spine than in the thoracic spine. In the cervical spine, the supraspinous ligament merges with the triangular ligamentum nuchae, the latter passing from the external occipital protuberance to the seventh cervical vertebra. Deep fibers of the ligamentum nuchae extend to the cervical spinous processes and the posterior tubercle of the atlas. Its role or function may be to assist in head position and control.[106]

MOVEMENTS OF THE VERTEBRAL COLUMN

The erect adult vertebral column has four anteroposterior curves, two of which are regarded as primary. An elongated curve, concave ventrally, extends throughout the thoracic spine. A second primary curve, also concave ventrally, is located in the sacral and coccygeal region. Secondary curves include a cervical curve, concave posteriorly, and a lumbar curve, also concave posteriorly.

The range of motion is slight between any two adjacent vertebrae due to the limited degree of deformation of the intervertebral disc, but the total vertebral movement is considerable.[1, 2, 83] Movements include flexion, extension, lateral bending, rotation, and circumduction. In flexion, the anterior longitudinal ligament is lax and the anterior aspect of the intervertebral disc is compressed. The posterior fibers of the intervertebral discs, posterior longitudinal ligament, and posterior spinal ligaments (ligamenta flava, interspinous and supraspinous ligaments) are stretched, although the fundamental limiting factor to flexion is the tension of the posterior vertebral muscles. During flexion, the space between adjacent laminae is widened, and the inferior articulating process of one vertebra moves superiorly on the superior articulating process of the vertebra below.

In extension, the vertebrae move backward on each other, particularly in the cervical and lumbar segments. During this movement, the anterior longitudinal ligament becomes taut, whereas the other ligaments of the vertebral column are relaxed. In lateral bending, which involves predominantly the cervical and lumbar segments, compression of the lateral aspects of the intervertebral discs is apparent.

Rotation, most prominent in the upper thoracic region, results in twisting of one vertebra in relation to the others, with tortional deformation of intervening intervertebral discs.

Regional differences exist in the degree and type of spinal movement. In the cervical spine, the upper inclination of the superior articulating facets allows considerable flexion and extension. This freedom of motion is accentuated by the relatively large size of the intervertebral discs compared to the length of the bony cervical column. Lateral flexion and rotation in the cervical spine occur simultaneously. In the thoracic spine, motion is limited because the intervertebral discs are relatively thin, the superior articulating facets lack an upward inclination, and adjacent bony structures such as ribs and sternum produce additional stability. Rotation is free, as the articular processes lie in an arch of a circle with its center at or near the center of the vertebral bodies.[107] In the lumbar spine, the intervertebral discs are prominent, allowing considerable flexion and extension. Rotation is somewhat restricted by the articular processes.

ATLANTO-AXIAL JOINTS

Osseous Anatomy

The ring-like first cervical vertebra, the atlas, does not possess a vertebral body or a spinous process (Fig. 3–35). It contains a small anterior arch, with a tubercle, a larger posterior arch with a corresponding tubercle, and two bulky lateral masses. The inferior surface of each lateral mass possesses a circular facet that is flat or slightly concave. This facet articulates with a corresponding facet on the superior articular process of the axis. The articular facet of the atlas is oriented inferiorly, medially, and slightly posteriorly. The medial portion of the lateral

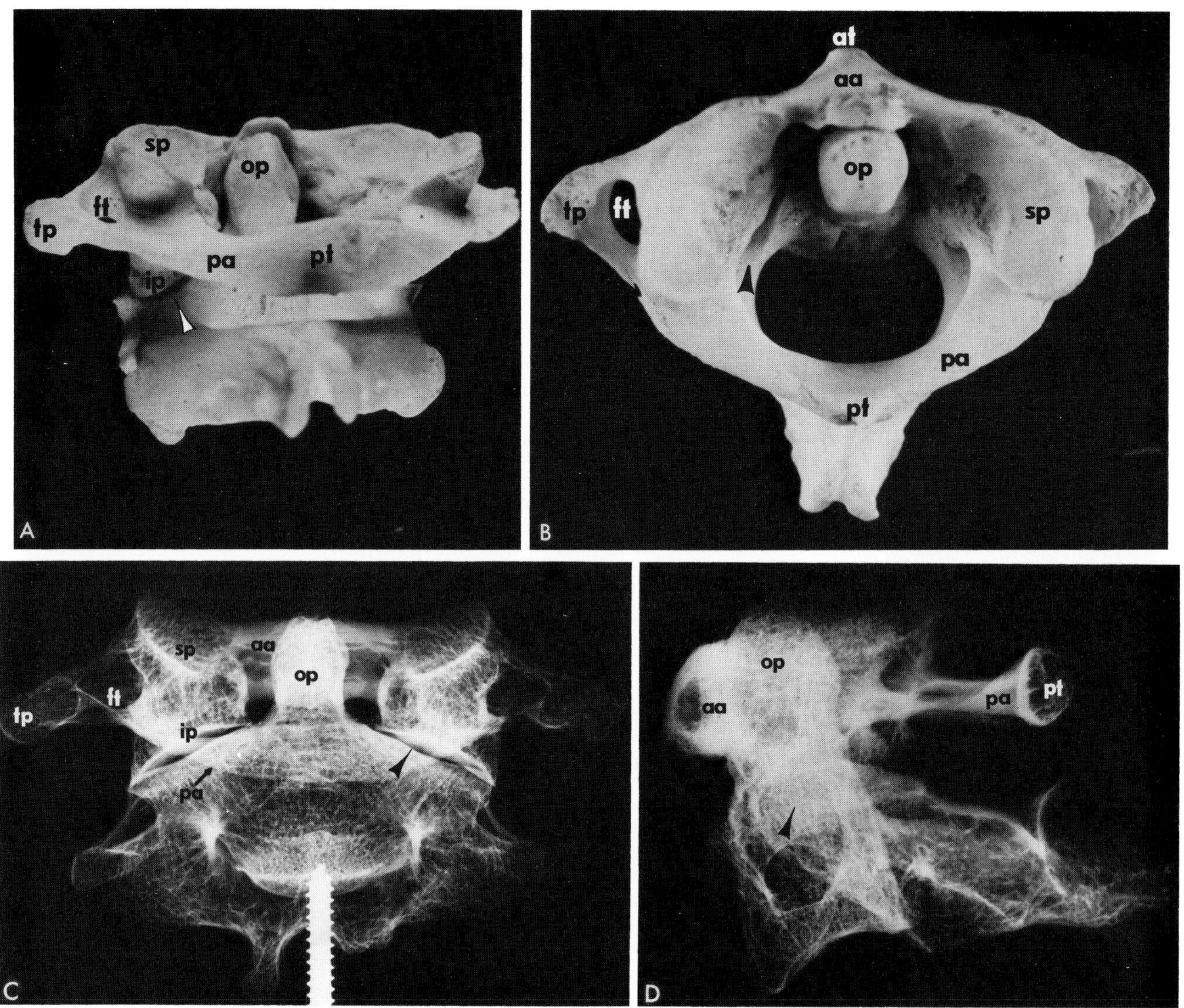

Figure 3–35. *Atlas and axis: Osseous anatomy.*

A, B *Posterior* **(A)** *and superior* **(B)** *views. Observe the anterior arch* (aa)*, posterior arch* (pa)*, anterior tubercle* (at)*, posterior tubercle* (pt)*, superior articular process* (sp)*, inferior articular process* (ip)*, transverse process* (tp)*, and foramen transversarium* (ft) *of the atlas, and the odontoid process* (op) *and superior articular process (arrowhead) of the axis.*

C, D *Frontal* **(C)** *and lateral* **(D)** *radiographs of atlas and axis.*

mass is roughened for the attachment of the transverse ligament of the atlas. The transverse processes of the atlas are long.

The second cervical vertebra, the axis, contains a superior peg of bone, the dens or odontoid process, which possesses a small oval facet for articulation with a facet on the posterior surface of the anterior arch of the atlas. On the posterior surface of the odontoid process is a groove for the transverse ligament of the atlas. The odontoid process is approximately 1.3 to 1.5 cm in length with flat sides and a pointed apex. The axis also possesses two slightly convex superior articular facets, facing superiorly and laterally, which are intimate with similar facets on the atlas. Posterior to the superior facets are inferior facets, which articulate with the third cervical vertebra. The transverse processes of the axis are small, with a single tubercle.

On lateral radiographs of the cervical spine, the normal space between the anterior arch of the atlas and the odontoid process of the axis in the adult is 1.238 − (0.0074 × age in years), plus or minus 0.90 mm in women, and 2.052 − (0.0192 × age in years), plus or minus 1.00 mm in men.[108] A useful rule is that this distance should not be greater than 2.5 mm in adults. In children the average distance between the anterior arch of the atlas and the odontoid process is 2.0 to 2.5 mm in extension and 2.0 to

3.0 mm in flexion.[109] This distance should not exceed 4.5 mm in children. An increase in distance between the anterior arch of the first cervical vertebra and the odontoid process is common in a variety of diseases, including articular and inflammatory disorders.

Soft Tissue Anatomy

Four synovial articulations occur between the atlas and axis: two lateral atlanto-axial joints, one on each side, between the inferior facet of the lateral mass of the atlas and the superior facet of the axis; two medial synovial joints, one between the anterior arch of the atlas and the odontoid process of the axis and a second between the odontoid process and the transverse ligament of the atlas (Fig. 3–36). In addition to these synovial articulations, syndesmoses between the atlas and axis include a continuation of the anterior longitudinal ligament anteriorly, and the ligamenta flava posteriorly.

LATERAL ATLANTO-AXIAL JOINTS. These synovial articulations exist on either side between the reciprocally curved cartilage-covered lateral masses of the atlas and axis, and are surrounded by thin, loose fibrous capsules. Each capsule is strengthened posteromedially by an accessory ligament, which extends from the body of the axis to the lateral mass of the atlas.

MEDIAN ATLANTO-AXIAL JOINTS. Two synovial articulations exist between the odontoid process of the axis and a ring formed by the anterior arch and transverse ligament of the atlas. The smaller of these two joints is located between a facet on the anterior surface of the odontoid and a second facet on the posterior surface of the anterior arch of the atlas. A weak, loose fibrous capsule surrounds this articulation. A second, larger joint lies between the cartilage-covered anterior surface of the transverse ligament of the atlas and the grooved posterior surface of the odontoid process. This articulation, which is also surrounded by a loose fibrous capsule, may be continuous with the articular cavity of one or both atlanto-occipital joints.[1, 110]

Movement at the atlanto-axial articulations occurs at all locations simultaneously. This movement results in rotation of the skull and atlas with respect to the axis. The lateral masses of the atlas glide on the upper articular facets of the axis. This rotation is accompanied by a slight vertical descent of the head related to the oblique character of the articular surfaces. Excessive rotation is limited by the alar ligaments (extending from the odontoid

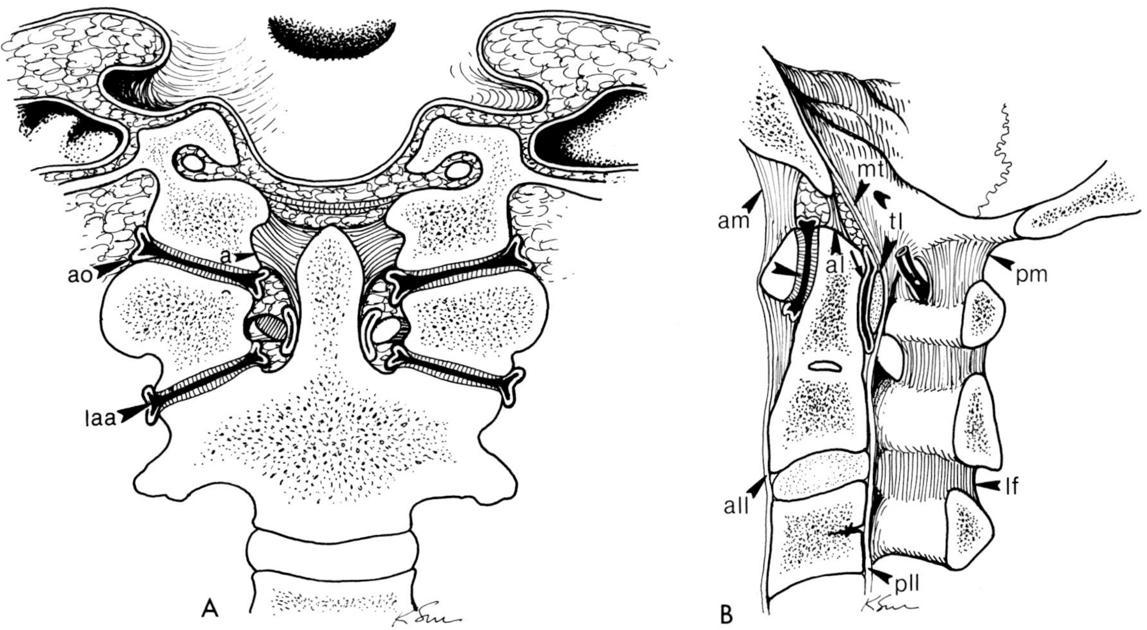

Figure 3–36. *Atlanto-axial and atlanto-occipital joints: Anatomy. Drawing of coronal* **(A)** *and sagittal* **(B)** *sections of the base of the skull and upper cervical spine. Note the lateral atlanto-axial joints* (laa), *atlanto-occipital synovial joints* (ao), *anterior median joint (arrowhead) between the odontoid process and anterior arch of the atlas, and posterior median joint (arrow) between the odontoid process and transverse ligament* (tl) *of the atlas. Additional structures are the anterior longitudinal ligament* (all), *posterior longitudinal ligament* (pll), *membrana tectoria* (mt), *anterior atlanto-occipital membane* (am), *posterior atlanto-occipital membrane* (pm), *apical ligament of odontoid process* (al), *alar ligament* (a), *and ligamentum flavum* (lf).

process to the occipital condyles) and, to a lesser extent, by the accessory atlanto-axial ligaments.

ATLANTO-OCCIPITAL JOINTS

Osseous Anatomy

The superior surface of each lateral mass of the atlas has a concave, kidney-shaped facet that articulates with the corresponding occipital condyle. This atlantial facet is oriented medially and superiorly. The occipital condyles are oval, located on the anterolateral aspect of the foramen magnum.

Soft Tissue Anatomy

The atlanto-occipital joints consist of a pair of synovial articulations between the articular facets of the atlas and the condyles of the occiput, and syndesmoses formed by the anterior and posterior atlanto-occipital membranes (Fig. 3–36).

ATLANTO-OCCIPITAL SYNOVIAL JOINTS. Reciprocally curved superior articular facets of the lateral mass of the atlas[111] and condyle of the occipital bone are separated by a synovial articulation surrounded by a fibrous capsule.[112] The capsule is particularly thick on its posterior and lateral surfaces but deficient medially, where it may allow communication of these joints with the synovial articulation between the odontoid process and the transverse ligament.[110]

ATLANTO-OCCIPITAL MEMBRANES. The anterior atlanto-occipital membrane is attached above to the anterior margin of the foramen magnum and below to the anterior arch of the atlas. Its central portion contains fibers continuous with those of the anterior longitudinal ligament. The posterior atlanto-occipital membrane is attached above to the posterior margin of the foramen magnum and below to the posterior arch of the atlas. The free border of this membrane arches over the vertebral artery and first cervical spinal nerve. This border may occasionally ossify.

Movement at the atlanto-occipital joints occurs as flexion, extension, and lateral bending and may produce changes elsewhere in the cervical spine.[113-115] No significant rotation is present between the occiput and the atlas.

OCCIPITAL-AXIAL SYNDESMOSES

Ligamentous structures connecting the axis and the occiput are the membrana tectoria, paired alar ligaments, and an apical ligament. The membrana tectoria appears as an upward continuation of the posterior longitudinal ligament, which extends from the axis to the occiput. The alar ligaments pass from the upper surface of the odontoid on each side to the medial sides of the occipital condyles. The apical ligament of the odontoid lies between the alar ligaments and runs from the tip of the process to the anterior margin of the foramen magnum. It blends both with the anterior atlanto-occipital membrane and with the cruciform ligament of the atlas.

OSSEOUS RELATIONSHIPS OF CERVICOBASILAR JUNCTION

The osseous relationships at the cervicobasilar junction have received considerable attention (Fig. 3–37). Chamberlain's line[219] can be drawn on a lateral radiograph from the posterior margin of the hard palate to the posterior border of the foramen magnum. In normal situations, the odontoid process should not extend more than 5 mm above this line. A modification of this line, McGregor's line,[224] utilizes the inferior surface of the occiput rather than the margin of the foramen magnum. In normal individuals, the odontoid tip does not extend more than 7 mm above this line. On frontal radiographs, a line connecting the mastoid tips is within 2 mm of the tip of the odontoid,[225] whereas a line connecting the digastric muscle fossae is located at the approximate level of the foramen magnum and above the odontoid process. The basilar angle is the angle of intersection of two lines, one drawn from the nasion to the tuberculum sellae and a second from the tuberculum to the anterior edge of the foramen magnum. This angle normally does not exceed 140 degrees. An atlanto-occipital joint angle is constructed on frontal tomograms by drawing a line along this articulation on either side. The angle formed by the intersection of these two lines should normally not exceed 150 degrees.

JOINTS OF THE SACRUM AND COCCYX

Included here are the lumbosacral, sacrococcygeal, and intercoccygeal joints. The sacroiliac joints will be discussed separately.

Osseous Anatomy

The fifth lumbar vertebra resembles the other lumbar vertebrae, although it has a larger transverse process and body and a smaller spinous process (Fig. 3–38). Although the superior articular processes are

Text continued on page 100

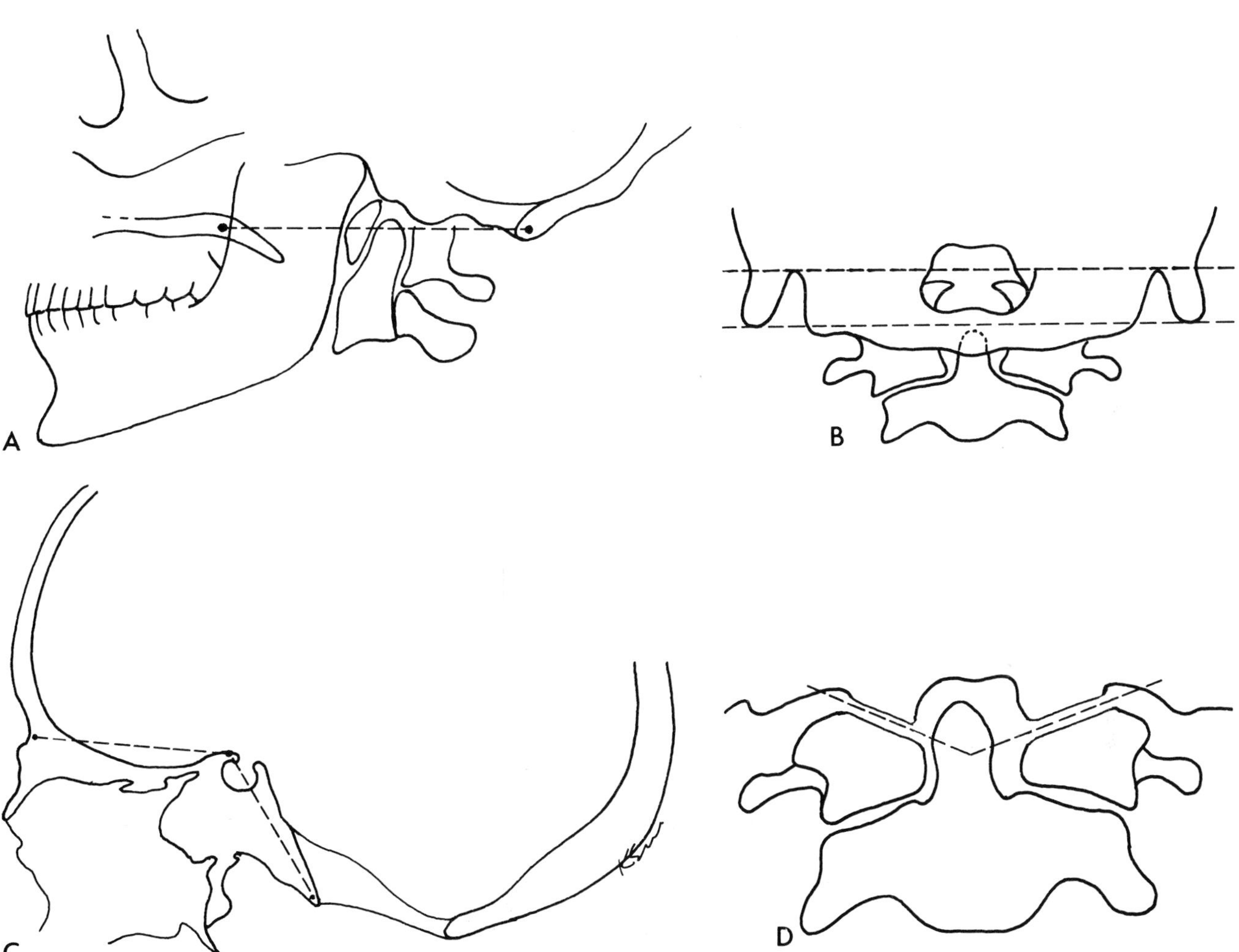

Figure 3–37. *Cervicobasilar junction: Normal osseous relationships.*

A *Chamberlain's line is drawn from the posterior margin of the hard palate to the posterior border of the foramen magnum. The odontoid process does not normally extend more than 5 mm above this line.*

B *The bimastoid line (lower line) connecting the tips of the mastoids is normally within 2 mm of the odontoid tip. The digastric line (upper line) connecting the digastric muscle fossae is normally located above the odontoid process.*

C *The basilar angle, which normally exceeds 140 degrees, is formed by the angle of intersection of two lines, one drawn from the nasion to the tuberculum sellae and a second from the latter structure to the anterior edge of the foramen magnum.*

D *An atlanto-occipital joint angle, constructed on frontal tomograms by the intersection of two lines drawn along the axes of these articulations, normally is not greater than 150 degrees.*

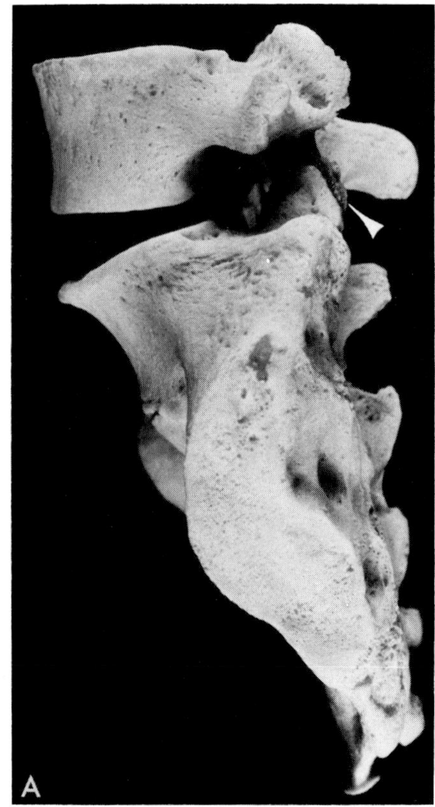

Figure 3–38. *Sacrum: Osseous anatomy.*

A *Lumbosacral junction. Note the synovial joint (arrowhead) between the inferior articular process of the fifth lumbar vertebra and the superior articular process of the sacrum.*

Illustration continued on the opposite page

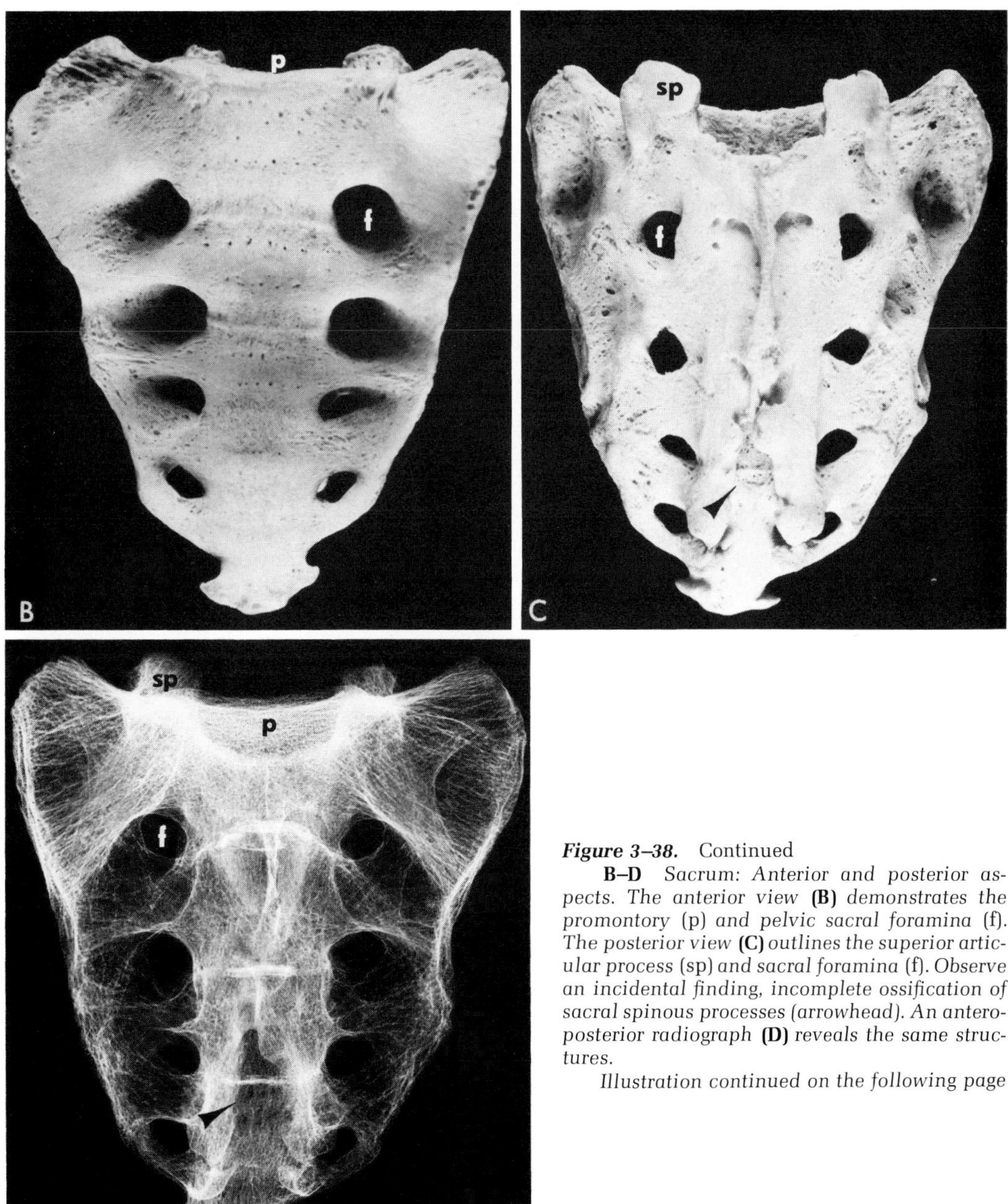

Figure 3–38. Continued

B–D *Sacrum: Anterior and posterior aspects. The anterior view* **(B)** *demonstrates the promontory* (p) *and pelvic sacral foramina* (f). *The posterior view* **(C)** *outlines the superior articular process* (sp) *and sacral foramina* (f). *Observe an incidental finding, incomplete ossification of sacral spinous processes (arrowhead). An anteroposterior radiograph* **(D)** *reveals the same structures.*

Illustration continued on the following page

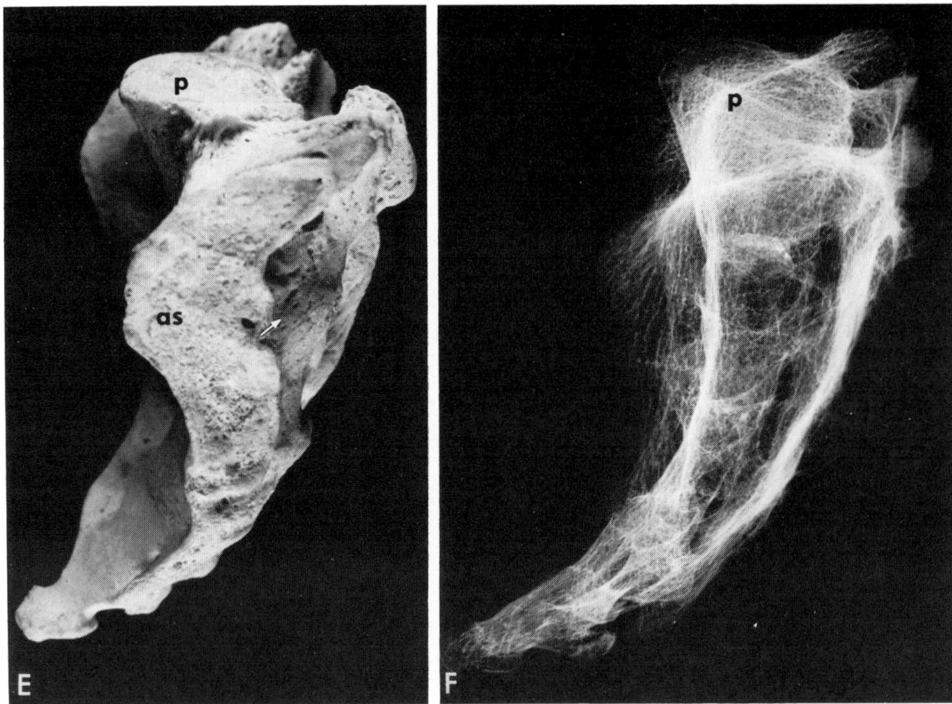

Figure 3–38. Continued
E, F *Sacrum: Lateral aspect. The promontory* (p) *and auricular articular surface* (as) *are observed. Areas of ligamentous attachment (arrow) are located behind the articular surface.*

wider than the inferior articular processes in the upper lumbar region, these processes are of approximately equal size in the fifth lumbar vertebra.

The sacrum is a large triangular bone (Fig. 3–38). The superiorly located base of the sacrum articulates with the fifth lumbar vertebra, creating the sacrovertebral angle. This angle represents the most abrupt change of alignment in the vertebral column and, as such, is subject to shearing forces. Measurement of this angle in both normal and abnormal situations has been undertaken. In a lateral projection with the spine parallel to the table, the angle of intersection of two lines, one drawn along the inclination of the first sacral surface, and a second, a line of the horizontal, is normally less than 34 degrees.[116]

The concave superior articular processes of the sacrum project upward to articulate with the inferior articular processes of the fifth lumbar vertebra. These sacral processes face posteriorly and medially.

Transitional type vertebral bodies are not infrequent at the lumbosacral junction. Expanded transverse processes of the fifth lumbar vertebra articulate with the top of the sacrum in either a unilateral or bilateral distribution, or the entire vertebra may be incorporated into the sacrum. This process is termed sacralization of the fifth lumbar vertebra. Similarly, lumbarization represents elevation of the first sacral segment above the sacral mass so that it assumes the shape of a lumbar vertebra. As the radiographic appearance of sacralization and lumbarization is similar, an accurate diagnosis may require investigation of the entire vertebral column. The reported incidence of transitional type situations at the lumbosacral junction has varied from 0.6 to 25 per cent of individuals.[84] When the transverse processes of the transitional vertebra are connected to the lateral mass of the sacrum by means of an articulation, true joints with cartilaginous surfaces, articular capsules, supporting ligaments, and even bursae are present.

The apex of the sacrum represents the inferior surface of the body of the fifth sacral vertebrae. An oval facet that articulates with the coccyx is apparent. The coccyx consists of three to five rudimentary vertebrae. Its upper surface or base contains an oval facet that articulates with the sacrum. Lateral to this facet are two processes, the coccygeal cornua, which are analogous to superior articular processes and pedicles of the more cephalad vertebrae. These cornua extend superiorly to articulate with the sacral cornua.

Soft Tissue Anatomy

Lumbosacral Joints. The fifth lumbar vertebra and the first sacral segment are united by a series of articulations that resemble those present at other levels of the vertebral column. These articulations include a symphysis (intervertebral disc), syndesmoses (anterior and posterior longitudinal ligaments, ligamenta flava, interspinous and supraspinous ligaments), and synovial joints (articular processes). One additional syndesmosis peculiar to this region is the iliolumbar ligament. This strong ligament extends from its medial attachment to the fifth lumbar transverse process (and occasionally to the fourth lumbar transverse process) to the pelvis. Two pelvic attachments are apparent. An upper band attaches to the iliac crest and a lower band attaches to the anterosuperior aspect of the sacrum, which blends with the ventral sacroiliac ligament.

The synovial articulations at the lumbosacral junction, consisting of articular facets on the fifth lumbar vertebra and sacrum, are suited for some degree of rotatory movement, although the iliolumbar ligaments certainly inhibit this motion. These synovial articulations must resist forward and downward displacement of the fifth lumbar vertebral body in relation to the sacrum.

Sacrococcygeal Joint. This articulation contains a symphysis, between the apex of the sacrum and the base of the coccyx, surrounded by ventral, dorsal, and lateral sacrococcygeal ligaments. The central fibrocartilaginous disc is thicker anteriorly and posteriorly and thinner laterally. The sacrococcygeal joint may become partially or completely obliterated in advanced age. Rarely, a freely movable coccyx articulates with the sacrum by a synovial joint.[1]

Intercoccygeal Joints. In young individuals, symphyses consisting of thin fibrocartilaginous discs exist between the coccygeal segments. In adult men, these symphyses may become obliterated at a younger age than in adult women. Rarely, the articulation between the first and second coccygeal segments is synovial in type. Throughout life, the coccygeal segments are also connected by ventral and dorsal sacrococcygeal ligaments.

SACROILIAC JOINTS

Osseous Anatomy

The apposing osseous surfaces of the sacrum and the ilium are irregular in character and allow interdigitation of sacrum and ilium, which contributes to the strength of the articulation and to its restricted motion (Fig. 3–39). The laterally located L-shaped auricular surface of the sacrum articulates with the ilium. Irregular osseous pits, which are the

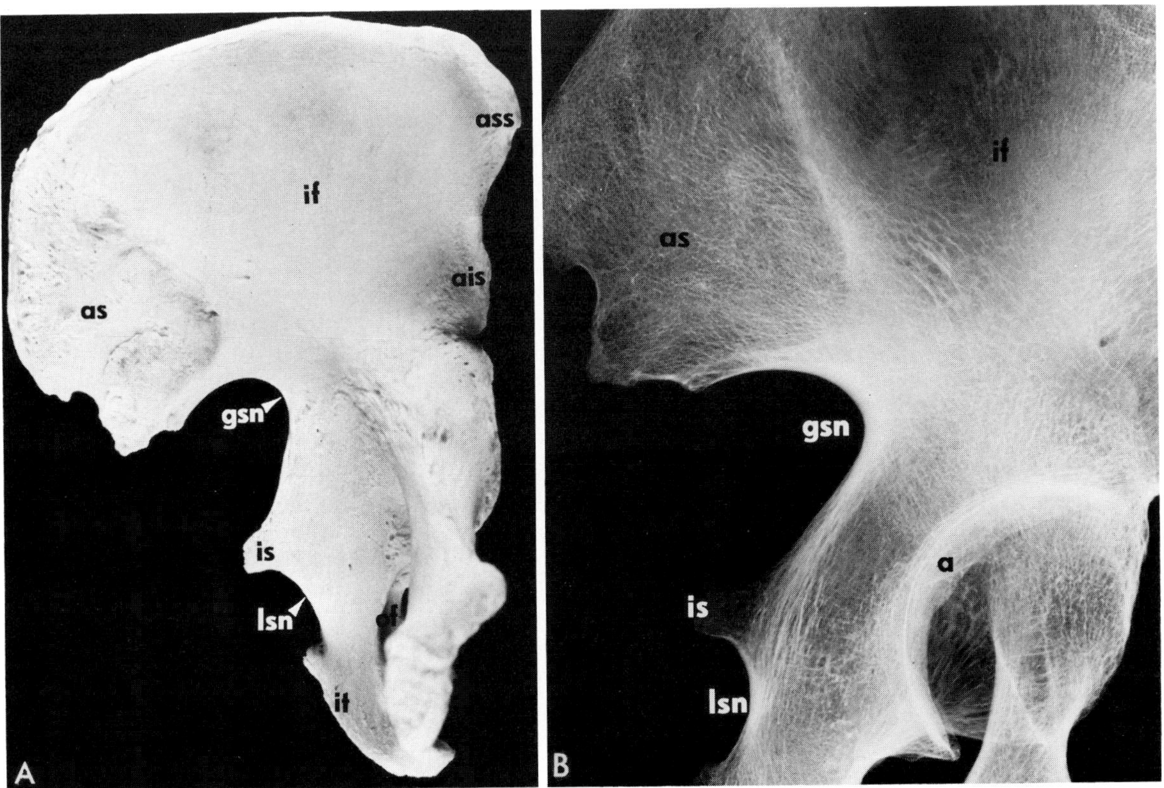

Figure 3–39. *Innominate bone: Osseous anatomy — internal (medial) aspect. Labeled structures are the auricular surface of ilium* (as), *iliac fossa* (if), *anterior superior iliac spine* (ass), *anterior inferior iliac spine* (ais), *ischial spine* (is), *lesser sciatic notch* (lsn), *greater sciatic notch* (gsn), *ischial tuberosity* (it), *obturator foramen* (of), *and acetabulum* (a).

site of attachment of various ligaments, are located posterior to the auricular surface. The auricular surface of the ilium is located on the medial aspect of the bone, inferior and anterior to the iliac tuberosity. The sharp anterior portion of the auricular surface is the site of attachment of the ventral sacroiliac ligament. This ligament also attaches to the preauricular sulcus, a groove at the inferior pelvic surface of the ilium, which is more prominent in women.

Soft Tissue Anatomy

The articulation between auricular surfaces of sacrum and ilium is synovial in type (Fig. 3–40). The auricular surface of the sacrum is covered with a thick layer of hyaline cartilage and that on the ilium is clothed by a thinner layer of fibrocartilage.[117, 118] This joint has a complete fibrous capsule, which is attached close to the margins of the adjacent surfaces of sacrum and ilium and is lined with synovial membrane. A joint cavity is apparent in younger individuals but with advancing age, fibrous and fibrocartilaginous adhesions may obliterate this cavity.[119-122]

A thin and broad band of tissue, the ventral sacroiliac ligament, is noted in front of the joint. Posteriorly, a deep thick interosseous sacroiliac ligament extends above the articular surface to fill the superior cleft between the sacrum and the ilium. The dorsal sacroiliac ligament courses superficially to the interosseous ligament, extending medially and inferiorly, some fibers running from the posterior superior iliac spine to the third and fourth sacral segments. These fibers may merge with a portion of the sacrotuberous ligament.[123]

Accessory synovial articulations are not uncommon between the lateral sacral crest and the posterior superior iliac spine and ilial tuberosity.[124]

Movement at the sacroiliac joint is limited, restricted by the undulating articular surfaces and thick dorsal sacroiliac ligaments.[125, 126] A slight degree of anterior and posterior rotary movement may occur.[123] This movement may be accentuated during pregnancy as hormonal influences result in softening and relaxation of the sacroiliac ligaments and symphysis pubis.[127, 128]

Radiographic evaluation of the sacroiliac joint is difficult.[129, 130] It is important to realize that only the lower one half to two thirds of the space between the sacrum and the ilium represents the synovial articulation; the superior aspect of this space is ligamentous. In young adults, the interosseous joint space is 2 to 5 mm, reflecting the combined thickness of sacral and ilial cartilage.[122, 131] Diminution of joint space is common in patients over 40 years of age and increases in frequency thereafter.[117] Bony ankylosis of the articulation has been reported in older patients.[117, 120, 122]

PELVIC-VERTEBRAL LIGAMENTS

In addition to the iliolumbar ligaments, other important ligaments connecting the pelvis and the vertebral column are the sacrotuberous and sacrospinous ligaments (Fig. 3–41). The sacrotuberous ligament extends from the posterior iliac spines, sacrum, and coccyx to the ischial tuberosity with some fibers running along the ischial ramus. The sacrospinous ligament runs from the ischial spine to the sacrum and the coccyx, where it merges with the fibers of the sacrotuberous ligament. These ligaments stabilize the lower portion of the sacrum and convert the sciatic notches into greater and lesser sciatic foramina.

SYMPHYSIS PUBIS

Osseous Anatomy

The medial aspect of the pubis, the symphyseal surface, articulates with its counterpart on the opposite side (Fig. 3–42). This surface is generally oval in shape, and the apposing bony margins are somewhat irregular in contour[132, 133]

Soft Tissue Anatomy

The symphysis pubis is a median cartilaginous articulation between the pubic bones (Fig. 3–42). Each pubic articular surface is clothed with a thin layer of hyaline cartilage united to its counterpart by a thick fibrocartilaginous disc, the interpubic disc. This disc may contain a cavity, probably related to softening and deformation of the cartilage. This cavity which begins in the posterosuperior aspect of the disc, rarely before the tenth year of life, may eventually extend throughout the cartilage.[1, 2] The cavity is more prominent in women and is not lined by synovial membrane. It may account for "vacuum" phenomena on radiographs in which radiolucent streaks of gas within the cavity become apparent.[134, 135]

A superior pubic ligament attached to the pubic crest and tubercles on each side strengthens the anterior aspect of the symphysis pubis. The arcuate pubic ligament connects the lower portion of the pubic bones.

Radiographic evaluation of the adult symphysis pubis reveals a mean transverse width of approximately 6 mm in men and 5 mm in women.[136] The width of the symphysis pubis may increase in pregnancy, averaging 7 mm.[135] This apparent increase in joint size during pregnancy probably relates to softening and relaxation of pelvic ligaments, accounting

Text continued on page 107

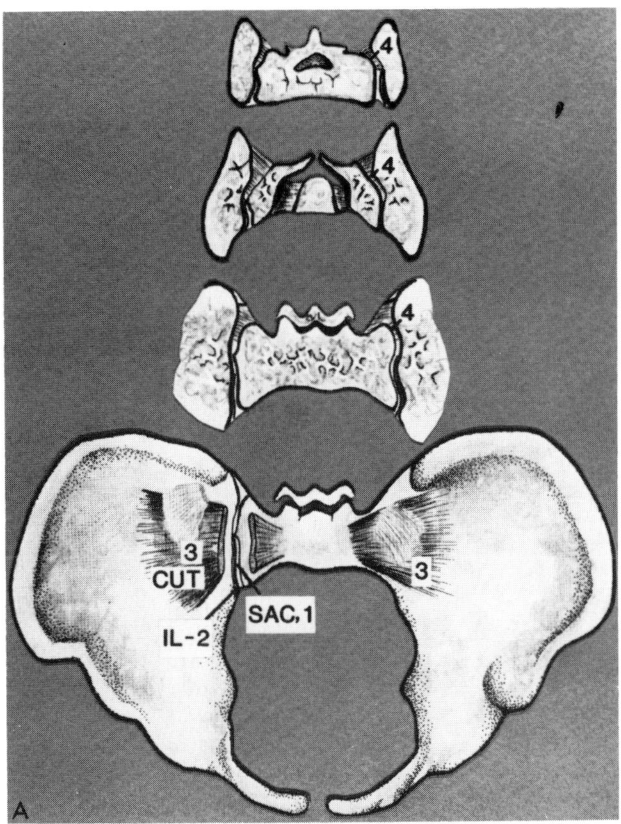

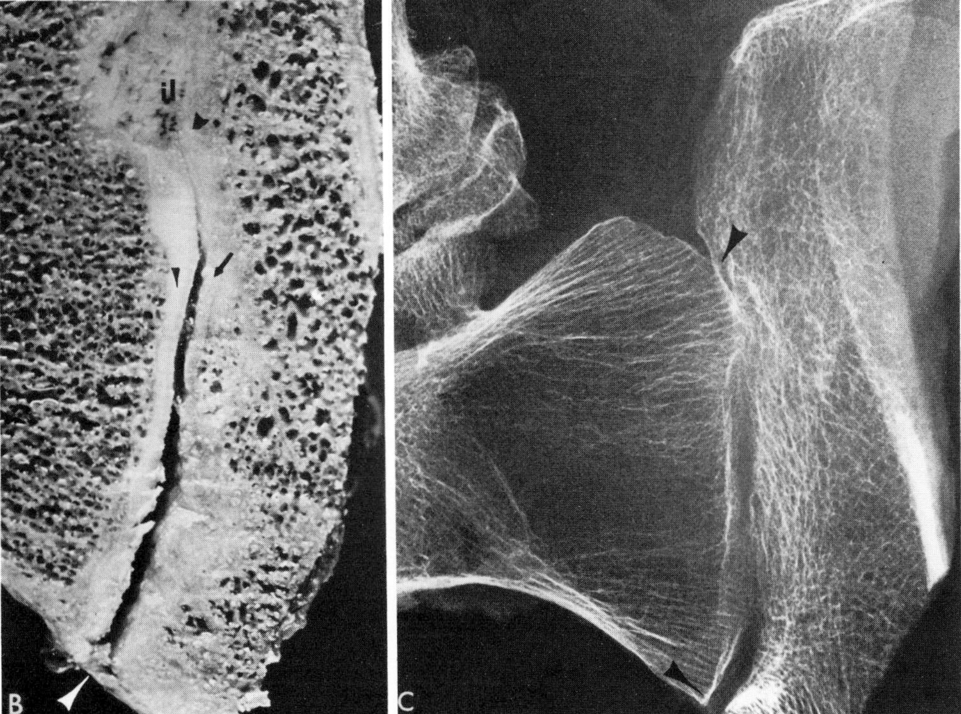

Figure 3–40. *Sacroiliac joint: Anatomy.*

A *Drawing of anterior aspect and coronal sections of articulation. Observe the ventral sacroiliac ligament (3), and interosseous ligament (4). When the ventral ligament is cut, thick sacral cartilage (1) and thinner iliac cartilage (2) are apparent. (From Resnick D, Niwayama G, Goergen TG: Invest Radiol 10:608–621, 1975.)*

B, C *Coronal section. Photograph and radiograph of two similar specimens reveal extent of synovial articulation (between large arrowheads), thick sacral cartilage (small arrowhead), and thinner iliac cartilage (arrow). Note the interosseous ligament (il) above the synovial joint.*

Illustration continued on the following page

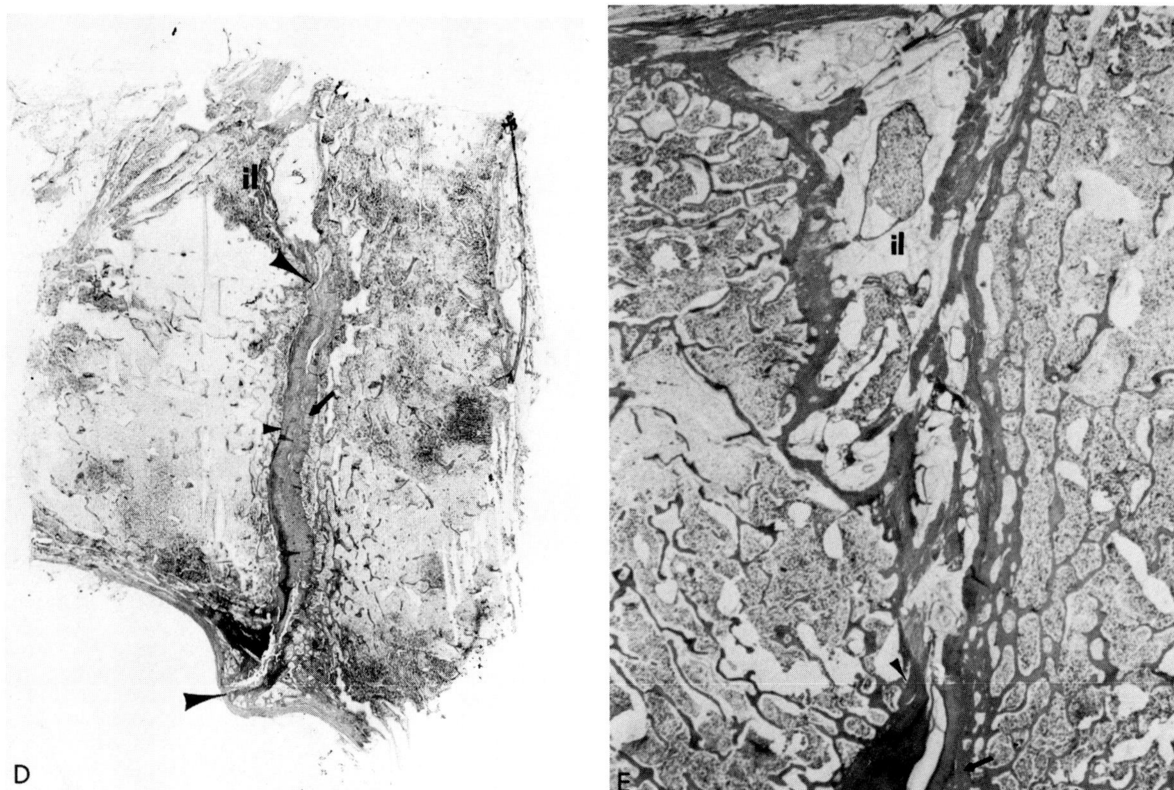

Figure 3–40. Continued

D *A photomicrograph (2×) of a coronal section demonstrating synovial joint (between large arrowheads), thick sacral cartilage (small arrowhead), thinner iliac cartilage (arrow), and interosseous ligament* (il).

E *At higher magnification (15×), these same structures are seen in a different coronal section.*

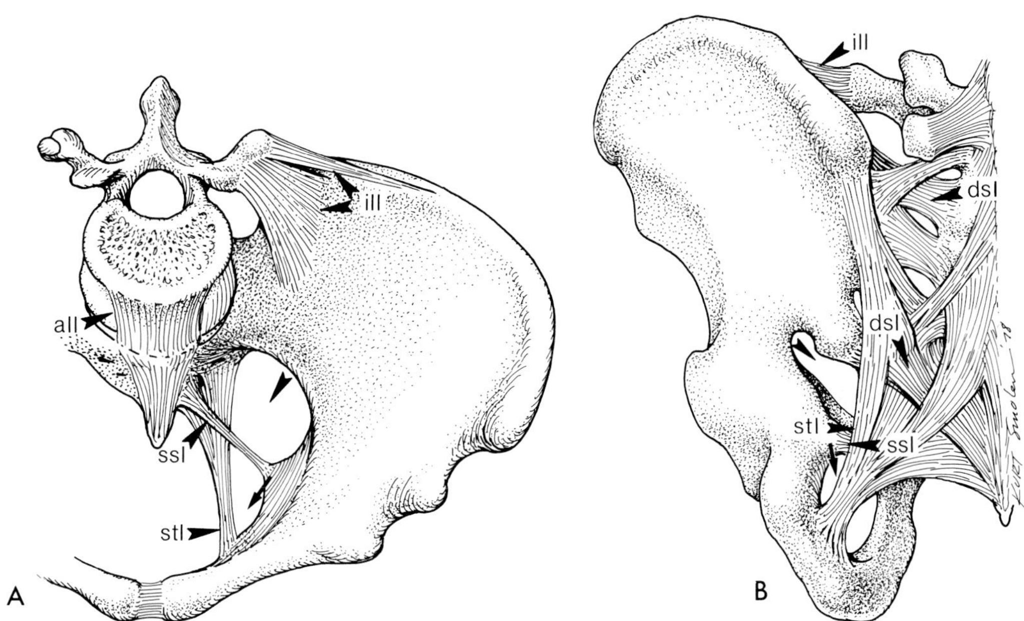

Figure 3–41. *Pelvic-vertebral ligaments: Anatomy.*

A *Anterior aspect. Visualized structures are the iliolumbar ligament (ill) with two pelvic attachments, sacrospinous ligament (ssl) sacrotuberous ligament (stl), anterior longitudinal ligament (all), and greater (arrowhead) and lesser (arrow) sciatic foramina.*

B *Posterior aspect. Observe the iliolumbar ligament (ill), short and long dorsal sacroiliac ligaments (dsl), sacrotuberous ligament (stl), sacrospinous ligament (ssl), and greater (arrowhead) and lesser (arrow) sciatic foramina.*

(From Warwick R, Williams P: Gray's Anatomy. 35th British Ed. Philadelphia, WB Saunders Co, 1973.)

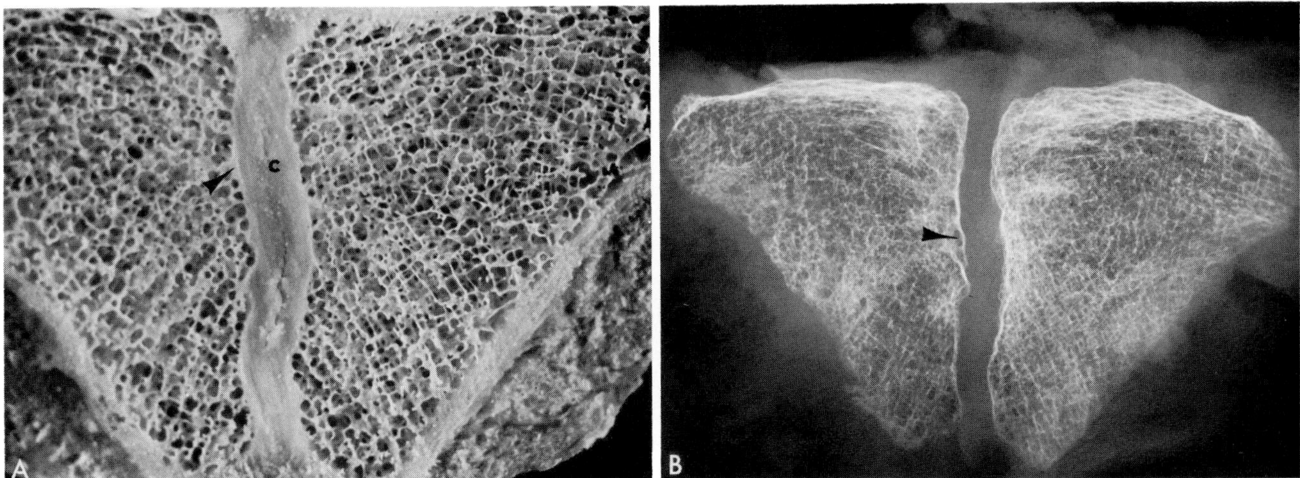

Figure 3–42. *Symphysis pubis: Anatomy.*

A, B *Coronal section. Observe the central cartilage (c) and the well-defined subchondral bone plate (arrowhead).*

Illustration continued on the following page

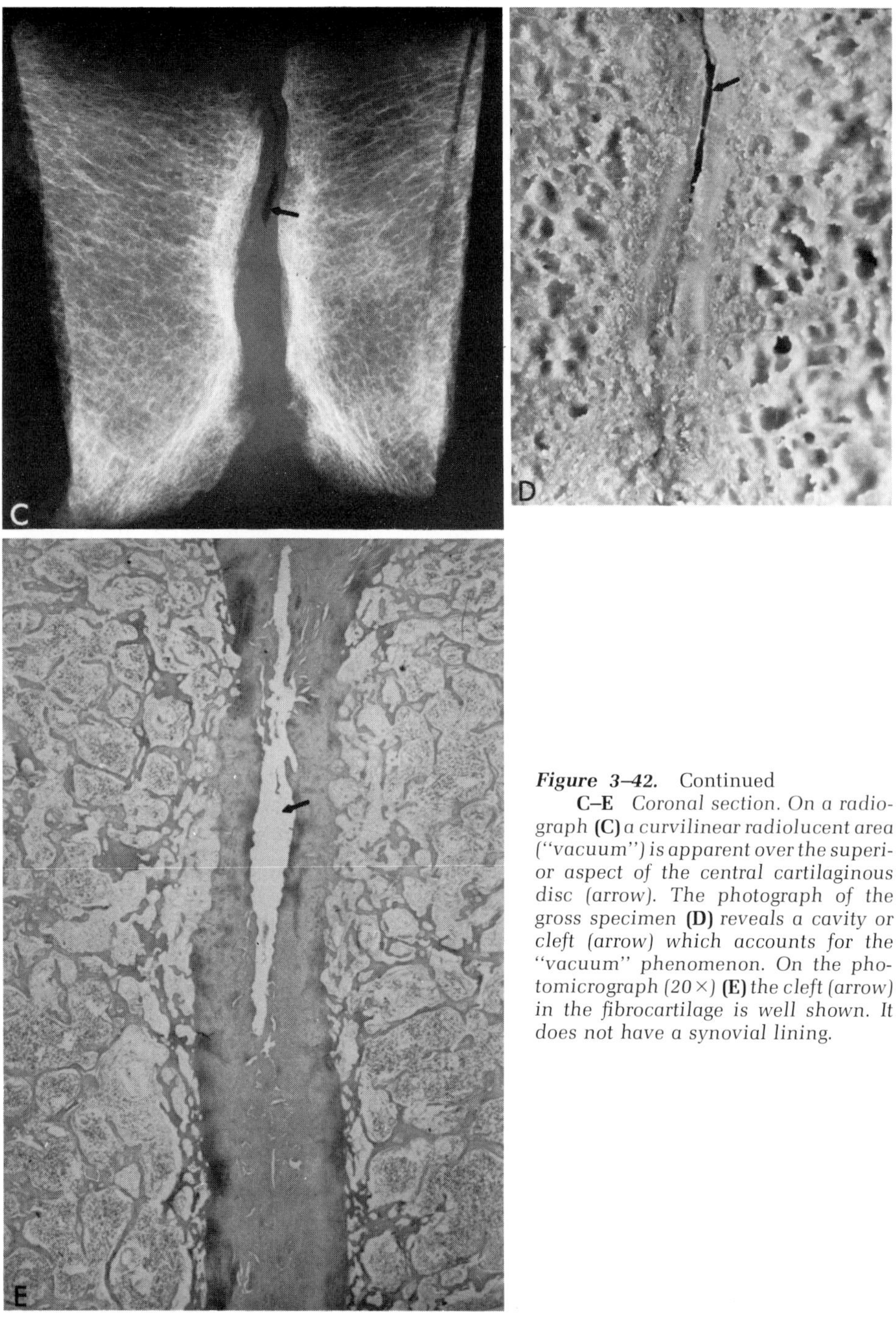

Figure 3–42. Continued

C–E *Coronal section. On a radiograph* **(C)** *a curvilinear radiolucent area ("vacuum") is apparent over the superior aspect of the central cartilaginous disc (arrow). The photograph of the gross specimen* **(D)** *reveals a cavity or cleft (arrow) which accounts for the "vacuum" phenomenon. On the photomicrograph (20×)* **(E)** *the cleft (arrow) in the fibrocartilage is well shown. It does not have a synovial lining.*

for increased movement at various pelvic joints,[127, 128] perhaps providing minor aid during childbirth.[137] There are several additional factors that allow greater movement of the pelvis in women and thereby assist in childbirth: less interlocking by reciprocal irregularities of bone about the sacroiliac joints; less fibrous ankylosis of the sacroiliac articulations; and decreased incidence of synostosis of coccygeal segments.[2]

HIP

Osseous Anatomy

At the hip, the globular head of the femur articulates with the cup-shaped fossa of the acetabulum. This latter structure develops in fetal life from ossification of the ilium, ischium, and pubis. At birth, the acetabulum is cartilaginous, with a triradiate stem extending medially from its deep aspect, producing a Y-shaped epiphyseal plate between ilium, ischium, and pubis.[1] Continued ossification results in eventual fusion of these three bones.

The fully developed acetabular cavity is hemispheric in shape and possesses an elevated bony rim (Fig. 3–43). This rim is absent inferiorly, the defect being termed the acetabular notch. A fibrocartilaginous labrum is attached to the bony rim, deepening the acetabular cavity. The acetabular floor above the notch, the acetabular fossa, is depressed and irregular. Between the rim and fossa is a smooth horseshoe-shaped articular lunate surface.

The hemispheric head of the femur extends superiorly, medially and anteriorly (Fig. 3–44). It is smooth except for a central roughened pit, the fovea, to which is attached the ligament of the head of the femur. The anterior surface of the femoral neck is intracapsular, as the capsular line extends to the intertrochanteric line; only the medial half of the posterior surface of the femoral neck is intracapsular, as the posterior attachment of the hip capsule does not extend to the intertrochanteric crest. The greater trochanter projects from the posterosuperior aspect of the femoral neck-shaft junction and is the site of attachment of numerous muscles, including the gluteus minimus, gluteus medius, and piriformis. The lesser trochanter is located at the posteromedial portion of the femoral neck-shaft junction. The psoas major and iliacus muscles attach to it.

Radiographic examination of normal osseous structures about the hip has received great attention, and various measurements have been determined. The acetabular angle, iliac angle, and angle of anteversion of the femoral neck are useful measurements, particularly in the young skeleton.[138-142] The CE angle of Wiberg[143] is an indication of acetabular depth (Fig. 3–45). It is the angle formed between a perpendicular line through the midportion of the femoral head and a line from the femoral head center to the upper outer acetabular margin. The normal CE angle is reported to be 20 to 40 degrees, with an average of 36 degrees.[144] This angle may be slightly larger in women and in older individuals.[145]

The pelvic radiograph is also useful in outlining certain normal lines and structures[145, 146] (Fig. 3–46). The acetabular rim appears as an osseous ring surrounding the outer aspect of the acetabulum. The posterior acetabular rim can be identified on radiographs exposed in various obliquities, but the 15 to 30 degree anterior oblique projection offers optimal visualization. The anterior acetabular rim is optimally visualized in the 30 to 45 degree posterior oblique projection. The ilioischial and iliopubic lines can also be identified. The ilioischial line is formed by that portion of the quadrilateral surface of the ilium that is tangent to the x-ray beam; the iliopubic line is simply the inner margin of the ilium, which forms a continuous line with the inner superior aspect of the pubis. Two columns of bone produce an arch, with the acetabulum located in the concavity of the arch. The ilioischial or posterior column is a thick structure that includes a portion of the ilium and extends to the ischial tuberosity. The iliopubic or anterior column consists of a portion of ilium and pubis and extends superolaterally to the anterior inferior iliac spine.

The "teardrop" is a U-shaped shadow medial to the hip joint that has been utilized to detect abnor-

Text continued on page 112

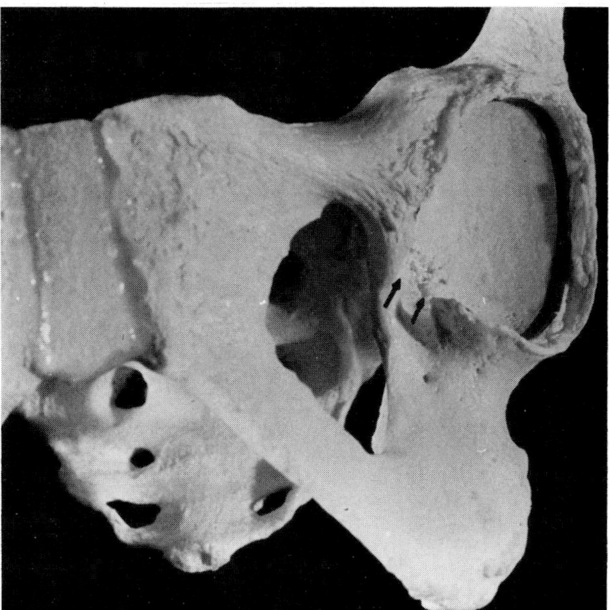

Figure 3–43. *Acetabular cavity: Osseous anatomy (anterior view). A metal marker (black strip) identifies the posterior acetabular rim. This rim is continuous except at the area of the acetabular notch inferiorly (arrows). (From Armbuster TG, et al: Radiology 128:1, 1978.)*

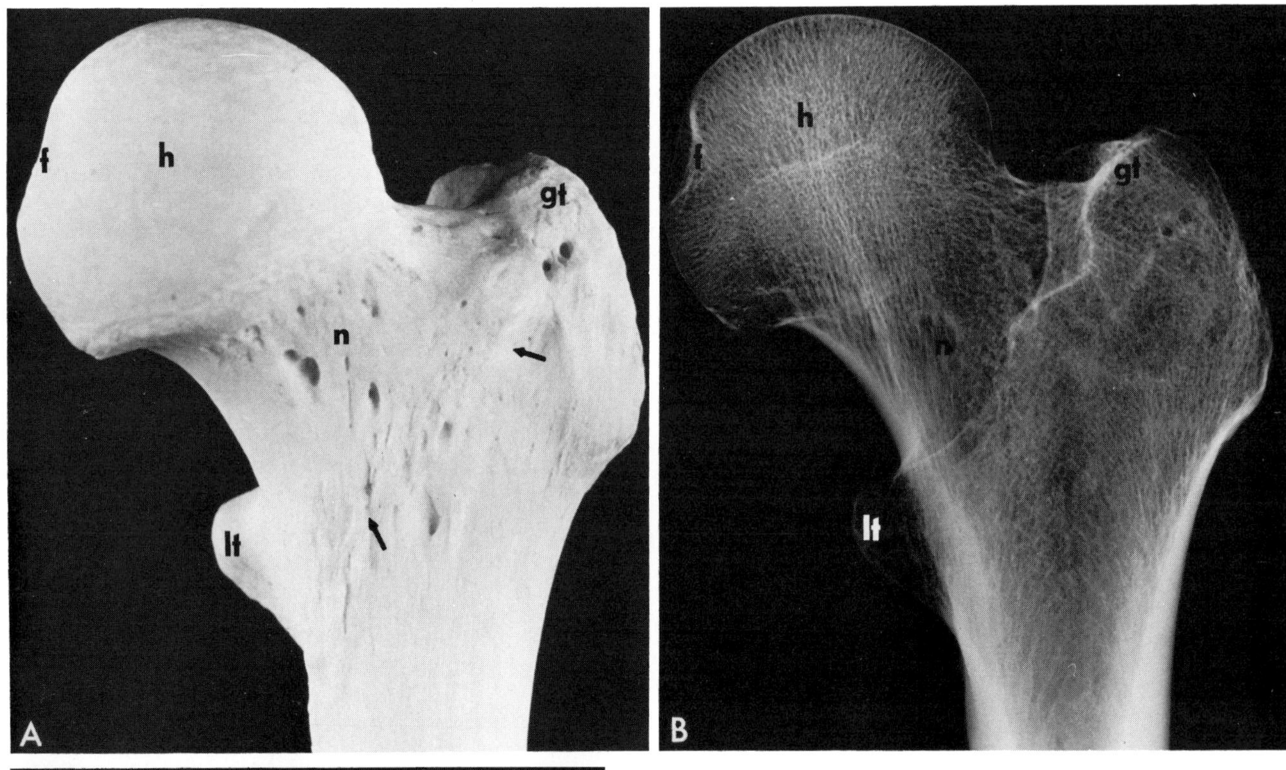

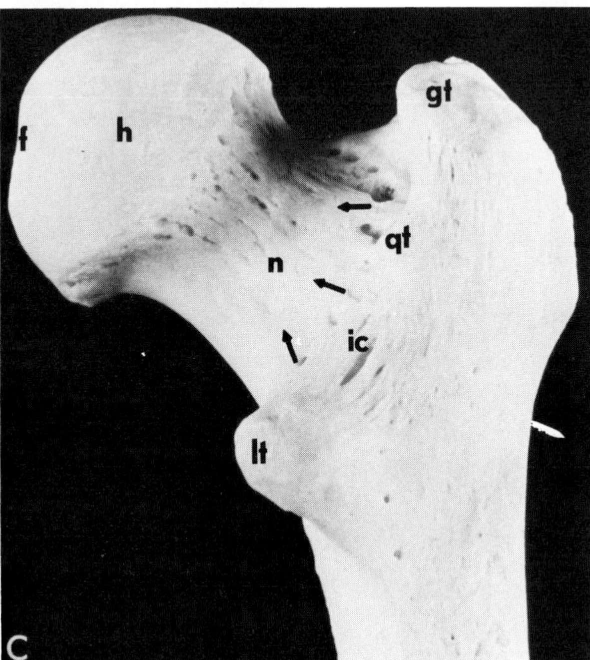

Figure 3–44. *Proximal femur: Osseous anatomy.*

A, B *Anterior aspect, neutral position. Observe the smooth femoral head (h), fovea (f), neck (n), greater trochanter (gt), and lesser trochanter (lt). The hip capsule attaches anteriorly to the intertrochanteric line (arrows).*

C *Posterior aspect, neutral position. The same structures as in* **A** *and* **B** *are identified. The intertrochanteric crest (ic) and quadrate tubercle (qt) are also indicated. Arrows point to the site of capsular attachment.*

Illustration continued on the opposite page

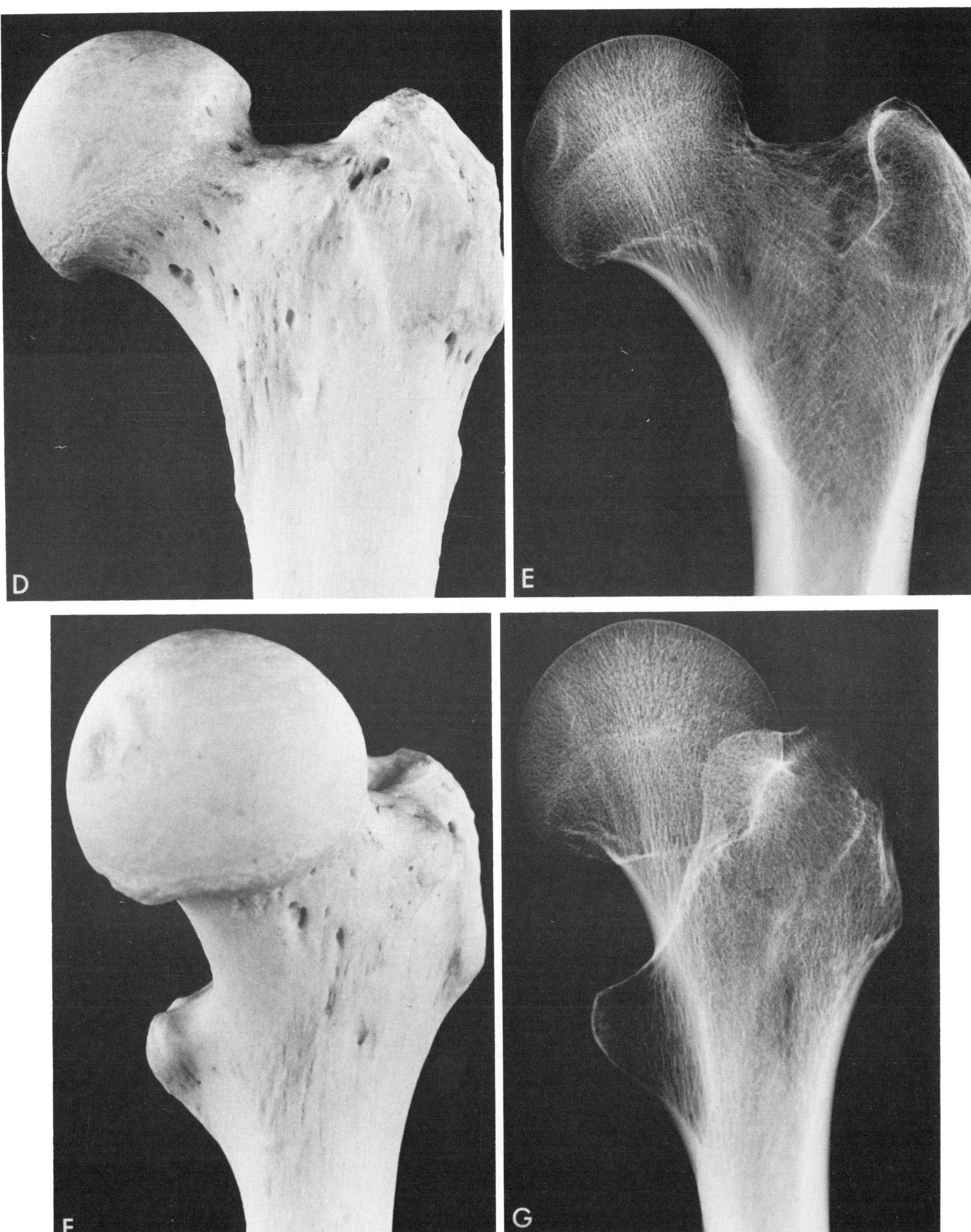

Figure 3–44. Continued
D, E *Anterior aspect, internal rotation. The femoral neck is elongated.*
F, G *Anterior aspect, external rotation. The femoral neck is foreshortened.*

Illustration continued on the following page

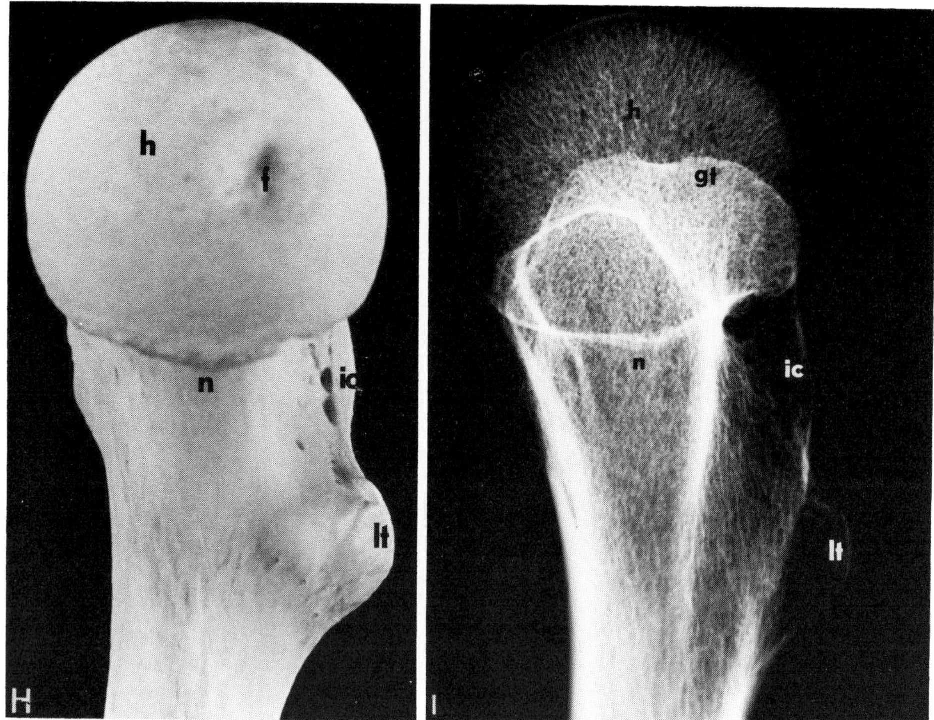

Figure 3–44. Continued
H, I *Medial aspect. Labels identify the femoral head* (h), *neck* (n), *fovea* (f), *greater trochanter* (gt), *lesser trochanter* (lt), *and intertrochanteric crest* (ic).

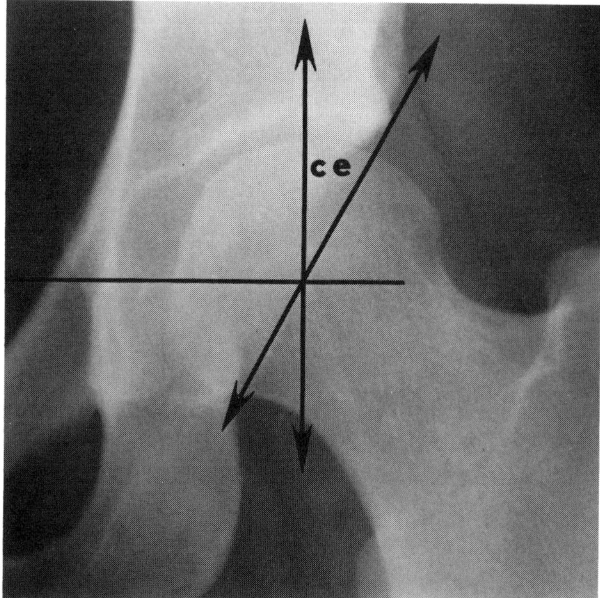

Figure 3–45. *CE angle of Wiberg. This is the angle formed by the intersection of a perpendicular line through the midpoint of the femoral head and a line from the femoral head center to the upper outer acetabular margin. The normal value for this angle is reported to be 20 to 40 degrees, with an average of 36 degrees. (From Armbuster TG, et al: Radiology 128:1, 1978.)*

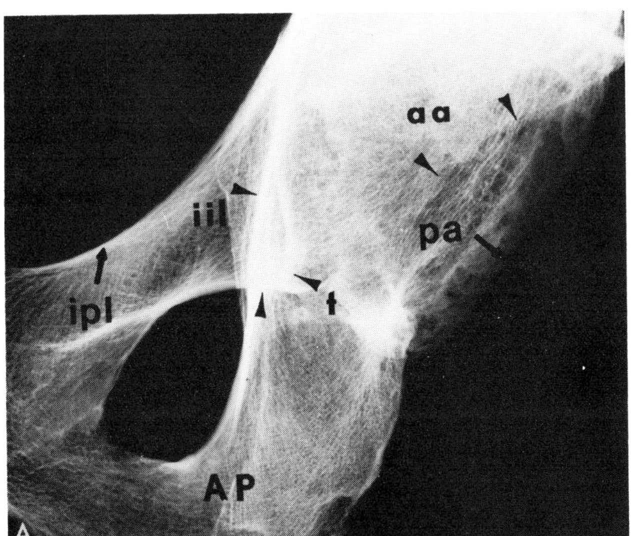

Figure 3–46. *Normal osseous landmarks of the pelvis.*

A, *Anteroposterior (AP) view. The posterior acetabular rim (pa) is more lateral than the anterior acetabular rim (aa). The ilioischial line (iil) is formed by that portion of the quadrilateral surface of the ilium that is tangent to the x-ray beam. The iliopubic line (ipl) is the inner margin of the ilium, which forms a continuous line with the inner superior surface of the pubis. The "teardrop" (t) is also labeled.*

B *Fifteen degree left posterior oblique (LPO) view. The quadrilateral surface (arrows) is observed.*

C *Thirty degree left posterior oblique (LPO) view. The 30 to 45 degree posterior oblique projection best delineates the ilioischial column (iic) and anterior acetabular rim (aa). The posterior acetabular rim (pa) is noted.*

Illustration continued on the following page

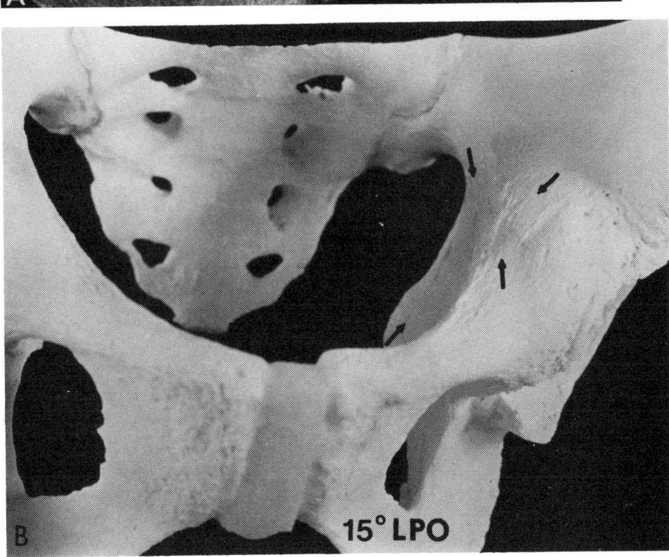

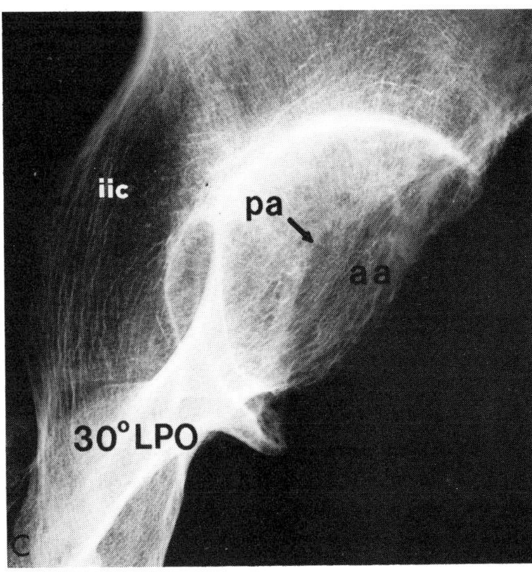

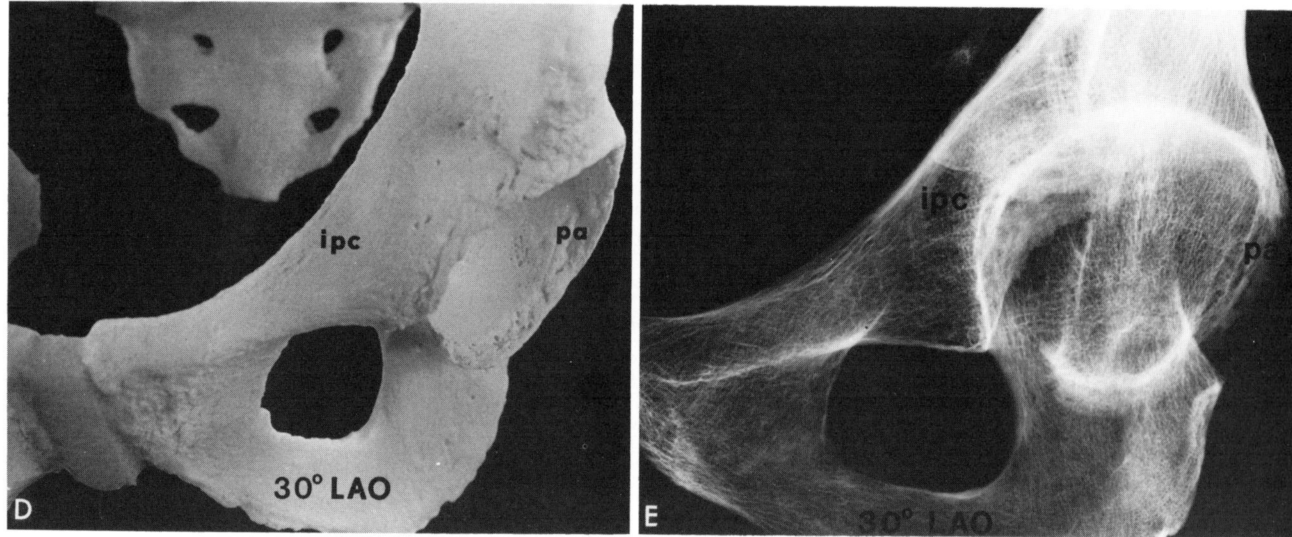

Figure 3–46. Continued
D, E *Thirty degree left anterior oblique (LAO) view. Well delineated are the iliopubic column* (ipc) *and posterior acetabular rim* (pa).
(From Armbuster TG, et al: Radiology 128:1, 1978.)

malities of acetabular depth, thereby establishing a diagnosis of acetabular protrusion (Fig. 3–47). The lateral aspect of the teardrop is the wall of the acetabular fossa, and the medial aspect is the anteroinferior margin of the quadrilateral surface. In the usual anteroposterior radiograph of the pelvis, the latter surface is parallel to the x-ray beam and is thereby projected as a typical "teardrop." However, the configuration of the teardrop varies in normal individuals. Furthermore, it is affected significantly by positioning the patient in oblique projections[145]; in a slight anterior oblique projection the teardrop is situated anterior to the ilioischial line creating a "crossed" appearance rather than the more usual "open" or "closed" position. With further anterior obliquity, the teardrop is situated medially to the ilioischial line, creating a "reversed" appearance. In the posterior oblique projection, the teardrop is located lateral to the ilioischial line.

Differentiation of normal acetabular depth and acetabular protrusion (protrusio acetabuli) can be accomplished by careful analysis of plain films in adults.[145] In the past, several different definitions of protrusio acetabuli have been utilized (Table 3–3): (1) a bony bulge on the inner aspect of the acetabulum; (2) the femoral head reaching the ilioischial line; (3) a CE angle of greater than 40 to 45 degrees; (4) "crossing" of the teardrop; (5) the acetabular line touching or crossing the ilioischial line.

These previous observations have certain limitations:

1. When protrusio acetabuli progresses to frank bulge of the acetabulum into the pelvis, the diagnosis is readily apparent. This is certainly not a reliable indicator of mild protrusio acetabuli.

2. The relationship of the femoral head to the ilioischial line is not adequate as a measurement of protrusio acetabuli because it introduces another variable, that is, the integrity of the joint space. If the joint space is decreased, the femoral head will reach the ilioischial line at an earlier stage than if the joint space is "normal."

3. The CE angle, originally described to evaluate congenital and dysplastic hips[143] was subsequently applied to the measurement of protrusio acetabuli, with varying degrees of enthusiasm and success.[144, 149-152] Our analysis reveals wide ranges in the value of the CE angle.[145] Although 40 degrees has been previously considered to be the upper limit of normal,[144] women over 40 years of age may have an average CE angle of greater than 40 degrees.[145] We have also made an attempt to correlate the CE angle with other parameters used in the diagnosis of protrusio acetabuli, and have found no significant relationship between the CE angle and the configuration of the teardrop or between the CE angle and the relative position of the acetabular and ilioischial lines.[145] This has led us to conclude that the CE angle is not a good indicator of protrusio acetabuli.

4. Most authors do not give a definition of a crossed teardrop but simply state that this is an indicator of protrusio acetabuli. We have defined a crossed teardrop as one that is crossed by the ilioischial line. As the teardrop configuration is affected by minimal amounts of rotation, slight anterior oblique projections can lead to crossing of the teardrop. Increasing the degree of anterior obliquity can even lead to a reversed teardrop. In addition, in normal situations on nonrotated pelvic radiographs, such crossing may be apparent; in 15 per cent of normal adult hips, radiographs reveal an acetabular line medial to the ilioischial line in association with an

Text continued on page 118

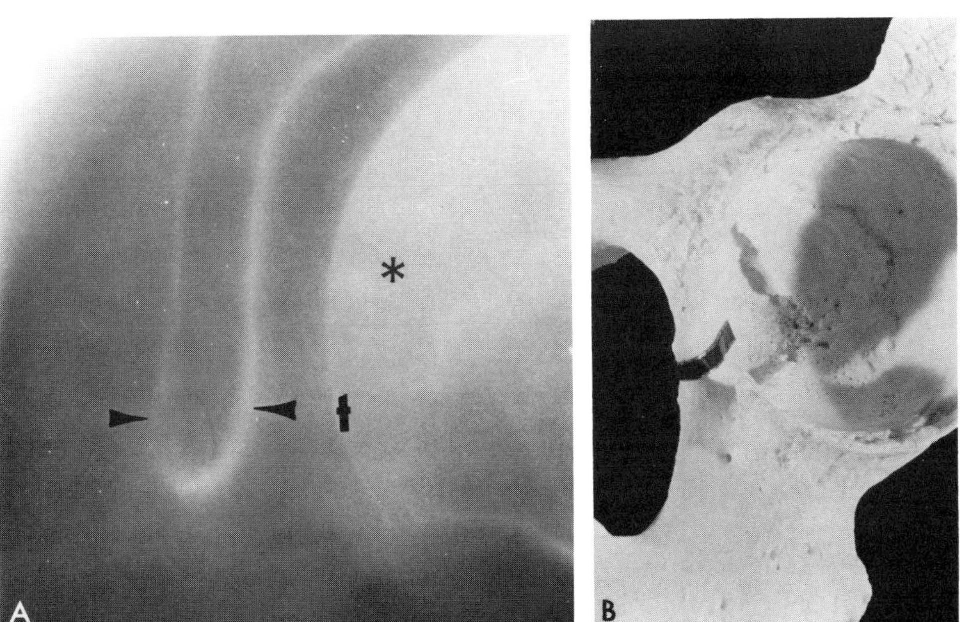

Figure 3–47. The "teardrop."

A *Anteroposterior tomogram. The "teardrop"* (t) *and femoral head (*) are seen. The lateral wall of the "teardrop" is the wall of the acetabular fossa. The medial wall is the anteroinferior margin of the quadrilateral surface.*

B *On a cadaveric specimen, a metal marker has been placed on the teardrop. The quadrilateral surface is not visualized in this projection.*

Illustration continued on the following page

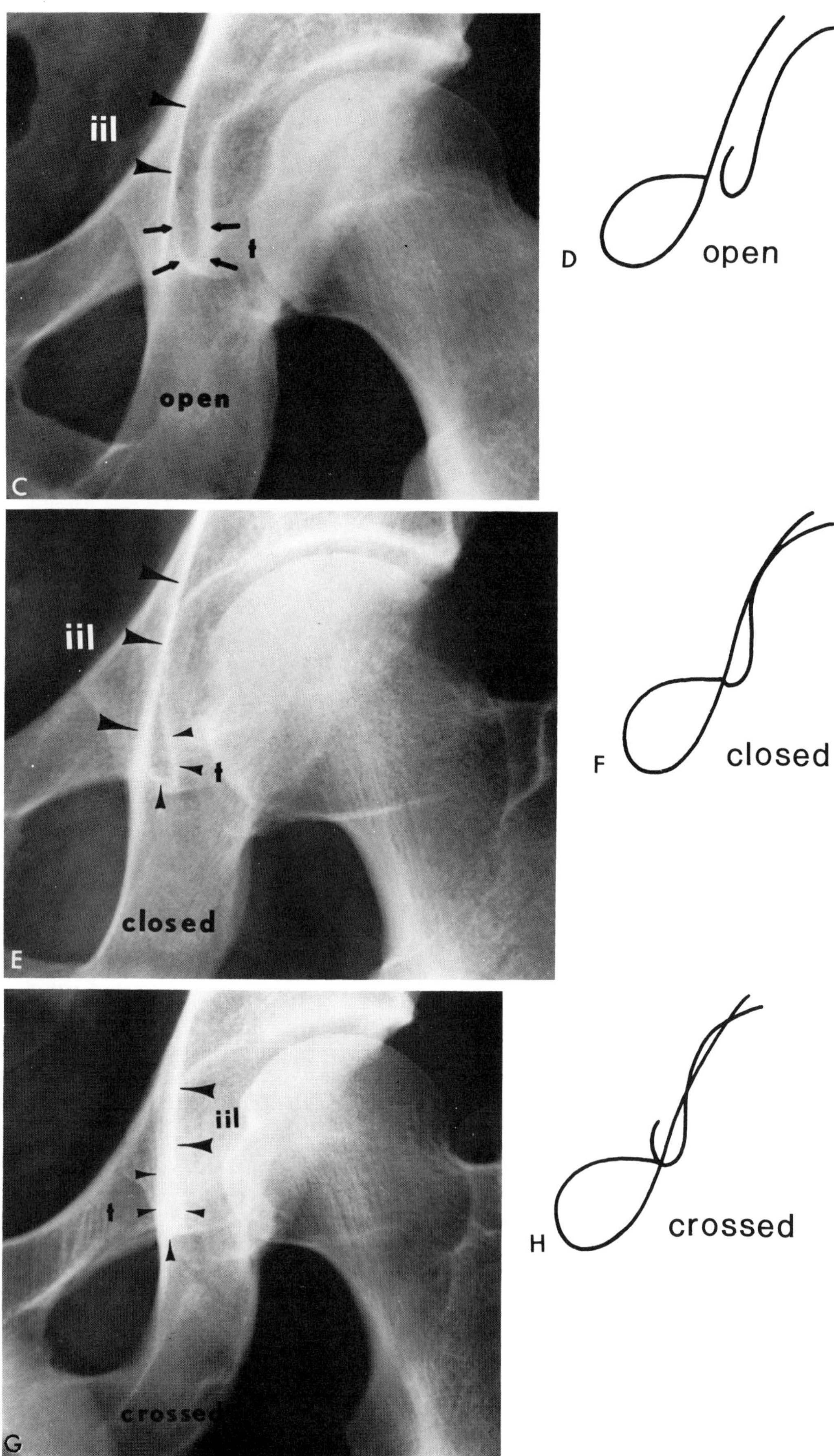

Figure 3–47. Continued

Illustration continued on the opposite page

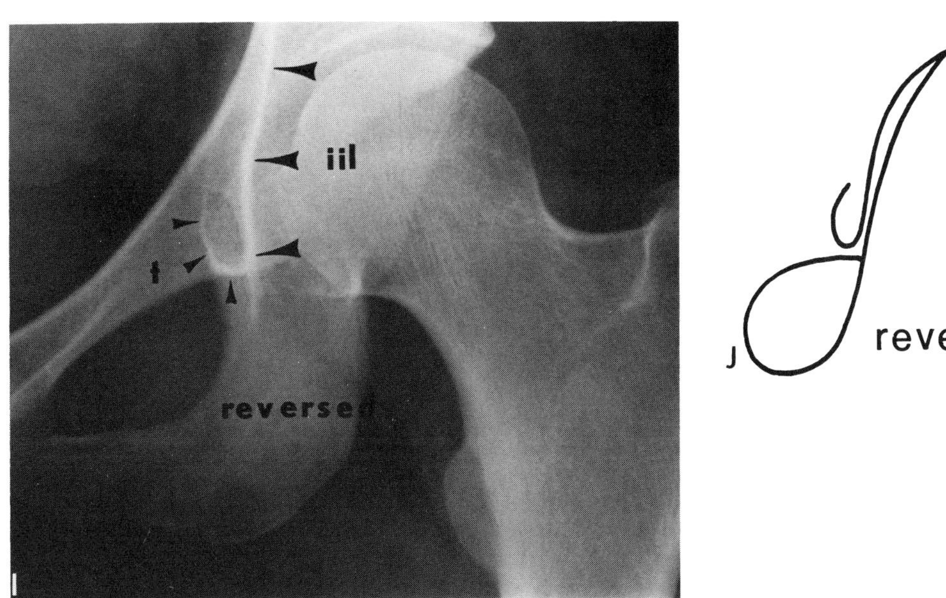

Figure 3–47. Continued

C–J *The different radiographic appearances of the teardrop* (t) *are illustrated. In the open type* **(C, D)**, *the entire teardrop is located lateral to the ilioischial line* (iil). *In the closed type* **(E, F)**, *the medial aspect of the teardrop touches the ilioischial line. In the crossed type* **(G, H)** *the teardrop is crossed by the ilioischial line. In the reversed type* **(I, J)** *the teardrop is entirely medial to the ilioischial line.*

Illustration continued on the following page

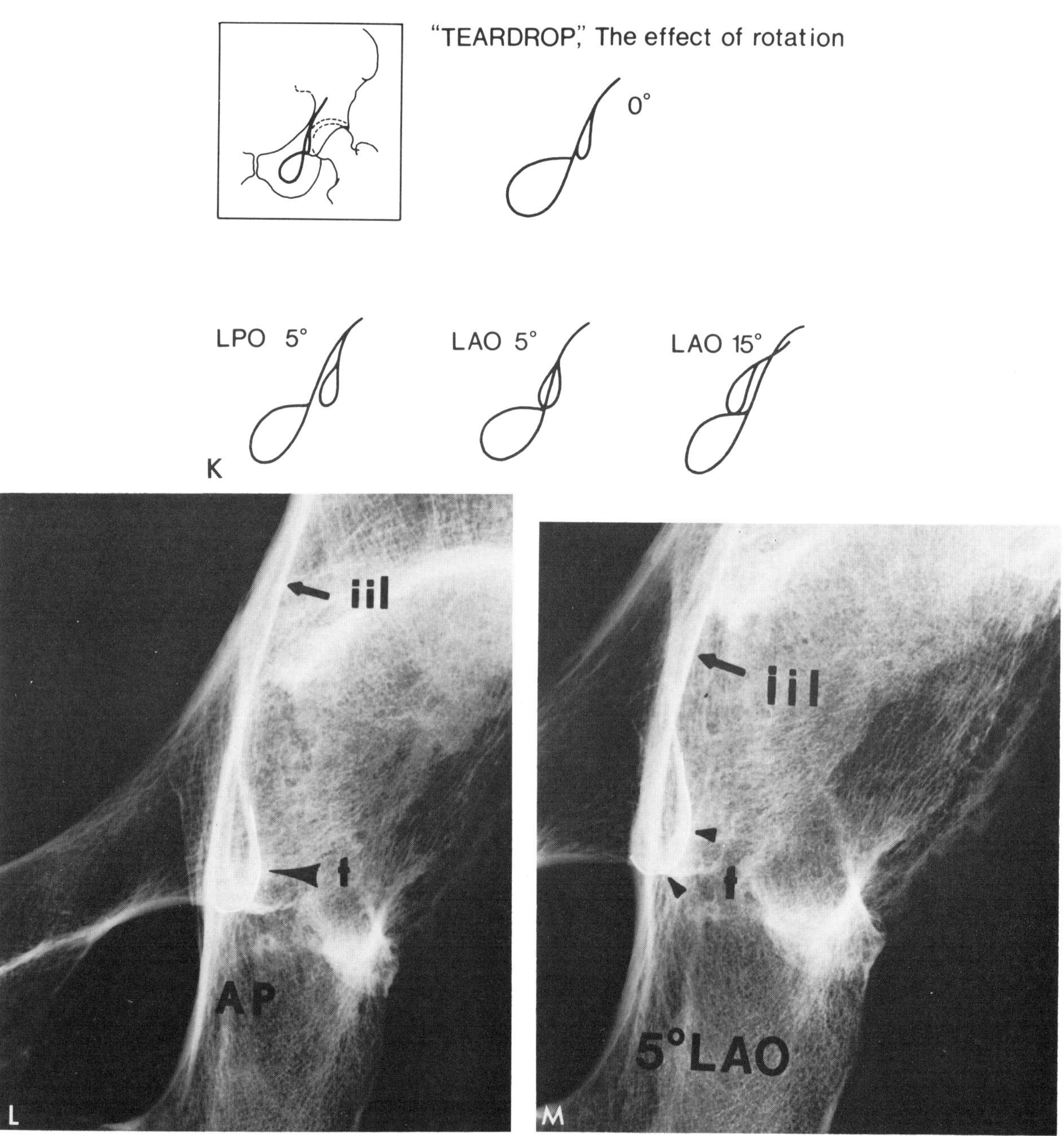

Figure 3–47. Continued

Illustration continued on the opposite page

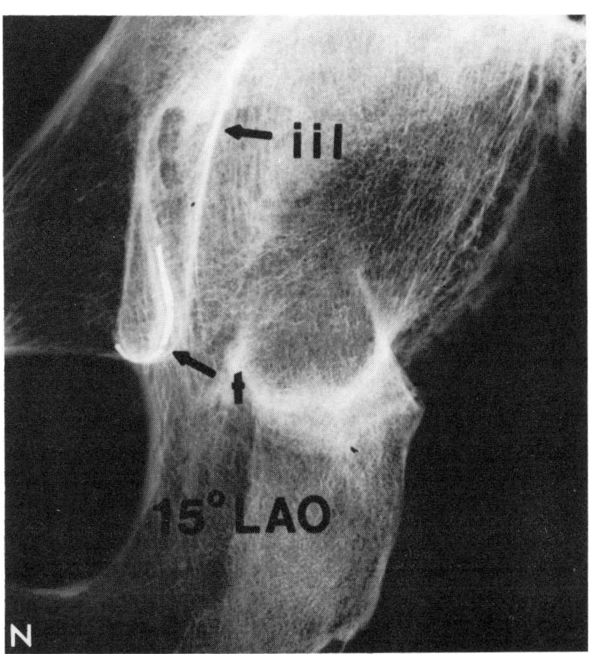

Figure 3–47. Continued

K–N *Effects of rotation on teardrop* (t) *configuration. A schematic representation* **(K)** *indicates that rotation changes significantly the appearance of the teardrop. Although the teardrop may appear open or closed on an anteroposterior radiograph* **(L)**, *it can assume a crossed appearance in a 5 degree left anterior oblique (LAO) projection* **(M)** *or a reversed appearance in a 15 degree LAO projection* **(N)**. *This changing appearance in different degrees of rotation relates to the anterior position of the teardrop and the posterior position of the ilioischial line.*

(From Armbuster TG, et al: Radiology 128:1, 1978.)

Table 3–3
PROTRUSIO ACETABULI

Date	Author	Criterion
1932	Pomeranz[147]	Dome-shaped mass projecting into pelvis
1935	Overgaard[148]	Acetabular line touching or crossing ilioischial line
1953	Friedenberg[149]	CE angle between 40 and 70 degrees
1965	Alexander[150]	Teardrop crossed on a well-centered film; femoral head reaching ilioischial line; bulge above pelvic brim
1969	Hubbard[151]	Acetabular line medial to ilioischial line
1971	Hooper and Jones[144]	Crossing of the teardrop
1971	MacDonald[152]	CE angle greater than 45 degrees

open or closed teardrop.[145] Therefore, the teardrop configuration is not a good index of protrusio acetabuli. Furthermore, the unqualified use of the term crossed teardrop is potentially misleading and unnecessary.

We prefer to use the relationship of the acetabular line to the ilioischial line as the index of protrusio acetabuli (Fig. 3–48). The acetabular line, which is the medial wall of the acetabulum, and the ilioischial line, which is a portion of the quadrilateral surface, are central structures whose relationships are little affected by minimal degrees of rotation. In examining and measuring these central structures, one minimizes any artifact caused by minor rotation in an anteroposterior pelvic radiograph. In fact, slight degrees of pelvic obliquity will create a crossed teardrop, while the relationship between the acetabular line and the ilioischial line remains normal. In addition, as protrusio acetabuli involves the central structures, it would seem appropriate to utilize their relative position to establish the diagnosis.

Although acetabular depth is a continuum from "shallow" to "normal" to "deep" to "protrusio acetabuli," our data[145] have led to the following conclusions:

1. Protrusio acetabuli is diagnosed when the acetabular line projects medial to the ilioischial line by 3 mm or more in adult men and by 6 mm or more in adult women.

2. The teardrop configuration is affected by minor degrees of rotation and therefore cannot be utilized as an indicator of protrusio acetabuli.

3. Measurement of the CE angle of Wiberg adds little to the diagnosis of protrusio acetabuli.

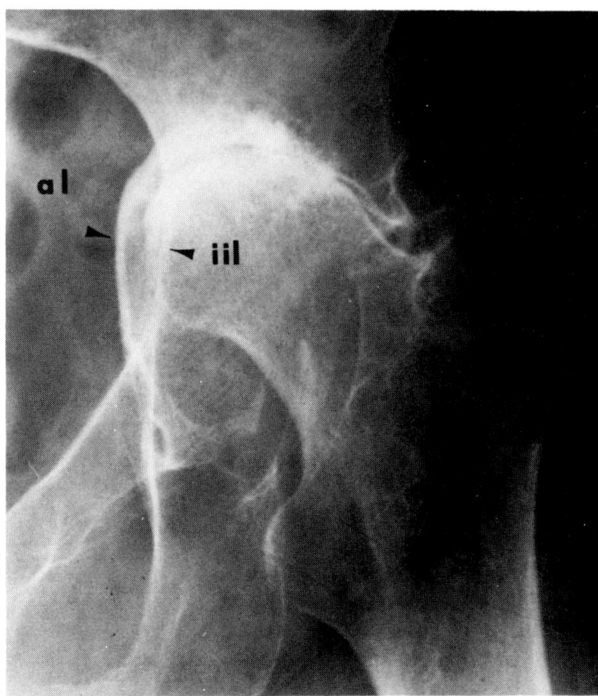

Figure 3–48. *Acetabular protrusion. A protrusio acetabuli deformity is present when the acetabular line (al) projects medial to the ilioischial line (iil) by 3 mm or more in adult men and by 6 mm or more in adult women. (From Armbuster TG, et al: Radiology 128:1, 1978.)*

The normal joint space on roentgenograms can be analyzed in adults by dividing it into three segments: superior, axial, and medial joint space[145] (Fig. 3–49). The superior and axial joint space measurements are usually quite similar, but the medial joint space measurement is normally greater because it includes the acetabular fossa, which adds synovium and fat to the joint space. Nevertheless, the medial measurement is meaningful since the same situation exists in all hips. The average medial joint space is 9 mm in men and 8 mm in women. The average axial and superior joint spaces are 4 mm in both men and women. Thus, in normal situations, the superior and axial spaces should be equal and approximately one half the medial joint space measurement. In pathologic situations, selective loss or gain of superior, axial, or medial joint space may aid in specific diagnoses.

Soft Tissue Anatomy

The femoral head is covered with articular cartilage, although a small area exists on its surface that is devoid of cartilage, to which attaches the ligament of the head of the femur (Fig. 3–50). The lunate surface is covered with articular cartilage; the floor of the acetabular fossa within this surface does not contain cartilage, but has a fibroelastic fat pad covered with synovial membrane.

A fibrous capsule encircles the joint and much of the femoral neck. The capsule attaches proximally to the acetabulum, labrum, and transverse ligament of the acetabulum. Distally it surrounds the femoral neck; in front, it is attached to the trochanteric line at the junction of the femoral neck and shaft; above and below, it is attached to the femoral neck close to the junction with the trochanters; behind the capsule extends over the medial two thirds of the neck. Because of these capsular attachments, the epiphyseal plate of the femur is intracapsular and the epiphyseal plates of the trochanters are extracapsular. The fibers of the fibrous capsule, although oriented longitudinally from pelvis to femur, also consist of a deeply situated circular group of fibers termed the zona orbicularis. The fibrous capsule is strengthened by surrounding ligaments, including the iliofemoral, pubofemoral, and ischiofemoral ligaments. The external surface of the capsule is covered by musculature and separated anteriorly from the psoas major and iliacus by a bursa. In this area, the joint may communicate with the subtendinous iliac bursa

Text continued on page 123

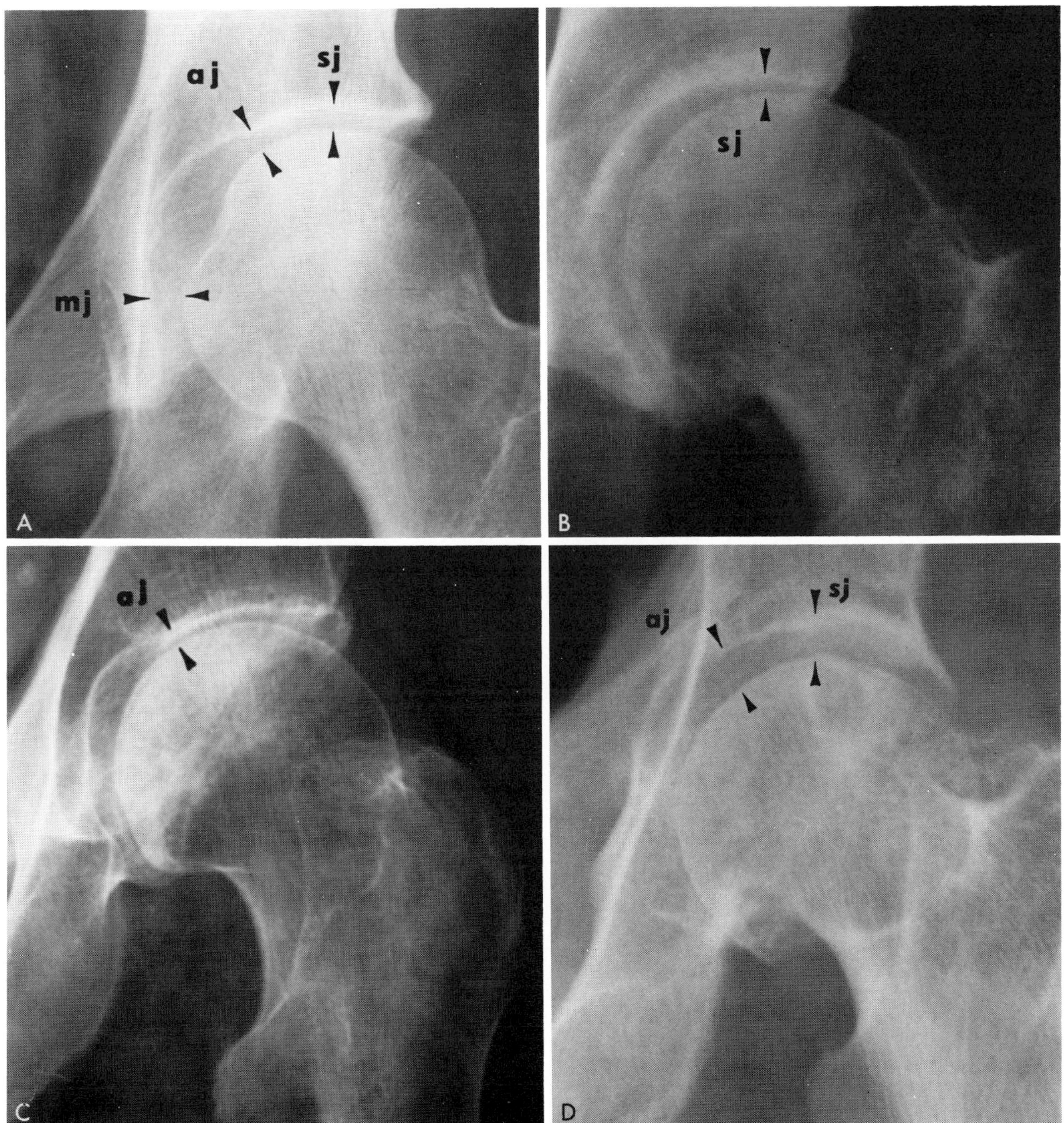

Figure 3–49. *Normal and abnormal joint space.*

A *The joint space measurement includes the intra-articular space and the thickness of the acetabular and femoral head cartilage. The axial joint space* (aj) *and superior joint space* (sj) *should be approximately one half the medial joint space* (mj).

B *Superior joint space* (sj) *loss is frequent in degenerative joint disease.*

C *Axial joint space* (aj) *loss may be apparent in disuse cartilage atrophy following paralysis.*

D *Increase of axial joint space* (aj) *and superior joint space* (sj) *can occur in acromegaly.* (*From Armbuster TG, et al: Radiology, 128:1, 1978.*)

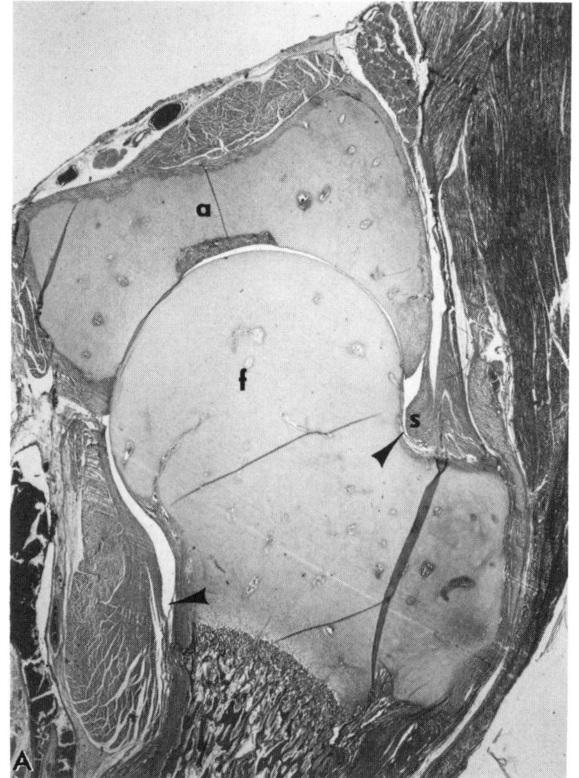

Figure 3–50. Hip joint: Normal development and anatomy.

A Photomicrograph (×20) of a coronal section through the hip reveals unossified acetabulum (a) and femoral head (f), synovium (s), and distal extent of articular cavity (arrowheads).

B Drawing of a coronal section through the hip.

Illustration continued on the opposite page

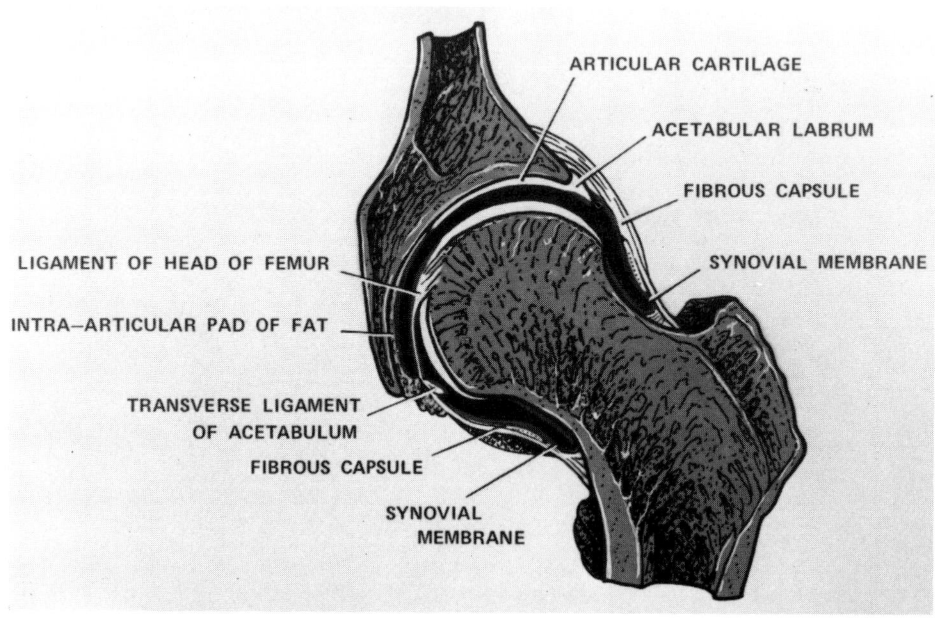

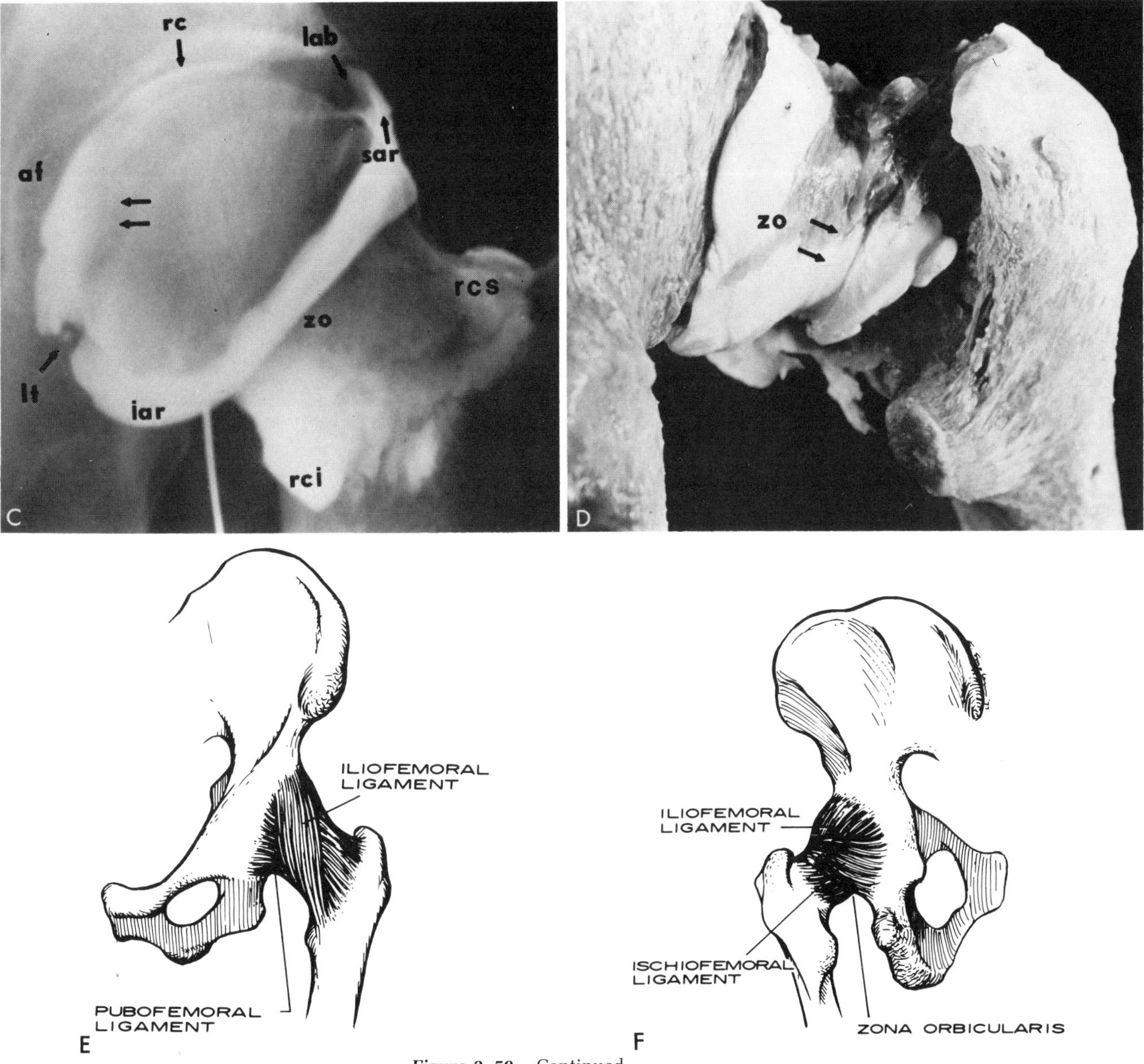

Figure 3–50. Continued

C *Normal left hip arthrogram. The recess capitus (rc) is a thin, smooth collection of contrast medium between apposing articular surfaces and is interrupted only where the ligamentum teres (double arrows) enters the fovea centralis of the femoral head. The ligamentum transversum (lt) is seen as a radiolucent defect adjacent to the inferior rim of the acetabulum. The ligamentum teres bridges the acetabular notch and effectively deepens the acetabulum. The inferior articular recess (iar) forms a pouch at the inferior base of the femoral head below the acetabular notch and ligamentum transversum (lt). The superior articular recess (sar) extends cephalad around the acetabular labrum (lab). The acetabular labrum is seen as a triangular radiolucency adjacent to the superolateral lip of the acetabulum. The zona orbicularis (zo) is a circumferential lucent band around the femoral neck, which changes configuration with rotation of the femur. The recess colli superior (rcs) and recess colli inferior (rci) are poolings of contrast material at the apex and base of the intertrochanteric line and are the most caudad extensions of the synovial membrane.*

D *Macerated specimen (posterior view) with prior barium-impregnated methylmethacrylate injection demonstrating the zona orbicularis (zo) as an impression made by the iliofemoral and ischiofemoral ligaments of the hip capsule.*

E *Capsular ligaments of hip, anterior view. The iliofemoral ligament extends anterior to the pubofemoral ligament. A gap may persist at this crossing, which allows communication between the iliopsoas bursa and the hip joint.*

F *Capsular ligaments of hip, posterior view. The iliofemoral and ischiofemoral ligaments are thick posteriorly and without inherent areas of weakness. The zona orbicularis is created by the crossing of the hip ligaments.*

G *Musculature, anterior aspect of hip. Observe the course of the iliacus and psoas muscles.*

Illustration continued on the following page

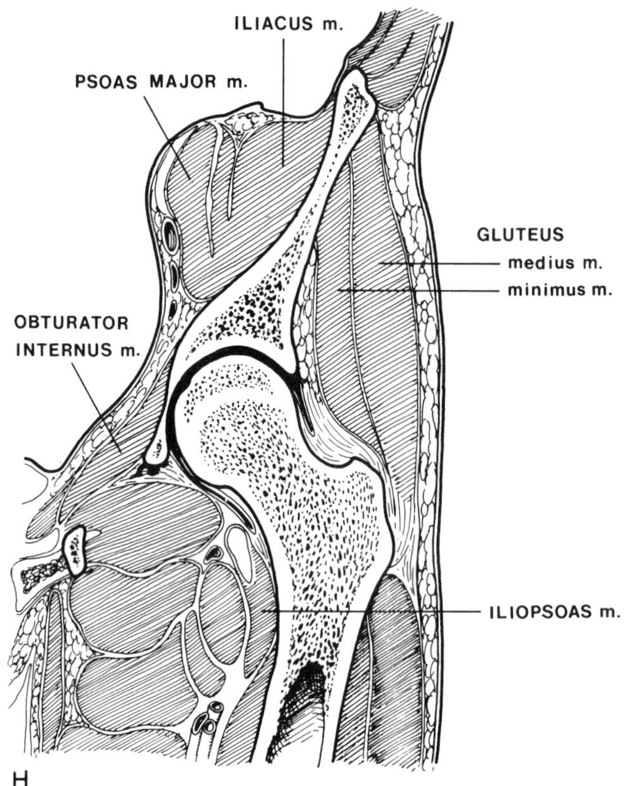

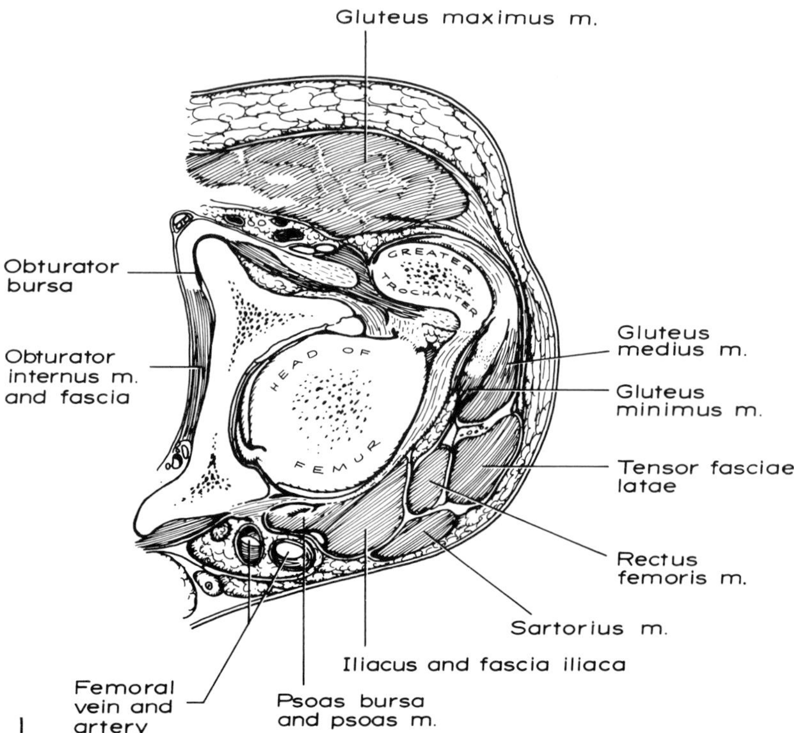

Figure 3–50. Continued
H *Musculature, coronal section of hip.*
I *Musculature, transverse section of hip. Anterior structures are located at the bottom of the drawing.*
*(**B–F**, From Guerra J Jr, et al: Radiology 128:11, 1978.)*

(iliopsoas bursa) beneath the psoas major tendon through an aperture between the pubofemoral and iliofemoral ligaments.[1, 2]

The extensive synovial membrane of the hip extends from the cartilaginous margins of the femoral head over intracapsular portions of the femoral neck. It is reflected beneath the fibrous capsule and covers the acetabular labrum, the ligament of the head of the femur, and the fat pad in the acetabular fossa.

Important ligaments include the iliofemoral, pubofemoral, and ischiofemoral ligaments, the ligament of the head of the femur, the transverse ligament of the acetabulum, and acetabular labrum. The strong iliofemoral ligament attaches proximally to the anterior inferior iliac spine and the adjoining part of the acetabular rim and distally to the intertrochanteric line on the femur. This ligament becomes taut in full extension of the hip. The pubofemoral ligament extends from the pubic part of the acetabular rim and the superior pubic ramus to the undersurface of the femoral neck, some of its fibers blending with the fibrous capsule. This ligament also becomes taut on hip extension. The ischiofemoral ligament is attached to the ischium below and behind the acetabulum and extends in a superolateral direction across the back of the femoral neck. Its fibers are continuous with those of the zona orbicularis or attach to the greater trochanter. This ligament, as the others, becomes taut in extension of the hip. The ligament of the head of the femur is a weak intra-articular ligament, which is attached to the margin of the acetabular fossa and the transverse ligament of the acetabulum. It extends to a pit on the femoral head. Between these areas of attachment, this ligament is clothed by a synovial sheath. In some individuals, the sheath alone is present, without the ligament, and in others, neither sheath nor ligament can be identified. The ligament is stretched when the thigh is flexed, adducted, and laterally rotated. The transverse ligament of the acetabulum is a portion of the acetabular labrum whose fibers extend across the acetabular notch. The acetabular labrum, the fibrocartilaginous rim about the acetabulum, is firmly attached to the bony rim and transverse ligament, is triangular on cross section, and has a free edge of apex that forms a smaller circle that closely embraces the femoral head.

Active movements of the hip are flexion, extension, adduction, abduction, circumduction, and medial and lateral rotation. Because of a close fit between acetabulum and femur and the intimacy of the acetabular labrum, the movements of the hip are restricted compared to those of the glenohumeral joint. No accessory movements occur in the hip.

Soft tissue anatomy about the hip has received great attention. A number of periarticular fat planes have been described that can be recognized on radiographs and which, when disturbed, may reportedly indicate significant intra-articular disease[153-158] (Fig. 3–51). Reichmann[159] reviewed the soft tissue anatomy about the hip joint. Four fatty layers were described, which could be identified on anteroposterior radiographs (Fig. 3–52):

Fat plane 1: On the pelvic surface of the acetabulum and pubis.

Fat plane 2: Medial to the femoral neck, extending to the lesser trochanter.

Fat plane 3: Lateral to the hip and extending to the greater trochanter.

Fat plane 4: Lateral to the hip and medial to fat plane 3, extending to the region of the greater trochanter.

Anatomic studies have revealed that fat plane 1 is medial to the obturator internus muscle[153, 160] and fat plane 2 is medial to the iliopsoas muscle.[160, 161] Fat plane 3 is between the gluteus medius (lateral) and the gluteus minimus (medial).[159-161] Fat plane 4 has been termed the "capsular" fat plane[161] although more recent evidence suggests that this fat pad is not related to the joint capsule.[159] Our investigation of adult hips[160] has supported the concept that this latter fat pad is indeed not true capsular fat. The bulk of this fat plane is intermuscular, lying between the rectus femoris and tensor fasciae latae muscles. This region is quite anterior to the hip capsule and it is here that this fat pad is widest. This fat plane (4) has an oblique orientation, and it becomes thinner dorsally as it changes from its intermuscular part to its pericapsular part between the superolateral aspect of the hip joint capsule and the medial aspect of the gluteus minimus muscle. The pericapsular portion of this fat plane is not discernible on routine hip radiography and, therefore, the "capsular" fat plane that is frequently seen on anteroposterior radiography is the intermuscular part of this fat plane and has no intimate relationship to the hip capsule. Although this plane does have a pericapsular extension, this latter extension is strongly reinforced by surrounding ligaments. Thus, one would not expect intra-articular fluid to create a noticeable change in this fat plane.

Our close evaluation of fat plane 2, the iliopsoas fat plane, has documented its periarticular course.[160] It is medial to the tendinous portion of the iliopsoas muscle. Anteriorly it blends with the fat of the femoral triangle just lateral to the femoral vessels. Posteriorly it reaches the superomedial portion of the hip capsule and inferomedial lip of the acetabulum. In its posterior course, it sends a fat plane laterally, posterior to the iliopsoas tendon. Here it makes intimate contact with the medial portion of the hip capsule adjacent to the femoral neck. This represents a point of weakness between the iliofemoral and iliopubic ligaments of the hip capsule. It is here that the iliopsoas bursa originates, a space

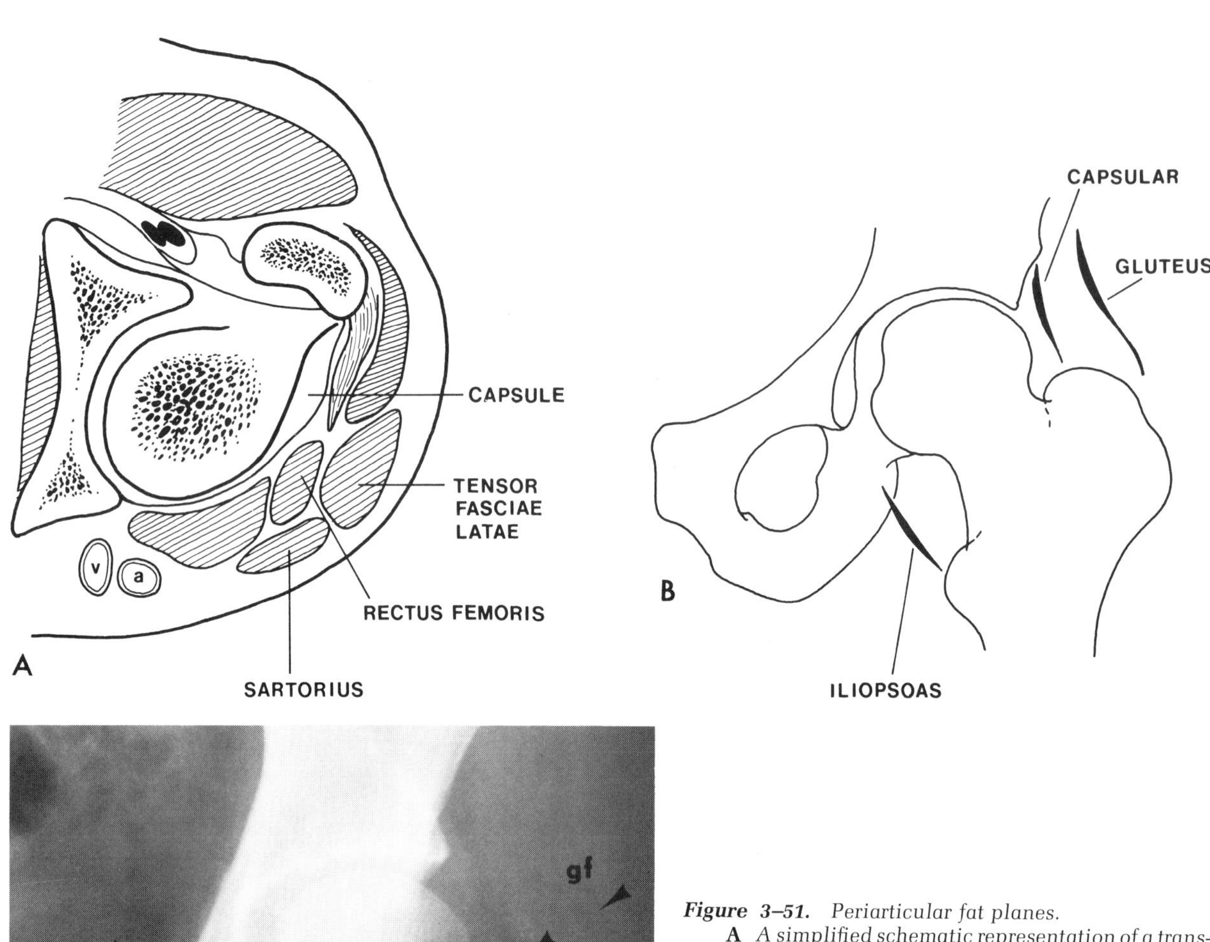

Figure 3–51. Periarticular fat planes.

A A simplified schematic representation of a transverse section through the hip.

B A drawing of three of the four fat planes that have been described.

C The fat planes include fat plane 1 (obturator internus fat plane, oif), fat plane 2 (iliopsoas fat plane, ipf), fat plane 3 (gluteus fat plane, gf), and fat plane 4 ("capsular" fat plane, cf). In each instance, arrowheads indicate distances of fat plane to adjacent osseous structures. (**C**, From Guerra J, Jr, et al: Radiology 128:11, 1978.)

that potentially could allow decompression of a joint in cases of elevated intra-articular pressure.[160] On radiographs, only the widest portion of the iliopsoas fat plane is seen on anteroposterior projections, a portion that is anterior to the medial aspect of the hip joint. Therefore, a small to moderate amount of intra-articular fluid should not displace the iliopsoas fat plane, although large amounts of fluid may alter it.

The iliopsoas and "capsular" fat planes (fat planes 2 and 4) are visible in a great percentage of hip radiographs, but measurements of the distance of these fat planes to bony landmarks in the pelvis vary.[160] The obturator internus fat plane (fat plane 1) is infrequently visualized and variable in its distance from the bony pelvis. The gluteal fat plane (fat plane 3) is neither frequently visualized nor constant in position. Additional characteristics of these fat planes are the following:

1. When one obturator internus fat plane is seen, the contralateral fat plane is also seen and has a similar appearance:
2. The iliopsoas fat plane is frequently well defined on one side and indistinct on the other, and may have either a neutral or "bulgy" appearance:
3. The "capsular" and gluteal fat planes vary in appearance when compared to their counterparts on the opposite side.

These factors diminish the reliability of radiographically discernible fat plane alterations in predicting hip disease, particularly in adults (Fig. 3–53). In children, intra-articular fluid may produce an increase in width of joint space between the femoral head and the medial acetabular wall. This sign may be more valuable than changes in the position and appearance of periarticular fat planes.

The iliopsoas bursa represents the largest and most important bursa about the hip. It is present in 98 per cent of hips, and is located anterior to the joint capsule.[162] It may extend proximally and communicates with the joint space in approximately 15 per cent of normal hips[163, 164] through a gap between the iliofemoral and pubofemoral ligaments.[1, 2, 165] Extension of hip disease into this bursa has been recognized in a variety of articular diseases, occasionally producing a mass in the ilio-inguinal region[166] with possible obstruction of the femoral vein (Fig. 3–53). One additional site that represents an inherent weak part of the hip capsule occurs at the crossing of the iliofemoral and iliopubic ligaments. At this site, fluid may extravasate into the fat plane of the obturator externus muscle.[160]

Bursae about the gluteus muscles may also be demonstrated anatomically and radiographically.[167] The bursa deep to the gluteus medius is larger than that deep to the gluteus minimus. Both bursae are intimate with the greater trochanter, and bursitis can lead to pain and soft tissue calcifications in this region.

KNEE

The knee joint is the largest and most complicated articulation in the human body.[1, 2, 168] In this articulation, three functional spaces exist: medial femorotibial space; lateral femorotibial space; and patellofemoral space.

Osseous and Soft Tissue Anatomy

The lower end of the femur contains a medial and lateral condyle, separated posteriorly by an intercondylar fossa or notch (Fig. 3–54). The medial condyle is larger than the lateral condyle, and possesses a superior prominence called the adductor tubercle for attachment of the tendon of the adductor magnus. Below this tubercle is a ridge, the medial epicondyle. The lateral condyle possesses a similar protuberance, the lateral epicondyle. The intercondylar fossa, between the condyles, stretches from the intercondylar line posteriorly to the lower border of the patellar surface anteriorly. The patella, the largest sesamoid bone of the body, is embedded within the tendon of the quadriceps femoris. It is oval in outline, with a pointed apex on its inferior surface. The ligamentum patellae, a continuation of the quadriceps tendon, is attached to the apex and adjacent bone of the patella.

Articular surfaces of the femur, tibia, and patella are not congruent. The articular surface of the femur comprises the condylar areas (femorotibial spaces) and the patellar surface (patellofemoral space). A shallow groove is present between each condylar surface and the patellar surface. As viewed from below, the outline of the femoral condylar surfaces generally conforms to that of the tibial articular surfaces. The surface on the lateral femoral condyle appears circular, whereas that on the medial femoral condyle is large and oval, elongated in an anteroposterior direction, with concavity extending laterally.

The tibial articular surfaces are the cartilage-clothed condyles, each with a central hollow and peripheral flattened area (Fig. 3–55). Between the condyles is the intercondylar area. The articular surface of the medial tibial condyle is oval, with its long axis in the sagittal plane, whereas the articular surface of the lateral tibial condyle is circular and smaller in size compared with the medial condyle.

The adjacent articular surfaces of the tibia and femur are more closely fitted together by the presence of the medial and lateral menisci (Fig. 3–56). The medial meniscus is nearly semicircular in shape, with a broadened or widened posterior horn. The anterior end of the medial meniscus is attached to the intercondylar area of the tibia anterior to the attachment of the anterior cruciate ligament. The posterior end of the medial meniscus is attached to the intercondylar area of the tibia between the at-

Text continued on page 135

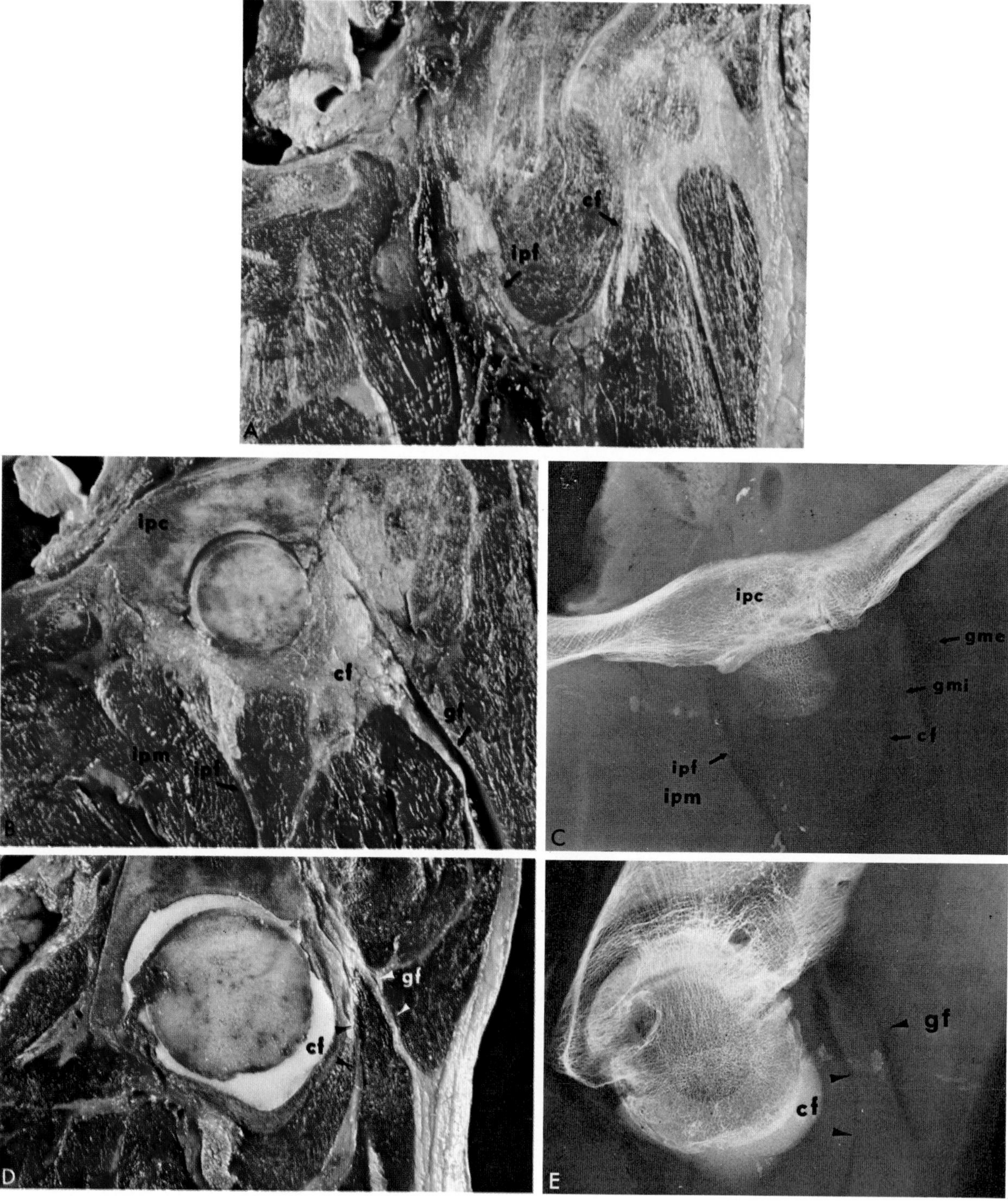
cf
ipf
A
ipc
cf
gf
ipm
ipf
B
ipc
gme
gmi
cf
ipf
ipm
C
gf
cf
D
gf
cf
E

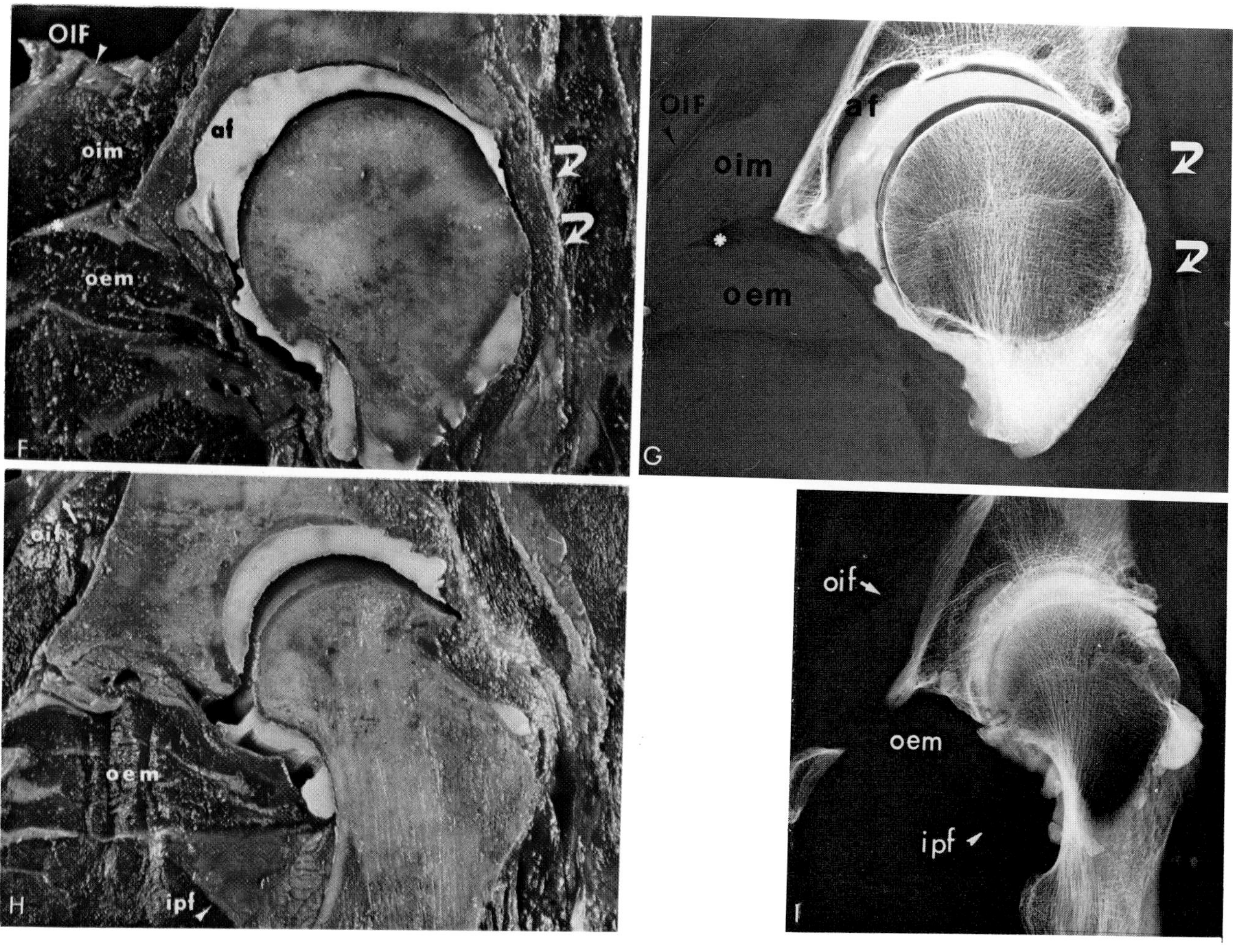

Figure 3–52. *Periarticular fat planes: cadaveric study.* ipf, *Iliopsoas fat;* cf, *capsular fat;* ipm, *iliopsoas muscle;* gf, *gluteal fat;* ipc, *iliopubic column;* oif, *obturator internus fat;* oim, *obturator internus muscle;* oem, *obturator externus muscle;* af, *acetabular fossa;* gme, *gluteus medius muscle;* gmi, *gluteus minimus muscle.*

A–I *Corresponding photographs and radiographs of 1 cm thick coronal sections through the hip with prior intra-articular injection of barium-impregnated methylmethacrylate. The sections from* **A** *to* **I** *proceed in an anterior to posterior direction. The obturator internus fat (oif) is medial to the obturator internus muscle (oim) in the pelvis* **(F, G, H, I).** *The obturator internus muscle (oim) is separated from the hip joint by the acetabulum and from the obturator externus muscle (oem) by the obturator membrane (asterisk)* **(F, G).** *The iliopsoas fat (ipf)* **(B, C)** *and iliopsoas muscle (ipm) are identified. Anteriorly the iliopsoas blends with the fat of the femoral triangle* **(A)** *(arrow) lateral to the femoral vessels. In its posterior course it sends a fat plane laterally to make contact with the hip capsule adjacent to the medial aspect of the femoral neck* **(H, I).** *This is the point of inherent weakness between the iliofemoral and pubofemoral ligaments, which may allow the iliopsoas bursa to communicate with the hip joint. Only the widest portion of the iliopsoas fat (ipf)* **(B, C)** *is seen on an AP radiograph, and this is anterior to the hip capsule. The most lateral fat plane is the gluteus fat (gf). It lies between the gluteus minimus and gluteus medius muscles and is most prominent in coronal sections through the femoral head (***B*** through* **E***). Its orientation is predominantly sagittal and it becomes thinner and less prominent as it proceeds dorsally. It has no definite connection with the immediate pericapsular region. The "capsular" fat (cf) is the more medial of the two lateral fat planes and is indirectly related to the hip capsule. The bulk of this fat plane is intermuscular and between the rectus femoris and tensor fasciae latae muscles anterior to the hip capsule (***A*** through* **C***). It is in this location that the fat plane is at its widest. It takes an oblique course similar to that seen on a routine anteroposterior radiograph of the hip. This fatty layer grows thinner dorsally as it changes from an intermuscular part to a pericapsular part between the superolateral aspect of the hip joint capsule and the medial aspect of the gluteus minimus muscle (gmi)* **(F, G).** *This true pericapsular fat (curved arrows) is visible on these coronal sections, but it is imperceptible on a routine anteroposterior radiograph of the hip. Furthermore, its orientation is dissimilar to that of the capsular fat plane. (From Guerra J, Jr, et al: Radiology 128:11, 1978.)*

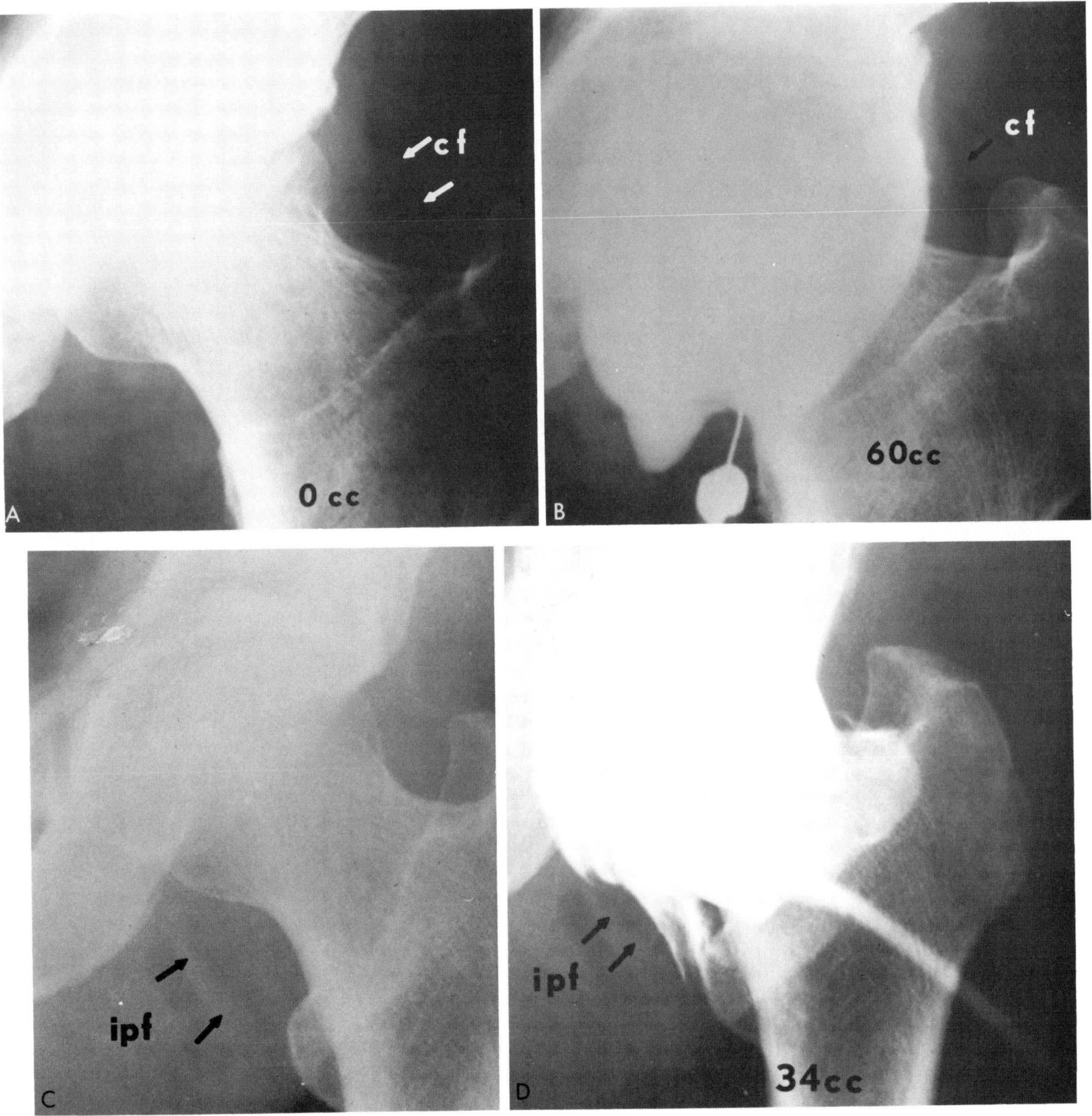

Figure 3–53. *Periarticular fat planes and bursae in disease.*

A, B *"Capsular" fat (cf). Introduction of 60 ml of contrast media fails to displace this fat plane.*

C, D *Iliopsoas fat (ipf). Introduction of 34 ml of contrast material fails to displace this fat plane.*

*(**A–D** from Guerra J Jr, et al: Radiology 128:11, 1978.)*

Illustration continued on the opposite page

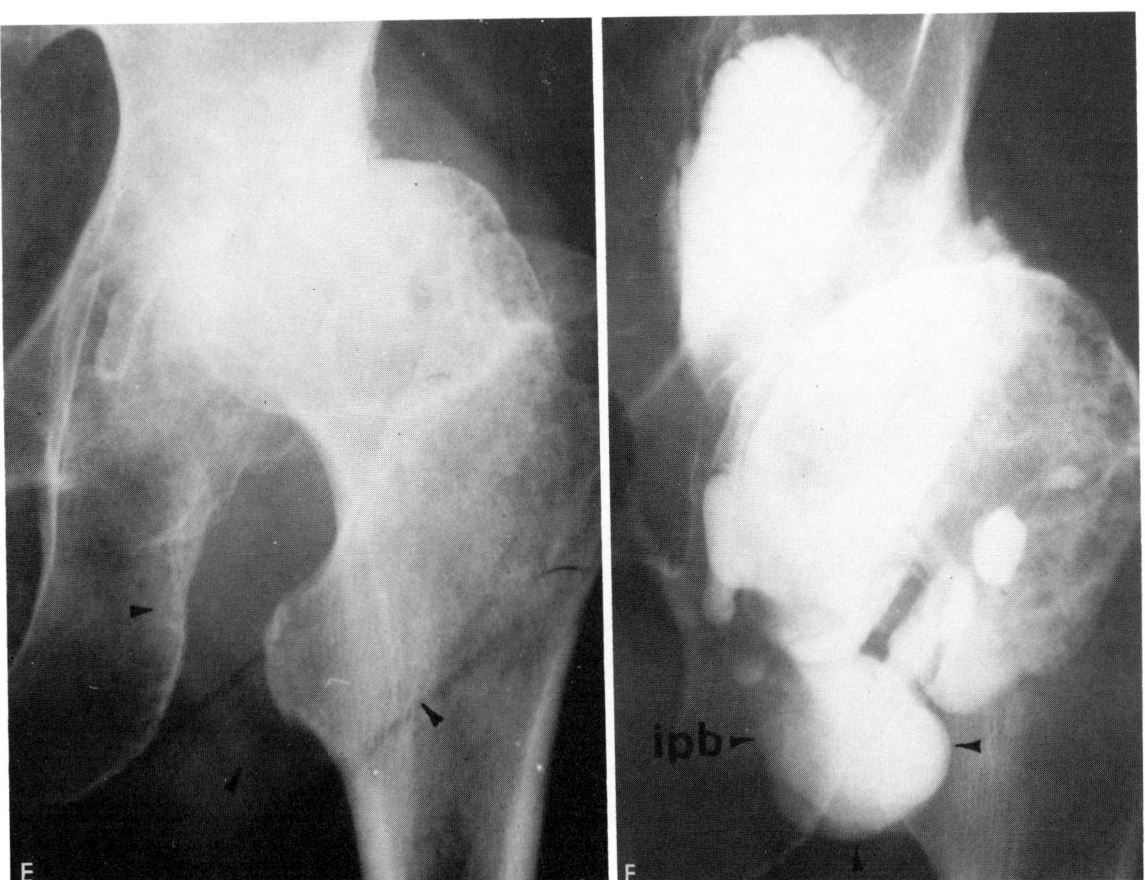

Figure 3–53. Continued

E, F *Osteoarthritis with enlarged iliopsoas bursa (ipb). The initial film demonstrates displacement of the iliopsoas fat (arrowheads). Arthrography reveals communication of the iliopsoas bursa (ipb) with the hip joint.*

(**E, F,** *From Warren R, et al: J Bone Joint Surg 57A:413, 1975.)*

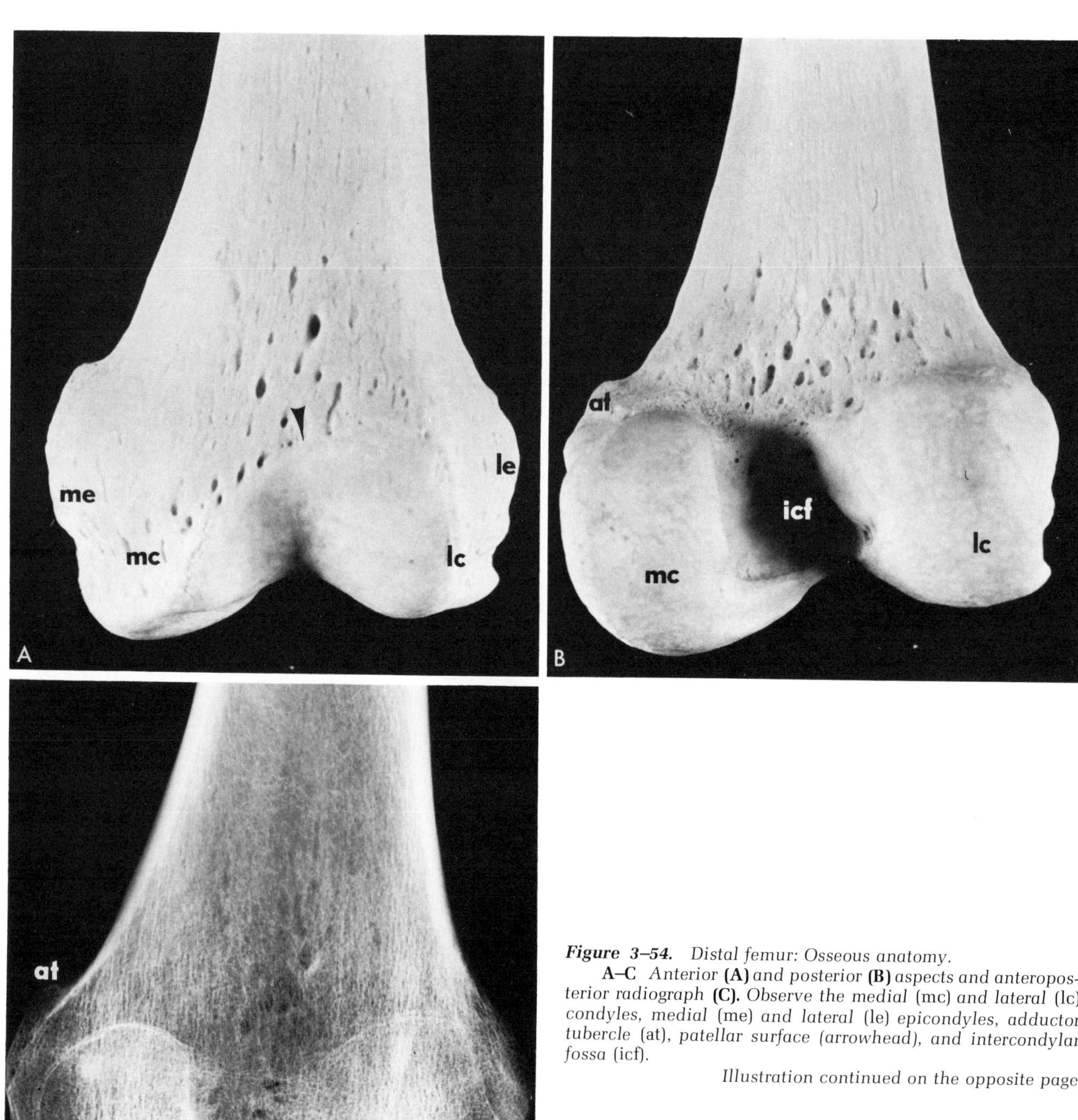

Figure 3–54. *Distal femur: Osseous anatomy.*

A–C *Anterior* **(A)** *and posterior* **(B)** *aspects and anteroposterior radiograph* **(C).** *Observe the medial* (mc) *and lateral* (lc) *condyles, medial* (me) *and lateral* (le) *epicondyles, adductor tubercle* (at), *patellar surface (arrowhead), and intercondylar fossa* (icf).

Illustration continued on the opposite page

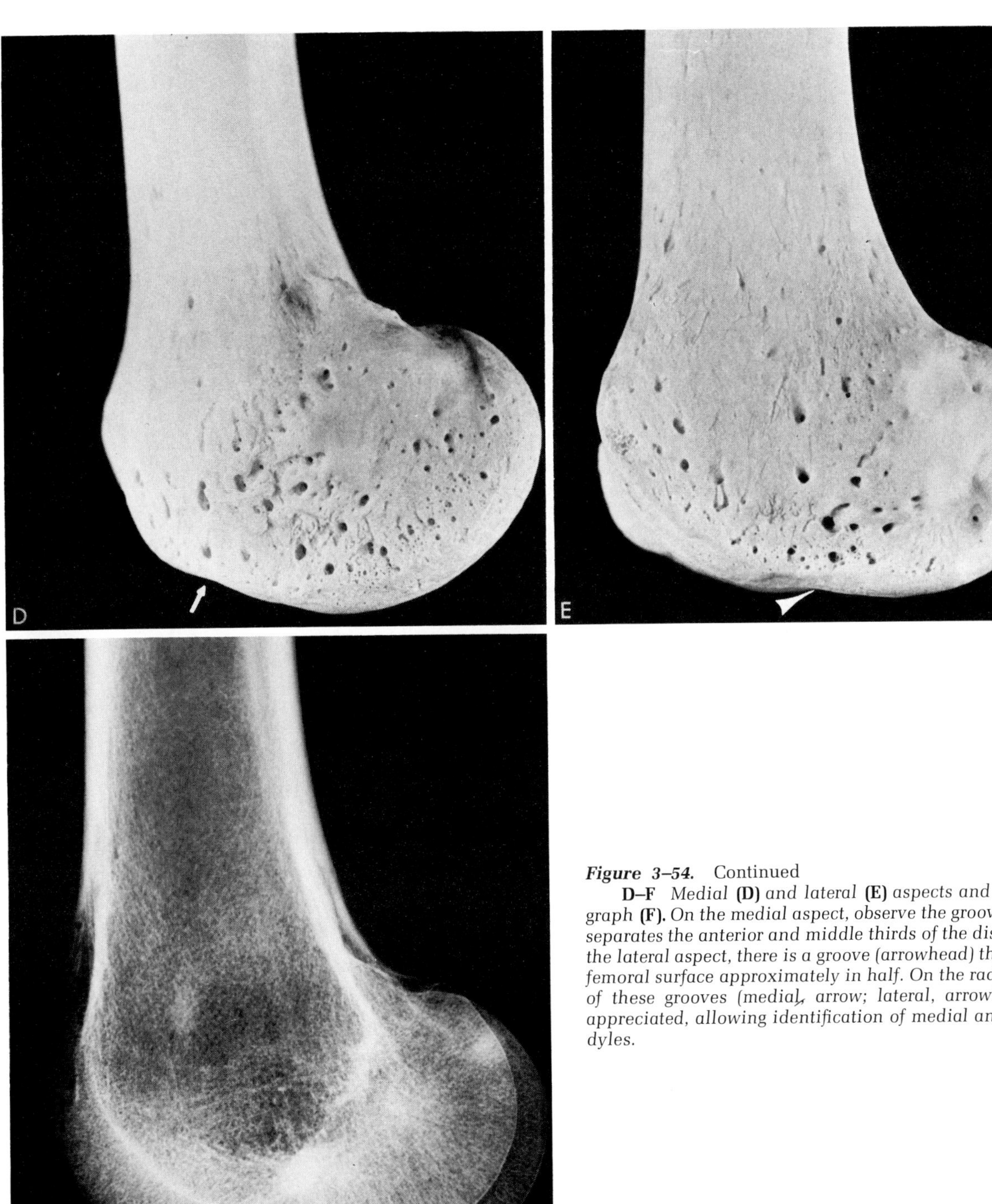

Figure 3–54. Continued

D–F *Medial* **(D)** *and lateral* **(E)** *aspects and lateral radiograph* **(F).** *On the medial aspect, observe the groove (arrow) that separates the anterior and middle thirds of the distal femur. On the lateral aspect, there is a groove (arrowhead) that divides the femoral surface approximately in half. On the radiograph, both of these grooves (medial, arrow; lateral, arrowhead) can be appreciated, allowing identification of medial and lateral condyles.*

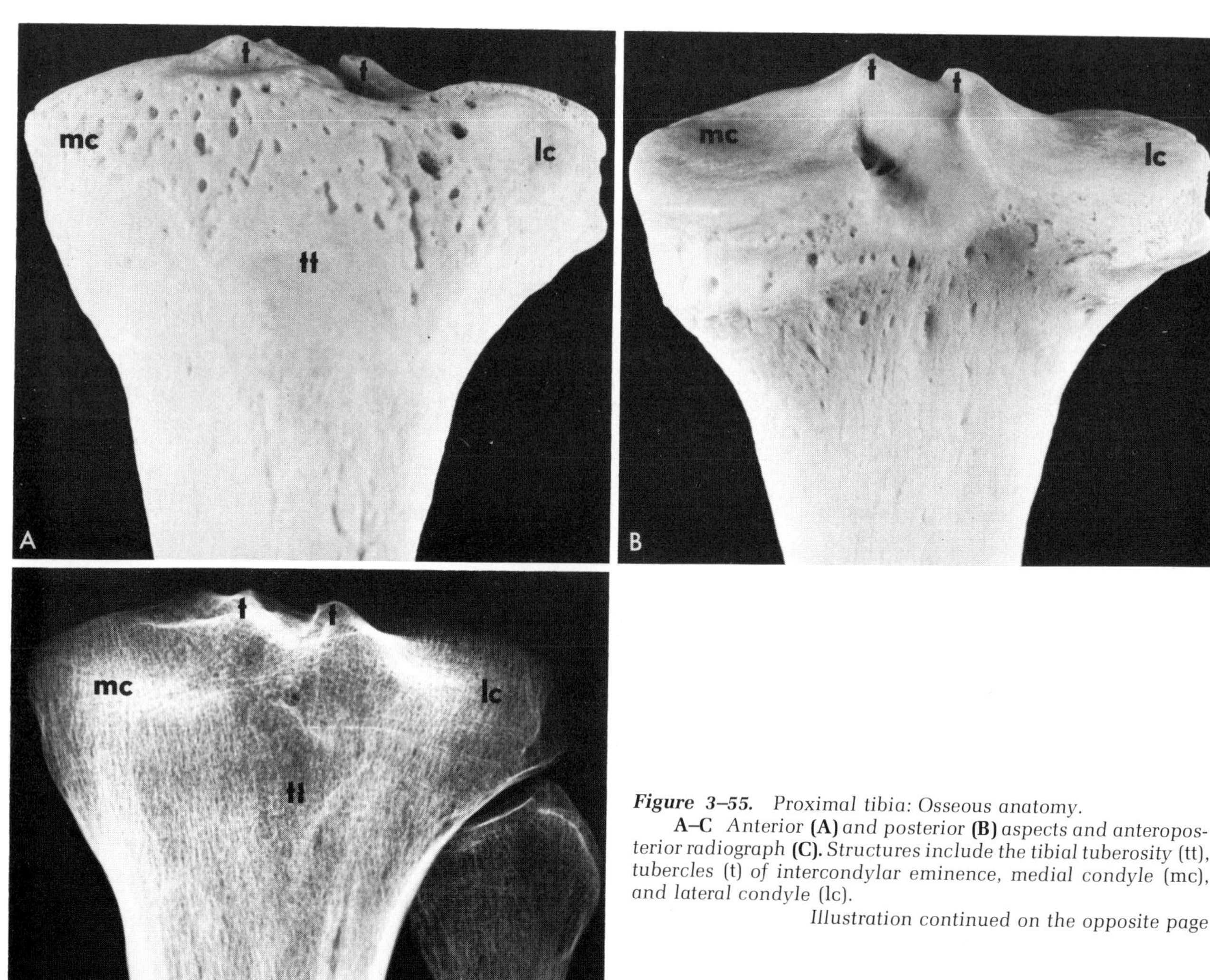

Figure 3–55. *Proximal tibia: Osseous anatomy.*

A–C *Anterior* **(A)** *and posterior* **(B)** *aspects and anteroposterior radiograph* **(C)**. *Structures include the tibial tuberosity (tt), tubercles (t) of intercondylar eminence, medial condyle (mc), and lateral condyle (lc).*

Illustration continued on the opposite page

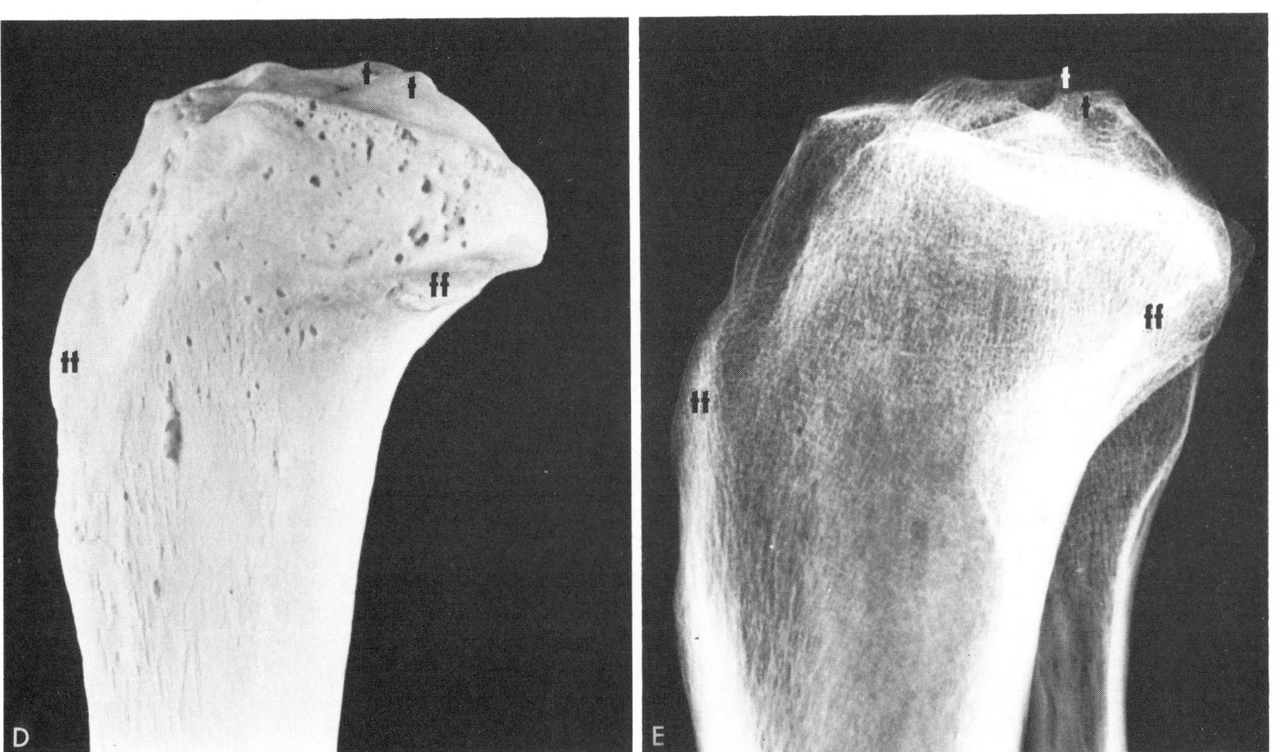

Figure 3–55. Continued

D, E *Lateral aspect* **(D)** *and lateral radiograph* **(E).** *Note the tibial tuberosity* (tt), *tubercles* (t) *of intercondylar eminence, and fibular facet* (ff).

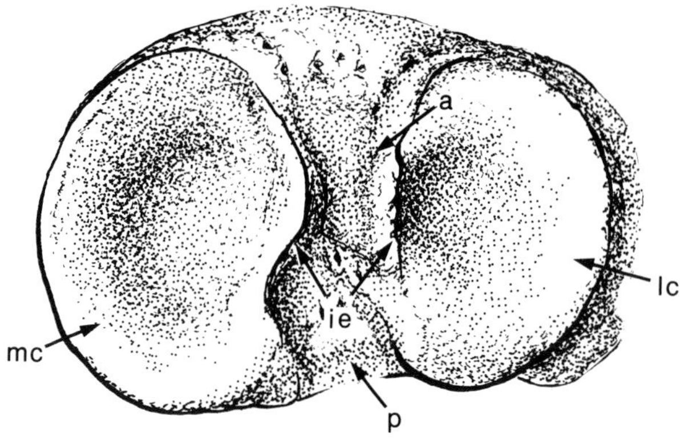

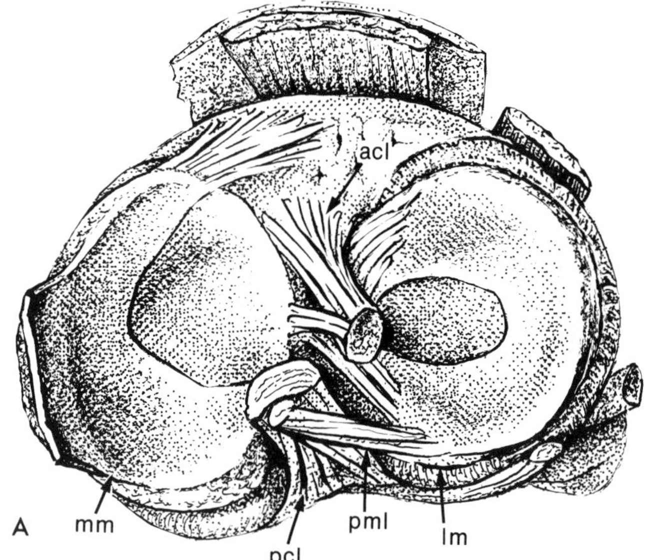

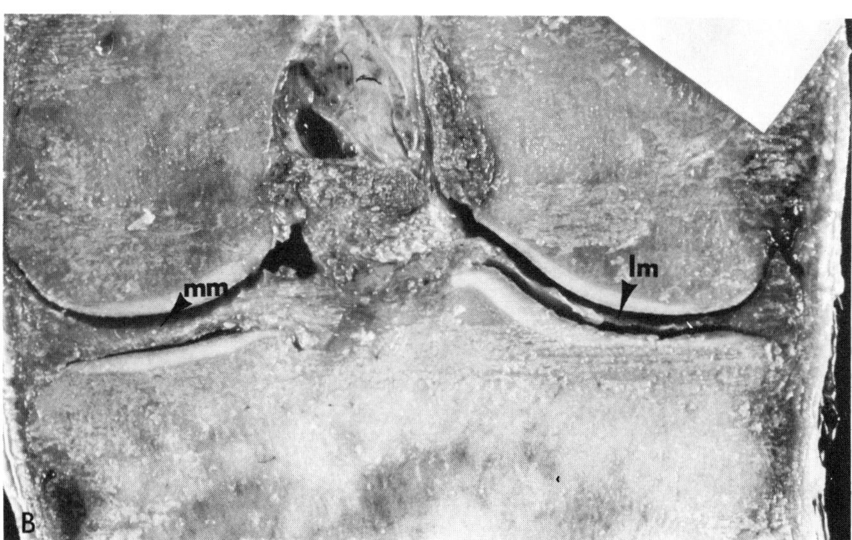

Figure 3–56. *Meniscal anatomy.*

A *Drawings of tibial articular surfaces without (upper) and with (below) the addition of soft tissue structures. Note the medial condyle (mc), lateral condyle (lc), intercondylar eminences (ie), anterior intercondylar area (a) and posterior intercondylar area (p). Soft tissue structures are the medial meniscus (mm), lateral meniscus (lm), posterior cruciate ligament (pcl), posterior meniscofemoral ligament (pml), and anterior cruciate ligament (acl).*

B *On a coronal section, the medial meniscus (mm) and lateral meniscus (lm) are identified between femur and tibia.*

tachments of the posterior cruciate ligament and lateral meniscus. Posterior fibers of the medial meniscus are continuous with the transverse ligament. The peripheral aspect of the medial meniscus is attached to the fibrous capsule and tibial collateral ligament. The lateral meniscus, which is of relatively uniform width throughout, resembles a ring. Its anterior aspect is attached to the intercondylar eminence of the tibia behind and lateral to the anterior cruciate ligament. Its posterior portion is attached to the intercondylar eminence of the tibia just anterior to the attachment of the medial meniscus. The lateral meniscus is grooved posteriorly by the popliteus tendon and its accompanying tendon sheath. Meniscofemoral ligaments, both anterior and posterior, represent attachments of the posterior horn of the lateral meniscus.

The articular surface of the patella is oval in shape and contains an osseous vertical ridge that divides it into a smaller medial area and a large lateral area[169] (Fig. 3–57). This patellar ridge fits into a corresponding groove on the anterior surface of the femur. The patellar articulating surface is subdivided still further by two ill-defined horizontal ridges of bone into three facets on either side. One additional vertical ridge of bone separates a narrow elongated facet on the medial border of the articular surface. Contact between these various patellar articular facets and the femur varies, depending upon the position of the knee. In full flexion, the most medial facet of the patella contacts the lateral portion of the medial femoral condyle, and the superior aspect of the lateral patellar facet contacts the anterior part of the lateral condyle. With extension of the knee, the middle facet of the patella becomes intimate with the lower portion of the femoral patellar surface, and in full extension, only the lowest patellar articular facets contact the femur.[1] During forced extension of the joint, there is a tendency for the patella to be displaced laterally, a tendency which is prevented by the action of adjacent musculature and the prominence of the lateral patellar surface of the femur.

The fibrous capsule of the knee joint is not a complete structure. Rather, the knee is surrounded by tendinous expansions, which reinforce the capsule. Between the capsule or tendinous expansions and synovial lining are various intra-articular structures, including ligaments and fat pads.

Anteriorly, the fibrous capsule is absent above and over the patellar surface. The ligamentous sheath in this area is composed mainly of a tendinous expansion from the rectus femoris and the vasti musculature, which descends to attach around the superior half of the bone. Superficial fibers continue to descend onto the strong ligamentum patellae. This structure, which represents the continuation of the quadriceps muscle, is attached above to the apex of the patella and below to the tibial tuberosity. Adjacent fibers, the medial and lateral patellar retinaculae, pass from the osseous margins of the patella to the tibial condyles. Superficial to these tendinous structures are the expansions of the fascia lata. Above the patella, deficiency of the fibrous capsule creates a suprapatellar bursa, which freely communicates with the articular cavity.

Posteriorly, capsular fibers extend from the femoral surface above the condyles and the intercondylar line to the posterior border of the tibia. This portion of the capsule is strengthened by the oblique popliteal ligament, which is derived from the semimembranosus tendon. Additional posterior reinforcement relates to the arcuate popliteal ligament, which emerges from the fibular head to blend with the capsular fibers.

Laterally, capsular fibers run from the femoral to the tibial condyles. In this area, the fibular collateral ligament is found, which is attached above to the lateral epicondyle of the femur and below to the fibular head. There is a space between capsular fibers and the fibular collateral ligament through which extend genicular vessels and nerves.

Medially, the capsule is strengthened by tendinous expansions from sartorius and semimembranosus muscles. These fibers pass upward to the tibial collateral ligament, which is attached above to the medial epicondyle of the femur and below to the medial tibial condyle and shaft. One or more bursae may separate the tibial collateral ligament from the fibrous capsule.[170] On its deep surface, the fibrous capsule connects the menisci and adjacent tibia, a connection which is termed the coronary ligament.

The tibial and fibular collateral ligaments reinforce the medial and lateral sides of the joint. They are taut in joint extension, and in this position, they prevent rotation of the knee.

The synovial membrane of the knee joint is the most extensive in the body and can be conveniently divided into several parts.[2] (Fig. 3–58).

Central Portion. This extends between the patella and the patellar surface of the femur to the cruciate ligaments. This portion lies between femoral and tibial condyles and, in addition, above and below the menisci. An infrapatellar fat pad below the patella, located deep to the patellar ligament, presses the synovial membrane posteriorly. In this area, a vertical infrapatellar synovial fold runs from the synovial surface of the fat pad to the intercondylar fossa. Horizontal alar synovial folds run from each side of the infrapatellar synovial fold.

Suprapatellar Synovial Pouch. This cavity, which develops separately from the knee joint but eventually communicates with it, extends vertically above the patella between the quadriceps muscle anteriorly and the femur posteriorly.

Posterior Femoral Recesses. These recesses lie behind the posterior portion of each femoral condyle, deep to the lateral and medial heads of the gastrocnemius muscle. Single or multiple bursae may be located between the muscular

Text continued on page 141

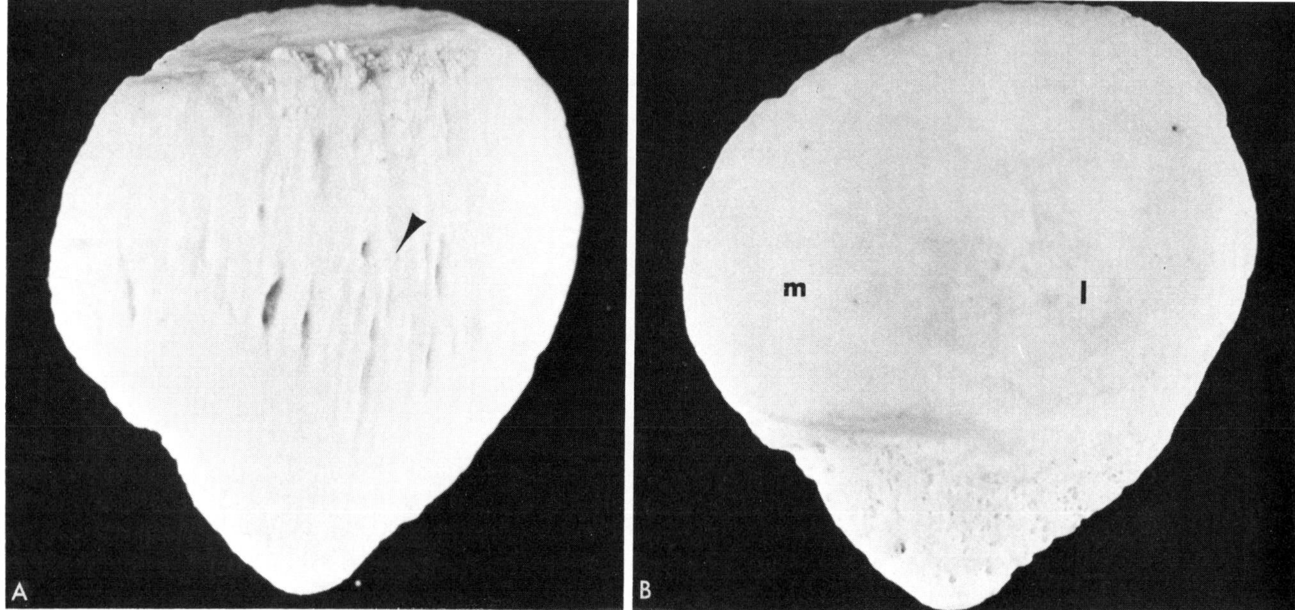

Figure 3–57. *Patella: Osseous anatomy.*

A, B *Anterior* **(A)** *and posterior* **(B)** *aspects. Note the irregular anterior patellar surface (arrowhead) to which attaches the quadriceps tendon. The posterior articular surface is divided into medial* (m) *and lateral* (l) *facets.*

Illustration continued on the opposite page

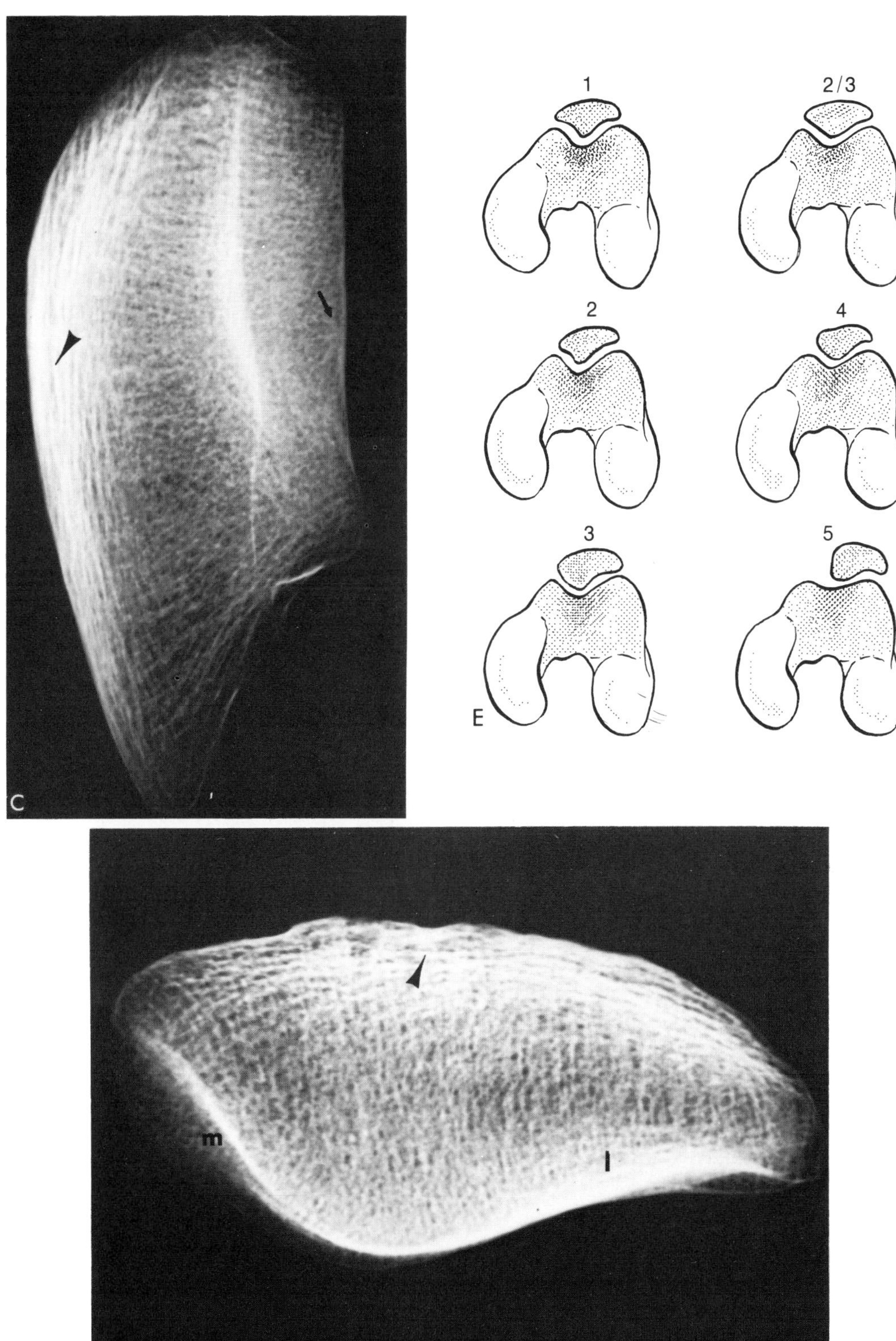

Figure 3–57. Continued

C, D *Lateral* **(C)** *and axial* **(D)** *radiographs of the patella outline thick anterior cortex (arrowhead) and smooth articular surface (arrow). Observe the medial* (m) *and lateral* (l) *facets.*

E *Patellar configurations have been delineated by Wiberg, Baumgarten, and other investigators and are summarized in this drawing. For each image, the medial condyle is depicted on the left and the lateral condyle is depicted on the right. Type 1 patellae have equal facets, which are slightly concave. Type 2 patellae are similar, with concave surfaces and a smaller medial facet. Type 3 patellae possess a small medial facet with a convex surface. Type 2/3 patellae have a flat medial facet. Type 4 patellae possess a small or absent medial facet. Type 5 (Jagerhut) patellae demonstrate no medial facet, no central ridge, and lateral subluxation.*

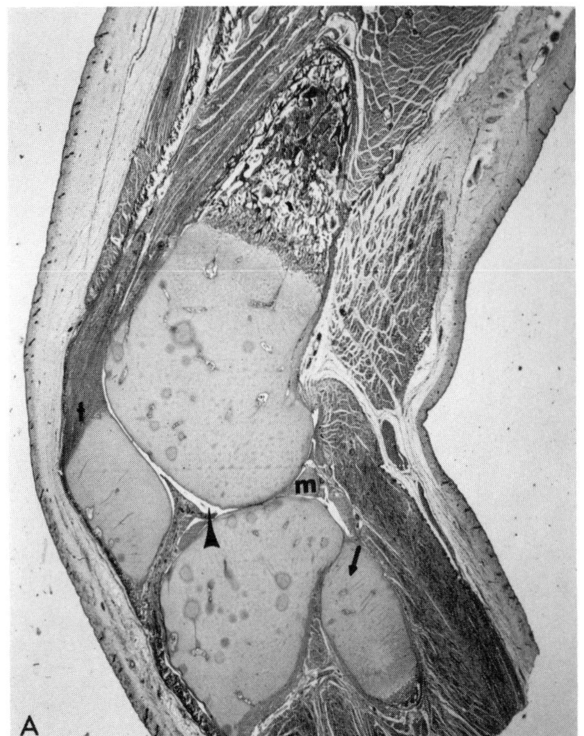

Figure 3–58. *Knee joint: Normal development and anatomy.*

A *A photomicrograph (×20) of a sagittal section depicting the developing joint (arrowhead) between unossified femur, tibia, and patella. Observe the proximal fibula (arrow), meniscus* (m), *and tendon* (t) *of the quadriceps femoris.*

B *Anterior aspect. The patella* (p) *has been divided to expose the joint interior. Observe the medial* (m) *and lateral* (l) *femoral condyles and alar folds* (af) *of synovium, which converge to form the infrapatellar fold* (if) *or ligamentum mucosum.*

C *Sagittal section. Drawing indicates femur, patella, and tibia, fibrous capsule* (FC), *prepatellar bursa* (pb), *deep infrapatellar bursa* (ib), *ligamentum patellae* (lp), *and suprapatellar pouch (arrowhead).*

Illustration continued on the opposite page

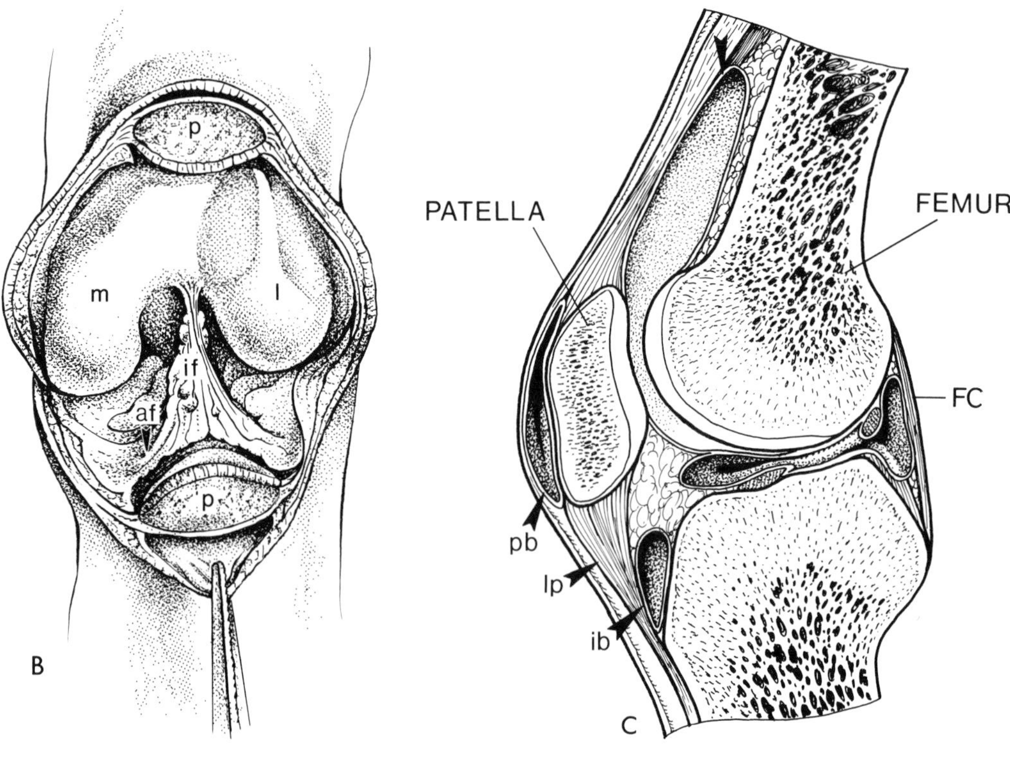

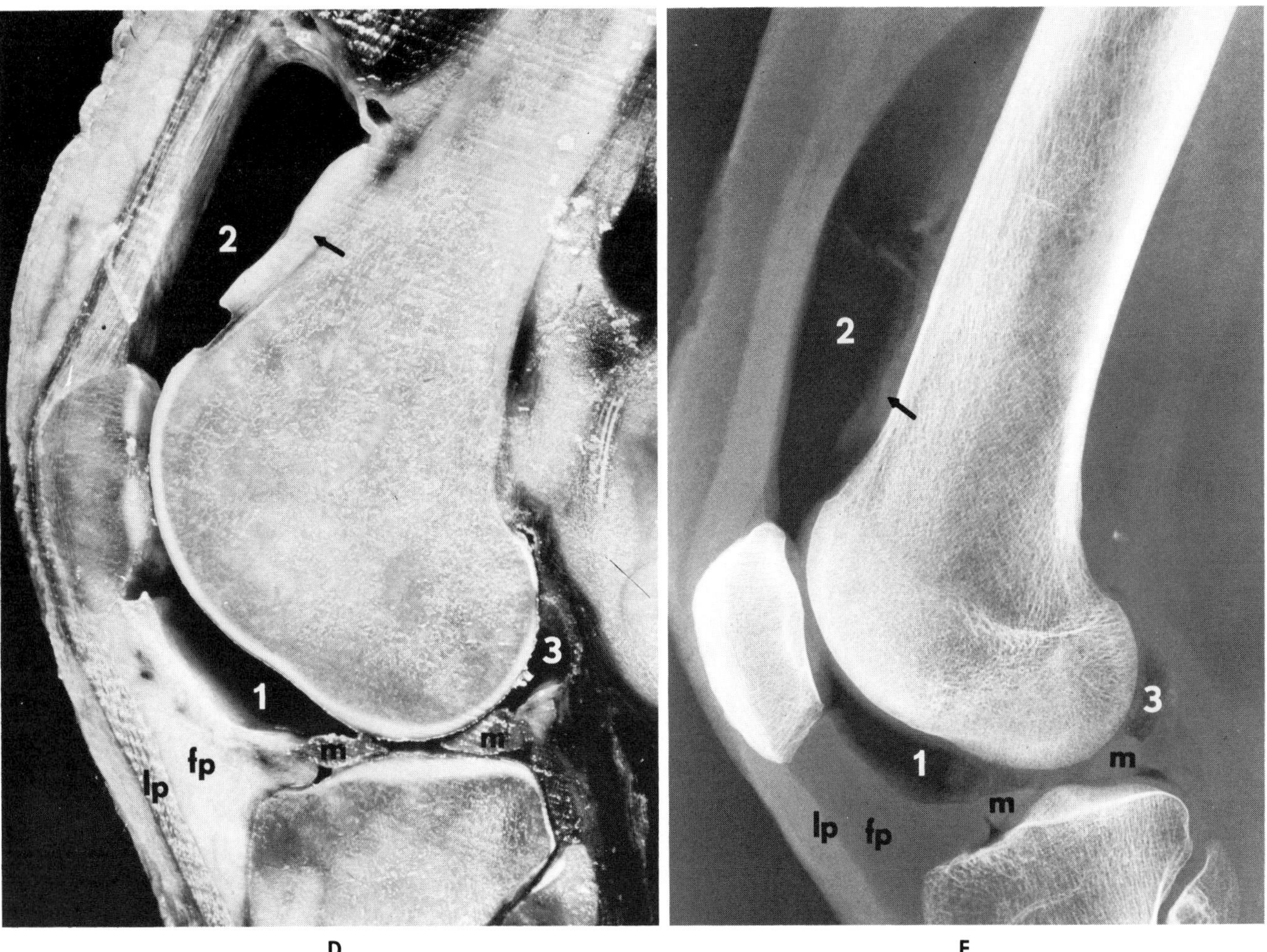

Figure 3–58. Continued

D, E *Sagittal section. Photograph and radiograph of an air-distended knee joint outlining ligamentum patellae* (lp), *infrapatellar fat pad* (fp), *and menisci* (m). *The articulation can be divided into a central portion* (1), *suprapatellar pouch* (2), *and posterior femoral recesses* (3). *Note fatty tissue (arrow), which is pressed against the anterior aspect of the femur.*

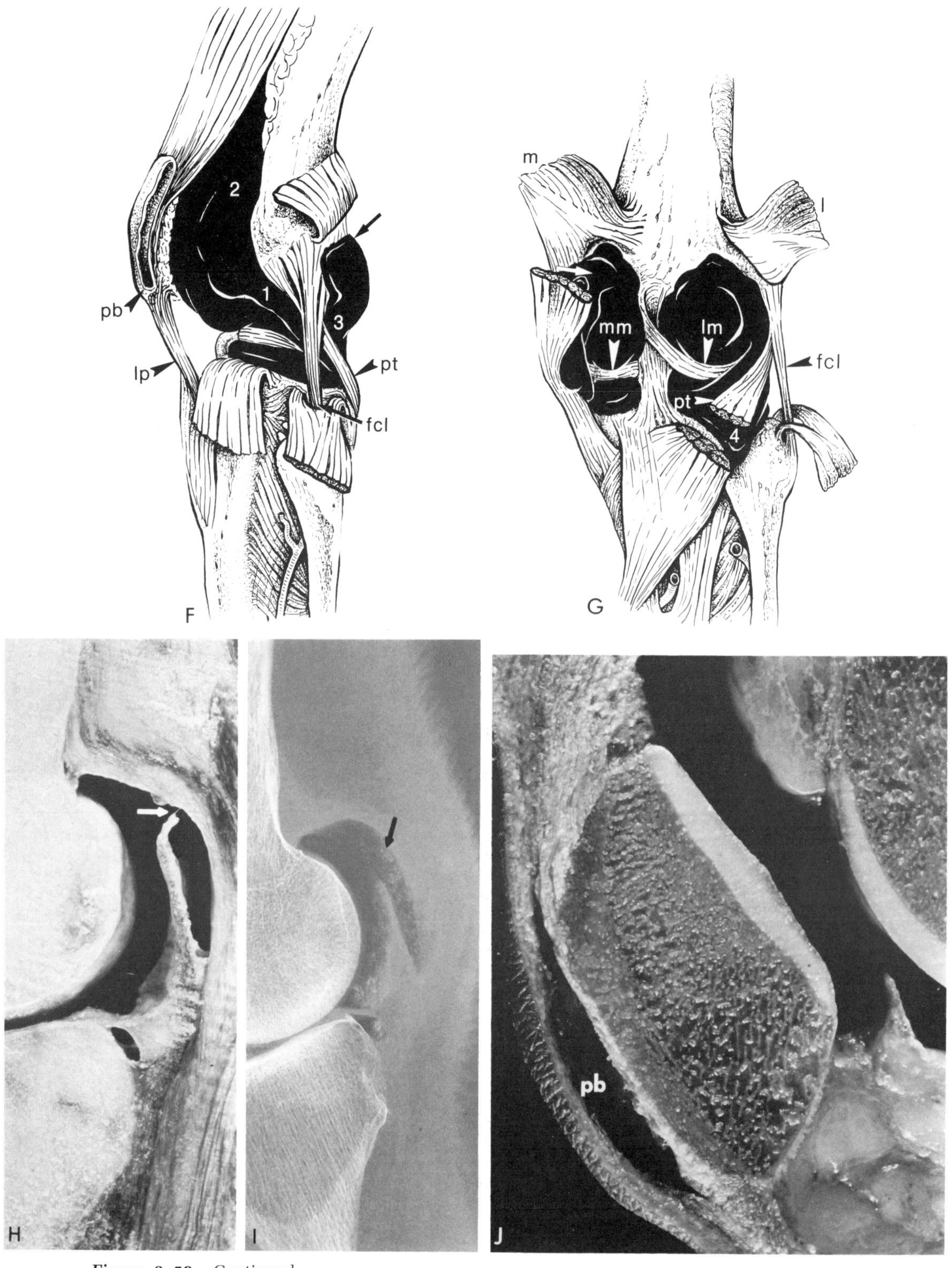

Figure 3–58. Continued

F *Lateral aspect. Distended joint is indicated in black. Observe the central portion* (1), *suprapatellar pouch* (2), *and posterior femoral recesses* (3). *The prepatellar bursa* (pb), *ligamentum patellae* (lp), *fibular collateral ligament* (fcl), *and popliteus tendon* (pt) *are indicated. The lateral head of the gastrocnemius muscle has been turned up, exposing a communicating bursa (arrow).*

G *Posterior aspect. The distended joint is indicated in black. The medial* (m) *and lateral* (l) *heads of the gastrocnemius have been sectioned. Note the bursa (arrow) beneath the lifted medial head, medial meniscus* (mm), *lateral meniscus* (lm), *popliteus tendon* (pt), *fibular collateral ligament* (fcl), *and subpopliteal recess* (4).

H, I *Photograph and radiograph of a sagittal section through the posterior aspect of the knee, revealing gastrocnemius-semimembranosus bursa (arrow) with communication with the knee joint.*

J *Sagittal section through the patella outlines the extent of the prepatellar bursa* (pb).

portions and the fibrous capsule, and may communicate with the articular cavity.[171-173] The medial and lateral posterior femoral recesses are separated by a thick central septum formed by a broad synovial fold around the cruciate ligaments, which may be continuous with the infrapatellar synovial fold.[174]

Subpopliteal Recess. A small synovial cul-de-sac lies between the lateral meniscus and the tendon of the popliteus, which may communicate with the superior tibiofibular joint in 10 per cent of adults.[175]

Additional Bursae. Numerous additional bursae may be found about the knee.[2, 172, 176-178] These include the subcutaneous prepatellar and subfascial prepatellar bursae anterior to the patella, deep infrapatellar bursa between the upper tibia and ligamentum patellae, anserine bursa between the tibial collateral ligament and tendons of the sartorius, gracilis, and semitendinosus muscles, and bursae between the semimembranosus tendon and tibial collateral ligament, and between the biceps tendon and fibular collateral ligament.

Intra-articular ligaments can be noted in the knee.[179-181] The anterior and posterior cruciate ligaments extend between the femur and the tibia. The anterior cruciate ligament attaches below to the anterior intercondylar area of the tibia and above to the medial side of the lateral femoral condyle. The posterior cruciate ligament extends from the posterior intercondylar area of the tibia to the lateral side of the medial femoral condyle. These ligaments prevent excessive posterior displacement (anterior cruciate ligament) or anterior displacement (posterior cruciate ligament) of the femur on the tibia.

The radiographic anatomy of the osseous structures about the knee has been reviewed. On anteroposterior radiographs, a line drawn along the mid-axis of the femoral shaft intersects a second line drawn tangent to the femoral articular surface with an average angle of 81 degrees (75 to 85 degrees) (femoral angle).[5] Similarly, a line drawn along the mid-axis of the tibial shaft intersects a second line drawn tangent to the tibial plateau with an average angle of 93 degrees (85 to 100 degrees) (tibial angle).[5]

The shallow grooves in the distal articular surface of the femur can be recognized.[182-184] The groove on the medial condyle appears as a sulcus at the junction of the anterior and middle thirds of the articular surface on lateral radiographs. In the same projection, the groove on the lateral condyle is located at the center of the articular surface and is generally more prominent. Landmarks allowing identification of each of the tibial condyles on lateral radiographs have also been summarized.[183]

Trabecular architecture about the knee has been studied[185] and a line of Blumensaat is identified as a condensed linear shadow on the lateral radiograph representing tangential bone in the intercondylar fossa.[186, 187] The location and appearance of Blumensaat's line is extremely sensitive to changes in knee position.[183] In the past, Blumensaat's line has been used to provide an indication of the relative position of the patella in lateral projections. Elevation of the distal pole of the patella above this line with the knee flexed 30 degrees has been used as an indicator of patella alta or an elevated position of the patella. More recently, other measurements on lateral roentgenograms have been suggested as more reliable indicators of patellar position (Fig. 3–59). Determination of the ratio of patellar tendon length to greatest diagonal length of the patella has revealed that in the normal situation, both measurements are approximately equal, with a variation of about 20 per cent.[188, 189] Another method involves determining the distance between the lower articular surface of the patella and the tibial plateau line. The ratio of this value over the length of the patellar articular surface in normal individuals has been reported to be approximately 0.8.[190] The diagnosis of patella alta may have clinical significance, as an abnormally high position of the patella has been recorded in chondromalacia patellae and patellar subluxation or dislocation, whereas a high or low position of the patella has been noted in Osgood-Schlatter's disease.[191]

The normal relationships of the anterior surface of the femur and the patella have been studied utilizing axial radiographs (Fig. 3–59). Various radiographic projections and measurements have been suggested.

The radiographic anatomy of the knee related to soft tissue shadows has also been described. In the lateral projection, the collapsed suprapatellar pouch creates a sharp vertical radiodense line between an anterior fat pad superior to the patella (anterior suprapatellar fat) and a posterior fat pad in front of the distal supracondylar region of the femur (prefemoral fat pad) (Fig. 3–60). This line is generally less than 5 mm in width, but may be between 5 and 10 mm. Shadows of increased thickness suggest the presence of intra-articular fluid.[192] Distortion of soft tissue planes[192, 193] with the production of a piriform mass[194] in this projection and displacement of fat planes about the suprapatellar pouch on frontal projections[195] are additional but less sensitive signs of knee effusions. Intra-articular fluid in the knee may also cause displacement of the ossified fabella.[196]

In lateral projections, a thin layer of extrasynovial fat hugs the femoral condyles posteriorly.[177] This fat plane extends from the origin of the femoral condyles to the posterior aspect of the lateral tibial condyle, forming a double curve resembling the numeral 3. A fat plane about the posterior cruciate ligament may also be visible. These fat planes become distorted in the presence of intra-articular fluid.

Active movements of the knee are flexion, extension, and medial and lateral rotation. Accessory

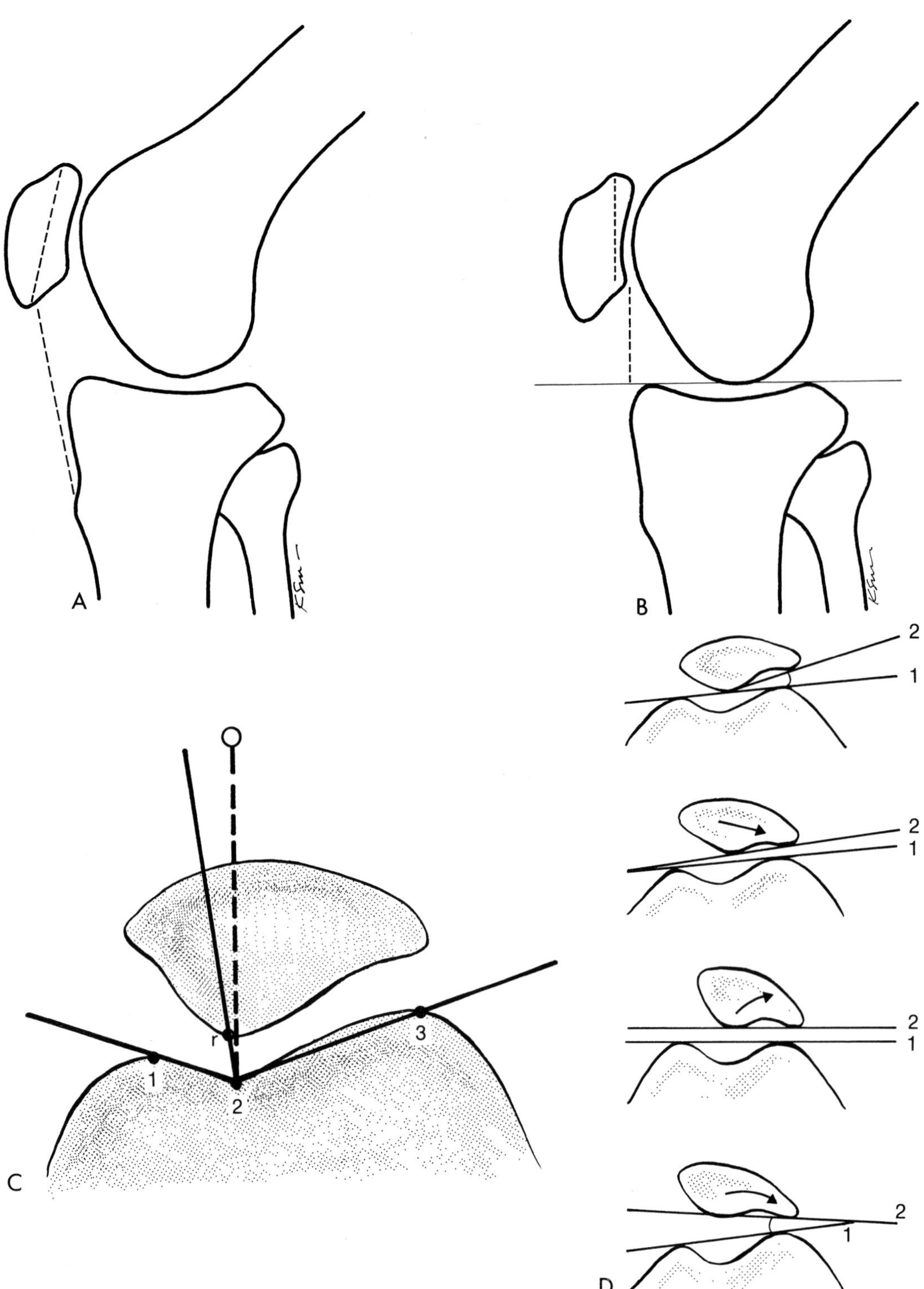

Figure 3–59. *Patellar position.*

A *The ratio of patellar tendon length to the greatest diagonal length of the patella may be used to diagnose patella alta.*

B *The ratio of the distance between the lower articular surface of the patella and the tibial plateau line to the length of the patellar articular surface has also been utilized for this purpose.*

C *On an axial radiograph, Merchant and co-workers (Merchant AC, et al: J Bone Joint Surg 56A:1391, 1974) have suggested that the line connecting the median ridge of the patella (r) and trochlear depth (2) should fall medial to or slightly lateral to a line (O) bisecting angle 1-2-3. Here the first line lies medial to line O, a normal finding.*

D *Laurin and co-workers have indicated other measurements that might be appropriate. The upper two diagrams reveal the normal situation; the lower two diagrams indicate the abnormal situation. On axial radiographs, normally an angle formed between a line connecting the anterior aspect of the femoral condyles (1) and a second line along the lateral facet of the patella (2) opens laterally. In patients with subluxation of the patella, these lines are parallel or the angle of intersection opens medially. (**D,** From Laurin CA, et al: J Bone Joint Surg 60A:55, 1978.)*

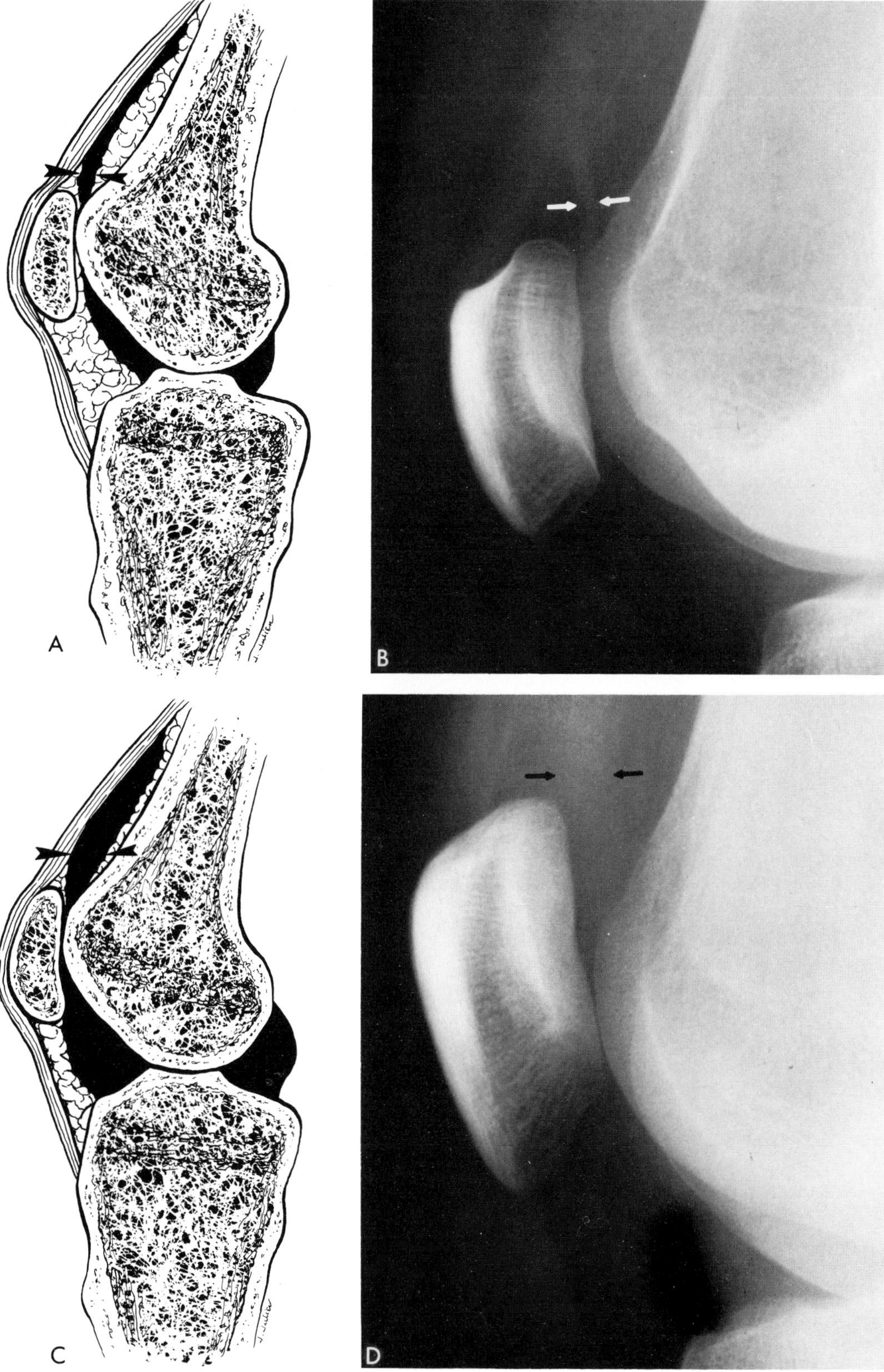

Figure 3–60. *Diagnosis of a synovial effusion in the knee.*

A, B *In normal situations, the collapsed suprapatellar pouch (arrowheads) creates a radiodense area (arrows) that is generally less than 5 mm in width but may be between 5 and 10 mm in width.*

C, D *In the presence of intra-articular fluid, distention of the pouch (arrowheads) creates a radiodense region of increased thickness with blurred margins (arrows).*

movements are increased rotation, backward and forward gliding, abduction, adduction, and separation of tibia and femur.

TIBIOFIBULAR JOINTS

Osseous and Soft Tissue Anatomy

Articulations uniting the tibia and the fibula are the proximal (superior) tibiofibular joint (synovial), the crural interosseous membrane (syndesmosis), and the distal tibiofibular joint (syndesmosis).

Proximal Tibiofibular Joint. The head of the fibula contains a circular facet that faces superiorly, anteriorly, and medially (Fig. 3–61). The styloid process of the fibular head is an upward protuberance on the lateral aspect of the posterior portion of the bone. The fibular facet on the lateral condyle of the tibia is directed downward, posteriorly, and laterally. The popliteus tendon creates a groove on the fibula superiorly and medially to the articular facet.

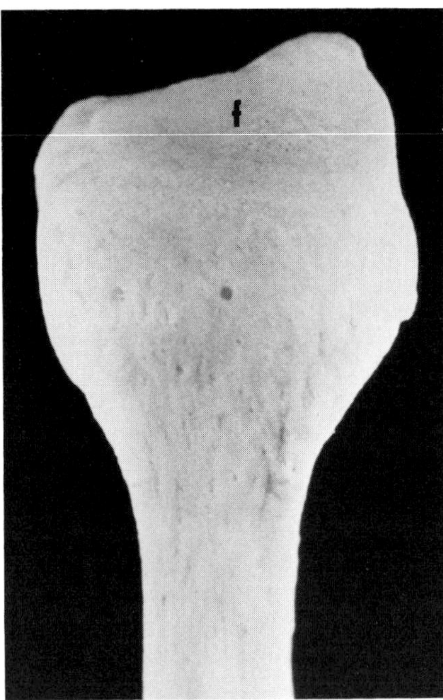

Figure 3–61. Proximal fibula: Osseous anatomy (medial aspect). A circular facet (f) is present on the fibular head.

The normal radiographic anatomy of the proximal tibiofibular joint has been outlined[175] (Fig. 3–62). Either of two types of articulations may be apparent[197]: a horizontal articulation (less than 20 degrees of joint inclination) and an oblique articulation (greater than 20 degrees of joint inclination), although intermediate variations are also noted. The horizontal type is associated with increased rotatory mobility and more joint surface area than the oblique type of articulation. The major functions of the proximal tibiofibular joint are dissipating torsional stresses applied at the ankle and providing tensile rather than significant weight-bearing strength.[197]

On an anteroposterior radiograph the medial aspect of the fibular head, which is the actual articulating surface, crosses the lateral border of the tibia. On the lateral radiograph the fibular head overlies the posterior border of the tibia. Its proper position in this projection can be confirmed by identifying its relationship to the lateral tibial condyle. An important landmark on the lateral knee radiograph for locating the exact position of the fibular head is formed by the posteromedial portion of the lateral tibial condyle.[183] If a line is drawn in an anterior to posterior direction along the lateral tibial spine and continued inferiorly along the posterior aspect of the tibia, this line will identify a groove that separates the midportion of the tibial shaft from the bulk of the bone forming the supporting structure of the lateral tibial condyle posteriorly. The linear sloping radiodensity observed on the lateral knee radiograph proceeds first posteriorly and inferiorly to form an acute angle posteriorly, which identifies the most posteromedial portion of the lateral tibial condyle. The linear radiodensity then extends inferiorly and anteriorly from this point in the groove described above. Knowledge of the exact location of this line greatly assists in the interpretation of lateral knee radiographs in tibiofibular joint dislocations (Fig. 3–63).

The optimal view for visualizing the proximal tibiofibular joint is a radiograph exposed with the knee in 45 to 60 degrees of internal rotation[175] (Fig. 3–64). In this projection, the articulation is seen in profile, generally free of overlying osseous structures, and the width of the articular space and appearance of subchondral bone can be evaluated.

Before 12 weeks of fetal age, the proximal tibiofibular joint does not possess a cavity[198] (Fig. 3–65). Subsequently, narrow cavities are apparent, which may be separated from the lateral femorotibial joint by a small amount of loose fibrous or areolar tissue. Communication between the knee joint and proximal tibiofibular joint may be identified in some fetuses and exists in approximately 10 per cent of adult articulations. Subsequent development of the proximal tibiofibular joint includes the formation of articular cartilage, synovial tissue, synovial recesses, and fibrous capsule.

The fully developed articulation is approximately a plane joint, between the lateral condyle of the tibia and the head of the fibula (Fig. 3–66). Apposing bony facets are covered with articular cartilage, and the bones are connected by a fibrous capsule and anterior and posterior ligaments. The fibrous capsule, which is attached to the margins of the tibial and fibular articular facets, is much thicker anteriorly than posteriorly. The anterior ligament

Text continued on page 150

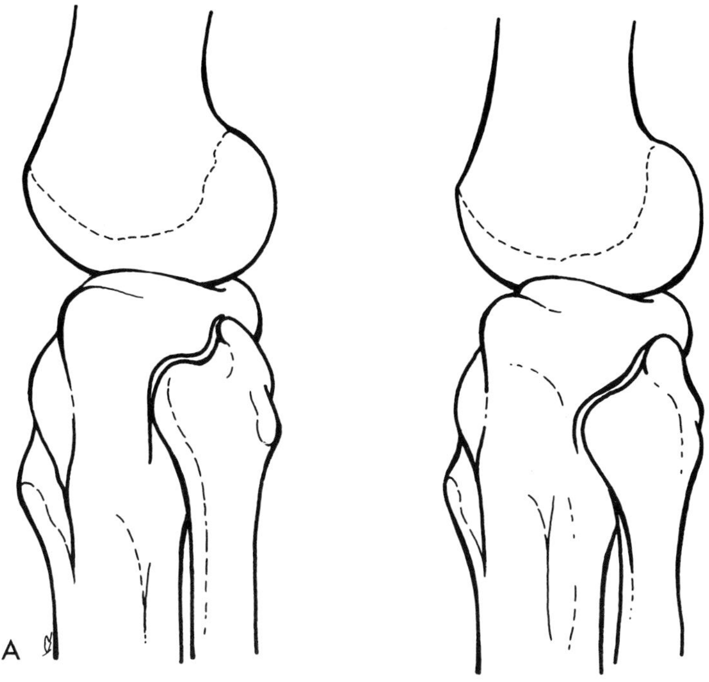

Figure 3–62. *Proximal tibiofibular joint: Osseous anatomy.*

A *Types of articulations. A horizontal (left) or oblique (right) type of articulation may be present.*

B *Anteroposterior radiograph outlining normal relationship of proximal tibia and fibula. Medial aspect of fibular head crosses lateral border of tibia (arrowheads).*

C *Lateral radiograph showing fibular head overlying posterior border of tibia. Note linear sloping radiodensity (arrowheads), which identifies the most posteromedial portion of lateral tibial condyle. This radiodense line is projected over the midportion of the fibular head.*

D *Posterior aspect of proximal tibia and fibula showing relationship of fibular head to posterior margin of tibia. Note groove (arrows) that separates midportion of tibial shaft from bulk of the bone forming the supporting structure of the lateral tibial condyle. This groove produces the linear sloping radiodensity on lateral knee radiographs.*

E *Steep oblique view showing relationship of proximal fibula and tibia. Again note groove (arrows).*

*(**B–E,** From Resnick D, et al: Am J Roentgenol 131:133, 1978. Copyright 1978, American Roentgen Ray Society.)*

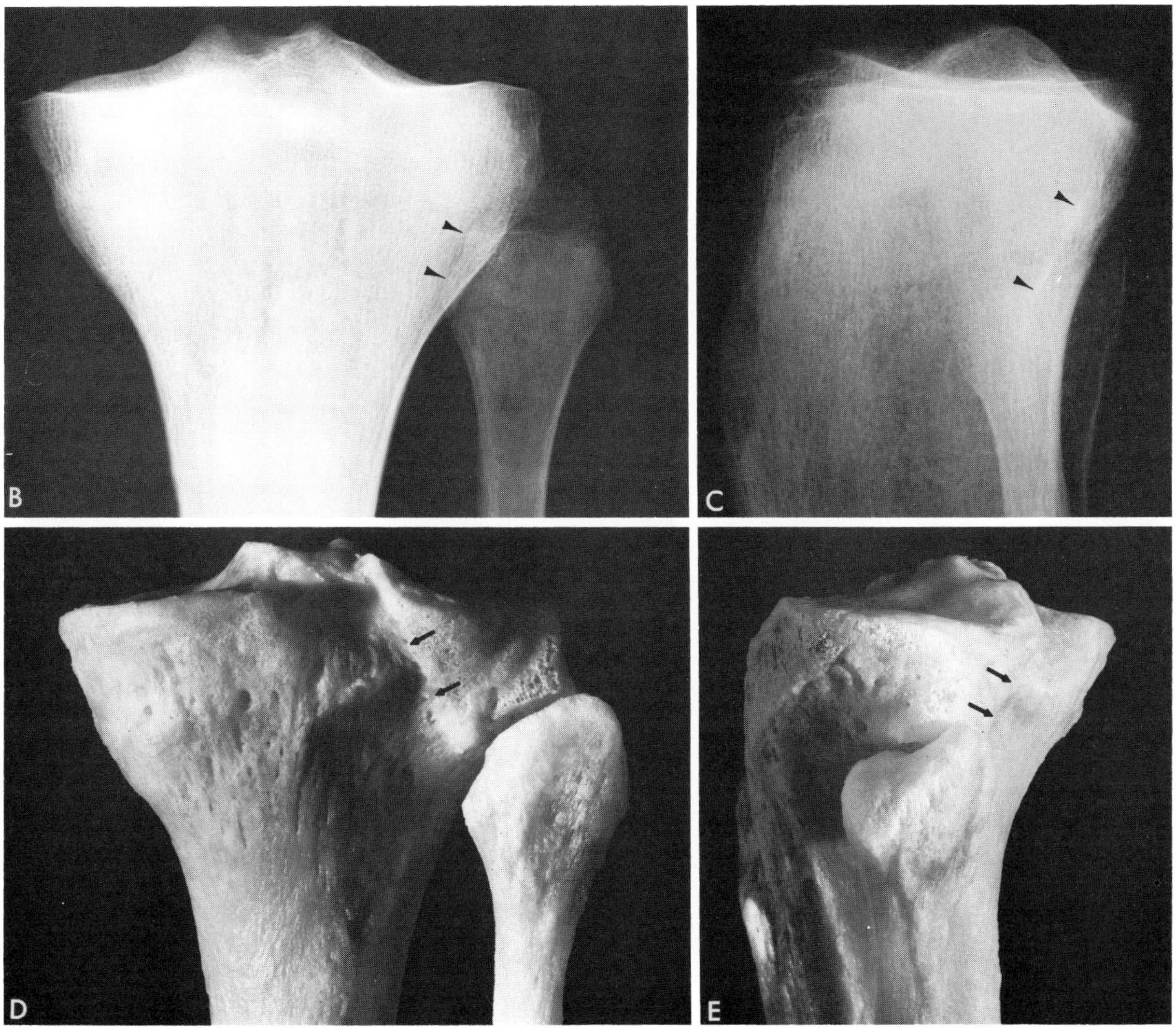

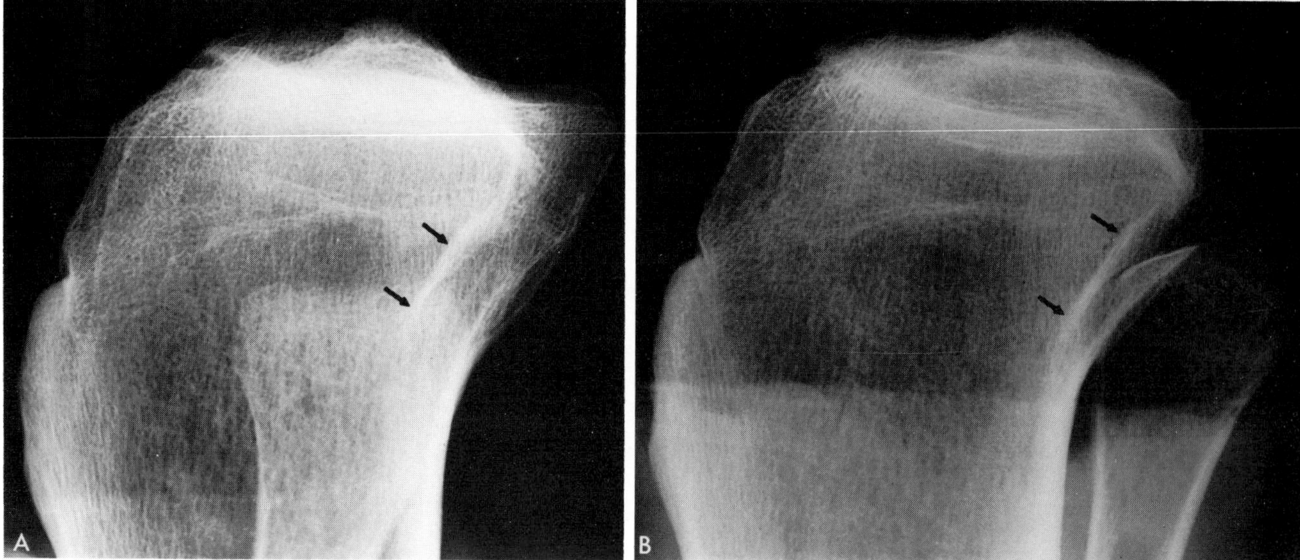

Figure 3–63. *Dislocation at proximal tibiofibular joint in cadaver.*

A *Anterolateral dislocation. Almost the entire fibular head is projected in front of sloping radiodense line (arrows).*

B *Posteromedial dislocation. There is little overlap between proximal tibia and fibula. Fibular head is projected entirely posterior to sloping radiodense line (arrows).*

(From Resnick D, et al: Am J Roentgenol 131:133, 1978. Copyright 1978, American Roentgen Ray Society.)

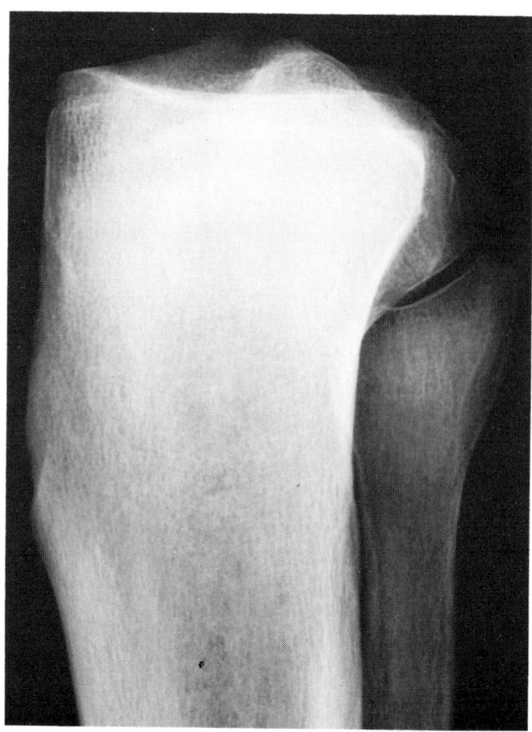

Figure 3–64. *The optimal view for visualizing proximal tibiofibular joint in profile. Radiograph is exposed in 45 to 60 degrees of internal rotation. (From Resnick D, et al: Am J Roentgenol 131:133, 1978. Copyright 1978, American Roentgen Ray Society.)*

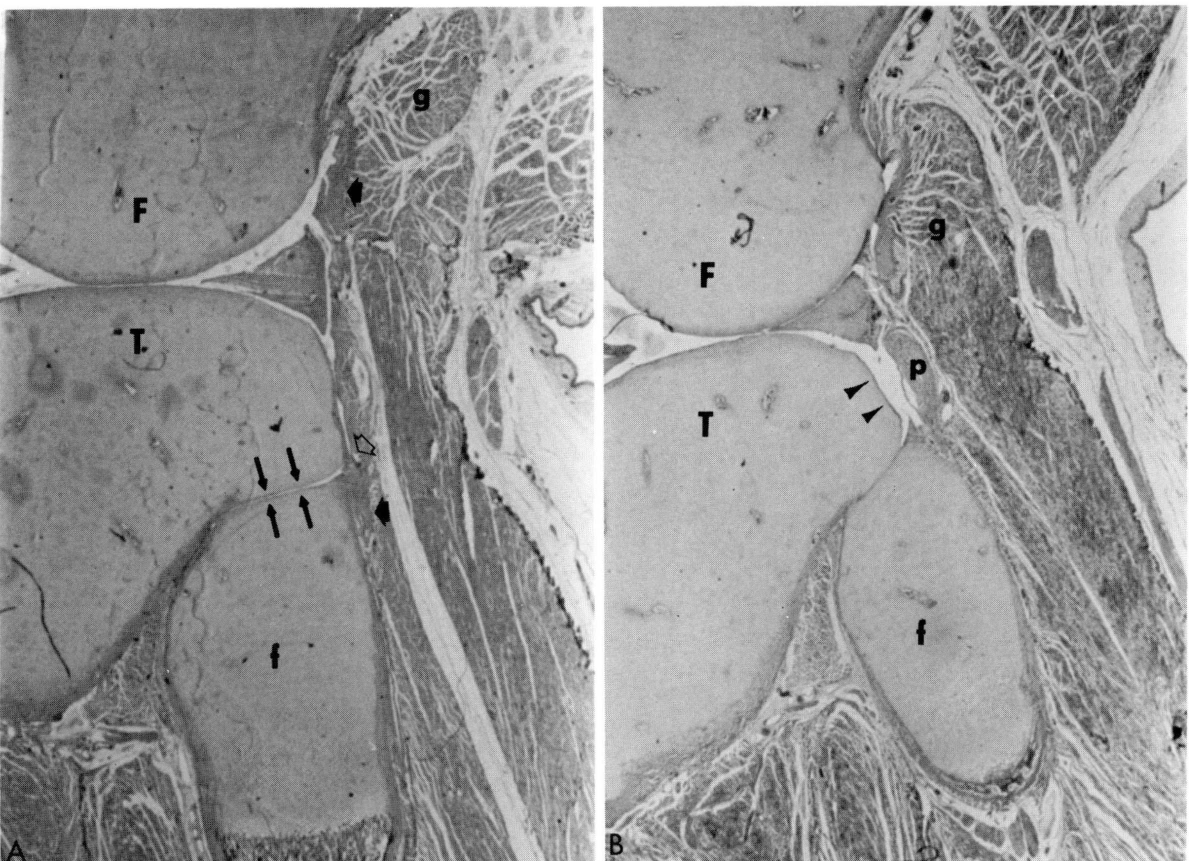

Figure 3–65. *Proximal tibiofibular joint: Normal developmental anatomy of proximal tibiofibular joint. Sagittal sections through articulation in embryos.* f, *Fibula;* T, *tibia;* F, *femur.*

A *Tibiofibular joint space (double arrows) is seen as a thin white line 1 mm wide. There are no articular recesses. Posterior horn of lateral meniscus is well developed. The posterior aspect of the knee joint capsule inserts on the fibula and femur (heavy arrows). The insertion of the lateral head of the gastrocnemius muscle* (g) *is noted at the posterior aspect of the lateral femoral condyle. A thin zone of fibrous tissue separates the femorotibial space from the proximal tibiofibular joint (open arrow).*

B *No central cavity is present within the proximal tibiofibular joint. Note prominent inferior recess beneath lateral meniscus (arrowheads) and direct communication between femorotibial and tibiofibular joints. Popliteus muscle* (p) *is cut in cross section. Lateral head of gastrocnemius muscle* (g) *is again noted.*

(From Resnick D, et al: Am J Roentgenol 131:133, 1978. Copyright 1978, American Roentgen Ray Society.)

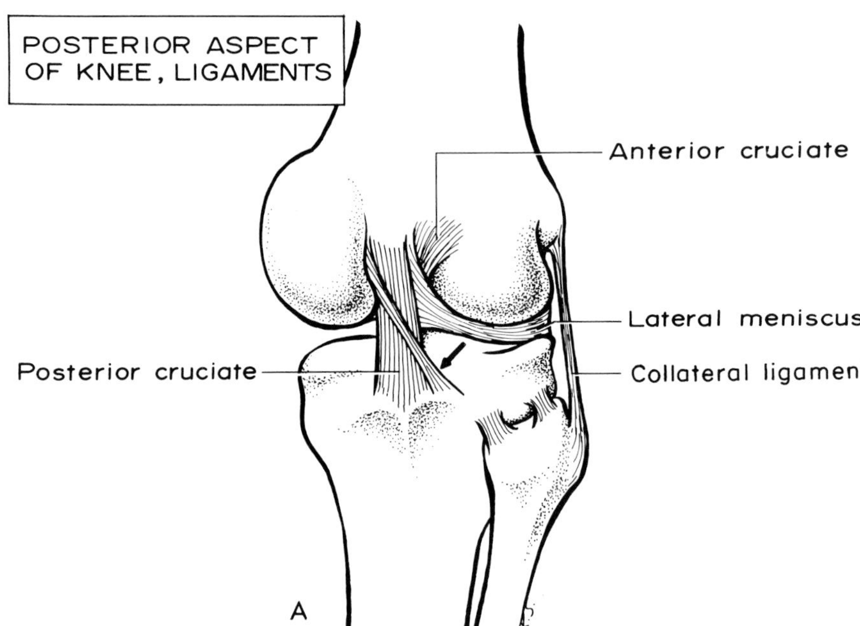

Figure 3–66. *Proximal tibiofibular joint: Articular anatomy.*

A *Anatomic features of fully developed proximal tibiofibular articulation. On posterior aspect of femur and tibia, two thick ligamentous bands pass obliquely from fibular head to posterior aspect of the lateral tibial condyle. Similar ligaments strengthen the anterior aspect of the tibiofibular joint (not shown). The fibular collateral ligament extends from the fibular head to the lateral femoral epicondyle. Posterior and anterior cruciate ligaments and the lateral meniscus are also indicated. Also note the posterior femoral meniscal ligament (ligament of Wrisberg, arrow).*

Illustration continued on the opposite page

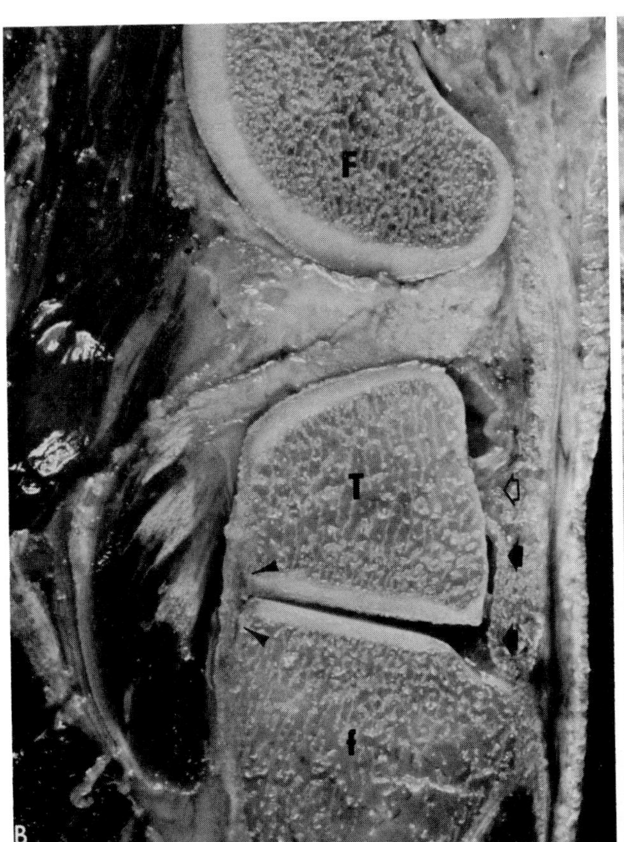

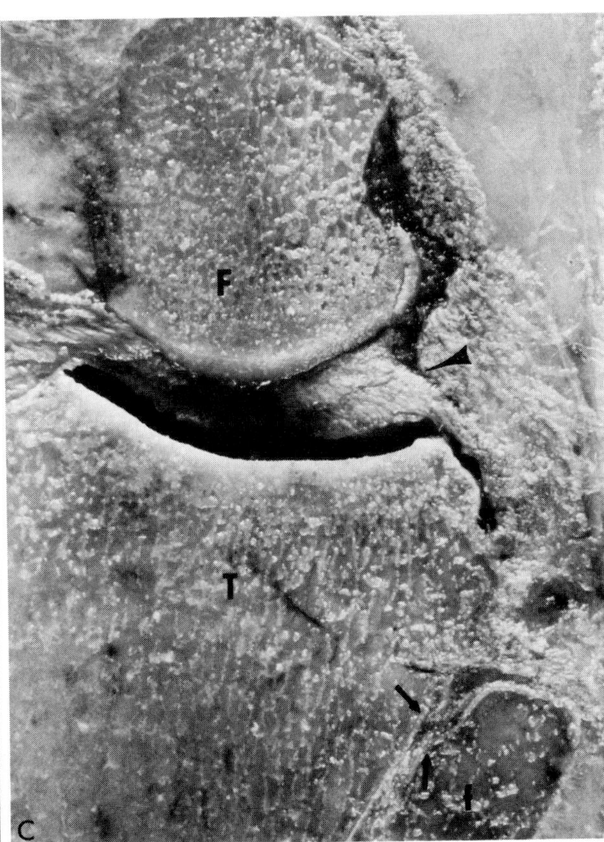

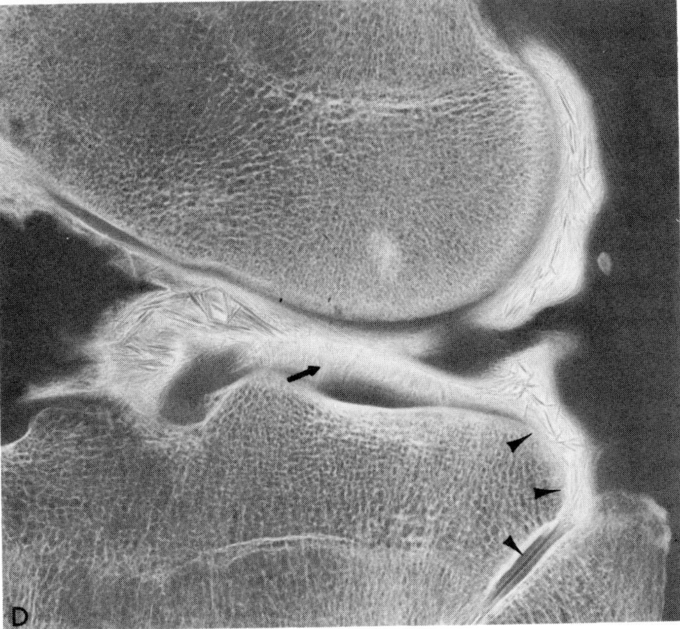

Figure 3–66. Continued

B, C *Coronal sections through two adult tibiofibular joints.* F, *Femur;* T, *tibia;* f, *fibula. Horizontal articulation* **(B)** *contains well-developed articular cartilage and joint space. The lateral recess (heavy arrows) is especially well developed, as is the joint capsule. The medial synovial recess is partially obliterated (arrowheads). Bands of fibrous and areolar tissue (open arrow) separate femorotibial and proximal tibiofibular articulations. The obliquely inclined joint is shown in* **C** *(arrows). An incidental finding is degeneration of the lateral meniscus (arrowhead).*

D *Radiograph of oblique section through knee joint after arthrography with methylmethacrylate. Contrast material is present within femorotibial space (arrow), continuous with small amount of contrast material within proximal tibiofibular articulation (arrowheads). Communication between these two articulations can be seen in about 10 per cent of adults. Note smooth cartilage of tibiofibular articulation.*

*(**B–D**, From Resnick D, et al: Am J Roentgenol 131:133, 1978. Copyright 1978, American Roentgen Ray Society.)*

passes obliquely upward from the front of the fibular head to the front of the lateral condyle of the tibia; the posterior ligament passes obliquely upward from the back of the fibular head to the back of the lateral condyle of the tibia. The posterior ligament is covered by the popliteus tendon. Superior support is provided by the fibular collateral ligament, extending from the lateral aspect of the fibular head to the lateral femoral epicondyle.

Crural Interosseous Membrane. This membrane is tightly stretched between the interosseous borders of tibia and fibula.[199] Its upper limit is just inferior to the proximal tibiofibular joint, and its lower limit contains fibers that blend with those about the distal tibiofibular joint. The oblique fibers in this membrane extend inferiorly and laterally from tibia to fibula. A large oval opening in the superior aspect of the membrane allows passage of the anterior tibial vessels; a smaller distal opening allows passage of the perforating branch of the peroneal artery.

Distal Tibiofibular Joint. This fibrous joint consists of a strong interosseous ligament that unites the convex surface of the medial distal fibula and the concave surface of the adjacent fibular notch of the tibia. Additionally, the anterior and posterior tibiofibular ligaments reinforce this articulation. Below this ligamentous joint, an upward prolongation of the synovial membrane of the ankle (talocrural joint) can extend 3 to 5 mm. This synovial recess may be associated with cartilaginous surfaces on tibia and fibula.

There is little movement between tibia and fibula. A small amount of lateral rotation of the fibula may be apparent during dorsiflexion of the ankle.[200]

ANKLE (TALOCRURAL JOINT)

This synovial articulation exists where the talus relates to the lower ends of the tibia and fibula and the inferior transverse tibiofibular ligament.

Osseous Anatomy

The distal end of the tibia contains the medial malleolus and articular surface (Fig. 3–67). The broad malleolus has an articular facet on its lateral surface, which is comma-shaped in configuration. On the posterior surface of the distal tibia is a groove, just lateral to the medial malleolus, related to the tendon of the tibialis posterior. The inferior surface of the tibia represents the articular area for the talus. It is smooth, wider anteriorly than posteriorly, concave anteriorly to posteriorly, and minimally convex medially to laterally. The articular surface on the inferior tibia is continuous with that on the medial malleolus. The triangular fibular notch is on the lateral side of the tibia. This notch represents the site of attachment of various ligaments that connect the distal tibia and fibula.

The distal end of the fibula contains the lateral malleolus (Fig. 3–67). This structure projects more inferiorly than the medial malleolus and contains a triangular facet on its medial surface for articulation with the talus, and an irregular surface above this facet for the interosseous ligament. Posterior to the convex articular facet is a depression, the malleolar fossa.

The dorsal surface of the talus contains the trochlear articular surface (Fig. 3–68). This surface is convex anteriorly to posteriorly and concave from side to side. The medial surface of the talar body possesses a facet that articulates with the medial malleolus. The lateral surface of the body contains a triangular articular facet that is intimate with the lateral malleolus.

Assessment of alignment of the ankle on radiographs is important in the evaluation of this joint following trauma. Small degrees of lateral displacement of the talus on the tibia may result in the rapid development of secondary degenerative arthritis. It has recently been shown that even 1 mm of lateral displacement of the talus reduces the tibiotalar contact areas by 42 per cent.[201] Incomplete ligament tears may result in relatively small amounts of displacement, which may be difficult to detect roentgenographically. This has stimulated investigators to propose radiographic criteria for assessment of tibiotalar alignment.[202]

A short, concave cortical line representing the posteromedial surface of the talus was utilized by some investigators in determination of tibiotalar displacement[203] (Fig. 3–68). However, this line actually delineates the insertion of the deep deltoid fibers and does not represent the true medial articular surface. In addition, this line cannot be accurately identified with moderate internal or external rotation of the talus, precluding accurate measurements on rotation roentgenograms. Our attempts to use these inconstant roentgenographic features to determine tibiotalar shift either by measurement of the so-called medial clear space or by determination of the central weight-bearing line of the talus[202, 203] utilizing ankle specimens with 0 to 3 millimeters of displacement have yielded markedly inconsistent results. The main pitfalls of these previously reported measurement techniques include (1) inability to accurately identify the posteromedial border of the talus with extreme degrees of rotation, (2) lack of an identifiable posterolateral talar landmark, and (3) variations in the weight-bearing line of the tibia with rotation, since this bone is not a true cylinder even above the metaphysis.

In the adult, the coronal plane of the ankle is

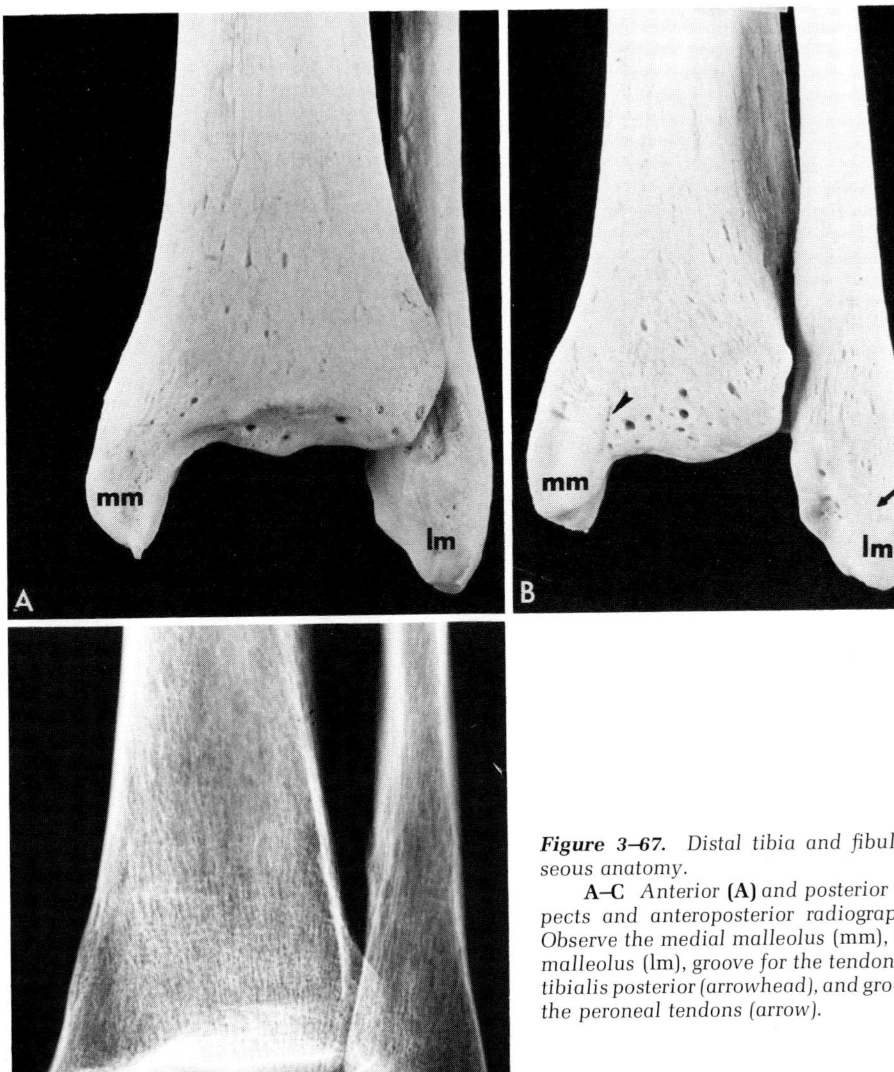

Figure 3–67. *Distal tibia and fibula: Osseous anatomy.*

A–C *Anterior* **(A)** *and posterior* **(B)** *aspects and anteroposterior radiograph* **(C)**. *Observe the medial malleolus* (mm), *lateral malleolus* (lm), *groove for the tendon of the tibialis posterior (arrowhead), and groove for the peroneal tendons (arrow).*

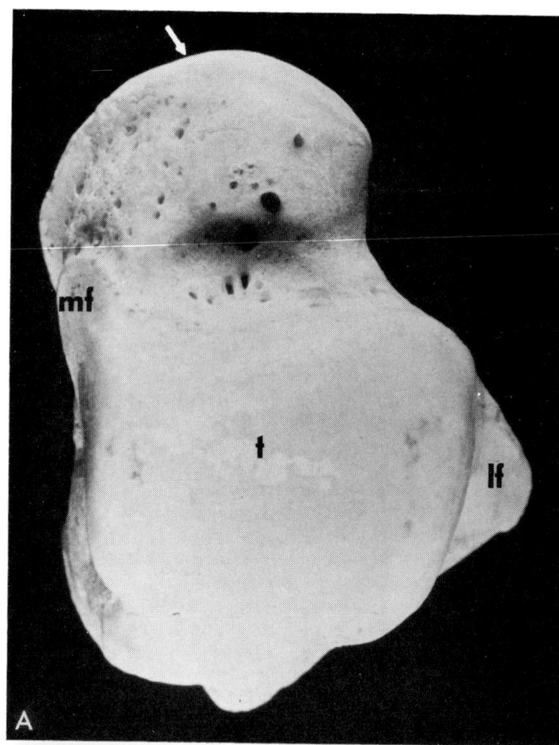

Figure 3–68. Talus: Osseous anatomy.

A *Dorsal aspect. Structures include the trochlear surface* (t), *medial facet* (mf) *for articulation with the medial malleolus, and lateral facet* (lf) *for articulation with the lateral malleolus. The distal surface (arrow) of the talus articulates with the tarsal navicular surface.*

B–D *Anteroposterior radiographs of the talus in 20 degrees of internal rotation* **(B)**, *0 degrees of rotation* **(C)** *and 15 degrees of external rotation* **(D)**. *With 20 degrees of internal rotation* **(B)**, *the medial articular surface, covered with lead foil, is seen in tangent (arrow). Lead strips cover the concave posteromedial surface (large arrowhead) and the posterolateral surface (small arrowhead). In 0 degrees of rotation* **(C)**, *the posteromedial surface is tangent and forms a border, the medial articular surface is not tangent and obscures the posteromedial surface, and the posterolateral surface is not tangent. In external rotation* **(D)**, *none of the identified structures is tangent.*

(**B–D**, From Goergen TG, et al.: J Bone Joint Surg 59A:874, 1977.)

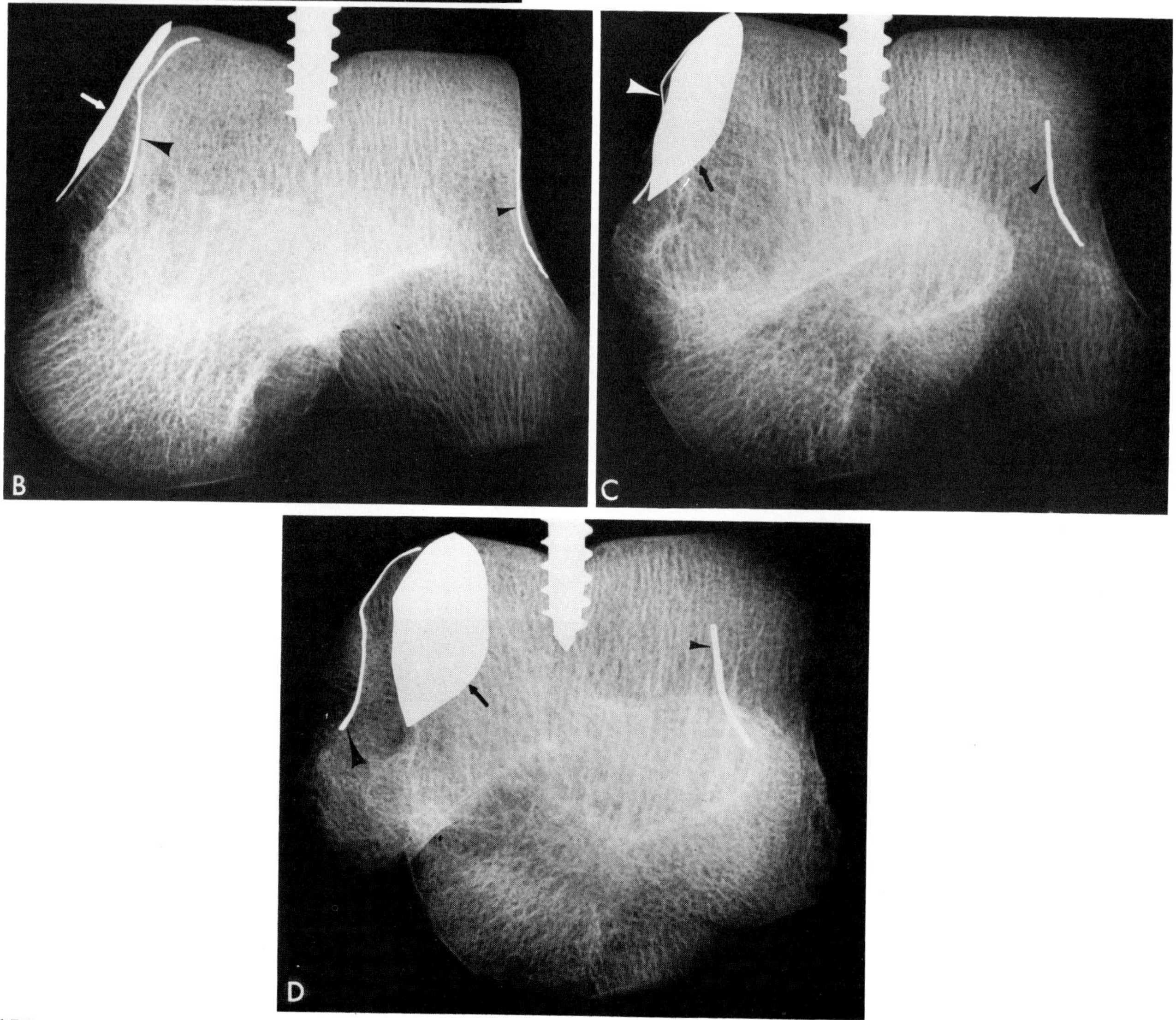

B

C

D

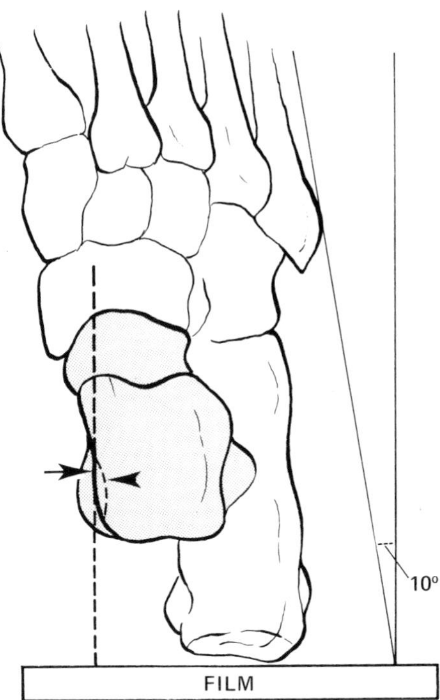

Figure 3–69. Mortise radiograph of ankle. By obtaining a radiograph in 10–15 degrees of internal rotation of the femur with respect to the fifth metatarsal, the medial articular surface of the talus (arrow) is tangential to the x-ray beam and the concave line representing the insertion of the deep deltoid ligament (arrowhead) falls slightly lateral to the articular surface. (From Goergen TG, et al: J Bone Joint Surg 59A:874, 1977.)

oriented in about 15 to 20 degrees of external rotation with reference to the coronal plane of the knee[204] and therefore the lateral malleolus is slightly posterior to the medial malleolus. To obtain a true anteroposterior roentgenogram of the tibiotalar articulation, the ankle must be positioned with the medial and lateral malleoli parallel to the tabletop; that is, in about 15 to 20 degrees of internal rotation, or the mortise view[205] (Fig. 3–69). This positioning places the medial articular surface tangent to the x-ray beam, and the short concave line representing the posteromedial surface of the talus falls slightly lateral to the medial articular surface. Utilizing this view, the roentgenographic medial clear space represents the actual width of the medial joint space.

The axial relationships of the ankle have been described.[5] The longitudinal axis of the tibia is perpendicular to the horizontal plane of the ankle joint and continuous with the longitudinal axis of the talus. The tibial angle, the angle formed by the intersection of one line drawn tangentially to the articular surface of the medial malleolus and a second drawn along the articular surface of the talus, averages 53 degrees (45 to 61 degrees). The fibular angle drawn in a corresponding way utilizing the lateral malleolus rather than the medial malleolus averages 52 degrees (45 to 63 degrees).

Soft Tissue Anatomy

The articular surfaces are cartilage-covered and the bones are connected by a fibrous capsule and the deltoid, the anterior and posterior talofibular, and the calcaneofibular ligaments (Figs. 3–70 and 3–71). The fibrous capsule is attached superiorly to the medial and lateral malleoli and tibia, and inferiorly to the talus. The talar attachment of the capsule is close to the margins of the trochlear surface except anteriorly, where the attachment to the neck of the talus is located at some distance from the articular margin. The capsule is weak both anteriorly and posteriorly, but it is reinforced medially and laterally by various ligments. A synovial membrane lines the inner aspect of the capsule and extends for a short vertical distance between the tibia and fibula. In this latter area, cartilage may be found on the osseous surfaces, continuous with that in the ankle joint.

Surrounding ligaments[206] include the deltoid, anterior and posterior talofibular, and calcaneofibular ligaments.

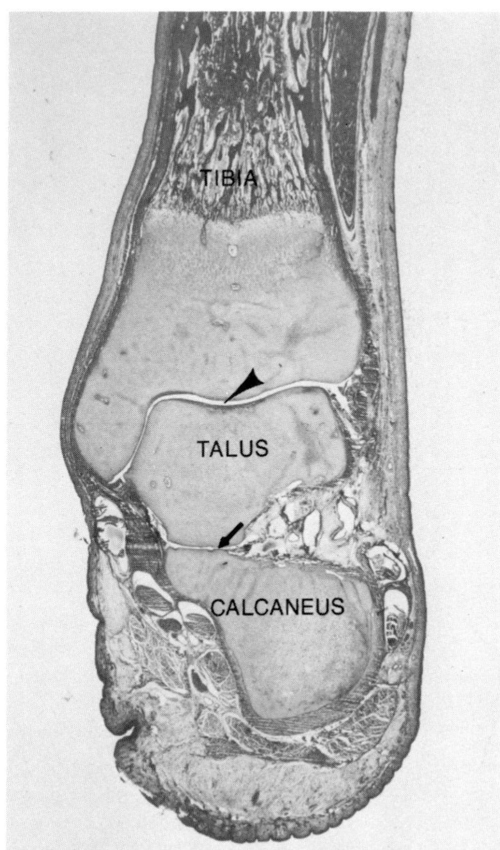

Figure 3–70. Ankle joint: Developmental anatomy (coronal section). Photomicrograph (20 ×) reveals the ankle joint (arrowhead) between the unossified portion of distal tibia and talus, and a portion of the talocalcaneonavicular joint (arrow) between the talus and sustentaculum tali of the calcaneus.

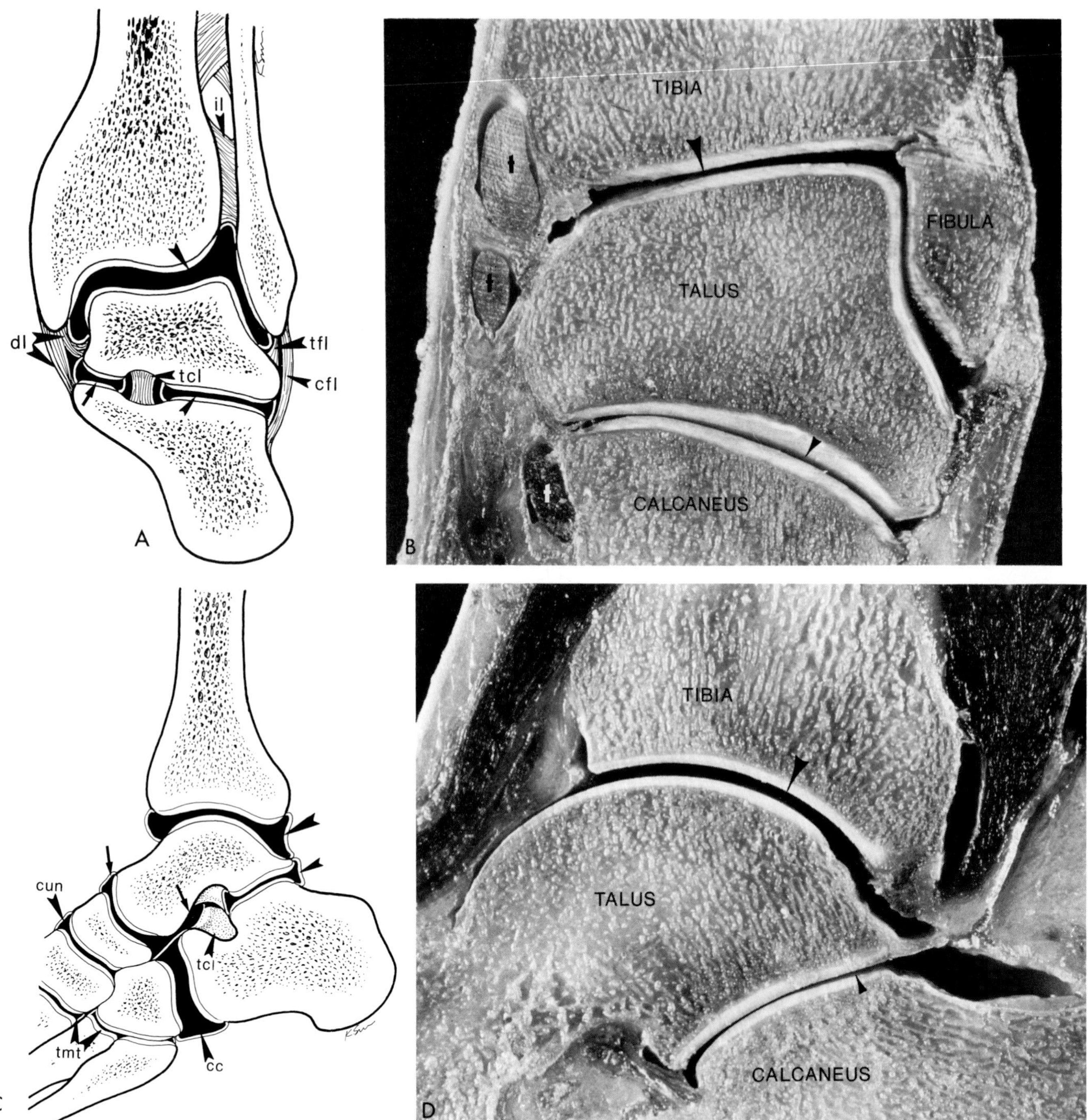

Figure 3–71. Ankle joint anatomy.

A, B *A drawing and photograph of a coronal section through the distal tibia, fibula, and talus, outlining the ankle joint (large arrowheads), interosseous ligament* (il) *of tibiofibular syndesmosis, interosseous talocalcaneal ligament* (tcl), portions of the deltoid ligament (dl), posterior talofibular ligament (tfl), *calcaneofibular ligament* (cfl), *surrounding tendons* (t), *subtalar joint (small arrowhead), and talocalcaneonavicular joint (arrow).*

C, D *Some of the same structures as in* **A** *and* **B** *can be identified in a drawing and photograph of a sagittal section of the ankle. Additional articulations that can be seen are the calcaneocuboid* (cc), *cuneonavicular* (cun), *and tarsometatarsal* (tmt) *joints.*

Deltoid Ligament. This medial ligament is triangular in shape and is attached above to the apex and the posterior and anterior borders of the medial malleolus. It contains superficial, middle, and deep fibers. Superficial fibers run anteriorly to the tuberosity of the tarsal navicular bone and blend with the plantar calcaneonavicular ligament. Middle fibers attach to the sustentaculum tali of the calcaneus, and posterior fibers pass to the medial talar surface, including its tubercle.

Anterior Talofibular Ligament. This ligament extends from the anterior margin of the lateral malleolus to the lateral articular facet on the neck of the talus.

Posterior Talofibular Ligament. This ligament attaches to the lateral malleolar fossa and extends horizontally to the lateral tubercle of the talus and medial malleolus.

Calcaneofibular Ligament. This structure extends from the lateral malleolus to the lateral surface of the calcaneus. It is crossed by the peroneus longus and peroneus brevis tendons. These three ligaments constitute the lateral ligament of the ankle.

Active movements of the ankle are dorsiflexion and plantar flexion. Accessory movements are a side to side gliding motion, rotation, abduction, and adduction.

TENDON SHEATHS AND BURSAE ABOUT THE ANKLE AND CALCANEUS

Tendons with accompanying tendon sheaths are intimate with the ankle joint.[207] Anteriorly, there are sheaths about the tibialis anterior, extensor hallucis longus, extensor digitorum longus, and peroneus tertius muscles. Medially, sheaths are present about the tibialis posterior, flexor digitorum longus, and flexor hallucis longus muscles. Laterally, the common sheath of the peroneus longus and peroneus brevis muscles may be appreciated.[208]

Important tendons, aponeuroses, and bursae are located about the calcaneus (Fig. 3–72). The plantar aponeurosis contains strong fibers that adhere to the posteroinferior surface of the bone. The Achilles tendon, which is the thickest and strongest human tendon, attaches to the posterior surface of the calcaneus approximately 2 cm below the upper surface of the bone. The retrocalcaneal bursa exists between the Achilles tendon and the posterosuperior surface of the calcaneus[209-212] (Fig. 3–73). This bursal space is lined with synovium, which extends over both the Achilles tendon and the inferior limit of the pre-achilles fat pad. The posterior surface of the calcaneus is covered with cartilage.

The normal radiographic features of these soft tissue landmarks about the calcaneus include the following[209]:

1. The Achilles tendon has a thickness of 4 to 8 mm at the level of the calcaneus or 1 to 2 cm above the top of the calcaneus (Fig. 3–74).

2. A vertical radiolucent area, the retrocalcaneal recess, of 2 mm or more in length, extends from the posterior aspect of the calcaneus behind the posterior portion of the bone, reflecting fat around the normal retrocalcaneal bursa (Fig. 3–75). The appearance of the retrocalcaneal recess can be influenced by severe dorsiflexion or plantar flexion of the foot.

Text continued on page 160

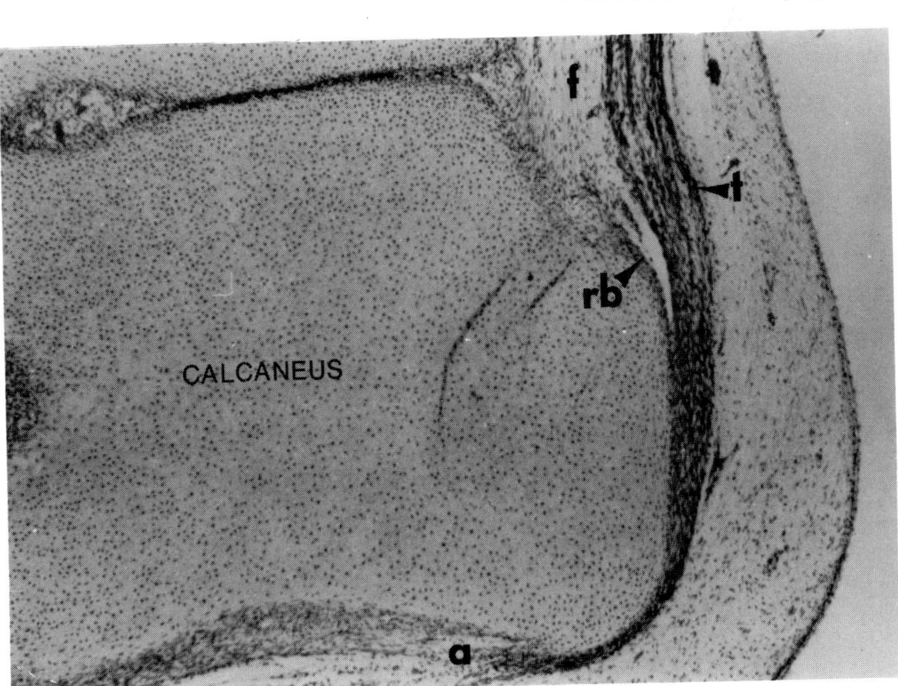

Figure 3–72. Soft tissues about the calcaneus: Developmental anatomy. A photomicrograph (20×) of a sagittal section through the calcaneus reveals the pre-achilles fat (f), Achilles tendon (t), retrocalcaneal bursa (rb), and plantar aponeurosis (a).

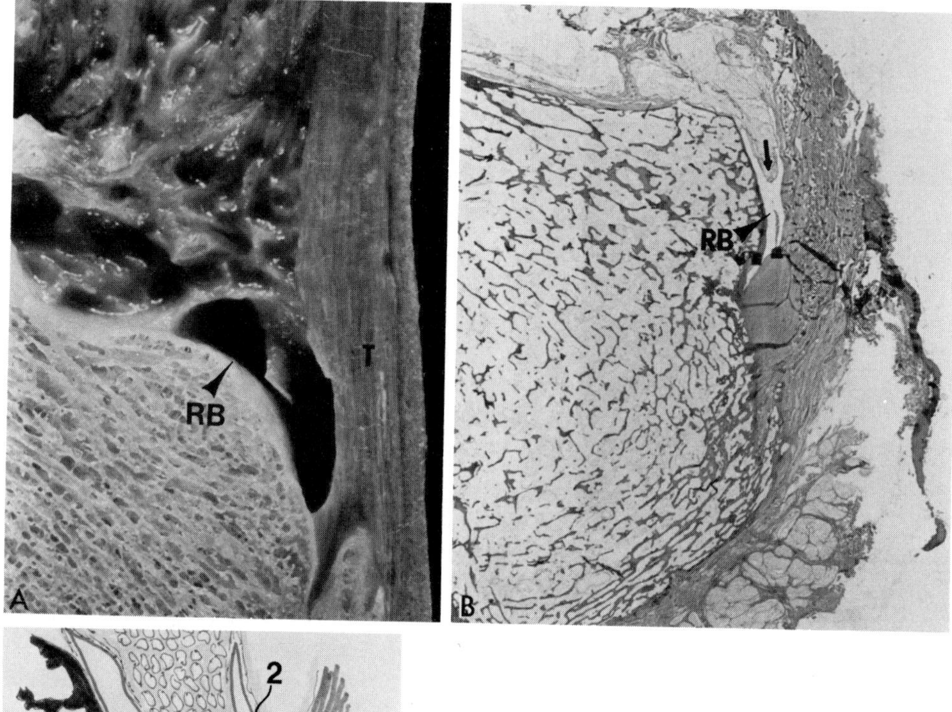

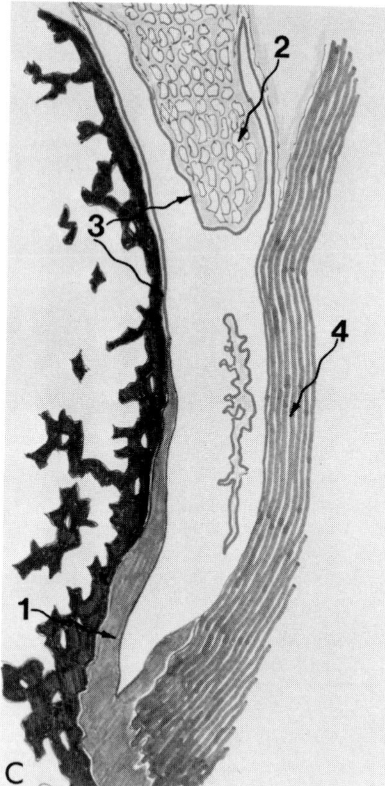

Figure 3–73. *Retrocalcaneal bursa: Anatomy.*

A *In this sagittal section, observe the retrocalcaneal bursa* (RB), *which is located between the Achilles tendon* (T) *and upper border of the calcaneus. Above the bursa, one can identify the pre-achilles fat pad.*

B *On this photomicrograph* (4 ×) *the retrocalcaneal bursa* (RB) *is enveloped in a synovial membrane that extends over the inferior limit of the pre-achilles fat pad (arrow).*

C *This drawing of the photomicrograph reveals calcaneal cartilage* (1), *the tip of the pre-achilles fat pad* (2), *synovium* (3) *lining the bursa, and the Achilles tendon* (4).

Illustration continued on the opposite page

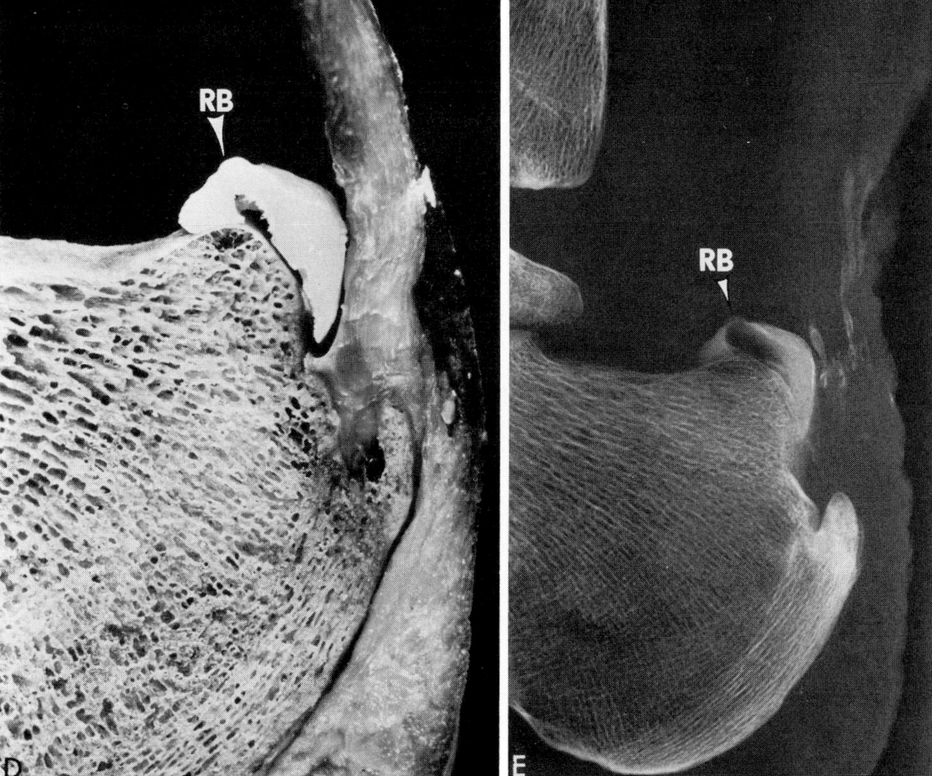

Figure 3–73. Continued

D, E *A photograph and radiograph of a sagittal section through the retrocalcaneal bursa* (RB), *which has been injected percutaneously with barium-impregnated methylmethacrylate, outlining the intimate relationship between the bursa and calcaneus.*

(From Resnick D, et al: Radiology 125:355, 1977.)

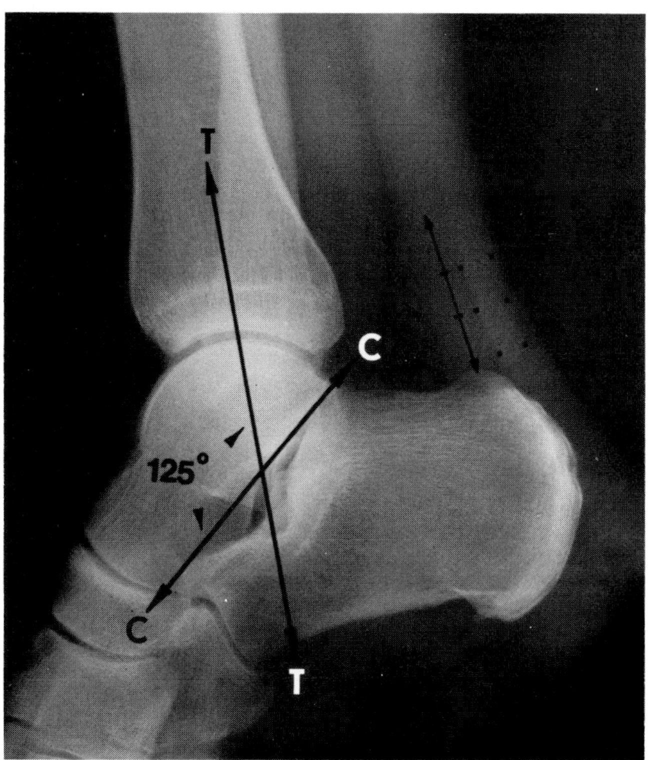

Figure 3–74. *Achilles tendon: Normal radiographic measurements. The thickness of the Achilles tendon is noted at the level of the calcaneus and at 1 and 2 cm above it. The determination of the calcaneal-talar angle guarantees that the radiograph has been taken in a "neutral" position. This angle is formed by the intersection of two lines, one drawn along the longitudinal axis of the tibia* (T) *and the second drawn along the top of the calcaneus* (C). *With proper positioning in normal individuals, this angle varies from approximately 90 degrees to 140 degrees. (From Resnick D, et al: Radiology 125:355, 1977.)*

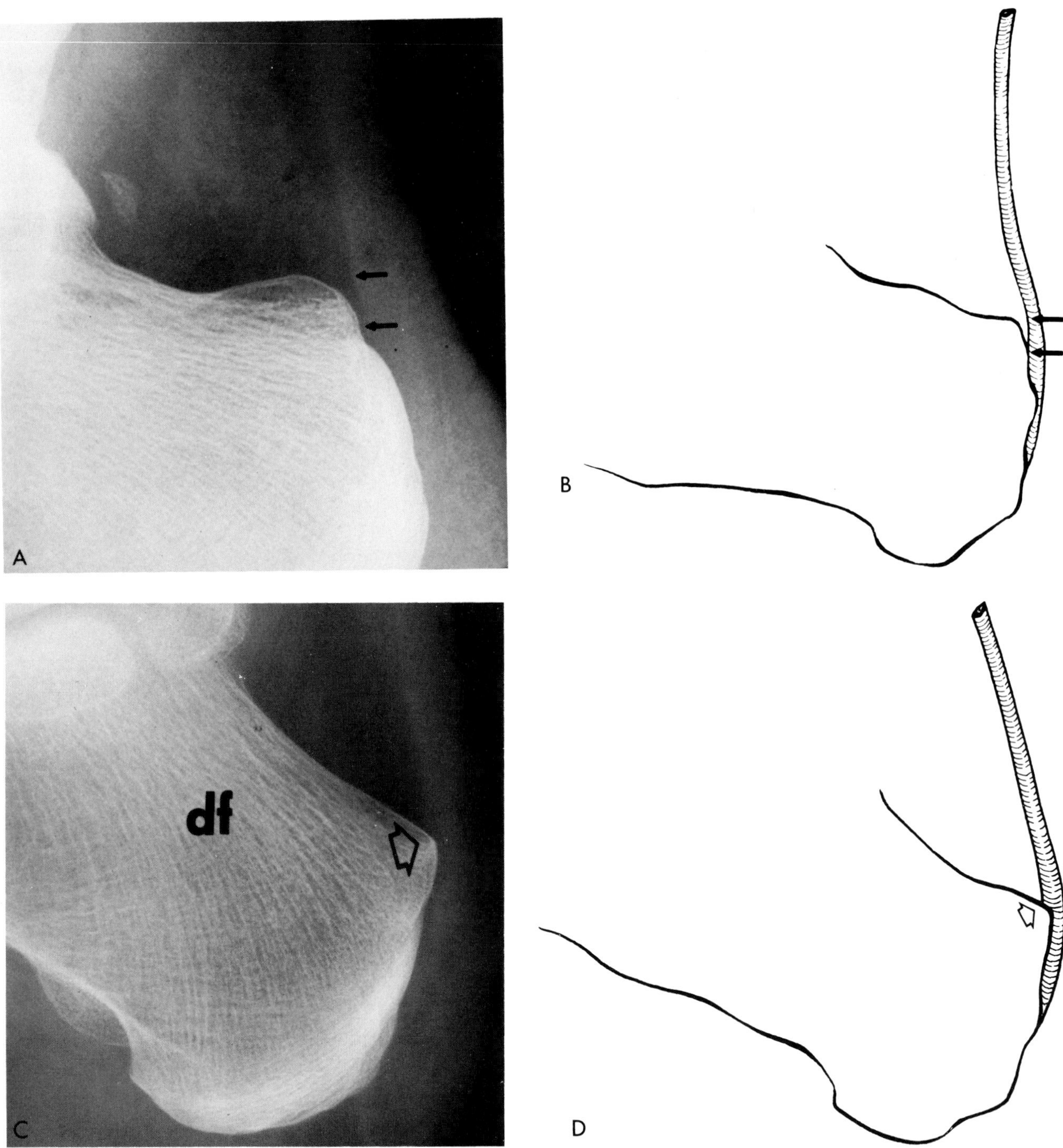

Figure 3–75. *Retrocalcaneal recess: Normal appearance.*

A, B *Neutral position. This recess appears as a triangular radiolucency between the Achilles tendon and calcaneus. It is normally 2 mm or more in length (between arrows).*

C, D *Dorsiflexion. In maximal dorsiflexion (df) of the foot, the retrocalcaneal recess may be obliterated (arrow).*

Illustration continued on the opposite page

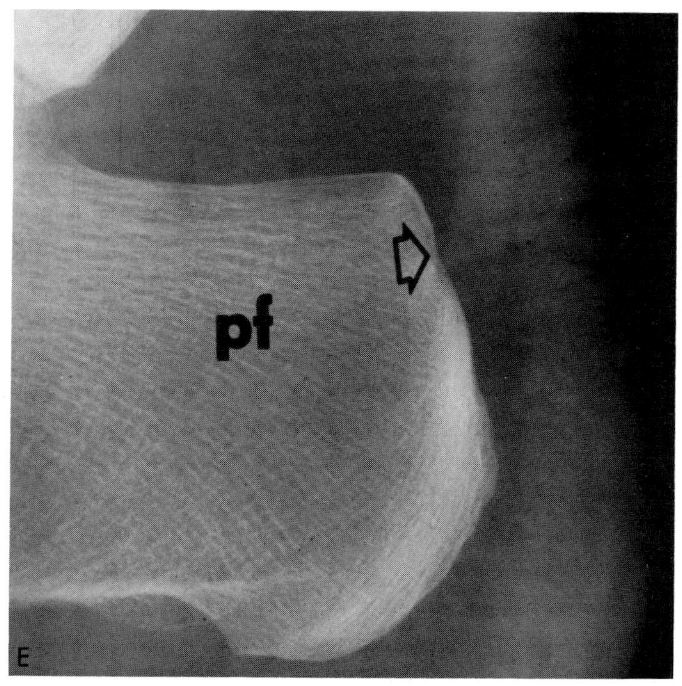

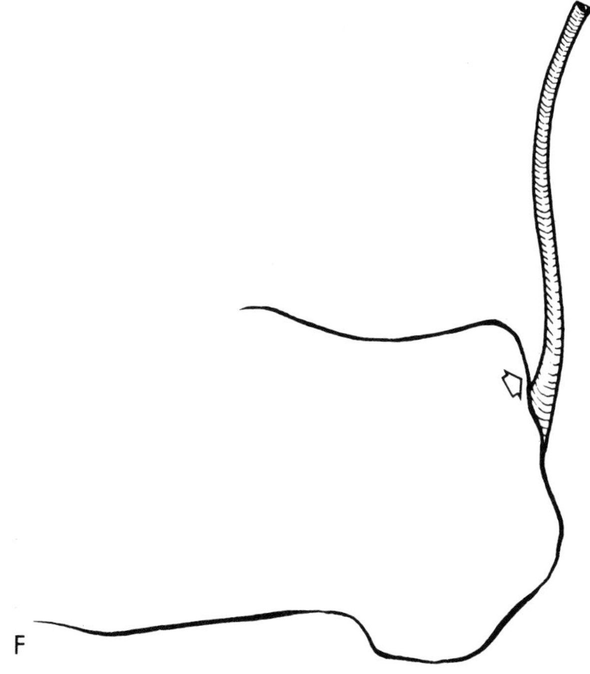

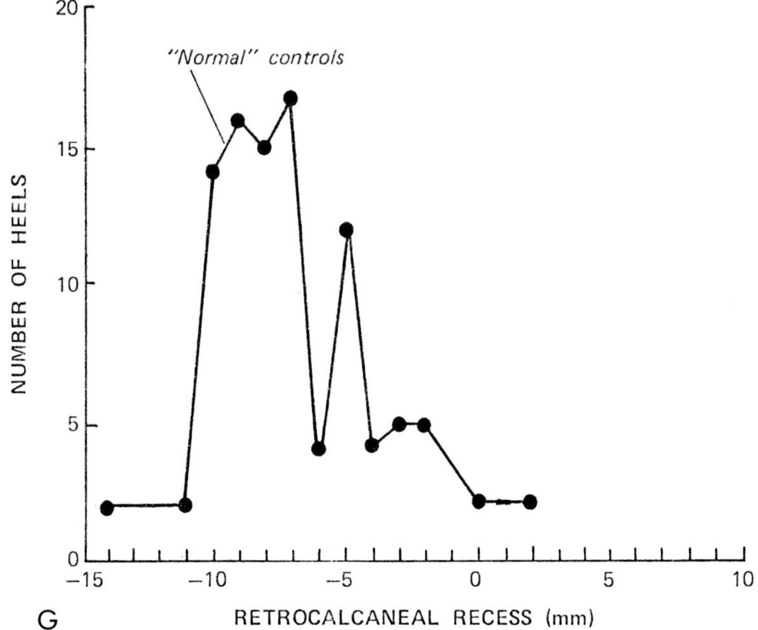

Figure 3–75. Continued

E, F *Plantar flexion. In maximum plantar flexion (pf) of the foot, the retrocalcaneal recess may be exaggerated (arrow).*

G *Neutral position. The size of the retrocalcaneal recess in a control population of 100 heels is indicated.*

*(**A, C, E, G,** From Resnick D, et al: Radiology 125:355, 1977.)*

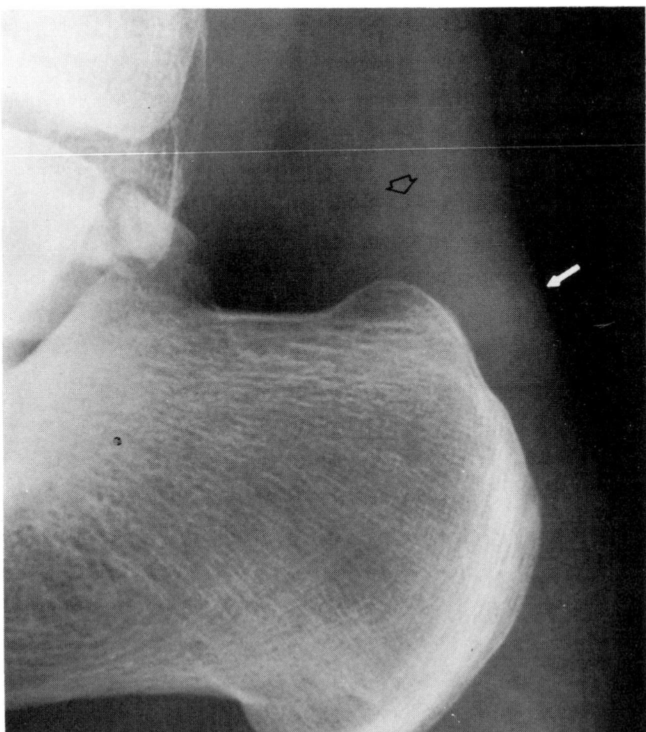

Figure 3–76. Retrocalcaneal recess: Abnormal appearance. Inflammation, synovial hypertrophy, and effusion result in an enlarged fluid-filled retrocalcaneal bursa which extends above the calcaneus as a radiodense area (open arrow). The Achilles tendon and surrounding tissue are also thickened (solid arrow).

Articular disorders may produce increased thickness and blurring of the Achilles tendon and obscuration of the retrocalcaneal recess (Fig. 3–76).

INTERTARSAL JOINTS

Osseous and Soft Tissue Anatomy

Numerous synovial articulations exist between the tarsal bones (Fig. 3–77).

TALOCALCANEAL JOINTS[213] **(Figs. 3–78, 3–79).** The talocalcaneal joints are two in number: the subtalar (posterior talocalcaneal or posterior subtalar) joint and the talocalcaneonavicular (anterior subtalar) joint. These articulations are separated by the tarsal canal and sinus and their contents.

The subtalar joint exists between the posterior talar facet of the calcaneus and the posterior calcaneal facet of the talus. The talar facet is oval and concave, and extends distally and laterally at an angle of approximately 45 degrees with the sagittal plane.[1] The posterior calcaneal facet is oval and convex anteroposteriorly. This synovium-lined joint, which may communicate with the talocrural or ankle joint in approximately 10 to 20 per cent of individuals[213-215], contains a capsule that contributes to the interosseous talocalcaneal ligament, the major bond between talus and calcaneus (Figs. 3–80 and 3–81). Additional structures binding talus and calcaneus are the anterior talocalcaneal ligament (extending from the lateral talar tubercle to the proximal medial calcaneus), the medial talocalcaneal ligament (extending from the medial talar tubercle to the sustentaculum tali), and the lateral talocalcaneal ligament (extending from the lateral surface of the talus to that of the calcaneus).

The talocalcaneonavicular joint is also a synovium-lined articulation, which exists between the head of the talus, the posterior surface of the navicular bone, the anterior articular surface of the calcaneus, and the proximal surface of the plantar calcaneonavicular ligament or "spring" ligament. The distal surface of the head of the talus is oval and convex, directed inferiorly and medially to articulate with the oval, concave proximal surface of the navicular bone. The plantar surface of the talar head has three articular areas separated by indistinct osseous ridges: the posterior area is large and oval, convex in shape, and articulates with the sustentaculum tali of the calcaneus; the second area, anterolateral to the posterior area, is flattened, articulating with the superior surface of the calcaneus; the navicular area, directed distally, is oval and convex, articulating with the tarsal navicular bone. The anterior articular surface of the talus also contacts the plantar calcaneonavicular ligament. This ligament has a central area that consists of fibrocartilage and bridges the triangular space between the anterior and middle talar facets of the calcaneus and navicular bone. The posterior surface of the joint capsule contributes to the interosseous ligament. On its medial side, this articulation is enlarged or deepened by a portion of the deltoid ligament, which is attached to the plantar calcaneonavicular ligament. Movements are coordinated between the talocalcaneonavicular and subtalar articulations, and include inversion and eversion of the foot.

CALCANEOCUBOID JOINT (Fig. 3–82). This joint is formed between apposing quadrilateral facets on the calcaneus and cuboid bones, and its capsule is reinforced by surrounding ligaments, including the long plantar ligament (extending from the plantar surface of the calcaneus to the cuboid and third through fifth metatarsals) and the plantar calcaneocuboid ligament (extending from calcaneus to cuboid). The calcaneocuboid and talocalcaneonavicular joints are often referred to collectively as the transverse tarsal joint. Movements at the calcaneocuboid articulation are limited to gliding and rotation.

CUNEONAVICULAR, INTERCUNEIFORM, CUNEOCUBOID, AND CUBOIDEONAVICULAR JOINTS (Fig. 3–82). The cuneonavicular joint is formed between the concave articular surfaces of the posterior portion of the three cuneiforms and the convex distal

Text continued on page 170

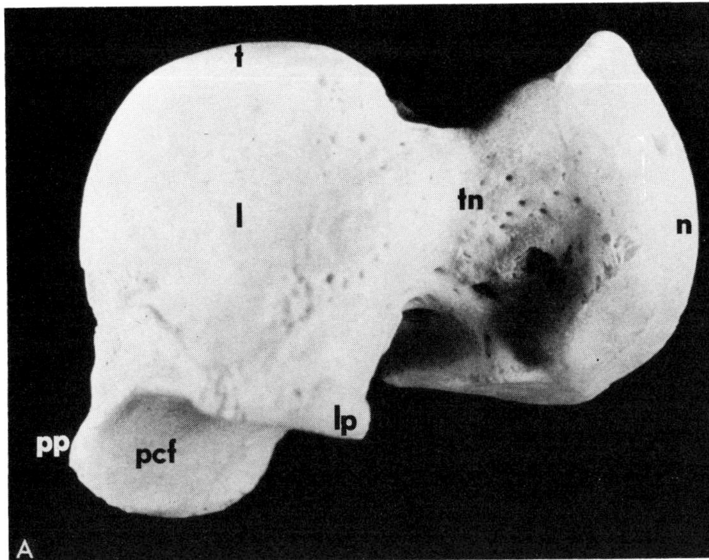

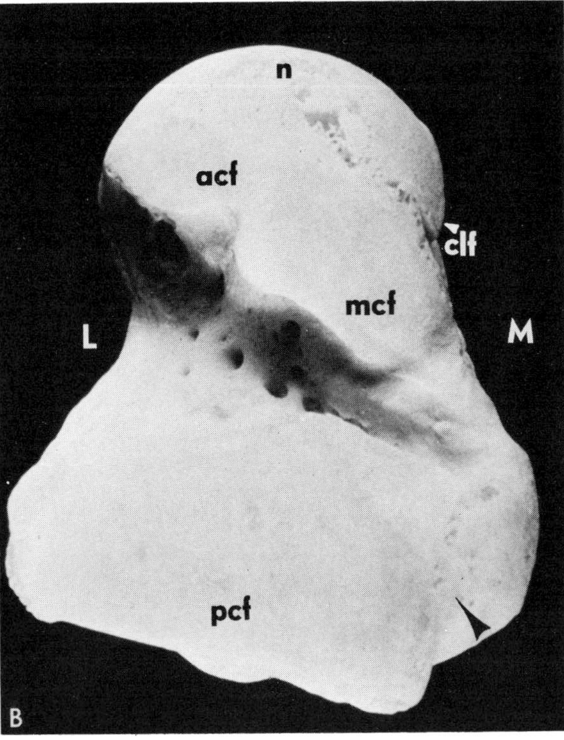

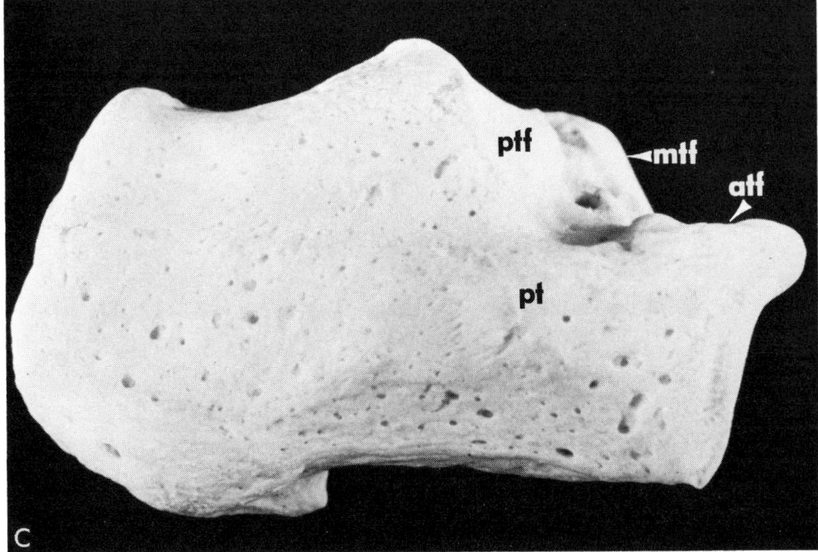

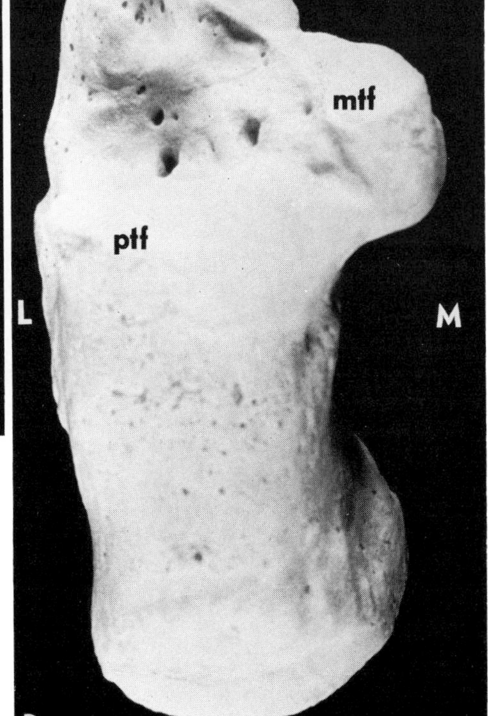

Figure 3–77. *Talus and calcaneus: Osseous anatomy.*

A *Talus: Lateral aspect. Structures include trochlear surface for tibia* (t), *articular surface for lateral malleolus* (l), *posterior process* (pp), *lateral process* (lp), *talar neck* (tn), *articular surface for navicular bone* (n), *and posterior calcaneal facet* (pcf).

B *Talus: Plantar aspect.* M, Medial; L, *lateral. Observe the posterior calcaneal facet* (pcf), *middle calcaneal facet* (mcf), *facet for the plantar calcaneonavicular ligament* (clf), *anterior calcaneal facet* (acf), *and facet for the navicular bone* (n). *Note the groove (arrowhead) for the flexor hallucis longus muscle.*

C *Calcaneus: Lateral aspect. Structures are the posterior talar facet* (ptf), *peroneal trochlea* (pt), *middle talar facet* (mtf), *and anterior talar facet* (atf).

D *Calcaneus: Superior aspect.* M, *Medial;* L, *lateral. The same structures as in* **C** *are identified.*

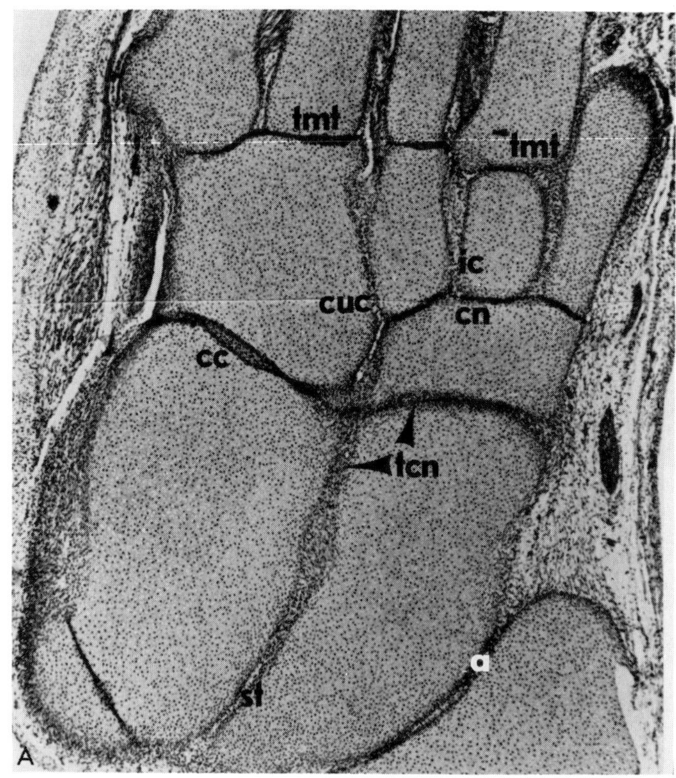

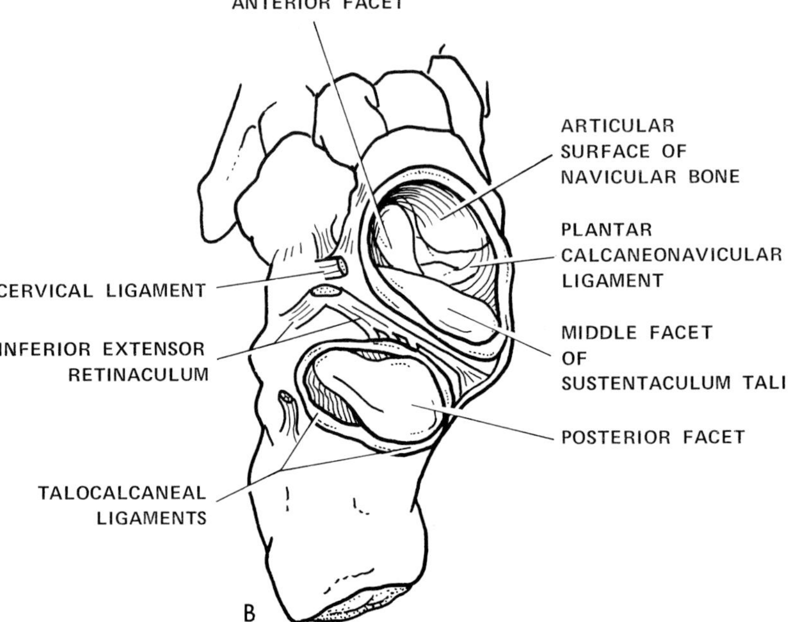

Figure 3–78. *Talocalcaneal joints: Normal development and anatomy.*

A *On this photomicrograph (20×) of an oblique section through the hindfoot and midfoot, developing articulations include the ankle* (a), *subtalar* (st), *talocalcaneonavicular* (tcn), *calcaneocuboid* (cc), *cuneonavicular* (cn), *cuneocuboid* (cuc), *intercuneiform* (ic), *and tarsometatarsal* (tmt) *joints.*

B *Superior surface of calcaneus. Note the broad convex posterior talar facet separated from the anterior and middle talar facets by the tarsal canal and its ligamentous structures. Two completely independent synovium-lined articulations are formed.*

Illustration continued on the opposite page

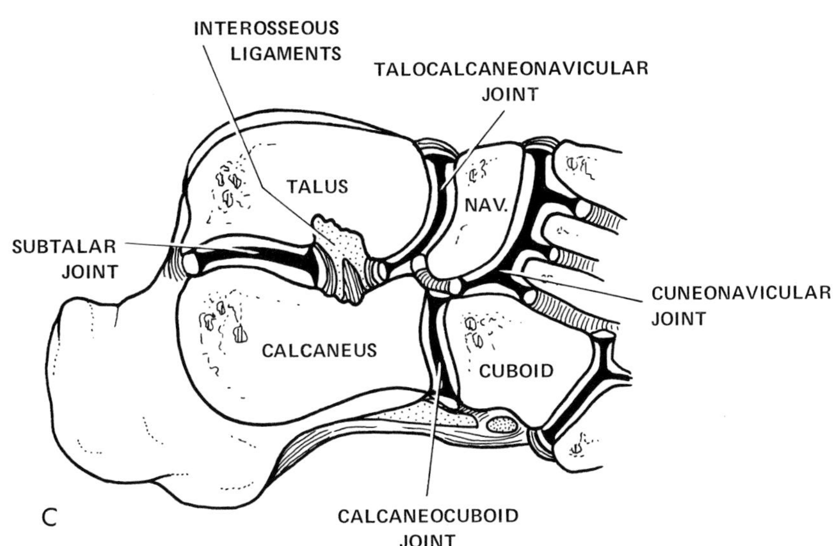

Figure 3–78. Continued

C *Oblique section of the foot. The interosseous ligaments between the talus and calcaneus are well shown, and the two separate talocalcaneal articulations are indicated. Note the independent calcaneocuboid and cuneonavicular joint cavities.*

*(***B, C,*** From Resnick D: Radiology 111:581, 1974.)*

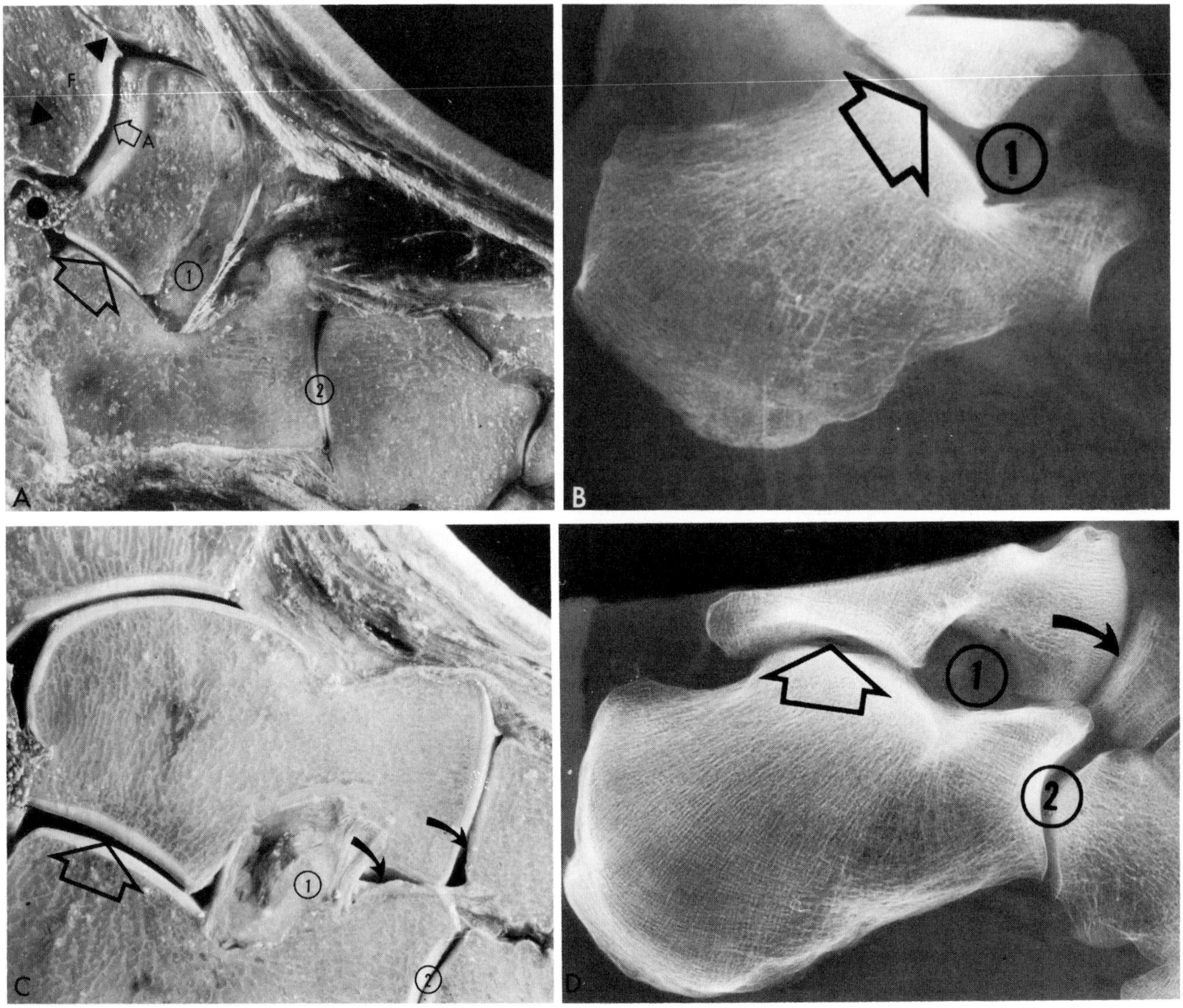

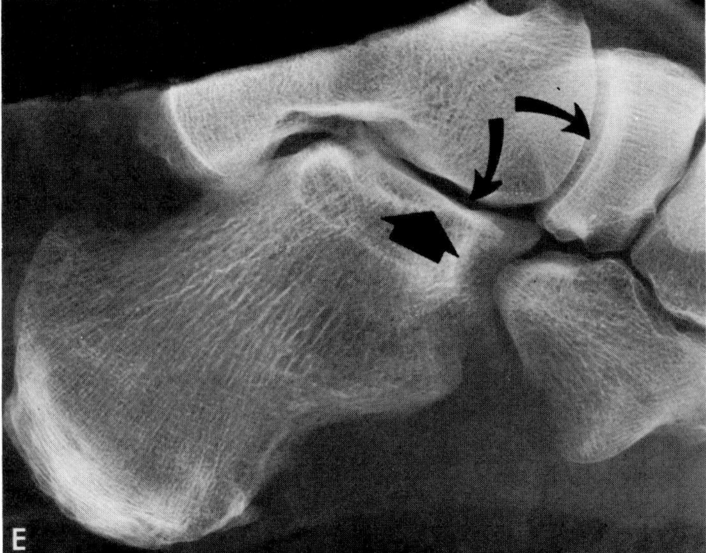

Figure 3–79. *Sagittal cross-sectional anatomy and radiography.*

A *A lateral sagittal section through the fibula (F) and ankle (A) demonstrates the subtalar articulation (open arrow) between the posterior facets of the talus and calcaneus. The tarsal sinus (1) and posterior talofibular ligament (black dot) are indicated. A separate calcaneocuboid joint (2) is evident.*

B *A radiograph of the section in* **A** *better reveals the posterior facets, subtalar joint (open arrow), and tarsal sinus (1).*

C, D *A more medial sagittal section and radiograph outline the talocalcaneonavicular (curved arrows) and subtalar (open arrow) joint cavities completely separated by the contents of the tarsal sinus (1). The calcaneocuboid articulation (2) is again indicated.*

E *A radiograph through a more medial section delineates the sustentaculum tali (heavy arrow) and anterior subtalar joint (curved arrows).*

(From Resnick D: Radiology 111:581, 1974.)

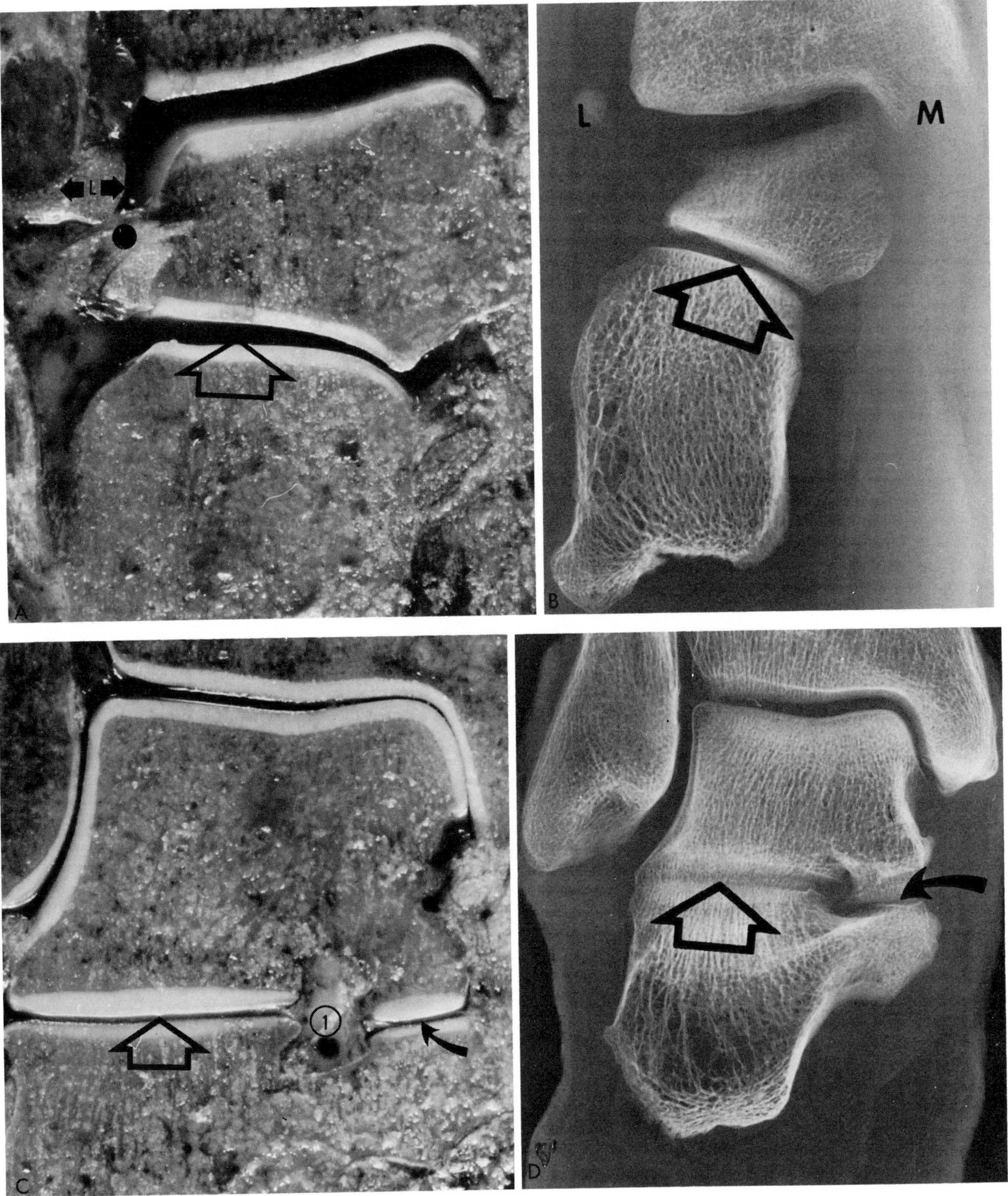

Figure 3–80. *Coronal cross-sectional anatomy and radiography.*

A, B *A section and radiograph through the subtalar articulation (open arrow) are shown. The lateral (L) and medial (M) malleoli, and posterior talofibular ligament (black dot) are indicated.*

C, D *A more anterior section and radiograph outline separate subtalar (open arrow) and talocalcaneonavicular (curved arrow) joints. The interosseous ligaments (1) are labeled.*

Illustration continued on the following page

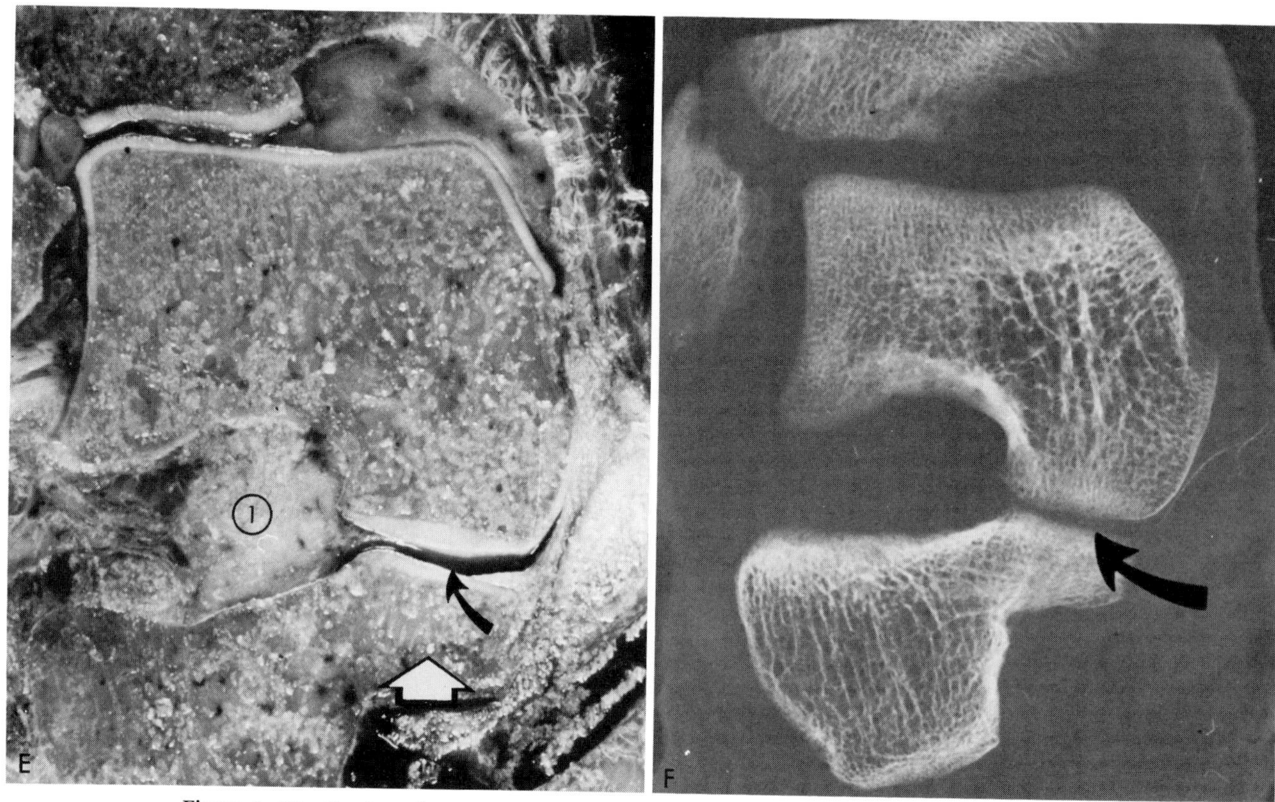

Figure 3–80. Continued

E, F *This most anterior section is through the sustentaculum tali (heavy arrow) and talocalcaneonavicular joint (curved arrow). The tarsal sinus (1) is well shown as it expands on the anterolateral aspect of the foot.*

(From Resnick D: Radiology 111:581, 1974.)

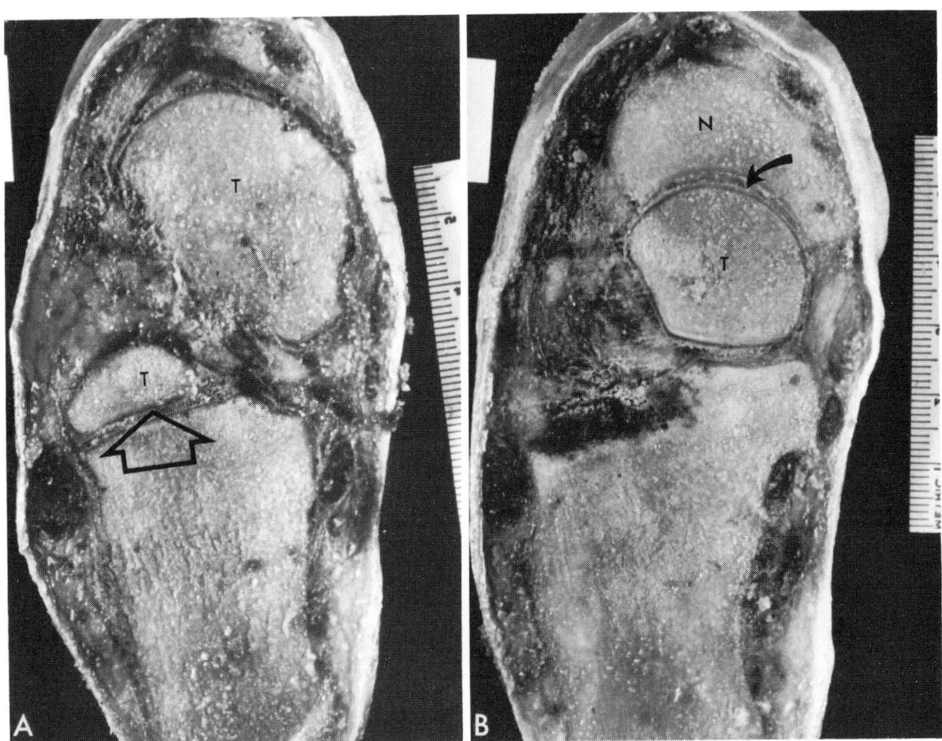

Figure 3–81. *Transverse cross-sectional anatomy and radiography.*

A *A dorsal section taken through the tarsal canal and sinus. Note how the latter is the expanded anterolateral section of the canal. The talus (T) has been cut twice, and its posterior aspect is separated from the calcaneus by the subtalar articulation (open arrow).*

B *A more plantar section outlines the anterior aspect of the talus (T) and navicular bone (N), with the intervening talonavicular portion of the talocalcaneonavicular joint (curved arrow).*

(From Resnick D: Radiology 111:581, 1974.)

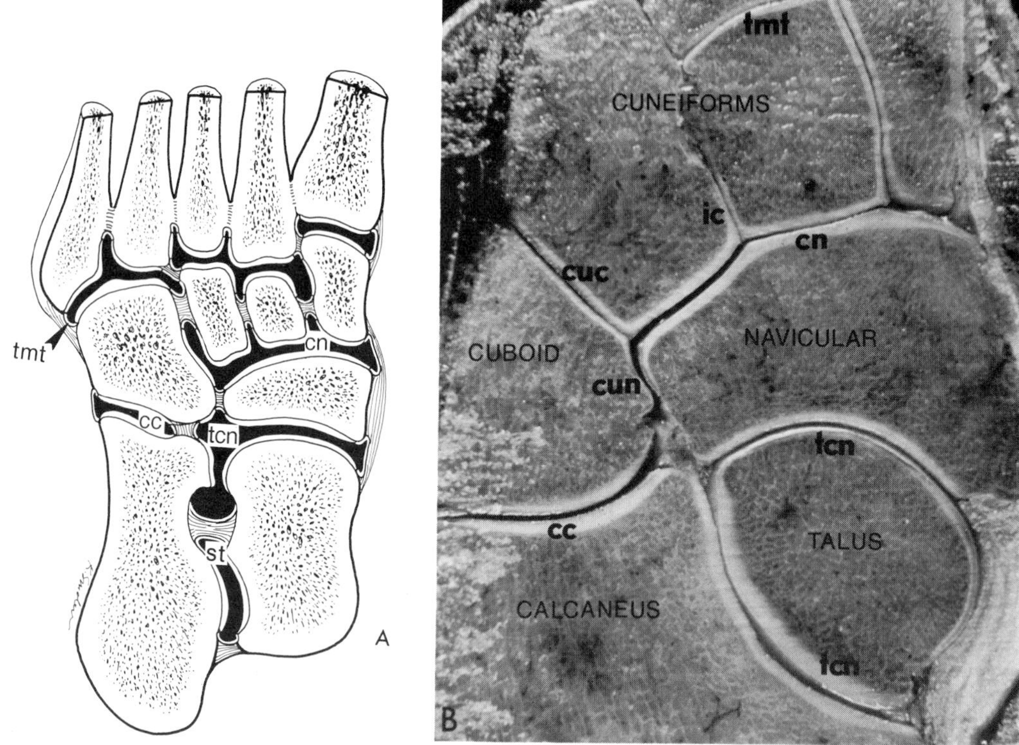

Figure 3–82. *Joints of the midfoot: Anatomy.*

A, B *Drawing and photograph of an oblique transverse section through the midfoot, outlining the following articulations: subtalar* (st), *talocalcaneonavicular* (tcn), *cuneonavicular* (cn), *calcaneocuboid* (cc), *cuboideonavicular* (cun), *cuneocuboid* (cuç), *intercuneiform* (ic), *and tarsometatarsal* (tmt) *joints.*

Illustration continued on the opposite page

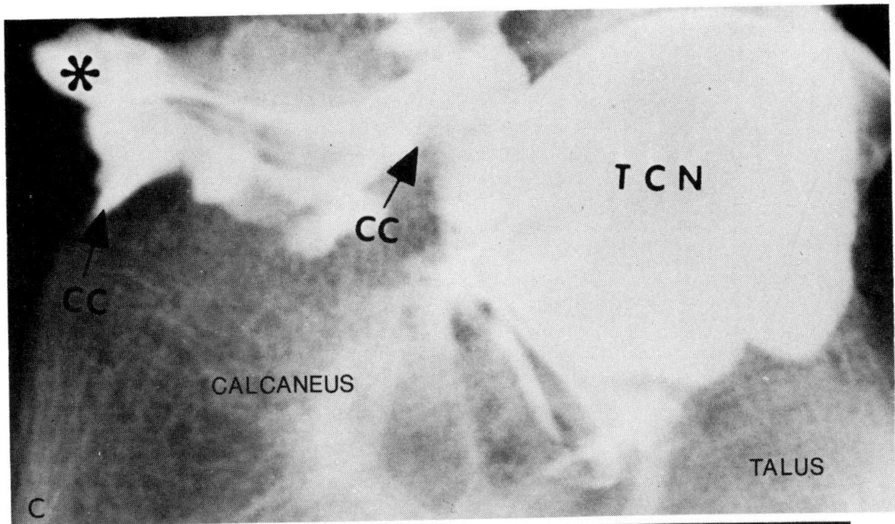

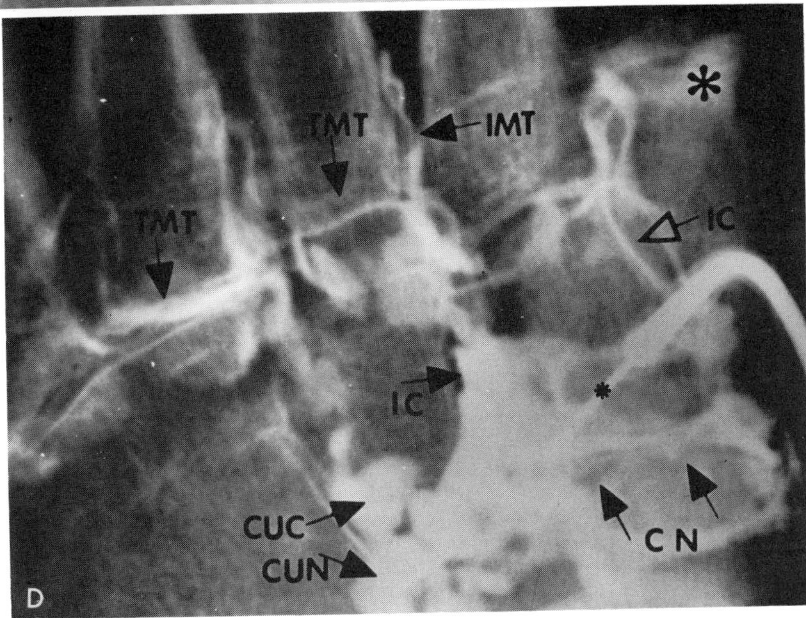

Figure 3–82. Continued

C, D *Arthrography. In* **C,** *contrast has been introduced into the talocalcaneonavicular* (TCN) *and calcaneocuboid* (CC) *cavities with two separate injections. A steep oblique radiograph reveals the extent of these two distinct synovial cavities. Note the plantar recess (asterisk) of the calcaneocuboid joint. In* **D** *contrast is introduced through a needle (small asterisk) in the cuneonavicular cavity between the intermediate and lateral cuneiform and navicular bones, outlining the extent of that joint* (CN) *and its frequent communication with the intercuneiform* (IC), *cuboideonavicular* (CUN), *cuneocuboid* (CUC), *tarsometatarsal* (TMT), *and intermetatarsal* (IMT) *cavities. The medial tarsometatarsal cavity between the medial cuneiform bone and first metatarsal is also filled (large asterisk).*

(**C–D,** *From Resnick D: J Can Assoc Radiol 27:9, 1976.*)

surface of the navicular. The articular capsule of this joint is continuous with two intercuneiform joints (small joint cavities between the proximal portions of the cuneiform bones), cuneocuboid joint (articulation between apposing facets on the cuboid bone and lateral cuneiform), and cuboideonavicular joint (inconstant cavity between cuboid and navicular bones). Movements at all of these joints occur simultaneously and include slight amounts of gliding and rotation of one bone on another.

TARSOMETATARSAL AND INTERMETATARSAL JOINTS

Osseous and Soft Tissue Anatomy

The medial cuneiform and first metatarsal possess an independent medial tarsometatarsal articulation (Fig. 3–82). The intermediate tarsometatarsal joint is located between the second and third meta-

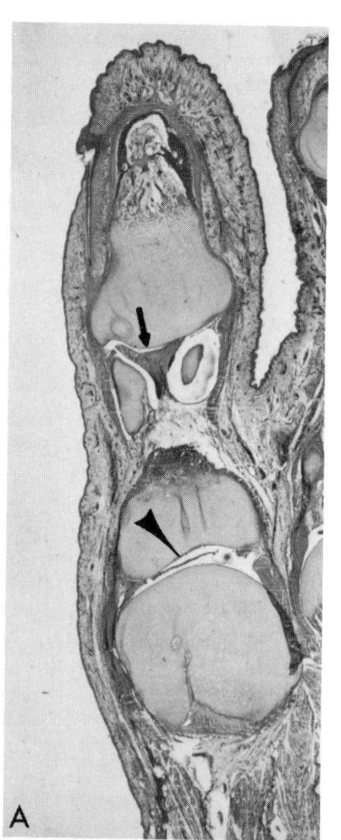

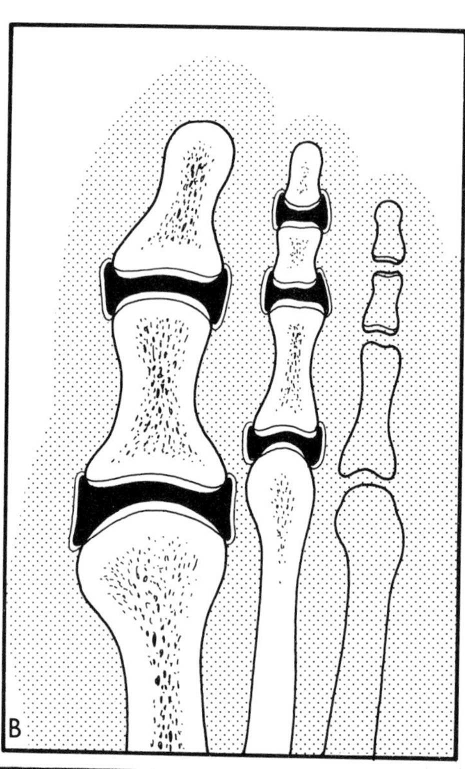

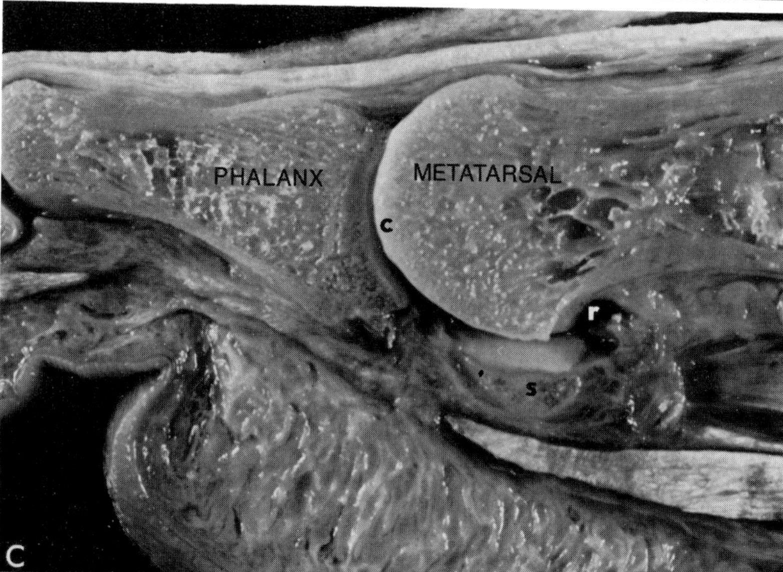

Figure 3–83. *Metatarsophalangeal and interphalangeal joints: Normal development and anatomy.*

A *A photomicrograph (20×) of the first digit reveals the first metatarsophalangeal joint (arrowhead) developing between the metatarsal head and proximal phalanx. Portions of the interphalangeal joint of the great toe (arrow) are also observed.*

B *A drawing of a transverse section of the foot outlining the capsular attachments of the metatarsophalangeal and interphalangeal articulations.*

C *A sagittal section through the first metatarsophalangeal joint revealing articular cartilage (c), proximal recesses (r), and a plantar sesamoid (s) bone.*

tarsals and the intermediate and lateral cuneiforms. This joint may communicate with the intercuneiform and cuneonavicular joints. The lateral tarsometatarsal joint exists between the distal aspect of the cuboid and the base of the fourth and fifth metatarsals. A limited amount of gliding motion may occur between tarsals and metatarsals, the motion being accentuated at the medial tarsometatarsal joint. The tarsometatarsal joints extend distally between the metatarsal bases as intermetatarsal joints. Slight gliding motion can occur at these latter articulations.

METATARSOPHALANGEAL JOINTS

Osseous and Soft Tissue Anatomy

These synovial articulations exist where the rounded heads of the metatarsals approximate the cupped surfaces of the proximal phalanges (Fig. 3–83). The articular portions of the metatarsal heads include the distal and plantar aspects of the bone, but do not include the dorsal surface. The plantar aspect of the first metatarsal is unique, containing two longitudinal grooves, separated by a ridge. Each groove may articulate with a sesamoid bone. Fibrous capsules surround these articulations. The thin dorsal portion of these capsules is frequently intimate with small bursae that separate the capsule from the extensor tendons. Ligaments about these joints include the plantar ligaments, the deep transverse metatarsal ligaments (which connect the plantar ligaments of adjacent metatarsophalangeal joints), and the collateral ligaments (which are located at each side of the joint and extend from the dorsal tubercle of the metatarsal head to the phalangeal base). Active movements at the metatarsophalangeal joints include extension, flexion, abduction, and adduction. Accessory movements are gliding and rotation of the phalanges.

INTERPHALANGEAL JOINTS OF THE FOOT

Osseous and Soft Tissue Anatomy

In each foot, these nine articulations (two in each of the four lateral digits and one interphalangeal joint of the great toe) separate phalanges and are surrounded by a capsule and two collateral ligaments (Fig. 3–83). The plantar ligament represents a fibrous plate on the plantar surface of the capsule. Active movements at the interphalangeal joints are flexion and extension. Accessory movements are rotation, abduction, and adduction.

REFERENCES

1. Warwick R, Williams PL: Grays's Anatomy. 35th British Ed. Philadelphia, WB Saunders Co, 1973, p 407.
2. Walmsley R: Joints. *In* GJ Romanes (Ed): Cunningham's Textbook of Anatomy. 11th Ed. London, Oxford University Press, 1972, p 214.
3. Shapiro JS: A new factor in the etiology of ulnar drift. Clin Orthop Rel Res *68*:32, 1970.
4. Resnick D: Inter-relationship between radiocarpal and metacarpophalangeal joint deformities in rheumatoid arthritis. J Can Assoc Radiol *27*:29, 1976.
5. Lusted LB, Keats TE: Atlas of Roentgenographic Measurement. 2nd Ed. Chicago, Year Book Medical Publishers, 1967, p 122.
6. Linscheid RL, Dobyns JH, Beabout JW, Bryan RS: Traumatic instability of the wrist. Diagnosis, classification and pathomechanics. J Bone Joint Surg *54*A:1612, 1972.
7. Arkless R: Cineradiography in normal and abnormal wrists. Am J Roentenol *96*:837, 1966.
8. Weston WJ, Kelsey CK: Functional anatomy of the pisi-cuneiform joint. Br J Radiol *46*:692, 1973.
9. Lewis OJ: The development of the human wrist joint during the fetal period. Anat Rec *166*:499, 1970.
10. Lewis OJ, Hamshere RJ, Bucknill TM: The anatomy of the wrist joint. J Anat *106*:539, 1970.
11. Vesely DG: The distal radio-ulnar joint. Clin Orthop Rel Res *51*:75, 1967.
12. Kaplan EB: Functional and Surgical Anatomy of the Hand. 2nd Ed. Philadelphia, JB Lippincott Co, 1965, p 114.
13. Resnick D: Arthrography in the evaluation of arthritic disorders of the wrist. Radiology *113*:331, 1974.
14. Kuczynski K: Carpometacarpal joint of the human thumb. J Anat *118*:119, 1974.
15. Liebolt FL: Surgical fusion of the wrist joint. Surg Gynecol Obstet *66*:1008, 1938.
16. Kessler I, Silberman Z: An experimental study of the radiocarpal joint by arthrography. Surg Gynecol Obstet *112*:33, 1961.
17. Harrison MO, Freiberger RH, Ranawat CS: Arthrography of the rheumatoid wrist joint. Am J Roentgenol *112*:480, 1971.
18. Resnick D: Rheumatoid arthritis of the wrist. The compartmental approach. Med Radiogr Photogr *52*:50, 1976.
19. Resnick D: Early abnormalities of the pisiform and triquetrum in rheumatoid arthritis. Ann Rheum Dis *35*:46, 1976.
20. Backdahl M: The caput ulnae syndrome in rheumatoid arthritis. A study of morphology, abnormal anatomy, and clinical picture. Acta Rheumatol Scand (Suppl) *5*:1, 1963.
21. MacConaill MA: The mechanical anatomy of the carpus and its bearings on some surgical problems. J Anat *75*:166, 1941.
22. Duparc J, De la Caffinière JY: A propos des mouvements du premier métacarpien. Presse Med *78*:833, 1970.
23. Harris H, Joseph J: Variation in extension of the metacarpophalangeal and interphalangeal joints of the thumb. J Bone Joint Surg *31B*:547, 1949.
24. Johnston HM: Varying positions of the carpal bones in the different movements of the wrist. Part I. J Anat Physiol *41*:109, 1907.
25. Johnston HM: Varying positions of the carpal bones in the different movements of the wrist. Part II. J Anat Physiol *41*:280, 1907.
26. Arkless R: Rheumatoid wrists. Cineradiography. Radiology *88*:543, 1967.
27. Terry DW Jr, Ramin JE: The navicular fat stripe. A useful roentgen feature for evaluating wrist traumå. Am J Roentgenol *124*:25, 1975.
28. MacEwan DW: Changes due to trauma in fat plane overlying pronator quadratus muscle: radiologic sign. Radiology *82*:879, 1964.
29. MacEwan DW, Dunbar JS: Early radiologic recognition of pus in joints of children. J Can Assoc Radiol *12*:72, 1961.
30. Yeh HC, Wolf BS: Radiographic anatomical landmarks of the metacarpophalangeal joint. Radiology *122*:353, 1977.
31. Gad P: The anatomy of the volar part of the capsules of the finger joints. J Bone Joint Surg *49B*:362, 1967.
32. Kuczynski K: The proximal interphalangeal joint. Anatomy and causes of stiffness in the fingers. J Bone Joint Surg *50B*:656, 1968.

33. Weston WJ, Palmer DG: Soft Tissues of the Extremities. New York, Springer-Verlag, 1978, p 61.
34. Smith RJ: Balance and kinetics of the fingers under normal and pathological conditions. Clin Orthop Rel Res *104*:92, 1974.
35. Bledsoe RC, Izenstark JL: Displacement of fat pads in diseases and injury of the elbow. Radiology *73*:717, 1959.
36. Bohrer SP: The fat pad sign following elbow trauma. Its usefulness and reliability in suspecting "invisible" fractures. Clin Radiol *21*:90, 1970.
37. Kohn AM: Soft tissue alterations in elbow trauma. Am J Roentgenol *82*:867, 1959.
38. Jackman RJ, Pugh DG: The positive elbow fat pad sign in rheumatoid arthritis. Am J Roentgenol *108*:812, 1970.
39. Norell HG: Roentgenologic visualization of the extracapsular fat: its importance in the diagnosis of traumatic injuries to the elbow. Acta Radiol *42*:205, 1954.
40. Murphy WA, Siegel MJ: Elbow fat pads with new signs and extended differential diagnosis. Radiology *124*:659, 1977.
41. Martin BF: The annular ligament of the superior radio-ulnar joint. J Anat *92*:473, 1958.
42. Weston WJ: The synovial changes at the elbow in rheumatoid arthritis. Australas Radiol *15*:170, 1971.
43. Rogers SL, MacEwan DW: Changes due to trauma in the fat plane overlying the supinator muscle. A radiologic sign. Radiology *92*:954, 1969.
44. Weston WJ: The olecranon bursa. Australas Radiol *14*:323, 1970.
45. Saha AK: Dynamic stability of the glenohumeral joint. Acta Orthop Scand *42*:491, 1971.
46. Rothman RH, Marvel JP Jr, Heppenstall RB: Anatomic considerations in the glenohumeral joint. Orthop Clin North Am *6*:341, 1975.
47. Keats TE, Teeslink R, Diamond AE, Williams JH: Normal axial relationships of the major joints. Radiology *87*:904, 1966.
48. Arndt JH, Sears AD: Posterior dislocation of the shoulder. Am J Roentgenol *94*:639, 1965.
49. Moseley HF, Overgaard B: The anterior capsular mechanisms in recurrent anterior dislocation of the shoulder. J Bone Joint Surg *44B*:913, 1962.
50. Killoran PJ, Marcove RC, Freiberger RH: Shoulder arthrography. Am J Roentgenol *103*:658, 1968.
51. Weston WJ: Subdeltoid bursa. Australas Radiol *17*:214. 1973.
52. Weston WJ: The enlarged subdeltoid bursa in rheumatoid arthritis. Br J Radiol *42*:481, 1969.
53. Freedman L, Munro R: Abduction of the arm in the scapula plane: scapular and glenohumeral movements. J Bone Joint Surg *48A*:1503, 1966.
54. Inman VT, Saunders JB, Abbott LC: Observations on function of the shoulder joint. J Bone Joint Surg *26*:1, 1944.
55. Lucas DB: Biomechanics of the shoulder joint. Arch Surg *107*:425, 1973.
56. DePalma AF: Surgical anatomy of acromioclavicular and sternoclavicular joints. Surg Clin North Am *43*:1541, 1963.
57. DePalma AF: Degenerative Changes in the Sternoclavicular and Acromioclavicular Joints in Various Decades. Springfield, Ill, Charles C Thomas, 1957.
58. Weston WJ: Soft tissue signs in recent subluxation and dislocation of the acromioclavicular joint. Br J Radiol *45*:832, 1972.
59. Weston WJ: Arthrography of the acromioclavicular joint. Australas Radiol *18*:213, 1974.
60. Bearn JG: Direct observations on the function of the capsule of the sternoclavicular joint in clavicular support. J Anat *101*:159, 1967.
61. Cave AJE: The nature and morphology of the costoclavicular ligament. J Anat *95*:170, 1961.
62. Moseley HF: Shoulder Lesions. 3rd Ed. Edinburgh, E & S Livingstone Ltd, 1969, p 207.
63. Klima M: Early development of the human sternum and the problem of homologization of the so-called suprasternal structures. Acta Anat *69*:473, 1968.
64. Kozielec T: A roentgenometric study of the process of ossification of the human sternum. Folia Morphol *32*:125, 1973.
65. Spencer RP: Radiographically determined sternal ossification. An approach to skeletal maturity. Biol Neonat *14*:341, 1969.
66. Cameron HU, Fornasier VL: The manubriosternal joint — an anatomicoradiological survey. Thorax *29*:472, 1974.
67. Trotter M: Synostosis between manubrium and body of the sternum in whites and negroes. Am J Phys Anthropol *18*:439, 1934.
68. Ashley GT: The morphological and pathological significance of synostosis at the manubrio-sternal joint. Thorax *9*:159, 1954.
69. Jones DR, Bahn RC, Randall RV, Sullivan CR: The human costochondral junction. I. Patients without primary growth disturbances. Mayo Clin Proc *44*:324, 1969.
70. Semine AA, Damon A: Costochondral ossification and aging in five populations Hum Biol *47*:101, 1975.
71. Sanders CF: Sexing by costal cartilage calcification. Letter to the editor. Br J Radiol *39*:233, 1966.
72. King JB: Calcification of costal cartilages. Br J Radiol *12*:2, 1939.
73. Elkeles A: Sex differences in calcification of costal cartilages. J Am Geriat Soc *14*:456, 1966.
74. Navani S, Shah JR, Levy PS: Determination of sex by costal cartilage calcification. Am J Roentgenol *108*:771, 1970.
75. Gray DJ, Gardner ED: The human sternochondral joints. Anat Rec *87*:235, 1943.
76. Haines RW: Movements of the first rib. J Anat *80*:94, 1946.
77. Meyer PR: Contribution à l'étude des cavités articulaires costo-vertebrales. Arch Anat Histol Embryol Norm Exp *55*:283, 1972.
78. Gloobe, H, Nathan H: The costovertebral joint. Anatomical observation in various mammals. Anat Anz *127*:22, 1970.
79. Nathan H, Weinberg H, Robin GC, Aviad I: The costovertebral joints. Anatomical-clinical observations in arthritis. Arthritis Rheum *7*:228, 1964.
80. Goldthwait JE: The rib joints. N Engl J Med *223*:568, 1940.
81. Jones MD: Limitation of hypertrophic spur formation by the costovertebral articulations. Radiology *75*:584, 1960.
82. Hohmann D, Gasteiger W: Zur röntgendiagnostik der Costotransversalgelenke. Fortsch Geb Roentgenstr Nuklearmed *112*:783, 1970.
83. Rothman RH, Simeone FA: The Spine. Philadelphia, WB Saunders Co, 1975, p 19.
84. Schmorl G, Junghanns H: *In* EF Besemann (Ed): The Human Spine in Health and Disease. 2nd Ed. Edited New York, Grune & Stratton, 1971.
85. Hall MC: Luschka's Joint. Springfield, Ill, Charles C Thomas, 1965.
86. Compere EL, Tachdjian MO, Kernahan WT: The Luschka joints. Their anatomy, physiology and pathology. Orthopedics *1*:159, 1959.
87. François RJ, Dhem A: Microradiographic study of the normal human vertebral body. Acta Anat *89*:251, 1974.
88. Nachemson A, Lewin T, Maroudas A, Freeman AR: In vitro diffusion of dye through the end-plates and the annulus fibrosus of human lumbar inter-vertebral discs. Acta Orthop Scand *41*:589, 1970.
89. Peacock A: Observations on the postnatal structure of the intervertebral disc in man. J Anat *86*:162, 1952.
90. Walmsley R: The development and growth of the intervertebral disc. Edinburgh Med J *60*:341, 1953.
91. Inman VT, Saunders JB de CM: Anatomicrophysiological aspects of injuries to the intervertebral disc. J Bone Joint Surg *29A*:461, 1947.
92. Hendry NGC: Hydration of nucleus pulposus and its relation to intervertebral disc derangement. J Bone Joint Surg *40B*:132, 1958.
93. Walmsley R: The development and growth of the intervertebral disc. Edinburgh Med J *60*:341, 1953.
94. Coventry MB: Anatomy of the intervertebral disc. Clin Orthop Rel Res *67*:9, 1969.
95. Crock HV, Yoshizawa H, Kame SK: Observations on the venous drainage of the human vertebral body. J Bone Joint Surg *55B*:528, 1973.
96. Batson OV: The function of the vertebral veins and their role in the spread of metastases. Ann Surg *112*:138, 1940.
97. Brandner ME: Normal values of the vertebral body and intervertebral disk index in adults. Am J Roentgenol *114*:411, 1972.
98. Brandner ME: Normal values of the vertebral body and intervertebral disk index during growth. Am J Roentgenol *110*:618, 1970.
99. Whalen JP, Woodruff CL: The cervical prevertebral fat stripe. A new aid in evaluating the cervical prevertebral soft tissue space. Am J Roentgenol *109*:445, 1970.
100. Wholey MH, Bruwer AT, Baker HL Jr: Lateral roentgenogram of the neck. Radiology *78*:350, 1958.
101. Reichmann S: Tomography of the lumbar intervertebral joints. Acta Radiol *12*:641, 1972.
102. Hadley LA: Anatomico-roentgenographic studies of the posterior spinal articulations. Am J Roentgenol *86*:270, 1961.
103. Morton SA: Value of the oblique view in the radiographic examination of the lumbar spine. Radiology *29*:568, 1937.
104. Reichmann S: The postnatal development of form and orientation of the lumbar intervertebral joint surfaces. Z Anat Entwicklungsgesch *133*:102, 1971.
105. Kohler R: Contrast examination of the lumbar interspinous ligaments. Preliminary report. Acta Radiol *52*:21, 1959.
106. Fielding JW, Burstein AH, Frankel VH: The nuchal ligament. Spine *1*:3, 1976.
107. Davis PR: The medial inclination of the human thoracic intervertebral articular facets. J Anat *93*:68, 1959.
108. Hinck VC, Hopkins CE: Measurement of the atlanto-dental interval in the adult. Am J Roentgenol *84*:945, 1960.
109. Jackson H: The diagnosis of minimal atlanto-axial subluxation. Br J Radiol *23*:672, 1950.
110. Cave AJE: Anatomical Notes: On the occipito-atlanto-axial articulations J Anat *68*:416, 1934.

111. Singh S: Variations of the superior articular facets of atlas vertebrae. J Anat *99*:565, 1965.
112. Dirheimer Y, Ramsheyi A, Reolon M: Positive arthrography of the craniocervical joints. Neuroradiology *12*:257, 1977.
113. Jirout J: The dynamic dependence of the lower cervical vertebrae on the atlanto-occipital joints. Neuroradiology *7*:249, 1974.
114. Jirout J: Patterns of changes in the cervical spine on lateroflexion. Neuroradiology *2*:164, 1971.
115. Jirout J: The motility of the cervical vertebrae in lateral flexion of the head and neck. Acta Radiol *13*:919, 1972.
116. Ferguson AB: Roentgen Diagnosis of Extremities and Spine. New York, Paul B Hoeber Inc, 1939.
117. Resnick D, Niwayama G, Goergen TG: Degenerative disease of the sacro-iliac joint. Invest Radiol *10*:608, 1975.
118. Schunke GB: Anatomy and development of sacro-iliac joint in man. Anat Rec *72*:313, 1938.
119. Brooke R: The sacro-iliac joint. J Anat *58*:299, 1924.
120. Sashin D: A critical analysis of the anatomy and the pathologic changes in the sacro-iliac joints. J Bone Joint Surg *12*:891, 1930.
121. Carter ME, Loewi G: Anatomical changes in normal sacro-iliac joints during childhood and comparison with the changes in Still's disease. Ann Rheum Dis *21*:121, 1962.
122. Macdonald GR, Hunt TE: Sacro-iliac joints. Observations on the gross and histological changes in the various age groups. Can Med Assoc J *66*:157, 1952.
123. Weisl H: The articular surfaces of the sacro-iliac joint and their relation to the movements of the sacrum. Acta Anat *22*:1, 1954.
124. Trotter M: Accessory sacro-iliac articulations Am J Phys Anthropol *22*:247, 1937.
125. Colachis SC Jr, Worden RE, Bechtol CO, Strohm BR: Movement of the sacro-iliac joint in the adult male: a preliminary report. Arch Phys Med *44*:490, 1963.
126. Frigerio NA, Stowe RR, Howe JW: Movement of the sacro-iliac joint. Clin Orthop *100*:370, 1974.
127. Abramson D, Roberts SM, Wilson PD: Relaxation of the pelvic joints in pregnancy. Surg Gynecol Obstet *58*:595, 1934.
128. Thorp DJ, Fray WE: The pelvic joints during pregnancy and labor. JAMA *111*:1162, 1938.
129. Cohen AS, McNeill JM, Calkins E, Sharp JT, Schubart A: The "normal" sacro-iliac joint. Analysis of 88 sacro-iliac roentgenograms. Am J Roentgenol *100*:559, 1967.
130. Wilkinson M, Meikle JAK: Tomography of the sacro-iliac joints. Ann Rheum Dis *25*:433, 1966.
131. Casuccio C: Studio anatomico e radiografico sull'articolazione sacro-iliaco normale nell'adulto. Chir Organi Mov *20*:353, 1934.
132. Todd TW: Age changes in the pubic bone. Am J Phys Anthropol *4*:1, 333, 1921.
133. Brooks ST: Skeletal age at death: the reliability of cranial and pubic age indicators. Am J Phys Anthropol *13*:567, 1955.
134. Camiel MR, Aaron JB: Gas or vacuum phenomenon in pubic symphysis during pregnancy. Radiology *66*:548, 1956.
135. Williams JL: Gas in symphysis pubis during and following pregnancy. Am J Roentgenol *73*:403, 1955.
136. Vix VA, Ryu CY: The adult symphysis pubis: normal and abnormal. Am J Roentgenol *112*:517, 1971.
137. Young J: Relaxation of the pelvic joints in pregnancy: pelvic arthropathy of pregnancy. J Obstet Gynaecol Br Emp *47*:493, 1940.
138. Caffey, J, Ames R, Silverman WA, Ryder CT, Hough G: Contradiction of the congenital dysplasia–predislocation hypothesis of congenital dislocation of the hip through a study of the normal variation in acetabular angles at successive periods in infancy. Pediatrics *17*:632, 1956.
139. Caffey J, Ross S: Pelvic bones in infantile mongoloidism. Am J Roentgenol *80*:458, 1958.
140. Astley R: Chromosomal abnormalities in childhood, with particular reference to Turner's syndrome and mongolism. B J Radiol *36*:2, 1963.
141. Budin E, Chandler E: Measurement of femoral neck anteversion by a direct method. Radiology *69*:209, 1957.
142. Billing L: Roentgen examination of the proximal femur end in children and adolescents. Acta Radiol Suppl *110*:5, 1954.
143. Wiberg G: Studies on dysplastic acetabula and congenital subluxation of the hip joint — with special reference to the complication of osteoarthritis. Acta Chir Scand Suppl *58*:1, 1939.
144. Hooper JC, Jones EW: Primary protrusion of the acetabulum. J Bone Joint Surg *53B*:23, 1971.
145. Armbuster TG, Guerra J Jr, Resnick D, Goergen TG, Feingold ML, Niwayama G, Danzig LA: The adult hip: An anatomic study. Part I. The bony landmarks. Radiology *128*:1, 1978.
146. Judet R, Judet J, Letournal E: Fractures of the acetabulum: classification and surgical approaches for open reduction — preliminary report. J Bone Joint Surg *46A*:1615, 1964.
147. Pomeranz MM: Intrapelvic protrusion of the acetabulum (Otto pelvis). J Bone Joint Surg *14*:663, 1932.
148. Overgaard K: Otto's disease and other forms of protrusio acetabuli. Acta Radiol *16*:390, 1935.
149. Friedenberg ZB: Protrusio acetabuli. Am J Surg *85*:764, 1953.
150. Alexander C: The aetiology of primary protrusio acetabuli. Br J Radiol *38*:567, 1965.
151. Hubbard MJS: The measurement of progression in protrusio acetabuli. Am J Roentgenol *106*:506, 1969.
152. MacDonald D: Primary protrusio acetabuli: report of an affected family. J Bone Joint Surg *53B*:30, 1971.
153. Hefke HW, Turner VC: The obturator sign as the earliest roentgenographic sign in the diagnosis of septic arthritis and tuberculosis of the hip. J Bone Joint Surg *24*:857, 1942.
154. Jorup S, Kjellberg SR: The early diagnosis of acute septic osteomyelitis, periostitis and arthritis and its importance in the treatment. Acta Radiol (Diagn) *30*:316, 1948.
155. Drey L: A roentgenographic study of transitory synovitis of the hip joint. Radiology *60*:588, 1953.
156. Bartley O, Chidekel N: Roentgenologic changes in postoperative septic osteoarthritis of the hip joint. Acata Radiol (Diagn) *4*:113, 1966.
157. Lewis MS, Norman A: The earliest signs of postoperative hip infection. Radiology *104*:309, 1972.
158. Brown I: A study of the "capsular" shadow in disorders of the hip in children. J Bone Joint Surg *57B*:175, 1975.
159. Reichmann S: Roentgenologic soft tissue appearances in hip disease. Acta Radiol (Diagn) *6*:167, 1967.
160. Guerra J Jr, Armbuster TG, Resnick D, Goergen TG, Feingold ML, Niwayama G, Danzig LA: The adult hip: an anatomic study. Part II. The soft-tissue landmarks. Radiology *128*:11, 1978.
161. Lange M: Die Erleichterung der Frühdiagnose der Koxitis durch bisher wenig beachtete Veränderungen im Röntgenbild. Z Orthop Chir *48*:90, 1927.
162. Armstrong P, Saxton H: Iliopsoas bursa. Br J Radiol *45*:493, 1972.
163. Chandler SB: The iliopsoas bursa in man. Anat Rec *58*:235, 1934.
164. Staple TW: Arthrographic demonstration of the iliopsoas bursa extension of the hip joint. Radiology *102*:515, 1972.
165. Last RJ: Anatomy. Regional and Applied. 5th Ed. London, Churchill Livingstone, 1972, p 211.
166. Warren R, Kaye JJ, Salvati EA: Arthrographic demonstration of an enlarged iliopsoas bursa complicating osteoarthritis of the hip — a case report. J Bone Joint Surg *57A*:413, 1975.
167. Weston WJ: The bursae deep to gluteus medius and minimus. Australas Radiol *14*:325, 1970.
168. Smillie IS: Injuries of the Knee Joint. 4th Ed. Baltimore, Williams & Wilkins, 1970, p 23.
169. Ficat RP, Hungerford D: Disorders of the Patello-Femoral Joint. Baltimore, Williams & Wilkins, 1977, p 3.
170. Brantigan OC, Voshell AF: The tibial collateral ligament: Its function, its bursae, and its relation to the medial meniscus. J Bone Joint Surg *25*:121, 1943.
171. Doppman JL: Baker's cyst and the normal gastrocnemio-semimembranosus bursa. Am J Roentgenol *94*:646, 1965.
172. Wilson PD, Eyre-Brook AL, Francis JD: A clinical and anatomical study of the semimembranosus bursa in relation to popliteal cyst. J Bone Joint Surg *20*:963, 1938.
173. Wolfe RD, Colloff B: Popliteal cysts. An arthrographic study and review of the literature. J Bone Joint Surg *54A*:1057, 1972.
174. Dalinka MK, Garofola J: The infrapatellar synovial fold: A cause for confusion in the evaluation of the anterior cruciate ligament. Am J Roentgenol *127*:589, 1976.
175. Resnick D, Newell JD, Guerra J Jr, Danzig LA, Niwayama G, Goergen TG: Proximal tibiofibular joint: Anatomic-pathologic-radiographic correlation. Am J Roentgenol *131*:133, 1978.
176. Weston WJ: The deep infrapatellar bursa. Australas Rad *17*:212, 1973.
177. Weston WJ: The extrasynovial and capsular fat pads on the posterior aspect of the knee joint. Skel Radiol *2*:87, 1977.
178. Lindgren PG, Willén R: Gastrocnemio-semimembranosus bursa and its relation to the knee joint. Acta Radiol *18*:497, 1977.
179. Kennedy JC, Weinberg HW, Wilson AS: The anatomy and function of the anterior cruciate ligament. J Bone Joint Surg *56A*:223, 1974.
180. Brantigan OC, Voshell AF: The mechanics of the ligaments and menisci of the knee joint. J Bone Joint Surg *23*:44, 1941.
181. Robichon J, Romero C: The functional anatomy of the knee joint with special reference to the medial collateral and anterior cruciate ligaments. Can J Surg *11*:36, 1968.
182. Harrison RB, Wood MB, Keats TE: The grooves of the distal articular surface of the femur — a normal variant. Am J Roentgenol *126*:751, 1976.
183. Jacobsen K: Landmarks of the knee joint on the lateral radiograph during rotation. Fortschr Geb Roentgenstr Nuklearmed *125*:399, 1976.

184. Ravelli A: Zum Roentgenbild des menschlichen Kniegelenkes. Fortschr Geb Roentgenstr Nuklearmed *71*:614, 1949.
185. Takechi H: Trabecular architecture of the knee joint. Acta Orthop Scand *48*:673, 1977.
186. Blumensaat C: Die Lageabweichungen und Verrenkungen der Kniescheibe. Ergebn Chir Orthop *31*:149, 1938.
187. Jacobsen K, Bertheussen K, Gjerloff CC: Characteristics of the line of Blumensaat. Acta Orthop Scand *45*:764, 1974.
188. Insall J, Salvati E: Patella position in the normal knee joint. Radiology *101*:101, 1971.
189. Jacobsen K, Bertheussen K: The vertical location of the patella. Fundamental views on the concept of patella alta, using a normal sample. Acta Orthop Scand *45*:436, 1974.
190. Blackburne JS, Peel TE: A new method of measuring patellar height. J Bone Joint Surg *59B*:241, 1977.
191. Lancourt JE, Cristini JA: Patella alta and patella infera. J Bone Joint Surg *57A*:1112, 1975.
192. Hall FM: Radiographic diagnosis and accuracy in knee joint effusions. Radiology *115*:49, 1975.
193. Lewis RW: Roentgenographic study of soft tissue pathology in and about the knee joint. Am J Roentgenol *65*:200, 1951.
194. Bachman AL: Roentgen diagnosis of knee-joint effusion. Radiology *46*:462, 1946.
195. Harris RD, Hecht HL: Suprapatellar effusions. A new diagnostic sign. Radiology *97*:1, 1970.
196. Friedman AC, Naidich TP: The fabella sign: fabella displacement in synovial effusion and popliteal fossa masses. Radiology *127*:113, 1978.
197. Ogden JA: The anatomy and function of the proximal tibiofibular joint. Clin Orthop Rel Res *101*:186, 1974.
198. Gray DJ, Gardner E: Prenatal development of the human knee and superior tibiofibular joints. Am J Anat *86*:235, 1950.
199. Minns RJ, Hunter JAA: The mechanical and structural characteristics of the tibiofibular interosseous membrane. Acta Orthop Scand *47*:236, 1976.
200. Barnett CH, Napier JR: The axis of rotation at the ankle joint in man. Its influence upon the form of the talus and the mobility of the fibula. J Anat *86*:1, 1952.
201. Ramsey PL, Hamilton W: Changes in tibiotalar area of contact caused by lateral talar shift. J Bone Joint Surg *58A*:356, 1976.
202. Skinner EH: The mathematical calculation of progress in fractures at the ankle and wrist. Surg Gynecol Obstet *18*:238, 1914.
203. Joy G, Patzakis MJ, Harvey JP Jr: Precise evaluation of the reduction of severe ankle fractures. Technique and correlation with end results. J Bone Joint Surg *56A*:979, 1974.
204. Hutter CG Jr, Scott W: Tibial torsion. J Bone Joint Surg *31A*:511, 1949.
205. Goergen TG, Danzig LA, Resnick D, Owen CA: Roentgenographic evaluation of the tibiotalar joint. J Bone Joint Surg *59A*:874, 1977.
206. Kaye JJ, Bohne WHO: A radiographic study of the ligamentous anatomy of the ankle. Radiology *125*:659, 1977.
207. Palmer DG: Tendon sheaths and bursae involved by rheumatoid disease at the foot and ankle. Australas Radiol *14*:419, 1970.
208. Resnick D, Goergen TG: Peroneal tenography in previous calcaneal fractures. Radiology *115*:211, 1975.
209. Resnick D, Feingold ML, Curd J, Niwayama G, Goergen TG: Calcaneal abnormalities in articular disorders. Rheumatoid arthritis, ankylosing spondylitis, psoriatic arthritis and Reiter syndrome. Radiology *125*:355, 1977.
210. Bywaters EG: Heel lesions of rheumatoid arthritis. Ann Rheum Dis *13*:42, 1954.
211. Sutro CJ: The os calcis, the tendo-achillis and the local bursae. Bull Hosp Joint Dis *27*:76, 1966.
212. Weston WJ: The bursa deep to the tendo achillis. Australas Radiol *14*:327, 1970.
213. Resnick D: Radiology of the talocalcaneal articulations. Anatomic considerations and arthrography. Radiology *111*:581, 1974.
214. Mehrez M, el-Geneidy S: Arthrography of the ankle. J Bone Joint Surg *52B*:308, 1970.
215. Olson RW: Arthrography of the ankle: its use in the evaluation of ankle sprains. Radiology *92*:1439, 1969.
216. Youm Y, McMurthy RY, Flatt AE, Gillespie TE: Kinematics of the wrist. I. An experimental study of radial-ulnar deviation and flexion-extension. J Bone Joint Surg *60A*:423, 1978.
217. Candardjis G, DeBosset PH, Saudan Y: L'articulation manubriosternale normale. Technique d'examen et étude des variantes. J Radiol Electrol *59*:89, 1978.
218. Cockshott WP: The coracoclavicular joint. Radiology *131*:313, 1979.
219. Chamberlain WE: Basilar impression (platybasia). Yale J Biol Med *11*:487, 1939.
220. Gradoyevitch B: Coracoclavicular joint. J Bone Joint Surg *21*:918, 1939.
221. Nutter PD: Coracoclavicular articulations. J Bone Joint Surg *23*:177, 1941.
222. Liberson F; The role of the coracoclavicular ligaments in affections of the shoulder girdle. Am J Surg *44*:145, 1939.
223. Wertheimer LG: Coracoclavicular joint. J Bone Joint Surg *30A*:570, 1948.
224. McGregor M: The significance of certain measurements of the skull in the diagnosis of basilar impression. Br J Radiol *21*:171, 1948.
225. Eischgold H, Metzger J: Etude radiotomographique de l'impression basilaire. Rev Rhum Mal Osteoartic *19*:261, 1952.
226. Ogden JA, Conlogue GJ, Bronson ML, Jensen PS: Radiology of postnatal skeletal development. II. The manubrium and sternum. Skel Radiol *4*:189, 1979.
227. Ogden JA, Conlogue GJ, Bronson ML: Radiology of postnatal skeletal development. III. The clavicle. Skel Radiol *4*:196, 1979.
228. Brower AC, Woodlief RM: Pseudarthrosis at the first sternocostal synchondrosis. Amer J Roentgen *135*:1276, 1980.
229. Küsswetter W: Die membrana interossea antebrachii — das gemeinsame gelenkband der radioulnargelenke. Z. Orthop *117*:767, 1979.

4

ARTICULAR CARTILAGE PHYSIOLOGY AND METABOLISM IN HEALTH AND DISEASE

by Wayne H. Akeson, M.D.
and David H. Gershuni, M.D., F.R.C.S.

The purpose of this chapter is to summarize existing knowledge of the composition, metabolism, and function of articular cartilage. Where possible, the relationships among these factors in health and disease will be described.

Articular cartilage is a unique tissue in many respects, but especially with regard to its structural, metabolic, and functional interactions. Articular cartilage possesses unparalleled functional efficiency. This efficiency is derived from design features that are marveled at by physicians and engineers attempting to design substitutes for diseased joints. For example, the articular cartilage lubrication efficiency is at least an order of magnitude superior to the best bearing surfaces known to modern engineering. Such efficiencies are achieved in spite of stringent limitations imposed upon the tissue, such as the lack of blood supply and a tissue thickness that measures only a few millimeters at the most. Couple these points with a limited repair capability and the consequent requirement that the tissue survive a lifetime of use, and one is forced to ask "How can synovial joints survive as long as they do?" rather than "Why do these joints fail?" The first task of this chapter will be to describe the morphologic, biochemical, and physiologic interactions of the cartilage matrix in order to gain insight into the answer to the first question.

AN OVERVIEW OF CARTILAGE FUNCTION

Before considering details of morphology and biochemistry of articular cartilage matrix it will be helpful for those who are reviewing joint physiology for the first time, or who are coming back to it after a period of disuse, to consider a simple scheme describing the interrelationship of these elements. A useful analogy with articular cartilage is the air tent seen in parts of the country as a cover for recreational areas such as swimming pools and tennis courts or as a temporary cover for exhibitions (Fig. 4–1). The requirements for the tent are a membrane (fabric cover), an inflation medium (air), and an energy source to keep the tent inflated (fan). These elements are interrelated, and a deficiency of any of them will result in failure of the system, with collapse of the tent. If the fabric has a tear, an air leak occurs, for which the pump may not be able to compensate, and the tent will collapse. Or, if the pump fails, the tent will gradually collapse as pressurized air leaks through the pores of the fabric. The tent obviously could not work in an environment such as the moon, which has no atmosphere to permit inflation of the space under the fabric.

Articular cartilage is analogous to the air tent in a number of respects. There is a fabric-like structure at the cartilage surface which consists of fine collagen fibrils packed tightly in a matted pattern, much different from that seen in the deeper layers, where fibers become thicker, the orientation becomes vertical, and the spaces between the fibers increase. The surface "fabric" of cartilage has tiny pores that permit fluid and small molecules access to and egress from the tissue but block movement of large molecules. The inflation medium in articular cartilage is, of course, fluid, not air. The cartilage fluid is in equilibrium with the synovial fluid, which in turn is essentially an ultrafiltrate of plasma. The fluid in articular cartilage is significantly pressurized. Calculations by Ogston[1] led him to conclude that articular cartilage is inflated to "motor tire pressure." The pump for this pressurized system is not intuitively obvious, but its presence has been established without doubt by modern techniques of rheology and biophysics.

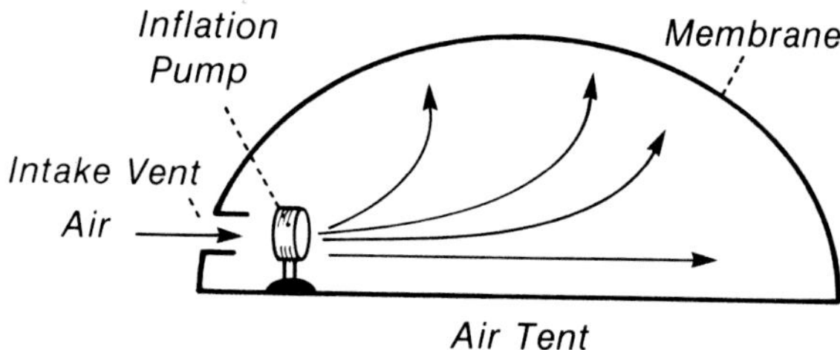

Figure 4–1. Air tent articular cartilage analogy. It is conceptually useful to think of cartilage as a pressurized structure such as exemplified by an air tent. The system requires a pump, which must be working constantly to maintain inflation of the system because of leaks through the fabric. In the case of cartilage, the surface membrane is the fine collagen fibril network concentrated at the surface. The inflation pump is the proteoglycan molecules, and the inflation medium is an ultrafiltrate of synovial fluid. In cartilage, of course, there is no single intake vent for the inflation medium to enter; rather, the fluid that inflates the tissue enters through the same fabric pores at the surface from which it exits when compressed (see text).

The pump for the articular cartilage system is chiefly the proteoglycan (PG) and the proteoglycan aggregate molecules, large macromolecules fixed within the articular cartilage fibrillar matrix as a result of their large size and volume. They are much too large to move between the fibrils of collagen and much much too large to exit through the small pores in the matted capsule-like surface of the articular cartilage. Side-arm branches of these molecules contain many negative surface charges that repel each other, causing the molecules to attempt to unwind and enlarge their domain within the cartilage. In addition, the protein polysaccharides have a large number of hydroxyl groups, which attract water molecules by a phenomenon called hydrogen bonding. These reactions collectively cause fluid to be pulled into articular cartilage through the matrix pores and cause the collagen matrix of the system to be expanded. This tendency to imbibe water creates a swelling pressure within the enclosed cartilage space. The collagen fibers are therefore placed under tension as the fluid pressure rises. In this manner the cartilage is pressurized and the collagen "fabric" is inflated. The equilibrium state reached is a balance that can be upset by external applied pressure. If the external pressure exceeds the internal pressure, fluid will be caused to flow outward until a new equilibrium is reached. This fluid movement will be of great interest to us later in this chapter, as it explains the mechanism of several indispensible elements of the articular cartilage system, such as lubrication, load-bearing, and nutrition.

The collagen matrix of cartilage, the proteoglycan and proteoglycan aggregate, and the movement of fluid within cartilage will be described below in greater detail with respect to morphologic, biochemical, metabolic, and functional aspects.

COLLAGEN

Morphology of the Collagen Framework

The pattern of collagen fibrils within articular cartilage is well suited to the functional requirements of the tissue. The air tent analogy described earlier requires that a pressurized internal medium

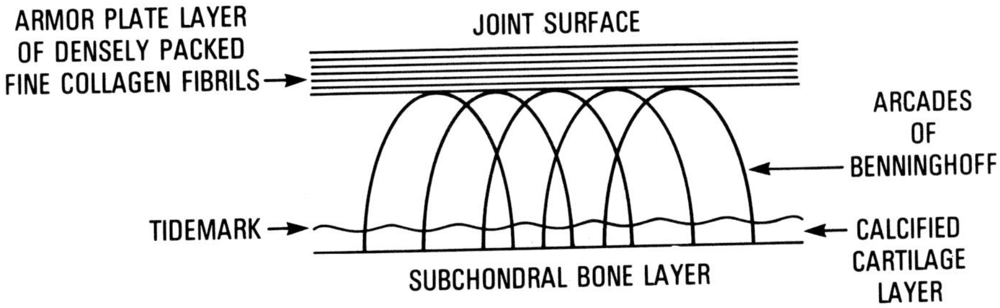

Figure 4–2. *Schematic diagram of the collagen fibril orientation within articular cartilage. The fibrils are tightly packed near the articular surface in a tangential layer that has been termed the "armor plate" layer. Fibrils in the deeper layers become progressively larger as they progress toward the subchondral bone layer. The fibrils are also more widely spaced in the deeper layers of cartilage. The change in orientation from tangential to perpendicular in the deeper layers creates a pattern which Benninghoff[2] termed an arcade. Although this is an idealized conception and the fibrils of cartilage are not so precisely ordered, the concept is still useful in visualizing the fundamental interaction of cartilage with other constituents of cartilage. The collagen fibrils anchor into the subchondral bone layer after traversing the calcified cartilage, which is demarcated by a change in staining properties termed the "tidemark line." The anchoring of these fibrils into bone is analogous to the continuation of ligamentous attachments into bone termed Sharpey's fibrils.*

be constrained from expansion by a membrane. A matted surface layer of collagen fibrils provides this membrane-like function.

The collagen pattern at the cartilage surface is morphologically quite different from the pattern in deeper layers. Benninghoff[2] described an arcade pattern of articular cartilage collagen organization in 1925 (Fig. 4–2). This pattern has been subsequently challenged with respect to the precise accuracy of the proposed scheme.[3] However, with respect to functional understanding, the concept is useful and at least partially correct. Certainly the surface fiber characteristics differ from those in deeper layers. The surface collagen fibrils are smaller (30 to 32 nm in diameter), and more closely packed than in the middle and deeper layers.[4] The heterogeneity of concentration of the principal cartilage constituents — collagen and proteoglycan — by dry weight is seen in Figure 4–3. The collagen concentration is greatest at the surface, where the small fibrils are compacted tangential to the surface. This arrangement creates an effective pore size, which has been calculated by McCutchen[5] to be about 6 nm. The largest molecule that can traverse a pore of this dimension is hemoglobin. Therefore, the surface pores readily admit most of the synovial fluid molecules, which are essentially an ultrafiltrate of plasma. Small ions and glucose, for example, easily traverse these pores, but larger molecules such as proteins and hyaluronic acid do not enter cartilage in significant amounts under normal conditions.

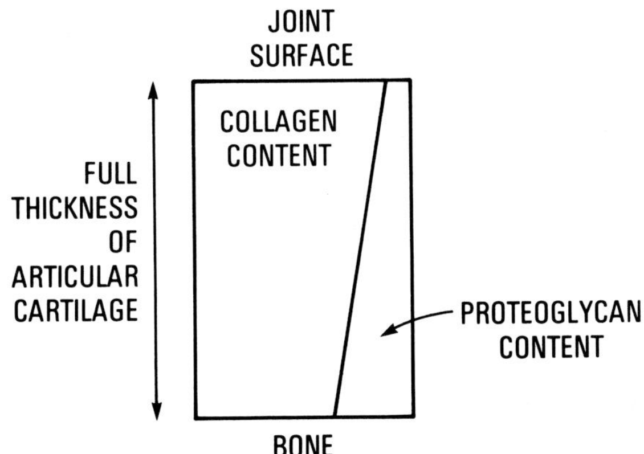

Figure 4–3. *Relative amounts of collagen and proteoglycan in cartilage. Collagen is the predominant organic constituent by weight in articular cartilage and is most concentrated at the surface layer. In contrast, proteoglycan is most concentrated in the deeper layers. The functional importance of the two constituents is more equal than these percentages might suggest, both constituents being essential for normal cartilage function.*

Collagen fibers in the intermediate layers no longer are oriented principally tangential to the surface but are obliquely or randomly directed. They are larger than the surface fibrils, most ranging between 40 and 100 nm.[4] The deepest fibrils are the largest in cartilage. They are perpendicularly disposed relative to the joint surface. They perforate the calcified basal layers of cartilage through the tidemark regions and eventually enter the subchondral bone layer, where they are firmly attached, much as in the case of Sharpey's fibers of cortical bone.

This anatomic arrangement is the key to the secure structural anchorage of cartilage to the bone that it overlies. The surface collagen fibrils possess characteristics that create the necessary functional barrier to fluid movement. However, this movement is rate-limited by the small pore size of the collagen meshwork of the cartilage surface, an important factor that prevents all the fluid from being expressed, as, for example, when an individual stands for hours at a time.

The surface pattern of the collagen framework described has been implicitly recognized for decades by the term "armor plate layer," referring to the tough resilient cartilage surface. It has been well demonstrated clinically that loss of the densely packed collagen mat at the surface of cartilage in weight-bearing regions is the prelude to fibrillation, thinning, and ensuing degenerative arthritis. This seems completely logical, as the coarse, widely spaced fibrils in deeper layers that are oriented principally vertically are poorly suited to constraining the swelling forces generated by the matrix proteoglycans. The term "fibrillation" describes the tendency of these fibrils to be split vertically all the way to their subchondral attachment, much as wood splits along the grain of its fibers. The villus-like strands so exposed collectively resemble a shag rug, and the individual strands are prone to tear off at the base when mechanically loaded and exposed to shear stresses. It is clear that the "armor plate" term applies well to the normal surface mat of collagen fibrils, but that loss of this layer no longer permits the cartilage to function as a pressurized unit suited to weight-bearing.

Evidence of the fibril pattern of collagen derives from several types of observation, including routine histology, transmission electron microscopy, scanning electron microscopy, and the demonstration of Hultkrantz lines.[6] The latter are typically observed on the surface of cartilage and are analogous to the Langer's lines of skin.[7] The Hultkrantz lines become visible when the surface of cartilage is pricked with a pin that is circular in cross section. The defect so created is emphasized by coating the cartilage with India ink and then wiping it dry. Hultkrantz noted many years ago that the puncture holes appeared as slits rather than round holes. Furthermore, the slits have an axis that is generally perpendicular to the principal axis of movement of the joint. Hultkrantz lines are therefore different for each joint of the body. Mechanical tensile tests have shown that the Hultkrantz lines indicate the preferred orientation of the collagen fibrils at the surface of the joint because the specimens are found to be strongest when the long axis of the specimen is parallel to the Hultkrantz lines. Bullough and Goodfellow[8] have shown this characteristic of joint surfaces very elegantly in experiments illustrated in Figures 4–4 and 4–5. Notice that in deeper layers the slits disappear, indicating that the fibril orientation is more random or more vertical, or both. Electron microscopy has also been used to show a preferred orientation of these fibrils at the surface and to characterize the dimensions of the fibrils at different depths from the surface.[4, 8]

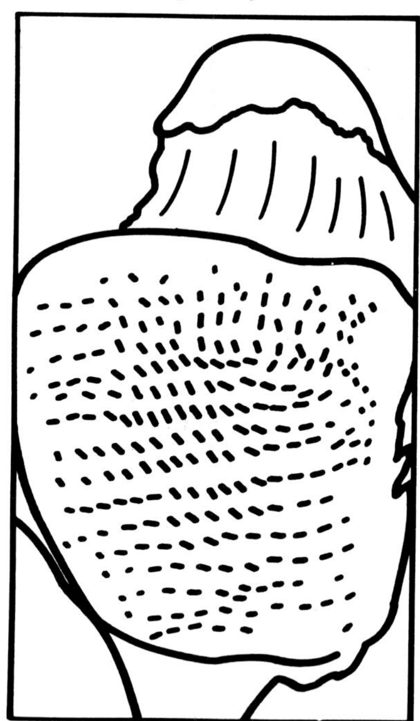

Figure 4–4. Hultkrantz lines. This figure illustrates the pattern of split lines on the surface of the human talus. The split lines are created by a pin pushed through the surface in a perpendicular direction. The lines are typically made more obvious by coating the surface with India ink and subsequently wiping it dry. The pattern of the defect is a slit rather than a circle because of the predominant orientation of the underlying collagen fibrils of the surface layers. The split line phenomenon is similar to that seen in skin (Langer's lines). Hultkrantz lines run predominantly perpendicular to the main axis of motion of the particular joint. (Redrawn after Bullough P, Goodfellow J: J Bone Joint Surg 50B:852, 1968.)

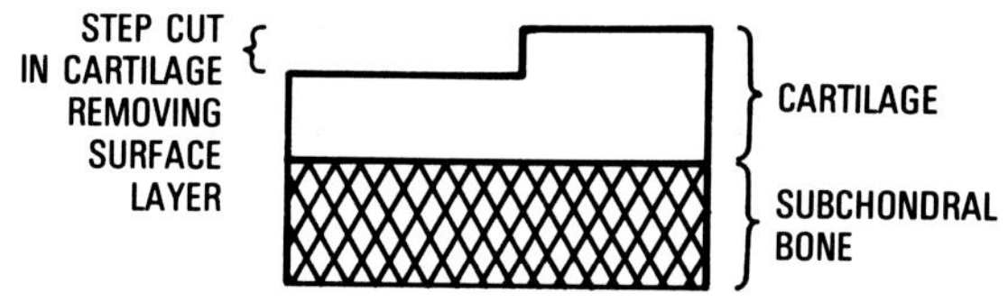

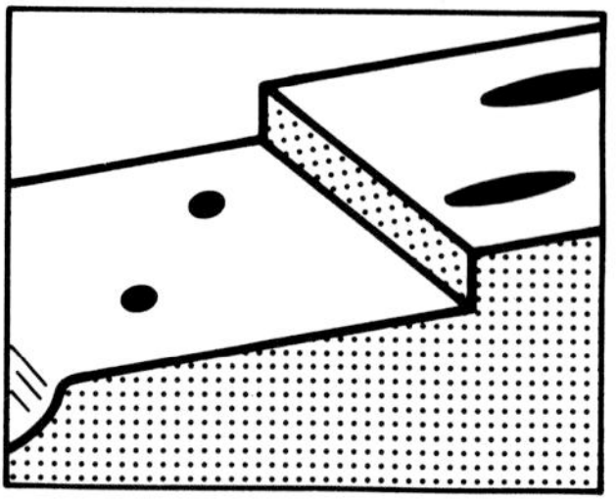

Figure 4–5. Hultkrantz lines. This figure shows the change in pattern of the Hultkrantz split lines in deeper layers of cartilage compared with the surface. If a step cut is made in cartilage, removing the surface layer after the Hultkrantz lines have been established, a different pattern is seen in the deeper layers. A circle rather than a split is the typical pattern made by a penetrating pin. The reason for the difference is that in the deeper layers there is no preference of direction of fibrils in the tangential plane. (Redrawn after Bullough P, Goodfellow J: J Bone Joint Surg 50B:852, 1968.)

Routine histology does not show the collagen fibrils of cartilage well because they tend to be masked by the abundant proteoglycan that is intertwined within the fibril network. The proteoglycan contains dense electronegative charges that are responsible for many of the observed staining characteristics of cartilage, such as metachromasia. However, the collagen fibril pattern can be inferred by viewing sections with polarized light, since a fibrillar pattern of preferred orientation will alter the polarized light characteristically. Examples of cartilage sections viewed with polarized light are seen in Figures 4–6 and 4–7. A key paper by Bullough and Goodfellow on cartilage fibril patterns describes the interpretation of this type of photomicrograph.[8]

Collagen Chemistry

The molecular structure of collagen has been of considerable interest for over a century, since it is the principal structural protein by mass for all mammals. It constitutes 65 to 80 per cent of the mass by dry weight of such specialized connective tissues as tendons, ligaments, skin, joint capsules, and cartilage. It is the only protein with significant tensile

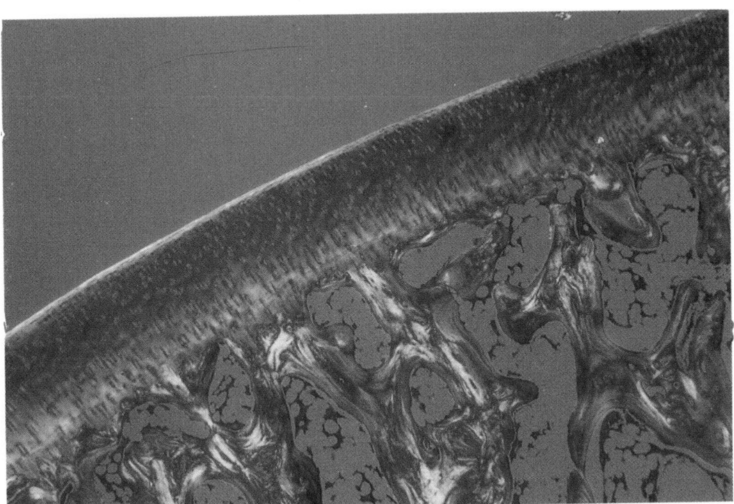

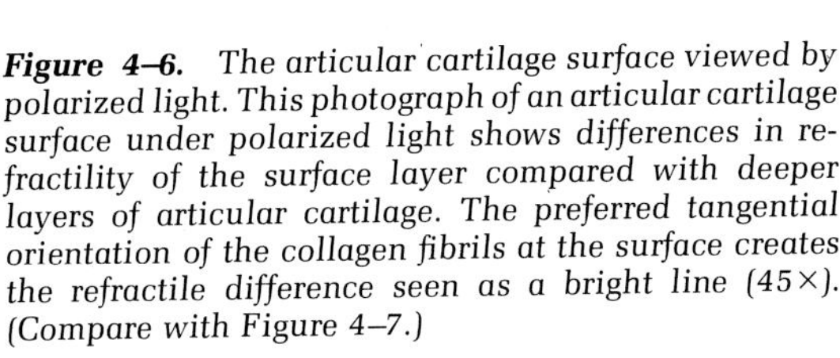

Figure 4–6. *The articular cartilage surface viewed by polarized light. This photograph of an articular cartilage surface under polarized light shows differences in refractility of the surface layer compared with deeper layers of articular cartilage. The preferred tangential orientation of the collagen fibrils at the surface creates the refractile difference seen as a bright line (45×). (Compare with Figure 4–7.)*

force–resisting properties with the exception of elastin, whose functional role is insignificant in comparison. Therefore, collagen is the key protein in musculoskeletal stability: It provides the mechanical properties imparting the "connect" ability in connective tissue.

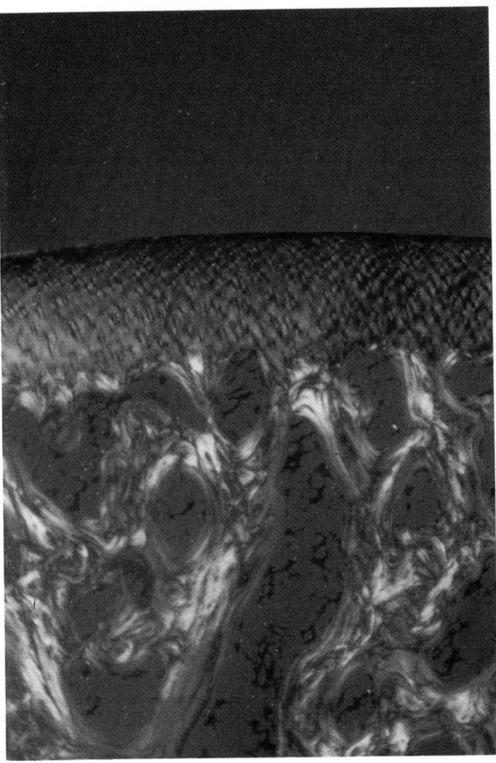

Figure 4–7. *The articular cartilage surface (same section as in Figure 4–6 with polarizing filter rotated 90 degrees). If the polarizing filter is rotated 90 degrees, a marked change is observed in the refractile pattern. The surface now is dark rather than bright because of the predominant orientation of the tangential layer of fibrils. The "arcade" pattern in the deeper layers can also be perceived with the filter in this rotation, in contrast to Figure 4–6. The polarized-light technique used in this way identifies areas in the tissue where a predominant orientation exists, in comparison with a random pattern of fibrils.*

The tensile force–resisting properties of cartilage derive from the precise molecular configuration of the collagen macromolecule. This molecule is one of the largest in the body, forming a rod-like structure whose dimensions are 300 nm in length and 1.5 nm in diameter. These rods are termed tropocollagen. They are assembled in a three-dimensional array in the extracellular environment, being somehow influenced by environmental stresses and additional biologic factors the details of whose nature are as yet unclear. The sum of the extracellular influences somehow affects the orientation and size of fibrils that are assembled from the tropocollagen units. The assembly is typically patterned in a quarter stagger (Fig. 4–8), which is seen as a 64 nm subbonding on transmission electron micrographs. A small gap that exists between the head to tail linear assembly of the tropocollagen units may be of functional importance in bone with respect to nucleation of apatite crystals in the process of matrix mineralization of osteoid.[9]

The individual tropocollagen units are made up of three chains that are synthesized independently intracellularly in the manner of other proteins (Fig. 4–8). The length of the messenger RNA molecule required for the synthesis is extraordinary, as each chain contains about 1000 amino acids. Most of the chains (called alpha chains) are precisely ordered with a general sequence of glycine-proline-hydroxyproline, glycine-proline-x-, or glycine-x-proline-, where x is another amino acid.[10] The higher percentages of the amino acids glycine, proline, and hydroxyproline are unique to collagen. Glycine is the smallest amino acid and permits the close packing necessary for the assembly of the three alpha chains into tropocollagen. Proline and hydroxyproline are cyclic amino acids whose structure presumably imparts rigidity to the final triple helix configu-

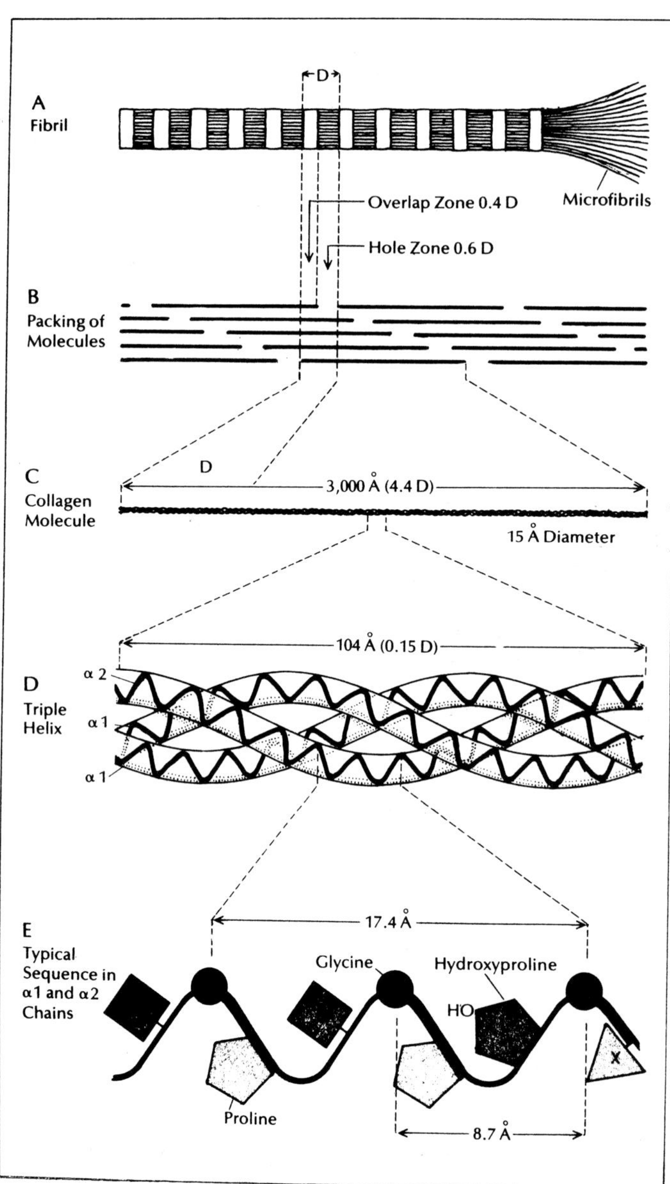

Figure 4–8. *This figure shows the relationship between the single strand protein of the alpha chain to the triple helix, the collagen molecule, and the fully developed fibril. The characteristic feature of the collagen molecule is its rigid, very long, narrow, rod-like structure, which is created by the tight winding of three alpha chains into a triple helix termed tropocollagen. (Reprinted, by permission, from Prockop DJ, et al: N Engl J Med 301:13, 1979.)*

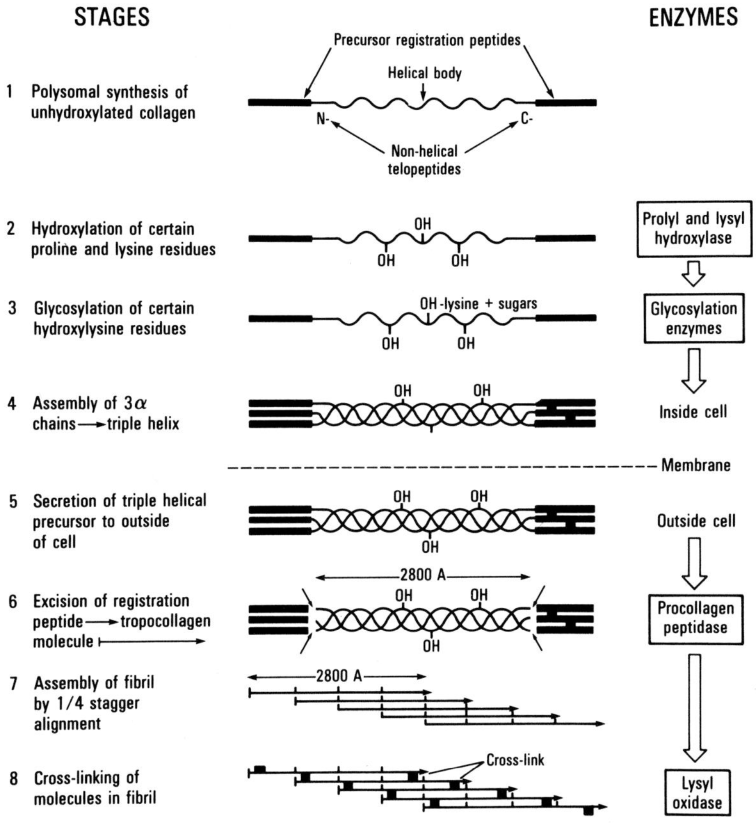

Figure 4–9. *The enzymatic stages in maturation of collagen. Several enzymatic steps are necessary for creation of the final collagen molecule and its maturation into a collagen fibril. These enzymatic steps take place partly within the cell and partly outside the cell. Even those steps that occur inside the cell are post-translational, that is, they are not directly under genetic control. However, they are very essential for the proper development of the final structure. Defects in many of the steps have been identified in a variety of heritable disorders of connective tissues. The final aggregation of collagen into a structure that becomes cross linked is essential in order to produce the requisite tensile stress–resistant properties characteristic of mature connective tissue. (From Levene CI: J Clin Pathol, Suppl 12:82, 1978.)*

ration. Further details of the collagen molecular arrangement are presented in recent reviews.[10-14] Collagen undergoes numerous modifications following ribosomal assembly, which are initiated by intracellular or extracellular enzymes. Examples of these processes include hydroxylation of proline or lysine and glycosylation of lysine. These modifications are termed "secondary features," as distinguished from the direct-coded structure (Fig. 4–9).

The assembly of the three alpha chains into tropocollagen is facilitated by a group of amino acids at the end of each alpha chain that are called registration peptides. The triple helix plus its registration peptide is larger than the tropocollagen mole-

Table 4–1

STRUCTURALLY AND GENETICALLY DISTINCT COLLAGENS*

Type	Tissue Distribution	Molecular Form	Chemical Characteristics
I	Bone, tendon, skin, dentin, ligament, fascia, artery and uterus	$[\alpha1(I)]_2\alpha2$	Hybrid composed of two kinds of chains. Low in hydroxylysine and glycosylated hydroxylysine
II	Hyaline cartilage	$[\alpha1(II)]_3$	Relatively high in hydroxylysine and glycosylated hydroxylysine
III	Skin, artery, and uterus	$[\alpha1(III)]_3$	High in hydroxyproline and low in hydroxylysine; contains interchain disulfide bonds
IV	Basement membranes	$[\alpha1(IV)]_3$	High in hydroxylysine and glycosylated hydroxylysine; may contain large globular regions
V	Basement membranes and perhaps other tissues	αA and αB	Similar to Type IV

*Reprinted, by permission, from Prockop DJ, et al: N Engl J Med *301*:13, 1979.

cule and is called procollagen. Once the assembly of the triple helix is completed, the registration peptides are no longer of utility and are cleaved by an enzyme, procollagen peptidase, as the procollagen passes through the cellular membrane into the extracellular space.

The alpha chains are not identical among species or within a single species. Early data on mammalian skin collagen showed two types of alpha chain, $\alpha 1$ and $\alpha 2$, present in a ratio of 2:1. Three types of alpha chains were identified in codfish skin collagen, $\alpha 1$, $\alpha 2$, and $\alpha 3$.[15] Many studies on typing of collagen soon followed. Miller and Matukas[16] were the first to show that cartilage possesses a collagen different in composition from that in most fibrous connective tissue. This collagen contains a different type of $\alpha 1$ chain, which they termed $\alpha 1$, Type II. The collagen in most cartilages consists of three such identical chains and the abbreviated nomenclature now used is $(\alpha 1[II])_3$ or Type II collagen.

A summary of the makeup and distribution of four collagen types accepted at present is given in Table 4–1.

Collagen Cross Links

Stabilization of collagen occurs extracellularly after assembly into the quarter stagger arrays that make up filaments, fibrils, and fibers. The stabilization and ultimate tensile strength of the structure are thought to result mainly from the development of intramolecular and intermolecular cross links. The former occur between alpha chains of the same tropocollagen molecule, the latter between adjacent tropocollagen molecules. The cross links result from enzyme-mediated reactions involving mainly lysine and hydroxylysine. The lysine and hydroxylysine molecules have secondary amine groups on terminal projections extending lateral from the alpha chain, which are available for the cross-linking reaction. The initial reaction in this process is the oxidative deamination of the terminal amine to an aldehyde by the enzyme lysyl oxidase (Fig. 4–10). These reactions have general similarity to the reactions that stabilize elastin. The resulting allysyl residues condense with one another to form an aldol condensation product[17] characteristic of intramolecular cross links[18, 19] (Fig. 4–11). Intermolecular cross links characteristically form from the reaction of allysine with lysine or hydroxylysine to form a Schiff base (delta semialdehyde) (Fig. 4–11). These aldol condensation and Schiff base reaction products possess double bonds that apparently are reduced to more stable forms in vivo with the passage of time. Most studies on cross linking of collagen in the past decade have utilized the presence of the double bond of the unsaturated compound to label the "reducible" cross links with tritium. Typically this has been done by reducing the aldol condensation product or delta-semialdehyde with tritium-labeled sodium borohydride. The reduced product is thereby labeled with tritium and can be detected following acid hydrolysis and column chromatography utilizing separation systems similar to those used in amino acid analysis. The details of the bifunctional, trifunctional, or quadrifunctional cross links so detected are beyond the scope of this chapter, but are presented in several reviews.[11, 20, 21]

The significance of the Type II collagen to cartilage is not yet known. The principal differences between this collagen and the more common Type I found in fibrous connective tissue consist in the number of hydroxylysine molecules present and the presence of a small number of residues of cysteine. Table 4–1 summarizes the principal differences between Type I and Type II collagen.

The fundamental process of formation of collagen by the chondroblasts and chondrocytes is apparently nearly identical to the process of synthesis by the fibroblast and fibrocyte. The steps in synthesis are outlined in Figure 4–9. The several posttranslational transformations are notable. The collagen turnover in cartilage proceeds at a rate not unlike that seen in connective tissue of the fibrous type. Since significant synthesis occurs in adult cartilage, it is clear that control processes for spatial orientation of the product are crucial.

It is notable that attempts to achieve cartilage repair, as in surgical arthroplasty, are seldom completely satisfactory clinically. This is probably because the collagen architecture of the arthroplasty surface is disordered, and the surface of the arthroplasty lacks the membrane-like characteristics of the surface layer of articular cartilage. Details of the repair process are described later in this chapter.

PROTEOGLYCANS OF ARTICULAR CARTILAGE

The extraordinary size of the proteoglycan aggregate molecules of articular cartilage is achieved by supra-assembly of three different types of linear chain molecular species: (1) sulfated glycosamin-

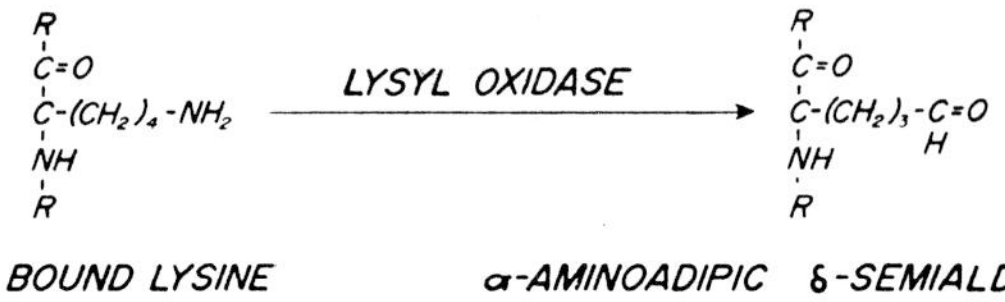

R–C=O–C–$(CH_2)_4$–NH_2–NH–R —LYSYL OXIDASE→ R–C=O–C–$(CH_2)_3$–C(=O)H–NH–R

PEPTIDE BOUND LYSINE — α-AMINOADIPIC δ-SEMIALDEHYDE

Figure 4–10. *The reaction that precedes formation of the collagen cross links illustrated in Figure 4–9 is given here in more detail. The enzyme lysyl oxidase is required for the cleavage of the terminal (secondary) amino group of lysine and the formation of an aldehyde. The aldehyde, in turn, reacts with another lysine or lysine-derived aldehyde to form a cross link (see Fig. 4–11* ***A, B****).*

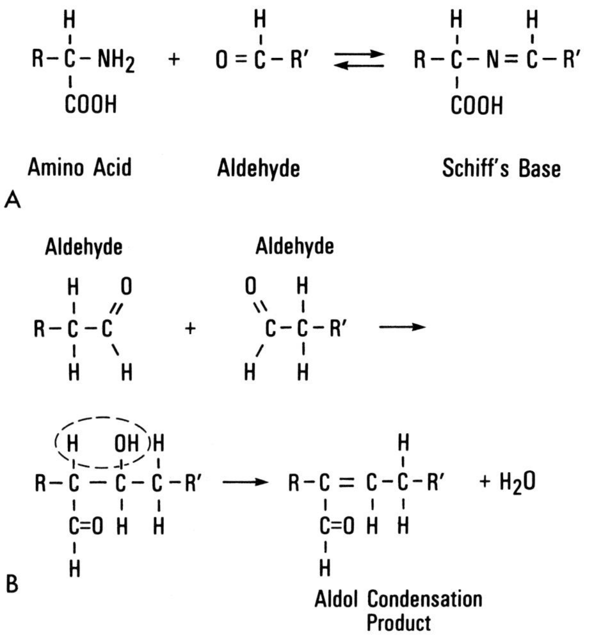

Amino Acid Aldehyde Schiff's Base

A

Aldehyde Aldehyde

B

Aldol Condensation Product

Figure 4–11. **A**, *This figure shows the reaction of lysine with a lysine aldehyde to form a Schiff's base by splitting out water and creating a double bond between the secondary amine of lysine and the terminal carbon of the aldehyde. This is the principal reaction between adjacent tropocollagen molecules, which produces intermolecular crosslinks.* **B**, *This is the complement to the reaction in* **A**. *In this case, two aldehydes derived from lysine react with each other in such a way as to split out water and create (through an intermediate step) an aldol condensation product. A double bond configuration results between the terminal carbon of one molecule and the carbon adjacent to the terminal carbon on the second molecule. This is the principal intramolecular cross link between alpha chains within a tropocollagen molecule. The reactions shown in* **A** *and* **B** *can also participate in more complex tri- and tetramolecular cross links, as cataloged by Tanzer.*[21]

oglycans, (2) the core protein, and (3) hyaluronic acid (a nonsulfated glycosaminoglycan). The proteoglycans of articular cartilage serve as the "pump" of the highly pressurized cartilage system. The characteristics of the proteoglycan molecules that permit this crucial function include their very large size and hence their immobility within the collagen fibril meshwork, their densely concentrated, fixed negative charges, and their large number of hydroxyl groups. These characteristics collectively serve to attract water and small ions into the cartilage. The sum of this attraction is termed the swelling pressure and consists of osmotic forces, ionic forces, and Donnan forces. The purpose of this section is to briefly describe the chemical structure of the functionally vital proteoglycan and its aggregate and to illustrate the manner in which the functional role derives from the chemical structure.

Glycosaminoglycans (GAG)

The terminology for this class of molecules has undergone complete change in recent years. A review of the modifications in terminology is offered in a recent review by Mathews.[22] The earlier term applied to this group of molecules was acid mucopolysaccharides. The more precise chemical term "glycosaminoglycans" has been accepted as preferable, although references are still occasionally found to the older term. Furthermore, there is not complete unanimity with respect to this terminology, and the

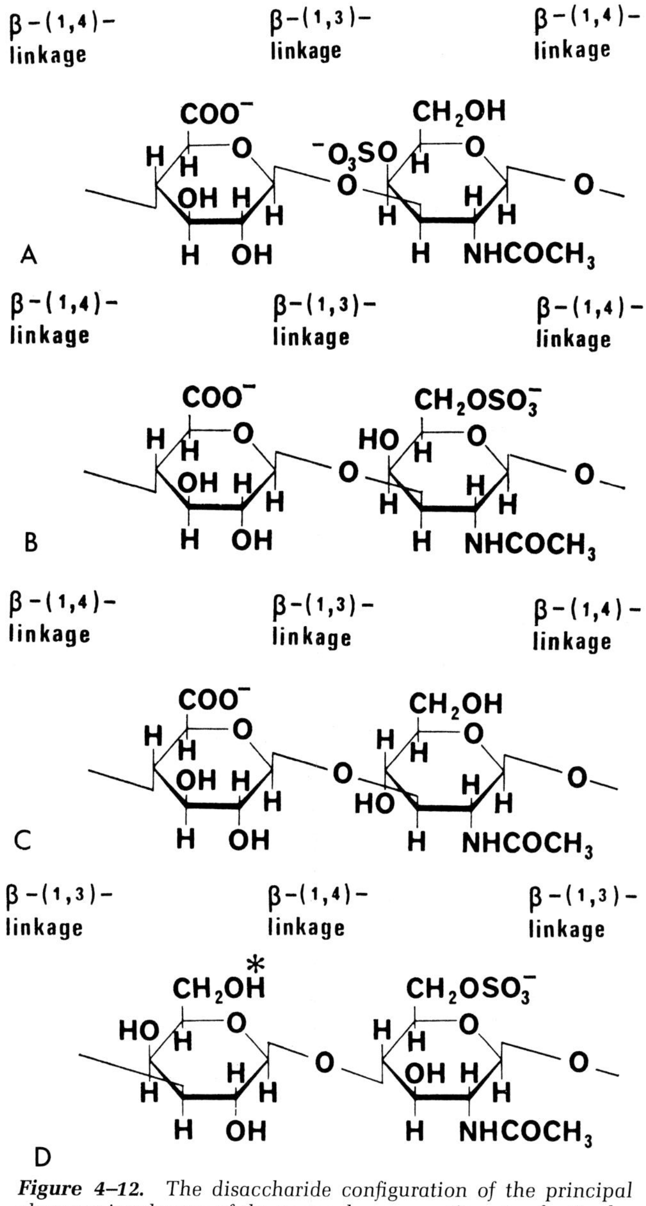

A: β-(1,4)-linkage β-(1,3)-linkage β-(1,4)-linkage

B: β-(1,4)-linkage β-(1,3)-linkage β-(1,4)-linkage

C: β-(1,4)-linkage β-(1,3)-linkage β-(1,4)-linkage

D: β-(1,3)-linkage β-(1,4)-linkage β-(1,3)-linkage

Figure 4–12. *The disaccharide configuration of the principal glycosaminoglycans of the proteoglycan constituents of articular cartilage.*

A *The molecular configuration of chondroitin-4-sulfate. This differs from chondroitin-6-sulfate* **(B)** *only in the location of the sulfate group on the hexosamine molecule. Both contain alternating glucuronic acid and galactosamine sugars.*

B *Chondroitin-6-sulfate.*

C *Hyaluronic acid contains alternating molecules of glucosamine and glucuronic acid but lacks a sulfate group.*

D *Keratan sulfate contains galactose rather than a uronic acid moiety in the disaccharide. The hexosamine is glucosamine, which is sulfated in the C6 position.*

term "polyanionic glycans" is also applied to these molecules.[2] The "acid" part of the earlier term refers to the large number of carboxyl and sulfate groups, which possess negative charges and which confer many predictable characteristics in chemical and staining reactions to the tissue. The prefix "muco-" refers to the gross physical characteristics of this molecular class, members of which are typically quite viscous and gel-like. Finally, the "polysaccharide" part of the term refers to the chemical structure of the molecule — it is made of many hexose units assembled linearly into long chains in a manner roughly analogous to the assembly of glucose into glycogen, but in this case the chains are unbranched.

In most of the glycosaminoglycan molecules, hexosamine alternates with another sugar polymerized in a repeating dissacharide pattern. The predominance of the amine group in this configuration is the reason for the occurrence of "amino-" in the term glycosaminoglycan. Figure 4–12 shows the disaccharide repeating unit for the glycosaminoglycans of articular cartilage: chondroitin-4-sulfate, chondroitin-6-sulfate, hyaluronate, and keratan sulfate. The common features of the group are obvious at first glance. In particular, the location of the N-acetyl-amine group at the number two carbon (C2) of the hexosamine is common to all the disaccharides shown. The hexosamine is galactosamine in three of the four cases; keratan sulfate possesses glucosamine as the alternating hexosamine. All except hyaluronate are sulfated at the C4 or C6 position of the hexosamine. Each disaccharide contains at least three hydroxyl groups. All except keratan sulfate contain uronic acid as the second element of the disaccharide, with a carboxyl terminal at C6. Keratan sulfate possesses galactose rather than uronic acid as the second half of the disaccharide.

The glycosaminoglycans are covalently bound to core protein in a pattern that locates keratan sulfate side arms preferentially close to the linkage region to hyaluronate. Therefore, a keratan sulfate–rich region exists in the protein polysaccharide, as illustrated in Figure 4–13, which therefore contains little chondroitin sulfate. The keratan sulfate molecules are characteristically of lower molecular weight than the chondroitin sulfate chains, as indicated by the diagrammatic representation in Figure 4–13.

Proteoglycan Aggregate

The ability of proteoglycan to aggregate further by combining with hyaluronic acid was described by Hardingham and Muir,[23] who elaborated on the dissociation and association experiments of Sajdera and Hascall[24] to establish the mechanism of formation of aggregate (Fig. 4–14). It has since been demonstrated that the formation of proteoglycan aggregate is facilitated and stabilized by a small protein termed *link protein.*[25-27] Much attention has been given recently to the degree of proteoglycan aggregate formation in various tissues and in various pathologic conditions. Clearly, the ability of the proteoglycan molecule to form aggregates of even greater molecular size amplifies its physiologic functional properties as the "pump" of the system. This is true because the aggregate formed will create even greater fixation of the proteoglycan molecules, locking them more securely within the interstices of the collagen framework of the tissue, ensuring fixation of the negative charges and assuring the cartilage of an adequate swelling pressure to maintain expansion of that matrix.

Nature of the Aggregate Linkage

As distinguished from the covalent linkage of GAG to core protein in proteoglycan subunit (PGS), the linkage of PGS to hyaluronate is noncovalent. The linkage is facilitated and strengthened by a low molecular weight protein termed link protein. The linkage can occur without the presence of link protein, but the latter has been found in all cartilages so far examined.[28] The noncovalent linkage of PGS

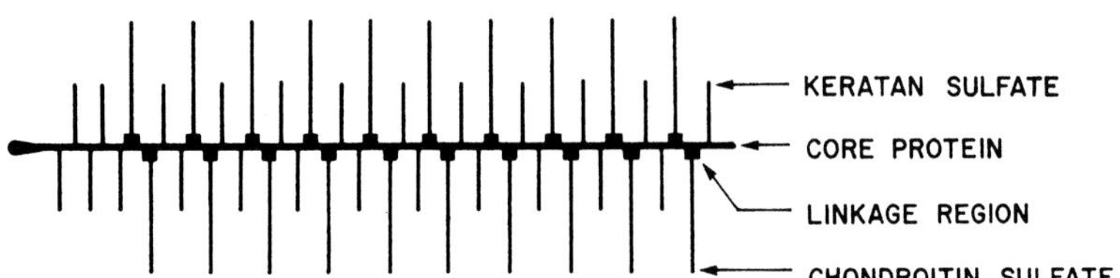

Figure 4–13. *Proteoglycan. This diagram of the proteoglycan molecule demonstrates the method of aggregation of chondroitin-4-sulfate, chondroitin-6-sulfate, and keratan sulfate to the core protein. The linkage regions indicated are composed of highly specific molecular configurations (see text). The attachment site of the core protein to hyaluronic acid at which an aggregate is created is seen at the far left of the diagram. There is typically a high concentration of keratan sulfate, a shorter chain glycosaminoglycan, near the attachment site of the core protein to hyaluronic acid, symbolized by the shorter side arms in that location. (From Rosenberg L: Structure of cartilage proteoglycan. In WH Simon [Ed]: The Human Joint in Health and Disease. Philadelphia, University of Pennsylvania Press, 1978.)*

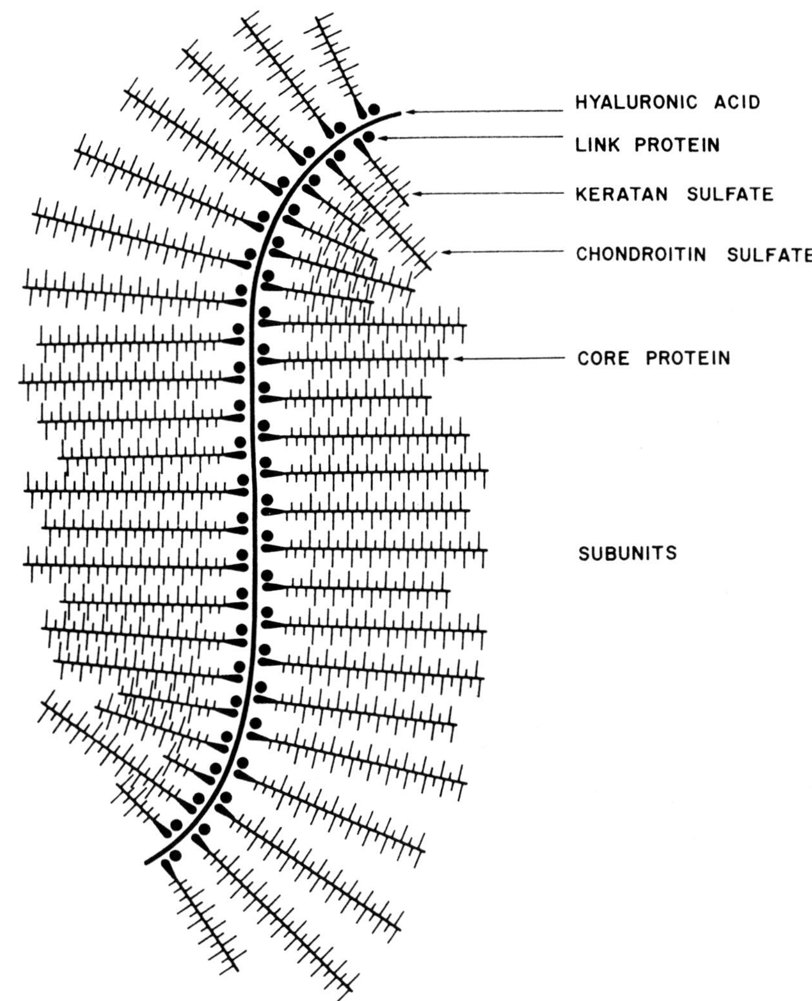

Figure 4–14. *This figure illustrates the pattern of aggregate formed by a complex of proteoglycan and hyaluronic acid. The aggregate is stabilized in part by a glycopeptide called* link protein *at the junction site. The spectacular augmentation in molecular weight from the original glycosaminoglycan weight of approximately 50,000 daltons to that of proteoglycan, reaching millions of daltons, and further increase to a structure with molecular weight of many millions of daltons by aggregate formation with hyaluronic acid is well illustrated by this diagram. (From Rosenberg L: Structure of cartilage proteoglycan. In* WH Simon *[Ed]: The Human Joint in Health and Disease. Philadelphia, University of Pennsylvania Press, 1978.)*

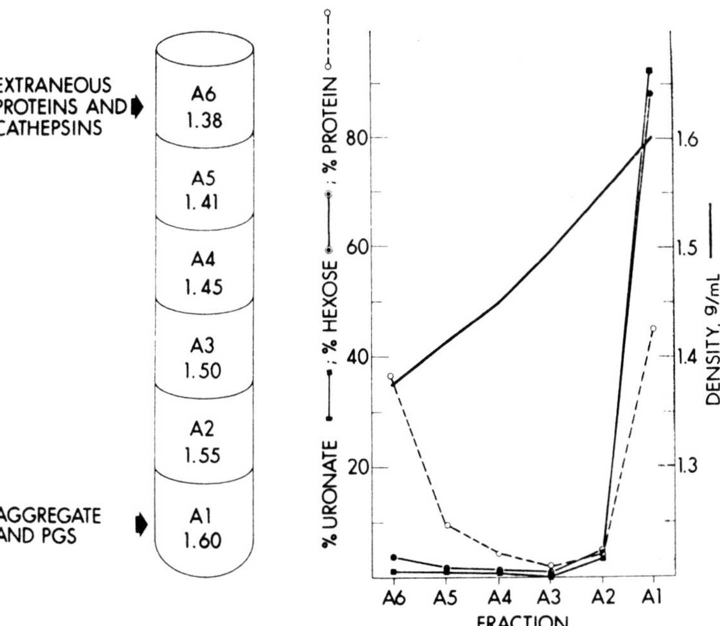

Figure 4–15. *This figure illustrates the separation of components of aggregate extracted from cartilage with guanidinium hydrochloride. When placed in an ultracentrifuge in a cesium chloride solution, the heavier molecules such as aggregate and the proteoglycan subunit (PGS) are forced to the bottom of the tube, whereas the lighter molecules, including extraneous proteins and cathepsins, remain in the upper layers. The contents of the tube can then be separated into several fractions as illustrated at the right of the figure. One can see that the uronate-containing material making up the glycosaminoglycans, which is part of the proteoglycan and aggregate, is located almost entirely in the A1 fraction. Similarly, hexose (the galactose moiety of keratan sulfate) is also in the A1 fraction. (From Rosenberg L: Structure of cartilage proteoglycan. In* WH Simon *[Ed]: The Human Joint in Health and Disease. Philadelphia, University of Pennsylvania Press, 1978.)*

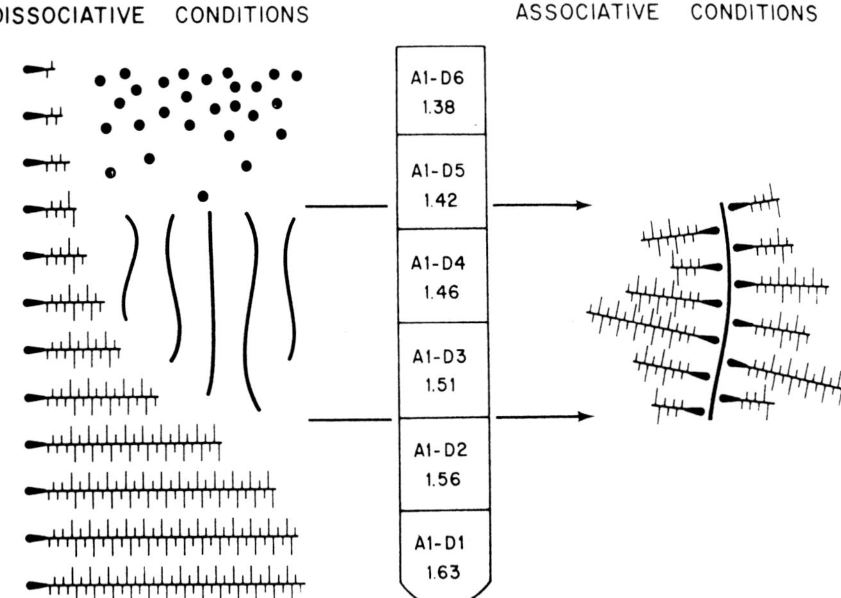

Figure 4–16. *If the A1 fraction (see Fig. 4–15) is separated into its components using dissociative techniques, these constituents can be arbitrarily separated further into six fractions, as seen on the left. In the uppermost layers are found very short fragments consisting of proteoglycans along with link protein. In the middle layers are hyaluronic acid and the intermediate-sized fragments of proteoglycan. At the bottom of the gradient are found the heaviest fragments of proteoglycan. The conditions for this separation of aggregate (dissociative conditions) are achieved with high concentrations of guanidinium hydrochloride or magnesium chloride. Under associative conditions, in which the salt concentrations of guanidinium hydrochloride or magnesium chloride are reduced, the proteoglycan and hyaluronic acid reaggregate, as seen on the right side of this figure. (From Rosenberg L: Structure of cartilage proteoglycan. In WH Simon [Ed]: The Human Joint in Health and Disease. Philadelphia, University of Pennsylvania Press, 1978.)*

and hyaluronate can be dissociated by concentrated solutions of guanidinium hydrochloride, calcium chloride, or magnesium chloride.[24] The dissociated components can be reassociated by the reduction of the concentration of the dissociative solvents. This process has been the key technique in unraveling the chemical structure of PGS and aggregate and in understanding the nature of their association as well as the role of link protein. A diagrammatic representation of the landmark experiments of Sajdera and Hascall[24] and of Hardingham and Muir[23] is shown in Figures 4–15 and 4–16. As is illustrated in these figures, a high concentration (approximately 4 molar) of guanidinium hydrochloride cancels the attraction charges of proteoglycan to hyaluronic acid. Under these conditions, density gradient centrifugation results in separation of the higher and lower molecular weight constituents. This step permits a characterization of the molecular species of differing molecular weights. Under conditions of about 0.5 M guanidinium hydrochloride, the three elements hyaluronic acid, link protein, and proteoglycan reassociate to form the aggregate once again. Cartilages from different sources possess differing percentages of aggregation of proteoglycan, but factors controlling this process are not yet fully understood.

THE FLUID OF ARTICULAR CARTILAGE

As was noted in the air tent analogy described earlier, the inflation medium of articular cartilage is synovial fluid. This is essentially an ultrafiltrate of plasma plus hyaluronic acid. The latter molecules are too large to enter cartilage through its 6 nm diameter surface pores, but most of the remaining ions and molecules of normal synovial fluid, such as water, sodium, potassium, and glucose, are sufficiently small to pass easily through these pores. Movement of fluid into and out of cartilage occurs to some extent by diffusion, but, as will be noted in the discussion on cartilage nutrition, diffusion does not seem adequate in and of itself to provide for cartilage health. Most of the fluid of articular cartilage is water, of course. The percentage of water in cartilage ranges from over 60 to nearly 80 per cent.[29-31] The water is bound by a variety of weak forces, such as hydrogen bonding to proteoglycan and collagen or simple hydration shell formation, but it is sufficiently mobile that clearance studies indicate essential equivalence in behavior between labeled water and urea.[32] The latter is uncharged and is not subject to hydrogen bonding, so that equivalence of movement of the water and urea molecules suggests that the binding forces holding water are extremely weak, and molecular exchange occurs readily.

Mankin and Thrasher[31] performed additional experiments that appeared to demonstrate that a small fraction, about 6 per cent, of water of articular cartilage is not easily exchangeable. After equilibration with tritiated water for 20 days, a small percentage of water remained in cartilage after drying with mild to severe methods. Net flow into and out of cartilage is induced by the normal weight-bearing function of synovial joints. Maroudas[33] has calculated that for normal articular cartilage the sum of swelling pressures is greatly exceeded (10 ×) by loading conditions such as walking. The implications of this fact would seem to be that under loading conditions cartilage would be rapidly and completely compressed, much as a wet sponge is compressed by a weight. However, the rate of fluid movement permitted by the small surface pore size and the

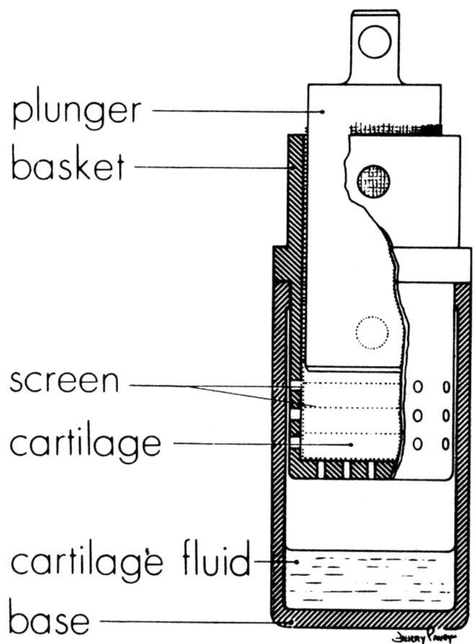

Figure 4–17. *Illustration of a device used by Linn and Sokoloff to express fluid from articular cartilage. The device consists of a perforated basket within a centrifuge collecting system. A plunger within the basket effectively compresses cartilage at the bottom of the basket when the system is spun in the centrifuge. Time and pressure can be controlled by the duration and speed of the centrifuge operation. This technique permits the amount and composition of cartilage fluid expressed to be analyzed (see Fig. 4–18). (From Linn FC, Sokoloff LH: Arthritis Rheum 8:481, 1965.)*

cartilage microarchitecture is sufficiently slow that cartilage is only partially compressed even after loading for hours. The elegant experiments of Linn and Sokoloff illustrate this point well. To study this problem these authors used an apparatus designed to fit into a centrifuge capable of forcing fluid out of cartilage into a receptacle[34] (Fig. 4–17). The cartilage fits into a porous basket-like container into which a plunger rests. The unit is placed into a centrifuge and the faster the centrifuge revolves, the greater the pressure on the cartilage in the basket. In this way the effect of varying loads over varying periods of time on the rate of fluid expression from cartilage can be evaluated. It was shown by these experiments that the amount of fluid that can be expressed (30 per cent) is extremely small in relation to the total water content (see Fig. 4–18). Subsequent experiments by Linn using an animal joint demonstrated the processes of fluid movement in cartilage more directly.[35] The device constructed for this experiment was termed an arthrotrypsometer (Fig. 4–19). By developing the necessary design criteria it was possible to vary loading conditions as to amplitude of load and as to stationary versus cyclic conditions. The joint was immersed in synovial fluid during testing. Deformation versus time is seen to be greater for stationary than for cyclic loads. The explanation for this observation is that in the cyclic condition, partial recovery occurs owing to the effect of swelling pressure in pulling fluid back into cartilage during the phase of the cycle when the cartilage is unloaded. This unparalleled system of load bearing by articular cartilage is dependent for its effectiveness on functional integrity and detailed interaction of each of the architectural, biomechanical, and biochemical elements within the system.

The fluid movement that occurs during the loading process described appears to be important for lubrication of the joint surfaces as well as for load carriage. On the basis of calculations obtained from complex mathematical models, Mow has proposed that fluid is expressed out of cartilage in front of the advancing contact surfaces of cartilage.[36] This process provides a fluid film that minimizes cartilage-cartilage contact, thus also minimizing wear. Indeed, if this analysis is correct, we walk on water! Further discussion of the lubrication mechanism of articular cartilage will be presented in Chapters 5 and 69.

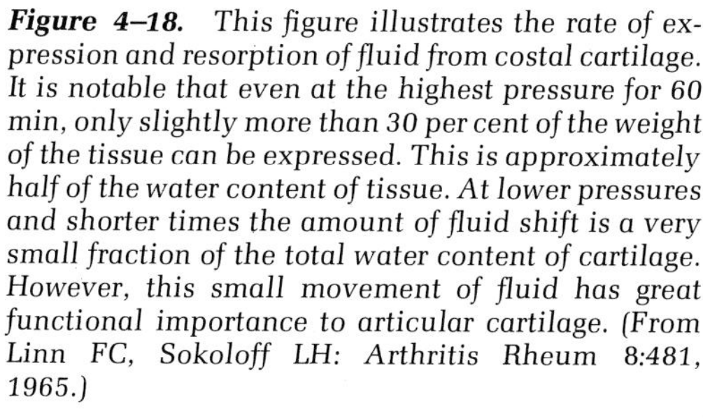

Figure 4–18. *This figure illustrates the rate of expression and resorption of fluid from costal cartilage. It is notable that even at the highest pressure for 60 min, only slightly more than 30 per cent of the weight of the tissue can be expressed. This is approximately half of the water content of tissue. At lower pressures and shorter times the amount of fluid shift is a very small fraction of the total water content of cartilage. However, this small movement of fluid has great functional importance to articular cartilage. (From Linn FC, Sokoloff LH: Arthritis Rheum 8:481, 1965.)*

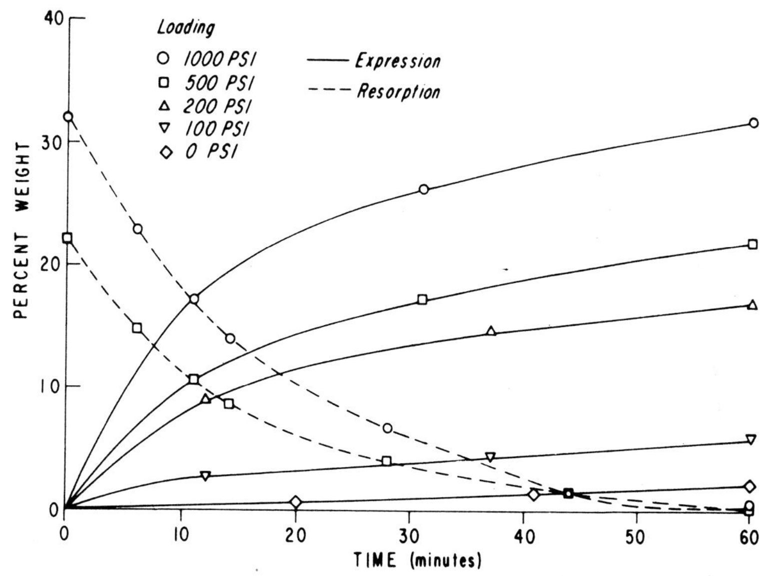

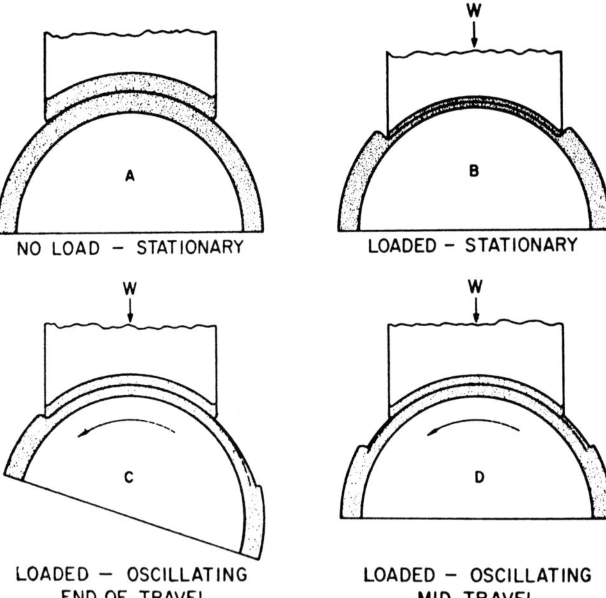

Figure 4–19. *This figure illustrates the effect of loading on articular cartilage. A stationary load, as illustrated in example B, shows significant cartilage compression after a period of time. However, when oscillation occurs using the same loading condition, the compressive effect for a given time is considerably less. Since the cartilage is unloaded a portion of the time, it resorbs some of the fluid that had been expressed during loading. (From Linn FC: J Bone Joint Surg 49A:1079, 1967.)*

NUTRITION

Fluid movement is necessary not only for load carriage and lubrication but also for nutrition of the chondrocytes. Students of articular cartilage generally agree that in the adult very little of the chondrocytic nutritional requirement is satisfied from subchondral vessels of bone. Rather, cartilage nutrition derives almost entirely from synovial fluid.[37] The pumping action of fluid into and out of cartilage during loading and unloading appears to be a key to this process. Joints that are immobilized suffer relatively quickly in a number of important respects. The metabolic activity of cells appears affected, as loss of proteoglycan and an increase in water content are soon observed.[38] The normal white, glistening appearance of the cartilage changes to a dull, bluish color, and the cartilage thickness is reduced. How much of this process is due to nutritional deficiency and how much is due to an upset in the stress-dependent metabolic homeostasis is not yet clear. The process is of sufficient significance, in any case, that it adds weight to the arguments for early remobilization of injured extremities.

METABOLISM OF ARTICULAR CARTILAGE

It should come as no surprise that this highly specialized, functionally complex tissue should be active metabolically. The specialized functional structures of cartilage, the collagen fabric and the proteoglycan pump, require constant maintenance and renewal. The protein synthesis necessary to maintain these elements requires much the same complex synthetic apparatus as that present in other cells of the body. Indeed, one is struck more by the metabolic similarities than the dissimilarities of chondrocytes compared with other mammalian cell types.

However, early anatomists and physiologists tended to the view that articular cartilage had an insignificant metabolic rate. This was reinforced by histologic studies showing the avascular nature of the tissue and its sparse cellular population. In addition, early metabolic experiments seemed to support this concept.[39] However, corrections for cell density expressing metabolic activity in relation to cellular volume altered that perception.[40] By most measures of cellular activity, cartilage cells are nearly equally active metabolically to other cell types from relatively avascular tissue sources.[41]

Some distinctive metabolic features of chondrocytes can be discerned with modern metabolic pathway analysis. Chondrocytes utilize anaerobic pathways for the most part,[39, 42] a choice well suited to the relative isolation of the cells, their lack of cell-to-cell contact, and their remote situation from capillary beds. Mankin and co-workers[41] used autoradiographic techniques to demonstrate that ^{3}H-cytidine is incorporated into cells and that the messenger RNA inhibitor actinomycin D inhibited this incorporation dramatically. This evidence was adduced to show another similarity of chrondrocytes to the general pattern of mammalian cellular metabolism.

Proteoglycan aggregation and collagen cross linking both occur outside the cell. In this respect the chondrocyte is able to avoid a very troublesome problem, that of exporting and properly locating molecules much too large to diffuse through cartilage matrix. As it is, proteoglycan and procollagen are among the largest molecules mammalian cells are called upon to synthesize. Each chain of procollagen has over 1000 amino acids, for example. The messenger RNA is therefore necessarily one of the largest in the cellular protein synthetic apparatus. The schemata for synthesis of collagen and proteoglycan are summarized in Figures 4–9 and 4–20. Each of these pathways is intricate. The general mode of synthesis for the proteoglycans involves primary formation of the protein core followed by addition of polysaccharide elements. This is thought to result from a step-wise glycosyl transfer from nucleotide sugars, beginning with transfer to a specific monosaccharide, xylose, to a specific amino acid sequence of the protein. Usually this sequence includes serine or threonine. Chain growth of the polysaccharide then occurs through a series of glycosyl transfer steps in which sugars are transferred to the nonreducing terminal monosaccharide of the lengthening polysaccharide side chain. Studies of the subcellular localization of biosynthesis of cartilage proteoglycans show that the enzymes catalyzing the transfer of the three sugars adjacent to the carbohydrate-protein linkage are found in highest concentration in the rough endoplasmic reticulum. Polymerizing enzymes necessary for the formation of disaccharide repeating units are more uniformly distributed between rough and smooth subcellular membrane fractions. It is as yet uncertain whether the monosaccharide transfers occur exclusively one by one to the growing polysaccharide chain, or whether part of the process might take place by assembly of an oligosaccharide chain on a lipid intermediate prior to transfer to the proteoglycan molecule in a manner analogous to certain synthetic steps that occur in glycoprotein synthesis. It is clear that the enzymes involved in these steps are highly specific. For example, the steps involved in assembly of chondroitin sulfate are shown in Figure 4–20 and require six specific enzymes. Further details of collagen and proteoglycan synthesis are beyond the scope of this chapter, and the interested reader is referred to more detailed reviews on the subject.[43-46]

THE ENZYMES OF ARTICULAR CARTILAGE

The continuation of normal function of articular cartilage is dependent upon the special properties of the cartilage matrix constituents and maintenance of their normal concentration within the matrix. There is thus a constant turnover of the components of the matrix. If the normal rate of degradation is increased or if synthesis of new matrix is interfered with, the concentration of the various articular cartilage components will change, and this is manifested by a particular disease process. The production, release and actions of the various enzymes acting on articular cartilage are preeminent in most articular cartilage diseases. Naturally occurring inhibitors exist in the synovial fluid or serum that can modify the actions of the matrix-degrading enzymes. The inhibitors, however, are relatively large molecules and cannot reach the enzymes in the matrix unless the latter diffuse out of the matrix or until degradation of the matrix has caused an increase in its normal impermeability to molecules above approximately 50,000 daltons in molecular weight, into which group the inhibitors fall.

The enzymes active on articular cartilage matrix may be divided into endogenous enzymes peculiar to the cartilage itself and exogenous enzymes arising in the synovium, polymorphonuclear leukocytes, macrophages, or blood serum.

Endogenous Enzymes

Lysosomes are intracytoplasmic vacuoles enclosed by a lipoprotein membrane that contains a number of enzymes responsible for the digestion of the proteoglycan and collagen molecules of articular cartilage matrix.[47] Chondrocytes may be stimulated to release the lysosomal enzymes to the exterior of the cell, where initial degradation of the macromolecules occurs. Subsequent diffusion of products from the matrix for intracellular digestion in the secondary or digestive lysosomes then occurs.[47] In this group are the cathepsins, which have maximal activity at acid pH and little or no activity at the neutral pH of the cartilage matrix.[48-51] Only the cathepsins occurring in human articular cartilage will be described.

Cathepsin D is capable of degrading proteoglycan at pH 4.5 to 5.0. It has been shown by electrophoresis to exist in six multiple forms.[52] Extracellular cathepsin D is mainly found in the immediate pericellular region of the chondrocytes,[53] which may in fact have a lower pH than the remainder of cartilage matrix. Cathepsin D splits the polypeptide backbone of proteoglycan without attacking the polysaccharide side chain. The products of this cleavage, the peptide fragments with polysaccharide chains attached, are then able to diffuse into the cells for completion of degradation. Although it is incapable of degrading collagen even at acid pH, cathepsin D is the most important autolytic enzyme in articular cartilage. Cathepsin D activity in the chondrocytes of guinea pig articular cartilage was found to decrease during growth and midlife and to increase during the later part of life.[54] The range of activity during the life of the animals was narrow, which suggests that the process of degradation influenced by cathepsin D proceeds at a relatively uniform rate throughout life in normal cartilage.

Cathepsin B_1 has a maximal activity at pH 6, at which it can degrade both proteoglycans[55] and collagen.[56] Unlike cathepsin D, it is still active at neutral pH[57] and thus may be more important in the normal

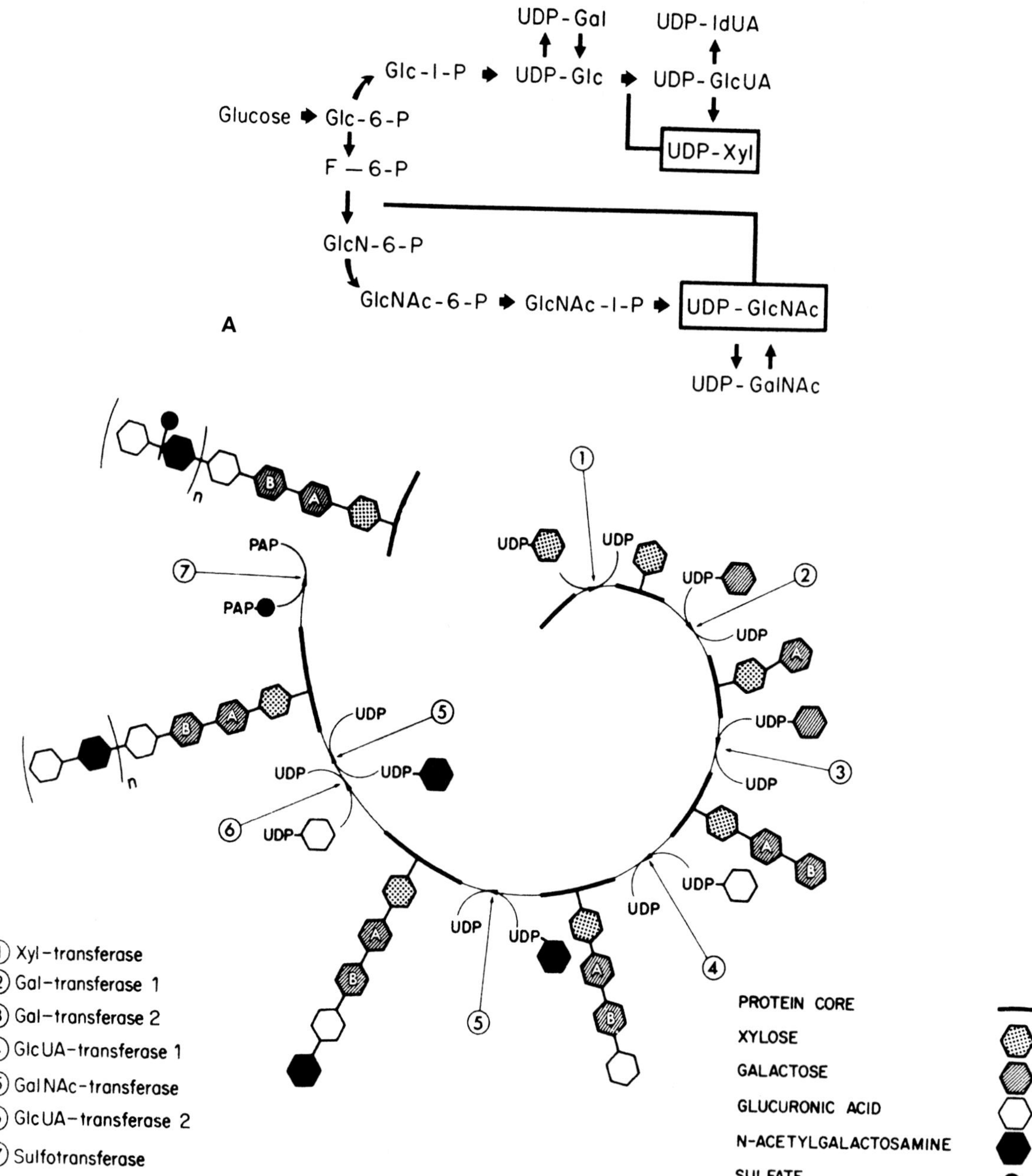

Figure 4–20. *Proteoglycan synthesis.* **A,** *The pathways taken by uridine nucleotide sugars involved in mucopolysaccharide synthesis.* **B,** *The pathway of biosynthesis of a typical glycosaminoglycan, chondroitin-4-sulfate. (From Dorfman A, Matlon R: The mucopolysaccharidoses. In Stanbury JB, et al: The Metabolic Basis of Inherited Disease. 3rd Ed. New York, McGraw-Hill Book Co, 1972.)*

physiologic turnover of proteoglycans. Both cathepsins B_1 and D show greater activity in the surface layers of articular cartilage compared with progressively deeper layers,[55] and there appears to be a progressive decrease of cathepsin B_1 activity with increasing age.

Cathepsin F also is present in cartilage, but its function is at present not well known.[58, 59]

It has been found that pepstatin inhibits the action of cathepsin D, and this action has been used to demonstrate that other acid and neutral proteases are capable of degrading proteoglycan.[52] Thus, one neutral and two acid metalloproteinases have been isolated from human articular cartilage and have been shown to degrade purified nasal septum proteoglycan.[60] The neutral metalloproteinase is optimally active at pH 7.25. The acid metalloproteinases are distinct from cathepsins B, D, and F and digest proteoglycan subunit at pH 4.5 and 5.5. Neutral proteases may be implicated as mediators of physiologic turnover of ground substance and in pathologic processes such as osteoarthritis.

Arylsulfatase is also capable of initiating the degradation of proteoglycan,[61] and levels of this enzyme have been shown to be elevated in experimental degenerative articular disease.[62] In addition, Vitamin E appears to inhibit arylsulfatase in chondrocyte cultures.[63]

Acid and alkaline phosphatases are also found in the lysosomes[64, 65] and alkaline phosphatase is found in extracellular matrix vesicles. Alkaline phosphatase is found only in the deeper cells of articular cartilage[66, 67] and may be related to a continuous process of remodeling at the osteochondral junction. Aging changes of enzyme activity have been examined in guinea pigs.[68] It has been found that the activity of alkaline phosphatase steadily declined over 2 weeks to 5¾ years, whereas the activity of the glycolytic enzymes in individual chondrocytes increased with advancing age. Acid phosphatase activity showed no consistent pattern of change with aging.

Collagenases are capable of degrading native collagen at physiologic pH and cleaving the helical part of the molecule into an amino terminal 75 per cent fragment and a carboxy terminal 25 per cent fragment.[69] The two smaller fragments spontaneously denature and in their uncoiled state are susceptible to digestion by extracellular proteases. Type II collagen (which is the normally occurring type in articular cartilage) is less susceptible to collagenase than is interstitial Type I collagen.[70-72] Cross-linked collagen is very much less sensitive to specific collagenase than it is to non–cross-linked collagenase,[73, 74] and this helps to explain why recently synthesized collagen is especially susceptible to degradation.[75] Conversely, as articular cartilage ages, the formation of intermolecular cross links of the collagen may make the tissue more resistant to breakdown by enzymes.[76, 77] Collagenase has not been demonstrated in normal articular cartilage but is present in osteoarthritic cartilage.[78]

Cathepsin D and collagenase have been shown to affect the hydraulic permeability of articular cartilage.[79] Thus, the flow of essential metabolites from the matrix, or the exposure of chondrocytes to toxins and immunoglobulins normally excluded from the cell, may further aid in degradation of the articular cartilage.

Lysozyme, first described by Fleming and Allison in 1922,[80] belongs to the glycosidase group of enzymes capable of carbohydrate hydrolysis. It is found in numerous locations in the human body, and articular cartilage is one site at which it occurs. It is synthesized in the chondrocytes and is then released immediately into the territorial matrix, without prior storage in the lysosomes.[81, 82] Lysozyme is found mainly in the deepest layer of articular cartilage.[83] It may be of importance in the final stages of polymer breakdown. Beta-glucuronidase[84] and N-β acetyl glucosaminidase[85] have also been demonstrated histochemically in cartilage and are considered to be involved in polysaccharide depolymerization. Hyaluronidase, which theoretically could attack the hyaluronic acid core of the proteoglycan molecule, has not been found in normal or diseased articular cartilage.[86, 87]

Exogenous Enzymes

The exogenous enzymes affecting articular cartilage matrix may arise from the synovium of the joint and then are secreted into the synovial fluid from lysosomes of both Type A and Type B lining cells. Enzymes in this category include protease, collagenase, and hyaluronidase.[52, 88] In addition in pathologic situations, when polymorphonucleocytes and macrophages reach the joint cavity, they may secrete a collagenase,[89] lysozyme,[47] or neutral protease,[90-93] the latter being distinguished from the proteases occurring in the synovial membrane. Recent studies further indicate that polymorphonuclear leukocytes contain three enzymes, β-glucuronidase, β-N-acetylgalactosaminidase, and a sulfatase, which act synergistically to further degrade cartilage-derived chondroitin sulfate into monosaccharides and inorganic sulfate.[94]

Collagenases have been implicated in several types of arthritis and have been detected in the synovium in rheumatoid arthritis and nonspecific inflammatory synovial conditions, respectively. All synovial tissues have the capacity to produce collagenase; however, it is likely that only in states of chronic proliferative synovitis and inflammation is collagenase produced in sufficient quantities to bring about the destruction of articular tissue. Although Type II collagen is a poorer substrate for collagenase than interstitial Type I collagen, cleavage can be significantly augmented by raising the temperature above the normal range of 33° to 36° C. Thus, in the inflamed joint affected by rheumatoid arthritis in which the joint temperature is raised,[95] the rate of cartilage degradation by collagenase would be increased.

Finally, in this group of exogenous enzymes is plasmin, a proteolytic enzyme derived from the blood. Plasmin is activated from plasminogen by several factors, including the kinases of streptococci and staphylococci. It normally acts as a fibrinolytic agent but when present in excess could theoretically attack the protein of cartilage matrix.[96, 97] However, cartilage degradation caused by this enzyme has not been substantiated as occurring in vivo.[62, 98]

ENZYMES IN ARTICULAR CARTILAGE DISEASE PROCESSES

The avascular nature of adult cartilage has a bearing on its limited capacity to respond to various insults, whether inflammatory, mechanical, or biomechanical. Thus, although adult joint cartilage has some potential for repair, a given insult will usually result in a degenerative lesion mediated by endogenous or exogenous enzymes.

Osteoarthritis

The cause of articular cartilage destruction in osteoarthritis may certainly be mechanical, but part of the matrix degradation is most likely due to enzymatic action. There may be an increase in the activity of enzymes involved in the normal turnover of the matrix, or the degradation may be due to production and release of special enzymes. The fact that secondary lysosomes are rare in normal articular cartilage but are readily found in the chondrocytes of osteoarthritic cartilage[99, 100] adds weight to this theory. The degradation process is mainly extracellular, but it may be completed within the cell.[101]

Several of the endogenous enzymes mentioned previously have been implicated in osteoarthritis. Cathepsin D was thought to be important in the process,[49-51 102] but since its greatest activity is at pH 4.5 to 5, it is difficult to accept it as a significant factor in the neutral pH environment of the matrix of articular cartilage. Nevertheless, cathepsin D levels are elevated in intracellular and extracellular situations in osteoarthritic cartilage, although this may be explained to some extent by the increased cellularity of osteoarthritic cartilage.[51, 55, 103] It may be that the microenvironment around the chondrocyte cell is more acid than the rest of the cartilage matrix, and it is mainly in this situation that cathepsin D is found and acts.[47] Since osteoarthritic synovial fluid only contains one fiftieth as much cathepsin D activity as cartilage, it is thought that the chondrocytes are the major or only source of this enzyme.[51] The focal nature of the increased cathepsin D activity in articular cartilage has also been demonstrated.[103]

The discovery of neutral proteases in human osteoarthritic articular cartilage provides an explanation for the initiation of cartilage degradation at neutral pH.[52, 104] Arylsulfatases A and B are lysosomal enzymes that may also be incriminated in the degradation of proteoglycan in osteoarthritic cartilage.[61, 105] Their activity helps to explain the increased sulfate levels in the joint fluid and loss of chondroitin sulfate from the affected cartilage of patients with osteoarthritis. Levels of both arylsulfatases A and B are elevated in osteoarthritic cartilage but that of arylsulfatase B to a greater extent. The role of arylsulfatase B in chondroitin sulfate degradation is possibly substantiated by the increased activity of this enzyme in Hurler's disease.[106]

Although a collagenase capable of splitting the collagen molecule has not been found in normal cartilage it is present in osteoarthritic human cartilage and is believed to be extralysosomal in origin. It is probably present in minute quantities and its demonstration necessitated prior removal of an inhibitor.[78] Collagenase does occur in the synovial tissue of joints affected by osteoarthritis[107] and has been produced by synovial explants from joints affected by osteoarthritis but in lesser amounts than in rheumatoid arthritis.[108] Neither the hydroxyproline content nor the extractability of collagen is affected in osteoarthritis.[86] However, in severe osteoarthritis, total loss of articular cartilage occurs.

In osteoarthritic cartilage, a rise in the levels of acid and alkaline phosphatase activities has been found.[103] In addition, a direct relationship between acid phosphatase levels and the severity of the osteoarthritic process was noted.[64] The same workers demonstrated an even higher level of phosphatase activity in the cartilage of marginal osteophytes than in that of more central lesions, and the level of acid phosphatase in chondrocyte cultures derived from osteoarthritic cartilage was observed to be elevated in comparison with normal chondrocytes grown under identical conditions.[109]

Bollett and Nance[110] reported a decrease in glycosaminoglycan chain length in osteoarthritic articular cartilage and suggested the presence of an hyaluronidase-like enzyme as part of the degenerative process. This logical theory has not been substantiated by finding hyaluronidase in normal or arthritic articular cartilage.[111] Lack and Rogers[96] suggested that plasmin activated by joint damage could attack cartilage proteoglycan and therefore be a factor in degenerative arthritis. This theory could not be substantiated in an experiment in which the intra-articular injection of large doses of plasmin was not followed by articular cartilage damage. This result may be explained by the normal presence of antiplasmin in synovial fluid.[112, 113]

Lysozyme has also been implicated in the osteoarthritic lesion by the finding of significant elevations of the enzyme in hip and knee joint cartilage affected by osteoarthritis.[114] The lysozymal levels were higher in early than in late lesions. It was thought that lysozyme had a hyaluronidase-like activity and could affect link protein.

One additional aspect of enzyme effects in the osteoarthritic process is the nature of the matrix synthesis response of chondrocytes to lysosomal enzymes. Thus, although the collagen content of osteoarthritic cartilage does not change, the cartilage synthesizes Type I collagen in addition to the usual Type II collagen. Deshmukh and Nimni[115] demonstrated that lysosomal enzymes could produce the same effect on articular cartilage in vivo. Thus, the enzymes altered the function of chondrocytes, causing them to synthesize nonspecific collagen molecules, which might lead to weakening of the mechanical structure of the cartilage and its subsequent mechanical destruction.

Rheumatoid Arthritis

Rheumatoid arthritis is characterized by destruction of articular cartilage. An as yet unknown stimulus to the synovial lining cells is involved in this disease and causes hyperplasia and hypertrophy of the cells. The resulting pannus growing over and under the articular cartilage is thought to release greatly increased numbers of intracellular lysosomal enzymes, which irreversibly destroy proteoglycan and collagen to produce the erosive focal lesion in the cartilage.[53, 116-118] A considerable increase in activity of many of the lysosomal enzymes, such as acid phosphatase, β-glucuronidase, β-acetylglucosaminidase, cathepsin D, and collagenase, has been found in the synovium and synovial fluid of patients with rheumatoid arthritis and provides evidence for their role in the cartilage erosion that occurs in this disease.[93, 107, 118-121] Woolley and coworkers[118] showed by an immunofluorescent technique the specific localization of collagenase to a 20 to 60 per cent length of the cartilage-pannus interface and only minimal distribution of collagenase to areas remote from the erosion front. Harris and McCroskery[71] have explained how synovial collagenase, once in contact with the cartilage, can degrade articular cartilage collagen in rheumatoid arthritic joints. Another cathepsin-type enzyme, leucine aminopeptidase, has been demonstrated in synovial lining cells, in pannus and in cartilage in rheumatoid arthritis; it may be a significant factor in cartilage damage.[122]

The levels of β-acetylglucosaminidase and cathepsin D were also found to be raised in rheumatoid articular cartilage, but these levels did not correlate with the levels of these same enzymes in the synovial membrane.[123] Poole and associates,[53] although not precluding the possibility that chondrocytes secrete the enzyme, thought that cathepsin D was essentially restricted to synovial and pannus tissue. Activity of the rheumatoid process was found not to be correlated with enzyme levels by Collins and Cosh, [124] although, conversely, Granda and associates[125] found close correlation between cathepsin D activity and an increased severity of the rheumatoid process. Other cellular sources for lysosomal enzyme release are the polymorphonuclear leukocytes and lymphocyte clusters that are present in large numbers in the inflamed synovial cavity and in the synovium, respectively, in rheumatoid arthritis.[93, 126] In addition, the levels of lysozyme in serum and synovial fluid are increased in rheumatoid arthritis patients and may accompany the loss of cartilage glycosaminoglycans seen in this disease.[82] In contradistinction, in the arthritis of systemic lupus erythematosus, in which usually no cartilage destruction occurs, normal serum lysozyme levels are seen.[127] The fact that continued inflammation hastens cartilage lysis implies that, in treatment, inflammation should be suppressed to reduce lysosomal protease accumulation and synovial collagenase production.

Pyogenic Arthritis

The result of untreated pyogenic arthritis is a severe and rapid destruction of joint cartilage,[88] which invariably evolves into an osteoarthritic process or possibly leads to fibrous or bony ankylosis. The extensive proteoglycan degradation of cartilage is due to the action of several proteinases, which may be derived from neutrophil leukocytes. The leukocytes can release their lysosomal enzymes on encountering bacteria or following eventual death of the leukocytes[93] The proteinases incriminated are elastase, cathepsin G, and collagenase, all of which are active at neutral pH.[91, 128, 129] The proteinases elastase and cathepsin G could attack first the proteoglycan molecule and subsequently the collagen molecule.[91] Lazarus and colleagues[130] described how the collagenase and a proteinase found in polymorphonuclear leukocytes can act synergistically to achieve maximal collagen breakdown. Final confirmation of this mode of cartilage destruction in vivo is awaited. In the body, there are various inhibitors secreted into the synovial fluid that can prevent the extracellular activity of these above-mentioned enzymes. It does, however, seem logical that in the treatment of septic joints removal of polymorphonuclear leukocytes by operation or aspiration is essential to minimize cartilage destruction.[131]

The fibrinolytic enzyme plasmin is produced in synovial fluid by the action of staphylococcal and streptococcal kinases and disrupted leukocytes on plasminogen. Plasmin could then degrade the proteoglycan of articular cartilage matrix.[96, 97, 132] Plasmin may then be an additional factor in cartilage destruction in pyogenic arthritis, but not in tuberculosis, because the tubercle bacillus does not produce an activator of plasminogen similar to the kinases of staphylococci and streptococci.

SUMMARY

This chapter reviews the structure of articular cartilage in relation to its special functions. The components of the matrix, in which the chondrocytes are dispersed, are described in detail with regard to their chemistry, synthesis, maturation, and unique interactions that allow articular cartilage to fulfill those special functions. The mechanisms for load carriage, lubrication, and nutrition and their interrelationships are explained. Some of the distinctive metabolic activities relating to chondrocyte function in the maintenance of the cartilage matrix are described. Finally, the endogenous and exogenous enzymes of articular cartilage and their role in maintaining tissue health and in provoking disease are discussed.

REFERENCES

1. Ogston AG: The biological functions of the glycosaminoglycans. *In* EA Balazs (Ed): Chemistry and Molecular Biology of the Intercellular Matrix. Vol 3. London, Academic Press, 1970, p 1231.
2. Benninghoff A: Form und Bau der Gelenkknorpel in ihren Beziehungen zur Funktion. Z Anat Entwicklungsgesch *76*:43, 1925.
3. Little K, Pimm LH, Trueta J: Osteoarthritis of the hip: An electron microscope study. J Bone Joint Surg *40B*:123, 1958.
4. Weiss C, Rosenberg L, Helfet AJ: An ultrastructural study of normal young adult human articular cartilage. J Bone Joint Surg *50A*:663, 1968.
5. McCutchen CW: The frictional properties of animal joints. Wear *5*:1, 1962.
6. Hultkrantz W: Über die Spaltrichtungen der Gelenkknorpel. Verhandlungen der Anatomischen Gesellschaft, *12*:248, 1898.
7. Langer C: Zur Anatomie und Physiologie der Haut. Sitzungsb d k Acad Wissensch *45*:223, 1861.
8. Bullough P, Goodfellow J: The significance of the fine structure of articular cartilage. J Bone Joint Surg *50B*:852, 1968.
9. Glimcher MJ, Krane SM: The organization and structure of bone, and the mechanism of calcification. *In* BS Gould (Ed): Treatise on Collagen. Vol 2, Biology of Collagen. New York, Academic Press, 1968, p 67.
10. Mathews MB: Collagen. *In* Connective Tissue: Macromolecular Structure and Evolution. New York, Springer-Verlag, 1975, p 15.
11. Serafini-Fracassini A, Smith, JW: Collagen. *In* The Structure and Biochemistry of Cartilage. Edinburgh, Churchill Livingstone, 1974, p 29.
12. Nimni ME: Molecular structure and function of collagen in normal and diseased tissue. *In* PMC Burleigh, AR Poole (Eds): Dynamics of Connective Tissue Macromolecules. New York, American Elsevier Publishing Company, 1975.
13. Lane JM, Weiss C: Review of articular cartilage collagen research. Arthritis Rheum *18*:553, 1975.
14. Miller EJ: The collagen of the extracellular matrix. *In* JW Lash, MM Burger (Eds): Cell and Tissue Interactions. New York, Raven Press, 1977.
15. Piez KA: Characterization of a collagen from codfish skin containing three chromatographically different α chains. Biochemistry *4*:2590, 1965.
16. Miller EG, Matukas VJ: Chick cartilage collagen: A new type of α1 chain not present in bone or skin of the species. Proc Natl Acad Sci USA *64*:1264, 1969.
17. Piez KA: Cross-linking of collagen and elastin. Ann Rev Biochem *37*:547, 1968.
18. Franzblau C: Elastin. *In* M Florkin, EH Stotz (Eds): Comprehensive Biochemistry. Vol 13. Amsterdam, Elsevier, 1971, p 659.
19. Kang AH, Gross J: Relationship between the intra- and intermolecular cross-links of collagen. Proc Natl Acad Sci USA *67*:1307, 1970.
20. Gallop PM, Blumenfeld OO, Seifter S: Structure and metabolism of connective tissue proteins. Ann Rev Biochem *41*:617, 1972.
21. Tanzer ML: Cross-linking of collagen (endogenous aldehydes in collagen react in several ways to form a variety of unique covalent cross-links). Science *180*:561, 1973.
22. Mathews MB: Polyanionic proteoglycans. *In* Molecular Biology, Biochemistry, and Biophysics Series, Vol. 19. Connective Tissue: Macromolecular Structure and Evolution. New York, Springer-Verlag, 1975, p. 93.
23. Hardingham TE, Muir H: The specific interaction of hyaluronic acid with cartilage proteoglycans. Biochem Biophys Acta *279*:401, 1972.
24. Sajdera SW, Hascall VC: Protein-polysaccharide complex from bovine nasal cartilage. A comparison of low and high shear extraction procedures. J Biol Chem *244*:77, 1969.
25. Gregory JD: Multiple aggregation factors in cartilage proteoglycan. Biochem J *133*:383, 1973.
26. Heinegaard D, Hascall VC: Aggregation of cartilage proteoglycans. III. Characteristics of the proteins isolated from trypsin digests of aggregates. J Biol Chem *249*:4250, 1974.
27. Hascall VC, Sajdera SW: Protein polysaccharide complex from bovine nasal cartilage: The function of glycoprotein in the formation of aggregates. J Biol Chem *244*:2384, 1969.
28. Rosenberg L: Structure of cartilage proteoglycans *In* WH Simon (Ed): The Human Joint in Health and Disease. Philadelphia, University of Pennsylvania Press, 1978.
29. Campo RD, Tourtellotte CD: The composition of bovine cartilage and bone. Biochem Biophys Acta *141*:614, 1967.
30. Eichelberger L, Akeson WH, Roma M: Biochemical studies of articular cartilage. I. Normal values. J Bone Joint Surg *40A*:142, 1958.
31. Mankin HJ, Thrasher AZ: Water content and binding in normal and osteoarthritic human cartilage. J Bone Joint Surg *57A*:76, 1975.
32. Jaffe FF, Mankin HJ, Weiss C, Varins A: Water binding in the articular cartilage of rabbits. J Bone Joint Surg *56A*:1031, 1974.
33. Maroudas A: Physicochemical properties of articular cartilage. *In* MAR Freeman (Ed): Adult Articular Cartilage. London, Pitman, 1973.
34. Linn FC, Sokoloff LH: Movement and composition of interstitial fluid of cartilage. Arthritis Rheum *8*:481, 1965.
35. Linn FC: Lubrication of animal joints. I. The Arthrotripsometer. J. Bone Joint Surg *49A*:1079, 1967.
36. Mow VC, Mansour JM, Redler I: The movement of interstitial fluid through normal and pathological cartilage during articulation. *In* JA Brighton, S Goldman (Eds): Advances in Bioengineering: Transactions of the American Society of Mechanical Engineers, p 177, 1974.
37. Lotke PA: Diffusion in cartilage *In* WH Simon (Ed): The Human Joint in Health and Disease. Philadelphia, University of Pennsylvania Press, 1978.
38. Akeson WH, Eichelberger L, Roma M: Biochemical studies of articular cartilage. II. Values following denervation of an extremity. J Bone Joint Surg *40A*:153, 1958.
39. Bywaters ECL: The metabolism of joint tissues. J Path Bacteriol *44*:247, 1937.
40. Rosenthal O, Bowie MA, Wagoner G: Studies on the metabolism of articular cartilage. I. Respiration and glycolysis of cartilage in relation to its age. J Cell Comp Physiol *17*:221, 1941.
41. Mankin HJ: The metabolism of articular cartilage in health and disease. *In* PMC Burleigh, AR Poole (Eds): Dynamics of Connective Tissue Macromolecules. New York, American Elsevier, 1975, p 327.
42. Tushan FS, Rodnan GP, Altman M, Robin ED: Aerobic glycolysis and lactate dehydrogenase (LDH) isoenzymes in articular cartilage. J Lab Clin Med *73*:649, 1969.
43. Roden L, Schwartz NB: Biosynthesis of connective tissue proteoglycans. *In* WJ Whelan (Ed): MTP International Review of Science: Bio-

chemistry Section. Biochemistry of Carbohydrates. Baltimore, University Park Press, 1975.

44. Muir H: Structure and function of proteoglycan of cartilage and cell-matrix interactions. *In* JW Lash, MM Burger (Eds): Cell and Tissue Interactions. New York, Raven Press, 1977.
45. Prockop DJ, Kivirikko KI, Tuderman L, Guzman N: Biosynthesis of collagen and its disorders. Part I. N Engl J Med *301*:13, 1979.
46. Prockop DJ, Kivirikko KI, Tuderman L, Guzman N: Biosynthesis of collagen and its disorders. Part II. N Engl J Med *301*:77, 1979.
47. Dingle, JT: The role of lysosomal enzymes in skeletal tissues. J Bone Joint Surg *55B*:87, 1973.
48. Fessel JM, Chrisman OD: Enzymatic degradation of chondromucoprotein by cell free extracts of human cartilage. Arthritis Rheum *7*:398, 1964.
49. Ali SY, Evans L, Stainthorpe E, Lack CH: Characterization of cathepsins in cartilage. Biochem J *105*:549, 1967.
50. Woessner JF: Cartilage cathepsin D and its action on matrix components. Fed Proc *32*:1485, 1973.
51. Sapolsky AI, Altman RD, Howell DS: Cathepsin D activity in normal and osteoarthritis human cartilage. Fed Proc *32*:1489, 1973.
52. Sapolsky AI, Howell DS, Woessner JF: Neutral proteases and Cathepsin D in human articular cartilage. J Clin Invest *53*:1044, 1974.
53. Poole AR, Hembry RM, Dingle JT, Pinder I, Ring EFJ, Cosh J: Secretion and localization of Cathepsin D in synovial tissues removed from rheumatoid and traumatized joints. Arthritis Rheum *19*:1295, 1976.
54. Silberberg R, Lesker PA: Enzyme activity in aging articular cartilage. Experientia *27*:133, 1971.
55. Bayliss MT, Ali SY: Studies on Cathepsin B in human articular cartilage. Biochem J *171*:149, 1978.
56. Burleigh MC, Barrett AJ, Lazarus GS: A lysosomal enzyme that degrades native collagen. Biochem J *137*:387, 1974.
57. Morrison RIG, Barrett AJ, Dingle JT, Prior D: Cathepsins B_1 and D: Action on human cartilage proteoglycans. Biochim Biophys Acta *302*:411, 1973.
58. Barrett AJ: The enzymic degradation of cartilage matrix. *In* PMC Burleigh, AR Poole (Eds): Dynamics of Connective Tissue Macromolecules. New York, American Elsevier, 1975, p 189.
59. Blow AMJ: Detection and characterization of Cathepsin F,a cartilage enzyme that degrades proteoglycan. Ital J Biochem *24*:13, 1975.
60. Sapolsky AI, Keiser H, Howell DS, Woessner JF: Metalloproteases of human articular cartilage that digest cartilage proteoglycan at neutral and acid pH. J Clin Invest *58*:1030, 1976.
61. Schwartz ER, Ogle RC, Thompson RC: Aryl sulfatase activities in normal and pathologic human articular cartilage. Arthritis Rheum *17*:455, 1974.
62. Thompson RC, Clark I: Acid hydrolases in slices of articular cartilage and synovium from normal and abnormal joints. Proc Soc Exp Biol Med *133*:1102, 1970.
63. Schwartz ER: Action of Vitamin E on enzymes and sulfated proteoglycans in human articular cartilage. Transactions of the 25th Annual Meeting, Orthopaedic Research Society, San Francisco, California, Feb 20–22, 1979, p 43.
64. Ehrlich MG, Mankin HJ, Treadwell BV: Acid hydrolase activity in osteoarthritic and normal human cartilage. J Bone Joint Surg *55A*:1068, 1973.
65. Ali SY, Bayliss MT: *In* SY Ali, MW Elves, DH Leaback (Eds): Normal and Osteoarthrotic Articular Cartilage. London, Institute of Orthopaedics, 1974, p 189.
66. Zorzoli A: The histochemical localization of alkaline phosphatase in demineralized bones of mice of different ages. Anat Rec *102*:445, 1948.
67. Shaw NE, Martin BF: Histological and histochemical studies on mammalian knee joint tissues. J Anat *96*:359, 1962.
68. Silberberg R, Stamp WG, Lesker PA, Hasler M: Aging changes in ultrastructure and enzymatic activity of articular cartilage of guinea pigs. J Gerontol *25*:184, 1970.
69. Gross J, Nagai Y: Specific degradation of the collagen molecule by tadpole collagenolytic enzyme. Proc Natl Acad Sci USA *54*:1197, 1965.
70. Woolley DE, Glanville RW, Lindberg KA, et al: Action of human skin collagenase on cartilage collagen. FEBS (Fed Eur Biochem Soc) Lett *34*:267, 1973.
71. Harris ED Jr, McCroskery PA: The influence of temperature and fibril stability on degradation of cartilage collagen by rheumatoid synovial collagenase. N Engl J Med *290*:1, 1974.
72. Woolley DE, Lindberg KA, Glanville RW, Evanson JM: Action of rheumatoid synovial collagenase on cartilage collagen. Eur J Biochem *50*:437, 1975.
73. Harris ED Jr, Farrell ME: Resistance to collagenase: A characteristic of collagen fibrils cross-linked with formaldehyde. Biochem Biophys Acta *278*:133, 1972.
74. Steven FS: Observations on the different substrate behaviour of tropocollagen molecules in solution and intermolecularly cross-linked tropocollagen within insoluble polymeric collagen fibrils. Biochem J *155*:391, 1976.
75. Gross J, Bruschi AB: The pattern of collagen degradation in cultured tadpole tissues. Dev Biol *26*:36, 1971.
76. Jolma VH, Hruza Z: Differences in properties of newly formed collagen during aging and parabiosis. J Gerontol *27*:178, 1972.
77. Lust G, Pronsky W: Glycosaminoglycan metabolism in normal and arthritic cartilage. Fed Proc *31*:883A, 1972.
78. Ehrlich MG, Mankin HJ, Jones H, Wright R, Crispen C, Vigliani G: Collagenase and collagenase inhibitors in osteoarthritic and normal human cartilage. J Clin Invest *59*:226, 1977.
79. Lotke PA, Granda JL: Alterations in the permeability of articular cartilage by proteolytic enzymes. Arthritis Rheum *15*:302, 1972.
80. Fleming A, Allison VD: Observations on a bacteriolytic substance (lysozyme) found in secretions and tissues. Br J Exp Pathol *3*:252, 1922.
81. Kuettner KE, Eisenstein R, Soble LW, Arsenis C: Lysozyme in epiphyseal cartilage: IV. Embryonic chick cartilage lysozyme — its localization and partial characterization. J Cell Biol *49*:450, 1971.
82. Greenwald RA, Josephson AS, Diamond HS, Tsang A: Human cartilage lysozyme. J Clin Invest *51*:2264, 1972.
83. Kuettner KE, Guenther HL, Ray RD, Schumacher GFB: Lysozyme in preosseous cartilage. Calcif Tissue Res *1*:298, 1968.
84. Gubisch W, Schlager F: Fermente im Knochen- und Knorpel-gewebe. III. Mitteilung: β-D-Glucuronidase. Acta Histochem *12*:69, 1961.
85. Pugh D, Walker PG: Localization of N-acetyl-β-glucosaminidase in tissues. J Histochem Cytochem *9*:242, 1961.
86. Bollett AJ, Bonner WM, Nance JL: The presence of hyaluronidase in various mammalian tissues. J Biol Chem *238*:3522, 1963.
87. Wasteson A, Amado R, Ingmar B, Heldin CH: *In* H Peeters (Ed): Protides of the Biological Fluids. New York, Pergamon Press, 1975, p 431.
88. Weissmann G, Spilberg I: Breakdown of cartilage proteinpolysaccharide by lysosomes. Arthritis Rheum *11*:162, 1968.
89. Lazarus GS, Daniels JR, Brown RS, Bladen HA, Fullmer HM: Degradation of collagen by a human granulocyte collagenolytic system. J Clin Invest *47*:2622, 1968.
90. Ziff M, Gribetz HJ, Lospalluto J: Effect of leukocyte and synovial membrane extracts on cartilage mucoprotein. J Clin Invest *39*:405, 1960.
91. Barrett AJ: The possible role of neutrophil proteinases in damage to articular cartilage. Agent Actions *8*:11, 1978.
92. Janoff A, Blondin J: Depletion of cartilage matrix by a neutral protease fraction of human leukocyte lysosomes. Proc Soc Exp Biol Med *135*:302, 1970.
93. Weissmann G: Lysosomal mechanisms of tissue injury in arthritis. Seminars in Medicine of the Beth Israel Hospital, Boston *286*:141, 1972.
94. Buermann CW, Horowitz MI, Oronsky AL: Degradation of chondroitin-4-sulfate by human polymorphonuclear leukocyte enzymes. Transactions of the 25th Annual Meeting, Orthopedic Research Society, San Francisco, California, Feb 20–22, 1979, p 44.
95. Horvath SM, Hollander JL: Intra-articular temperature as a measure of joint reaction. J Clin Invest *28*:469, 1949.
96. Lack CH, Rogers HJ: Action of plasmin on cartilage. Nature *182*:948, 1958.
97. Lack CH: Chondrolysis in arthritis. J Bone Joint Surg *41B*:384, 1959.
98. Chrisman OD, Southwick WO, Fessel JM: Plasmin and articular cartilage. Yale J Biol Med *34*:524, 1962.
99. Roy S, Meachim G: Chondrocyte ultrastructure in adult human articular cartilage. Ann Rheum Dis *27*:544, 1968.
100. Zimny ML, Redler I: An ultrastructural study of patellar chondromalacia in humans. J Bone Joint Surg *51A*:1179, 1969.
101. Fell HB: Role of biological membranes in some skeletal reactions. Ann Rheum Dis *28*:213, 1969.
102. Barrett AJ: Cathepsin D: Purification of isoenzymes from human and chicken liver. Biochem J *117*:601, 1970.
103. Ali SY, Evans L: Enzymic degradation of cartilage in osteoarthritis. Fed Proc *32*:1494, 1973.
104. Nagase H, Woessner JF Jr: Neutral protease from bovine nasal cartilage that digests proteoglycan. Arthritis Rheum *20*:77, 1977.
105. Gold EW, Anderson LB, Miller CW, Schwartz ER: Effect of salicylate on the surgical inducement of joint degeneration in rabbit knees. J Bone Joint Surg *58A*:1012, 1976.
106. Austin J, McAfee D, Armstrong D, et al: Abnormal sulfatase activities in two human diseases (metachromatic leucodystrophy and gargoylism). Biochem J *93*:15C, 1964.
107. Evanson JM, Jeffrey JJ, Krane SM: Human collagenase: Identification and characterization of an enzyme from rheumatoid synovium in culture. Science *158*:499, 1967.
108. Harris ED Jr, Cohen GL, Krane SM: Synovial collagenase: Its presence

in culture from joint disease of diverse etiology. Arthritis Rheum *12*:92, 1969.
109. Schwartz ER, Adamy L: Effect of ascorbic acid on arylsulfatase activities and sulfated proteoglycan metabolism in chondrocyte cultures. J Clin Invest *60*:96, 1977.
110. Bollett AJ, Nance JL: Biochemical findings in normal and osteoarthritic articular cartilage. II. Chondroitin sulfate concentration and chain length, water and ash content. J Clin Invest *45*:1170, 1966.
111. Lust G, Pronsky W, Sherman DM: Biochemical studies on developing canine hip joints. J Bone Joint Surg *54A*:986, 1972.
112. Chrisman OD, Southwick WO: Sulfate metabolism in cartilage. III. The effects of various adjuvants of sulfate exchange in cartilage slices. J Bone Joint Surg *44A*:464, 1962.
113. Curtiss PH Jr, Klein L: Destruction of articular cartilage in septic arthritis. J Bone Joint Surg *47A*:1595, 1965.
114. Howell DS, Pita JC, Sorgente N, Kuettner K: Possible role of lysozyme in degradation of osteoarthritic cartilage. Trans Assoc Am Physicians *87*:169, 1974.
115. Deshmukh K, Nimni ME: Effects of lysosomal enzymes on the type of collagen synthesized by bovine articular cartilage. Biochem Biophys Res Comm *53*:424, 1973
116. Krane SM: Joint erosion in rheumatoid arthritis. Arthritis Rheum *17*:306, 1974.
117. Kobayashi I, Ziff M: Electron microscopic studies on the cartilage-pannus junction in rheumatoid arthritis. Arthritis Rheum *18*:475, 1975.
118. Woolley DE, Crossley MJ, Evanson JM: Collagenase at sites of cartilage erosion in the rheumatoid joint. Arthritis Rheum *20*:1231, 1977.
119. Luscombe M: Acid phosphatase and catheptic activity in rheumatoid synovial tissue. Nature *197*:1010, 1963.
120. Wegelius O, Klockars M, Vainio K: Acid phosphatase activity in rheumatoid synovia. Acta Med Scand *183*:549, 1968.
121. Harris ED Jr, Evanson JM, DiBona DR, Krane SM: Collagenase and rheumatoid arthritis. Arthritis Rheum *13*:83, 1970.
122. Vainio U: Leucine aminopeptidase in rheumatoid arthritis. Ann Rheum Dis *29*:434, 1970.
123. Muirden KD, Deutschmann P, Phillips M: Articular cartilage in rheumatoid arthritis: Ultrastructure and enzymology. J Rheumatol *1*:24, 1974.
124. Collins AJ, Cosh JA: Temperature and biochemical studies of joint inflammation. Ann Rheum Dis *29*:386, 1970.
125. Granda JL, Ranawat CS, Posner AS: Levels of three hydrolases in rheumatoid and regenerated synovium. Arthritis Rheum *14*:223, 1971.
126. Wood GC, Pryce-Jones RH, White DD, Nuki G: Chondromucoprotein degrading neutral protease activity in rheumatoid synovial fluid. Ann Rheum Dis *30*:73, 1971.
127. Josephson AS, Greenwald RA, Gerber DA: Serum lysozyme and histidine in rheumatoid arthritis (Abstr) Clin Res *19*:444, 1971.
128. Lazarus GS, Daniels JR, Brown RS, Bladen HA, Fullmer HM: Degradation of collagen by a human granulocyte collagenolytic system. J Clin Invest *47*:2622, 1968.
129. Murphy G, Reynolds JJ, Bretz U, Baggiolini M: Collagenase is a component of the specific granules of human neutrophil leucocytes. Biochem J *162*:195, 1977.
130. Lazarus GS, Daniels JR, Lian J, Burleigh MC: Role of granulocyte collagenase in collagen degradation. Am J Pathol *68*:565, 1972.
131. Harris ED Jr, Faulkner CS II, Brown FE: Collagenolytic systems in rheumatoid arthritis. Clin Orthop Relat Res *110*:303, 1975.
132. Curtiss PH Jr, Klein L: Destruction of articular cartilage in septic arthritis. J Bone Joint Surg *45A*:797, 1963.

5

BIOMECHANICS OF JOINTS

by Peter S. Walker, Ph.D.

Mechanics deals with force and motion and the effects that they have. A force applied to a fixed object will deform the object and will induce stresses in the material. If the object is free to move, it will accelerate in the direction of the force. A moving object has energy that can be dissipated in heat or in permanently deforming the material if it suddenly strikes an obstruction. The mechanical properties of materials describe their elasticity, their strength in tension and compression, or their resistance to wear. Whenever two surfaces are in motion relative to each other with a force between them, there is a frictional resistance to the motion, and wear of one or both surfaces will ensue. Lubricants usually reduce both the friction and the wear.

Described in this fashion, mechanics deals largely with everyday materials such as metal, wood, plastic, water, and oil, and with everyday structures from workshop tools and appliances to automobiles and airplanes. The human body can be evaluated in a similar way, but there are a number of complicating factors. The body materials are not homogeneous but display significant directional properties, usually because of an aligned fibrous collagen component. The materials are neither purely elastic nor linear, but have a complex rheology which is time and strain-rate dependent. The properties of the materials within one structure can vary considerably, such as in osseous or cartilaginous layers. The structures themselves are not uniform in shape. Furthermore, the forces imposed on the structures depend upon the type of activity and the existence and location of surrounding muscular and ligamentous tissues. Finally, over long periods of time, the shape and the properties of the structures themselves can change owing to the imposition of external forces and motions.

This phenomenon, the response of biologic structures to forces and motions, is perhaps the most significant way in which "biomechanics" differs from "mechanics," and is a fascinating and challenging area, which encompasses biology, mechanics, and electricity as well. It is particularly relevant to the analysis of joint replacement, in which prosthetic components must work in harmony with the remaining osseous and soft tissue structures. Frequently, the match is imperfect, and failure of the implant eventually occurs that is either due to an adverse biologic reaction to the component, which leads to loosening, or due to a resulting mechanical failure of the components themselves.

This chapter will deal with the mechanics of articulations and the changes in mechanics that occur when artificial joints are implanted.

FORCES AND MOMENTS

Definitions

A force is defined by its *magnitude* (size), its *direction*, and its *point of application*. Thus, force is a *vector*. The units of force that are employed are often confusing, because the international standard unit is the *newton*, whereas, colloquially, pounds and

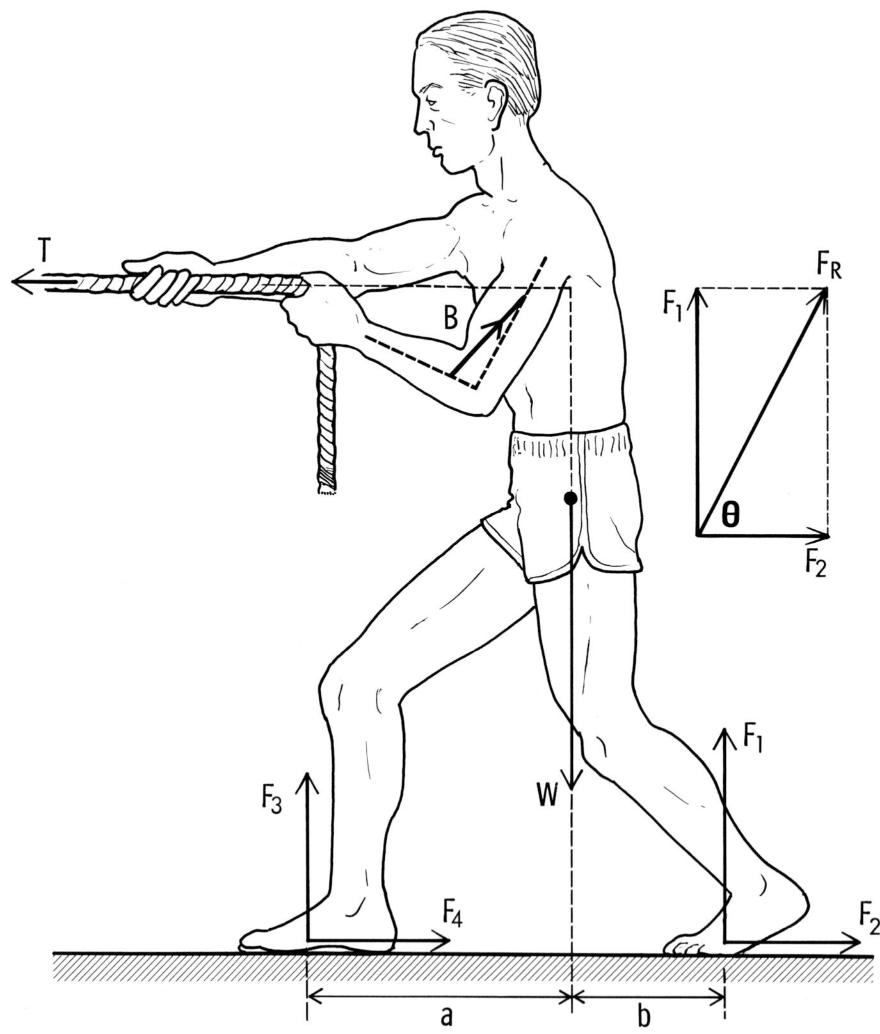

Figure 5–1. *Examples of forces on the body. The inset at the right shows combination and resolution of forces.*

kilograms are more commonly used and are more familiar. The conversion values are 1 newton (N) = 0.102 kilogram-force (kgf) = 0.225 pound-force (lbf). An average man weighing about 75 kg or 165 lb exerts a downward force of about 750 N; or, "one body weight of force" is about 750 N. The concept of a force acting on an object can be visualized by the law stating "for every action there is an equal and opposite reaction." If an object is resting on a fixed surface, there is a downward force on the surface, and an equal upward force on the object.

Examples of forces applied to and in the body are shown in Figure 5–1, in which a man is pulling a rope. There is a tensile force in the rope acting along the rope. Several forces are acting on the hands; the magnitude of the combined forces is equal to that of the tensile force in the rope. In order to maintain flexion in the elbow, there is a tensile force in the brachialis muscle. The body exerts a downward force due to its mass, acting through the center of mass. There are two vertical forces acting on the feet, the sum of which balances the body weight. To counter the horizontal pull of the rope, there are horizontal forces at the feet as a result of friction between the soles and the ground.

It is noted that there are two *components* of force acting on each foot. Any two components can be combined into a single *resultant* by drawing a parallelogram of forces (in this case a rectangle). In Figure 5–1, the resultant is the diagonal of the parallelogram. When the forces are *orthogonal* (at right angles), the resultant can be calculated by pythagorean theorem:

$$F_R{}^2 = F_1{}^2 + F_2{}^2$$

Conversely, if the resultant force F_R is given, the two components F_1 and F_2 can be easily calculated from the following simple equations:

$$F_2 = F_R \cos \theta$$
$$F_1 = F_R \sin \theta$$

With respect to the man, the forces at the hands and feet and the body weight are *external forces*, whereas the brachialis force is an *internal force*. This is an important distinction, which relates to the idea of a "free body." A *free body* is the object that is being analyzed within a defined boundary. An external force crosses the boundary of the free body and exerts a force at a point or over an area of the free body. An internal force affects only the interior of the free body.

If a free body is in equilibrium, the *resultant external forces in any direction must be zero*. Thus, in the example of Figure 5–1, consider the forces in a vertical direction; or, in other words, *resolve the forces in a vertical direction*:

$$F_1 + F_3 - W = 0$$

Similarly, *resolve the forces in a horizontal direction*:

$$F_4 + F_2 - T = 0$$

Note that the force in the brachialis muscle (B) does not appear in these equations because it is an internal force. In order to determine B, the forearm must be considered as a free body, and certain geometric data around the elbow joint must be known.

We now consider the concept of *moments* (Fig. 5–2). The *moment of a force* (F) about any point (P) is the *magnitude of the force multiplied by the perpendicular distance*. For the simply supported bone in Figure 5–2, the reaction forces R_1 and R_2 can be determined by the application of the resolution of forces and the moments of force:

Resolve vertically: $R_1 + R_2 - W = 0$

Take moments about the left support: $R_2\,(a + b) - Wa = 0$

$$R_2 = W\frac{a}{a+b}$$

and $$R_1 = W\frac{b}{a+b}$$

In general, to determine the equilibrium equations of a free body in a plane, resolve the forces in two perpendicular directions and take moments about any point in the plane.

Returning to the example of Figure 5–1, assume that T and W are known, and it is required to calculate F_1 and F_3.

Resolve vertically: $F_3 + F_1 - W = 0$

Take moments about right foot (h = height of rope): $F_1\,(a + b) + Th - Wa = 0$

$$F_1 = \frac{Wa - Th}{a+b}$$

and $$F_3 = W - F_1 = \frac{Wb + Th}{a+b}$$

It is a basic law in mechanics that *any system of forces and moments acting in a plane can be reduced to a single resultant force acting in a certain direction plus a moment in the plane*, or, alternatively, to two forces along orthogonal axes plus a moment about each of these axes. In three dimensions, any system of forces can be resolved into a single force and a single moment, or, alternatively, into three orthogonal force components along three axes plus three moments about these axes. An example of moments in the upper femur is shown in Figure 5–3. If there are forces F and M acting on the femoral head and the trochanter, respectively, with respect to the centerline of the femoral shaft, there is a vertical force of ($F - M$) and a moment of ($Fa - Mb$).

Another important concept is that of *a moment* or *a torque*. When a moment is applied to a body in a plane, there is a pure turning effect but no resultant linear force in the plane of moment. Examples are the turning action on a screw by a screwdriver, or the action of removing a lid from a jar (Fig. 5–3).

So far, only parallel forces have been considered. Observe the case in Figure 5–4, where it is required to calculate the resultant force at the tibiotalar joint at "toe-off" in level walking. The ground-to-foot reaction force G, the distance from G, and the

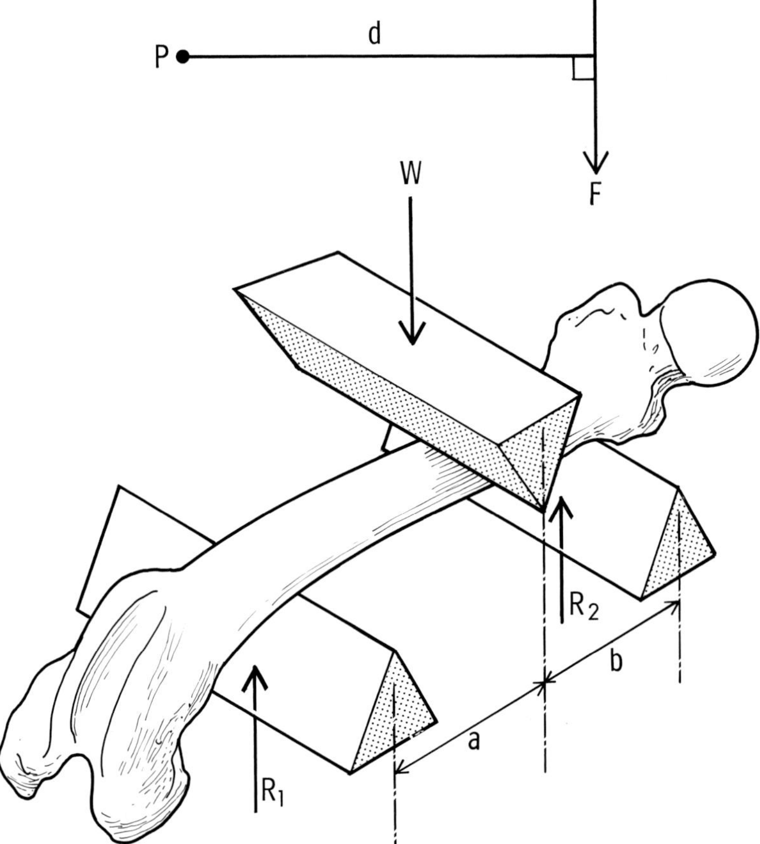

Figure 5–2. *Moments of force. In the diagram at the top, the moment of force F about P is equal to F × d. The lower diagram shows a simply supported bone in a three-point bending test.*

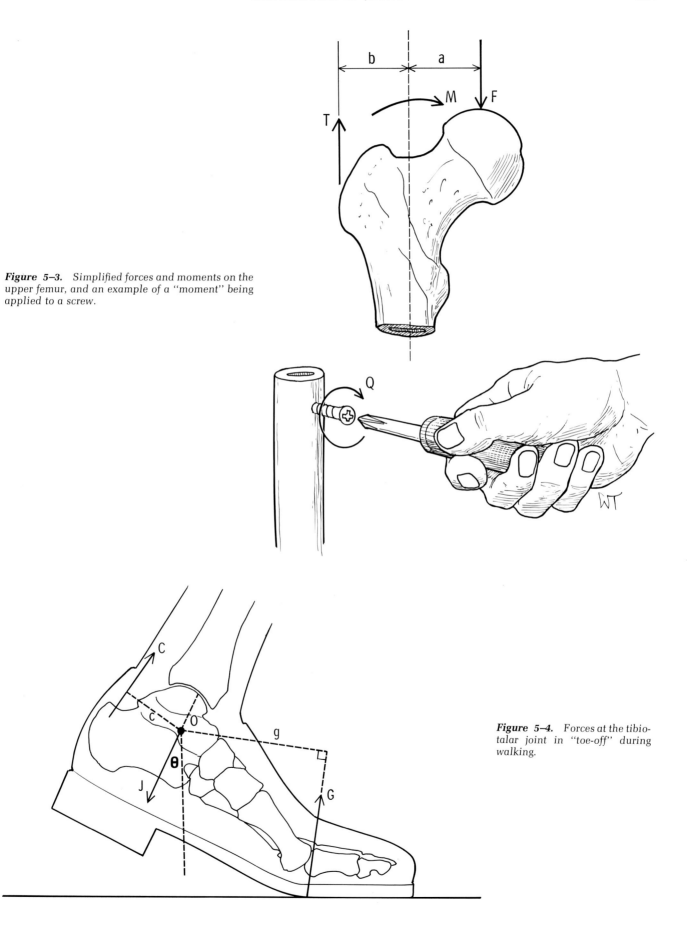

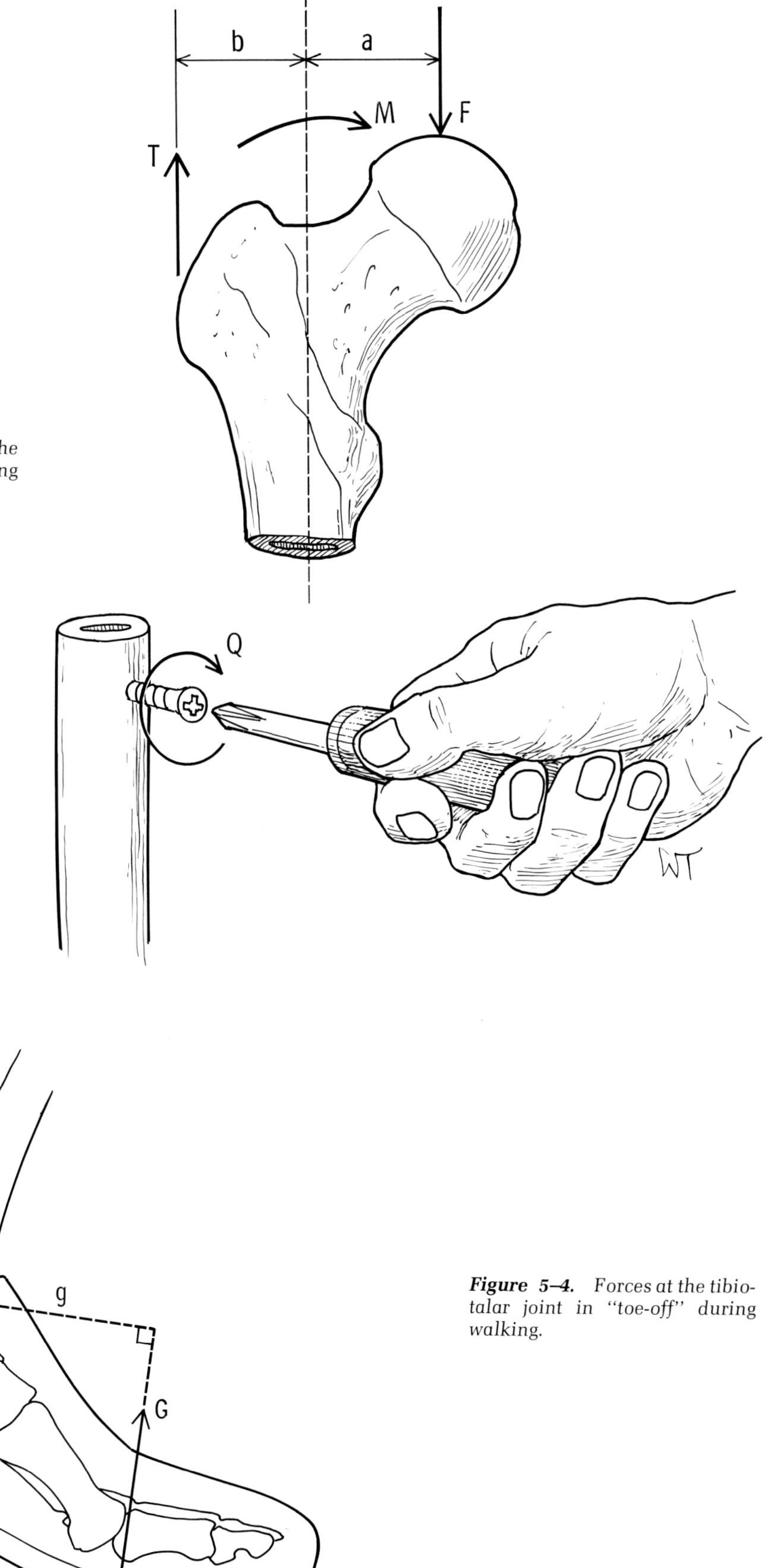

Figure 5–3. *Simplified forces and moments on the upper femur, and an example of a "moment" being applied to a screw.*

Figure 5–4. *Forces at the tibiotalar joint in "toe-off" during walking.*

distance from G to the center of the ankle are all known. C, the force in the Achilles tendon, is known in direction and location but not in magnitude. The free body is defined by a boundary through the ankle joint and around the foot. The forces crossing the boundary are G, C, and the unknown resultant force at the joint J. Because the joint surfaces are assumed to be frictionless, there is no torque around the articulation. Other muscular and ligamentous forces are ignored in this problem. There are three unknowns: C, J, and O. Solution requires three equations, which are obtained by resolving the forces horizontally and vertically and by taking moments about a point. Let the vertical and horizontal components of G, C, and J be denoted by suffixes V and H, respectively.

Resolve vertically:	$C_V + G_V - J_V = 0$
Resolve horizontally:	$C_H + G_H - J_H = 0$
Moments about 0:	$C \times c - G \times g = 0$

Values for a particular example are G_V = 1.15 BW (BW = body weight), G_H = 0.18 BW, G = 132 mm, and c = 61 mm. The solution is J_V = 3.26 BW and J_H = 1.50 BW, giving an overall resultant J = 3.59 BW ($J^2 = 3.26^2 + 1.50^2$).

Before analyzing forces and moments acting in human joints, it will be useful to explain some additional terminology. *Compressive forces* are those pressing two surfaces together or acting longitudinally within a structure. *Tensile forces* act to pull apart two surfaces or to distract the material in a structure. *Shearing forces* act in a tangential direction to two surfaces. As explained above, if the friction is extremely low, as is the case in healthy human joints, there can be no shearing forces across the articular surfaces: Such forces can only be supported by ligaments, muscles, and "containment" of the joint surfaces themselves. The analysis of forces in joints requires definition of the directions of the force components, and this is conveniently done by introducing *an origin*, O, and a set of *orthogonal axes*, x, y, and z, which are fixed with respect to one of the bones. A planar analysis need consider only x and y axes and is useful and accurate in many situations. However, a complete three-dimensional analysis requires x, y, and z axes; this analysis is necessary in the study of forces in the hip during gait or of obliquely applied forces in the upper extremity. The steps in the analysis are as follows: At the particular instant in time—

1. Define the free body — e.g., the shank of the leg if knee forces are required (Fig. 5–5).
2. Define the geometry of the free body from radiographs, photographs, etc.
3. Measure the external forces acting on the free body, in this case the foot-to-ground force (the inertia forces and moments need also be determined from analysis of the gait cycle) (Fig. 5–6).
4. Determine which muscles are active from electromyogram records, and draw the lines of action of these muscle forces, in this case the hamstrings.
5. Define axes as required, such as those that are parallel and perpendicular to the long axis of the tibia.

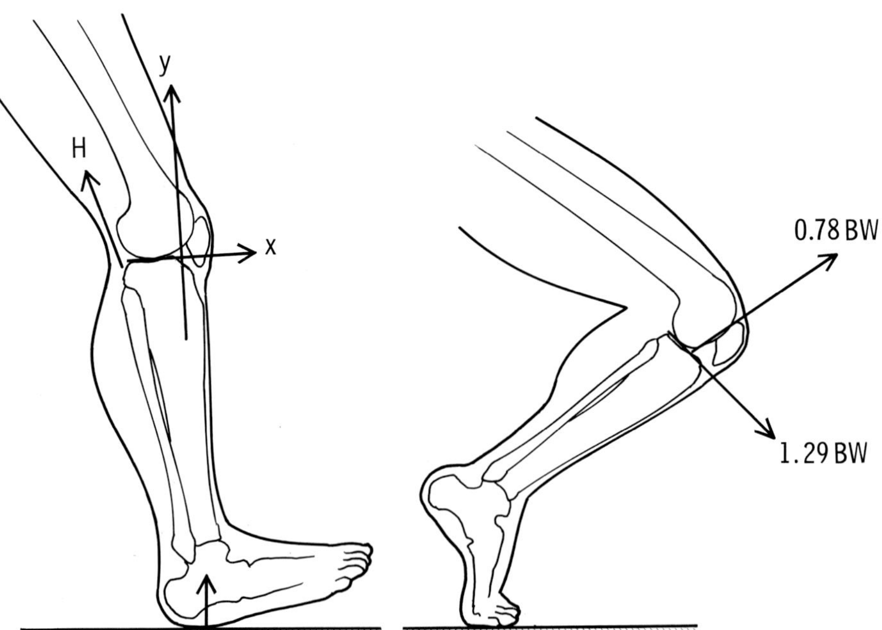

Figure 5–5. *Compressive and shear forces across the knee joint for walking and for full knee bend. The force vectors shown for full knee bend are those acting on the femur.*

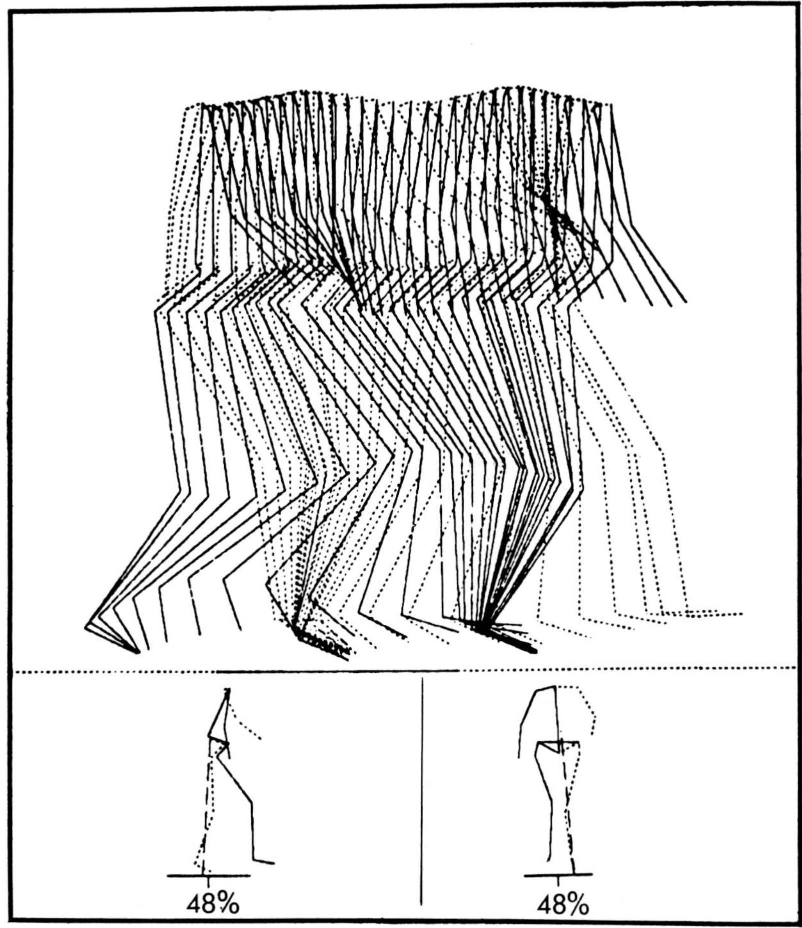

Figure 5–6. *Gait analysis using the Selspot technique. Below is shown the line of action of the foot-to-ground reaction force. (Courtesy of S Simon, MD, Children's Hospital, Boston.)*

6. Resolve the forces in two directions and take moments about any point.

The calculations will yield a single resultant through O (or components along x and y), and a moment about O. These are the *resultant forces and moments at the joint*. Frequently, however, there are more unknowns than equations owing to the fact that several muscles are acting simultaneously and that ligamentous forces are also operational. The consequence is that there is no single or unique solution for the joint forces and moments, and the same action in the same individual could well be accomplished with different forces. To obtain a likely solution (or any solution at all), certain assumptions need to be made. These include the assigning of maximum forces for given muscles based upon their areas, the weighing of muscle forces according to the integrated electromyogram signals, and the assumption that the joint minimizes the total resultant, the shear component, the torque component, or the weighted combinations.

To determine the meaning of the resultant force and the moment with respect to a particular joint, determinations must be made about which structures are carrying the force and the moment. In the knee (Fig. 5–5) the y component of force will be direct compression across the joint surfaces, while the shear component along x will be carried by a combination of the slight dishing of the medial joint surfaces and of one of the cruciate ligaments.

The key to determining lower limb forces is the foot-to-ground force, conveniently described in three orthogonal components. In level walking, the vertical component peaks at heel-strike and at toe-off at 110 to 130 per cent of body weight. The point of application begins close to the heel at heel-strike, and moves steadily forward during swing phase, reaching the ball of the foot at toe-off. The fore and aft shear forces peak at about 15 to 20 per cent of body weight, being backward on the foot at heel-strike and forward at toe-off. The lateral shear forces are usually small. The vertical peaks in an activity such as running up and down stairs can reach over twice the body weight.

An elegant method of visualizing the forces on the foot in relation to the lines joining the centers of the joints has been developed and an example is shown in Figure 5–6. The force vector is displayed in real time as the subject is undergoing the activity, and the moments of the force about any joint in the frontal or sagittal planes can be readily seen. Consider, for example, the knee: In the sagittal plane, if the line of force is anterior, there is an extending moment and the hamstring or the gastrocnemius muscles would be needed for balance; conversely, a posterior line of action constitutes a flexing moment, which can be balanced by the quadriceps muscles. It is most important to realize that although external forces, including body weight, will produce a compressive force across a joint, *the greater portion of the total joint force is usually due to the muscle action that is needed to stabilize the joint.*

Forces on Human Joints

Some examples of studies on actual joint forces will now be given. The forces in the tibiotalar joint during walking were calculated by Stauffer and co-workers,[24] analyzing the sagittal plane and accounting for the forces in the anterior tibial and Achilles tendons. The compressive force component had peaks at heel-strike and toe-off of 3 and 4.7 times body weight, respectively, the latter being related to the action of the Achilles tendon in plantar flexion of the foot. The shear forces were significant, particularly the aft force, which peaked at 0.68 BW through heel-strike and foot-flat. This shear force would normally be supported by the congruity of the joint surfaces.

Paul[18] summarized the various studies from Strathclyde University on the forces in the knee joint for certain activities. In level walking, there were three stance phase force peaks corresponding to activity in the hamstrings, the quadriceps, and the gastrocnemius muscles. The maximum force for fast walking was 4.3 BW. The peaks of forces for ascending and descending stairs were 4.4 and 4.9 BW, respectively. The anterior cruciate ligament was most highly loaded during the activity of walking down a ramp. However, the highest cruciate forces were encountered in the posterior cruciate ligaments in walking up a ramp, down stairs, or up stairs (highest force of all: 1220 N). Seireg and Arvikar,[23] using a more complex approach, discovered a peak force of 7.1 BW in the double leg support phase of level walking; these investigations included an analysis of antagonistic muscle activity (Paul did not account for this). In an earlier study, the same investigators[22] calculated a compressive component of 0.78 BW and a forward shearing force of the femur on the tibia of 1.29 BW for a full knee bend (stooping position) (Fig. 5–5). Of interest in this regard are the clinical observations that many meniscal injuries occur when the patient rises from such a position, and that the posterior aspect of the tibia, particularly on the lateral side, often shows cartilaginous ulceration.

In level walking, the forces that are generated at the patellofemoral joint will be relatively low, because even when the quadriceps force is high, the component of this force and that of the patella tendon (which will have a magnitude of force close to that in the quadriceps tendon), operating in a direction that is perpendicular to the contact region, will be small. However, in stair climbing, peak forces of about 3 BW will be encountered.[20]

The compressive force in the hip joint during the stance phase of level walking shows two peaks at heel-strike and toe-off[7, 17] and a possible additional peak just prior to toe-off.[23] The average of these peaks, as determined by these three studies, was 3.6, 4.3, and 4.8 BW. However, it is significant to consider the three orthogonal components of force because of the separate effects they will have on the femur.

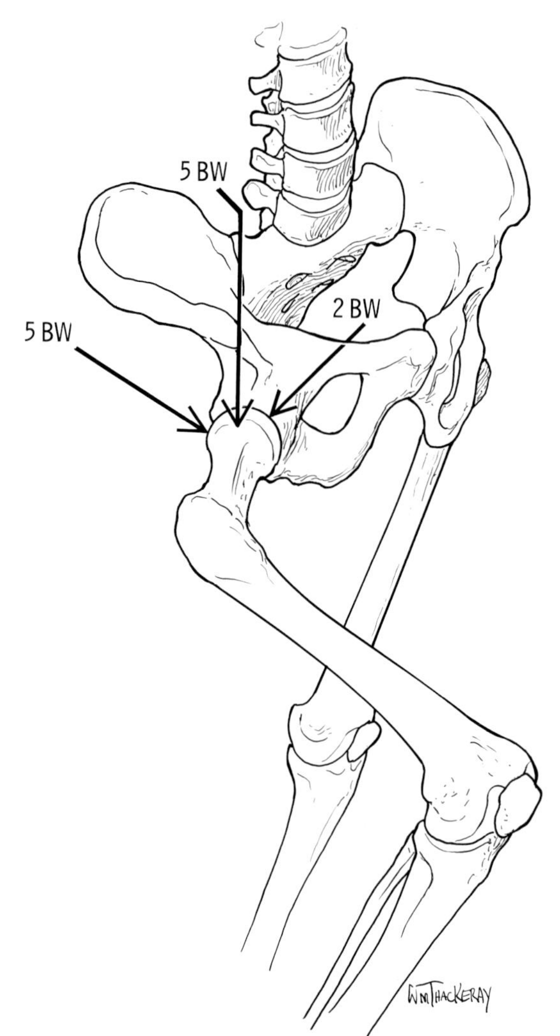

Figure 5–7. *Force components acting on the femoral head in ascending stairs. (Data from Crowninshield RD, et al: J Biomechanics 9:387, 1978.)*

For example, Crowninshield and associates[7] calculated the force components that developed during the ascent of stairs in relation to axes in the pelvis. The forces shown in Figure 5–7 are those acting on the femoral head. Assuming for simplicity that the femur lies in a horizontal plane, the vertical force component will produce a large moment about the long axis of the femur. If a hip prosthesis were in place, this moment would produce a torque about the axis of the prosthetic stem and the cement-bone interface. The horizontal force component would produce an overall bending moment on the femur, similar to that illustrated in Figure 5–3.

The forces in the joints of the upper extremity are usually much less than those of the lower extremity because the body weight component is absent and the other external forces are seldom so high. Furthermore, the upper extremity is used primarily to position the hand for manipulative activities rather than for power activities. However, the frequency of upper extremity forces may be more or less than that of lower extremity forces, depending upon the occupation and the activities of the individual.[8]

External forces acting on the fingers were measured by Walker and co-workers[26] (Fig. 5–8) in an attempt to define, as a tool for clinical evaluation, the forces and manipulation ability in different activities. The average maximum values in men were: grip strength, 153 N; pulp, key, chuck, and lateral pinch, 70 to 90 N; and extension, radial, and ulnar forces, 10 to 18 N. The standard deviation of results in any test was about 25 per cent and men were stronger than women by about 50 per cent. Arthritic patients displayed strengths of approximately 20 per cent of normal. Chao and colleagues[6] used biplanar radiographs and sectional geometric studies to calculate joint and tendon forces. They expressed the forces and the moments along three orthogonal axes that were set in each joint. The forces in the metacarpophalangeal joints (MCP) were the highest, and in any joint the compressive component was greater than either shear component. In terms of a unit external force, the compressive and downward shear forces in the MCP joint were 8.0 N and 2.7 N, respectively, in pinch; the values were 11.4 N and 4.2 N in grasp. In view of these experimental data, it is obvious that very high forces are generated at the joints of the fingers. In fact, Berme and co-workers[1] calculated that compressive and shear forces at the MCP joint were 170 N and 46.5 N, respectively, much of the compressive component being derived from the high loading in the collateral ligaments.

The determination of forces at the wrist requires a three-dimensional analysis as well as knowledge of the mechanical properties at the radial and ulnar bearing surfaces. Although it appears likely that the radius will carry most of the forces, there are no available data on this subject at the present time.

The elbow joint presents a complex problem because there are three articulations, some of the major muscles have broad osseous attachments (brachialis on the humerus) or transmit their force through an extensive membrane (biceps aponeurosis), and force directions are altered as the radius rotates. A simple three-dimensional analysis of forces generated while lifting an object in the hand was carried out by Walker and Novick in 1977. For a 1 kg weight and the elbow flexed at 90 degrees, the humeroulnar force was 215 N directed along the humeral axis at its distal end. Without any weight in the hand, the forces were reduced by 50 per cent; for an additional 1 kg weight, the joint force increased by 50 per cent. The forces at 45 degrees of flexion were about twice those at 90 degrees because the lever arms of the muscles were reduced. Hue and co-workers[12] determined that the force had an anterior component on the humerus at low flexion angles and a posterior component after about 30 degrees of flexion (0 degrees of flexion is defined as a straight arm). The implication of these results in prosthetic elbow surgery is that the humeral component will be toggled back and forth, a fact which may explain the high incidence of loosening found clinically in postoperative patients. A detailed study of elbow forces in eating, reaching, table-pull, and seat-rise was reported by Nicol.[15] In seat-rise with arm-assist, the humeroulnar force increased from 500 N to 1800 N during the course of the activity, whereas there was a 600 N lateral ligament force throughout. Note that if a rigid hinge prosthesis were in place, this ligament force would be carried as a varus bending moment on the prosthesis.

In isometric abduction of the arm in the plane of the scapula, the maximum resultant force at the glenohumeral joint may reach 0.89 BW, whereas the maximum shearing force component up the face of the glenoid may reach 0.42 BW at 60 degrees of abduction.[19] With a 1 kg weight in the hand, these forces can be increased by 60 per cent; with the elbow flexed to 90 degrees the forces may be reduced by 30 per cent. Figure 5–9 illustrates some of the mechanical aspects of the forces in abduction. The upward shearing components at 30 degrees and 60 degrees of abduction are due to the directions of force in the supraspinatus and deltoid musculature. At 90 degrees of abduction and beyond, however, the line of the deltoid pull is more perpendicular to the face of the glenoid, and the actions of the subscapularis and infraspinatus muscles produce a resultant force close to the center of the glenoid cavity.

In the previous description, the forces and the moments in joints have been considered as vectors with magnitude, line of action, and point of application. However, it is known that the resultant force within articulations is not transmitted at a single point but instead is spread over a wide area. In other words, the resultant force is *distributed* over an area, such that at any location there is a certain force

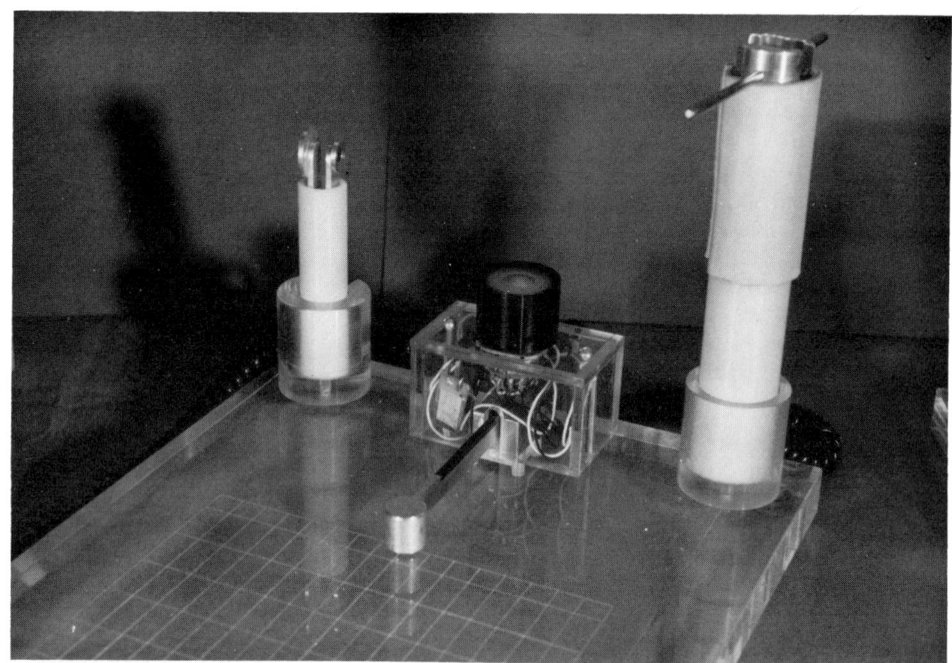

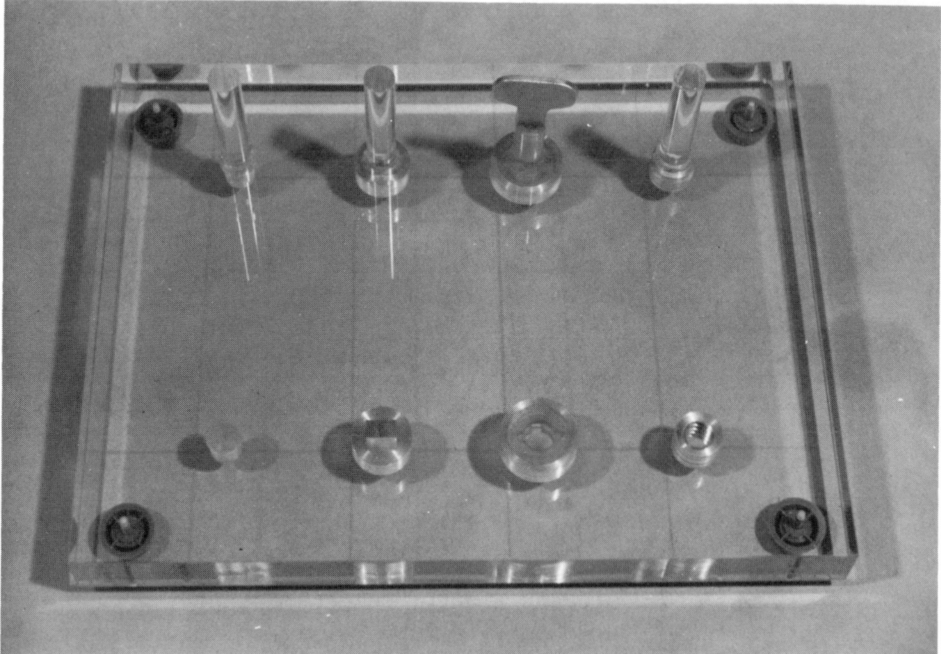

Figure 5–8. *Apparatus to measure the function of the hand. Top, left to right: pinch meter, lateral and extension force meter, and grip meter. Bottom, manipulation tester.*

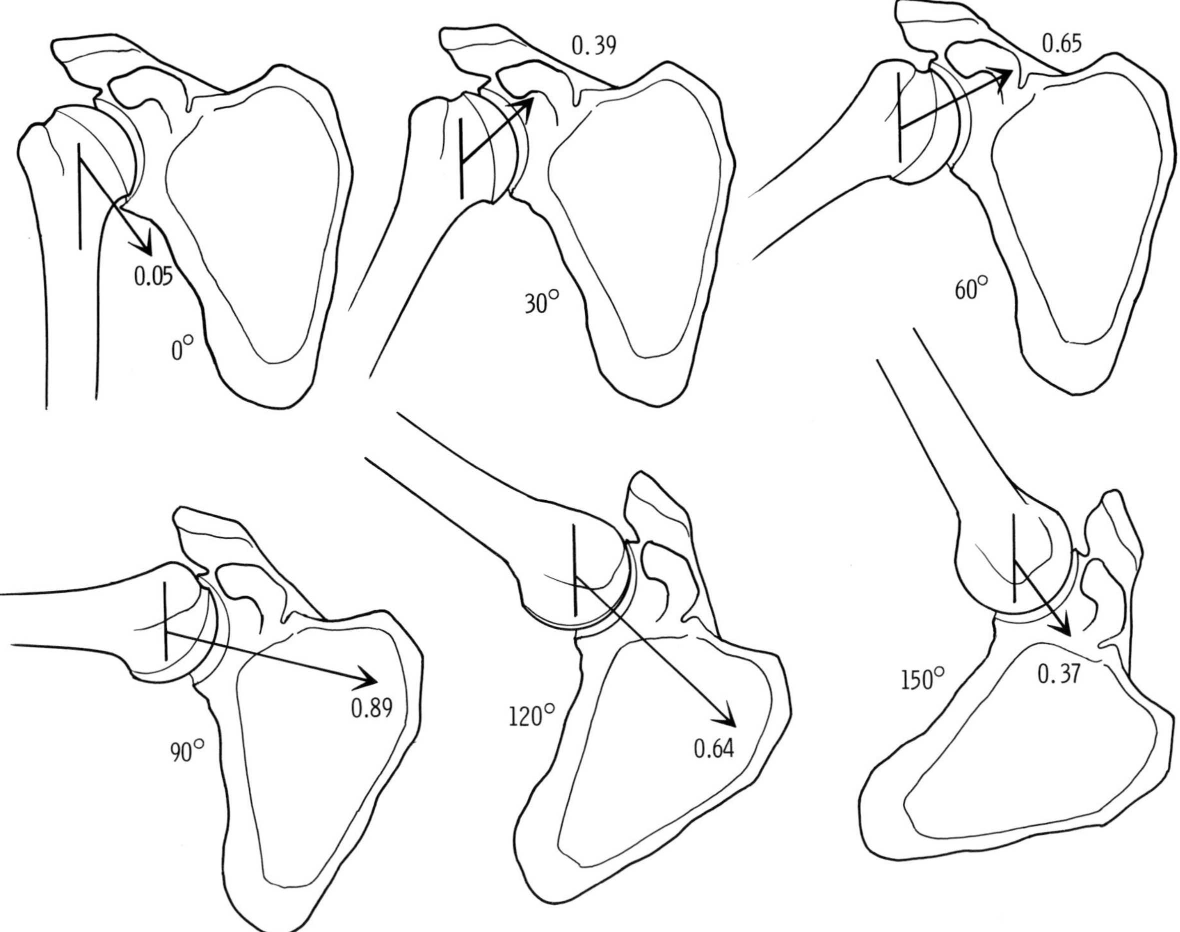

Figure 5–9. *The forces across the glenohumeral joint as a fraction of body weight for abduction in the plane of the scapula. The relative positions of the humerus and scapula are also shown.*

density, or *force per unit area*. This force per unit area is known as *pressure* or *contact stress*.

When resultant force is applied to the articular surfaces or to individual structures, the effects will be a stress in the material and a distortion or strain. The effects of forces on the materials and the structures of the joints will now be discussed.

STRESSES AND STRAINS

Definitions

If a force P is applied longitudinally to a uniform bar of area A, a *direct tensile stress* or a *direct compressive stress* is generated, which is of magnitude $P \div A$. If the lower end of the bar is clamped, and P is applied transversely, *shear stress* will be generated, again of magnitude $P \div A$, across any section. With longitudinal forces, there are also shear stresses acting on nontransverse planes which are maximum on planes at 45 degrees to the long axis. *Pressure* is usually used to describe stresses on a surface and is also measured as force per unit area. *Hydrostatic pressure* is the force per unit area acting within a fluid, and it is generated equally in all directions. In general, to express the state of stress at a point in an object, a small element is selected (Fig. 5–10). The direct stresses and the shear stresses are shown acting on the faces of the element; there are one direct stress and two shear stresses on each face. There are three independent direct stresses, denoted σ_x, σ_y, and σ_z and three independent shear stresses, denoted τ_{xy}, τ_{yx}, and τ_{zx}. These six independent quantities are the components of stress at the point and completely describe the state of stress at that point. Another way to describe the state of stress is to use *principal stresses*. Taking the three-dimensional element, it is possible to orient the element such that the shear stresses on the faces are zero. At this orientation, only direct tensile and compressive stresses are operational, and these stresses are called the principal stresses. Considering any plane, such as the xy plane, the stresses in the x and y directions will be the *maximum and minimum direct stresses*.

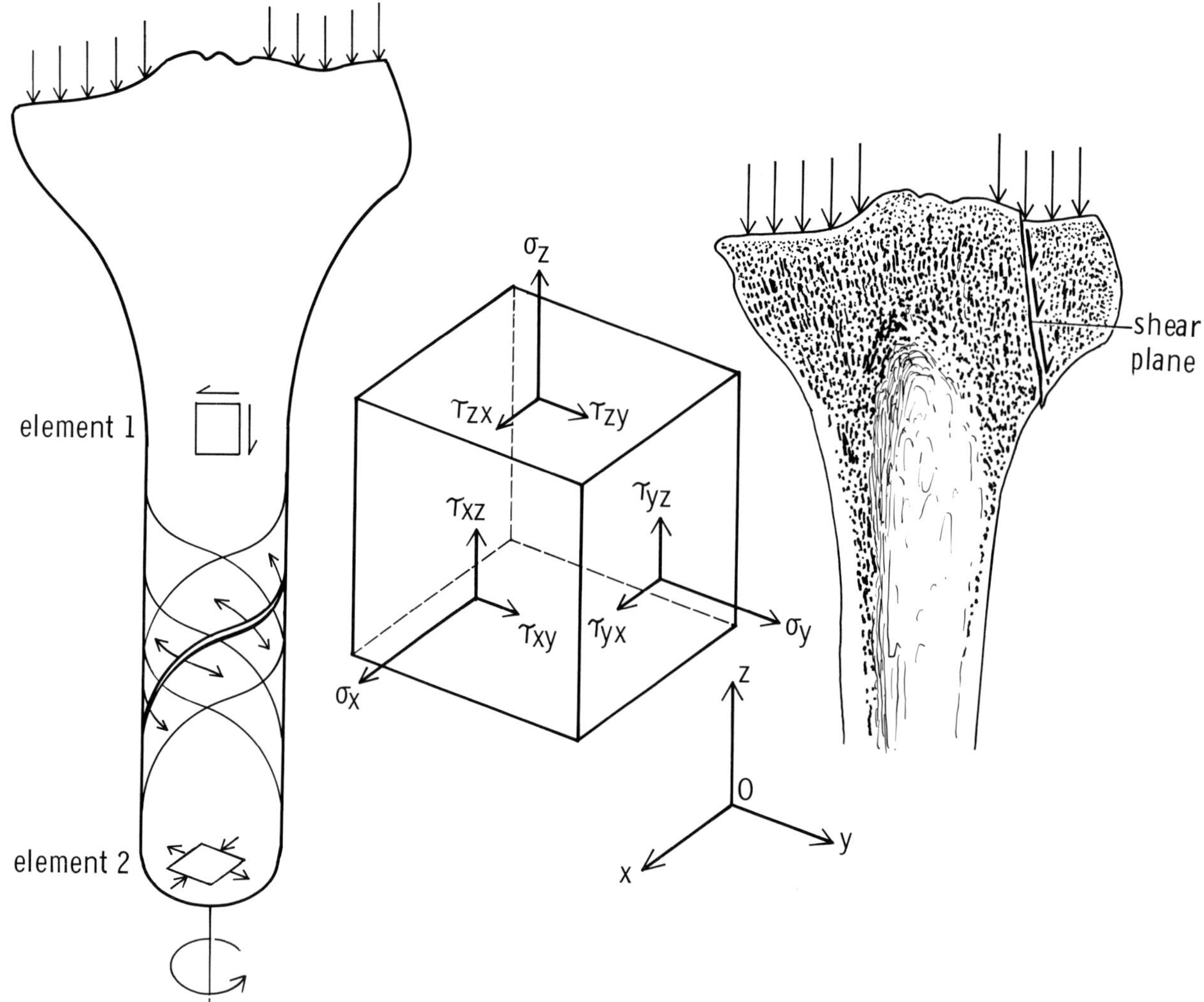

Figure 5–10. *The faces of a cubical element have a direct stress and two shear stresses acting. On the tibia, in torsion, principal shear planes are shown at element 1 and principal direct stress planes at element 2. Shear planes at different angles occur for loading of the upper tibial surface.*

In stress analyses of a section, the directions of the principal stresses can be determined at numerous points, and these points can then be connected to produce contour lines of the principal stresses. There is good evidence that the trabeculae in joints are aligned in the directions of the principal stresses. Usually, the density or strength of trabeculae in one direction is much greater than that in the other. The "high-density" direction will be aligned according to the maximum stress, usually compressive, whereas the "low-density" direction will be aligned according to the minimum stress (which could be either a low compressive stress or a tensile stress).

Consider the loading situation of Figure 5–7, in which, in addition to a longitudinal force and a bending moment on the femur, there is a force that twists the femur about its long axis. The effect of this force is to apply a torque to the femur. If an element is chosen with sides parallel to the bone, the torque produces *pure shear stresses* of equal magnitude on adjacent sides. These are the maximum shear stresses. An element at 45 degrees to the axes of the bone has pure tensile and compressive stresses as shown in Figure 5–10. The shear stresses on the faces of this element are zero and, therefore, the element is aligned in the direction of the maximum principal stresses. For the tibia as a whole, the lines of maximum stress are on 45 degree spirals, as shown in Figure 5–10. Most spiral fractures that are evident in long bones are likely to be the result of torsion, in which failure occurs by tension along the 45 degree lines.

Bending stresses usually refer to the stresses that exist in a beam of some sort as a result of loads or moments acting transversely to the long axis of the beam. A simple example is a circular bar which is fixed rigidly at one end, with a force *P* applied at its free end (Fig. 5–11). The overall effect of the force is

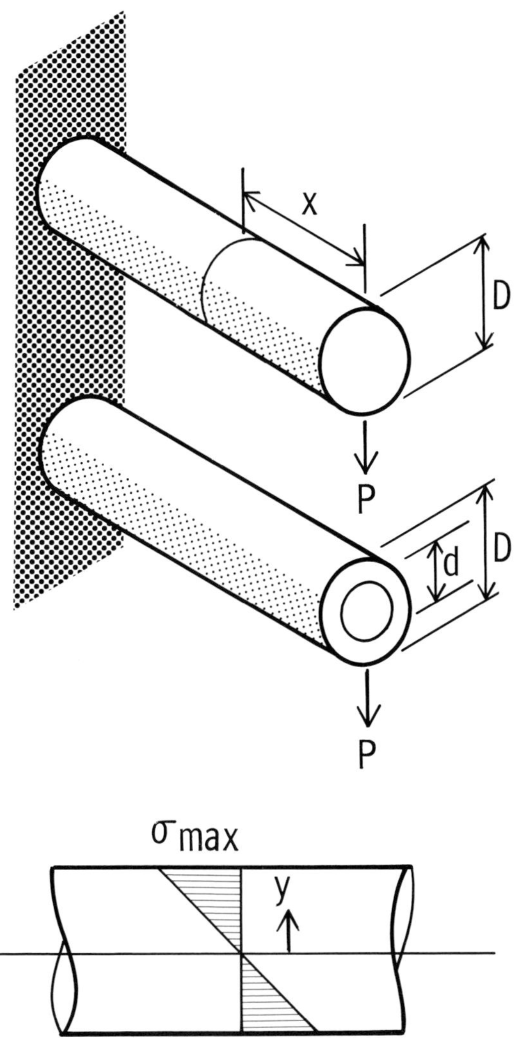

Figure 5–11. Bending stresses on a circular bar or tube.

to stretch the upper fibers and compress the lower fibers, whereas along the center, there will be no stress. The central line is called the neutral axis. At a section that is located at distance x from the free end, the bending moment is force times distance = $P \times x$. The stresses in the material at that section are calculated from the equation:

$$\sigma = \frac{M\ y}{I}$$

where M is the moment, y is the distance from the neutral axis, and I is the section modulus or moment of inertia of the section. Values of I for sections of different shape are given in standard engineering textbooks, but for a circular bar, $I = \pi\ d^4/64$. Most often, it is the maximum stress σ_{max} at the extreme fibers that is of interest, where $y = \frac{1}{2} D$. Substituting these various values in the stress equation gives:

$$\sigma = \frac{PxD\ (64)}{2\ \pi\ D^4} = \frac{32\ Px}{\pi\ D^3}$$

Thus, for a circular bar, the maximum stress is inversely proportional to the cube of the diameter. An increase in diameter by less than 30 per cent will halve the maximum stresses. For the round beam shown in Figure 5–11, the moment Px increases linearly with the distance from the suspended end, so that it is a maximum at the fixed end. For a uniform section and material, the stresses would be maximum at this point, and this would be the most likely area of breakage. For a tubular section, which is an approximation of the situation in most bones, the equation for I is:

$$I = \frac{\pi\ (D^4 - d^4)}{64}$$

Compare a solid bar of diameter D with a hollow bar of outer and inner diameters D and $\frac{1}{2}D$. For the same applied moment, the stresses in the hollow bar are only 7 per cent greater than in the solid bar. To determine I accurately for a bone, a graphic integration method can be used, as described by Minns and co-workers,[14] who applied it to the tibia. The shank of the femur can be regarded as a hollow circular tube.

Tests

Bending tests can be used to determine the strength of a bone or of a sample of material in the form of a bar. The type of bending that is used during the test is very important in obtaining meaningful and reproducible results. *Three-point bending* refers to a test in which the bar is supported at each end and loaded in the center (Fig. 5–2). The maximum bending moment is directly beneath the central load, but the stress pattern will be distorted owing to the localized load application. It is preferable, when possible, to use a *four-point bending* test, in which the load is applied at two points equidistant from the center. In this situation the central section is in pure and uniform bending, free from localized distortions. It is a general rule that stress patterns are complex in the vicinity of the loading point, but they are uniform at some distance from it.

Consider the example in Figure 5–12, in which the femur is subjected to a resultant force H on the femoral head. The problem is to analyze the stresses at section A. The first stage is to determine the compressive and bending components of force. The compressive force is H cos 50° and the bending force is H cos 40.° The *theory of superposition* states that

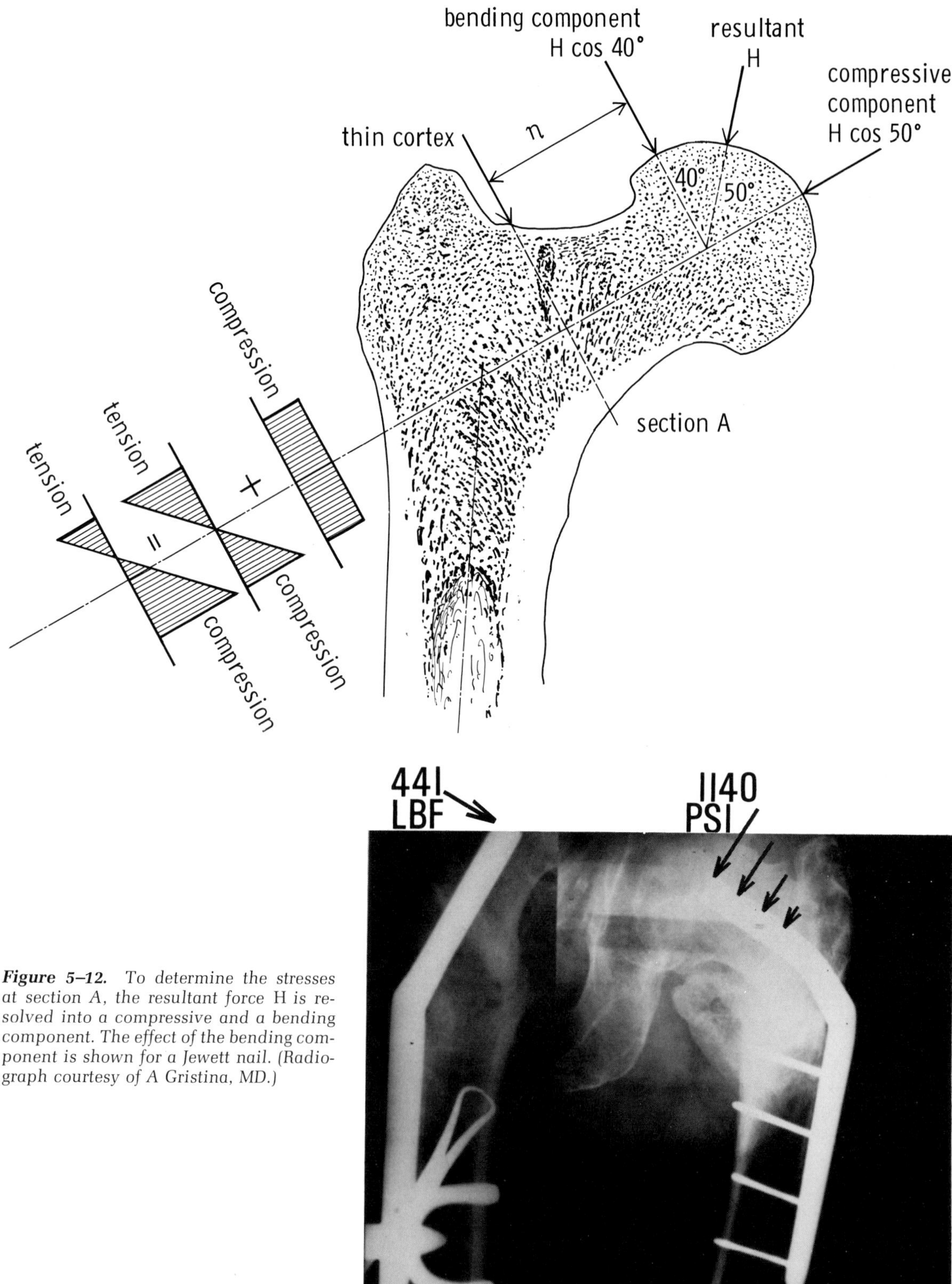

Figure 5–12. To determine the stresses at section A, the resultant force H is resolved into a compressive and a bending component. The effect of the bending component is shown for a Jewett nail. (Radiograph courtesy of A Gristina, MD.)

the total effect of separate forces and moments is the sum of the separate effects. The stresses due to each of the forces are determined separately and are then combined. Note that, as is frequently the case, the bending stresses in this example are greater than the direct stresses.

The effects of the bending component are illustrated for a Jewett nail, applied to stabilize an intertrochanteric fracture. Calculations have been made of the force needed to bend the nail, which, if applied at the tip, is 441 lbf (200 kgf, 1960 N), almost three times the body weight of an average man! It is notable that the face of the nail has not appreciably cut into the bone. Assuming a triangular stress distribution as shown, the stress (load per unit area) on the bone close to the tip is 1140 psi (7.9 N/mm^2), a considerable stress, but one that is resisted by the trabecular bone in the normal femoral head.[2]

One method of testing the stress of a hip prosthesis was used by Burstein and Wright.[5] It involved supporting the stem just beneath the collar and laterally at the tip, and applying a force V at the femoral head. A force analysis is shown in Figure 5–13. The tip support is assumed to be frictionless; thus, all the vertical force is supported under the collar. There will also be equal and opposite forces H at the collar and the tip. Taking moments about the collar gives the relation between V and H:

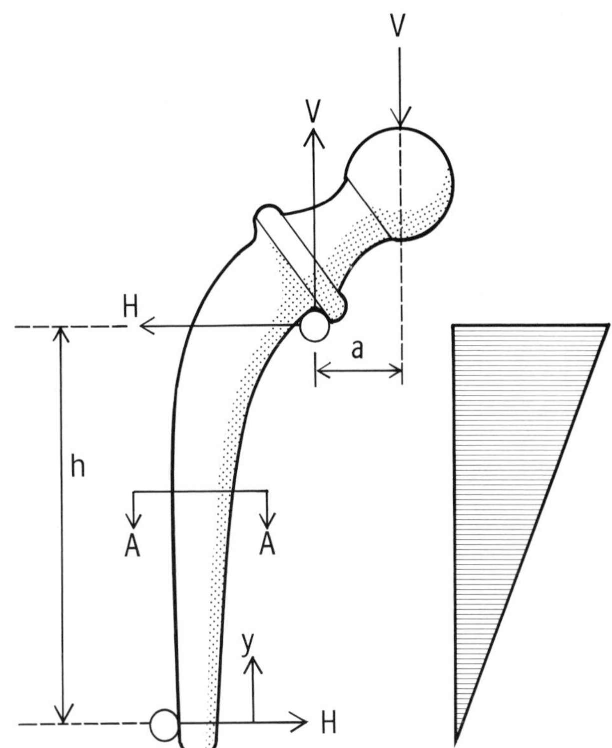

Figure 5–13. *A method for loading a femoral component to measure the strains in the material on the lateral surface.*

$$Va = Hh$$

$$H = V\frac{a}{h}$$

Considering any section A, and looking distally, the bending moment is Hy. Thus, the bending moment increases linearly from 0 at the tip to Hh just below the collar. Because of the geometry of most contemporary stems, the maximum tensile stresses on the lateral side will occur in the middle third, providing a useful test method.

If a stem is cemented into a femur, the system is called a *composite beam*. For a given bending moment M acting across a given section, the bone, the cement, and the stem will each carry a portion of the bending moment, the sum being M. The separate portions can be calculated using composite beam theory, which does require, however, that there be perfect bonding at the interfaces. An elastic property of each of the materials must be known — namely E, *Young's modulus of elasticity*, or more simply, the *elastic modulus*. E is a measure of the stiffness of the material. The ratios of the bending moments for each of the materials are: M (bone): M (cement): M (stem) = EI (Bone): EI (cement): EI (stem).

For the case in which the outer and inner bone diameters are 25 mm and 14 mm, and in which the stem diameter is 10 mm, the percentages of the bending moment that are carried are: bone, 69 per cent; cement, 1 per cent; stem, 30 per cent. Thus, the bone carries only 69 per cent of the bending moment and will consequently be stressed only 69 per cent of its normal level. The cement layer carries a negligible portion of the bending moment but serves to transmit shearing stresses along the stem-cement and cement-bone interfaces. This situation is typical of stem-cement–cortical bone systems. Analysis of the proximal part of the femur (or of any site) in which the geometry is complex and in which cancellous bone is also involved is quite complicated. Both experimental and finite-element analytic methods are applicable in this situation.

Experimental methods using strain gauge techniques have the advantage that actual bone and prosthetic specimens can be used but the practical limitations that each bone is different and that the strain can be measured at only a finite number of locations. Analytic methods, on the other hand, can never reproduce the actual situation in terms of material properties, geometry, and boundary conditions. These methods have the advantage that parametric analysis can be utilized to assess the effect of changing any one variable.

To investigate the strains in the bone and the stem before and after inserting a hip prosthesis, Oh and Harris[16] used a strain gauge study. They found that the longitudinal strain in the femoral neck was only about 10 per cent of normal and that this was increased by only 5 to 10 per cent if the prosthesis had a collar. This finding has been confirmed by

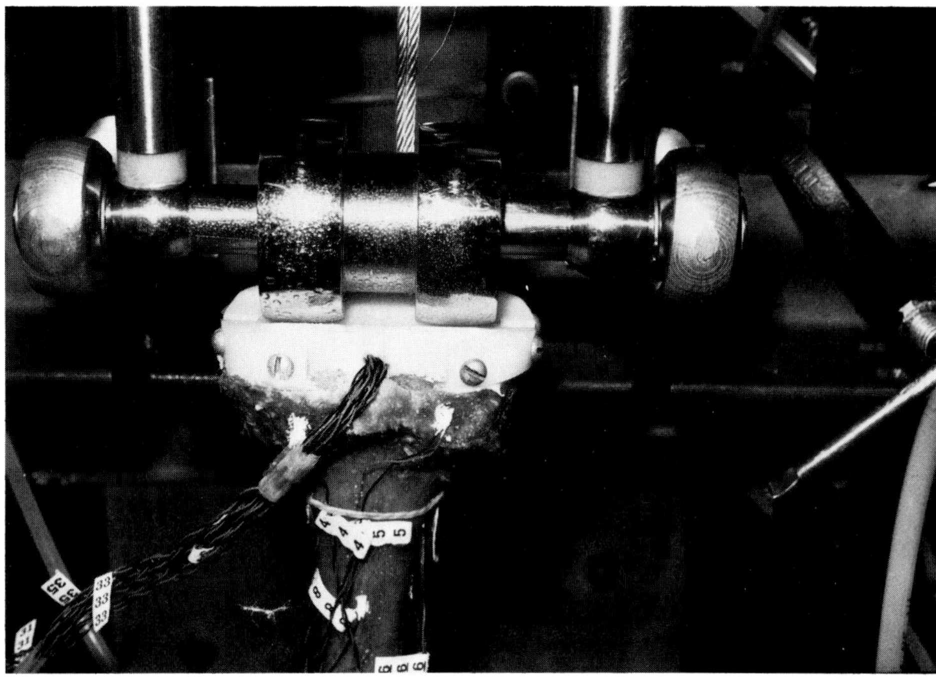

Figure 5–14. *Method for measuring the strains on the tibia and on a tibial component under different loading conditions. The results are relevant to the design of knee prostheses. (Reilly, Walker, and Ben-Dov; unpublished data.)*

others using experimental and theoretic methods, and the additional information has been obtained that the tensile stresses in a circumferential direction (hoop stresses) are higher than normal. Both of these factors are probably responsible for the osteoporosis that occurs in the proximal femoral neck–calcar area in many cases a number of years following hip replacement.

An example of a strain gauge study on a knee joint is shown in Figure 5–14. The aim of the study is to measure strains in the normal tibia at different angles of flexion and loading situations, and then to determine the strain patterns after the insertion of a prosthetic component. The component variables include the presence or absence of a metal support for the plastic, the complete or partial contact on the upper surface, and the stem length. The information is important initially for determining the stresses in the materials and predicting possible fixation failure. For example, excessive bending stresses in the acrylic cement will be deleterious. In the long run, if the strains on certain areas of bone, particularly proximal segments, are significantly lower than normal, osteoporosis could result. The latter situation might apply, for example, to the use of long metallic stems, in which much of the load at the upper surface would be transmitted directly to the cortex, bypassing the proximal cancellous bone.

There have been many finite-element analysis studies of the hip, and more recently of the knee. In general terms, the method of investigation is as follows. The geometry is drawn, and the structures are divided into small elements in the shape of squares, rectangles, or triangles. (For a three-dimensional analysis, cubes or other solid shapes are used.) The element size can be made smaller in

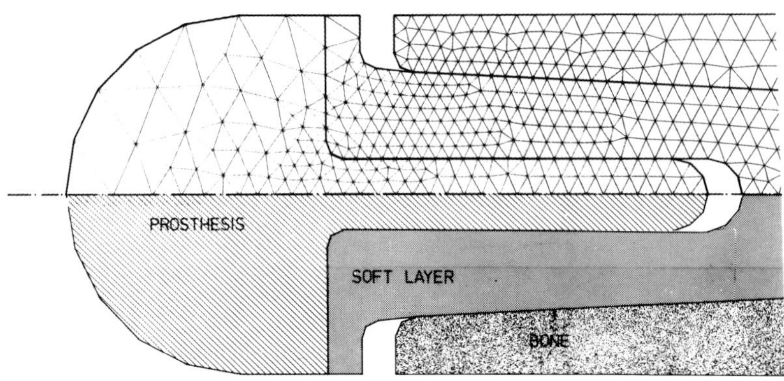

Figure 5–15. *A finite element model of a particular design of finger prosthesis. (From Huiskes R, et al: 1979.)*

critical areas (Fig. 5–15). Geometric and material properties are specified for each element, and the external forces are defined. The analysis yields the stress and strain components at each element and along each interface. The problem then is to determine the significance of these components, and to correlate them with known bone properties in the case of normal joints, or with prosthetic design in the case of artificial joints. Some parts of the stress information will be of more importance than others. In a total hip prosthesis (Fig. 5–16), the tensile stress on the lateral surface of the stem (*A*) is important with regard to stem breakage. After a long period of time, stems frequently drift into a more varus position; this is due to the bending effect of the force on the femoral head, producing high compressive stresses on the cement (*B*) in combination with the low compressive stresses in the neck-calcar area (*C*), which are weakening the bone. Tensile stresses located laterally (*D*) will likely exceed the strength of the cement-bone bond. Sinkage is another possible complication of prosthetic surgery, indicated by tensile stresses in the distal cement (*E*) and shear stresses at the cement-bone and cement-stem interfaces (*F*). Around the acetabular component, high compressive stresses at *G* and tensile stresses at *H* can lead to migration of the prosthesis. As a general rule, the stresses in the materials and at the interfaces should be within their known strength limit.

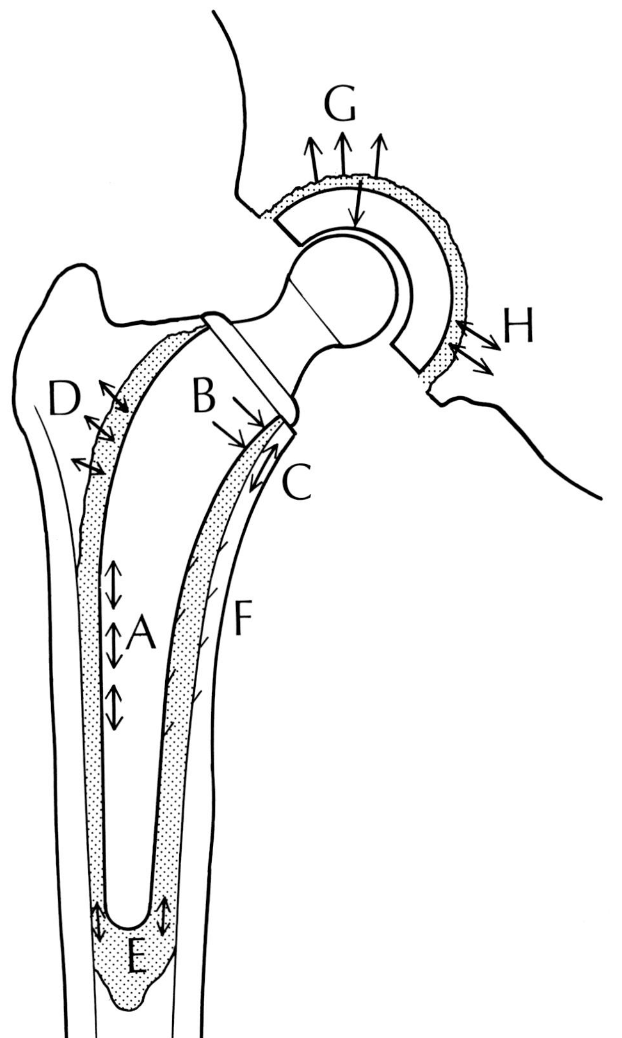

Figure 5–16. *Areas in a stem type of total hip prosthesis that are known to be of clinical significance.*

Stresses on Normal and Artificial Joint Surfaces

As noted earlier, the forces across joints are usually transmitted over a large surface area. This clearly reduces the force per unit area on the cartilage and the trabecular bone, provides stability to the joint, and encourages fluid film lubrication. The surface stress patterns are determined by the loads that are acting on the articulation, the relative geometry of the joint surfaces, and the elastic properties of the materials. In general, the greater the congruity and the lower the elastic modulus of the materials (i.e., the materials are more deformable), the greater the contact area and the lower the contact stresses.

Greenwald and Haynes[9] determined that in the acetabulum, the load-bearing area was concentrated around the periphery and on the anterior and posterior horns at loads up to about one fourth of body weight, but, at higher loads, spread to include the remaining areas of the acetabular surface. The load-bearing areas on the femoral head were obviously equivalent to those on the acetabulum. This mechanism of load-bearing would impart a "springiness" to the joint, reducing the impact forces.

The knee is more complicated than the hip because of the presence of the menisci (Fig. 5–17). The menisci are clearly in contact with both joint surfaces, but whether or not they are weight-bearing has remained a controversial issue. Recently, however, it has been shown that at light loads, the menisci transmit most of the force. As the force is increased during weight-bearing activities, the load-bearing includes more and more of the exposed cartilaginous surfaces, but the menisci still transmit as much as half the load.[3, 21, 27] As in the hip, there will be a certain "springiness" effect under direct loads and a similar effect at the extremes of motion. Owing to the mobility of the menisci, transverse rotations are possible without reduction in contact area. Also, the varus-valgus stability of the knee is enhanced because the loads are carried directly to each side.

Each of the joints can be considered in a similar fashion. Generally the articular surfaces are almost congruent, such that most of the available surface area of the concave side of the joint comes into contact with the opposite side under load-bearing,

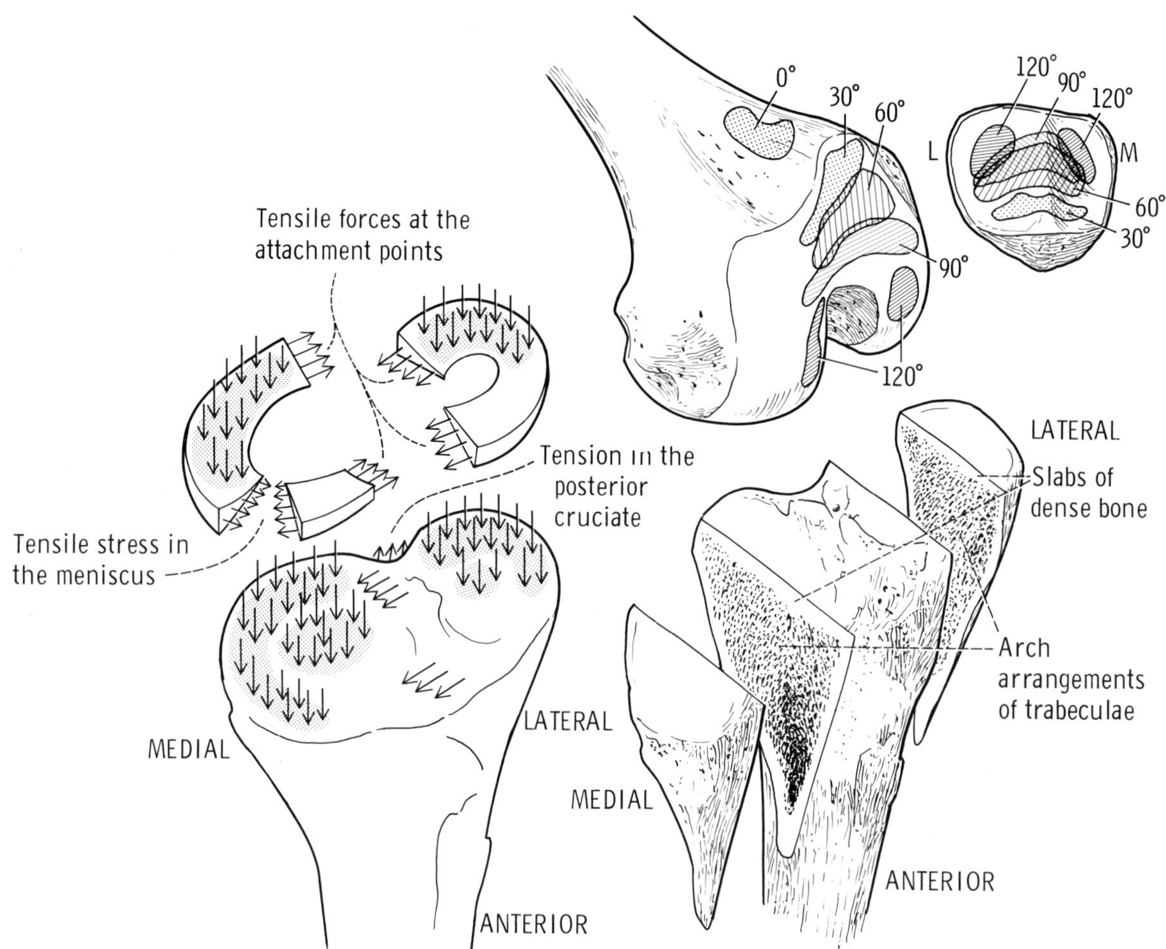

Figure 5–17. *The stresses across the knee joint during typical load-bearing activities.*

but the slight lack of congruity ensures some force damping. Spreading of the load and force damping, which occur at the extremes of the motion, appear to be accomplished by "menisci" in the glenohumeral, hip, knee, and other joints.

Various types of artificial joints, however, are only partially conforming. Because of this configuration and the hardness of the materials, they will have only small areas of contact (e.g., the condylar replacement knee prosthesis). The contact areas can be determined experimentally by coating the plastic surfaces with a colored medium (e.g., engineers' blue), loading the prostheses, then measuring the contact patches. Alternatively, hertzian contact theory can be used, which requires knowledge of the geometry, the elastic properties of the materials, and the loads. The contact areas have been determined for several contemporary metal-plastic prostheses, ranging from the relatively conforming designs, such as the Geometric and Freeman-Swanson prostheses, to the nonconforming designs, such as the Anametric and Modular prostheses. In flexion of the knee, in which the stresses are greater owing to tighter femoral curvature, at a load of three times body weight, the contact areas ranged from 40 to 400 mm^2, giving average stresses of from 5 to 56 N/mm^2. As the stresses approach and exceed the yield limit of the material (in the region of 20 to 30 N/mm^2), *permanent deformation* of the plastic surfaces will occur as well as an increase in wear rate due to the localized stress failure of the material.

Friction and Wear

When two loaded surfaces are in relative motion, there is a resistance to the motion, called *friction*. The friction forces are due to molecular, adhesive, or plowing interactions at the localized contact points. The *friction coefficient* is defined as the shear resistance divided by the normal (i.e., compressive) force: $\mu = F \div W$. For metals and plastics, the friction coefficients are usually between 0.1 and 0.3. However, if two surfaces are smooth and a thin film of fluid is between them, the resistance to sliding can be exceedingly small. In healthy synovial joints, the friction coefficient is in the range of about 0.01 and 0.001, which is due to the presence of a complex lubrication mechanism involving fluid films of synovial fluid, fluid exchange in and out of the cartilage, and a macromolecular boundary protection at the high points of the surfaces. The friction coefficient between polished metal and polyethylene in a joint is between 0.1 and 0.05, still quite low, although this can increase by several times if acrylic particles are present. Cobalt-chrome on cobalt-chrome, used in McKee-Farrar hips and in Guepar knees, has a coefficient of 0.15 and an extremely low wear rate, probably due to the adsorption of proteins on the metallic surfaces.

Wear is defined as the removal of material from one or both surfaces. It can be of three types: adhesive, at the localized contact points, which can produce small particles; abrasive, in which the rough points on a hard material cut into the soft material, or in which a third material is interposed between the two surfaces (an example being fragments of acrylic cement in a metal-plastic prosthesis); and fatigue, in which high surface stresses lead to microcracking and eventual release of large particles. Penetration of the surface due to permanent deformation can contribute to wearing out of a prosthetic component. The penetration rate in typical metal-plastic artificial hip and knee joints is about 1 mm over a 10 to 20 year period.

MATERIALS

Definitions and Properties

The mechanical properties of materials are characterized according to various standard tests. The most common test is stress-strain, obtained by stretching a sample of the material at a prescribed rate. *Stress* is a load divided by the original area, and *strain* is change in length divided by the original length. For very deformable materials, which stretch a great deal, stress at a certain level can refer to load divided by the actual area. Basic stress-strain graphs are shown in Figure 5–18. Graph *A* displays a linear relation with fracture at *F*. Strain is proportional to stress up to the fracture point and this is a *linearly elastic material*, where the *modulus* of *elasticity* is defined as stress divided by strain. If the material fractures at the end of its linear portion, it is termed a *brittle* material, examples of which are glass or ceramics. The opposite of brittle is *ductile*, illustrated in curve *B*. In this condition the material is linear up to point *Y*, the *yield point*, where it begins to stretch a great deal. After this point, only a small amount of additional force is needed to cause large strains, and finally the material fractures at point *F*. The segment of the curve up to point *Y* is the *elastic region*, which means that the deformation disappears on removal of the load. Beyond *Y* is the *plastic region*: If the load is removed, the deformation returns as on the thin line on the graph, leaving a *permanent deformation* or *set*. Examples of ductile materials are metals such as *stainless steel* and polymers such as polyethylene. *Cobalt-chrome alloy* and *titanium alloy* are ductile but not to the same extent as stainless steel. Even bone exhibits some ductility.[4] Silicone rubber is not ductile, even though it elongates several hundred per cent before breaking, because at any point up to its breakage, the material snaps back to its original shape. Curve *C* is an example of a *strain stiffening* material. As stress is applied, the slope of the stress-strain curve increases, meaning that the effective modulus of elasticity increases with strain. Some materials, such as tendon and ligament, exhibit a *toe* beyond which the slope does not greatly increase. Fracture is preceded by a "yield" zone, in which failure of different parts of the material occurs. Fiber-reinforced materials typically reveal this behavior.

The *energy absorbed* in deforming a sample of material is equal to the area under the stress-strain curve times the volume of material. Thus, in a joint, even though the articular cartilage may have a large strain (deflection divided by original length), the energy absorbed by the cancellous bone will be greater because of its much larger volume. Stainless steel has a high energy-absorbing capability because of its plasticity, although it may permanently bend (see Jewett nail in Fig. 5–12). It can be seen from Figure 5–18 that once stainless steel is in the plastic region, the area under the curve is large. *Toughness* is a measure of the energy-absorbing capacity of a material under an *impact load*. The standard impact test involves striking a notched bar with a swinging pendulum and measuring the energy absorbed by the diminution in the subsequent swing of the pendulum.

Some of these material properties are illustrated by the samples shown in Figure 5–18, which were all tested in direct compression. The tall cylinder of acrylic (left) has buckled and undergone tensile failure at the center of the left side. Internal cracks indicate failure in shear. However, the short column of acrylic (second from left) has been deformed permanently without failure. The material has passed its yield point and is into its plastic region, with permanent deformation. Third from the left is a short cylinder of orthopedic acrylic cement, which has also yielded, but which has suffered tensile failure on a longitudinal line. The properties of acrylic within bone cement are not the same as solid dense acrylic, mainly because of the multitude of voids in the material, reducing the tensile strength and the amount of plastic deformation before fracture. The specimen on the right, high-molecular-

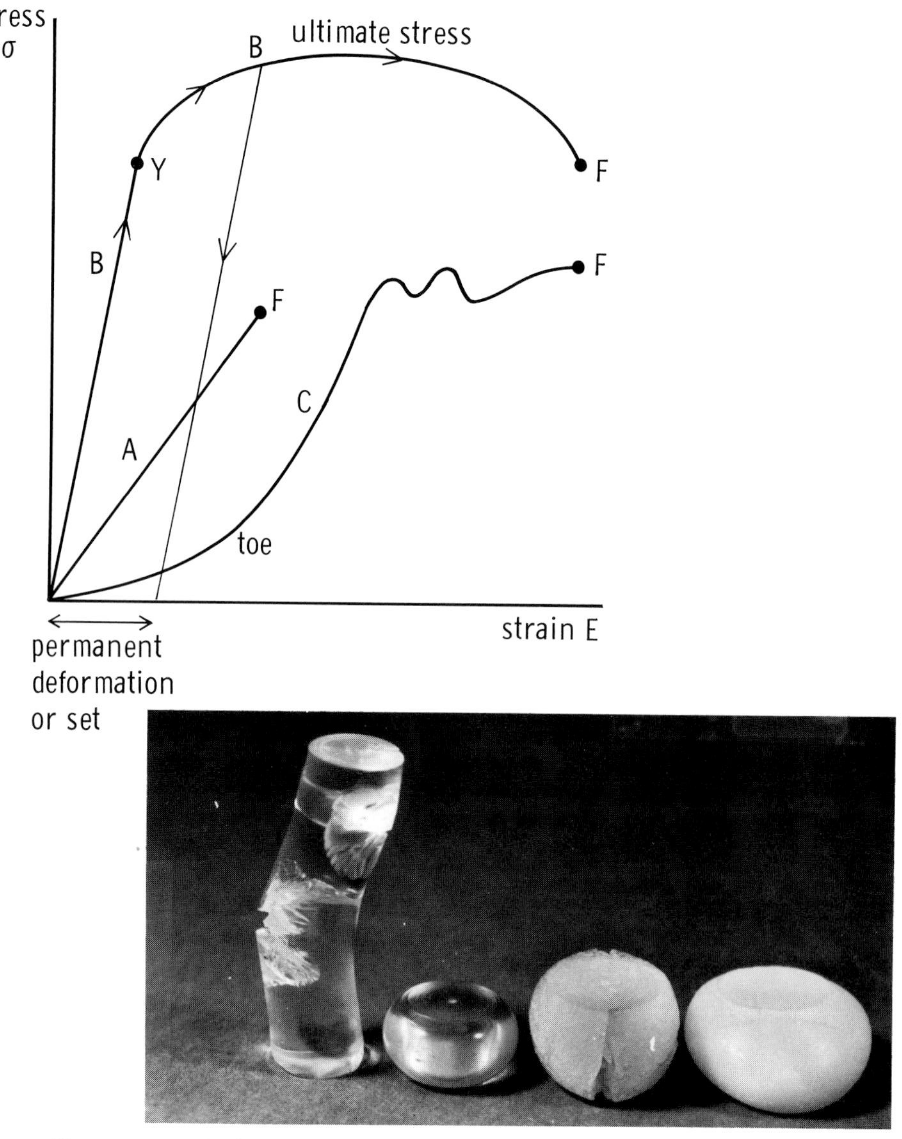

Figure 5–18. *Stress-strain curves illustrating different properties of materials.*

weight polyethylene, is capable of a great deal of permanent deformation (often called *cold flow*) before failure. Cold flow is often regarded as "failure"; although it implies that the material has been overstressed, cold flow is far preferable to fracture.

For all the materials in the body, the effect of time must be considered; the stress-strain curve and the apparent modulus of elasticity depend upon the rate of loading. Consider a specimen of articular cartilage subjected to a given compressive stress, or a ligament subjected to the sudden application and maintenance of a tensile stress. A graph of deflection versus time (Fig. 5–19) will show an initial deflection followed by a gradually increasing deflection called *creep*. An asymptotic limit will generally be reached. When the stress is removed, there will be a rapid recovery of part of the deflection and an eventual return to zero deflection with time. If these specimens are now subjected to a stress and the deflection is maintained at a constant level, there will be a fall-off in the stress with time, which is termed *stress relaxation*.

Such properties are characteristic of *viscoelastic* materials. Conceptually their behavior can be visualized by mechanical analogues. A spring represents perfect elasticity and a dashpot represents perfect viscosity. A combination of these two elements is viscoelastic. The model that most closely expresses body materials is a spring in series with a parallel spring and dashpot. This is called the *three-element model*.

Bone is almost elastic in nature in that its stress-strain properties vary only slightly with the rate of loading. This is probably due to its high content of hydroxyapatite bound with a dense collagenous matrix with relatively little fluid content. Articular cartilage, on the other hand, is strongly viscoelastic owing to its high fluid content. At high strain rates, such as occur in walking, cartilage exhibits primarily elastic behavior because the fluid has insufficient time to flow in or out, except perhaps at the bearing surfaces. Under slow or sustained loading, however, fluid flows from high to low pressure, and the deformation increases considerably, until the elasticity of the collagen matrix supports most of the load. In a similar way, ligaments and tendons are primarily elastic in behavior for the rates of loading encountered during activity. However, the elasticity is not linear; the initial stiffness is low up to the point at which the waviness in the collagen fibers has become aligned, after which the stiffness is high. The forces necessary to rupture ligaments can be high. For example, in the knee joint, rupturing forces of the cruciate and collateral ligaments are in the range of 400 to 800 N.[25] However, because of the small volume of the ligaments, their energy-absorbing capability is low, making them susceptible to rupture under high-energy impact conditions. Synovial fluid is mainly viscous but when present in thin films, it does display an elastic behavior under rapid loading conditions owing to the macromolecular constitution of hyaluronic acid–protein complex.

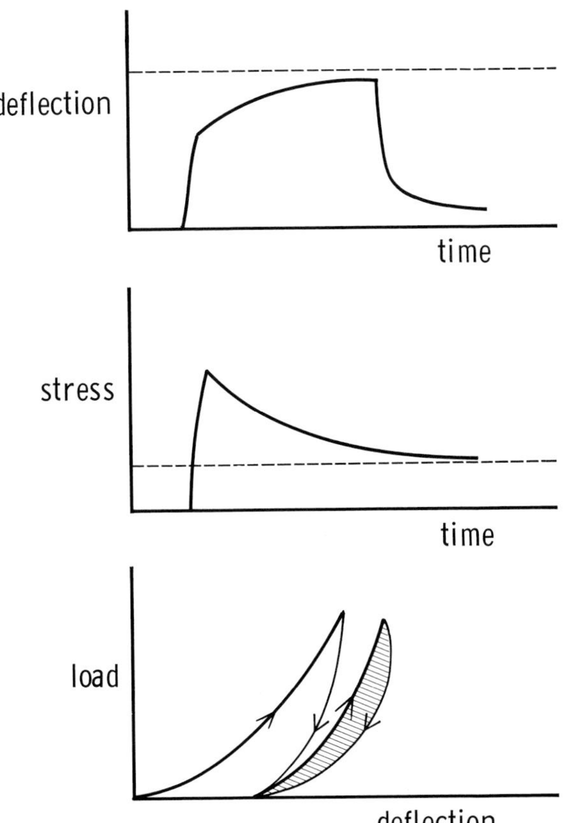

Figure 5–19. *Graphs illustrating the time dependence of material properties. Top, Creep after an initial stress is applied. Center, Stress relaxation after an initial deflection is applied. Bottom, Hysteresis loops for cyclic load applied to a viscoelastic material.*

Another important characteristic of material is *isotropy*. An *isotropic* material is one in which the mechanical properties are equal in all directions. The metals and plastics used in artificial joints reveal isotropy. However, this is not the case for the materials that constitute joints.

Since the classic work of Koch, it has been generally accepted that the density and mechanical properties of cancellous bone are demonstrated in proportion to the stresses that are imposed. The trabeculae carry a uniform stress regardless of their location. This explains the orientation of the trabeculae in the directions of principal stress and the high trabecular density evident at sites at which the maximum stress density occurs. However, there is evidence to suggest that trabecular bone can be subject to *fatigue failure* under normal stresses over an extended period of time. Microfractures are believed to occur at locations of stress concentration in the complex osseous architecture and to aid in energy absorption. The resulting callus will lead to local trabecular thickening, a situation that increases the area's ability to resist the stress.

Fatigue failure is a well-known phenomenon in metals. The failure of total hip stems is an example of such fatigue. Assume that the yield stress of the material for a single loading is Y. If the material is repeatedly subjected to stresses just below Y, it will fail after a certain number of cycles. The lower the value of applied stress, the greater the number of cycles that will be needed for failure to occur. The stress at which an indefinite number of cycles will not induce failure is called the *endurance limit*. This is an important property of any material that is to be used in total joint replacements, and it should represent the maximum design stress. Local defects in a material will naturally reduce the endurance limit, so that inspection standards in certain joint replacements must be rigorous. Any scratch, corner, or hole will lead to *stress concentration*. Implant designs must avoid stress-concentrating features in order to protect the component as well as the adjacent cement or bone.

ARTIFICIAL JOINTS

Indications

The most common surgical indication for joint replacement is severe pain, but, almost invariably, there is also a serious loss of function due to mechanical disruption of the articular structures. Destructive changes can include erosion of the cartilaginous surfaces, distortion of the normal osseous anatomy, breakage or attenuation of ligaments, and weakening of the muscles. A general surgical principle is that the joint replacement should substitute for only the articular deficiencies. In the knee, for example, there are six modes of loading with respect to the axis of the tibia: direct compression, anteroposterior (AP) forces, mediolateral forces, varus-valgus moments, transverse rotational moments, and flexion-extension moments. In most patients, a condylar replacement is satisfactory, with slight "dishing" of the tibial component and preservation of the posterior or both cruciate ligaments. Even in the absence of cruciate integrity, exaggerated "dishing" can be sufficient to absorb the AP forces. Only exceptionally is it necessary to incorporate varus-valgus stability into the prostheses.

Historical Aspects

The surgical treatment of arthritis and other disabling conditions of joints began at the end of the nineteenth century, when Gluck in 1891 reported his experience with implantation of various joints; he even used a cement made from pumice for fixing prosthetic stems into the medullary canal. Early in the 1900s, Jones utilized gold foil to separate the roughened surfaces of arthritic joints. These two basic concepts, replacement of one or both sides of the joint and interposition of a material, have been used in one form or another up to the present day.

A spectacular example of interposition was the hip cup of Smith-Petersen, who began this work in 1923. From 1937, the cups were made from cobalt-chrome alloy, and, in many thousands of patients, the results were generally satisfactory and enduring.

The success of joint replacements was hampered by the difficulty in fixing the components to the bones. In the 1920s and 1930s, Groves and Bohlman experimented with various replacements for the femoral head. As early as 1938, Wiles performed six total hip replacements. In these replacements, the femoral component resembled a hip nail with a ball for the head, while the acetabular socket was a metallic shell; although both components were screwed to the underlying bone, loosening and breakage unfortunately occurred. In 1947, Judet began implanting a femoral head replacement made initially from acrylic. Many hundreds of these prostheses were used subsequently in various medical centers, and although in most cases the initial results were good, these prostheses soon deteriorated owing to breakage or loosening and settling of the device. It was not until 1951 that successful femoral head replacements were developed, notably the Austin Moore and the Thompson prostheses. These were made from cast cobalt-chrome alloy, and consisted of a femoral ball on an intramedullary stem. They are still used extensively today. McKee's metal-to-metal total hip prosthesis was utilized from 1950 to 1960, incorporating screws for fixation, but many of these loosened.

It was clear that the problem of adequate fixation of prostheses was related to transmission of the forces from the device to the bone without incurring interfacial micromovements or areas of excessively high or low stresses, all of which could lead to bone resorption. One method of disseminating the forces over a wider area was to cement the components in place. Apart from Gluck, the first recorded attempt at cement fixation was that of Haboush in 1951. This investigator used self-curing methyl methacrylate, a substance then utilized for the repair of skull defects.

Current Prostheses

Charnley began his work with methyl methacrylate in 1959 in England. From 1960 onward, he used this material for cementing in his total hip prosthesis, utilizing a stainless steel femoral component and a polytetrafluoroethylene acetabular component; he later changed the acetabular material to high-molecular-weight polyethylene. The vast majority of total joint replacements used today consist of cobalt-chrome alloy or stainless steel for one component, high-molecular-weight polyethylene for the other component, and methyl methacrylate cement, cured in situ, for fixation. It has been estimated that currently (1980) in the United States, about 80,000 total hip replacements, 40,000 total knee replacements, and 10,000 replacements of other joints are implanted annually.[11] Some typical examples of prostheses are shown in Figure 5–20.

The total hip stem has rounded corners to avoid stress concentrations, and a "tear drop" shape to enhance its bond to the adjacent cement. The collar is intended to impart some direct force to the neck of the bone but its role is controversial. If the overhang of the femoral head (or neck angle) is anatomic, the bending moment on the stem-bone composite is high. If the overhang is small, greater abductor forces are required, and there is a higher risk of dislocation.

Surface replacements are being used with increasing frequency, especially in younger patients. Although less resection of bone is necessary with these replacements, fundamental problems such as the adequacy of long-term fixation and the avoidance of femoral head fracture or bony resorption have yet to be solved. Recently, "floating cup" hip replacements have been introduced; these are apparently associated with slower penetration of the acetabulum, and can readily be revised to a total hip prosthesis if necessary.

The "variable axis" knee allows an axis of rotation along any line parallel to the surface of the upper tibia, providing complete rotatory freedom.

The metallic container for the tibial component and the intramedullary stem are intended for long-term fixation.

Elbow joint replacement can be of three types: a fixed hinge, a loose hinge, and a surface replacement (Fig. 5–20). A loose hinge prosthesis allows a proportion of the force or moment to be carried by muscles and ligaments. Replacement of the shoulder can be provided by either a nonlinked surface prosthesis or a linked hinge design. The latter can be given enhanced motion before impingement by utilizing a double ball-in-socket arrangement. Fixation of the glenoid component is a major problem encountered in all shoulder replacements.

The success of joint replacement is measured in various ways, including relief of pain, adequacy of function, and longevity of the prosthetic component, but even current devices are far from perfect. Many designs, such as those for the hip, the elbow, and the knee, use a cemented intramedullary stem for fixation. Fatigue fracture of the prosthetic stem has not been uncommon in the hip, owing to the bending stresses generated by the large repetitive forces (three to four times body weight) in combination with the overhang of the femoral head. A typical failure mode exists when the distal part of the stem is well cemented in the bony tube but the proximal support is inadequate. The upper part of the stem is then effectively cantilevered.

In the hinge types of knee joint replacement,

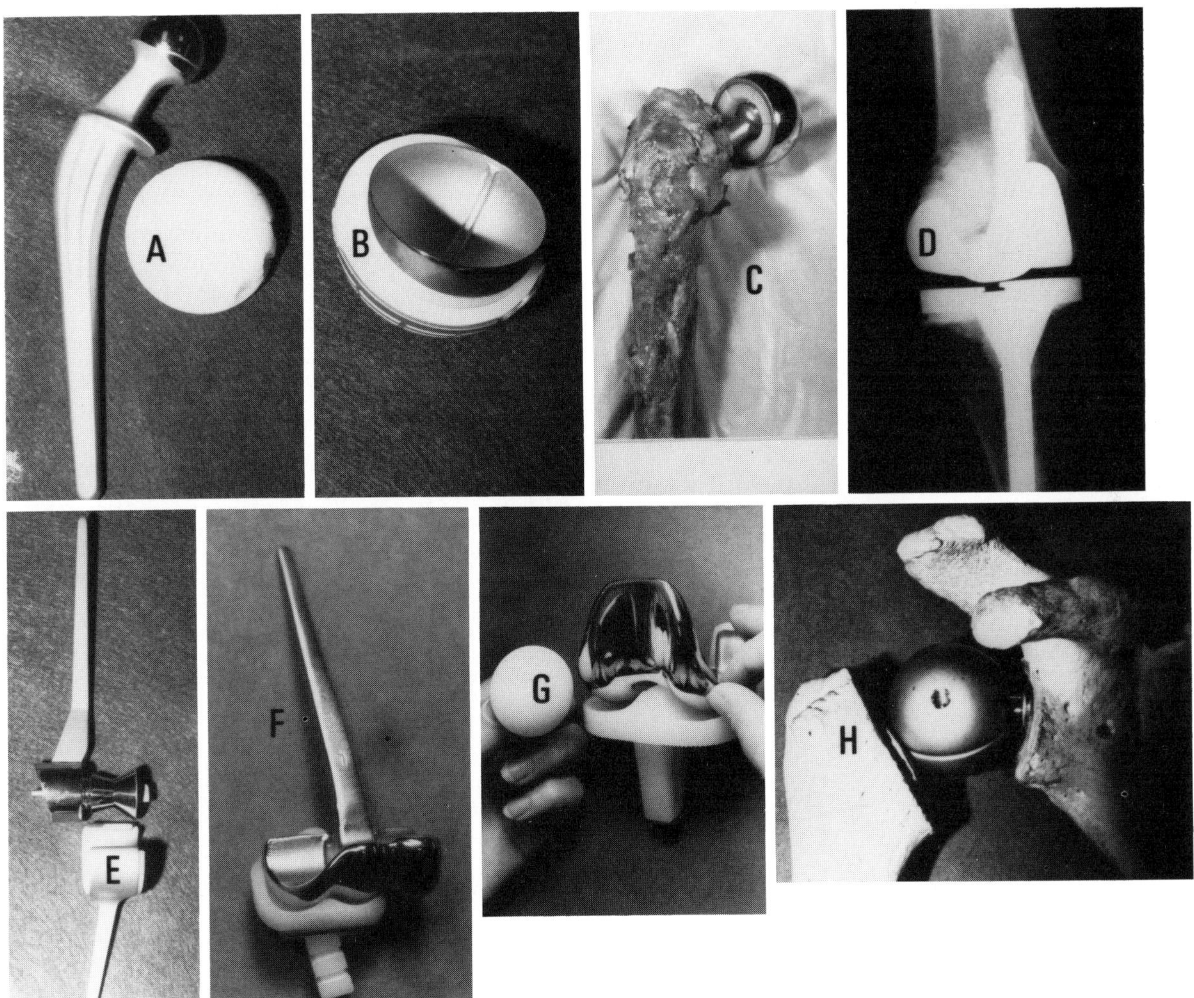

Figure 5–20. *Examples of present-day artificial joints.*
A *HD-2 Total Hip.*
B *Aufranc Surface Replacement.*
C *Bateman Femoral Prosthesis.*
D *"Variable Axis" Knee.*
E *Mayo Elbow.*
F *Ewald Elbow.*
G *Total Condylar Knee.*
H *Trispherical Shoulder.*

fractures of the intramedullary stems have occurred, probably due to a varus or valgus "thrust" in most cases. It is known that in the knee, the line of action of the force is disposed to the medial side of the joint; if the cement or bony support on this side is lacking, a cantilever effect can again result.

A number of methods have been employed in order to reduce the stresses, including the reduction of the offset distance of the femoral head, the provision of a stem of optimum thickness, the placement of the stem in valgus, and the improvement of techniques of cement fixation. The utilization of cement that is closely interdigitated with bone and stem reduces the stresses in the metal and thus improves stress transmission to the bone. This technique, together with the recent introduction of "super-strong" alloys, should considerably reduce some of the potential problems of joint replacement. However, loosening of prosthetic components remains the most frequent and serious of the postoperative problems, which is fundamentally related to the lack of a reliable method for fixation of the prosthesis. Loosening in either cemented or uncemented components leads to resorption of bone around all or part of the interface. Although heat necrosis from the cement or the chemical effect of monomers may contribute to prosthetic loosening, excessive compression or tensile stresses, coupled with interfacial micromovements, appear to be the most important reasons for this complication.

REFERENCES

1. Berme N, Paul JP, Purves WK: A biomechanical analysis of the metacarpophalangeal joint. J Biomech *10*:409, 1977.
2. Brown TD, Ferguson AB Jr: Spatial and directional variations in the mechanical properties of the cancellous bone of the human proximal femur. Pittsburgh, University of Pittsburgh, Department of Orthopaedic Surgery, 1978.
3. Burke DL, Ahmed AM, Miller J: A biomechanical study of partial and total medial meniscectomy of the knee. Proceedings of the Orthopaedic Research Society, Dallas, Texas, February 1978.
4. Burstein AH, Currey JD, Frankel VH, Reilly DT: The ultimate properties of bone tissue. J Biomech *5*:35, 1972.
5. Burstein AH, Wright JM: Mechanical performance of three new materials in total hip stems. 25th Annual Meeting of the Orthopaedic Research Society, San Francisco, February 1979.
6. Chao EYS, Opgrande JD, Axmear FE: Three-dimensional force analysis of finger joints in selected isometric hand functions. J Biomech *9*:387, 1976.
7. Crowninshield RD, Johnston RC, Andrews JG, Brand RA: A biomechanical investigation of the human hip. J Biomech *11*:75, 1978.
8. Davis PR: Some significant aspects of normal upper limb functions. Joint Replacement of the Upper Limb. London, Institution of Mechanical Engineers, 1977, p 1.
9. Greenwald AS, Haynes DW: Weight-bearing areas in the human hip joint. J Bone Joint Surg *54B*:157, 1972.
10. Grood ES, Noyes FR, Miller EH: Comparative mechanical properties of the medial collateral and capsular structures of the knee. Proceedings of the Orthopaedic Research Society, Las Vegas, Nevada, February 1977.
11. Hori RY, Lewis JL, Zimmerman JR, Compere CL: The number of total joint replacements in the United States. Clin Orthop *132*:46, 1978.
12. Hue FC, An KN, Chao, EYS: Three-dimensional force analysis of the elbow under isometric functions. Proceedings of the Biomechanics Symposium, American Society of Mechanical Engineers, New York, 1977.
13. Huiskes R, Heck JV, Walker PS, Greene DJ: A three-dimensional stress analysis of a new intramedullary fixation system. Proceedings of the Orthopaedic Research Society, Las Vegas, Nevada, February 1977.
14. Minns RJ, Bremble GR, Campbell J: The geometrical properties of the human tibia. J Biomech *8*:253, 1975.
15. Nicol AC: Elbow joint prosthesis design: biomechanical aspects. Thesis, Department of Bioengineering, University of Strathclyde, Glasgow, Scotland, 1977.
16. Oh I, Harris WH: Proximal strain distribution in the loaded femur. J Bone Joint Surg *60A*:75, 1978.
17. Paul JP: Forces transmitted by joints in the human body. Proceedings of the Institution of Mechanical Engineers. Conference on Total Hip Replacement, London, 1966.
18. Paul JP: Force actions transmitted in the knee of normal subjects and by prosthetic joint replacements. *In* Total Knee Replacement. Proceedings of the Conference of the Institution of Mechanical Engineers. London, Mechanical Engineering Publications, 1975, p 92.
19. Poppen NK, Walker PS: Forces at the glenohumeral joint in abduction. Clin Orthop *135*:165, 1978.
20. Reilly DT, Martens M: Experimental analysis of the quadriceps muscle force and patello-femoral joint reaction force for various activities. Acta Orthop Scand *43*:126, 1972.
21. Seedhom BB, Dowson D, Wright V: The load-bearing function of the menisci. *In* OS Ingwersen et al (Eds): The Knee Joint: Recent Advances in Basic Research and Clinical Aspects. Proceedings of the International Congress on the Knee, New York, American Elsevier Publishing Co, 1974.
22. Seireg A, Arvikar RJ: A mathematical model for evaluation in lower extremities of the musculo-skeletal system. J Biomech *6*:313, 1973.
23. Seireg A, Arvikar RJ: The prediction of muscular load-sharing and joint forces in the lower extremities during walking. J Biomech *8*:89, 1975.
24. Stauffer RN, Chao EYS, Brewster RC: Force and motion analysis of the normal diseased and prosthetic ankle joint. 23rd Annual Meeting of the Orthopaedic Research Society, Las Vegas, February 1977.
25. Trent PS, Walker PS, Wolf B: Ligament length patterns, strength and rotational axes of the knee joint. Clin Orthop *117*:263, 1976.
26. Walker PS, Davidson W, Erkman MJ: An apparatus to assess function of the hand. J Hand Surg *3*:189, 1978.
27. Walker PS, Erkman MJ: The role of the menisci in force transmission across the knee. Clin Orthop *109*:184, 1975.

6

NATURALLY OCCURRING ARTHROPATHIES OF ANIMALS

by Niels C. Pedersen, D.V.M., Ph.D.,
Roy R. Pool, D.V.M., Ph.D.,
and Timothy R. O'Brien, D.V.M., Ph.D.

NONINFLAMMATORY JOINT DISEASE
- *DEGENERATIVE JOINT DISEASE*
- *DEVELOPMENTAL ARTHROPATHIES*
- *ARTHROPATHIES OCCURRING SECONDARY TO INBORN ERRORS OF METABOLISM*
- *DIETARY ARTHROPATHIES*
- *NEOPLASTIC ARTHROPATHIES*

INFLAMMATORY JOINT DISEASE
- *INFECTIOUS ARTHRITIS*
- *NONINFECTIOUS ARTHRITIS*
  - Deforming or Erosive Arthritis
  - Periosteal Proliferative Arthritis
  - Nondeforming or Nonerosive Arthritis
  - Crystal-induced Arthritis

Rheumatologists specializing in human diseases classify joint disorders in a number of different ways. One nomenclature and classification scheme was compiled by the American Rheumatism Association.[13] There are 13 major etiologic groups of rheumatic disorders in this classification, most of which have joint disease as a primary or secondary manifestation. Although it is certain that animal analogues will be recognized for most of these disorders, the state of knowledge in veterinary medicine makes adoption of this type of classification premature. Given the present knowledge of joint disorders in animals, the following scheme is most appropriate in reviewing naturally occurring arthropathies.

I. Noninflammatory Joint Disease

A. Degenerative Joint Disease (Osteoarthrosis, Osteoarthritis)

B. Developmental Arthropathies
C. Arthropathies Occurring Secondary to Inborn Errors of Metabolism
D. Dietary Arthropathies
E. Neoplastic Arthropathies

II. Inflammatory Joint Disease

A. Infectious
B. Noninfectious

NONINFLAMMATORY JOINT DISEASE

Noninflammatory joint disorders of animals are characterized by the absence of synovial membrane inflammation, normal or near normal synovial fluid, and lack of systemic signs of illness such as depression, malaise, anorexia, fever, leukocytosis, hyperfibrinogenemia, or elevated erythrocyte sedimentation rate.

Degenerative Joint Disease

Degenerative joint disease is the most common noninflammatory arthropathy of animals. It is a disorder of movable joints that is characterized grossly by fragmentation and loss of articular cartilage and radiographically by narrowing of the joint space, sclerosis of subchondral bone, and osteophyte production at the joint margins.[112] Until recently it has commonly been held that most cases of degenerative joint disease of animals were secondary to a predisposing condition, and primary degenerative joint disease was not an important entity. Clinical impressions do not support this belief, and it is apparent that at least a portion of the cases of degenerative joint disease in animals are primary or idiopathic in origin.

Primary degenerative joint disease is the most common articular cartilage problem of humans. At autopsy, people over 40 years of age frequently have gross changes in weight-bearing articular surfaces.[96] Discoloration and fibrillation of articular cartilage with periarticular osteophytes are commonly identified in older animals of several species, even though signs of lameness may not be noticeable. One study of the canine stifle joint revealed that 20 per cent of randomly selected dogs had degenerative changes at autopsy, and of these dogs, 61 per cent had no identifiable predisposing causes.[157] We have also seen dogs examined because of stiffness or lameness that develops insidiously with age, tends to involve the larger weight-bearing joints, and has radiographic signs characteristic of degenerative joint disease, but without clinical, anatomic, or radiographic evidence of any predisposing problem. The radiographic findings of disease in these dogs resemble those of primary degenerative joint disease in humans. Widespread degenerative joint disease is also found in aged cats, but clinical signs are often not associated with the disorder unless the condition is severe.

Degenerative joint disease is frequent in cattle, and in many cases it appears to be primary in origin.[165] The disease in cattle also tends to affect larger weight-bearing joints, such as the hips, stifles (knees), carpi, and tarsi.[160, 164, 165] There is an osteoarthrosis of the stifle joint of the Jersey and Holstein breeds that becomes clinically apparent around 5 years of age, and progresses at varying speeds thereafter.[65] Pedigree studies suggest that the condition might be an autosomal recessive trait. A strongly heritable coxofemoral arthropathy has also been recognized mainly in young bulls.[53, 54, 121] It may not be primary in origin, as there is a suggestion that it is similar to hip dysplasia of dogs.[121] Degenerative joint disease in particular strains of laboratory rodents has also been recognized, and this joint disease has been used as a model for the human disease.[4, 44, 175]

Secondary degenerative joint disease is much more common in animals than it is in humans. Any condition that damages cartilage directly, causes an unstable joint, or subjects the joint surfaces and underlying bone to excessive or abnormal forces can cause degenerative joint disease. The net result of these factors is to hasten the rate of cartilage loss, stimulate marginal bone production, and damage the synovial lining. Conditions that predispose the joint to degenerative changes are varied and numerous. They may be classified as follows:

1. Damage to cartilage surfaces
   a. Traumatic
   b. Sequelae to inflammatory joint disease
2. Damage to supporting structures of the joint
3. Neuropathies
4. Conformational abnormalities
5. Steroid arthropathy
6. Developmental disorders
   a. Osteochondrosis
   b. Failure of ossification centers to fuse (e.g., ununited anconeal and coronoid processes of the elbow of dogs and horses)
   c. Abnormal development of joints (e.g., hip dysplasia, medial and lateral patellar luxation)
   d. Ectopic ossification centers in the synovium

Damage to articular cartilage can occur as a result of acute or chronic trauma to the joint. In small animals such as the dog and cat, the trauma is usually an acute one, most often from being hit by an automobile, gunshot wounds, fights with larger animals, or abuse from people. In such instances, cartilage damage frequently occurs with fractures of bone. The cartilage damage often is not detected or its importance is minimized. Even with good fracture repair, degenerative joint disease frequently develops months or years later. In contrast to small animals, joint trauma in larger animals is more likely to be chronically sustained.

Traumatic joint disease is very common in the horse, especially those animals that are used for racing. The repeated stress associated with training and racing can cause extensive articular and periarticular changes in several diarthrodial joints. Thoroughbred and Standardbred horses train daily and race regularly as 2 year olds in the United States, and severe joint disease often develops by 4 to 6 years of age. The metacarpophalangeal (fetlock) joints of the thoracic limbs develop signs at an early age and are typically the most severely affected joints of the horse. This is probably due to the greater range of motion of this joint, and to the fact that animals bear a larger percentage of their body weight on their forelimbs. Gross pathologic findings in the metacarpophalangeal and other ginglymus joints begin as long superficial scoring or wear lines on the major weight-bearing regions of the joint surfaces. These lines run parallel to the plane of motion of the joint. Erosion of the articular cartilage progresses from focal superficial lesions to large, deep defects extending into the subchondral bone. The latter defects are manifested radiographically as narrowing of the width of the joint space with subchondral sclerosis and cysts. Periarticular osteophytes can become very large in horses that continue to race with the aid of anti-inflammatory and analgesic drugs (Fig. 6–1). Fractures of these large osteophytes are common sequelae.

Horses that perform strenuous work, such as racing, or are used in such activities as roping or cutting cattle can also develop fractures from joint trauma that in turn lead to the development of severe degenerative changes. Overextension of the carpal and metacarpophalangeal joints often results in chip, corner, or slab fractures of the carpal bones or of the proximal first phalanx. Repeated trauma to these damaged joints results in extensive degeneration of the articular cartilage and subchondral bone adjacent to the fracture. Radiographic signs of extensive secondary joint disease are identified within 3 or 4 months if the horse is forced to exercise (Fig. 6–2).

Radiographic signs of chronic secondary degenerative joint disease in cattle tend to be more exaggerated than in other animal species. Periosteal and periarticular reaction to trauma can be most pronounced.

Inflammatory joint disease can predispose a joint to degenerative changes. Infectious arthritis in the neonatal period is a common predisposing cause in sheep, pigs, cattle, and horses, but is an infrequent predisposing cause in dogs and cats. Canine rheu-

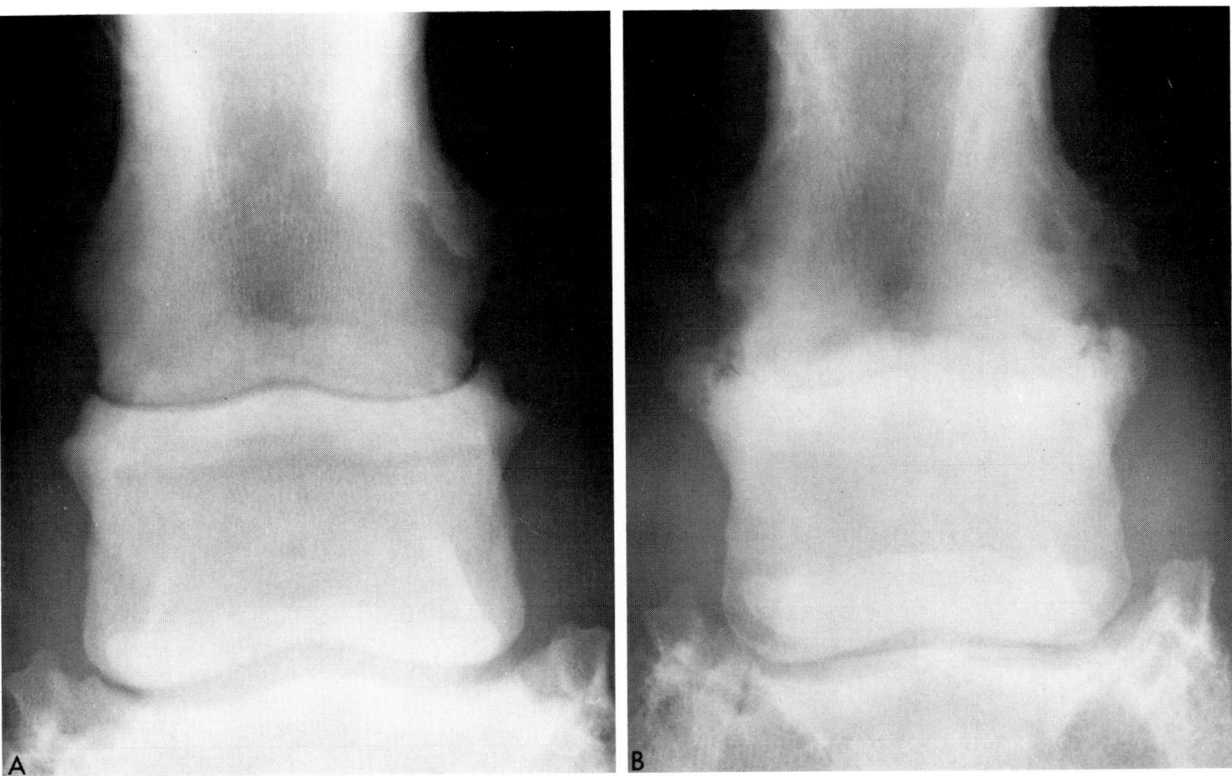

Figure 6–1. *Degenerative joint disease.* **A,** *This noninflammatory arthropathy commonly occurs within the proximal interphalangeal joint of the horse and is recognized radiographically in the early stages by narrowing of the joint space and presence of periarticular osteophytes.* **B,** *The radiographic signs of this disease are dramatic following 16 months of forced exercise.*

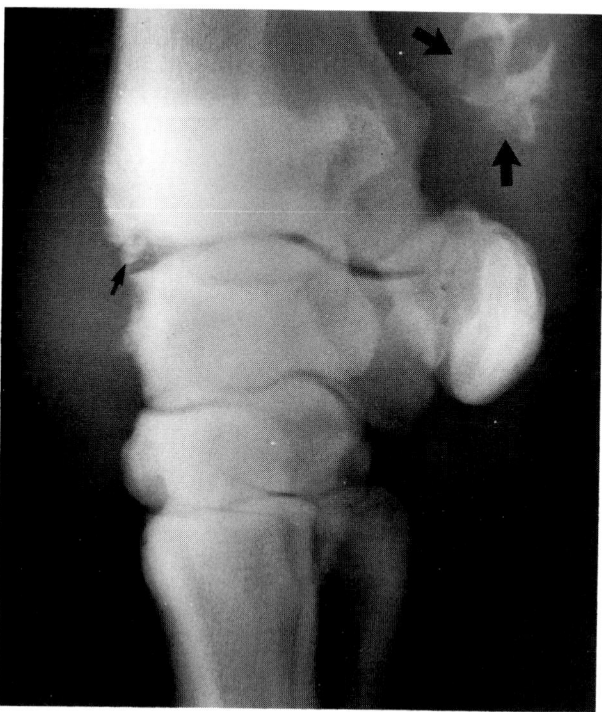

Figure 6–2. *Severe degenerative joint disease. A long-standing intra-articular fracture (small arrow) is a common cause of severe joint disease in the horse. Destruction of the subchondral bone adjacent to the fracture of the distal radius and across the joint space on the carpal bone results. Periosteal new bone production dorsally and ossification in the palmar aspect of the joint capsule (large arrows) can be identified.*

matoid arthritis, if advanced when therapy is instigated, will predispose the joints to degenerative changes even after the inflammatory component of the disease is eliminated. The nondeforming, noninfectious arthritides of dogs will induce minimal degenerative changes in some individuals after a long duration of disease. This can be confusing to veterinarians who mistakenly diagnose the cause of the lameness as degenerative joint disease solely on the basis of radiographic appearance.

Damage to supporting structures of the joint that leads to instability is frequently implicated as a cause of degenerative joint disease in dogs, cattle, and horses. Degeneration and eventual rupture of the anterior cruciate ligament of the knee occurs commonly in dogs,[156, 179] resulting in a "drawer-like" movement of the tibia in relation to the femur. Rupture of the anterior cruciate ligament has also been described in breeding bulls and some older cows.[47, 160] Traumatic damage to menisci leading to degenerative joint disease is found in dogs, cattle, and horses. This is rarely an isolated event, but usually occurs concurrently with rupture of the collateral or cruciate ligaments.

Traumatic luxation of the metacarpophalangeal and tarsometatarsal joints in the horse results in a very extensive fibrosis of the joint capsule and severe secondary degenerative joint disease that usually terminates in ankylosis. Likewise, traumatic hip luxation seen frequently in the dog and cat leads to severe degenerative joint disease.

Neuropathic arthritis is uncommonly observed in animals. When this form of joint disease is identified, it is generally secondary to extensive trauma resulting from diminished pain and proprioceptive reflexes that lead to a relaxation of supporting structures, chronic instability, and hypermobility of affected joints. Animals are frequently destroyed soon after developing severe neurologic deficits, which may explain why neuropathic arthropathies seem to have a much lower incidence in animals than in humans.

Neurectomy of the posterior digital nerves is a common procedure in horses that is done to relieve the pain and gait abnormalities resulting from degeneration of the navicular bone, an elongated sesamoid bone located at the palmar or plantar aspect of the distal interphalangeal joints. This bone has an articular surface and a nonarticular flexor surface. In the normal state the deep digital flexor tendon glides over the smooth layer of fibrocartilage that forms the flexor surface of the navicular bone. Severe degeneration of the navicular bone leads to fibrillation and ulceration of the fibrocartilage of the flexor surface, which in turn often results in the development of adhesions between the deep digital flexor tendon and navicular bone. Neuropathic arthritis does not result from the neurectomy per se, but secondary joint disease can develop at an accelerated rate if the horse is kept in use. Degeneration of the navicular bone is one of the most common and severe orthopedic problems of horses.[61, 106]

Conformational abnormalities can predispose joints to secondary degenerative joint disease. These abnormalities may be genetically controlled, in which case they are present at birth or become noticeable during growth. Varus deformities of the carpal joints are seen in some Doberman Pinscher dogs, and such animals often develop degenerative disease in these joints later in life. Some breeds of dogs, such as the Boxer, have straight stifle joints, and this predisposes the stifle and hock joints to degenerative changes. Poor tarsal joint conformation is a major cause of tarsal osteoarthrosis in younger cattle.

Chondrodystrophy is an inherited trait in many breeds of dogs, and was once a severe economic problem in some bloodlines of Hereford and Angus cattle. Chondrodystrophic breeds include the Bulldog, Basset Hound, Lhasa Apso, Pekingese, Pug, and similar breeds. In these breeds the conformational abnormalities associated with chondrodystrophy are accepted as "normal," whereas in other breeds, e.g., Malamute, in which dwarfism is a recessive trait, it is considered highly undesirable. Chondrodystrophic animals, like chondrodystrophic human dwarfs, demonstrate angular deformities of the limb joints, and the cartilage surfaces vary greatly in structure. These changes predispose the joints to degenerative changes. Fortunately, most chondrodystrophic breeds of dogs are not working animals and often lead rather sedate lives. This slows the progression of joint disease.

Good conformation is especially important to the function of the mature horse. Poor conformation contributes greatly to degenerative joint disease and other disorders. Fractures in bones forming the carpal, metacarpophalangeal, and tarsal joints are often attributed to excessive or abnormal stresses produced by poor conformation. The mature horse must also have proper trimming and shoeing to insure correct function of joints. Incorrect foot care results in abnormal joint stress, which is often exaggerated by poor conformation and forced exercise.

Conformational abnormalities can also result from damage to the growing epiphyses. Trauma to the distal ulnar epiphysis in fast-growing puppies can cause premature closure of the epiphysis and cessation of growth in the distal ulna.[108, 109, 122] Because the distal radial physis continues to grow, curvature of the forelimb occurs. The conformational defect, if not surgically corrected, causes great stress at the carpal and elbow joints, which can result in degenerative joint disease (Fig. 6–3). A similar problem is recognized in foals. The condition in foals results from a difference in the growth rate between the medial and lateral regions of the distal radial physis. Contracture of tendons of the digital flexor muscles, laxity of the ligaments at the carpal or metacarpophalangeal joints, or aseptic necrosis of bones of the carpus or tarsus (Fig. 6–4) can also cause distal forelimb deformities in the foal. Signs of secondary degenerative joint disease are complicated in these cases by the development of abnormally shaped bones and subluxation.

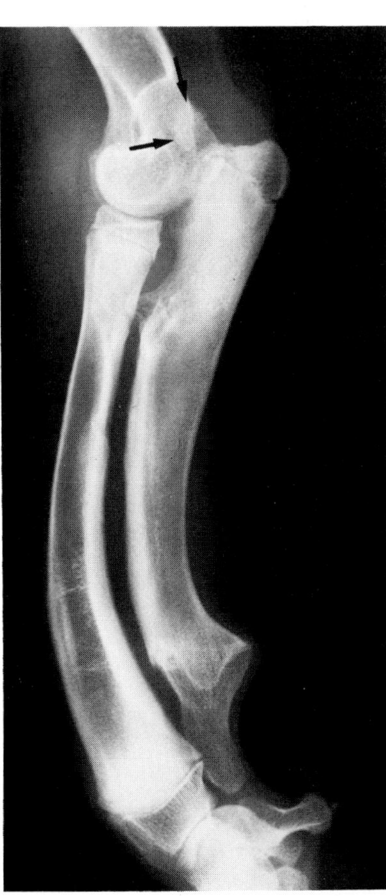

Figure 6–3. *Acquired conformational defect. Premature closure of the distal ulnar growth plate in the young dog leads to a valgus deformity of the distal extremity and secondary joint disease of the elbow and carpus. Continued growth of the radius resulted in luxation of the distal humerus and displacement of the anconeal process (arrows).*

Collapsing or folding fractures, if not properly treated, can result in a shortening of the limb upon healing. This is more commonly a problem in dogs, in which fractures of major limb bones are treated. Large animals are usually killed when such fractures occur. To compensate for the limb shortening, the angulations of the pelvic or thoracic girdle and of the distal and proximal joints are altered, which in turn predisposes these joints to degenerative changes. This is analogous to the long leg–short leg syndrome of humans. Similarly, if fractures are repaired so that rotation of the distal segment occurs upon healing, degenerative changes can occur in distal and proximal joints.

Steroid arthropathy is a condition that is almost unique to racing and working horses. In an attempt to alleviate lameness resulting from early degenerative joint disease and to prolong working life, veterinarians may inject glucocorticoids directly into the synovial cavity. The injected joint often undergoes severe structural alteration, leading to narrowing of the articular cartilage, dystrophic calcification of periarticular soft tissues, bone production within the joint capsule, and subchondral cystic lesions (Fig. 6–5). Morphologic changes resemble those of degenerative joint disease but the structural alterations develop at an accelerated rate. Repeated intra-articular injections and forced exercise can lead to limitations of the range of motion of the affected joint. Eventually the horse will be unable to perform, and it will be retired.

Developmental arthropathies include osteochondrosis, failure of ossification centers to fuse, abnormal development of joints, and ectopic ossification centers in the synovium. In the early stages they may be clinically inapparent or may be manifested by gait abnormalities and lameness. Degenerative changes occur later in life in affected joints, at which time the clinical signs may differ in nature and severity. These disorders will be discussed in greater depth in a subsequent section.

The clinical signs of degenerative joint disease in animals are essentially the same as those described in humans. In cases that are secondary to some predisposing cause, lameness and gait abnormalities may precede signs referable to degenerative joint disease by months or years. The earliest sign of

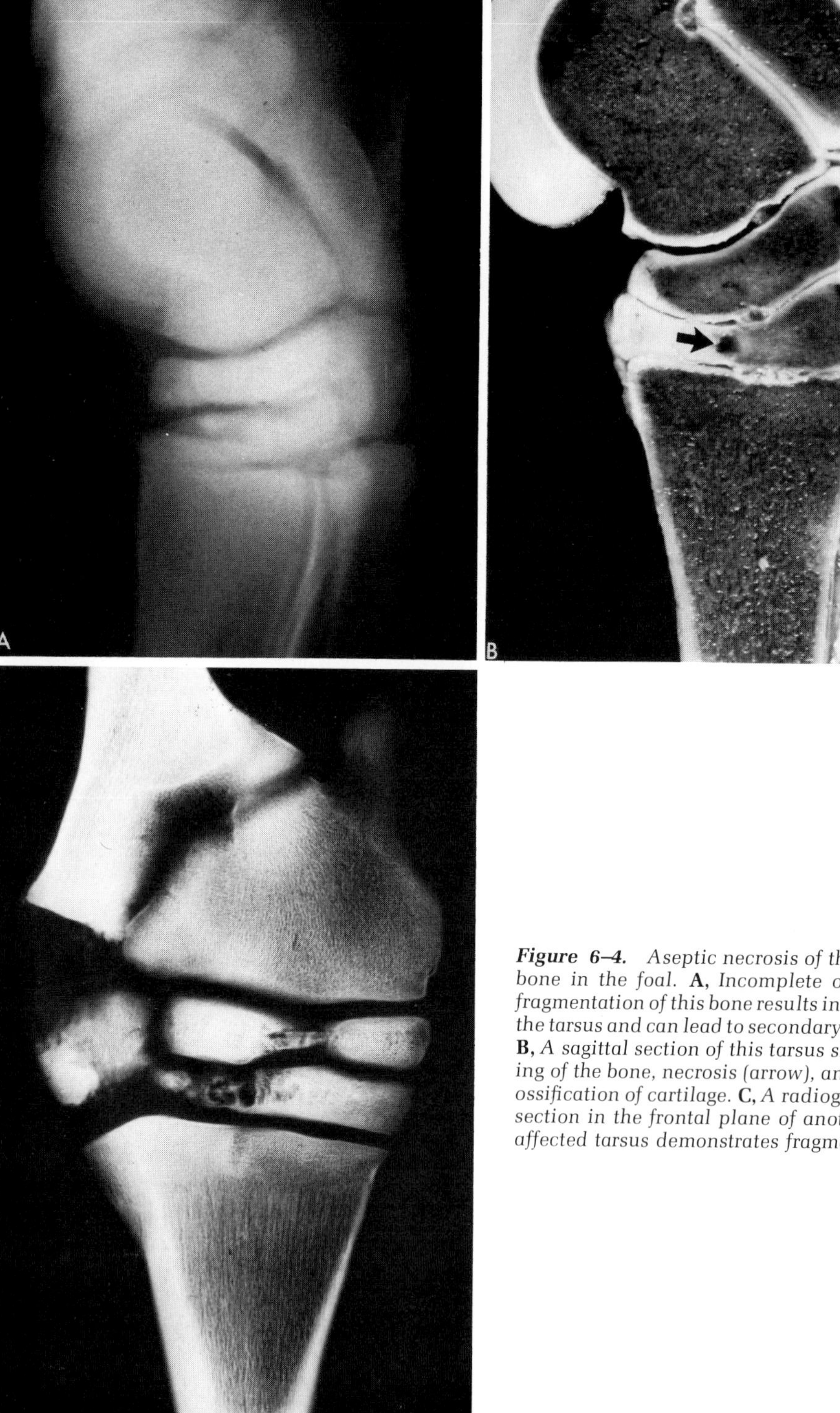

Figure 6–4. *Aseptic necrosis of the third tarsal bone in the foal.* **A,** *Incomplete ossification or fragmentation of this bone results in angulation at the tarsus and can lead to secondary joint disease.* **B,** *A sagittal section of this tarsus shows narrowing of the bone, necrosis (arrow), and incomplete ossification of cartilage.* **C,** *A radiograph of a slab section in the frontal plane of another similarly affected tarsus demonstrates fragmentation.*

degenerative joint disease is a reluctance of the animal to perform certain tasks or maneuvers, without more obvious signs of stiffness or lameness. The discomfort is apparently felt only when certain stressful forces are applied to the subclinically damaged joints. In the next stage, lameness and stiffness frequently are seen following periods of sustained activity or overexertion. After several days of rest, the clinical signs often disappear. As the degeneration becomes more severe, stiffness may be most pronounced following periods of rest, and with movement the animals appear to "warm" out of their lameness or stiffness. Cold and damp weather often increases the severity of clinical signs. In the final stages of the disease, stiffness and lameness are fairly constant features, although the severity of signs may still be influenced by environmental factors. Carnivores, such as dogs, may show signs of increased irritability and reclusiveness, and may snap or bite when approached or touched. Unfortunately, this type of behavior is often directed against children. The owners may not appreciate that the continuous pain caused by the joint disease is responsible for the abnormal behavior.

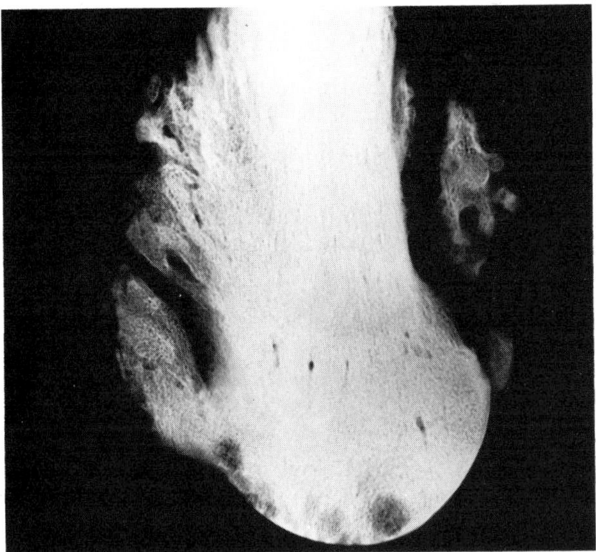

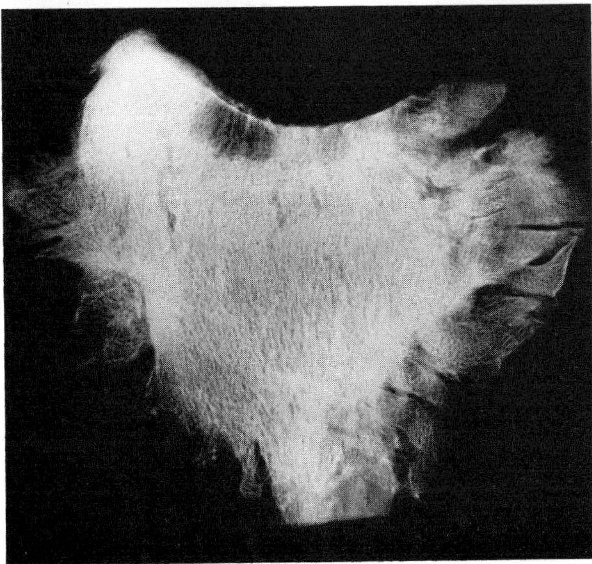

Figure 6–5. *Steroid arthropathy. Glucocorticosteroids injected intra-articularly into a damaged equine joint can result in severe degenerative joint disease within a few months. Radiographs of 1 cm thick midsaggital bone sections of the distal third metacarpus and first phalanx forming part of the joint illustrate extensive periarticular and periosteal new bone with subchondral cysts.*

Marked gross deformities of the joints are uncommon in primary degenerative joint disease. In contrast, animals with predisposing congenital or acquired deformities often develop pronounced gross joint changes. Gross deformities consist of an increase in the dimensions of the joint due to the marginal new bone formation and thickening of the joint capsule. Destruction of articular surfaces and ankylosis of the joint are uncommon. Palpable swellings of the joints due to effusions occur in horses with severe arthritis, but are uncommon in small animals. Joint distention is less pronounced than the swelling accompanying inflammatory joint problems. Likewise, redness and heat in the area of the joint are usually not present.

The earliest lesion seen in an affected joint is an area of dullness in the articular cartilage accompanied by a color change from the normal flat white of mature cartilage to a mottled gray-white or yellow hue. Irregular fissure lines (Fig. 6–6) or a velvety disruption (Fig. 6–7) of the articular surface may be visible grossly. As the articular cartilage deteriorates, the mechanical forces of weight-bearing and movement are transferred directly to the underlying subchondral bone. This underlying subchondral bone reacts by becoming thicker and denser (sclerosis) (Fig. 6–8).

The earliest microscopic change seen in the degenerating articular cartilage is a roughening of

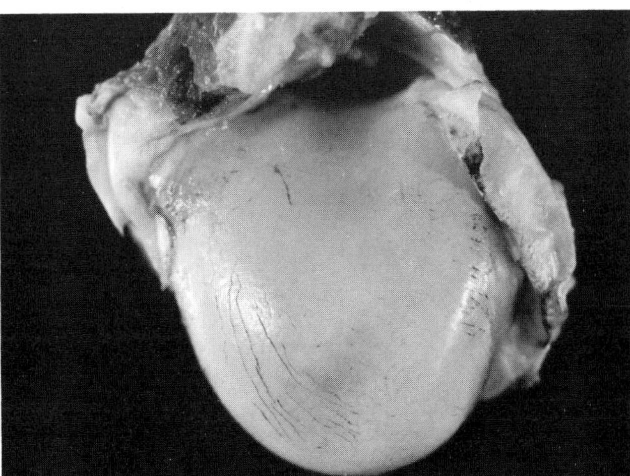

Figure 6–6. *Proximal humerus of a 12 year old dog with primary degenerative joint disease. Fissures in the surface were emphasized by rubbing the articular cartilage with carbon.*

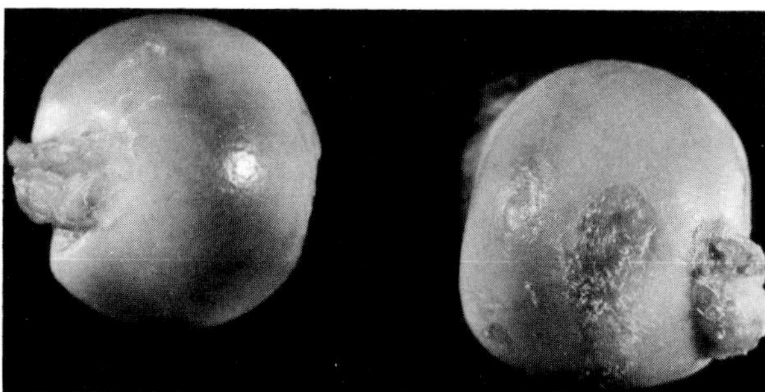

Figure 6–7. *Femoral heads of a 6 month old dog 2 months following fracture of the right acetabulum. The left femoral head is normal. The right femoral head shows effects of secondary degenerative joint disease. Note the alteration in shape and size. Several areas of the articular surface are discolored and have a velvety appearance.*

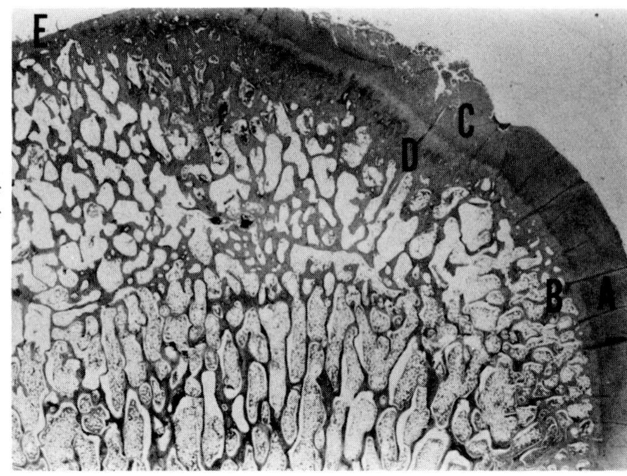

Figure 6–8. *Microscopic changes in degenerative joint disease. Observe the loss of normal structure of the joint, beginning at the junction of the normal cartilage (A) and subchondral bone (B) with the area of cartilage degeneration (C) and subchondral bone sclerosis (D), which becomes progressively more severe until the surface is eburnated (E).*

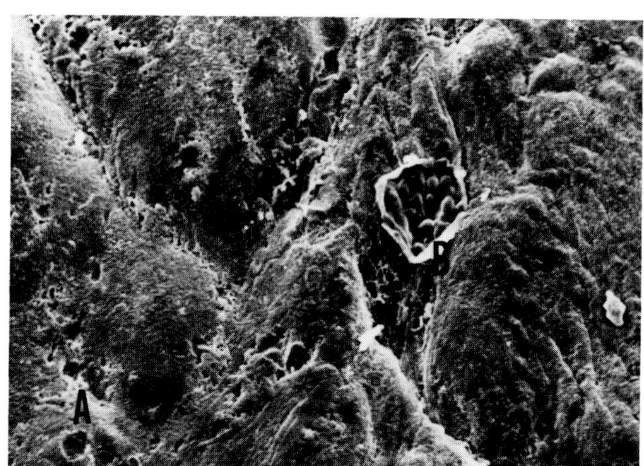

Figure 6–9. *Scanning electron micrograph of early changes in a degenerating articular surface. The entire surface shows roughening and irregularity. Microulcerations (A) may be of sufficient depth to expose chondrocytes (B) of the tangential zone to the joint surface.*

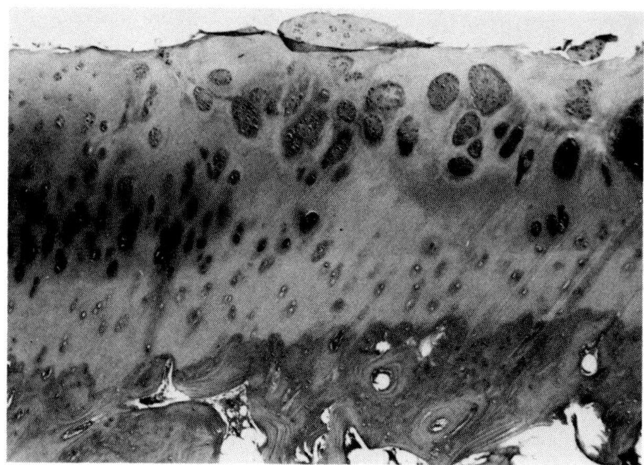

Figure 6–10. *Loss of the superficial layer and proliferation of nests of chondrocytes in the transitional and radial zones in an ineffectual attempt at repair.*

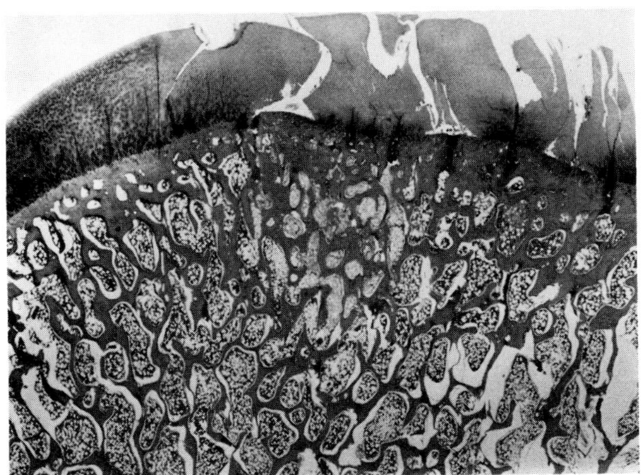

Figure 6–11. Fissures extend completely through the layer of degenerative cartilage and reach the subchondral bone.

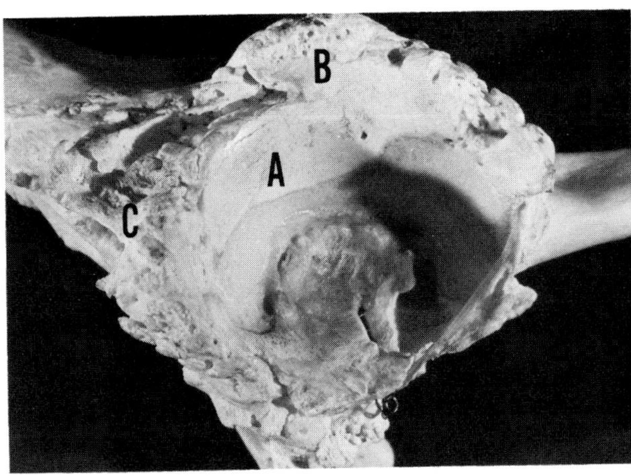

Figure 6–13. Severe secondary degenerative joint disease following chronic luxation of the hip. A, Eburnated (polished) rim of the acetabulum. Osteophytic bone production is seen at the joint margin (B) and along the joint capsule insertion (C).

the surface fiber layer, followed by the exposure and loss of underlying chondrocytes (Fig. 6–9). Chondrocytes in these areas appear to be damaged or dead, and there is a generalized loss of normal staining properties of the surrounding cartilage matrix. As the degenerative process becomes more severe, the most superficial layer of cartilage is worn away, exposing the deeper layer of chondrocytes in the transitional zone. In an attempt at repair, chondrocytes in the area proliferate, but are unable to separate and differentiate in the firm chondroid matrix of mature cartilage (Fig. 6–10). These clones of newly formed chondrocytes produce a soft, imperfect matrix that wears more quickly than normal matrix. Fissures develop in the damaged cartilage, and these fissures may extend through to the subchondral bone (Fig. 6–11). Chondrocytes immediately adjacent to the fissure lines make an abortive attempt at repair (Fig. 6–12). Where fissures reach the subchondral bone, separation at the osteochondral junction occurs along with varying amounts of hemorrhage and necrosis. The resulting osteochondral defect heals with granulation tissue and fibrocartilage. With continued cartilage loss, the sclerotic subchondral bone becomes progressively exposed (Fig. 6–13) and is polished by the opposing articular surface (eburnation).

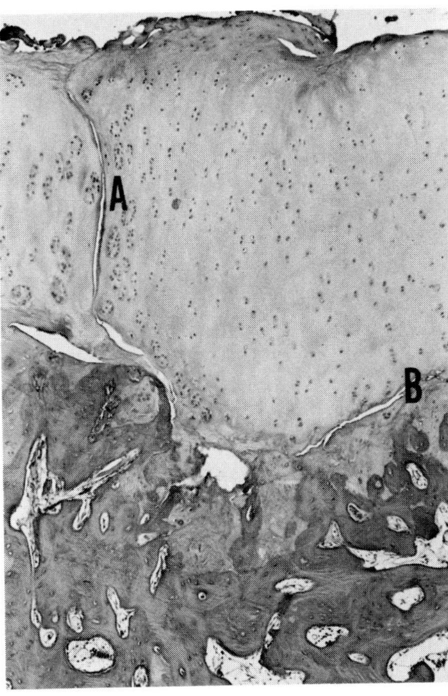

Figure 6–12. Chondrocytes adjacent to fissure lines proliferate (A) in an abortive attempt at repair. Note the continuation of the fissure line with the line of osteochondral separation (B).

Changes in the articular cartilage and subchondral bone lead to loss of normal contour of the articular surfaces, and this predisposes the joint to further abnormal movement. In an attempt to respond to these new stresses, and to contain the abnormal motion, the borders of the articular surfaces undergo remodeling and extend the articular surface area (Fig. 6–13). Typically this is accompanied by bone proliferation (osteophytes) on the periarticular bone surfaces adjacent to or within the insertion line of the joint capsule (Fig. 6–14).

Changes in the joint capsule of animals with degenerative joint disease are stereotyped. There is a generalized increase in fibrous connective tissue in the synovium. Condensations of collagen occur immediately beneath the surface layer of the synovium, and there is collagenization of the adventitia of the small caliber vessels that form the superficial plexus in the synovium. Hyalinization of the subsynovial connective tissue with chondroid metaplasia and dystrophic calcification is sometimes present. These changes are not necessarily accompanying features of osteoarthrosis because identical changes can also be seen in the joint capsule of aging animals

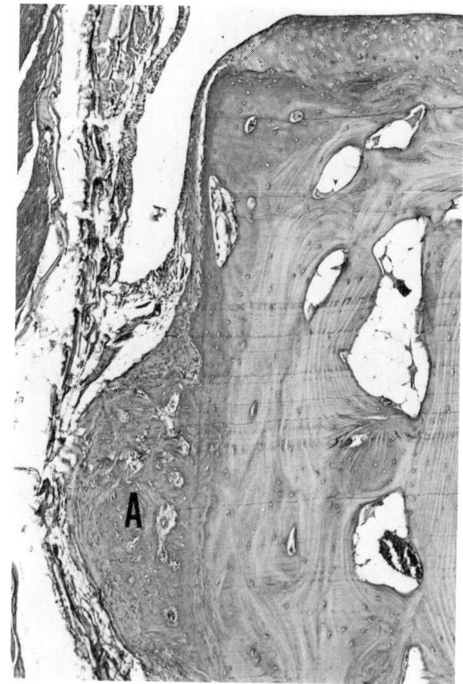

Figure 6–14. Formation of a periarticular osteophyte (A).

without changes in their joint surfaces. Villous hypertrophy occurs more commonly in larger animals and mainly in larger joints that are severely affected. Inflammation in the synovium is usually absent, although mild chronic inflammatory changes centered on cartilaginous debris in the synovial recesses are occasionally seen. In horses with severe chronic osteoarthrosis, sustained edema in the fibrous layer of the joint capsule is organized by fibroblasts. This results in a permanent thickening of the joint capsule and a reduction in range of motion for the joint.

Developmental Arthropathies

As the name implies, arthropathies of this type develop in the preadolescent and adolescent stages of life. They may have a genetic basis, but the full genetic expression of the abnormality is often greatly influenced by environmental factors.

Osteochondrosis is an important cause of both transient and permanent lameness in dogs,[111] swine,[40-42, 142] horses,[124] cattle,[123] turkeys,[87, 149] and broiler chickens.[119, 124, 125] The clinical, radiographic, etiologic, and pathologic features of this condition in dogs, swine, and poultry have been extensively reviewed. A similar condition occurs in children,[145] although much more seems to be known about the cause and effect of the disease in animals.

Osteochondrosis most commonly is identified in shoulder joints of dogs, where the lesion occurs on the caudal aspect of the humeral head. Osteochondrosis, however, does affect a number of other joints, with the incidence of such lesions in the stifle being great in dogs,[130] horses, turkey poults, and broiler chickens. The lateral and medial femoral condyles are affected in the dog, but only the medial condyle is affected in the horse (Fig. 6–15). Recently osteochondrosis has been recognized as an important cause of lameness involving the medial condyle of the humerus, the femoral trochlea (Fig. 6–16), and the medial ridge of the talus of the dog and horse.

Osteochondrosis first becomes clinically apparent at about 4 to 5 months of age in the dog and swine, at 1 year of age in the horse, and at 4 to 8 weeks of age or younger in broiler chickens and turkey poults. The actual lesion, however, begins to appear much earlier in life. It may cause clinical signs of lameness or subtle gait abnormalities, or it may remain clinically inapparent. Clinical signs may persist for weeks or months if the lesion resolves, or permanent lameness may develop over a longer period of time as a result of secondary joint disease. There is a strong tendency for the condition to occur more frequently in strains or breeds of animals that are genetically selected for large size and rapid growth.[72, 111, 126] Males, which tend to grow faster than females, and animals on rapid growth promoting diets, are more often affected.[42, 72, 111, 123, 126]

Bone formation occurs as a result of the orderly mineralization and ossification of the growing cartilage model. Osteochondrosis is believed to be caused by disturbances in this normal endochondral ossification,[111] which in turn may be due to an imbalance between the growth and sex hormones.[82] In osteochondrosis the articular cartilage in affected sites becomes thicker than normal because endochondral ossification does not keep pace with cartilage growth in these fast-growing individuals. The initial lesion is necrosis of chondrocytes in the deeper layers of the articular cartilage, which may be due to an inability of these deeply situated chondrocytes to receive adequate nutrients by diffusion from the synovial fluid or subchondral capillaries. Because of the death of these deeply situated chondrocytes, the surrounding cartilage matrix fails to mineralize. Blood vessels from the subchondral bone will not invade the area of unmineralized articular cartilage as they normally would. Consequently, the osteogenic mesenchyme that accompanies these vessels does not penetrate the cartilage, and normal ossification fails to occur.

All changes in the osteochondritic lesion subsequent to the development of the area of chondromalacia are secondary events. At one extreme in this morphologic spectrum are those animals that are able to resolve the lesion spontaneously. The subchondral capillary bed is able to surround, bridge over, and bypass the area of chondromalacia and re-establish normal endochondral ossification superficial to the lesion. The result is a delay in modeling

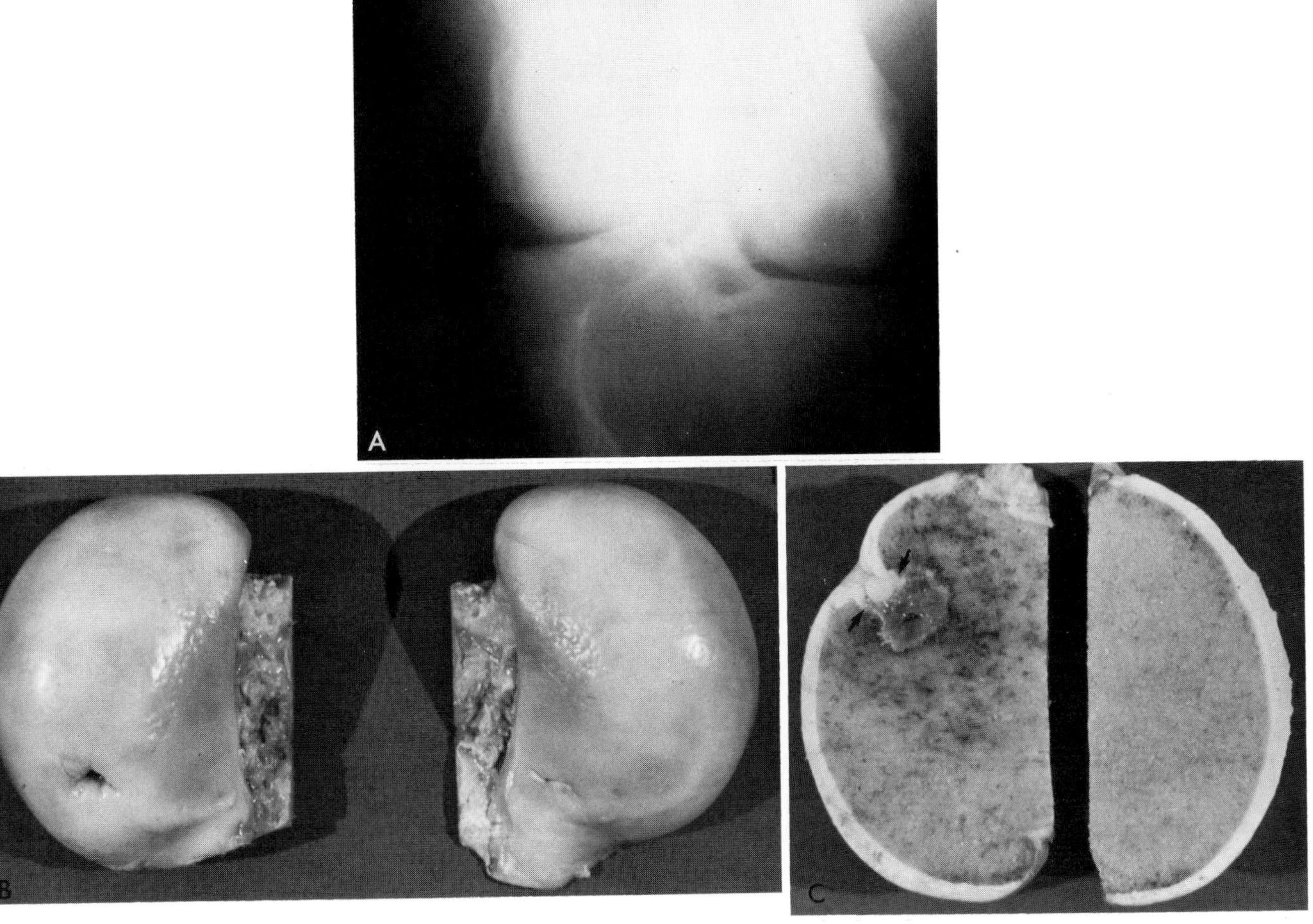

Figure 6–15. Osteochondrosis. **A,** *A cystic lesion of the medial condyle of the femur is a common radiographic finding in the young horse with osteochondrosis. The normal (right) and abnormal (left) medial condyles before* **(B)** *and after* **(C)** *sectioning demonstrate the lesion. Most lesions have irregular margins and undermining of the subchondral bone instead of a lining of articular cartilage (arrows), as is shown in this example.*

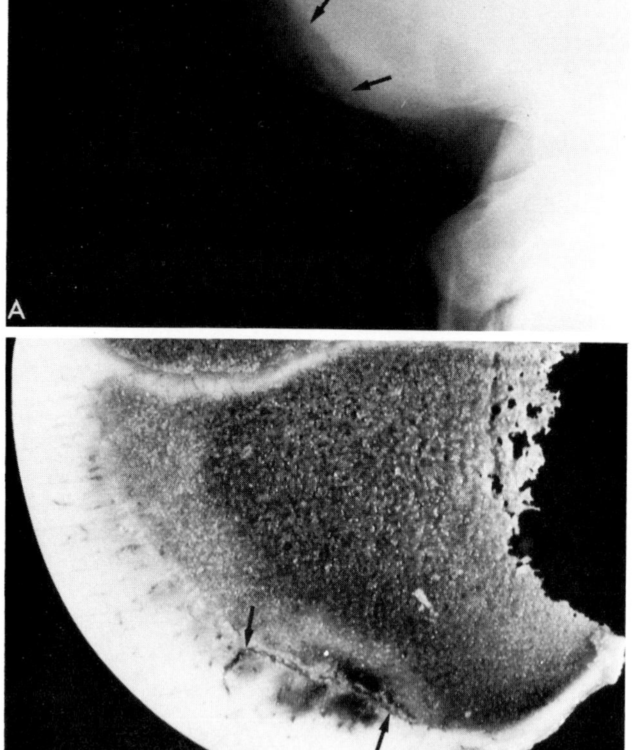

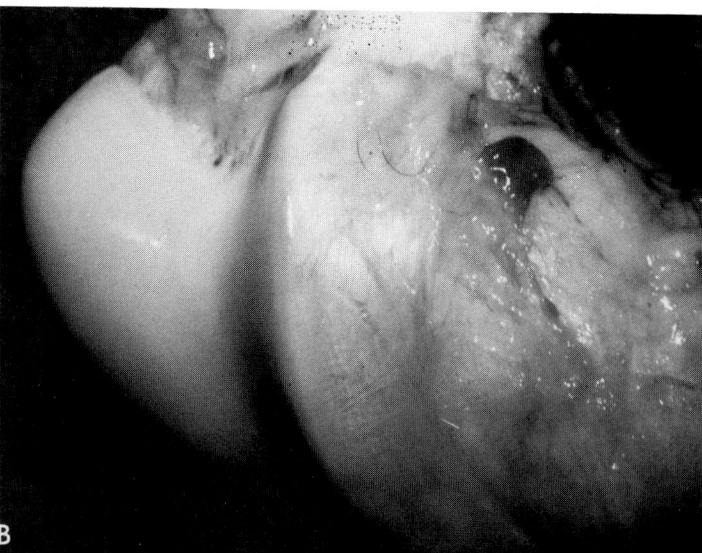

Figure 6–16. *Osteochondrosis of the femoral trochlea.* **A,** *Osteochondrosis of the femoral trochlea in the horse most commonly is identified within the lateral ridge (arrows). The articular surface may appear normal and intact at necropsy* **(B)**, *but a sagittal section may reveal an underlying lesion (arrows,* **C**) *in the subchondral bone.*

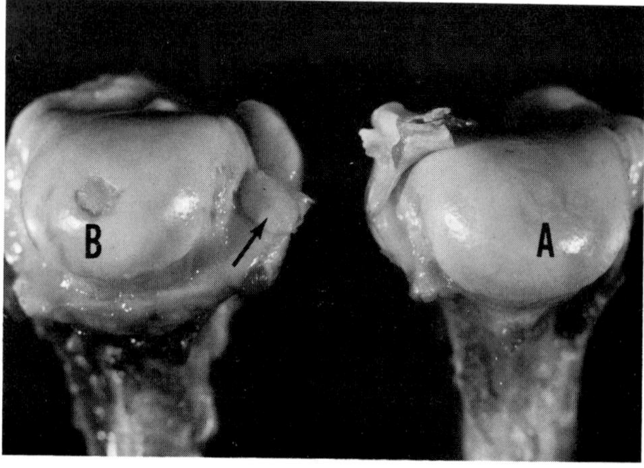

Figure 6–17. *Osteochondrosis of the humeral head. Early lesion* (A) *has smooth articular surface but is outlined by discoloration of the cartilage. Advanced lesion* (B) *shows defect that has partially filled with fibrocartilage. Note that the detached piece of cartilage (arrow) has grown to be larger than the original defect.*

of the developing articular surface, as witnessed by a flattening of the subchondral bone as seen in clinical radiographs. Grossly, the early lesion is outlined by a discoloration of the cartilage in the affected area (Fig. 6–17). Percussion of the area is normal and indicates that there has been no separation of the cartilage from the subchondral bone. At the other extreme, the area of chondromalacia becomes separated from the subchondral bone. This loosened area of cartilage usually tears partially away from the articular surface and forms a flap. Complete separation can occur, in which case the detached piece of cartilage becomes a joint body (Fig. 6–17). In either event, the animal is apt to show clinical signs of lameness. Healing of the defect occurs by granulation tissue arising from the subchondral bone. This granulation tissue eventually becomes fibrocartilage.

Synovial fluid from involved joints is normal, except for a minimal increase in neutrophils and macrophages in some severe cases. Radiographic signs of a lesion are an irregular subchondral surface, a destructive focal defect in the subchondral bone, and varying degrees of increased density surrounding the defect. The defect may not have a distinct zone of increased density surrounding it, or the zone may be 1 to 3 mm. thick. The subchondral defect may have a small distinct opening at the surface of the joint or appear as a large, crater-like lesion. Free fragments are sometimes identified on survey radiographs, but a cartilage flap with underlying subchondral bone is more commonly seen on survey radiography and arthrography. Secondary joint disease and abnormal shape of the affected epiphysis are seen in the chronic stages of the clinical disorder.

The treatment of osteochondrosis in the dog and horse involves either rest alone or rest combined with surgical curettage of the lesion. Milder cases can often be managed successfully by strict rest for 4 to 8 weeks, followed by an equal period of limited exercise. Surgery is indicated when the devitalized cartilage defect is impeding healing or has broken partially or completely free. Following surgical curettage and removal of cartilage debris from the joint cavity, the animal is rested for an extended period of time to allow the defect to undergo fibrocartilaginous repair. Failure to treat the problem appropriately in the early stages can lead ultimately to debilitating secondary degenerative joint disease.

Ununited coronoid and anconeal processes (Figs. 6–18 and 6–19) may be additional manifestations of osteochondrosis.[111] These lesions tend to occur in the same breeds of dogs and under similar conditions of rapid growth and genetic predisposition.[10, 27] The histologic lesion is characterized by degeneration of cartilage along the base of the developing coronoid and anconeal processes. This can delay the bony union of these processes with the shaft of the ulna, and eventual avulsion from the

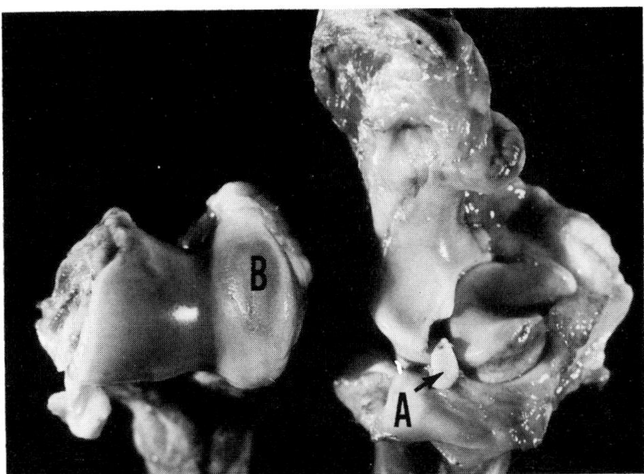

Figure 6–18. *Ununited coronoid process (A) has caused secondary degenerative disease in the elbow joint. Note the abraded surface of the medial condyle of the humerus (B) apposing the loose coronoid process.*

ulnar shaft can occur. After separation the processes may remain loosely attached in situ and retain a blood supply, or, in the case of the anconeal process, can become completely detached. In either event, joint instability results, and this can lead to secondary degenerative joint disease with time (Fig. 6–19).

Hypoplasia of the coronoid process of the dog is an uncommon clinical disorder. Hypoplasia may result from trauma or sustained pressure to the developing coronoid process. The entire thickness of

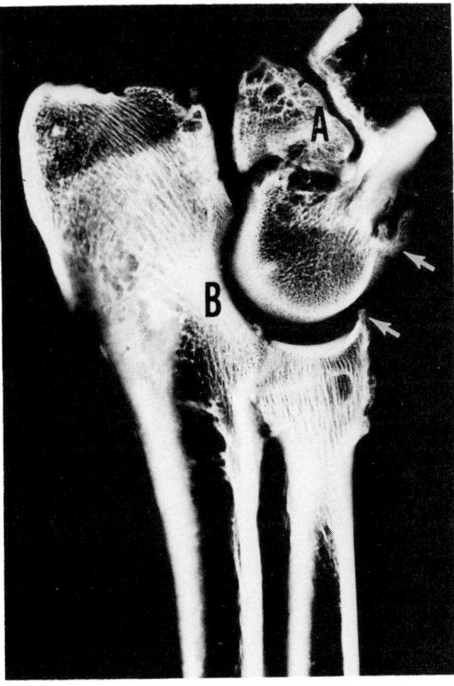

Figure 6–19. *Ununited anconeal process (A) is lodged in the olecranon fossa. Secondary degenerative joint disease of the elbow is characterized by subchondral bone sclerosis in the trochlear notch of the ulna (B) and the formation of periarticular osteophytes (arrows).*

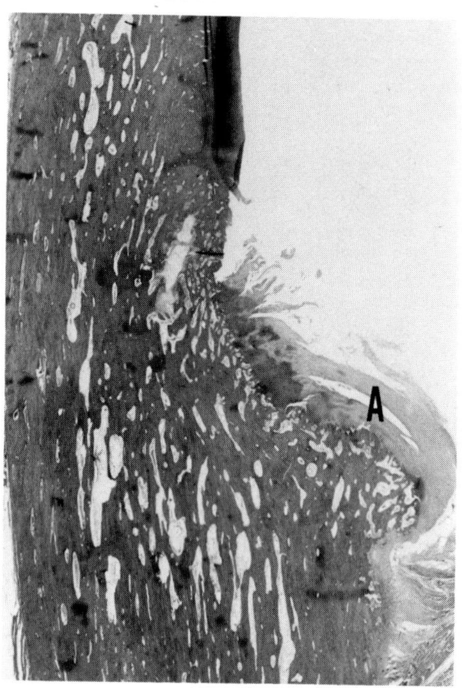

Figure 6–20. Hypoplasia of the coronoid process. Necrosis and fibrillation of the entire layer of articular cartilage (A).

the articular cartilage over the coronoid process is necrotic, and no germinative cells remain to initiate regrowth of the process (Fig. 6–20).

An *ectopic ossification center* resembling a sesamoid bone has been observed medial to the head of the radius in the joint capsule of the elbow of some young dogs (Fig. 6–21).[43, 120, 158] In some cases a lameness may result from the presence of the ossification center, and in other cases it is only an incidental radiographic finding in clinically normal animals. The lameness begins at 8 to 11 months of age, and occurs most frequently in certain breeds of dogs, e.g., Labrador Retrievers, German Shepherds, Burmese Mountain Dogs, Newfoundlands, and Rottweilers. The elbow disorder can be bilateral or unilateral and may predispose the joint to degenerative changes. The lameness ceases when the ectopic ossification center is removed. A similar ectopic ossification center can occasionally be seen over the dorsocranial aspect of the acetabulum of dogs. This condition does not produce clinical signs.

Hip dysplasia is a developmental disease identified in most breeds of dogs, but tends to occur more frequently in larger, well-fed, faster-growing breeds.[84, 85] The development of hip dysplasia is strongly influenced by genetic factors, and it affects both sexes of dogs with equal frequency. Coxofemoral arthropathy of cattle may represent a similar condition,[19, 53, 54, 121, 174] and similar genetic and environmental factors appear to be related to the evolution of the disease in both species. A similar disorder has been less frequently described in cats[95] and horses.[45, 60] The relationship of hip dysplasia in animals to familial joint laxity and acetabular dysplasia[83, 177] of humans is not precisely known. Acetabular dysplasia of humans resembles hip dysplasia of animals in its genetic basis.[177]

The clinical progression of the disorder has been best documented for dogs, but the evolution of the changes in all species appears to be rather stereotyped. Dysplastic dogs are born with normal hip joints that subsequently undergo progressive structural alterations. The following structural findings are identified pathologically or radiographically: joint laxity; shallow acetabular cavities; subluxation; swelling, fraying, and rupture of the teres ligament; erosion of the articular cartilage with eburnation of the subchondral bone; remodeling of the acetabular rim and flattening of the femoral head; and periarticular osteophyte production (Figs. 6–22 and 6–23). There are considerable variations in the severity of the clinical signs, time of onset of structural changes, age at which clinical signs occur, rate of disease progression, and degree of pain and impaired mobility. Gait abnormalities without overt lameness or stiffness may precede the degenerative changes by months or years. Degenerative joint disease may occur within the first year of life, but many animals show no clinical signs until 2 to 6 years of age. There may be a poor correlation between clinical and radiographic signs.

The precise etiology of hip dysplasia in the dog remains in question, although genetic, environmental, and nutritional factors all seem to be involved.[50, 64] There is debate as to whether the fundamental cause is intrinsic or extrinsic to the hip joint. Proponents of an intrinsic cause believe that the primary change occurs in the developing coxofemoral joint,[71, 84] and one suggestion is that hip dysplasia is another example of osteochondrosis.[111] Proponents of an extrinsic cause believe that the hip abnormalities occur secondary to alterations or inadequacies in the muscles that support the coxofemoral joint during development.[128] Whatever the cause, the end effect is a joint that is unstable and predisposed to degenerative joint disease.

Patellar luxation is an orthopedic problem of frequent occurrence in certain toy breeds of dogs. It is less frequently seen in the horse and cat.[34] The trochlear ridge of the distal femur, which forms the patellar groove, appears to be unusually flattened. The patella disengages from the patellar groove either laterally or medially, but medial luxation is more common in the dog and horse. When this happens, acute lameness results until the patella "pops" out of abnormal position. With time the patella moves either more laterally or medially, and the corresponding trochlear ridge becomes progressively flattened, which allows even more lateral or medial movement of the patella. Eventually the patella is located completely outside of the groove (Fig. 6–24). The pull of the straight patellar ligaments on their insertion at the tibial crest causes a

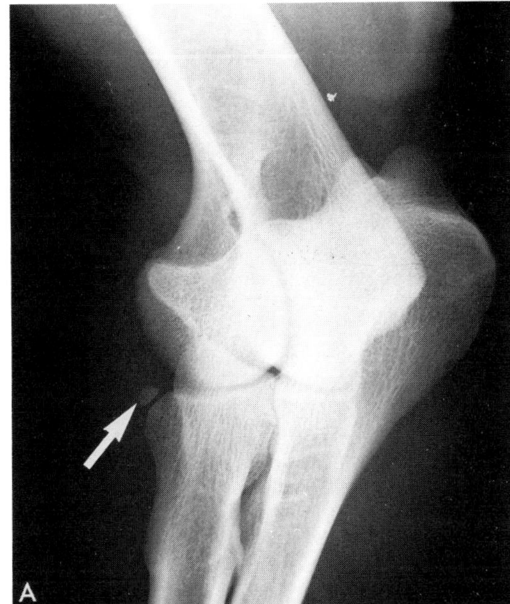

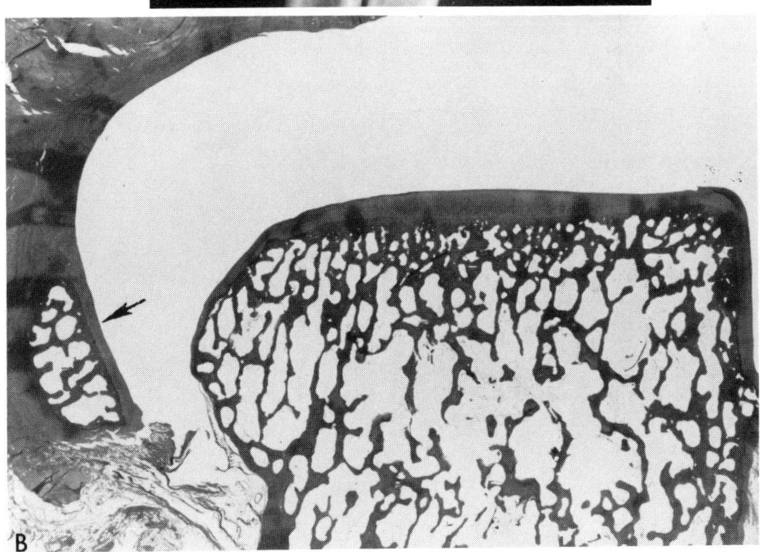

Figure 6–21. **A**, *Ectopic ossification center in the medial joint capsule of a canine elbow. This small ossicle has a body of spongy bone that is covered by hyaline cartilage (arrow), which articulates with the head of the radius* **(B)**.

repositioning of the tibial crest to the side of the luxated patella. With time the knee joint becomes deformed in a valgus or varus position and is predisposed to degenerative changes.

Aseptic necrosis of the femoral head frequently occurs without apparent predisposing cause in adolescent dogs of toy and small breeds.[73, 81] For some undetermined reason a major portion of the blood supply to the capital epiphysis of the femur is compromised, and the ischemic portion of the developing epiphysis undergoes necrosis (Fig. 6–25). This condition is probably similar to Legg-Calvé-Perthes disease of children.[73, 81] Aseptic necrosis of the capital epiphysis has also been described as a feature of osteochondrosis in growing pigs and has been observed in cattle.[31] Such necrosis can also occur following traumatic fractures through the femoral neck or through the epiphysis itself. Following disruption of its blood supply, the affected area of epiphyseal spongiosa undergoes necrosis (Fig. 6–26), while the overlying cartilage, which receives its nutrition from the synovial fluid, remains viable. The body tries to repair the defect with granulation tissue and new cancellous bone arising from intramembranous ossification (Fig. 6–27). Unfortunately, the amount of bony repair is often insignificant, and occurs too late to prevent collapse of the unsupported articular cartilage. Collapse of the femoral head affects congruity of the articular surfaces and predisposes the joint to secondary joint disease.

The condition is manifested by slight to severe lameness. Femoral head ostectomy is the accepted treatment.

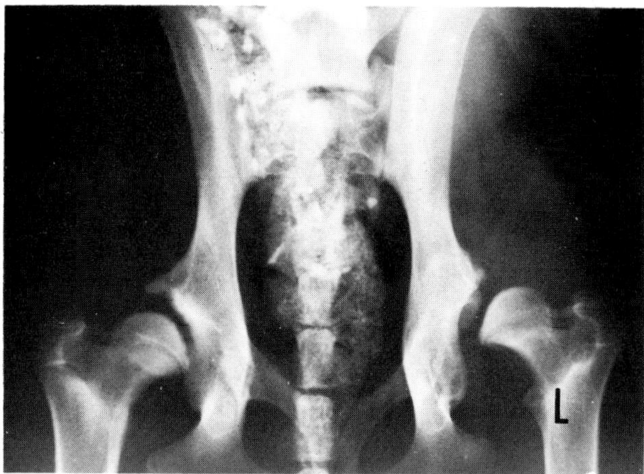

Figure 6–22. A dog with severe bilateral hip dysplasia, as evidenced by lesions characteristic of chronic secondary degenerative joint disease. Severe subluxation of the left hip (L) with an abnormally shallow acetabulum is demonstrated. Note the abnormal contours of the femoral heads and periarticular new bone formation.

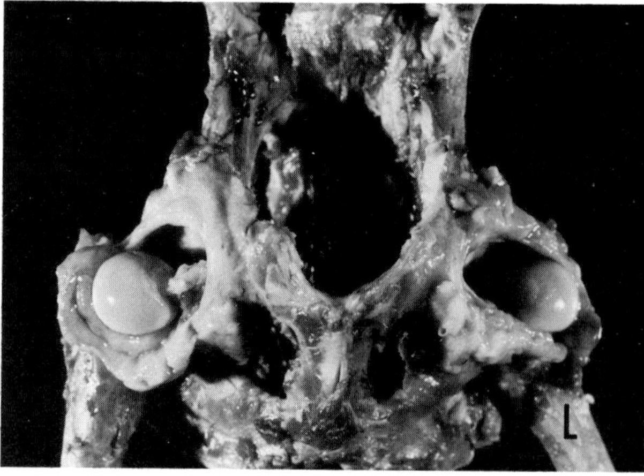

Figure 6–23. Gross tissues of the same dog as in Figure 6–22. Note the thickened joint capsules. The ligament of the head of the right femur was thickened and frayed, while the ligament of the left femur (L) was ruptured. Note that the left femoral head has an abnormal shape and that the articular surface is irregular.

Arthropathies Occurring Secondary to Inborn Errors of Metabolism

Lameness is one of the most common complaints of humans and dogs with congenital coagulation defects. In fact, *hemophilia A* of the dog can lead to an arthropathy indistinguishable from that occurring in people with congenital coagulation defects.[154] The arthropathy is caused by chronic hemorrhage into the joint, which is induced by clinical and subclinical trauma. The effusion of blood into the joint cavity resulting from synovial or subsynovial hemorrhage provokes an acute inflammatory reaction. The synovial membrane becomes thickened and undergoes villous hypertrophy, and there is hyperplasia of the intimal layer of the synovium and infiltration of lymphocytes, macro-

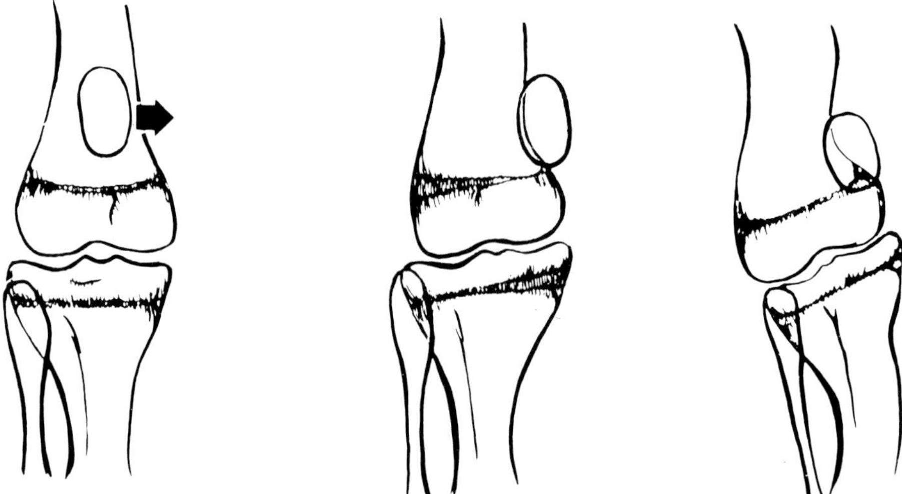

Figure 6–24. Medial patellar luxation in the dog. Medial patellar luxation in the puppy leads to abnormal growth in the physes on either side of the joint. The joint space is more angulated and secondary joint disease with cruciate and collateral ligament damage can result.

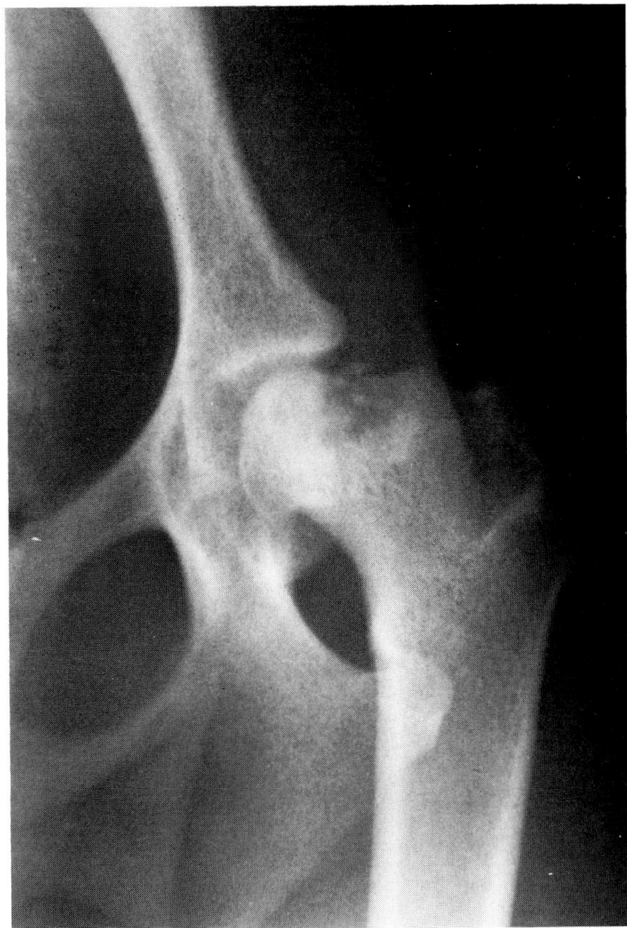

Figure 6–25. Aseptic necrosis. Radiographic appearance of typical aseptic necrosis of the femoral head in a small dog. The condition was bilateral.

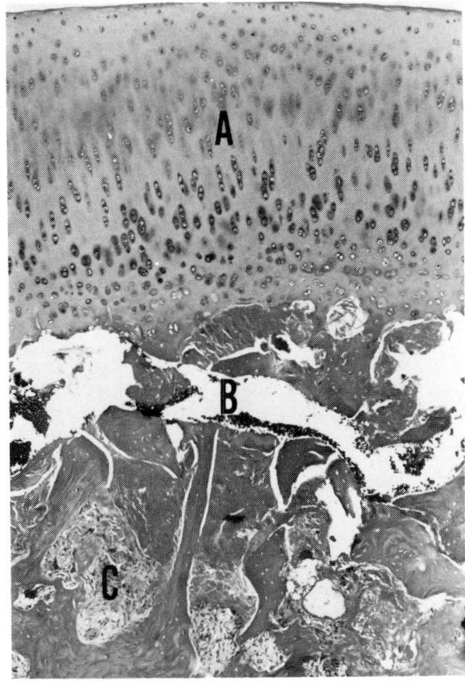

Figure 6–26. Aseptic necrosis of the femoral head. Acute lesion shows normal articular cartilage (A), necrosis, and hemorrhage in the subchondral bone and adjacent epiphyseal spongiosa (B). Granulation tissue (C) arises in the marrow spaces along the border of the infarct.

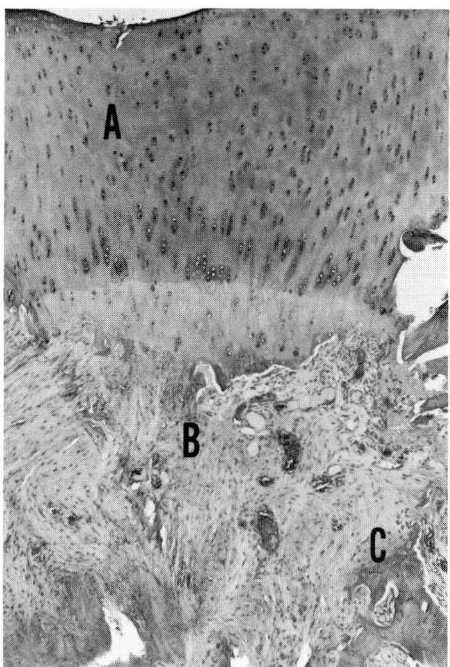

Figure 6–27. *Aseptic necrosis of the femoral head. Healing lesion shows abnormal articular cartilage (A), maturing granulation tissue replacing the area of bone necrosis (B), and attempts at intramembranous bone formation (C) in the fibrous connective tissue response.*

phages, and plasma cells. The reaction subsides after several days to weeks, but each subsequent hemorrhagic episode leads to further synovial fibrosis and hemosiderosis. The fibrosis causes rigidity of the joints and contributes to the clinical signs. However, the most significant sites of injury are the articular cartilage and subchondral bone. Injury to the articular cartilage is caused by granulation tissue arising from the synovium and from the subchondral bone.

Arylsulfatase B enzyme deficiency, or mucopolysaccharidosis, has been identified as an autosomal recessive trait in cats.[59] The condition is analogous to Maroteaux-Lamy syndrome of humans. Because of the inability to degrade glycosaminoglycans properly, these materials build up in cellular lysosomes. Clinical signs in the cat include small stature, pectus excavatum, broad flattened face with drooping eyelids, mild diffuse corneal clouding, reluctance to walk, and rigid neck. Radiographs show bone proliferation and fusion of cervical vertebrae, shortened thoracic vertebrae, broad, oar-shaped ribs, irregular bony proliferations around the epiphyses of long bones, rarefaction of bone, and irregular articular surfaces. Bone proliferation often obscures the carpal and tarsal joints.

Dietary Arthropathies

Improper diets have been associated with *secondary hyperparathyroidism* and a rickets-like syndrome in cats fed diets composed mainly of beef heart[127, 135] and in bulls fattened on improper rations.[63] Demineralization of the skeleton from medullary bone resorption, subperiosteal new bone formation, and pathologic fractures are common sequelae. Pelvic lesions may cause mechanical bowel obstruction in the cat. Major limb joints may undergo ankylosis of opposing joint surfaces. Young

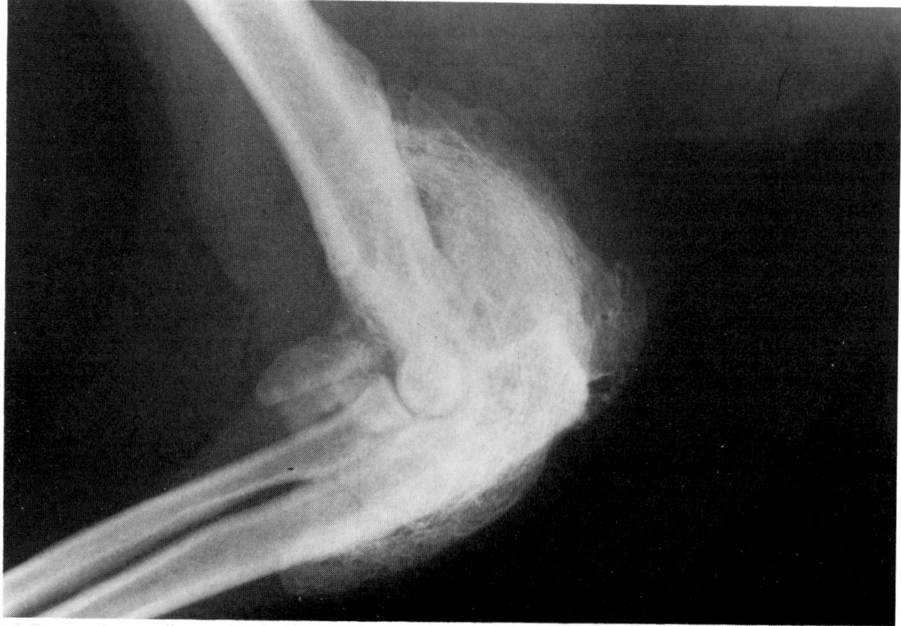

Figure 6–28. *Hypervitaminosis A. Severe proliferation of bone has resulted in ankylosis of the elbow in this cat with hypervitaminosis A.*

bulls on growth-promoting diets consisting of a high proportion of concentrates and low levels of roughage, especially if supplemented with a low calcium and high phosphorous salt mix, rapidly develop *degenerative joint disease.*[152] Degenerative changes in the articular cartilage are most pronounced in the carpal joints.

Hypervitaminosis A, a condition caused by feeding large amounts of raw liver, has been described as a naturally occurring entity of cats.[136] It is characterized by subperiosteal proliferation of new woven bone around the apophyseal joints of the cervical and thoracic vertebrae and proliferation of cartilage from the joint margin. The process overgrows the synovium and bridges the joint (Fig. 6–28).

The potentiating effect of growth-promoting diets on *osteochondrosis* has already been discussed. *Fluorosis* is an osteodystrophy mainly of herbivores, particularly in cattle that ingest high levels of fluoride in their food and drinking water.[62, 137] The most dramatic responses are dental disease and marked hyperostosis affecting the entire skeleton. Lameness and joint pain appear to be due to the encroachment of the proliferative bony response on tendon sheaths and ligaments, and to periarticular exostoses that may become so severe as to cause ankylosis of some joints.

Neoplastic Arthropathies

Neoplasms involving the joints are rare in animals, but a *synovial sarcoma* is by far the most common primary joint tumor in animals. These tumors occur most frequently in middle-aged dogs (7 to 8 years old).[79, 86] These tumors in dogs typically involve a major limb joint, most often the stifle or elbow joint. Radiographic signs include soft tissue swelling in all cases, and bone destruction with irregular periosteal response involving bones on either side of the affected joint in more than half of the dogs with this condition. Canine synovial sarcomas are characterized microscopically by the presence in varying proportions of two intermingled cellular components, a pleomorphic synovioblastic or "epithelioid" component and a spindle cell or "fibroblastic" cellular component. Synovial sarcomas associated with tendon sheaths are probably just as common but are usually diagnosed as undifferentiated sarcomas of the deeper soft tissues.

The *osteogenic sarcoma* is a frequent cause of lameness in large and giant breeds of dogs. The tumor arises in the metaphyseal area, and rarely crosses the epiphysis, and is therefore not technically a joint tumor. *Villonodular synovitis*, a condition of humans that has been classified variously as a benign tumor or a granulomatous reaction, has been described in the metacarpophalangeal joint of the horse.[102]

Tumors rarely metastasize to the joint. The exception is the arthropathy that occurs in some cattle with generalized lymphosarcoma.[162, 163] The synovial membrane is infiltrated with neoplastic lymphoid cells, and the amount of synovial fluid within the joint is increased. The condition appears to cause some cartilage degeneration and may precipitate or accelerate ongoing degenerative joint disease.

INFLAMMATORY JOINT DISEASE

This major form of joint disease is characterized by inflammatory changes in the synovial membrane and synovial fluid with systemic signs of illness, e.g., fever, leukocytosis, malaise, anorexia, and hyperfibrinogenemia. The etiology of inflammatory joint disease of animals is diverse and includes both infectious and noninfectious causes. A simple classification scheme for the common etiologies of inflammatory joint disorders of animals is:

1. Infectious (bacterial, mycoplasmal, chlamydial, viral, fungal, protozoal)
   a. Nonhematogenous
   b. Hematogenous
2. Noninfectious
   a. Arthritis of apparent immunologic cause
   b. Crystal-induced arthritis

Infectious Arthritis

Bacteria may gain entrance to the joint through penetrating wounds or from contiguous sites of infection in bone or soft tissue. Surgical contamination and unsterile injections are other sources of sepsis. Infection via penetrating wounds is much more frequent in large animals, such as sheep, swine, horses, and cattle. These animals inhabit environments that are often unclean and cluttered with hazardous objects. Infection can enter the interphalangeal, carpal, and tarsal joints when animals step on sticks, rocks, nails, wire, and similar sharp objects. Grass awns, especially from foxtail barley, may also penetrate the skin and subcutaneous tissue and enter the joint. Infection of the elbow joint has been seen in horses, and bacteria often enter through penetrating wounds on the lateral aspect, where there is very little tissue overlying the synovial cavity.[32] In other cases, especially in cattle[168] and horses,[167] the route of infection is unknown.

Bacteria may also gain access to the joints from infectious foci within blood vessels and on heart valves that shed organisms directly into the blood. Infection of the umbilical cord at birth is a very common cause of infection of the umbilical vein (omphalophlebitis).[7, 24, 118] Many young animals, especially farm animals, are born into unclean environments. In addition, the young animal often does not receive the postparturient umbilical cord care that human infants are given. Cats will sometimes chew off the umbilical cords of their newborn kittens too close to the abdominal wall. Normally, the umbilical cord is chewed off several centimeters or more from the abdomen, and the dried-up umbilical cord remnant forms an impermeable barrier that prevents bacteria from reaching the patent umbilical vein. These kittens invariably develop omphalophlebitis, usually from Pasteurella organisms that inhabit the mother's mouth. Tail biting among baby pigs, with subsequent infection of the tail stump, is another source of joint infection.[7] The bacteria probably enter the bloodstream via the vertebral veins and marrow spaces of the vertebral body. Subacute bacterial endocarditis occurs in all species of animals, and occasionally it may be manifested by septic arthritis. Staphylococci, streptococci, coliforms, and Erysipelothrix are the organisms most frequently isolated from joints, blood, and heart valves.

Septic arthritis is a common feature of many of the classic systemic bacterial diseases of animals. Systemic infections occur predominantly in neonates and preadolescent animals. In these diseases the bloodstream is a vehicle to carry the bacteria from the infected tissue to the synovial lining. Bacteria, as well as other microorganisms, may preferentially localize in the joint because of the rich blood supply to the joint and the phagocytic nature of the synovial membrane. The pathogenesis of all of these diseases is similar in that most of them began as a localized infection of the respiratory, enteric, or urogenital tract. Streptococcus,[118, 176] Staphylococcus,[91, 97, 144] Salmonella,[118] Hemophilus,[66, 101] Erysipelothrix, Corynebacteria,[17, 161] Pasteurella, coliform bacteria,[58, 118, 173] and other miscellaneous bacteria[1, 23, 92, 172, 178] are the usual offending organisms among all species of animals. The systemic spread of a localized bacterial infection may be enhanced in young animals that fail to receive adequate amounts of colostral antibodies during the first several days of life.[57, 118] Failure of passive transfer of maternal immunity is a common problem in the calf and foal. Systemic spread of infection may also be caused by stressful incidents that occur at the time the primary localized infection is taking place. Common precipitating causes include inclement weather, weaning, shipping, feedlot stresses, concurrent viral disease, overcrowding, and dietary changes.

Septic arthritis can cause permanent damage to the cartilage and predispose the joint to degenerative changes. Severe and extensive secondary joint disease limits the working ability of the horse. It has been estimated that only one half as many foals with septic arthritis go on to race successfully as do unaffected foals.[118]

One of the most interesting systemic diseases of swine is caused by *Erysipelothrix insidiosa (E. rhusiopathiae)*.[3, 15, 103, 104] The arthritis seen in the chronic stages of this disease has been linked to human rheumatoid arthritis.[2, 22, 139, 142] The acute or systemic stage of Erysipelothrix infection is manifested by high fever, depression, diamond-shaped hemorrhagic lesions of the skin, splenomegaly, hemorrhagic gastroenteritis, and focal hemorrhages in the kidneys. A suppurative polyarthritis may also occur in the acute stage of the infection. Pigs that recover from the acute phase of the disease often develop vegetative endocarditis and chronic polyarthritis. The arthritis is usually nonsuppurative in the chronic form and has a predilection for the carpal, tarsal, and interphalangeal joints. The resultant lameness is characterized by periods of clinical exacerbation and remission, and has been observed to persist for as long as 4 years or more after the acute infection.

The arthritis is characteristically a proliferative synovitis in the early stages. With time, there is pannus formation, marginal erosions of subchondral bone, fibrous adhesions between damaged articular surfaces, ossification and ankylosis in some cases, and gross deformities of the phalanges. Rheumatoid nodules are sometimes observed. Histopathologic changes resemble those seen in human rheumatoid arthritis.

Viable Erysipelothrix organisms cannot usually be cultured from the synovium during the chronic stage of the infection. Erysipelothrix antigen must persist somewhere in the body because plasma cells in the synovium often contain antibodies to the organism. Endocarditis may be an important source of antigen release. The tube agglutination titer to Erysipelothrix remains greatly elevated throughout the course of the disease. Pigs with chronic arthritis also develop titers of rheumatoid factor in their serum. The arthritis can also be reproduced by transfusing whole blood from diseased to nondiseased pigs.[141] The arthritis-producing factor can be found only in the cellular component of the donor blood, and organisms cannot be isolated from the donor blood or from the recipients. Recipient pigs do not develop high titers of erysipelas antibody, which makes the phenomenon even more intriguing.

Erysipelothrix insidiosa has been isolated from the blood of a woman with subacute bacterial endocarditis, and this isolate readily caused ankylosing spondylitis when inoculated into swine.[140] A rheumatoid arthritis–like condition has also been experimentally induced in dogs that were inoculated intra-articularly with *E. insidiosa*.[138] A naturally occurring infection of dogs causing endocarditis and arthritis has been described.[38]

Discospondylitis, often associated with septic arthritis in the shoulder, hip, or stifle joint, is seen in dogs. It is particularly common in young adults of large canine breeds such as the Great Dane and in German Shepherd dogs. The offending organism is often a Staphylococcus, although Streptococcus and coliform organisms can also be isolated from some animals. The usual source of the infection is the urinary tract, and in most cases the same organism can be isolated from the disc space, blood, joint, and bladder. It can be theorized that the bacteria pass retrogradely up the vertebral veins via the pelvic veins, or by way of lymphatics.

Mycoplasmas are normal inhabitants of the respiratory passages, nasal cavity, conjunctival membrane, urogenital tract, and mammary glands of many animal species. Each species of animal may be infected by a number of closely related strains of Mycoplasma. These various strains can cause similar

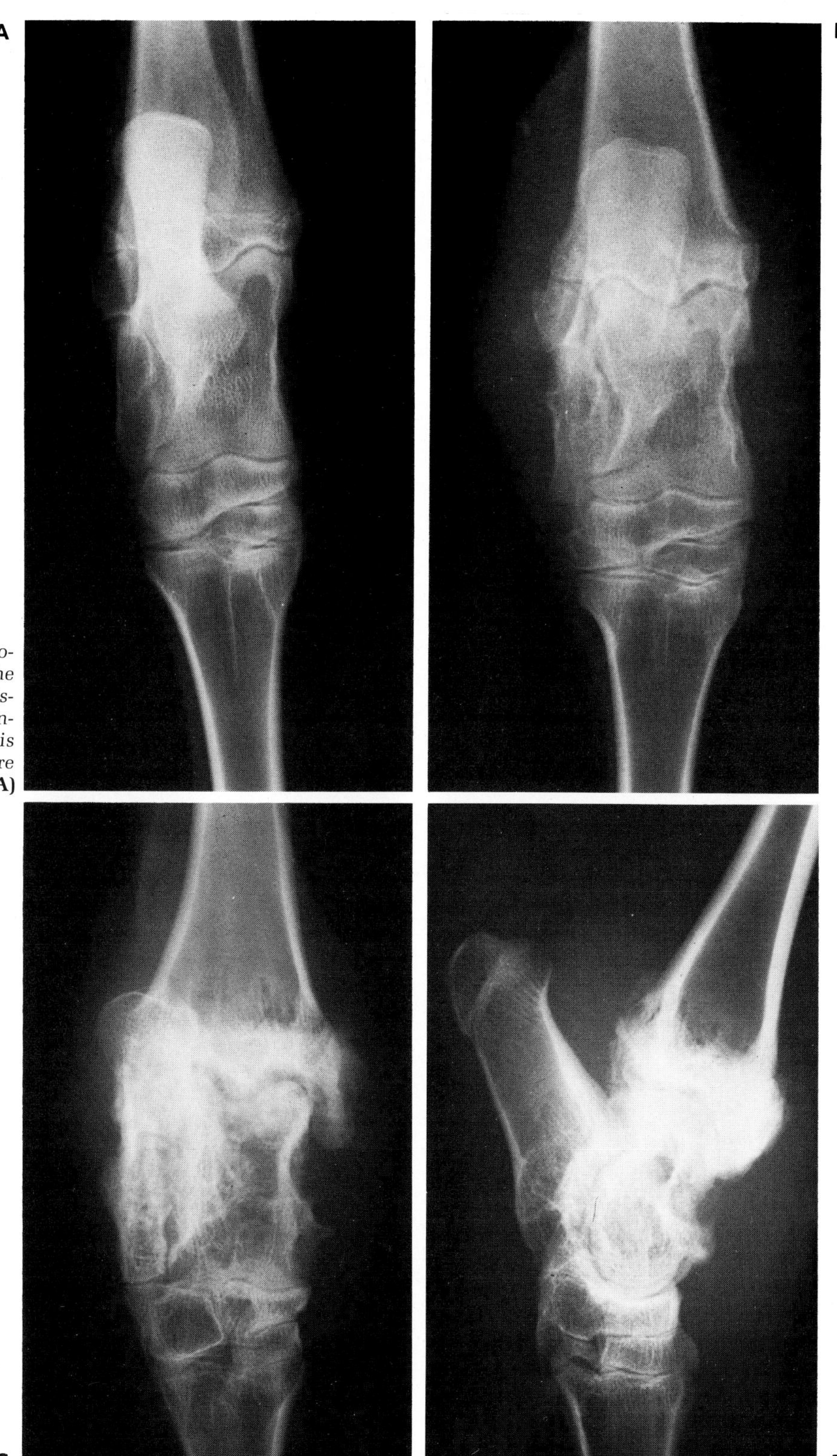

Figure 6–29. *Infectious arthritis. Progression of a mycoplasma infection of the tarsus is demonstrated. Extensive soft tissue swelling with small subchondral lucencies and periarticular osteophytes* **(B)** *is followed in 4 to 6 months by signs of severe joint disease* **(C–D)**. *The opposite tarsus* **(A)** *is included for a normal comparison.*

or greatly different types of disease. Mycoplasmas can produce localized disease in any of the areas that they normally inhabit and occasionally cause systemic illness. Clinical disease usually occurs following a severe primary infection, or from secondary flare-ups of a chronic latent infection. Mycoplasmas also act as secondary invaders in tissues infected initially with other pathogens.

A mycoplasmal arthritis is a frequent chronic sequela of the systemic spread of organisms from localized sites of infection (Fig. 6–29). Systemic disease occurs mainly in young or preadolescent animals, and it is often precipitated by some stressful situation that occurs at the time of the primary or recurrent infection. Mycoplasmal arthritis is a serious problem in swine, poultry,[18, 67, 69, 129, 134] goats,[98] sheep,[153] and both calves and older cattle.[11, 39, 51, 55, 70, 143, 147, 148] It has been less commonly seen in foals.[94] It is a common problem of laboratory rodents.[4, 49, 146]

Mycoplasmal arthritis of swine has been used as a model for human rheumatoid arthritis.[22, 146] *Mycoplasma hyorhinis* causes an acute systemic disease in young swine 3 to 10 weeks of age that is characterized by a polyserositis and polyarthritis.[7, 8, 9, 66, 146] In adolescent pigs the polyarthritis is the main clinical manifestation. *Mycoplasma hyosynoviae* produces a similar chronic polyarthritis in adolescent pigs.[131-133] *Mycoplasma hyoarthrinosa* produces a polyarthritis in adolescent and young pigs that is similar to the disease caused by *M. hyosynoviae*.[93] Unfortunately, isolates of *M. hyoarthrinosa* are no longer available.[133]

Similarly to Mycoplasma, *Chlamydia* frequently inhabits the conjunctival membrane and upper respiratory tracts of normal animals. Localized disease in these organs may occur following the primary infection or as a result of the activation of a chronic latent infection. Under certain conditions, Chlamydia can cause pneumonia and systemic disease, especially in young animals. Stress also appears to play an important role in precipitating illness. Subacute to chronic joint involvement is a common sequela of the systemic disease. Chlamydial arthritis is most prevalent in sheep[29, 30, 52, 105, 117, 150, 155] and cattle,[151] but has also been described in the foal.[88]

A fleeting arthropathy is a symptom of many acute *viral* diseases of humans. Because animals show signs of pain only when the joint inflammation is relatively severe, the degree to which arthropathy complicates viral diseases in animals is unknown. A chronic arthritis lasting up to 6 months has been observed in young Hereford bulls that were naturally infected with bovine virus diarrhea.[48] A synovitis caused by a reovirus has been recognized in chickens.[28, 37, 110, 169, 171] Bovine adenovirus, Type 5, has been associated with arthritis and weakness in calves.[26, 89]

Fungal arthritis is infrequent in animals. It can occur as an extension of a fungal osteomyelitis or as a primary granulomatous synovitis, with the former occurring more frequently (Fig. 6–30). *Coccidioides immitis, Blastomyces dermatitidis,* and *Cryptococcus neoformans* are the most frequently encountered organisms. Desert rheumatism, an arthropathy that accompanies the primary respiratory stage of coccidioidomycosis of humans, has also been seen in dogs.

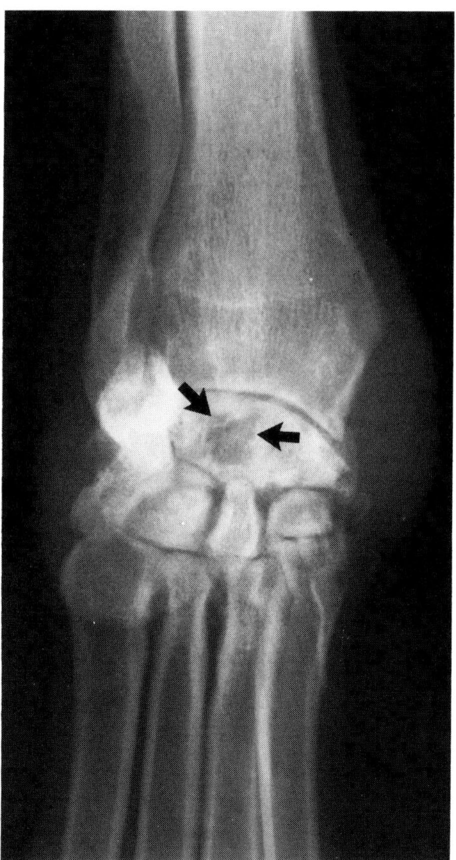

Figure 6–30. *Coccidioidomycosis. Osteomyelitis occasionally results in an arthritis, as seen in this dog with osteomyelitis of the radiocarpal bone (arrows). However, arthritis with a primary synovitis is rare in the dog with this infection.*

Visceral leishmaniasis (Leishmania donovani) is a chronic systemic reticuloendothelial proliferative disease of humans and some species of animals. The predominant presenting signs of the disease in dogs are fever, malaise, weight loss, dermatopathy, and polyarthritis. Generalized lymphadenopathy and hepatosplenomegaly are also seen. The synovial membrane is infiltrated by large numbers of macrophages that are filled with leishmanial bodies.

Noninfectious Arthritis

The noninfectious arthritides of animals can be classified into several groups, depending on the nature and etiology of the disorder:

1. Arthritis of Apparent Immunologic Cause
   a. Deforming or erosive
      (1) Canine rheumatoid arthritis

- (2) Polyarthritis of Greyhound dogs
- (3) Erosive form of feline progressive polyarthritis
- (4) Polyarthritis of rhesus monkeys
- (5) Miscellaneous

b. Periosteal proliferative
- (1) Feline chronic progressive polyarthritis

c. Nondeforming or nonerosive
- (1) Idiopathic
- (2) Associated with systemic lupus erythematosus
- (3) Associated with chronic infectious diseases
- (4) Enteropathic

2. Crystal-Induced Arthritis
   a. Gout
   b. Pseudogout

DEFORMING OR EROSIVE ARTHRITIS. *Canine rheumatoid arthritis* is a well-documented clinical entity.[46, 80, 99, 100, 114] It is a rare condition, with an incidence of approximately 2 per 25,000 dogs examined at our hospital. This disorder occurs mainly in small or toy breeds of dogs, and has an average age at onset of 4 years. The disease has been recognized in dogs as young as 8 months and as old as 8 years of age.

Canine rheumatoid arthritis is manifested initially as a shifting lameness with soft tissue swelling around involved joints. Within a period of several weeks or months, the disease localizes in particular joints, and characteristic radiographic signs develop. Joint involvement is more severe and is commonly seen in the carpal and tarsal joints, although in individual dogs the elbow, stifle, shoulder, and hip joints may show similar radiographic signs. Involvement of the apophyseal joints and the costovertebral articulations rarely progresses to the point of causing radiographic changes. The disease is often accompanied by fever, malaise, anorexia, and lymphadenopathy in the earlier stages.

The earliest radiographic changes consist of soft tissue swelling and a loss of trabecular bone density in the area of the joint. Lucent cyst-like areas are frequently seen in the subchondral bone. The prominent lesion is a progressive destruction of subchondral bone in the more central area as well as marginally at the attachment of the synovium.[12, 114] Both narrowing and widening of a joint space are identified radiographically as a result of cartilage erosion and destruction of subchondral bone (Fig. 6–31). Subluxation, luxation, and deformation occur most frequently in the carpal, tarsal, and phalangeal joints and occasionally in the elbow and stifle joints. Fibrous ankylosis can occur in advanced cases, particularly in the intercarpal and intertarsal joint space. Soft tissue calcification and atrophy accompany disuse osteoporosis and other radiographic findings.

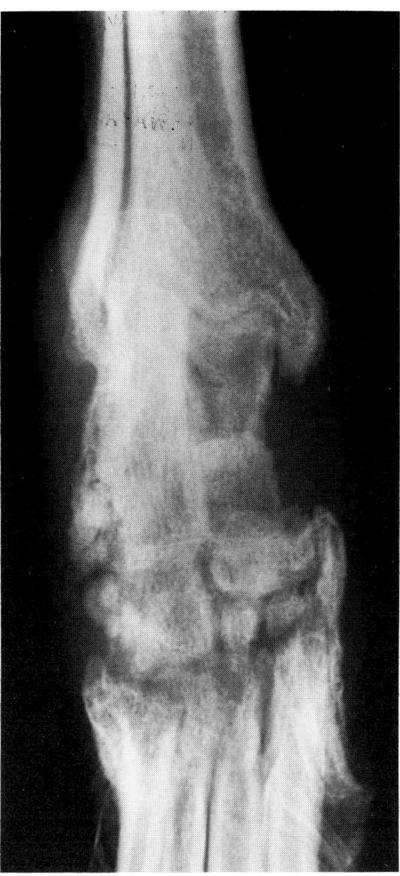

Figure 6–31. *Rheumatoid arthritis. Radiograph of severe rheumatoid arthritis of the tarsus demonstrates the destructive tendencies of this joint disease in the dog.*

Hemograms are either normal or reflect the generalized inflammatory process with a leukocytosis, neutrophilia, and hyperfibrinogenemia. Serum electrophoresis will show a variable hypoalbuminemia, and variable elevation in alpha-2 and gamma globulins. Unlike the situation in humans, serologic abnormalities in canine rheumatoid arthritis–like disease are often absent. Rheumatoid factor is present in comparatively low titer in about one quarter of the cases. LE cell preparations and fluorescent antinuclear antibody tests are usually negative. Synovial fluid changes are indicative of an inflammatory synovitis, with elevated total cell count, a high proportion of neutrophils in the synovial fluid cell population, and a variable decrease in the quality of the mucin clot. Ragocytes, as described in human rheumatoid arthritis, are not usually seen. A characteristic finding of canine rheumatoid arthritis is the presence in synovial fluid of mononuclear cells containing IgG with only rare cells containing C_3 protein. These mononuclear cells may be producing the immunoglobulin or ingesting it from the synovial fluid.

The characteristic pathologic lesions consist of a villous hyperplasia of the synovial membrane, lymphoid and plasma cell infiltrates in the synovium, and erosion of articular cartilage at the margins of

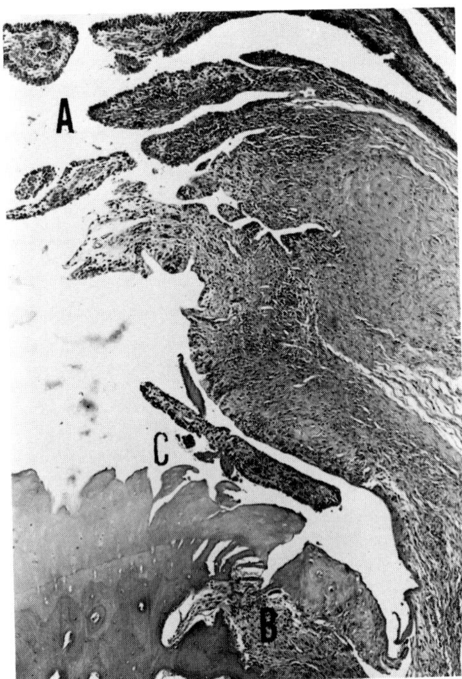

Figure 6–32. Joint margin from a dog with rheumatoid-like arthritis. Note the villous hypertrophy (A), destruction of the subchondral bone by granulation tissue arising from the inflamed synovium (B), and fibrillation of the articular cartilage (C).

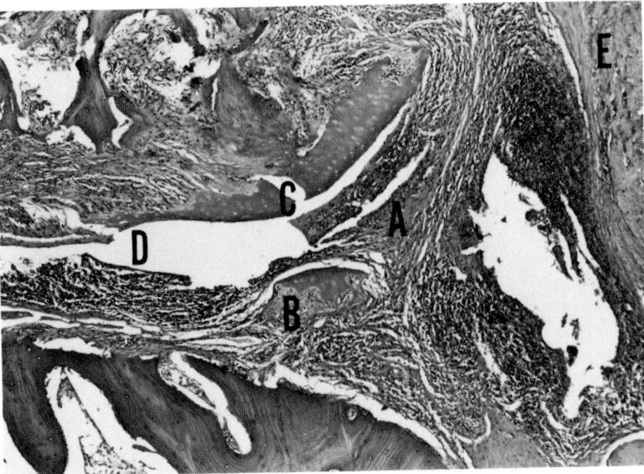

Figure 6–34. Joint margin from an advanced lesion of canine rheumatoid-like arthritis. Pannus (A) arising from the inflamed synovium has completely destroyed one articular surface (B), has nearly destroyed the opposing joint surface (C), and is beginning to fill the joint cavity (D) as a prelude to ankylosis of the joint. The fibrous layer of the joint capsule is shown (E).

the joint (Fig. 6–32). The dense lymphoid and plasma cell infiltrate in the synovium (Fig. 6–33) and the subchondral erosions differentiate this disease from the synovitis seen in the nonerosive types of arthritis, which will be discussed in the following section. The erosion of the articular cartilage at the margins of affected joints occurs as a result of two pathologic processes, i.e., granulation tissue from an inflamed synovium either extends across the articular surface as a pannus or undermines the cartilage by eroding subchondral bone (Fig. 6–34). In some instances, there is a loss of cartilage and subchondral bone in the central regions of the joint caused by an invasion of granulation tissue from the underlying marrow cavity (Fig. 6–35).

The pathogenesis of this disease in the dog is unknown. It is considered to be immunologic in nature because of the inability to culture bacteria, viruses, mycoplasmas, or chlamydiae from the affected joints, and because of its response to therapy with potent immunosuppressive drugs. Whether the etiology of the canine disease is identical to that of human rheumatoid arthritis remains to be established.

Canine rheumatoid arthritis–like disease responds only temporarily to systemic corticosteroids.

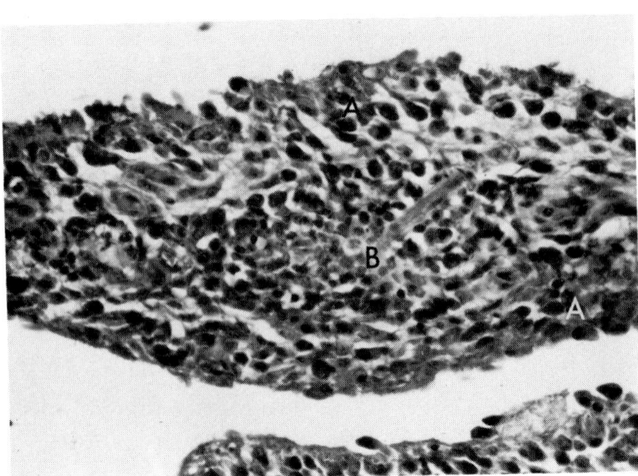

Figure 6–33. Synovial villus from a dog with rheumatoid-like arthritis showing hyperplasia of lining cells (A) and plasma cells and lymphocytes dispersed in the stroma or aggregated around small vessels (B).

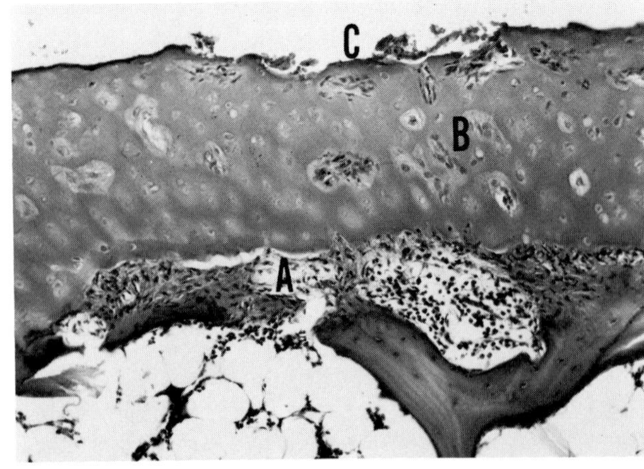

Figure 6–35. Cartilaginous defect in the trochlear groove of the femur of a dog with canine rheumatoid-like arthritis. Note the destruction of the subchondral bone by granulation tissue arising in the marrow spaces (A), extension of vessels through the articular cartilage (B), and destruction of the articular cartilage by a pannus originating in the marrow spaces of the subchondral bone (C).

There is an initial dramatic improvement, but this cannot be sustained even with high dosages. Aspirin has no appreciable therapeutic benefits in the dog, probably because the disease is much more severe and rapidly progressive in the dog. If the condition is recognized before severe joint damage occurs, it can usually be arrested with cyclophosphamide, azathioprine, and prednisolone given in combination. In dogs with advanced deformities, immunosuppressive drug therapy may have to be combined with arthrodesis of selected joints. Arthrodesis is not warranted if more than two joints need to be reconstructed, or if the disease process cannot first be successfully halted with drug therapy.

An *erosive polyarthritis of the Greyhound dog* has been described in different parts of the world.[20, 56] The disease appears in animals from 3 to 30 months of age, and most frequently attacks the proximal interphalangeal, carpal, tarsal, elbow, and stifle joints. The shoulder, hip, and atlanto-occipital joints are less frequently involved. A tenosynovitis may be an accompanying feature. The synovial membrane is edematous and hyperemic in the early course of the disease and may be covered with a fine layer of fibrin; the synovial fluid is cloudy, yellowish, and often contains fibrin tags. In later stages a lymphocyte and plasma cell infiltrate is seen in the synovial lining. Peripheral lymph nodes are enlarged and hyperactive. Pannus formation and marginal subchondral erosions are seen to a limited extent. Destruction of articular cartilage is accelerated in some joints, but often is not associated with pannus formation. Gross deformities and radiographic changes are not so apparent as those seen in canine rheumatoid arthritis, but appear more pronounced than those described for nonerosive joint disease.

Mycoplasmal and bacterial isolation has been unsuccessful, and dogs are serologically negative for Erysipelothrix and Chlamydia. Because of the custom of racing Greyhound breeders to destroy any unsound or diseased individuals, only a limited number of these dogs are seen by veterinarians. Discussions with Greyhound breeders indicate that the disease may be more frequent than is realized.

One form of *feline chronic progressive polyarthritis* is an erosive and deforming arthritis that appears similar to canine and human rheumatoid arthritis.[115] Like the canine disease, the incidence is relatively low. This form of the disease is a less common variant of feline chronic progressive polyarthritis than is the periosteal proliferative type.[116]

The deforming arthritis is recognized in the carpal, metacarpophalangeal, metatarsophalangeal, and interphalangeal joints (Fig. 6–36). Radiographic signs of erosion of the margins and central parts of

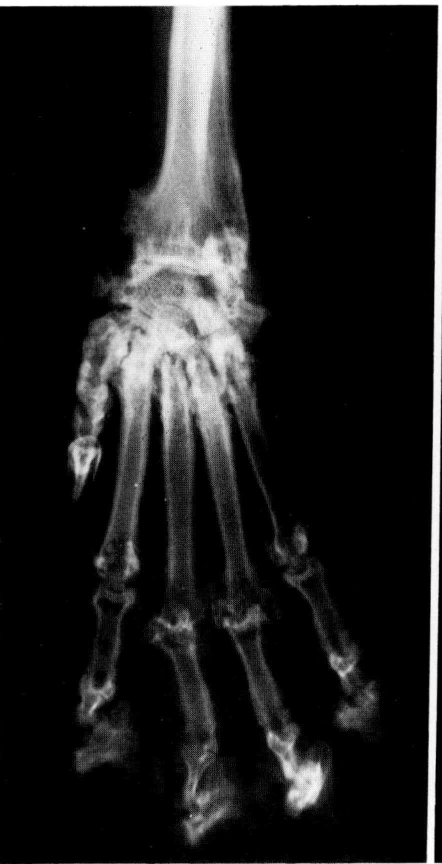

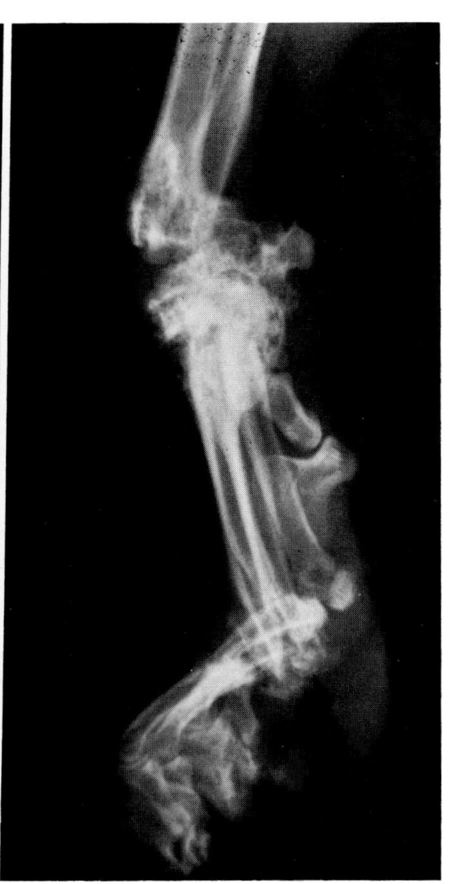

Figure 6–36. *Feline progressive polyarthritis. The deforming form of progressive polyarthritis in the cat is less common than the proliferative form. Severe joint disease with extensive erosion and instability is seen. Luxation of the carpus and the metacarpophalangeal and interphalangeal joints can be identified in this animal with the deforming form of arthritis.*

the subchondral bone in these joints precede joint instability and deformities. Proliferation of bone adjacent to affected joints can be identified, but proliferative bony findings are minor in degree, whereas destructive signs are excessive.

A *rheumatoid arthritis–like disease of rhesus monkeys* has been reported.[21, 107, 159] The condition is generally associated with amyloidosis in other organs, such as the spleen, and occasionally with chronic enterocolitis.[21] Tests for rheumatoid factor have been negative in some reports and positive in others. The etiology is somewhat obscured by the isolation of Shigella from the intestines of some of the monkeys with chronic enterocolitis[21] and by a rising mycoplasmal antibody titer in others.[107] In a report of monkeys with "rheumatoid arthritis," Mycoplasma was isolated from the joints of two in four animals.[159] The relationship of Shigella to Reiter's syndrome of humans and the similarity of chronic mycoplasmal arthritis in goats and pigs to rheumatoid arthritis make speculation on the classification of the disease in rhesus monkeys premature.

An erosive arthritis that fulfilled many of the criteria established for human rheumatoid arthritis has been described in a gorilla.[16] Mycoplasma was isolated from the joint, although its causal role was not determined.

Periosteal Proliferative Arthritis. *Feline chronic progressive polyarthritis* is the best example of a periosteal proliferative polyarthritis of animals.[115, 116] The disorder occurs exclusively in male cats with the common age at onset of 2 to 4½ years. There are two forms of the disease as determined by radiographic changes, the presence or absence of joint deformities, and the clinical course. The most prevalent form of the disease is characterized by osteoporosis and periosteal new bone formation surrounding a joint (Fig. 6–37). Periarticular erosions and collapse of the joint spaces with fibrous ankylosis occur with time, but gross joint deformities are not seen. The periosteal proliferative form of this disease in the cat resembles Reiter's syndrome of humans, while the erosive form is more typical of human rheumatoid arthritis. Histopathologic abnormalities are similar to those occurring in both chronic Reiter's syndrome and human rheumatoid arthritis.

Chronic progressive polyarthritis of cats is not caused by identifiable bacteria or Mycoplasma, but is etiologically linked to feline leukemia virus (FeLV) and feline syncytia-forming virus (FeSFV) infections. Feline syncytia-forming virus can be isolated from the blood or detected by serologic means in all cats with the disease, whereas FeLV is isolated from 70 per cent of the cats. The incidence of FeSFV infection in diseased cats is 2 to 4 times greater than age-matched healthy cats, whereas the incidence of FeLV infection is 6 to 10 times greater than expected. The arthritis cannot be reproduced, however, with infectious material from diseased cats. It is postulated that the arthritis is an uncommon disease manifestation of FeSFV infection that occurs in genetically predisposed male cats. Feline leukemia virus may not be directly involved in the disease, but acts in some way to potentiate the pathogenic effect of FeSFV. The actual joint disease is probably immunologically mediated, as evidenced by the dense lymphocytic and plasmacytic synovial infiltrate and the therapeutic response to immunosuppressive drugs.

Nondeforming or Nonerosive Arthritis. A nonerosive arthritis is identified in the dog, and although etiologically diverse, it is probably mediated by similar immunopathologic mechanisms.[113] The presenting clinical signs of this type of arthritis are similar with regard to the joint disease, whether it is idiopathic in origin or associated with secondary infectious disease, systemic lupus erythematosus (SLE), or inflammatory bowel disease. The joint disease tends to be cyclic in nature, has a predisposition for smaller distal joints, in particular the carpus and tarsus, and can occur in monoarticular, pauciarticular, or polyarticular forms. Radiographic changes, even after many months of joint disease, tend to be minimal or nonexistent. Biopsies of the synovial membranes show a sparse mononuclear cell infiltrate with moderate to severe superficial inflammation characterized by polymorphonuclear cell infiltrates and fibrin exudation. Villous hyperplasia, marginal erosions, and pannus formation are not prominent features in these diseases. Regardless of the overlying or underlying disease process that leads to the arthritis, the joint disease is believed to be due to deposition of immune complexes in the synovial membrane, with resultant immune-mediated inflammatory reactions.

Idiopathic nondeforming arthritis is by far the most common disorder of dogs manifesting this type of arthritis.[113] It is termed idiopathic because there is no evidence of a primary chronic infectious disease process, serologic abnormalities of SLE are absent, and joint disease is often the sole manifestation of illness. This condition occurs most commonly in large breeds of dogs, in particular German Shepherds, Doberman Pinschers, Retrievers, Spaniels, and Pointers. When seen in toy breeds, it most frequently occurs in toy Poodles, Lhasa Apsos, Yorkshire Terriers, and Chihuahuas, or mixes of these breeds. A similar condition has been rarely recognized in horses and cats.

The initial presenting history is one of a cyclic fever, during which time malaise, anorexia, lameness, or generalized stiffness is noted. In severe cases, periods of remission are usually incomplete, in which case the disease can be very debilitating.

Generalized muscle atrophy and disproportionate atrophy of the temporal and masseter muscles are frequently seen.

During the most severe stages of the disease, swelling and heat in distal joints are sometimes detected. Generalized lymphadenopathy is often present to varying degrees. During attacks, the dogs run high fevers and demonstrate leukocytosis with neutrophilia and hyperfibrinogenemia. The joint disease can be manifested as a single limb lameness in cases of monoarticular or pauciarticular involvement. When the disease is monoarticular in presentation, the elbow joint is often involved. The monoarticular form is much more common in Irish Setter dogs. Polyarticular involvement is the most common presentation, in which case the dogs will show

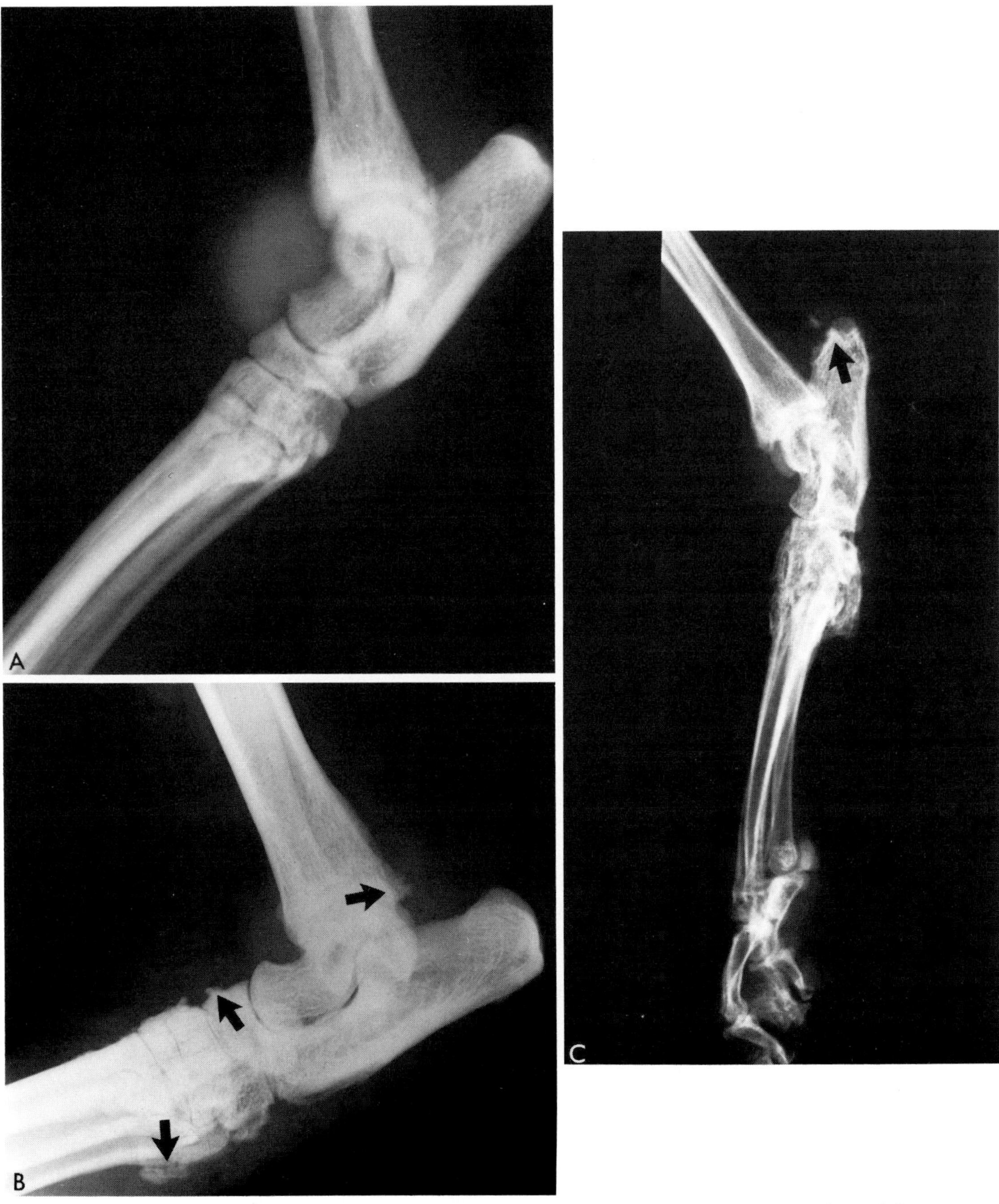

Figure 6–37. *Feline progressive polyarthritis. Radiographic signs of the proliferative form of this chronic joint disease of cats in the acute stage are joint capsule thickening and distention at the carpus and tarsus* **(A)** *with soft tissue swelling of tendon sheaths. Periosteal proliferation and soft tissue calcification (arrows) follow in the subacute* **(B)** *and chronic* **(C)** *stages. Remodeling of bone at tendinous (arrows) and ligamentous attachments is a common finding.*

generalized stiffness and reluctance to move the spine, tail, or limbs. Toy breeds, which often have severe generalized arthritis, can become virtually immobile, making it difficult to tell whether the joints are the source of the problem or if the immobility is due solely to depression.

Diagnosis is made by consideration of the clinical history of cyclic, antibiotic-unresponsive fever, malaise, and anorexia on which is superimposed the stiffness or lameness. Synovial fluid is inflammatory in nature and sterile for bacteria, viruses, Mycoplasma, and Chlamydia. Serologic abnormalities such as the LE cell phenomenon, antinuclear antibody, or rheumatoid factor are absent. Blood cultures are negative for bacteria. The treatment of this disorder involves corticosteroids or corticosteroids used in combination with more potent immunosuppressive drugs. A complete remission of signs can usually be achieved. About 30 to 50 per cent of the dogs will have recurrences of their illness after the drug therapy is discontinued.

A *nondeforming arthritis associated with chronic infectious diseases* has been described in dogs.[113] Infectious diseases that can be associated with this form of arthritis include chronic bacterial infections, chronic fungal infections, and occasionally parasitic infections. This type of arthritis is frequently associated with subacute bacterial endocarditis in dogs and chronic Actinomyces infections of the chest, abdomen, or paravertebral musculature. Joint involvement in this type of disorder is usually monoarticular or pauciarticular and has a predisposition for the carpal and tarsal joints. The fact that the offending organisms involved in the primary disease process cannot be identified in the synovial membrane makes it likely that this disease is also of immune complex origin, although a low-grade infection from which the organism cannot be recovered is also possible. A similar relationship between a sterile arthritis and chronic infections in other parts of the body has been recognized much earlier in humans.[25]

Canine SLE was initially defined as the triad of glomerulonephritis, thrombocytopenia, and hemolytic anemia associated with a salicylate-responsive arthralgia in some cases.[68, 78] It is apparent, however, that canine SLE is similar in its presentation to human SLE, i.e., articular, dermatologic, renal, and neuromuscular problems seem to be more common than hematologic abnormalities.[76, 113] Hematologic abnormalities in the dog, such as thrombocytopenia or hemolytic anemia, occur in only 10 to 20 per cent or less of the total cases of SLE that we have seen.

The arthritis of canine SLE is similar in every detail to that seen in cases of idiopathic nonerosive arthritis. Both conditions predominate in the same breeds, and, in fact, serologic abnormalities such as antinuclear antibodies are often the only thing that allows one to classify the condition as SLE. In cases in which other systemic manifestations of SLE are present with the arthritis, the diagnosis is more easily made. The joint disease is usually polyarticular or pauciarticular in nature.

There is currently a great deal of interest in canine SLE as a model for human SLE. Studies on the progeny of matings between affected dogs are currently in progress. Interestingly, about 95 per cent of the progeny of such matings develop serologic abnormalities consistent with SLE by 18 months of age.[77] Clinical signs of SLE are not seen, however. Attempts to explain this occurrence by genetic factors have been somewhat inconclusive, and it appears that if the serologic marker is genetically transmitted, it is not as a single gene. As a next step, experiments have been designed to determine whether such a phenomenon could be due to the transmission of an infectious agent from one generation to another. Cell-free filtrates of spleen from affected dogs, when passed into normal Beagle puppies and newborn CAF_1 mice, induce antinuclear antibodies and the LE cell phenomenon in a high percentage of individuals.[75] Moreover, the development of antinuclear antibodies in CAF_1 mice is often associated with the development of lymphoblastic leukemia, reticulum cell sarcomas, or plasma cell myelomas. All these tumors occur at a much higher incidence in inoculated than in uninoculated mice, and in culture all the tumors express murine leukemia virus. Antinuclear antibody and lymphomas can be regularly transmitted to syngeneic mice with cell-free extracts of the mouse lymphomas induced by the dog spleen filtrate. Finally, it is possible to show that some of the lymphocytes from the blood of a dog with SLE contain surface antigens similar to the 30,000 dalton interspecies antigen of feline leukemia virus.[74] The presence of an infectious agent in dogs with SLE, if confirmed, has important implications for humans. This is especially true in that no C-type virus has been demonstrated as a naturally expressed entity in either dog or human.

Enteropathic arthritis is frequently associated with diseases like ulcerative colitis and regional enteritis of humans.[33] The cause of the arthritis is unknown, but it can be postulated that the bowel and joint disease share a common etiology, or that antigenic products released into the blood from the inflamed bowel have some effect on the synovium. The frequency of enteropathic arthritis in the dog is unknown, although we have recognized polyarthritis in dogs with ulcerative colitis and in dogs with a more fulminating enterocolitis. Changes in the synovial membrane and synovial fluid are indistinguishable from those described for idiopathic polyarthritis or systemic lupus erythematosus of the dog. A similar sterile arthritis has been described in calves with acute and subacute enteric and respiratory infections.[166]

Crystal-Induced Arthritis. *Hyperuricemia* and *gout* have been recognized as naturally occurring entities in animals, including chickens, birds, and reptiles.[170] They are rare in mammalian species. By selectively breeding chickens with high blood uric acid levels, it has been possible to create a line of chickens that develop visceral and articular gout. In this condition there is an inherited defect in the ability of the kidney tubules to transport uric acid.[5, 6] In acute gouty arthritis of birds, urate crystals are deposited in the soft tissues of joints, tendon sheaths, and bursae, where they provoke an inflammatory response resembling the one seen in humans. The one report of gout in the dog was based on radiographic evidence but was not confirmed by pathologic studies.[90] Visceral and articular gout has been induced in chickens fed diets deficient in vitamin A.[14] Although the uric acid levels in the serum are normal, the level of uric acid in tissues such as the kidney is increased.

Pseudogout is a rare entity in animals. There is one reported case in the dog[36] and one in a turtle.[35]

REFERENCES

1. Ackerman LJ, Kishimoto RA, Emerson JS: Nonpigmented *Serratia marcescens* arthritis in a teju (*Tupinambis teguixin*). Am J Vet Res *32*:823, 1971.
2. Ajmal M: Experimental erysipelothrix arthritis. I. Observations on specific-pathogen-free and gnotobiotic pigs following systemic administration of live *E. rhusiopathiae* or intra-articular injection of non-living *E. rhusiopathiae* cells or cell wall fragments. Res Vet Sci *12*:403, 1971.
3. Ajmal M: *Erysipelothrix rhusiopathiae* and spontaneous arthritis in pigs. Res Vet Sci *10*:579, 1969.
4. Alspaugh MA, Van Hoosier GL Jr: Naturally occurring and experimentally induced arthritides in rodents: A review of the literature. Lab Anim Sci *23*:724, 1973.
5. Austic RE, Cole RK: Hereditary variation in uric acid transport by avian kidney slices. Am J Physiol *231*:1147, 1976.
6. Austic RE, Cole RK: Specificity of the renal transport impairment in chickens having hyperuricemia and articular gout. Proc Soc Exp Biol Med *146*:931, 1974.
7. Bailey JH: Swine arthritis (a review). Vet Med Small Anim Clin *67*:197, 1972.
8. Barden JA, Decker JL: *Mycoplasma hyorhinis* swine arthritis. Clinical and microbiologic features. Arthritis Rheum *14*:193, 1971.
9. Barthel CH, Duncan JR, Ross RF: Histologic and histochemical characterization of synovial membrane from normal and *Mycoplasma hyorhinis*-infected swine. Am J Vet Res *33*:2501, 1972.
10. Battershell D: Ununited anconeal process. J Am Vet Med Assoc *155*:35, 1969.
11. Bennett RH, Jasper DE: *Mycoplasma alkalescens*-induced arthritis in dairy calves. J Am Vet Med Assoc *172*:484, 1978.
12. Biery DN, Newton CD: Radiographic appearance of rheumatoid arthritis in the dog. J Am Anim Hosp Assoc *11*:607, 1975.
13. Blumberg BS, Bunim JJ, Calkins E, Pirani CL, Zvaifler NJ: Nomenclature of arthritis and rheumatism (tentative) accepted by the American Rheumatism Association. Bull Rheum Dis *14*:339, 1964.
14. Bokori J: Studies on nutritional gout in poultry. II. The aetiological role of A-avitaminosis in poultry gout. Acta Vet Acad Sci Hung *15*:421, 1965.
15. Bond MP: Polyarthritis of pigs in western Australia: The role of *Erysipelothrix rhusiopathiae*. Aust Vet J *52*:462, 1976.
16. Brown TM, Clark HW, Bailey JS, Gray CW: A mechanistic approach to treatment of rheumatoid type arthritis naturally occurring in a gorilla. Trans Am Clin Climatol Assoc *82*:227, 1970.
17. Burrows GE: *Corynebacterium equi* infection in two foals. J Am Vet Med Assoc *152*:1119, 1968.
18. Buys SB: The isolation of *Mycoplasma synoviae* from chickens with infectious synovitis and air-sacculitis in the Republic of South Africa. Onderstepoort J Vet Res *43*:39, 1976.
19. Carnaham DL, Guffy MM, Hibbs CM, Leipold HW, Huston K: Hip dysplasia in Hereford cattle. J Am Vet Med Assoc *152*:1150, 1968.
20. Castell MJ: Acute peri-arthritis in a kennel of greyhounds. Vet Rec *84*:652, 1969.
21. Chapman WL Jr, Crowell WA: Amyloidosis in Rhesus monkeys with rheumatoid arthritis and enterocolitis. J Am Vet Med Assoc *171*:855, 1977.
22. Christian CL: Experimental models of arthritis and related connective tissue diseases and some naturally occurring counterparts in animals. Arthritis Rheum *13*:621, 1970.
23. Clegg FG, Rorrison JM: *Brucella abortus* infection in the dog: A case of polyarthritis. Res Vet Sci 9:183, 1968.
24. Coffman JR: Joint ill in foals. Vet Med Small Anim Clin *65*:274, 1970.
25. Coggeshall HC, Bennett GA, Warren CF, Bauer W.: Synovial fluid and synovial membrane abnormalities resulting from varying grades of systemic infection and edema. Am J Med Sci *202*:486, 1941.
26. Coria MF, McClurkin AW, Cutlip RC, Ritchie AE: Isolation and characterization of bovine adenovirus type 5 associated with "weak calf" syndrome. Arch Virol *47*:309, 1975.
27. Corley EA, Sutherland TM, Carlson WD: Genetic aspects of canine elbow dysplasia. J Am Vet Med Assoc *153*:543, 1968.
28. Cullen GA: Teno-synovitis (viral arthritis) of chickens. *In* LE Glynn, HD Schlumberger (eds): Experimental Models of Chronic Inflammatory Diseases. Berlin, Springer Verlag, 1977, p 212.
29. Cutlip RC: Ultrastructure of the synovial membrane of lambs affected with chlamydial polyarthritis. Am J Vet Res *35*:171, 1974.
30. Cutlip RC, Smith PC, Page LA: Chlamydial polyarthritis of lambs: A review. J Am Vet Med Assoc *161*:1213, 1972.
31. Diplock PT: Legg-Perthes disease (coxa plana) in cattle. J Am Vet Med Assoc *141*:462, 1962.
32. Edwards GB, Vaughan LC: Infective arthritis of the elbow joint in horses. Vet Rec *103*:227, 1978.
33. Ferguson RH: Enteropathic arthritis. *In* JL Hollander, DJ McCarty (Eds.) : Arthritis and Allied Conditions. Philadelphia, Lea & Febiger, 1972, p 841.
34. Flecknell PA, Gruffydd-Jones TJ: Congenital luxation of the patellae in the cat. Feline Pract 9:18, 1979.
35. Frye FL, Dutra FR: Articular pseudogout in a turtle (*Chrysemys s. elegans*). Vet Med Small Anim Clin *71*:655, 1976.
36. Gibson JP, Roenigk WJ: Pseudogout in a dog. J Am Vet Med Assoc *161*:912, 1972.
37. Glass SE, Naqi SA, Hall CF, Kerr KM: Isolation and characterization of a virus associated with arthritis of chickens. Avian Dis *17*:415, 1973.
38. Goudswaard J, Hartman EG, Janmaat A, Huisman, GH: *Erysipelothrix rhusiopathiae* Strain 7, a causative agent of endocarditis and arthritis in the dog. Tijdschr Diergeneeskd *98*:416, 1973.
39. Gourlay RN, Thomas LH, Howard CJ: Pneumonia and arthritis in gnotobiotic calves following inoculation with *Mycoplasma agalactiae subsp. bovis*. Vet Rec *98*:506, 1976.
40. Grondalen T: Osteochondrosis, arthrosis and leg weakness in pigs. Nord Vet Med *26*:534, 1974.
41. Grondalen T: Osteochondrosis and arthrosis in pigs. VII. Relationship to joint shape and exterior conformation. Acta Vet Scand (Suppl) *46*: 1, 1974.
42. Grondalen T: Osteochondrosis and arthrosis in pigs. VI. Relationship to feed level and calcium, phosphorus and protein levels in the ration. Acta Vet Scand *15*:147, 1974.
43. Grondalen, J., Braut T: Lameness in two young dogs caused by a calcified body in the joint capsule of the elbow. J Small Anim Pract *17*:681, 1976.
44. Gupta BN, Conner GH, Meyer DB: Osteoarthritis in guinea pigs. Lab Anim Sci *22*:326, 1972.
45. Haakenstad LH: Studies on the pathologic dislocation of the hip joint in horses with special reference to the nature and etiological aspects of the lesions. Nord Vet Med *5*:884, 1953.
46. Halliwell RE, Lavelle RB, Butt KM: Canine rheumatoid arthritis — a review and a case report. J Small Anim Pract *13*:239, 1972.
47. Hamilton GF, Adams OR: Anterior cruciate ligament repair in cattle. J Am Vet Med Assoc *158*:178, 1971.
48. Hanly GJ, Mossman DH: Polyarthritis in hereford bulls associated with BVD-MD infection. NZ Vet J *25*:38, 1977.

49. Harwick JH, Kalmanson GM, Fox MA, Guze LB: Arthritis in mice due to infection with *Mycoplasma pulmonis*. I. Clinical and microbiologic features. J Infect Dis *128*:533, 1973.
50. Hedhammer A, Wu FM, Krook L, Schryver HF, DeLahunta A, Whalen JP, Kallfelz FA, Nunez EA, Hintz HF, Sheffy BE, Ryan, GD: Overnutrition and skeletal disease. An experimental study in growing Great Dane dogs. Cornell Vet *64*(Suppl 5):5, 1974.
51. Hjerpe CA, Knight HD: Polyarthritis and synovitis associated with *Mycoplasma bovimastitidis* in feedlot cattle. J Am Vet Med Assoc *160*:1414, 1972.
52. Hopkins JB, Stephenson EH, Storz J, Pierson RE: Conjunctivitis associated with chlamydial polyarthritis in lambs. J Am Vet Med Assoc *163*:1157, 1973.
53. Howlett CR: Pathology of coxofemoral arthropathy in young beef bulls. Pathology *5*:135, 1973.
54. Howlett CR: Inherited degenerative arthropathy of the hip in young beef bulls. Aust Vet J *48*:562, 1972.
55. Hughes KL, Edwards MJ, Hartley WT, Murphy S: Polyarthritis in calves caused by *Mycoplasma sp*. Vet Rec *78*:276, 1966.
56. Huxtable CR, Davis PE: The pathology of polyarthritis in young greyhounds. J Comp Pathol *86*:11, 1976.
57. Ivanoff MR, Renshaw HW: Weak calf syndrome: Serum immunoglobulin concentrations in precolostral calves. Am J Vet Res *36*:1129, 1975.
58. Janovski NA: Arthropathy associated with *Escherichia coli* septicemia in caged birds. J Am Vet Med Assoc *148*:1517, 1966.
59. Jezyk PF, Haskins ME, Patterson DF, Mellman WJ, Greenstein M: Mucopolysaccharidosis in a cat with arylsulfatase B deficiency. A model of Maroteaux-Lamy syndrome. Science *198*:834, 1977.
60. Jögi P, Norberg I: Malformation of the hip joint in a standardbred horse. Vet Rec *74*:421, 1962.
61. Johnson JH: The navicular syndrome. Mod Vet Pract *54*:69, 1973.
62. Jones WG: Fluorosis in a dairy herd. Vet Rec *90*:503, 1972.
63. Jonsson G, Jacobson SO, Stromberg G, Olsson SE, Bjorklund NE: Rickets and secondary nutritional hyperparathyroidism. A clinical syndrome in fattening bulls. Acta Radiol Suppl *319*:91, 1972.
64. Kasstrom H: Nutrition, weight gain, and development of hip dysplasia. An experimental investigation in growing dogs with special reference to the effect of feeding intensity. Acta Radiol Suppl *344*:136, 1975.
65. Kendrick JW, Sittmann K: Inherited osteoarthritis of dairy cattle. J Am Vet Med Assoc *149*:17, 1966.
66. King SJ: Porcine polyserositis and arthritis — with particular reference to mycoplasmosis and Glasser's disease. Aust Vet J *44*:227, 1968.
67. Kleven SH, Fletcher OJ, Davis RB: Influence of strain of *Mycoplasma synoviae* and route of infection in development of synovitis and air sacculitis in broilers. Avian Dis *19*:126, 1975.
68. Krum SH, Cardinet GH III, Anderson BC, Holliday TA: Polymyositis and polyarthritis associated with systemic lupus erythematosus in a dog. J Am Vet Med Assoc *170*:61, 1977.
69. Lamas Da Silva JM, Alder HE: Pathogenesis of arthritis induced in chickens by *Mycoplasma gallisepticum*. Pathol Vet 6:385, 1969.
70. Langford EV: *Mycoplasma agalactiae subsp. bovis* in pneumonia and arthritis of the bovine. Can J Comp Med *41*:89, 1977.
71. Larsen JS (Ed): Symposium workshop panel reports in canine hip dysplasia. *In* proceedings of Canine Hip Dysplasia Symposium and Workshop, St. Louis, Missouri, 1973, p 153.
72. Leach RM Jr, Nesheim MC: Nutritonal, genetic and morphological studies of an abnormal cartilage formation in young chicks. J Nutr *86*:236, 1965.
73. Lee R: A study of the radiographic and histological changes occurring in Legg-Calvé-Perthes disease (LCP) in the dog. J Small Anim Pract *11*:621, 1970.
74. Lewis RM: Evidence for a virus in canine systemic lupus erythematosus. *In* LE Glyn, HD Schlumberger (Eds): Experimental Models of Chronic Inflammatory Disease. Berlin, Springer Verlag, 1977, p 71.
75. Lewis RM, Andre-Schwartz J, Harris GS, Hirsch MS, Black PN, Schwartz RS: Canine systemic lupus erythematosus. Transmission of serologic abnormalities by cell free filtrates. J. Clin Invest *52*:1893, 1973.
76. Lewis RM, Hathaway JE: Canine systemic lupus erythematosus presenting with symmetrical polyarthritis. J Small Anim Pract *8*:273, 1967.
77. Lewis, RM, Schwartz RS: Canine systemic lupus erythematosus. Genetic analysis of an established breeding colony. J Exp Med *134*:417, 1971.
78. Lewis RM, Schwartz R, Henry WB Jr: Canine systemic lupus erythematosus. Blood *25*:143, 1965.
79. Lipowitz AJ, Fetter AW, Walker MA: Synovial sarcoma of the dog. J Am Vet Med Assoc *174*:76, 1979.
80. Liu SK, Suter PF, Fischer CA, Dorfman HD: Rheumatoid arthritis in a dog. J Am Vet Med Assoc *154*:495, 1969.
81. Ljunggren G: Legg-Perthes disease in the dog. Acta Orthop Scand (Suppl) *95*:1, 1967.
82. Ljunggren G, Reiland S: Osteochondrosis in adolescent animals: An endocrine disorder? Calcif Tissue Res (Suppl): 150, 1970.
83. Lloyd-Roberts GC: Osteoarthritis of the hip. J bone Joint Surg *37(B)*:8, 1955.
84. Lust G: Pathogenesis of degenerative hip joint disease in young dogs. *In* Proceedings of the Twenty-third Annual Gaines Veterinary Symposium, Pullman, WA, 1973, p 11.
85. Lust G, Geary JC, Sheffy BE: Development of hip dysplasia in dogs. Am J Vet Res *34*:87, 1973.
86. Madewell BR, Pool R: Neoplasms of joints and related structures. Vet Clin North Am *8*:511, 1978.
87. McCapes RH: Lameness in turkeys due to faulty bone formations. Ann Nutr Health *22*:17, 1967.
88. McChesney AE, Becerra V, England JJ: Chlamydial polyarthritis in a foal. J Am Vet Med Assoc *165*:259, 1974.
89. McClurkin AW, Coria MF: Infectivity of bovine adenovirus type 5 recovered from a polyarthritic calf with weak calf syndrome. J Am Vet Med Assoc *167*:139, 1975.
90. Miller RM, Kind RE: A gout-like syndrome in a dog. Vet Med Small Anim Clin *61*:236, 1966.
91. Miner ML, Smart RA, Olson AE: Pathogenesis of staphylococcal synovitis in turkeys: Pathologic changes. Avian Dis *12*:46, 1968.
92. Mohamed YS, Moorhead PD, Bohl EH: Natural *Streptobacillus moniliformis* infection of turkeys, and attempts to infect turkeys, sheep, and pigs. Avian Dis *13*:379, 1969.
93. Moore RW, Redmond HE, Livingston CW Jr: Pathologic and seriologic characteristics of a Mycoplasma causing arthritis in swine. Am J Vet Res *27*:1649, 1966.
94. Moorthy AR, Spradbrow PB, Eisler ME: Isolation of Mycoplasma from an arthritic foal. Br Vet J *133*:320, 1977.
95. Morgan JP: Radiology in Veterinary Orthopedics. Philadelphia, Lea & Febiger, 1972.
96. Moskowitz, RW: Clinical and laboratory findings in osteoarthritis. *In* JL Hollander, DJ McCarty (Eds): Arthritis and Allied Conditions. Philadelphia, Lea & Febiger, 1972, p 1032.
97. Nairn ME: Bacterial osteomyelitis and synovitis of the turkey. Avian Dis *17*:504, 1973.
98. Nakagawa M, Motoi Y, Iizuka M, Azuma, R: Histopathology of enzootic chronic polyarthritis of goats in Japan. Natl Inst Anim Health Q *11*:191, 1971.
99. Newton CD, Lipowitz AJ, Halliwell RE, Allen HL, Biery DN, Schumacher L: Rheumatoid arthritis in dogs. J Am Vet Med Assoc *168*:113, 1976.
100. Newton CD: RA in dogs. Arthritis Rheum *19*:970, 1976.
101. Nielsen R, Danielsen V: An outbreak of Glasser's disease. Studies on etiology, serology and the effect of vaccination. Nord Vet Med *27*:20, 1975.
102. Nickels FA, Grant BD, Lincoln SD: Villonodular synovitis of the equine metacarpophalangeal joint. J Am Vet Med Assoc *168*:1043, 1976.
103. Norrung V: Studies on *Erysipelothrix insidiosa s. rhusiopathiae*. 1. Morphology, cultural features, biochemical reactions and virulence. Acta Vet Scand *11*:577, 1970.
104. Norrung V: Studies on *Erysipelothrix insidiosa s. rhusiopathiae*. 2. Serological study. Acta Vet Scand *11*:586, 1970.
105. Norton WL, Storz J: Observations on sheep with polyarthritis produced by an agent of the *Psittacosis–lymphogranuloma venereum–trachoma* group. Arthritis Rheum *10*:1, 1967.
106. Numans SR, Van Der Watering CC: Navicular disease: *Podotrochlitis chronica aseptica podotrochlosis*. Equine Vet J *5*:1, 1973.
107. Obeck DK, Toft JD II, Dupuy D: Severe polyarthritis in a Rhesus monkey: Suggested Mycoplasma etiology. Lab Anim Sci *26*:613, 1976.
108. O'Brien TR: Developmental deformities due to arrested epiphyseal growth. Vet Clin North Am *1*:441, 1971.
109. O'Brien TR, Morgan JP, Suter PF: Epiphyseal plate injuries in the dog: A radiographic study of growth disturbance in the forelimbs. J Small Anim Pract *12*:19, 1971.
110. Olson NO, Solomon DP: A natural outbreak of synovitis caused by the viral arthritis agent. Avian Dis *12*:311, 1968.
111. Olsson S: Osteochondrosis — a growing problem to dog breeders. Gaines Dog Research Progress, Summer, 1976.
112. Olsson SE: Degenerative joint disease (osteoarthrosis): A review with special reference to the dog. J Small Anim Pract *12*:333, 1971.
113. Pedersen NC, Weisner K, Castles JJ, Ling GU, Weiser G: Noninfectious canine arthritis: The inflammatory, nonerosive arthritides. J Am Vet Med Assoc *169*:304, 1976.
114. Pedersen NC, Pool RR, Castles JJ, Weisner K: Noninfectious canine arthritis: Rheumatoid arthritis. J Am Vet Med Assoc *169*:295, 1976.
115. Pedersen NC, Pool RR, O'Brien T: Feline chronic progressive polyarthritis. Am J Vet Res *41*:522, 1980.
116. Pedersen NC, Pool RR, O'Brien T, Evans WR, Shatilla H: Chronic progressive polyarthritis of the cat. Feline Pract *5*:42, 1975.

117. Pierson RE: Polyarthritis in Colorado feedlot lambs. J Am Vet Med Assoc *150*:1487, 1967.
118. Platt H: Joint-ill and other bacterial infections on thoroughbred studs. Equine Vet J *9*:141, 1977.
119. Prasad S, Hairr WT, Dallas JT: Observations of abnormal cartilage formation associated with leg weakness in commercial broilers. Avian Dis *16*:457, 1972.
120. Price CJ, King SC: Elbow lameness in a young dog caused by an ossified disc in the joint capsule. Vet Rec *100*:566, 1977.
121. Radostits OM, Doige CE, Pharr JW: Coxofemoral arthropathy in a young bull. Can Vet J *17*:48, 1976.
122. Ramadan RO, Vaughan LC: Premature closure of the distal ulnar growth plate in dogs — a review of 58 cases. J Small Anim Pract *19*:647, 1978.
123. Reiland S, Stromberg B, Olsson SE, Dreimanis I, Olsson I: Osteochondrosis in growing bulls: Pathology, frequency and severity on different feedings. Acta Radiol Suppl *358*:179, 1978.
124. Rejnö S, Strömberg B: Osteochondroses in the horse. II. Pathology. Acta Radiol Suppl *358*:153, 1978.
125. Riddell C: The development of tibial dyschondroplasia in broiler chickens. Avian Dis *19*:443, 1975.
126. Riddell C: Studies on the pathogenesis of tibial dyschondroplasia in chickens. II. Growth rate of long bones. Avian Dis *19*:490, 1975.
127. Riser WH: Juvenile osteoporosis (osteogenesis imperfecta) in the dog and cat. J Am Vet Radiol Soc *3*:50, 1962.
128. Riser WH, Shirer JF: Correlation between canine hip dysplasia and pelvic muscle mass: A study of 95 dogs. Am J Vet Res *28*:769, 1967.
129. Roberts DH, Olesiuk OM: Serological studies with *Mycoplasma synoviae*. Avian Dis *11*:104, 1967.
130. Robins GM: A case of *Osteochondritis dissecans* of the stifle joints in a bitch. J Small Anim Pract *11*:813, 1970.
131. Ross RF: Predisposing factors in *Mycoplasma hyosynoviae* arthritis in swine. J Infect Dis *127*:84, 1973.
132. Ross RF, Switzer WP, Duncan JR: Experimental production of *Mycoplasma hyosynoviae* arthritis in swine. Am J Vet Res *32*:1743, 1971.
133. Ross RF, Duncan JR: *Mycoplasma hyosynoviae* arthritis of swine. J Am Vet Med Assoc *157*:1515, 1970.
134. Sato S, Shoya S, Horiuchi T, Nonomura I: An outbreak of synovitis caused by *Mycoplasma gallisepticum* in chickens. Natl Inst Anim Health Q *12*:54, 1972.
135. Scott PP, McKusick VA, McKusick AB: The nature of osteogenesis imperfecta in cats. J Bone Joint Surg *45*:125, 1963.
136. Seawright AH, English PB, Gartner RJW: Hypervitaminosis A of the cat. Adv Vet Sci Comp Med *14*:1, 1970.
137. Shupe JL, Miner ML, Greenwood DA: Clinical and pathological aspects of fluorine toxicosis in cattle. Ann NY Acad Sci *111*:618, 1964.
138. Sikes D, Causey EW, Jones TJ, Fletcher OJ Jr, Hayes FA: Electrophoretic and serologic changes of blood serum of arthritic (rheumatoid) dogs infected with *Erysipelothrix insidiosa*. Am J Vet Res *32*:1083, 1971.
139. Sikes D: Experimental production of rheumatoid arthritis of swine: Physiopathologic changes of tissues. Am J Vet Res *29*:1719, 1968.
140. Sikes D: Experimental production of ankylosing spondylitis in swine with an isolate of *Erysipelothrix insidiosa* of human origin. Am J Vet Res *28*:1437, 1967.
141. Sikes D, Fletcher O Jr, Papp E: Further studies on the pathologic alterations of tissues of swine given repeated whole blood transfusions from swine with rheumatoid-like arthritis. Am J Vet Res *28*:1413, 1967.
142. Sikes D, Fletcher O Jr, Papp E: Experimental production of pannus in a rheumatoid-like arthritis of swine. Am J Vet Res *27*:1017, 1966.
143. Singh UM, Doig PA, Ruhnke HL: Mycoplasma arthritis in calves. Can Vet J *12*:183, 1971.
144. Smart RA, Miner ML, Davis RV: Pathogenesis of *Staphylococcal synovitis* in turkeys: Cultural retrieval in experimental infection. Avian Dis *12*:37, 1968.
145. Smillie IS: Osteochondritis Dissecans. Edinburgh, E & S Livingstone, Ltd 1960.
146. Sokoloff L: Rheumatoid arthritis, animal model: Arthritis due to mycoplasma in rats and swine. Am J Pathol *73*:261, 1973.
147. Stalheim OH, Stone SS: Isolation and identification of *Mycoplasma agalactiae subsp. bovis* from arthritic cattle in Iowa and Nebraska. J Clin Microbiol *2*:169, 1975.
148. Stalheim OH, Page LA: Naturally occurring and experimentally induced mycoplasmal arthritis of cattle. J Clin Microbiol *2*:165, 1975.
149. Steinke FH: Osteodystrophy — nutritional and related factors. *In* Proceedings of Symposium on Leg Weakness in Turkeys, Ames, Iowa, 1970, p 30.
150. Stephenson EH, Storz J, Hopkins JB: Properties and frequency of isolation of chlamydiae from eyes of lambs with conjunctivitis and polyarthritis. Am J Vet Res *35*:177, 1974.
151. Storz J, Smart RA, Marriott ME, Davis RV: Polyarthritis of calves: Isolation of psittacosis agents from affected joints. Am J Vet Res *27*:633, 1966.
152. Studer E, Nelson JR: Nutrition-related degenerative joint disease in young bulls. Vet Med Small Anim Clin *66*:1007, 1971.
153. Swanepoel R, Efstratiou S, Blackburn NK: *Mycoplasma capricolum* associated with arthritis in sheep. Vet Rec *101*:446, 1977.
154. Swanton MC: The pathology of hemarthrosis in hemophilia. *In* KM Brinkhaus (Ed): Hemophilia and Hemophilioid Diseases. Chapel Hill, North Carolina, University of North Carolina Press, 1957, p 219.
155. Tammemagi L, Simmons GC: Psittacosis lymphogranuloma polyarthritis of sheep in Queensland. Aust Vet J *44*:585, 1968.
156. Tirgari M: Changes in the canine stifle joint following rupture of the anterior cruciate ligament. J Small Anim Pract *19*:17, 1978.
157. Tirgari M, Vaughan LC: Arthritis of the canine stifle joint. Vet Rec *96*:394, 1975.
158. Vaananen M, Skutnabb K: Elbow lameness in the young dog caused by a sesamoidal fragment. J Small Anim Pract *19*:363, 1978.
159. Valerio DA, Valerio MG, Ulland BM, et al: Clinical conditions and diseases encountered in a large simian colony. *In* Proceedings of the Third International Congress on Primatology. Vol 2. Zurich, 1970. Basel, S Karger, 1971, p 205.
160. Van Pelt RW, Olson DP, Gallagher KF: Chronic gonitis in cattle: Clinicopathologic findings and treatment. J Am Vet Med Assoc *163*:1378, 1973.
161. Van Pelt RW: Infectious arthritis in cattle caused by *Corynebacterium pyogenes*. J Am Vet Med Assoc *156*:457, 1970.
162. Van Pelt RW: Pathologic changes of joint disease associated with malignant lymphoma in cattle: Clinical, gross pathologic, and histopathologic observations. Am J Vet Res *28*:429, 1967.
163. Van Pelt RW: Pathologic changes of joint disease associated with malignant lymphoma in cattle: Comparative blood, serum and synovial fluid findings. Am J Vet Res *28*:421, 1967.
164. Van Pelt RW, Langham RF: Degenerative joint disease of the carpus and fetlock in cattle. J Am Vet Med Assoc *157*:953, 1970.
165. Van Pelt RW, Langham RF: Degenerative joint disease in cattle. J Am Vet Med Assoc *148*:535, 1966.
166. Van Pelt RW, Langham RF: Nonspecific polyarthritis secondary to primary systemic infection in calves. J Am Vet Med Assoc *149*:505, 1966.
167. Van Pelt RW: Monarticular idiopathic septic arthritis in horses. J Am Vet Med Assoc *158*:1658, 1971.
168. Van Pelt RW: Idiopathic septic arthritis in dairy cattle. J Am Vet Med Assoc *161*:278, 1972.
169. Walker ER, Friedman MH, Olson NO, DeNee PB: Ultrastructural study of avian synovium infected with an arthrotropic reovirus. Arthritis Rheum *20*:1269, 1977.
170. Wallach JD: Environmental and nutritional diseases of captive reptiles. J Am Vet Med Assoc 159:1632, 1971.
171. Walsum JV: Contribution to the aetiology of synovitis in chickens, with special reference to non-infective factor. III. Tijdschr Diergeneeskd *102*:793, 1977.
172. Watt DA, Bamford V, Nairn ME: *Actinobacillus seminis* as a cause of polyarthritis and posthitis in sheep. Aust Vet J *46*:515, 1970.
173. Waxler GL, Britt AL: Polyserositis and arthritis due to *Escherichia coli* in gnotobiotic pigs. Can J Comp Med *36*:226, 1972.
174. Weaver AD: Hip lameness in cattle. Vet Rec *85*:504, 1969.
175. Wilhelmi G, Faust R: Suitability of the C57 black mouse as an experimental animal for the study of skeletal changes due to aging, with special reference to osteo-arthritis and its response to tribenoside. Pharmacology *14*:289, 1976.
176. Wood RL, Cutlip RC, Shuman RD: Osteomyelitis and arthritis induced in swine by Lancefield's group A streptococci (*Streptococcus pyogenes*). Cornell Vet *61*:457, 1971.
177. Wynne-Davies R: Acetabular dysplasia and familial joint laxity: Two etiological factors in congenital dislocation of the hip. J Bone Joint Surg *52(B)*:704, 1970.
178. Yamamoto R, Clark GT: *Streptobacillus moniliformis* infection in turkeys. Vet Rec *79*:95, 1966.
179. The radiological examination for osteoarthritis and instability of the canine stifle. J Small Anim Pract 16:61, 1975.

SECTION II

RADIOGRAPHY AND RELATED MODALITIES IN THE EVALUATION OF BONE AND JOINT DISEASE

7

PLAIN FILM RADIOGRAPHY

by Donald Resnick, M.D.

The radiographic evaluation of articular disease begins in the x-ray room. Without high quality roentgenograms of properly positioned patients, the physician frequently is unable to detect significant abnormalities and thereby to establish a correct diagnosis. Although there is no substitute for a well-trained radiologic technician who is aware of methods and techniques of skeletal roentgenology, it is also imperative that both the referring physician and radiologist be familiar with these available techniques so that the proper radiographs are ordered and obtained.

This chapter summarizes various roentgenographic projections that are available for the evaluation of articulations.[1-3] Some are general projections that are used for the examination of patients with many types of disorders, including arthritis. Other projections have more limited indications. At the conclusion of the discussion of each region of the body, a recommended screening examination is included for the evaluation of a patient with symptoms or signs in that region. At the end of the entire chapter, a discussion of appropriate "arthritic surveys" is entertained. Specialized radiographic procedures and related examinations investigating the patient with articular disease are discussed in the following chapters.

FINGERS AND HAND

Adequate radiographic evaluation of the fingers requires posteroanterior and lateral projections (Fig. 7–1). The particular position employed for obtaining a lateral radiograph of one of the four ulnar digits will depend upon the specific digit being examined. Positioning of the thumb is unique because its axis differs from that of the other digits (Fig. 7–2). Stress views of the first metacarpophalangeal articulation may be required for evaluation of injuries of the ligaments of this joint.[4]

The radiographic examination of the hand utilizes posteroanterior, oblique and lateral projections (Fig. 7–3). Occasionally anteroposterior and lateral flexion roentgenograms may be useful to further evaluate the dorsum of the hand and the metacarpophalangeal articulations. Recently, the value of traction during roentgenography of the metacarpophalangeal joints (as well as the wrist) has been described.[105] During this procedure, the absence of release of intra-articular gas is indicative of an effusion. A similar technique has been utilized to evaluate the hip.

Basic Examination: Hand
Posteroanterior
Oblique
Lateral

WRIST

Frontal and lateral radiographs of the wrist are routine (Fig. 7–4). For the evaluation of arthritis, oblique projections are also necessary. These latter projections should include radiographs exposed with the wrist in both a semipronated oblique and a semisupinated oblique position.[5] In the latter view, the pisiform-triquetral joint is well seen.[6]

Roentgenograms obtained during radial and ulnar deviation of the wrist are useful for visualizing the carpal bones, particularly the scaphoid (ulnar deviation), and for assessing carpal mobility (Fig. 7–5). Similarly, lateral radiographs may be obtained in palmar flexion and dorsiflexion. Specialized projections for the scaphoid may be required for detection of fractures.[7-9] The "carpal tunnel" view (Fig. 7–5) delineates the osseous structures and soft tissues of the carpal canal, including the hook of the hamate, pisiform, trapezium, trapezoid, and tuberosity of the scaphoid.[10-13] A "carpal bridge" view (Fig. 7–5) demonstrates the osseous and soft tissue structures on the dorsum of the wrist.[14] Radiographs obtained by angulating the beam along the axis of the radiocarpal joint allow better visualization of this articulation; a lateral radiograph from the radial side of the joint should be obtained with the beam angulated 15 degrees proximally, and a posteroan-

Text continued on page 263

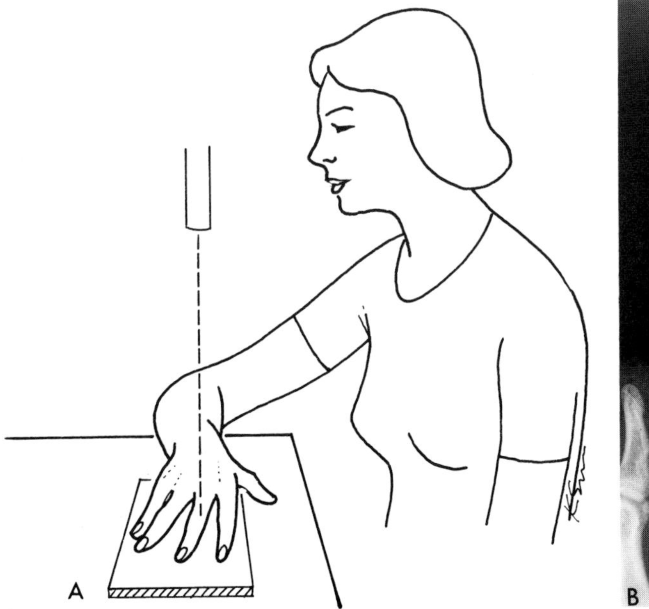

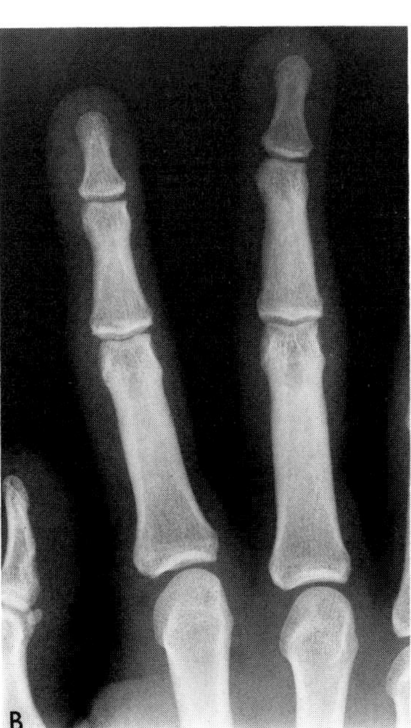

Figure 7–1. *Fingers: Routine radiographs.*
A, B *Posteroanterior radiograph: Normal. The fingers should be separated slightly to provide better visualization of the osseous and articular structures.*

Illustration continued on the following page

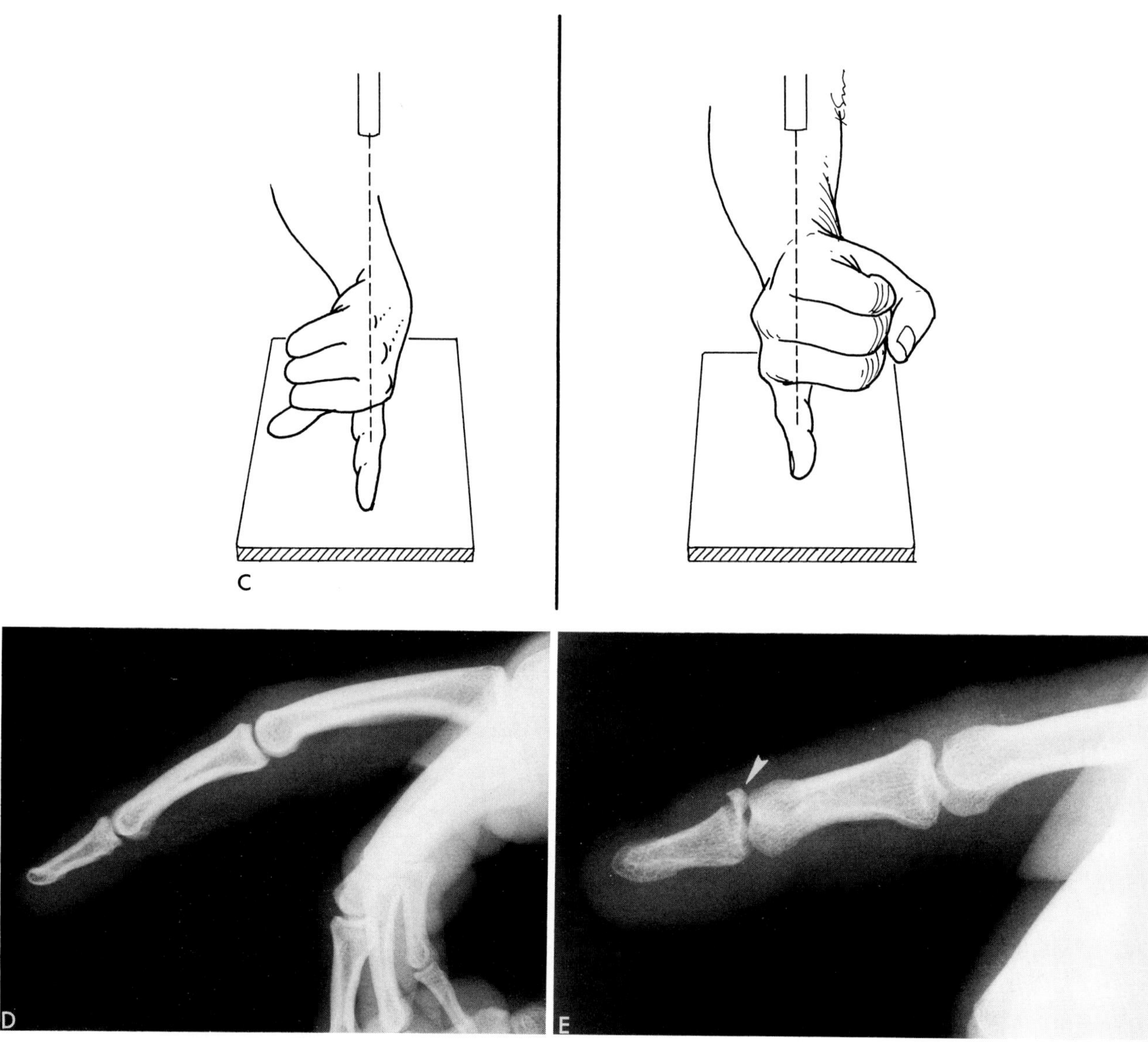

Figure 7–1. Continued

C, D *Lateral radiograph: Normal. Note that the position of the hand will vary depending upon which digit is being examined. The involved finger is extended and the remaining digits are folded into a fist.*

E *Lateral radiograph: dorsal fracture. The intra-articular fracture is well delineated (arrowhead).*

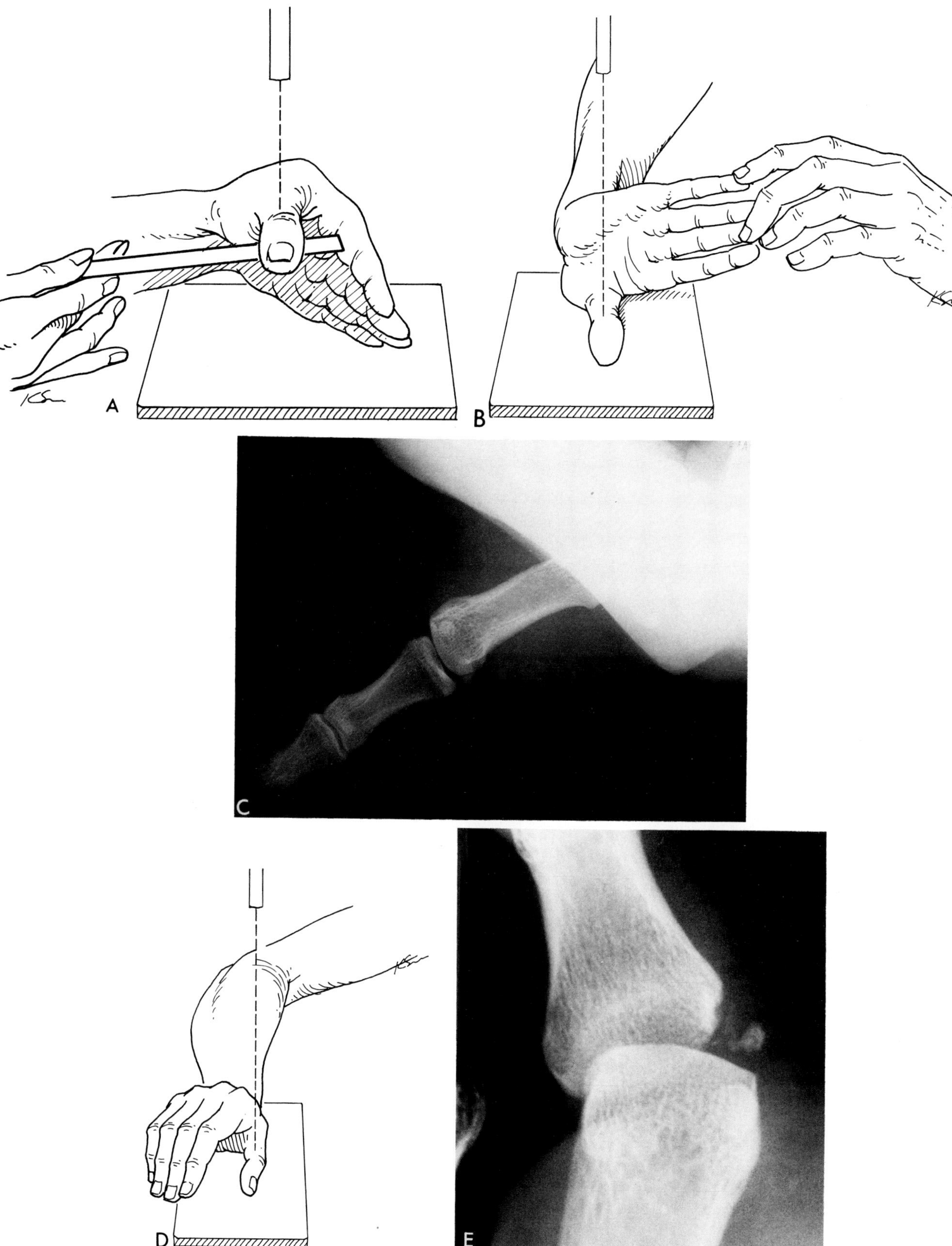

Figure 7–2. *Thumb: Routine radiographs.*

A, B *Posteroanterior* **(A)** *and anteroposterior* **(B)** *radiographs: Normal. Either view is satisfactory.*

C *Anteroposterior radiograph: Normal.*

D *Lateral radiograph.*

E *Stress radiograph of first metacarpophalangeal joint: "gamekeeper's thumb." With radial stress, laxity of the ulnar aspect of the articulation and chip fractures are observed.*

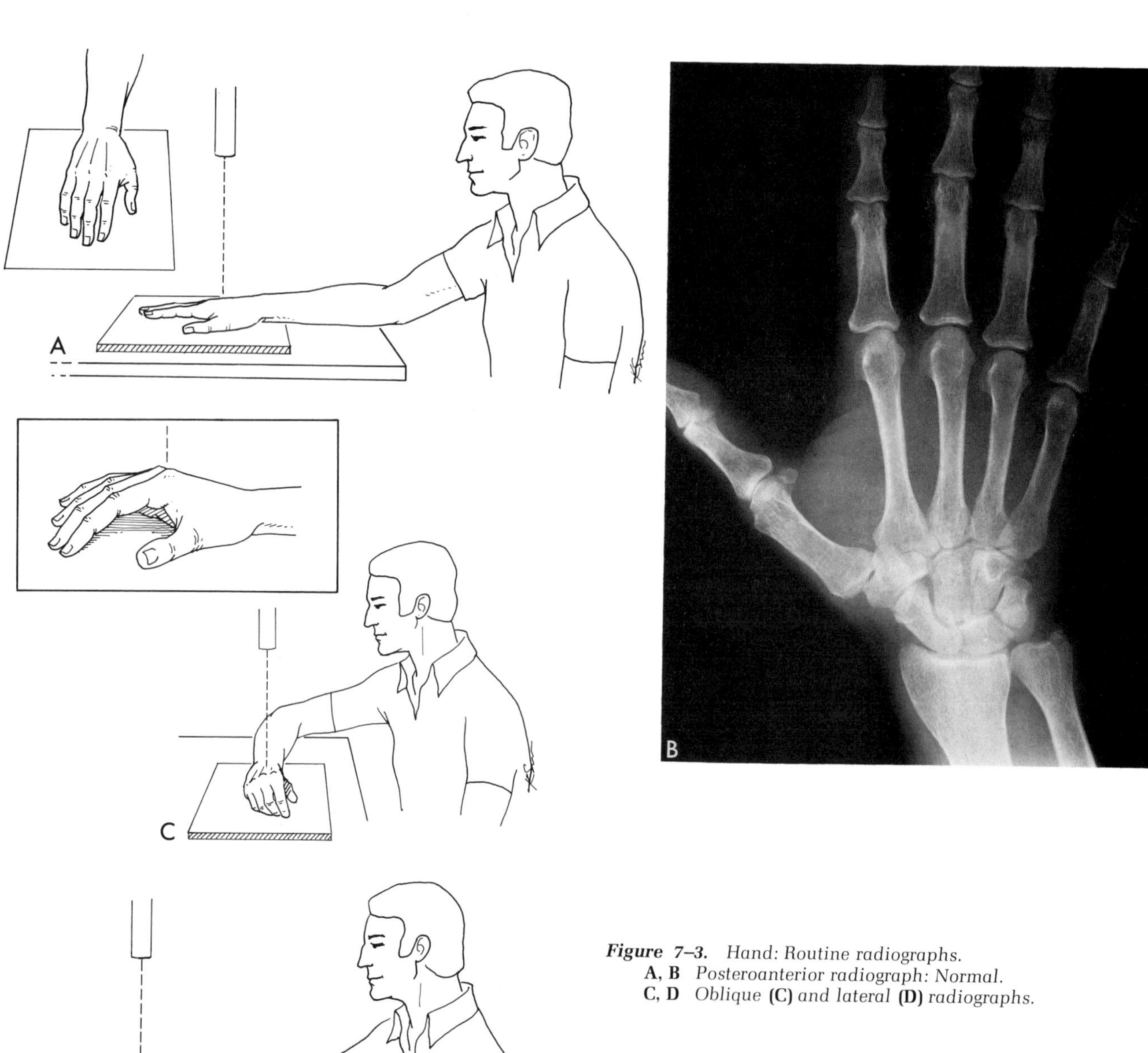

Figure 7–3. *Hand: Routine radiographs.*
A, B *Posteroanterior radiograph: Normal.*
C, D *Oblique* **(C)** *and lateral* **(D)** *radiographs.*

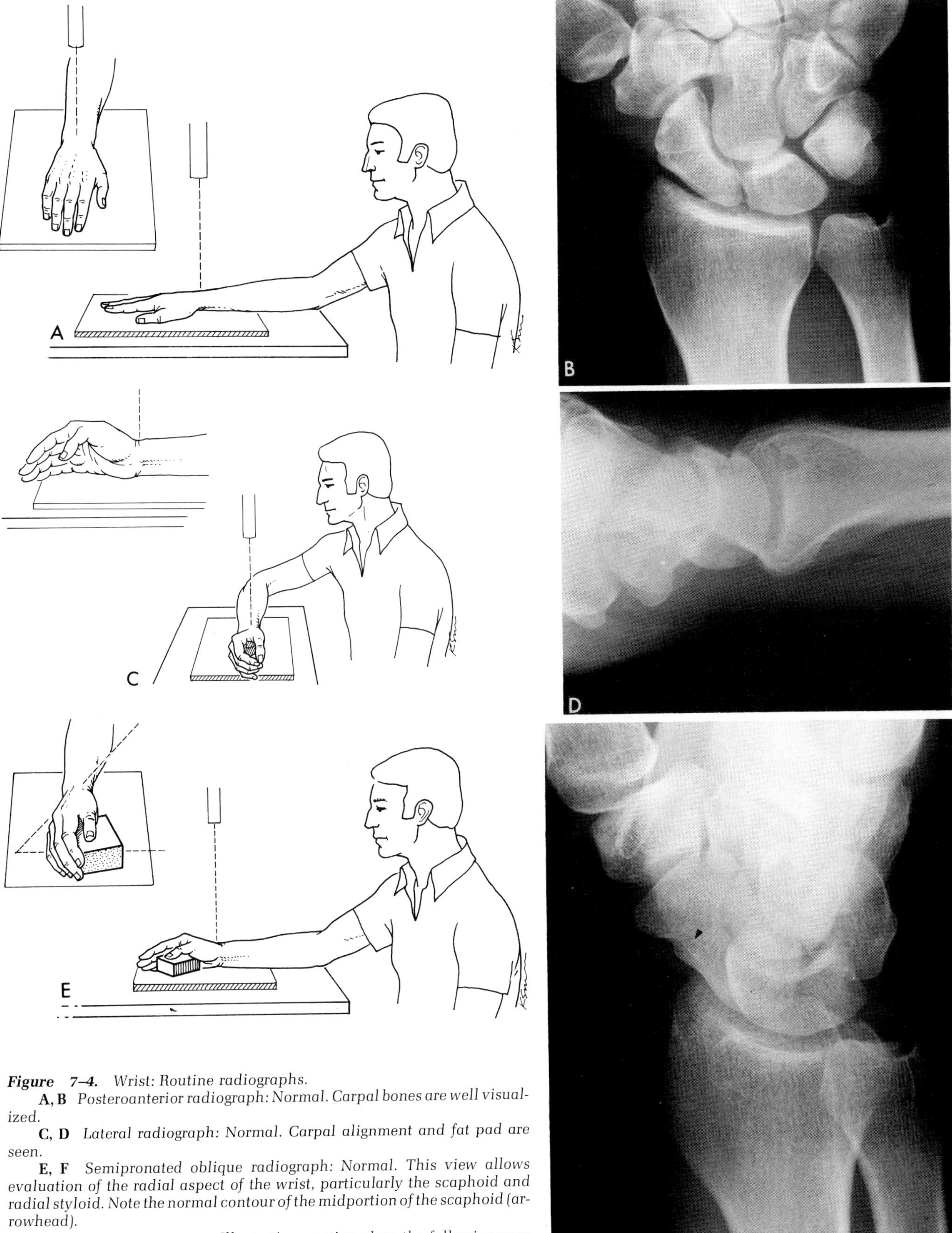

Figure 7–4. *Wrist: Routine radiographs.*

A, B *Posteroanterior radiograph: Normal. Carpal bones are well visualized.*

C, D *Lateral radiograph: Normal. Carpal alignment and fat pad are seen.*

E, F *Semipronated oblique radiograph: Normal. This view allows evaluation of the radial aspect of the wrist, particularly the scaphoid and radial styloid. Note the normal contour of the midportion of the scaphoid (arrowhead).*

Illustration continued on the following page

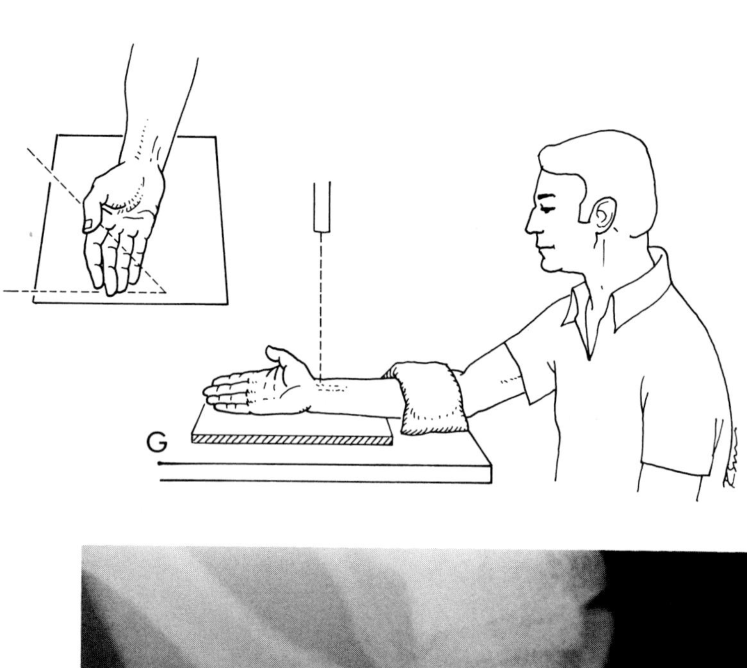

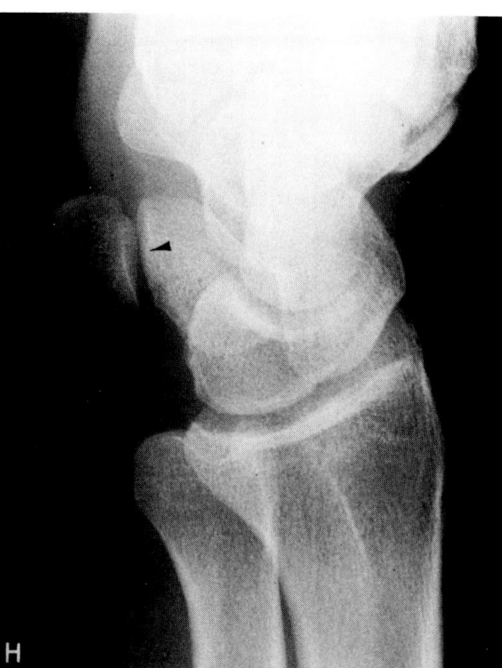

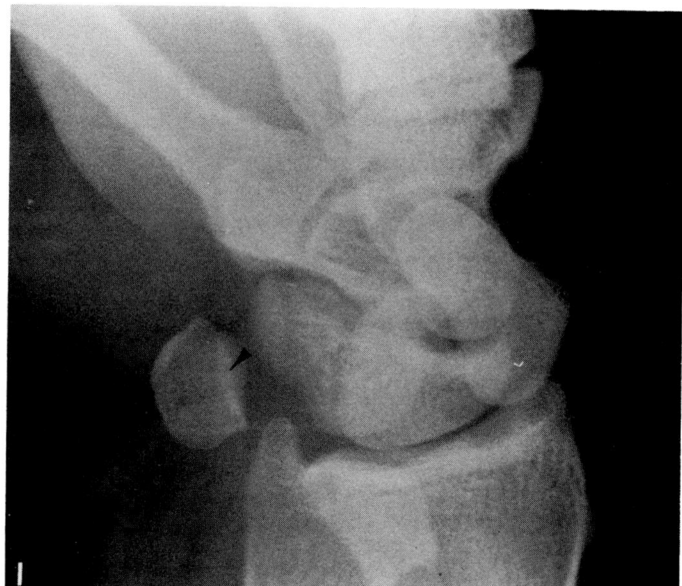

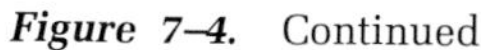

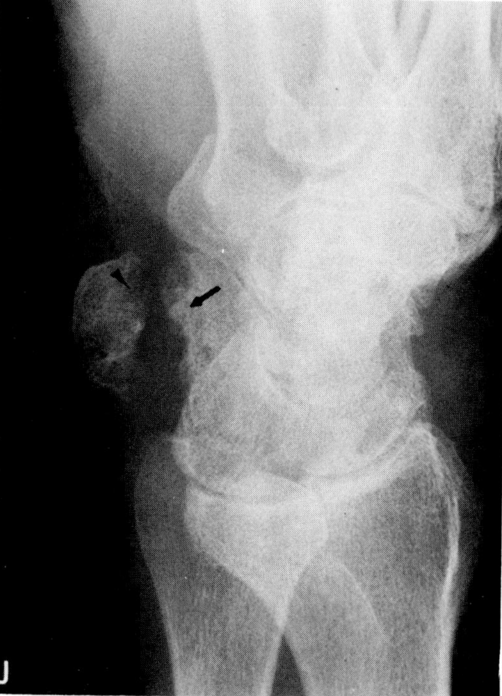

Figure 7–4. Continued

G, H *Semisupinated oblique radiograph: Normal. Observe the pisiform bone, which is separated from the remaining carpal bones, and the tangential view of the pisiform-triquetral joint (arrowhead).*

I *Semisupinated oblique radiograph in flexion. Note that the pisiform (arrowhead) can move proximally because of the normal laxity of the joint capsule.*

J *Semisupinated oblique radiograph: Rheumatoid arthritis. Characteristic erosions occur in the dorsal surface of the pisiform (arrowhead) and the volar surface of the triquetrum (arrow) related to synovitis in the pisiform-triquetral compartment.*

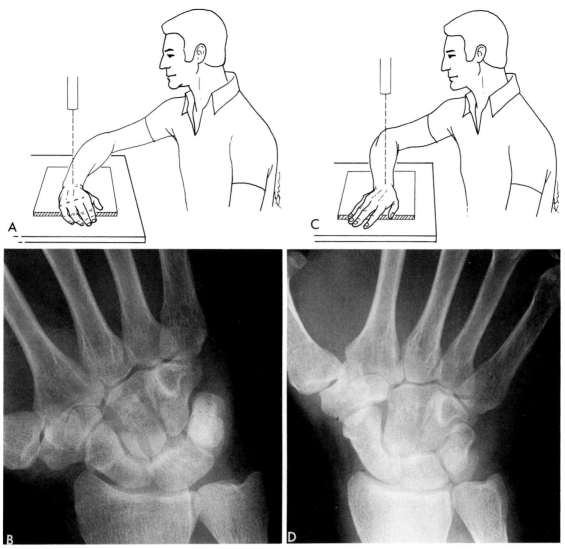

Figure 7–5. *Wrist: Additional radiographs.*

A–D *Radial* **(A, B)** *and ulnar* **(C, D)** *deviation. Observe the normal change in alignment of the carpal bones in the two projections. In radial deviation, palmar flexion of the proximal carpal row occurs and the distal scaphoid rotates into the palm; the proximal carpal row moves in an ulnar direction with respect to the distal radius. In ulnar deviation, the scaphoid-lunate space may increase slightly and the scaphoid is exposed in full profile.*

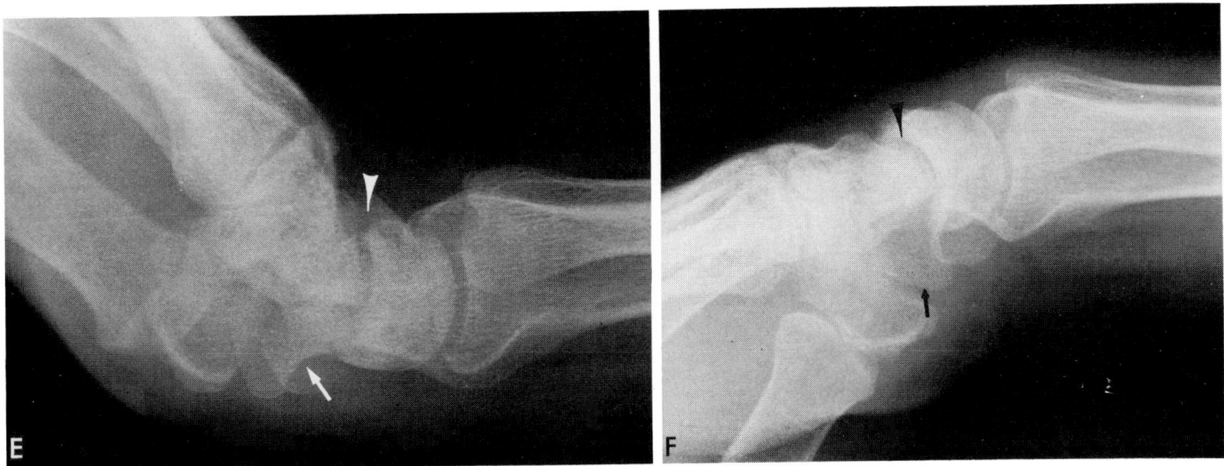

E, F *Dorsiflexion* **(E)** *and palmar flexion* **(F)**. *Motion at the lunate-capitate area (arrowheads) can be observed, and the scaphoid (arrows) is identified.*

Illustration continued on the following page

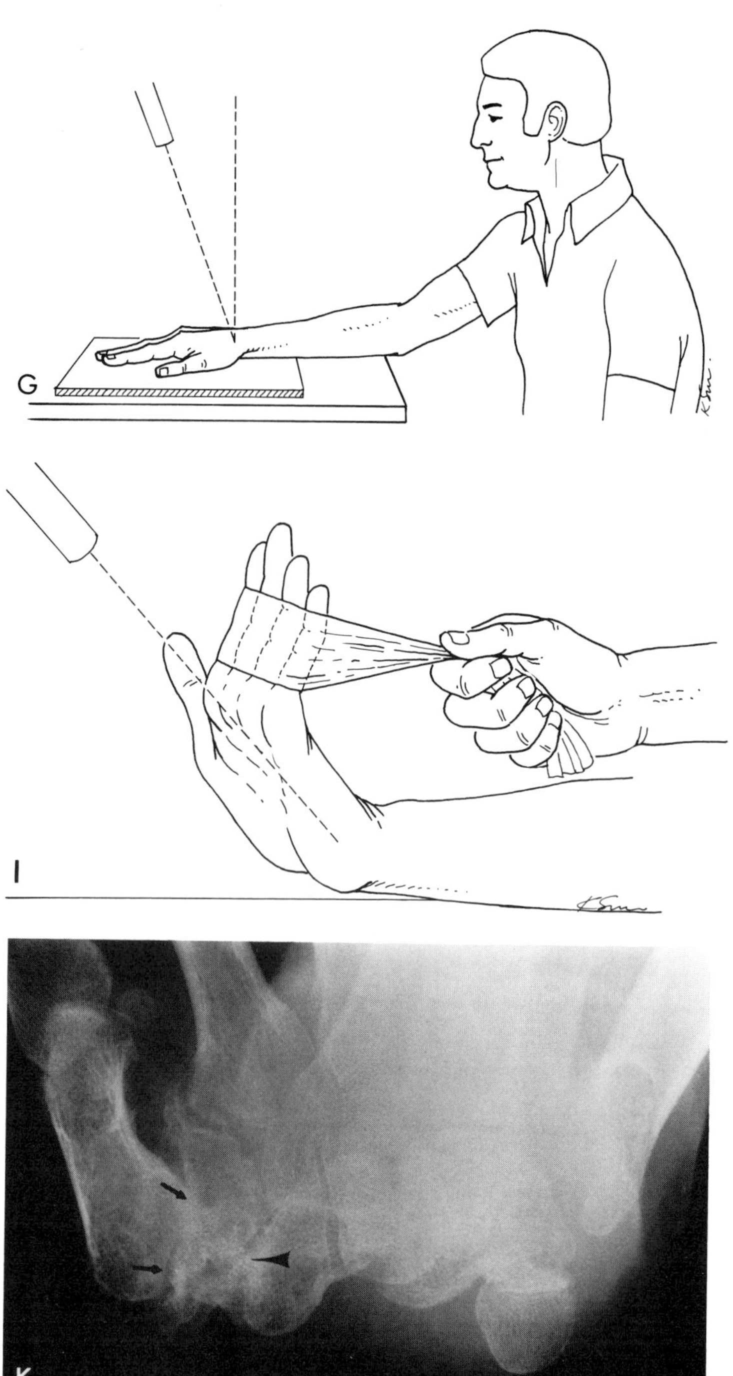

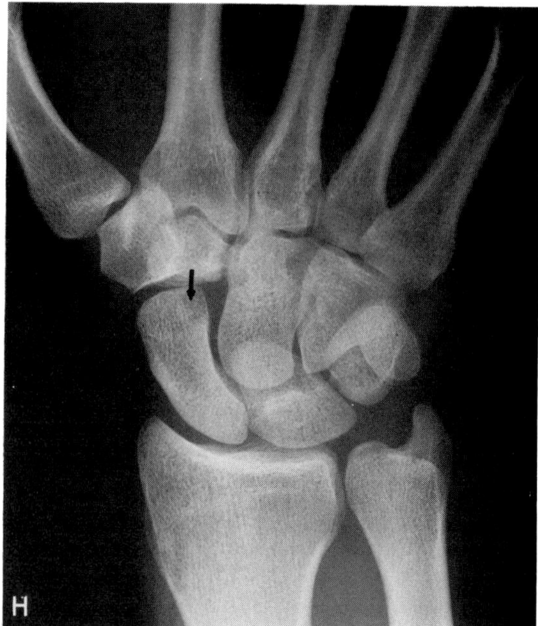

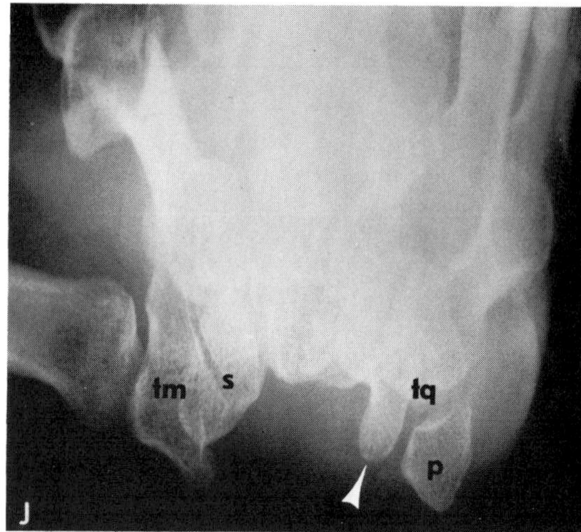

Figure 7–5. Continued

G, H *Scaphoid: Specialized view. The hand and wrist are placed horizontally on the film and the central ray is directed 20 degrees toward the elbow. The scaphoid (arrow) is projected free of adjacent osseous structures.*

I–K *"Carpal tunnel" view. The drawing* **(I)** *indicates that the long axis of the hand is placed in a vertical direction and the central ray is directed at an angle of 25 to 30 degrees to this long axis. In the normal situation* **(J),** *one can delineate the trapezium* (tm), *scaphoid* (s), *triquetrum* (tq), *pisiform* (p), *and hook of the hamate (arrowhead). In the abnormal situation* **(K),** *observe considerable degenerative disease at the first carpometacarpal joint (arrows) and trapezioscaphoid area of the midcarpal joint (arrowhead).*

Illustration continued on the opposite page

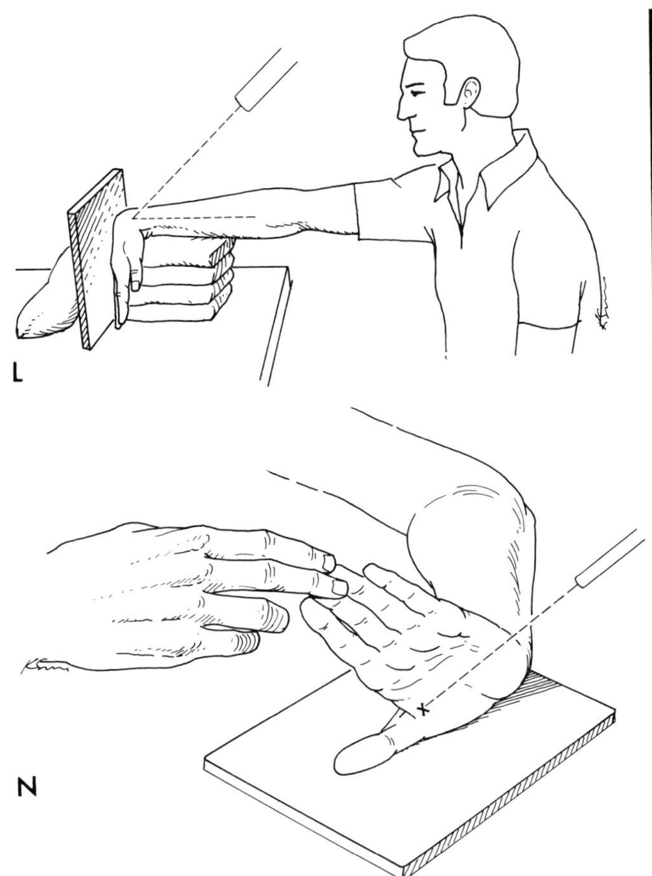

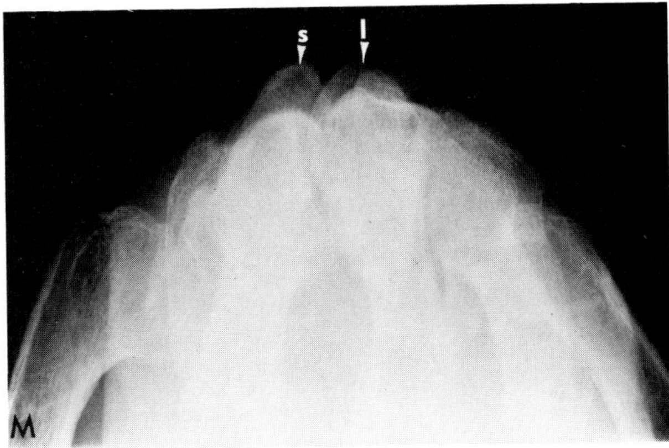

Figure 7–5. Continued

L, M *"Carpal bridge" view. The drawing indicates that the wrist is flexed to approximately 90 degrees and the central ray is angled at 45 degrees in a superor-inferior direction. This view demonstrates the scaphoid (s) and lunate (l) and is useful for diagnosing fractures, foreign bodies, and soft tissue swelling on the dorsal aspect of the wrist.*

N *First carpometacarpal joint: specialized view. The hand is hyperextended and the thumb is placed in a horizontal position. The central ray is angled approximately 45 degrees toward the elbow.*

terior roentgenogram should be obtained with the beam angulated 10 degrees proximally. A specialized anteroposterior projection with beam angulation has been utilized to define changes in the first carpometacarpal joint[15] (Fig. 7–5).

Basic Examination: Wrist
Posteroanterior
Lateral
Semisupinated Oblique
Semipronated Oblique

ELBOW

Standard examination of the elbow includes anteroposterior and lateral radiographs and, in many cases, an oblique roentgenogram (Fig. 7–6). The frontal radiographs should be obtained with supination of the hand so that rotation of radius and ulna does not occur. On the oblique roentgenogram, the coronoid process is well visualized, and the lateral projection, taken in elbow flexion, allows identification of the important fat pads about this articulation. Additional radiographs that occasionally are utilized are frontal roentgenograms with acute flexion of the elbow to visualize the olecranon process,[2] and angulated[16] and axial radiographs to better delineate the radial head[1,2] and olecranon process[17,18] (Fig. 7–7).

Basic Examination: Elbow
Anteroposterior
Lateral

GLENOHUMERAL JOINT

Anteroposterior radiographs are obtained in external and internal rotation (Fig. 7–8). The former reveals the greater tuberosity in profile and is useful in detecting calcification in the supraspinatus tendon. As the arm is rotated internally, the greater tuberosity is projected en face over the humerus, and the lesser tuberosity may overlie the glenohumeral joint. In this position, calcification in the infraspinatus and teres minor tendons is seen on the outer aspect of the humerus, and calcification in the subscapularis tendon is seen adjacent to the lesser tuberosity. These views may be obtained with 15 degrees of caudal angulation of the x-ray beam to better demonstrate the area of the subdeltoid bursa between humeral head and acromion.[19] Additional projections for detecting calcification in the teres

Text continued on page 271

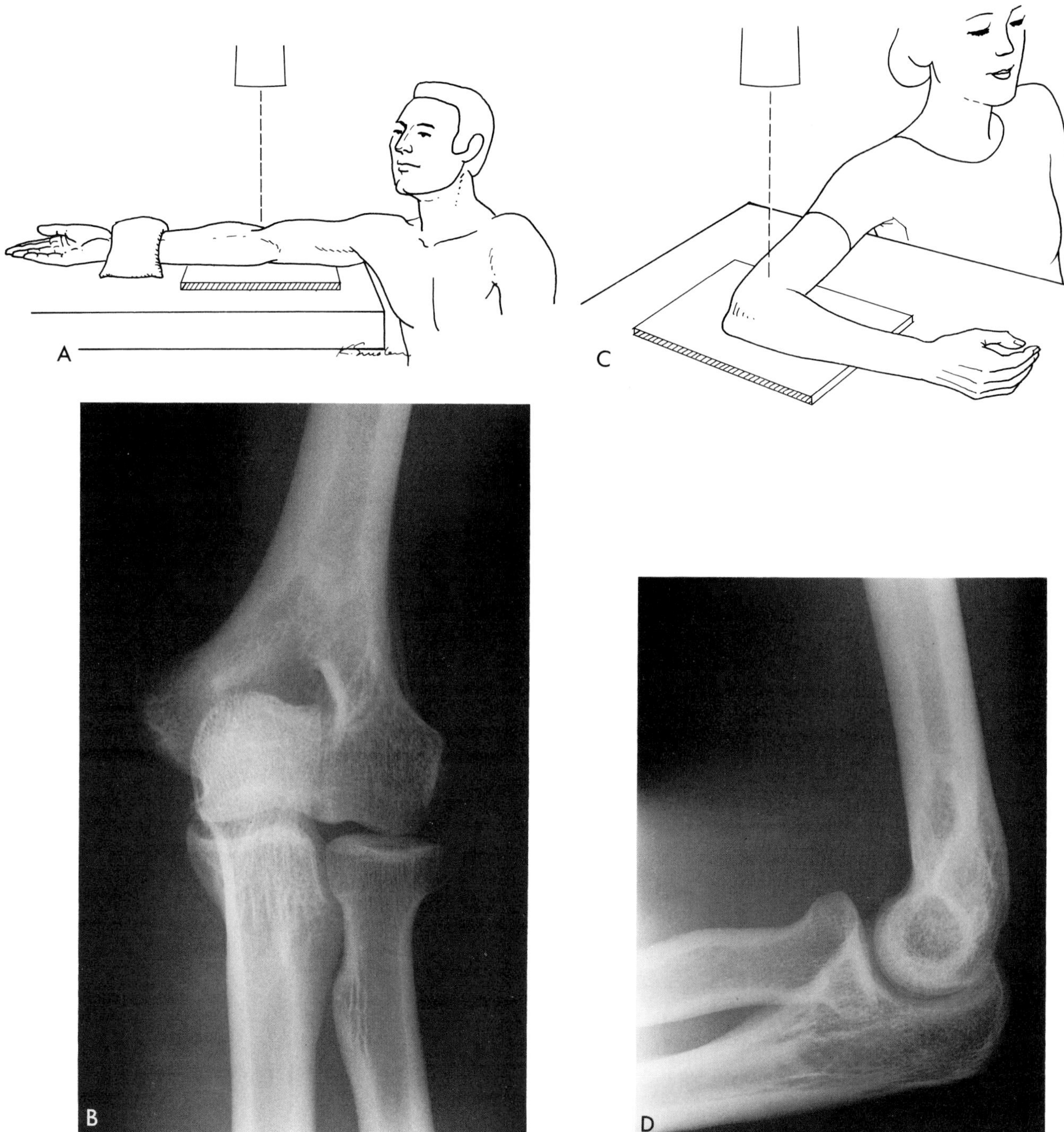

Figure 7–6. Elbow: Routine radiographs.
A, B *Anteroposterior radiograph: Normal.*
C, D *Lateral radiograph: Normal.*

Illustration continued on the opposite page

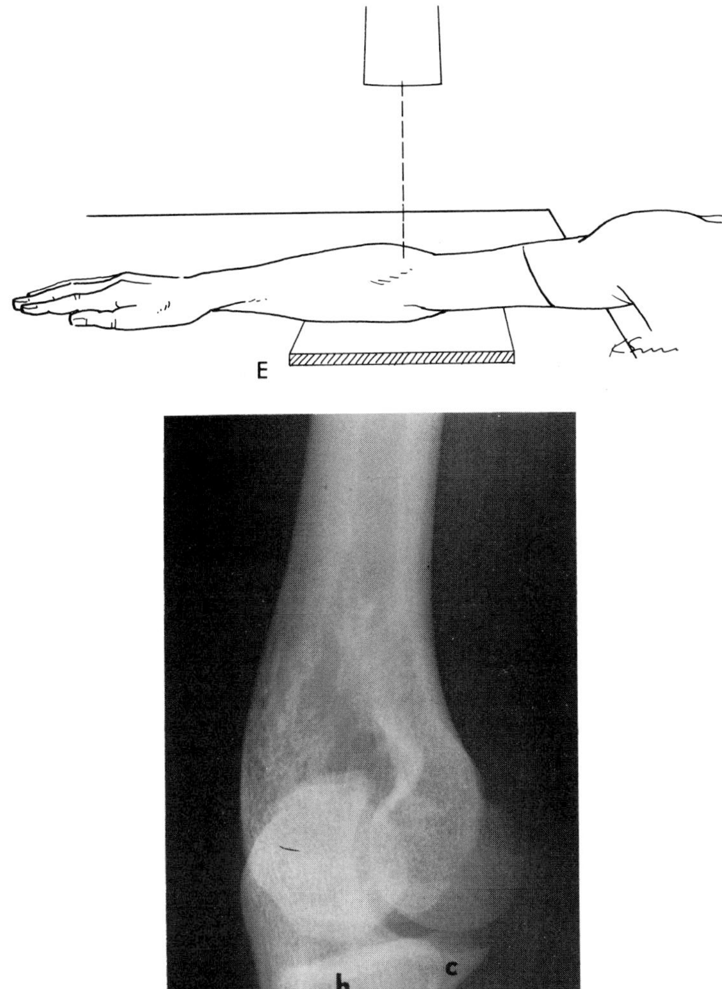

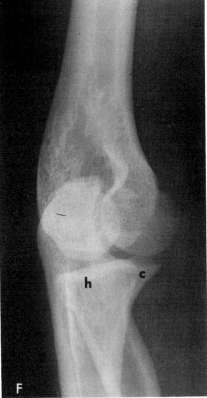

Figure 7–6. Continued
E, F *Oblique radiograph: Normal. Observe that the radial head (h) is superimposed on the proximal ulna, and the coronoid process (c) is well visualized.*

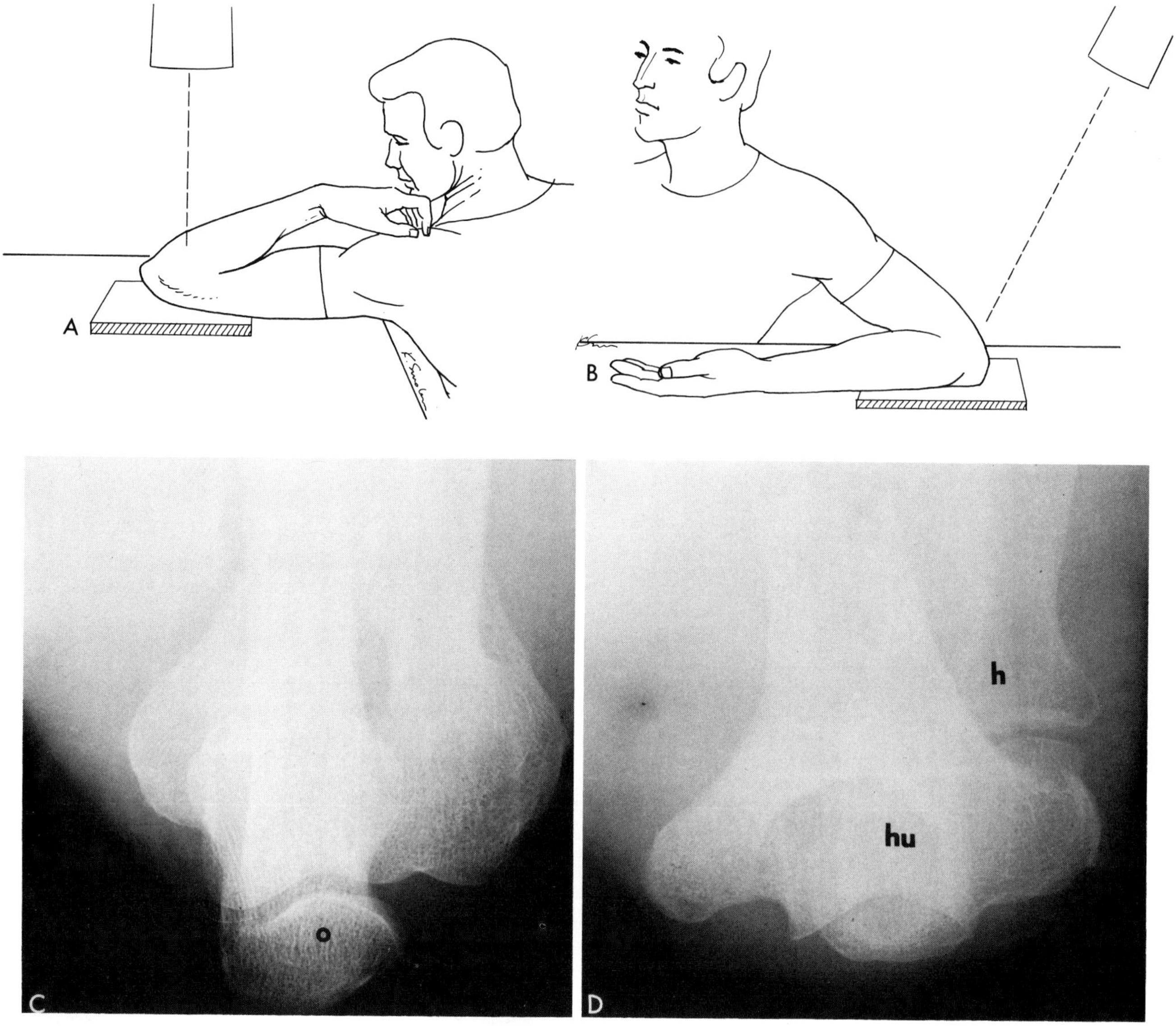

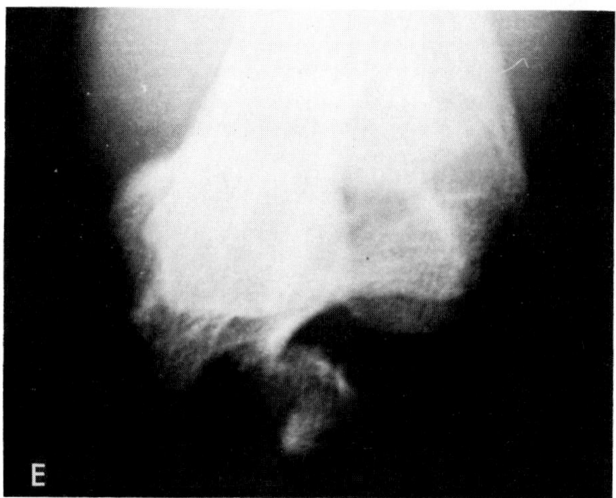

Figure 7–7. *Elbow: Additional radiographs.*

A–D *Flexion views: Normal. Radiographs obtained with elbow flexion allow visualization of the olecranon process* (o), *distal humerus* (hu), *and radial head* (h).

E *Flexion view: Olecranon fracture. The fracture fragment is well delineated.*

Illustration continued on the opposite page

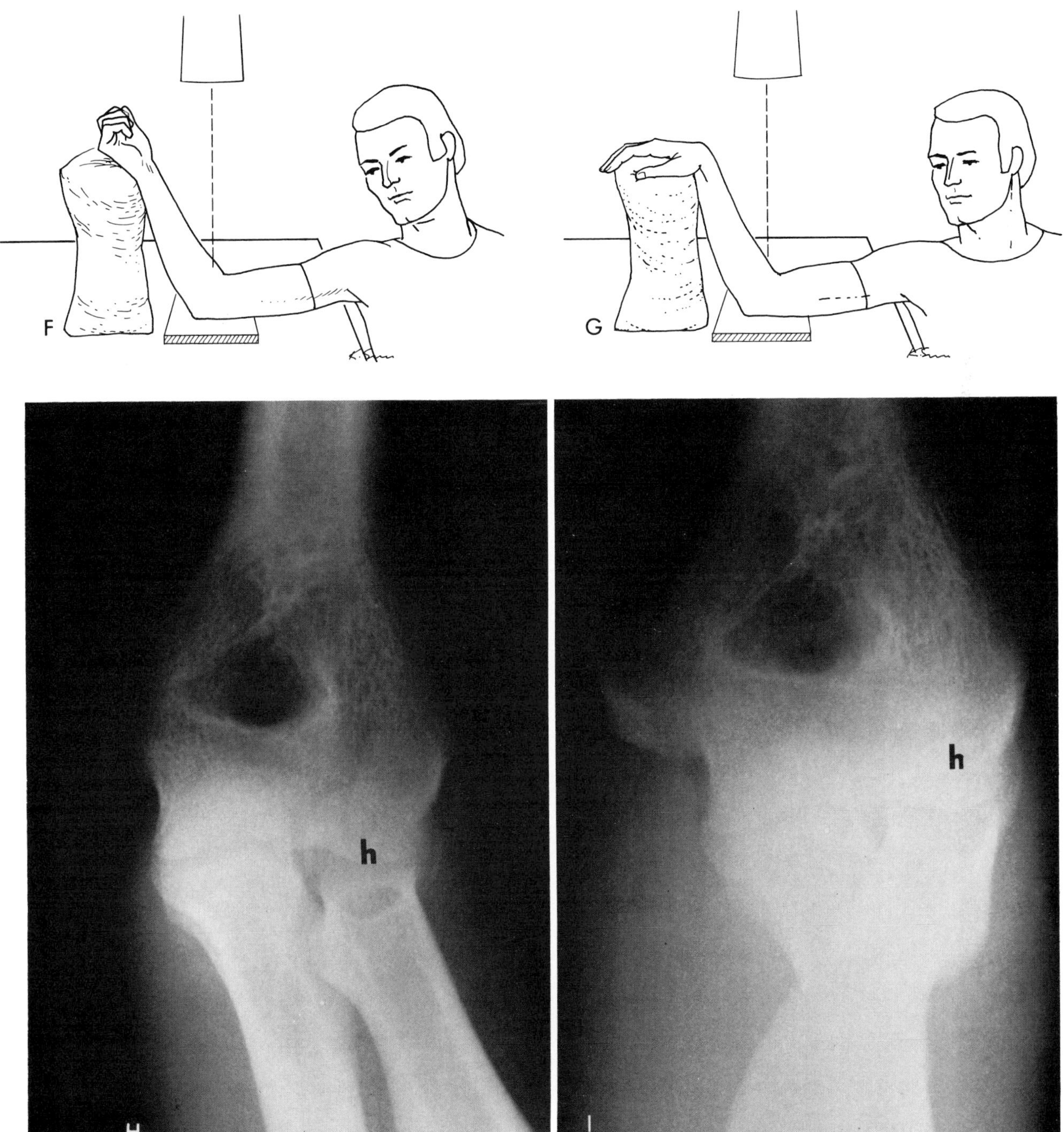

Figure 7–7. Continued
F–I *Radial head: Supinated and pronated flexion views of the elbow allow visualization of the entire surface of the radial head* (h).

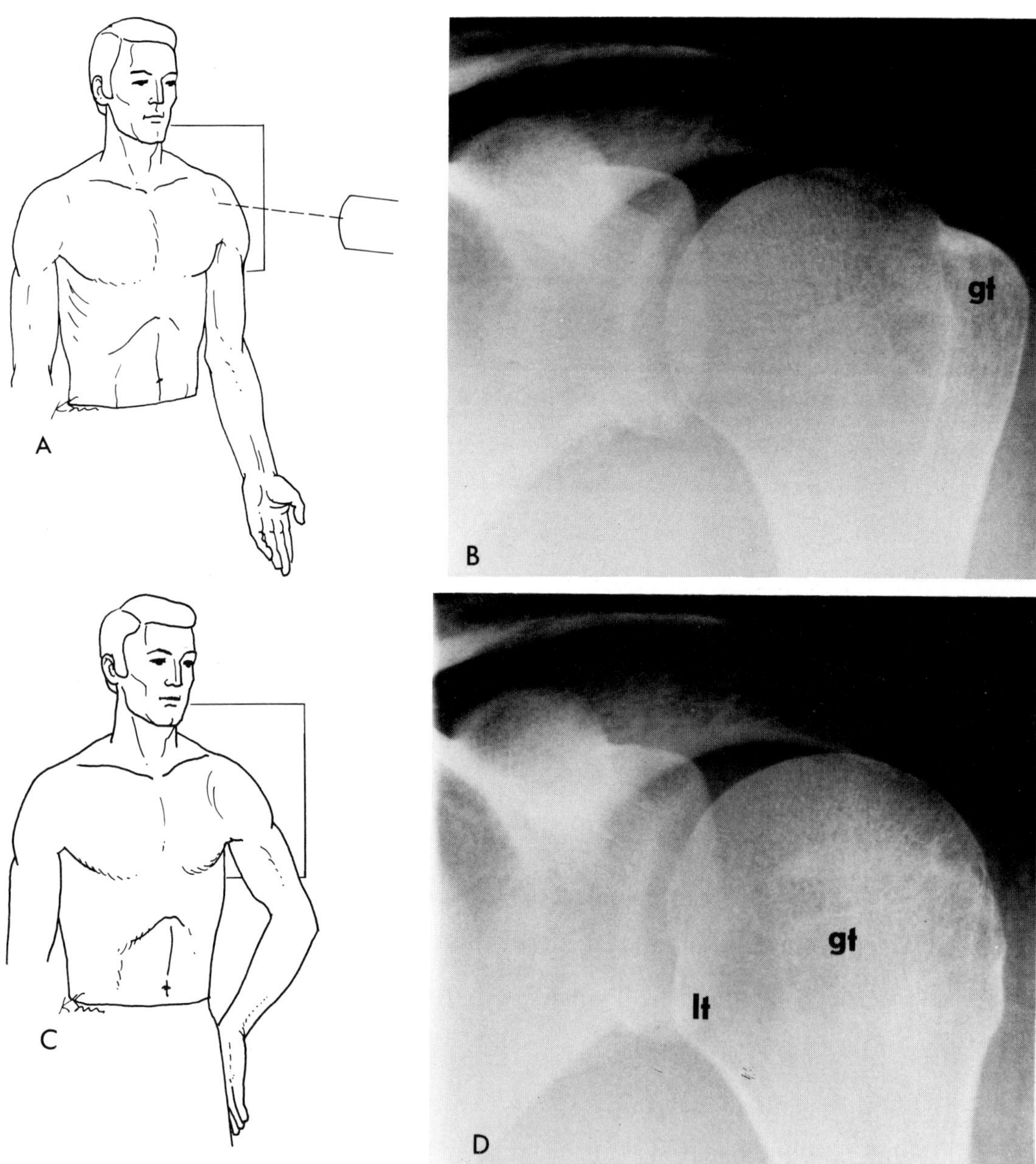

Figure 7–8. *Glenohumeral joint: Routine radiographs.*

A, B *External rotation: Normal. The greater tuberosity (gt) is seen in profile.*

C, D *Internal rotation. The greater tuberosity (gt) is now projected over the humerus and the lesser tuberosity (lt) is observed on the medial aspect of the humeral head.*

Illustration continued on the opposite page

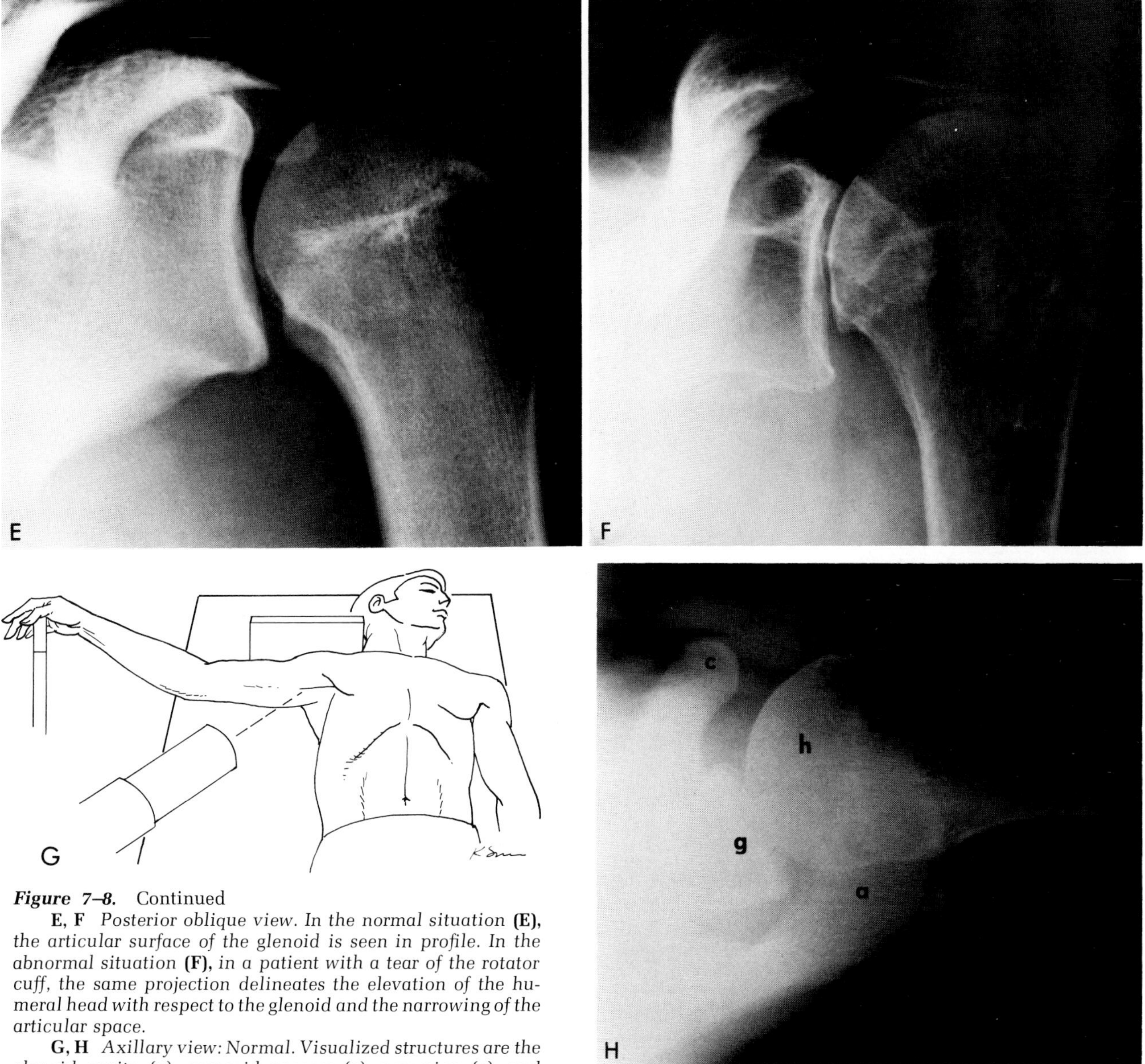

Figure 7–8. Continued

E, F *Posterior oblique view. In the normal situation* **(E)**, *the articular surface of the glenoid is seen in profile. In the abnormal situation* **(F)**, *in a patient with a tear of the rotator cuff, the same projection delineates the elevation of the humeral head with respect to the glenoid and the narrowing of the articular space.*

G, H *Axillary view: Normal. Visualized structures are the glenoid cavity (g), coracoid process (c), acromion (a), and humeral head (h).*

Illustration continued on the following page

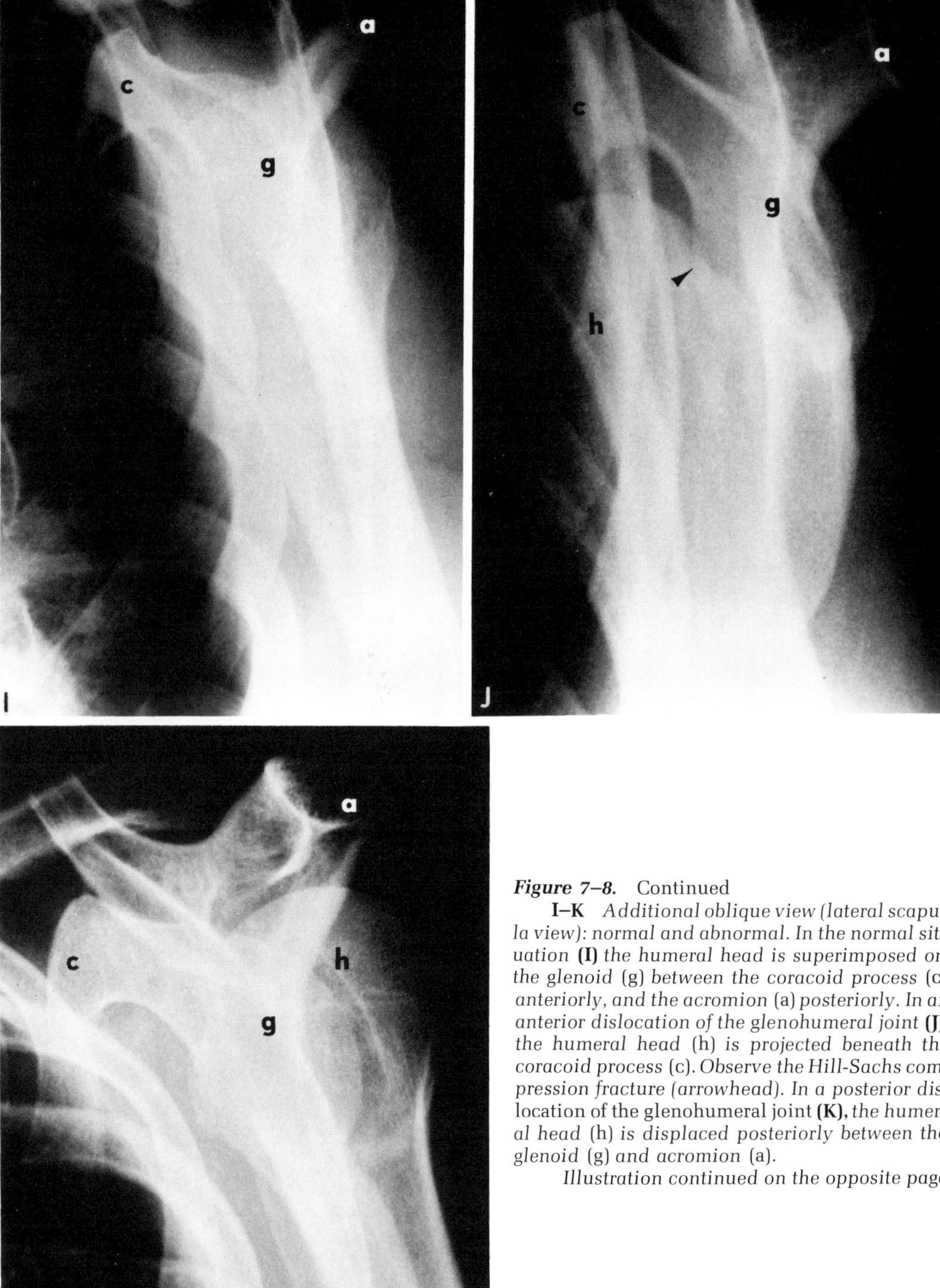

Figure 7–8. Continued

I–K *Additional oblique view (lateral scapula view): normal and abnormal. In the normal situation* **(I)** *the humeral head is superimposed on the glenoid* (g) *between the coracoid process* (c) *anteriorly, and the acromion* (a) *posteriorly. In an anterior dislocation of the glenohumeral joint* **(J)**, *the humeral head* (h) *is projected beneath the coracoid process* (c). *Observe the Hill-Sachs compression fracture (arrowhead). In a posterior dislocation of the glenohumeral joint* **(K)**, *the humeral head* (h) *is displaced posteriorly between the glenoid* (g) *and acromion* (a).

Illustration continued on the opposite page

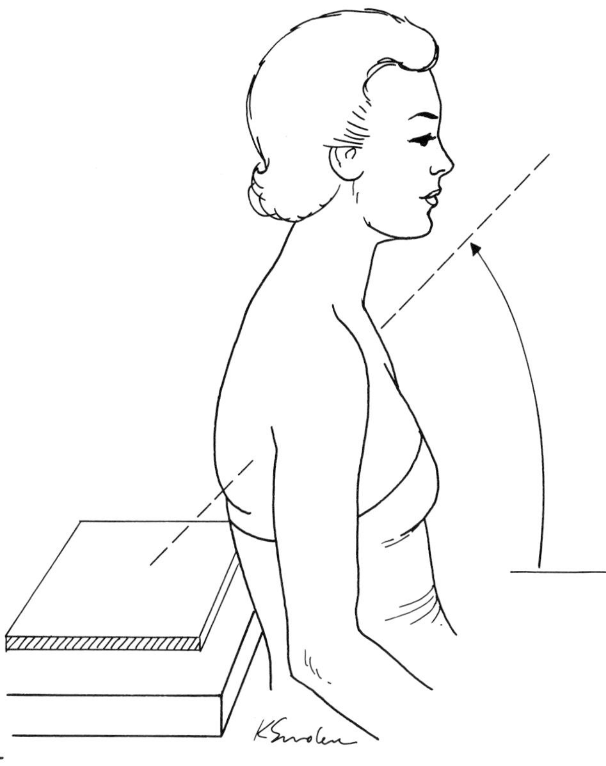

Figure 7–8. Continued
L *Semiaxial projection.*

minor and subscapularis tendons have been described.[2]

It should be recognized that an anteroposterior radiograph of the shoulder is not a true anteroposterior radiograph of the scapula nor does it allow adequate visualization of the glenohumeral joint space. A true anteroposterior radiograph of the scapula is obtained with the patient in a 40 degree posterior oblique position and is the most ideal projection for visualizing the joint, as this articulation is projected tangentially in this view (Fig. 7–8).[20, 21]

In evaluating the shoulder following trauma, it is mandatory to obtain an additional radiograph at approximately right angles to the frontal radiographs in order to determine the relative positions of the humeral head and glenoid. This can be accomplished in one of several ways. An axillary projection is particularly useful (Fig. 7–8),[113] and although it can be obtained in several different ways,[2] it may be difficult to acquire in patients with fractures and dislocations about the shoulder. A transthoracic projection has been utilized in some patients,[1] but it may be difficult to interpret. The most ideal view utilizes a true lateral projection of the scapula (Fig. 7–8), which is acquired with the patient in a 60 degree anterior oblique position.[22-24, 112] It may be obtained in an upright or recumbent position, whichever is more comfortable for the patient. The projection is superior to a semiaxial anteroposterior projection, which has been recommended by some investigators for evaluation of the glenohumeral joint.[2]

Several different roentgenographic projections have been described to evaluate patients with previous anterior dislocations of the glenohumeral joint (Fig. 7–9). These roentgenograms are utilized to delineate a typical compression fracture of the posterolateral aspect of the humeral head, the Hill-Sachs lesion, which is associated with such dislocations,[25] and include an angulated internal rotation projection,[26-27] Hermodsson's tangential projection,[24] the "notch" view of Stryker,[28] and the Didiee view.[29] A "West Point" projection is also described. Multiple radiographs obtained in varying degrees of internal rotation are also helpful in delineating this fracture.

In the diagnosis of posterior dislocation of the glenohumeral joint, additional radiographic projections have been utilized, including modified axillary and angle-up views[30] (Fig. 7–10). To visualize the bicipital groove, a roentgenogram obtained in a superoinferior projection is recommended[31] (Fig. 7–11).

Because of the density differences of the structures about the shoulder, equalization filters may be helpful.[110]

Basic Examination: Glenohumeral Joint
Anteroposterior (Internal Rotation)
Anteroposterior (External Rotation)
40 Degree Posterior Oblique

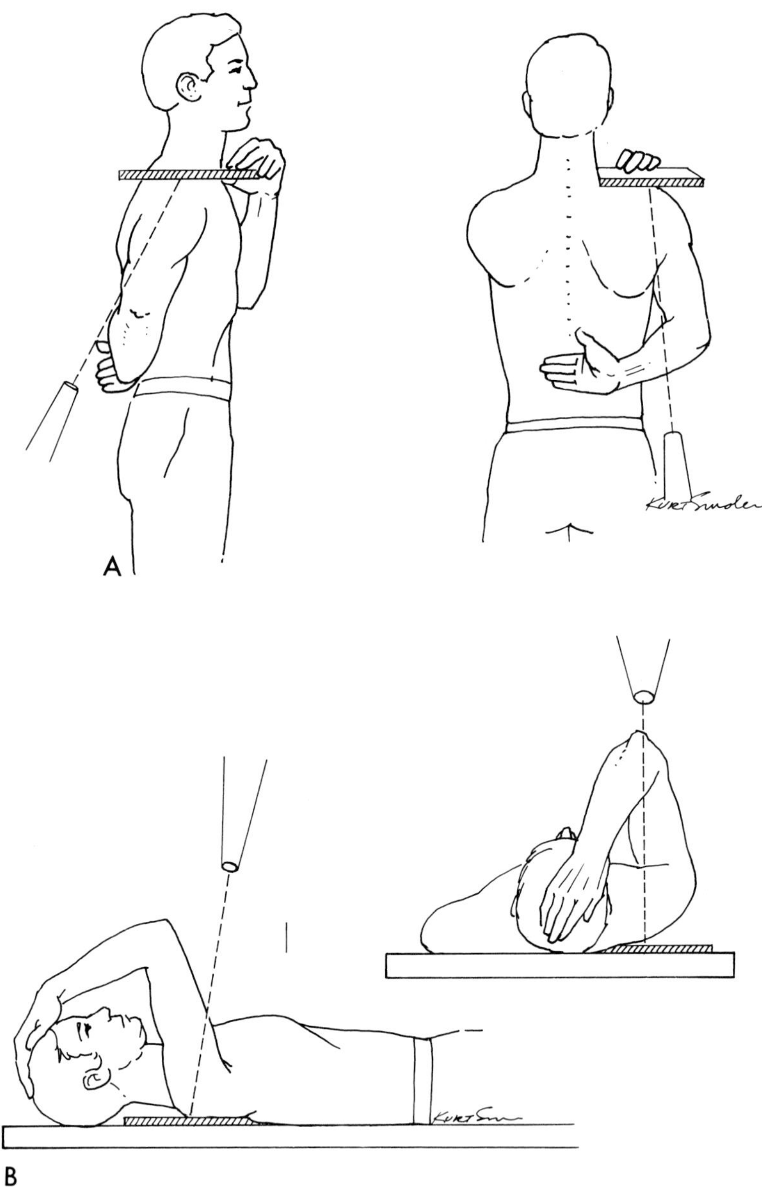

Figure 7–9. *Glenohumeral joint: Evaluation of patients with previous anterior dislocation of glenohumeral joint.*

A *Hermodsson view. The dorsum of the hand is placed over the upper lumbar vertebrae with the thumb pointing upward. The central ray is directed at a 30 degree angle from the vertical, with the film held on the shoulder, parallel to the floor.*

B *"Notch" view. The palm is placed on top of the head. The central ray is directed 10 degrees cephalad.*

Illustration continued on the opposite page

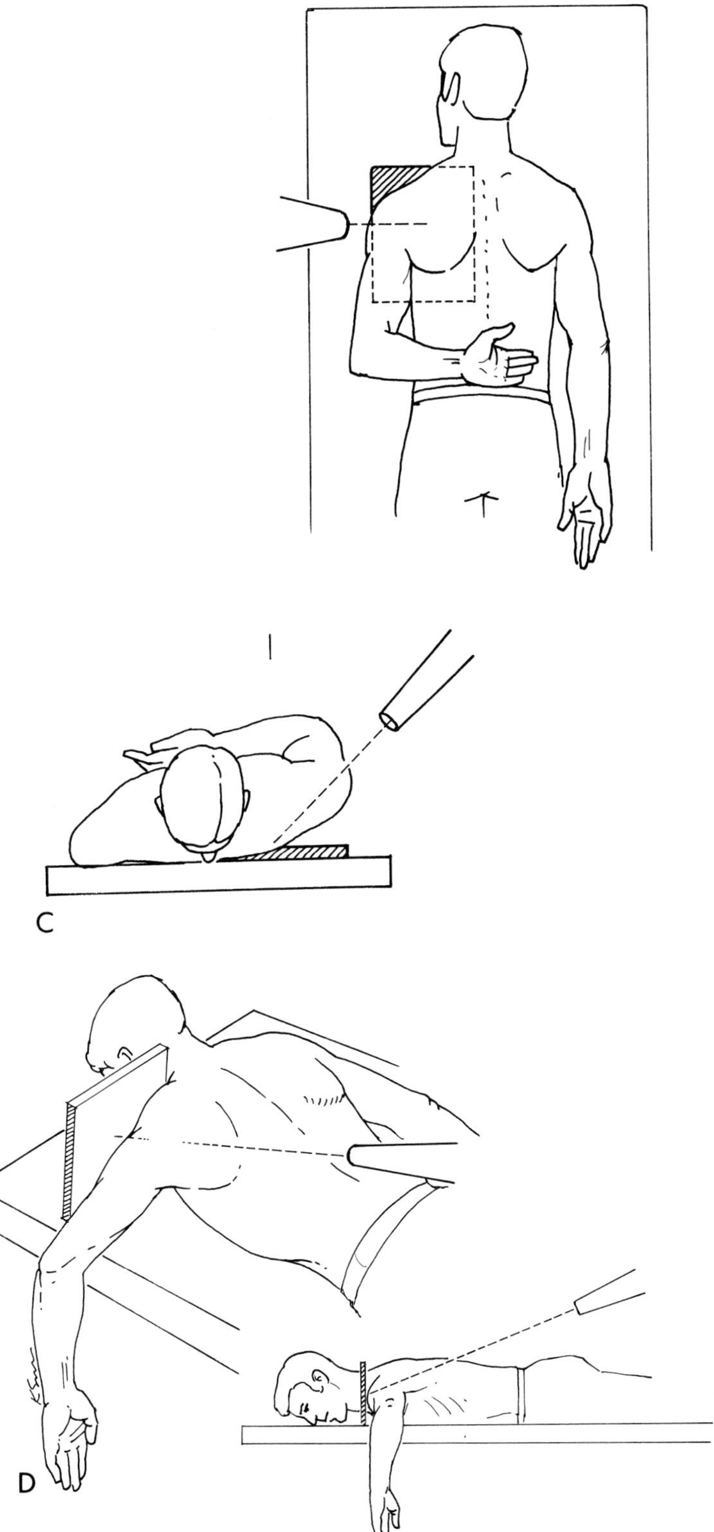

Figure 7–9. Continued

C *Modified Didiee view. The hand is placed on the iliac crest with the thumb directed upward. The central ray is angled 45 degrees in a lateral to medial direction.*

D *"West Point" view. In the prone position, the patient abducts the arm 90 degrees and the hand is placed over the end of the table. The central ray is angled 25 degrees in a cephalad direction and 25 degrees in a lateral to medial direction.*

Illustration continued on the following page

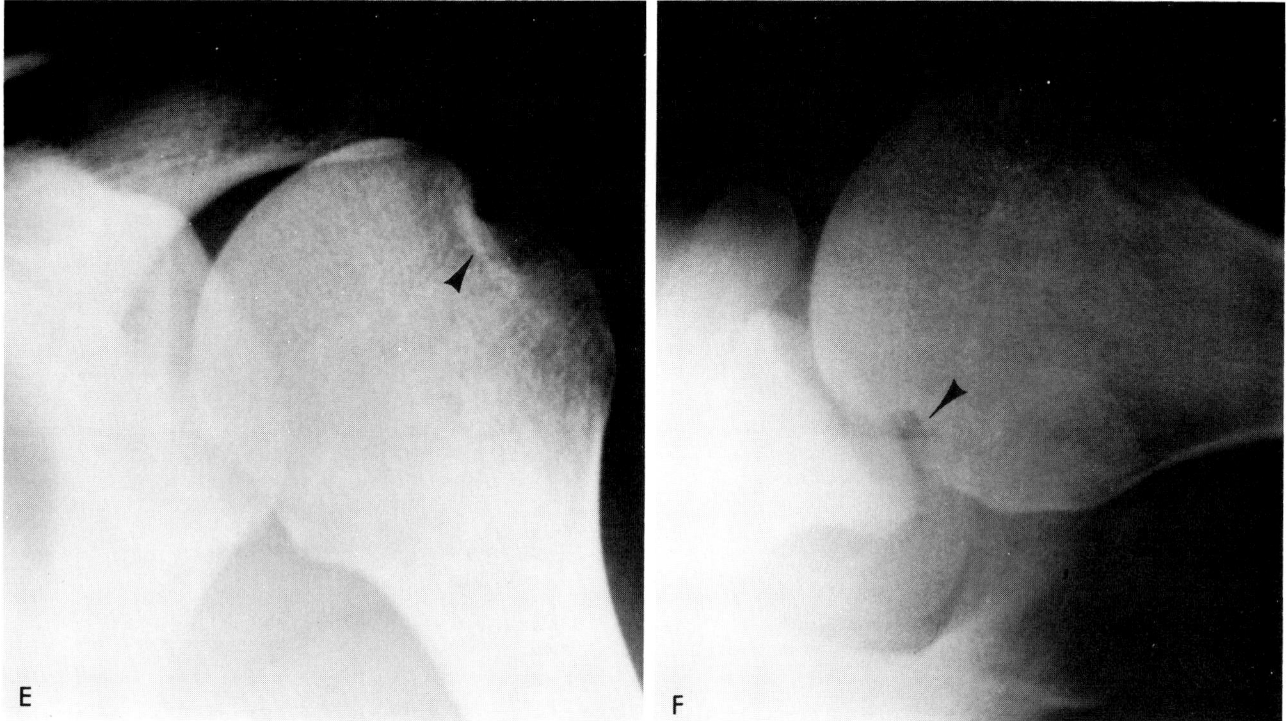

Figure 7–9. Continued

E, F *Hill-Sachs lesion. In this patient with previous anterior dislocation of the glenohumeral joint, a Hill-Sachs lesion (arrowhead) is identified in the superolateral aspect of the humeral head in internal rotation* **(E)** *and axillary* **(F)** *projections.*

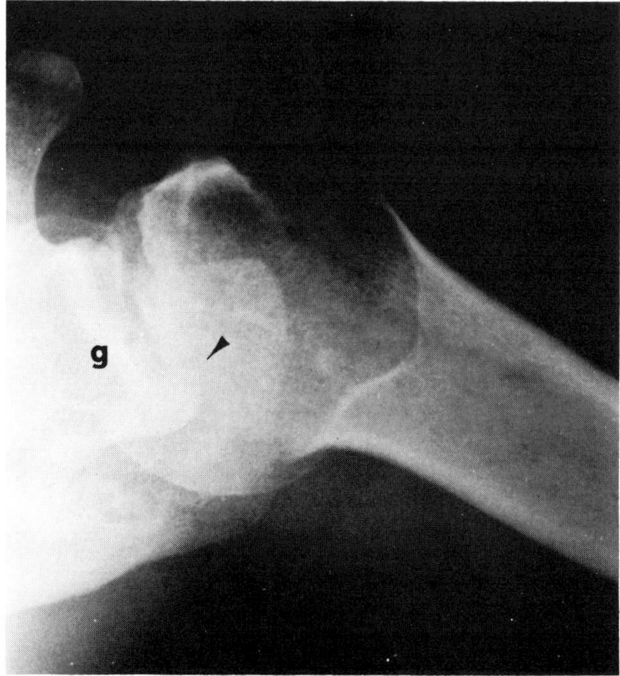

Figure 7–10. *Glenohumeral joint: Evaluation of patients with posterior dislocation of the glenohumeral joint. In a modified axillary projection, observe the subluxed humeral head, which is displaced posteriorly with respect to the glenoid (g). The latter structure is producing an impaction fracture of the humerus (arrowhead).*

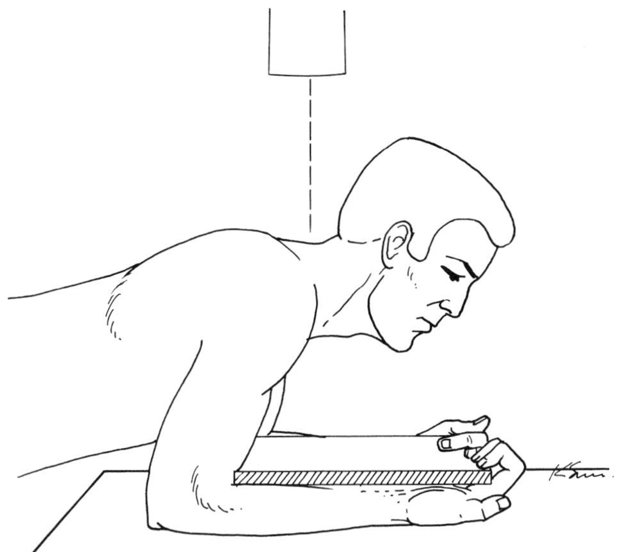

Figure 7–11. Glenohumeral joint: Bicipital groove view. The patient flexes the trunk across the table and holds the cassette on the forearms. The central ray is directed vertically.

ACROMIOCLAVICULAR JOINT

Although the acromioclavicular articulation is visualized in routine views of the shoulder, it may be superimposed on other osseous structures. Radiographs obtained in the frontal projection with cephalad tilt of the incident beam of approximately 15 degrees are superior in delineating abnormalities of this articulation[32, 33] (Fig. 7–12). A lateral projection of this joint has also been described,[2, 33] and an additional technique includes a frontal roentgenogram taken in a lordotic position.[2]

In order to diagnose acromioclavicular joint subluxation and dislocation, stress roentgenograms frequently are necessary. These are obtained by having the patient hold a 2.3 to 7 kg (5 to 15 lb) mass (weight) in the hand. If possible, it is beneficial to view both acromioclavicular articulations on a single film. This allows one to compare the two joints, carefully observing the distance between coracoid process and clavicle on both sides.[24, 34] A "shoulder forward projection" and an axial projection have been recommended as additional methods in diagnosing abnormalities of the clavicle and acromioclavicular joint subluxation.[35-37]

Basic Examination: Acromioclavicular Joint
Anteroposterior with 15 Degrees Cephalad Angulation

STERNUM AND STERNOCLAVICULAR JOINT

The radiographic evaluation of the sternum requires oblique and lateral projections. Long exposure times are useful, as the patient's breathing during several phases of respiration will produce blurring of overlying lung and rib shadows. The lateral projection can be obtained in an erect or a recumbent position.

Adequate roentgenograms of the sternoclavicular articulations are difficult to obtain. Oblique and frontal radiographs of the sternum frequently do not provide optimal visualization of this articulation (Fig. 7–13). Many special views have been recommended.[38-40] The Hobbs view, a superoinferior projection of the sternoclavicular joint[41] and lordotic projection[24] may both be helpful, particularly in evaluating an individual with a possible dislocation of the sternoclavicular joint (Fig. 7–14). One additional projection, the Heinig view, which is similar to Kurzbauer's lateral projection,[40] can also docu-

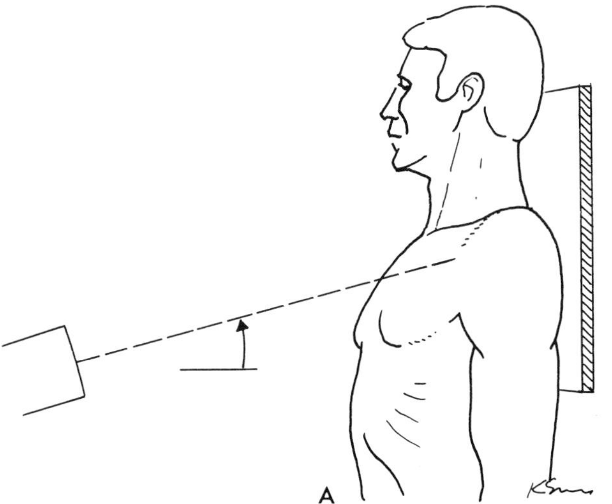

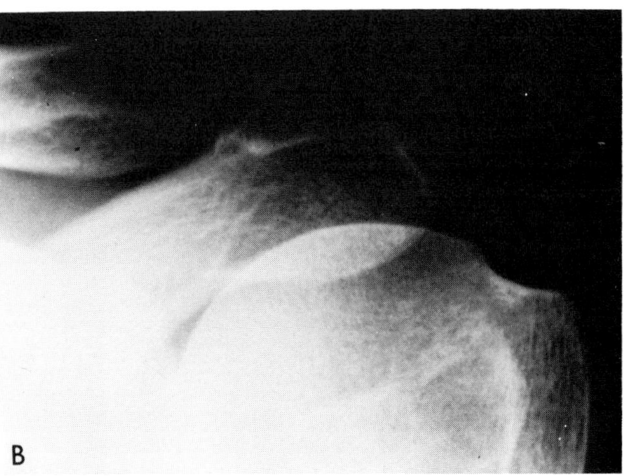

Figure 7–12. Acromioclavicular joint: Routine radiographs. Anteroposterior radiograph: Normal. The central ray is angled 15 degrees in a cephalad direction.

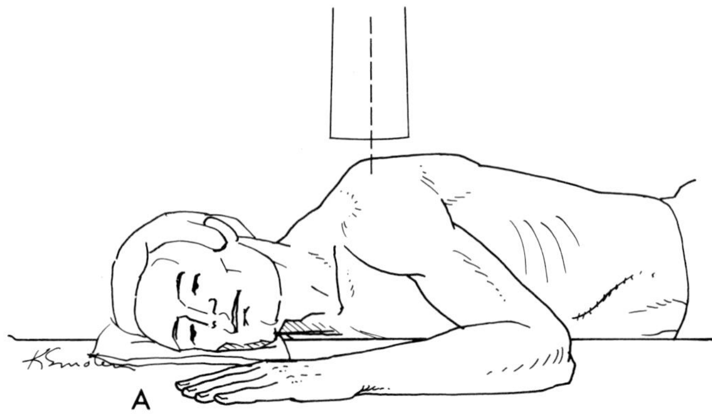

Figure 7–13. *Sternoclavicular joint: Routine radiographs.*
A, B *Oblique radiograph: Normal. Although the sternoclavicular joint can be seen (arrow), it is partially obscured by overlying shadows.*
C *Position for anteroposterior radiograph.*

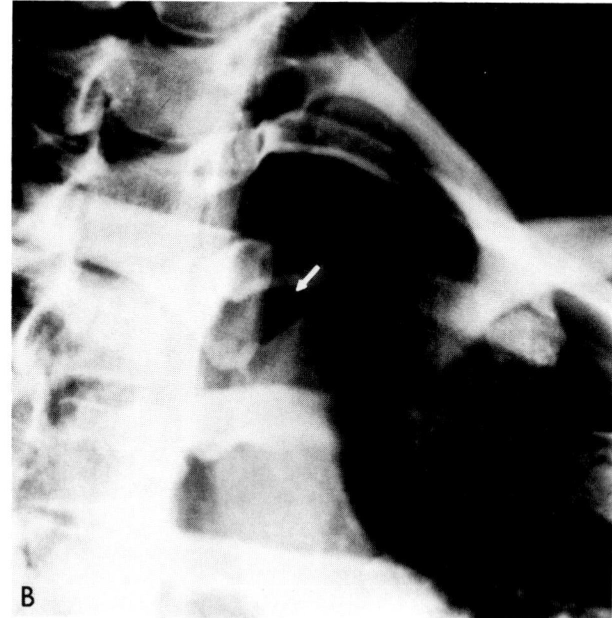

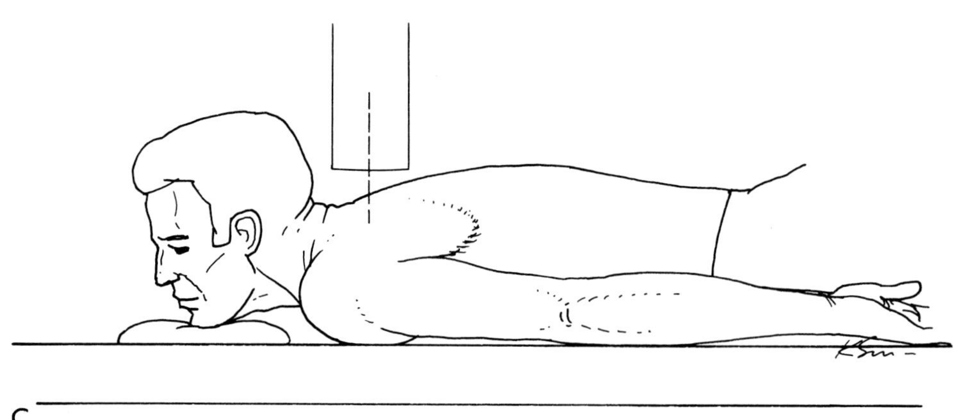

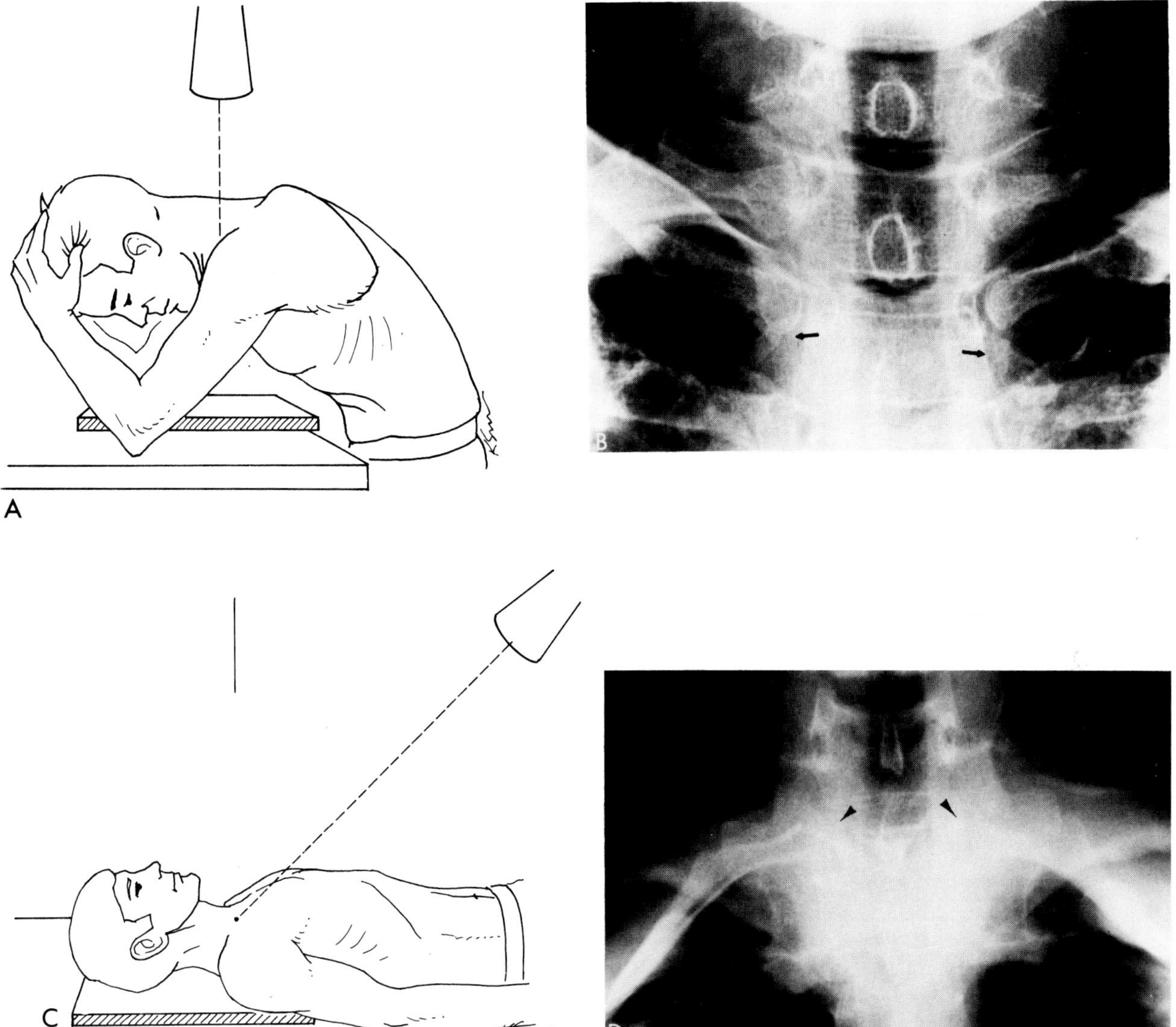

Figure 7–14. *Sternoclavicular joint: Additional radiographs.*

A, B *Hobbs' view: Normal. This radiograph is obtained with the patient bent over the table, hands placed on the head. The medial border of the clavicle can be identified and the sternoclavicular joints are projected at the same level (arrows).*

C, D *Lordotic view: Normal. The central ray is directed with a 40 to 50 degree cephalad tilt. The medial margins of the clavicles are at the same height (arrowheads).*

Illustration continued on the following page

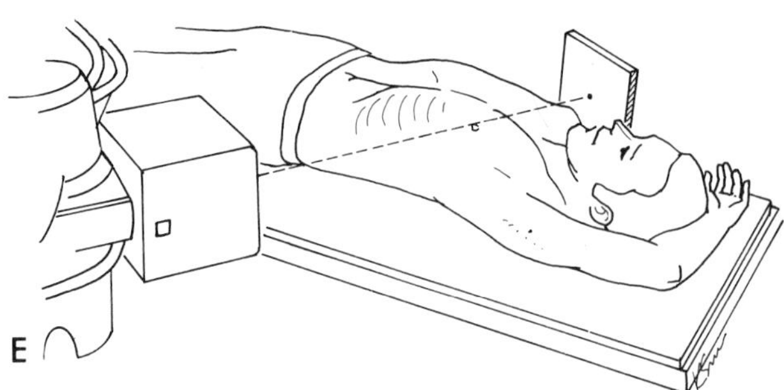

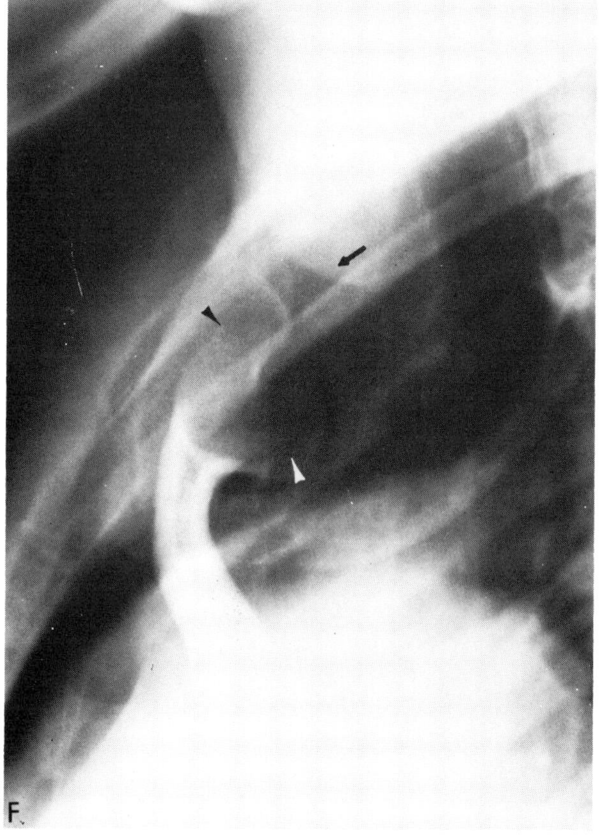

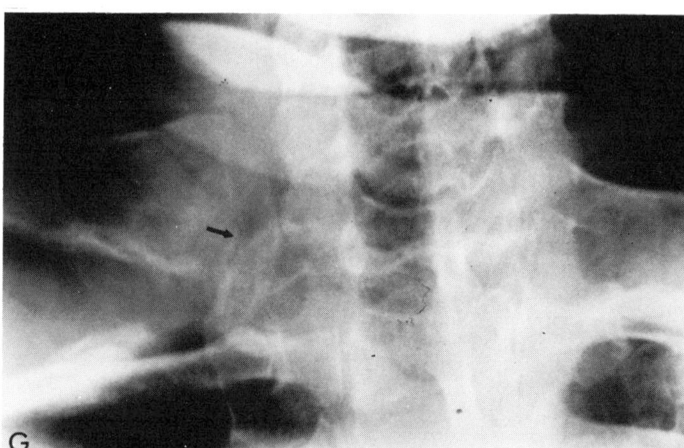

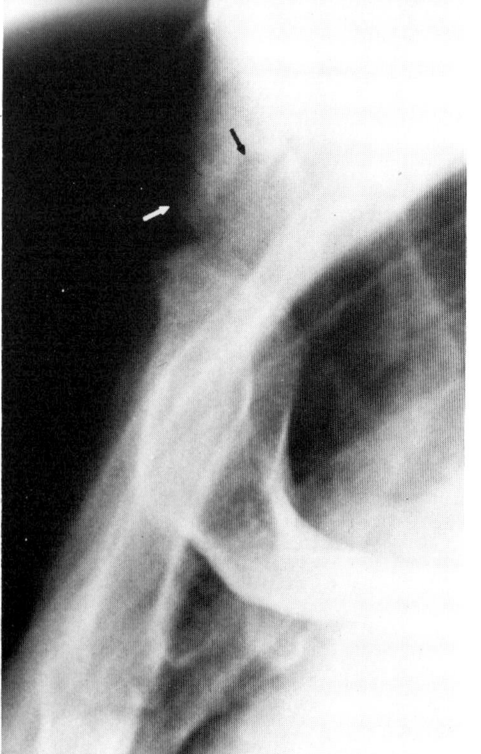

Figure 7–14. Continued

E, F *Heinig view: Normal. The patient is recumbent. The shoulder closest to the tube is abducted. The central ray is centered at the sternoclavicular joint and directed along the axis of the clavicle. On the normal Heinig projection, the medial end of the clavicle closest to the film is projected through the manubrium (arrowheads) and the medial end of the clavicle closest to the tube is in direct alignment with the top of the manubrium (arrow).*

G, H *Lordotic and Heinig views: Anterior fracture–dislocation of sternoclavicular joint. On the lordotic projection* **(G)**, *the medial end of the right clavicle is elevated (indicating an anterior dislocation) and a fracture can be visualized (arrow). In the Heinig view* **(H)**, *the anterior portion of the clavicle and fracture are again identified (arrows).*

ment dislocation of this joint.[42, 43] Utilization of an ultrafine focal spot tube and a short focal spot–patient distance allows differential magnification with projection of the sternoclavicular joints to either side of the thoracic spine on an anteroposterior projection.[106]

Basic Examination: Sternum and Sternoclavicular Joint
Posteroanterior
Oblique
Lateral

SPINE

The radiographic examination of the spine varies considerably, depending upon the vertebral segment being examined and the specific indication for the examination.

Cervical Spine

Although a screening examination of the cervical spine in a patient with widespread articular disease may require only anteroposterior and lateral flexion roentgenograms, a more complete evaluation may be necessary in a patient with neck pain and is mandatory in a patient who has sustained neck trauma.[44-48]

The standard examination of the cervical spine consists of multiple views (Fig. 7–15). A frontal radiograph is obtained with the patient either recumbent or erect in an anteroposterior projection with approximately 15 degrees to 20 degrees of cephalad angulation of the tube. Mandibular motion during the exposure allows more optimal visualization of the upper cervical vertebrae in this projection.[49] The lateral radiograph is usually obtained with the head in neutral position but may be supplemented with lateral roentgenograms obtained with head flexion and extension. Forty-five degree oblique projections are obtained with the patient sitting or standing. An anteroposterior open-mouth projection allows visualization of the atlas and axis.[50] A "pillar" view for demonstration of the vertebral arches is obtained in an anteroposterior or posteroanterior position with neck extension. In the former position, the central ray is angulated 25 to 30 degrees toward the feet[51]; in the latter position, the central ray is angulated 40 degrees cephalad. Certain modifications of the pillar view have been suggested.[48] One such technique employs turning the mandible to each side in order to eliminate overlying soft tissue and osseous structures that may obscure the cervical spine. We prefer to have the patient maintain a central position of the mandible as this position facilitates comparison between the two sides.

Following significant cervical spine trauma, initial radiographs should include cross-table lateral and anteroposterior views, which may be obtained without disturbing the patient. After this "screening" examination, further roentgenograms can be taken. The complete cervical spine examination in these patients should include those projections that have previously been noted: anteroposterior view with 20 degree cephalad angulation of the tube, open-mouth view, right and left 45 degree oblique views, lateral views in neutral position, flexion, and extension, and "pillar" view. Additionally, shallow oblique radiographs (approximately 20 degrees of obliquity) may be needed.

For certain portions of the cervical spine, additional roentgenograms are suggested (Fig. 7–16). Specific projections are designed for the cervicobasilar region.[2, 52] For the cervicothoracic region, recommended views include the "swimmer's" projection,[2] a lateral view with the arms pulled down,[47] "flying angel" projection with traction on a single arm,[47] and a supine oblique projection.[53] To better delineate alterations at the atlanto-axial articulation, multiple open-mouth views may be necessary.[54] These are obtained with the patient in the frontal position, with rotation of the head of 10 to 15 degrees to either side and with lateral tilting of the head to either side.

Basic Examination: Cervical Spine
Anteroposterior
"Pillar"
Lateral in Neutral Position and in Flexion
Open-mouth
Obliques

Thoracic Spine

A radiographic series of the thoracic spine should include anteroposterior and lateral roentgenograms and a swimmer's view of the lower cervical and upper thoracic vertebrae (Fig. 7–17). The anteroposterior projection places the spine adjacent to the x-ray film. Because of the normal thoracic kyphosis, diverging incident rays are relatively parallel to the upper and lower aspects of the vertebrae in this position. Certain modifications in the technique may allow more uniform density throughout the entire radiograph.[55] On the lateral radiograph nonsuspended respiration may blur the overlying shadows of the thoracic cage. Radiographs exposed with the patient positioned in slight obliquity allow visualization of the apophyseal joints of the thoracic spine.[2, 56, 57]

Basic Examination: Thoracic Spine
Anteroposterior
Lateral

Text continued on page 285

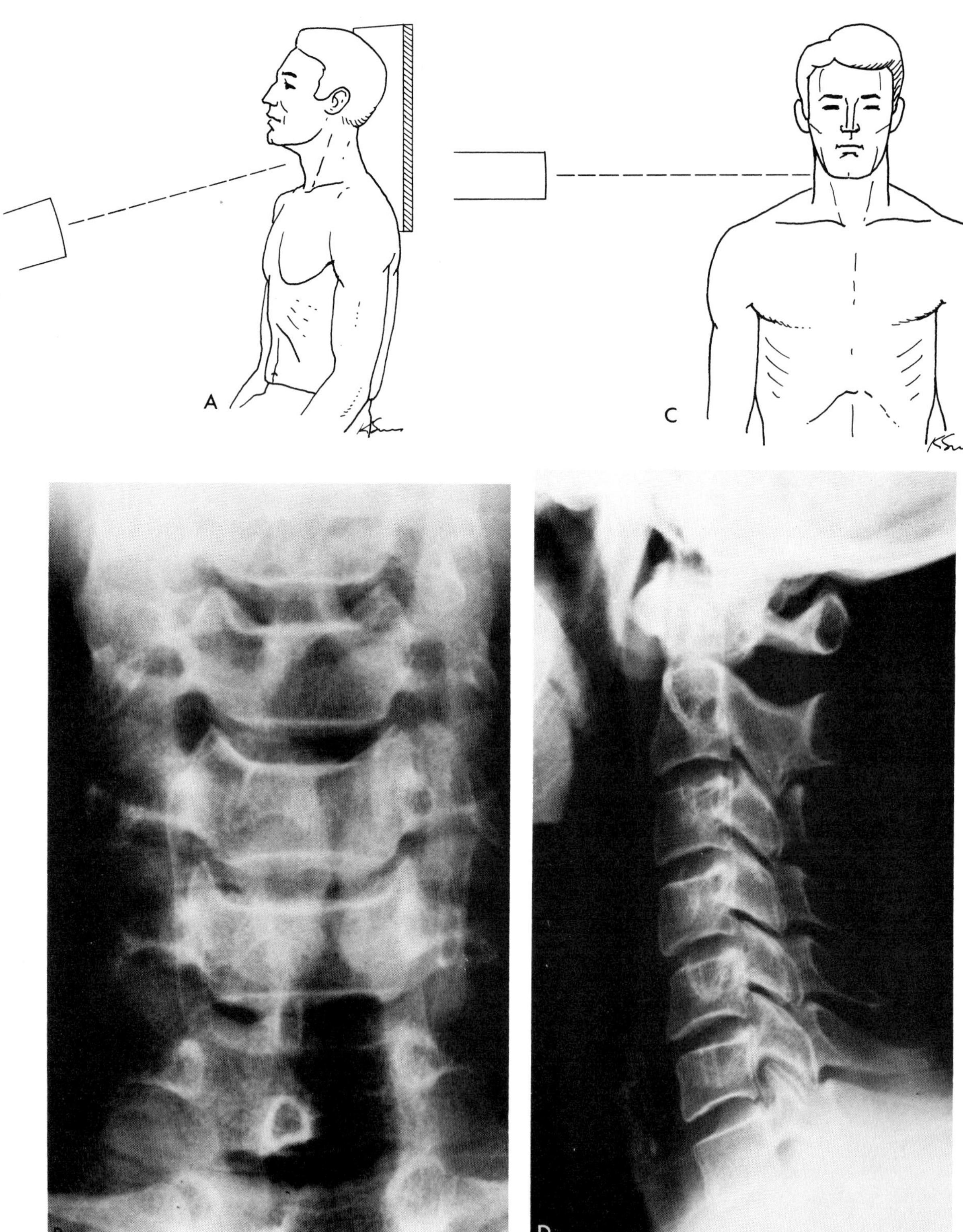

Figure 7–15. *Cervical spine: Routine radiographs.*
A, B *Anteroposterior radiograph: Normal.*
C, D *Lateral radiograph: Normal.*
Illustration continued on the opposite page

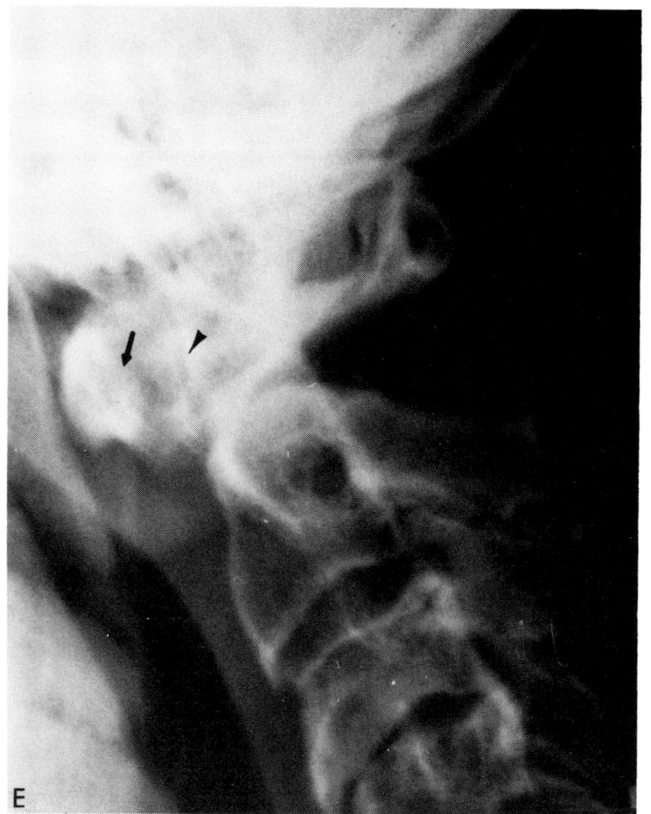

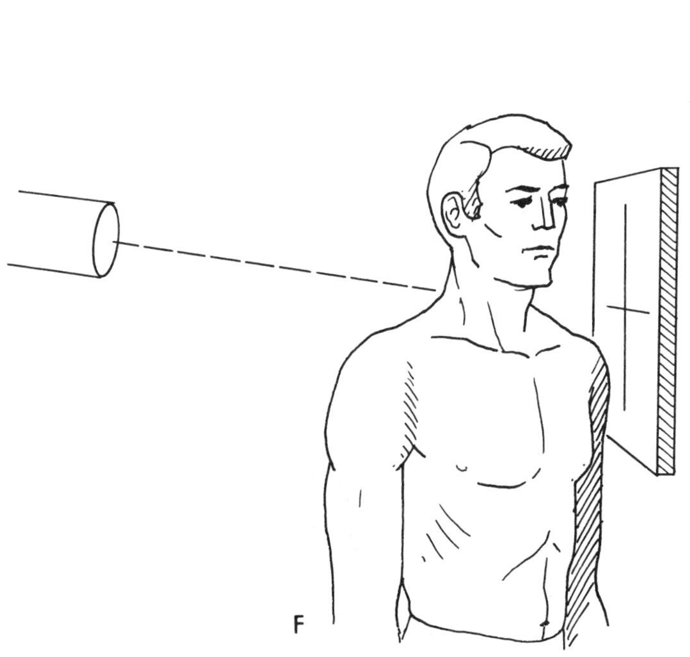

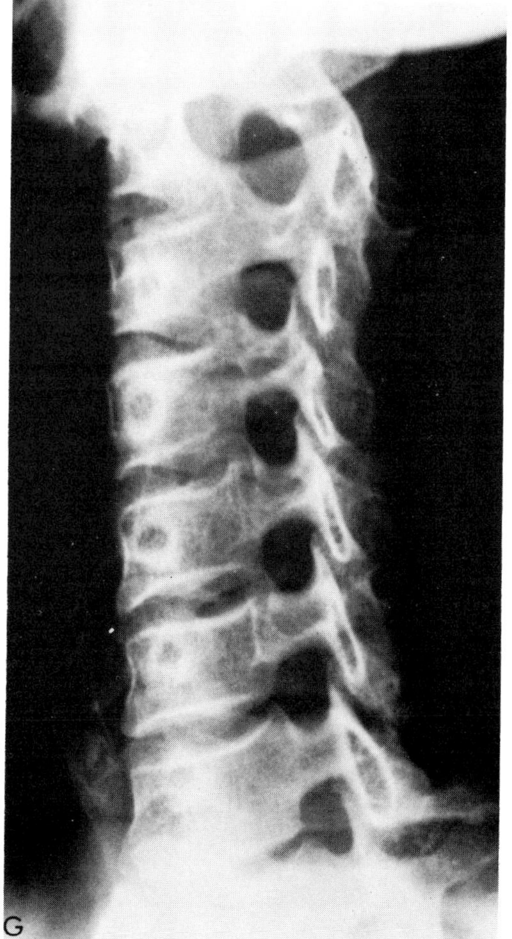

Figure 7–15. Continued

E *Lateral radiograph: Atlanto-axial subluxation in rheumatoid arthritis. Note the increased distance between the anterior arch of the atlas (arrow) and the anterior aspect of the odontoid process (arrowhead).*

F, G *Oblique radiograph: Normal. The neural foramina are well visualized.*

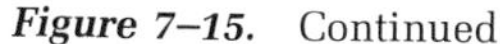

Illustration continued on the following page

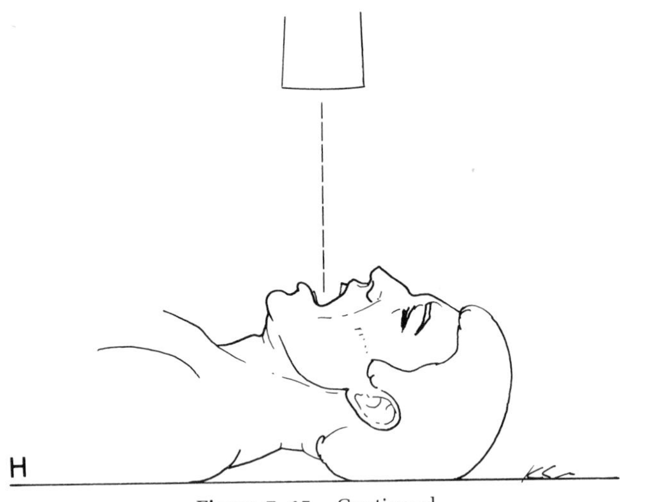
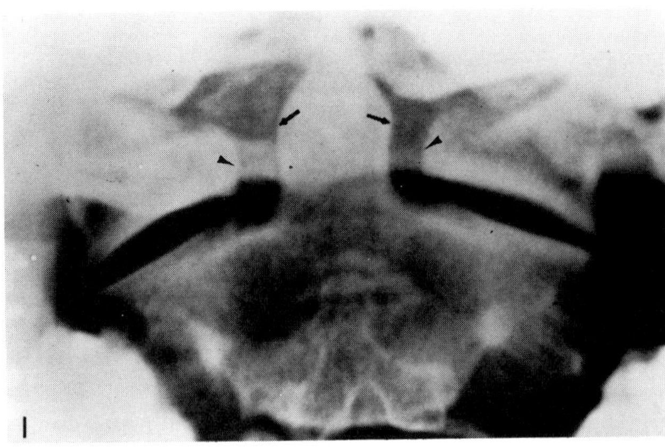

Figure 7–15. Continued
H, I Open-mouth radiograph: Normal, Observe the odontoid process (arrows) symmetrically placed between the lateral masses (arrowheads) of the atlas.

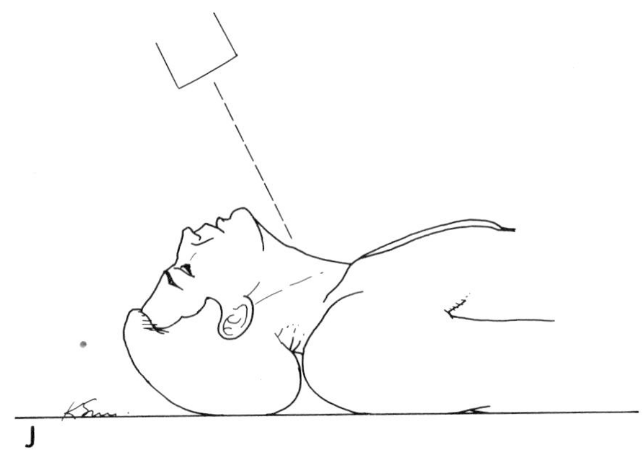
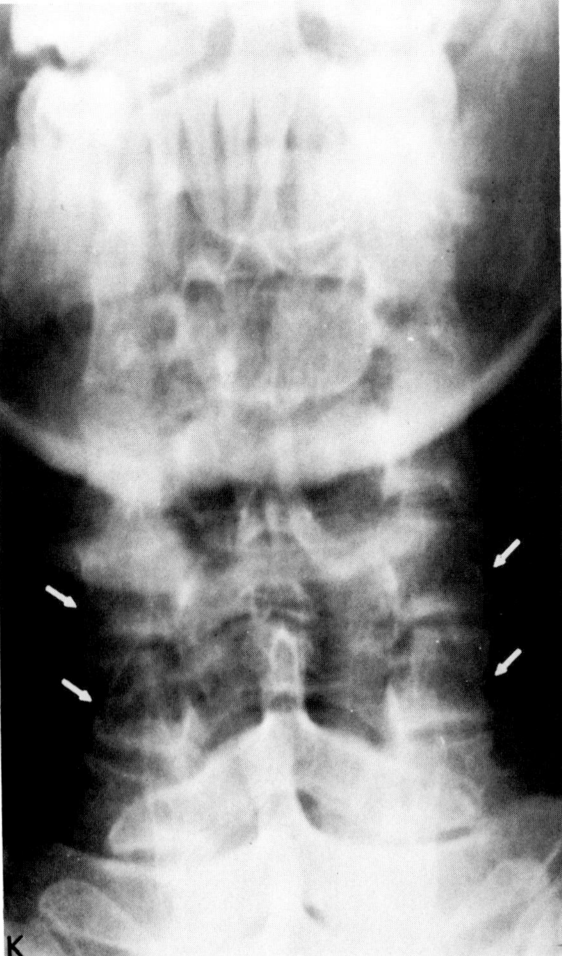

Figure 7–15. Continued
J, K "Pillar" radiograph: Normal. In an anteroposterior position, the central ray is angulated 25 to 30 degrees toward the feet. The lateral masses (arrows) are well shown.

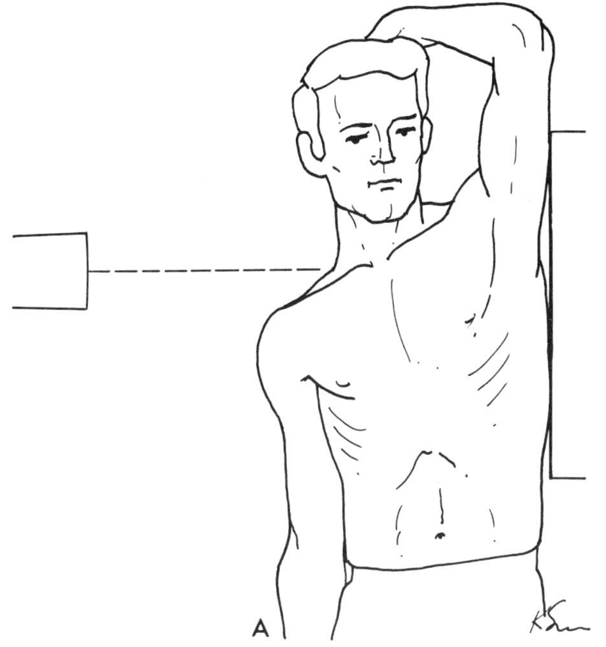
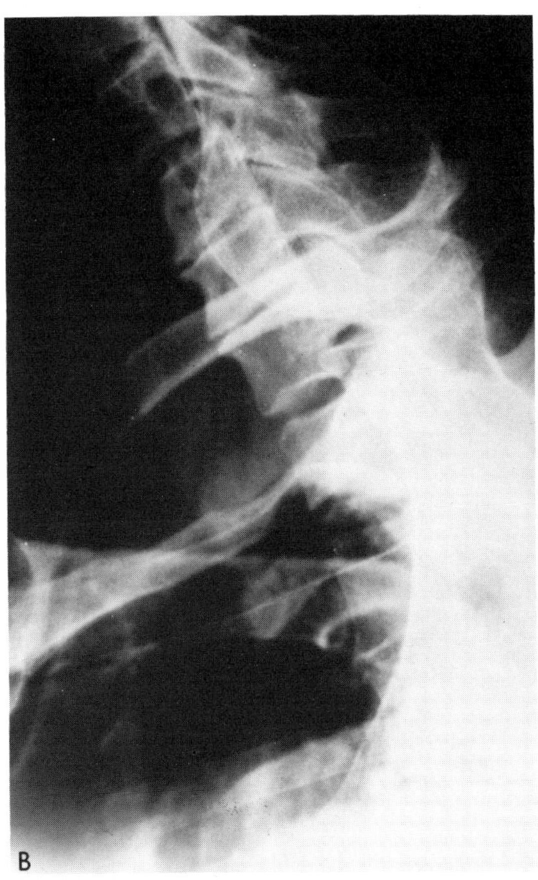
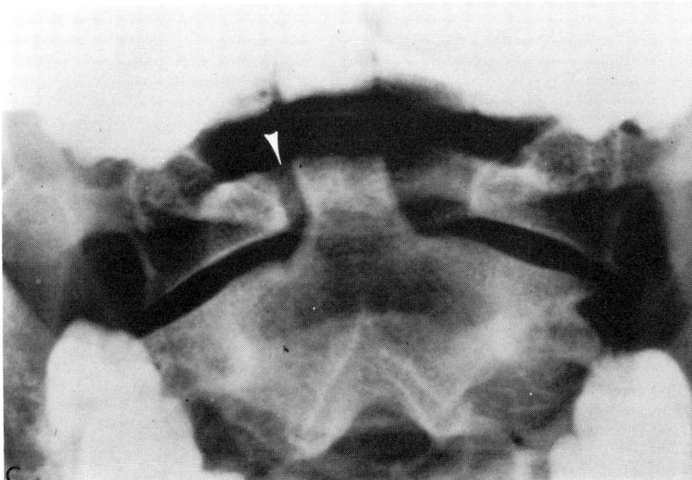
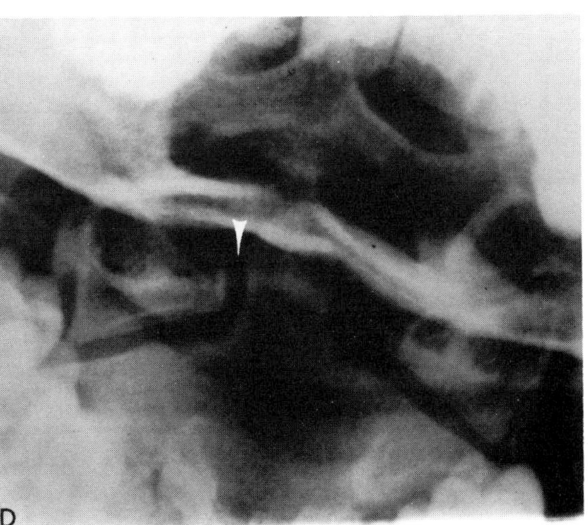

Figure 7–16. *Cervical spine: Additional radiographs.*

A, B *Swimmer's position radiograph: Abnormal. The lateral radiograph is obtained with one arm elevated. This allows evaluation of the cervicothoracic junction. Disc space narrowing is apparent.*

C, D *Open-mouth views: Rotary fixation of the atlas and axis. These two radiographs were taken with the patient tilting the head. They demonstrate persistent asymmetry at the atlanto-axial junction, with the odontoid more closely associated with the right lateral mass (arrowhead). This indicates rotary fixation at the atlanto-axial junction.*

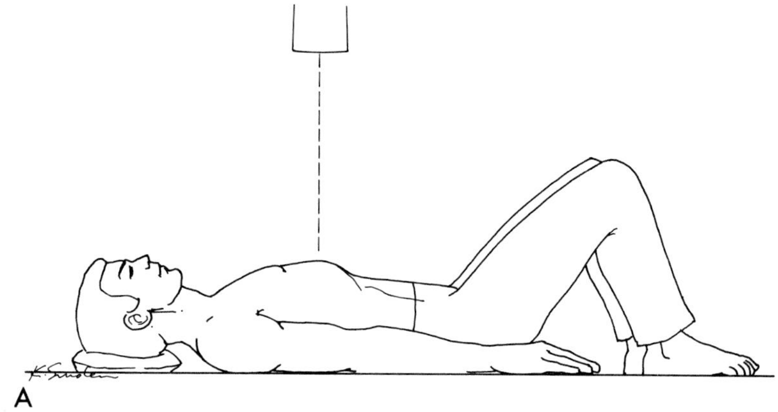

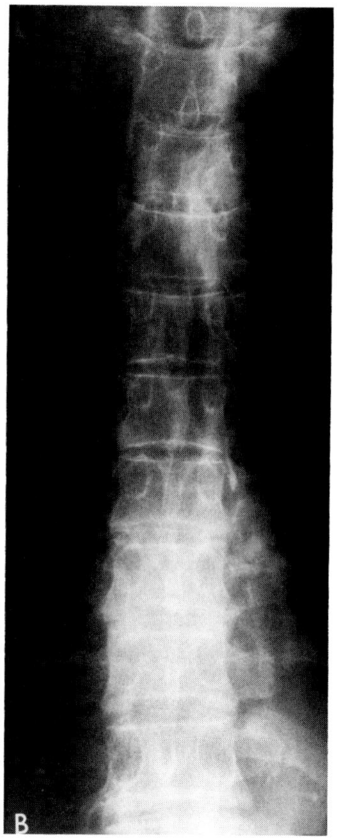

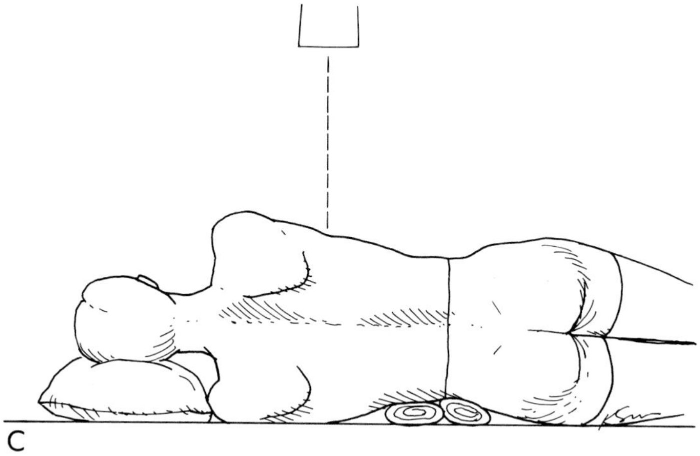

A

B

C

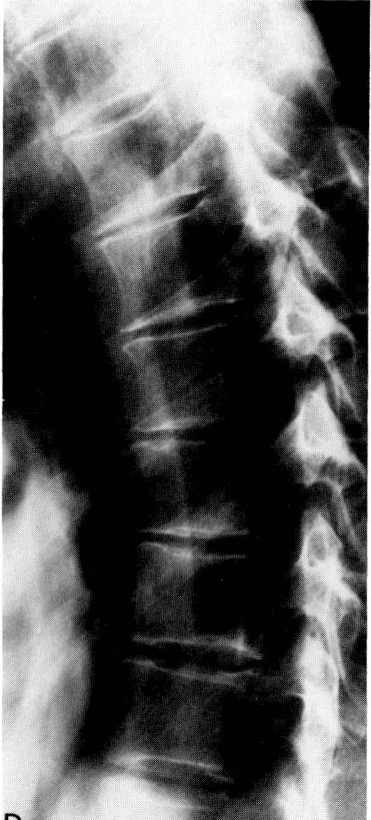

Figure 7–17. *Thoracic spine: Routine radiographs.*
A, B *Anteroposterior radiograph: Normal. The flexed position of the knees produces some straightening of the normal thoracic kyphosis.*
C, D *Lateral radiograph: Normal.*

Lumbar Spine

The frontal radiograph of the lumbar spine can be obtained in a posteroanterior or anteroposterior projection with the patient erect or recumbent (Fig. 7–18). The recumbent anteroposterior radiograph should be taken with the hips and knees flexed, which reduces the lumbar lordosis and better delineates the vertebral bodies and intervertebral discs. The lateral radiograph is also exposed with slight flexion of the hips and knees. A coned-down lateral projection of the lumbosacral junction is also included. Oblique roentgenograms allow evaluation of the posterior elements of the lumbar spine, although some regard the oblique projections as unnecessary.[111] These radiographs can be obtained in anteroposterior or posteroanterior positions by turning the patient 45 degrees. An anteroposterior view of the pelvis is generally included in the evaluation of the lumbosacral spine. To evaluate the laminae and articular processes in this region, an axial radiograph (in infants)[107] or an anteroposterior radiograph with 45 degrees of caudal angulation of the beam can be obtained.[58] An anteroposterior radiograph with the incident beam angled 15 to 30 degrees cephalad will allow visualization of tangential surfaces of the inferior aspect of the fifth lumbar vertebral body and the superior aspect of the first sacral segment.[2] An oblique semiaxial projection provides delineation of the inferior intervertebral foramina.[59]

Examination of motion of the lumbar spine may provide useful information.[60] To accomplish this, lateral radiographs may be obtained during flexion and extension and frontal roentgenograms may be obtained during lateral bending of the spine.

Basic Examination: Lumbar Spine
Anteroposterior
Lateral
Lateral Coned to L5-S1
Obliques
Anteroposterior of Pelvis

PELVIS

The standard radiographic view for the pelvis is obtained in an anteroposterior position with the

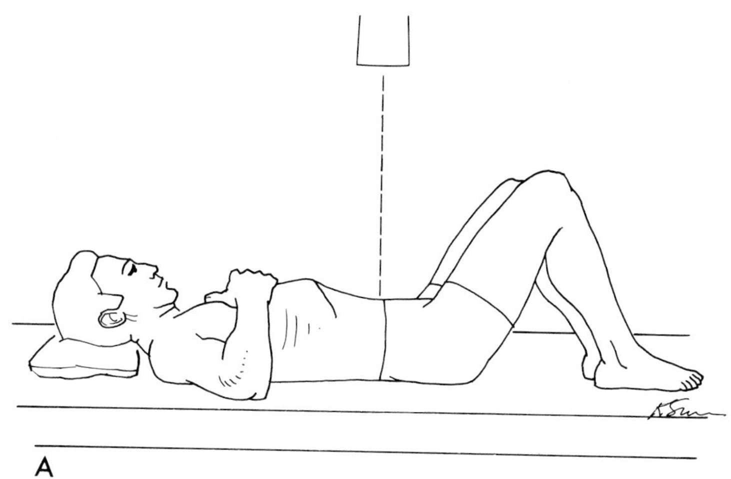
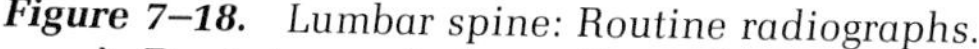

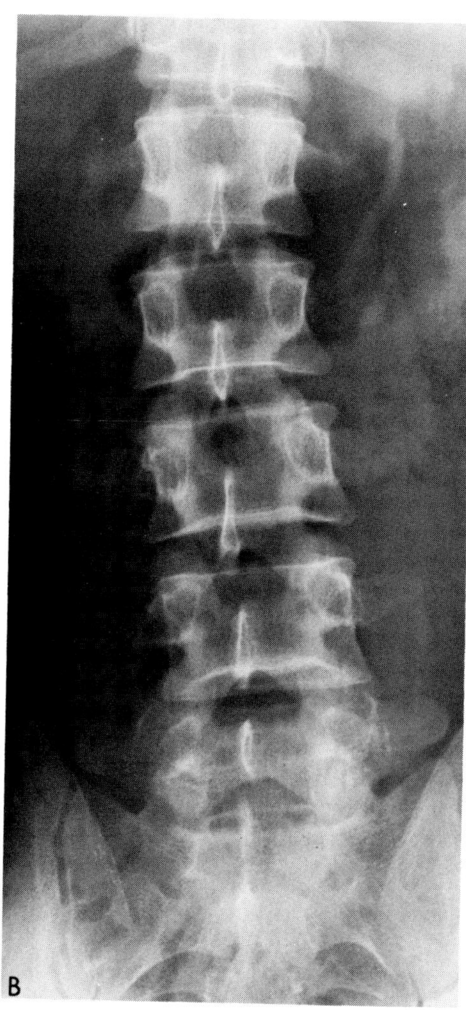

Figure 7–18. *Lumbar spine: Routine radiographs.*
A, B *Anteroposterior radiograph: Normal. The knees and hips are flexed to reduce the degree of lumbar lordosis. Mild angulation of the upper spine is seen.*

Illustration continued on the following page

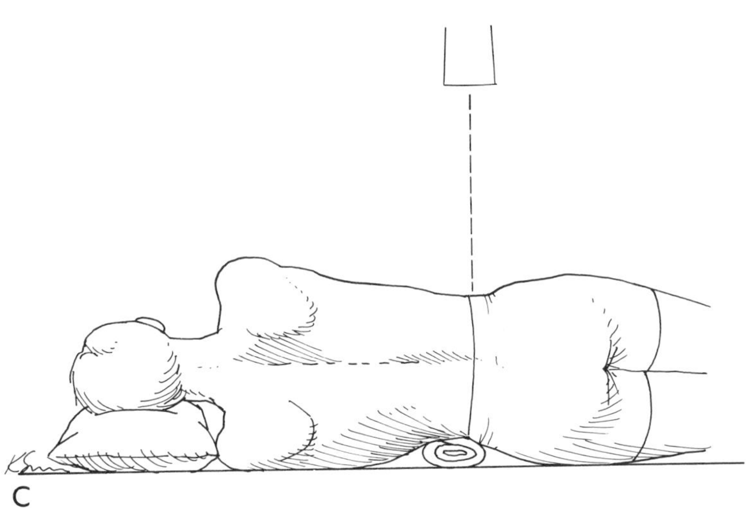

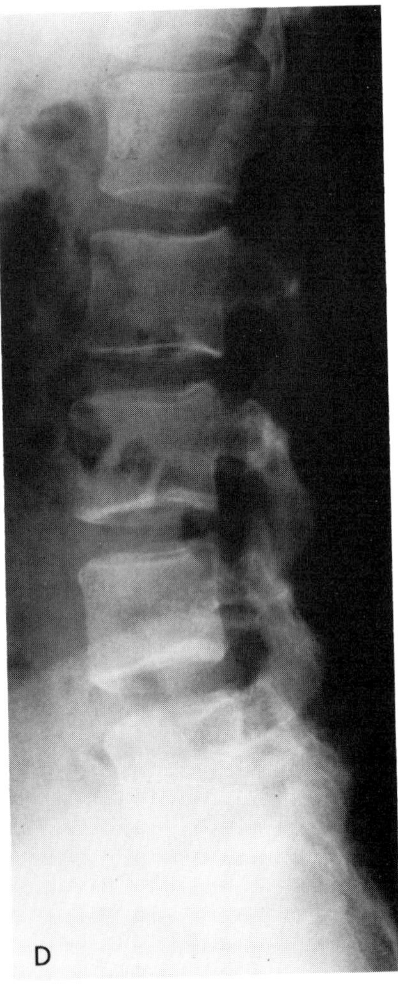

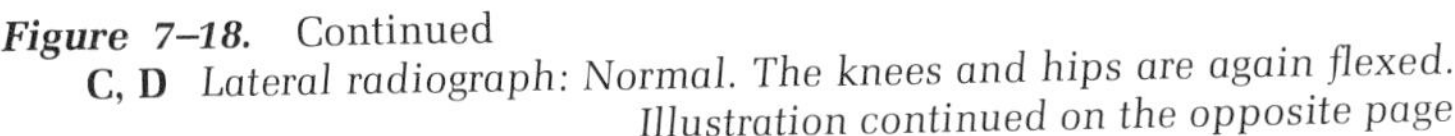

Figure 7–18. Continued
C, D *Lateral radiograph: Normal. The knees and hips are again flexed.*
Illustration continued on the opposite page

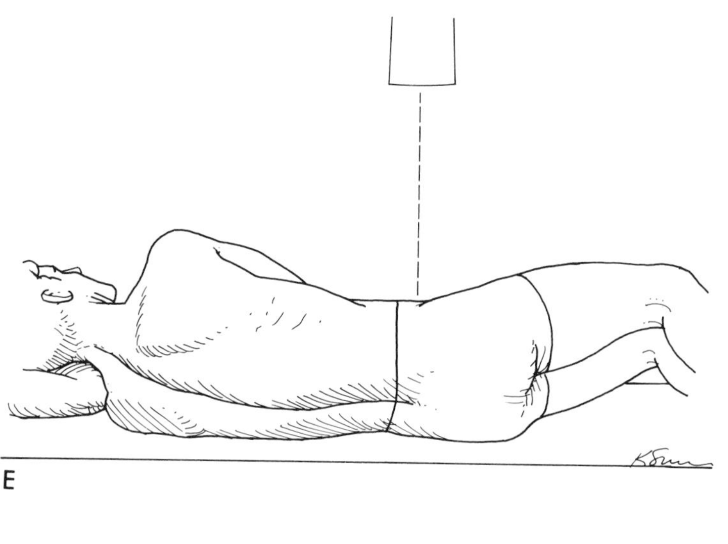

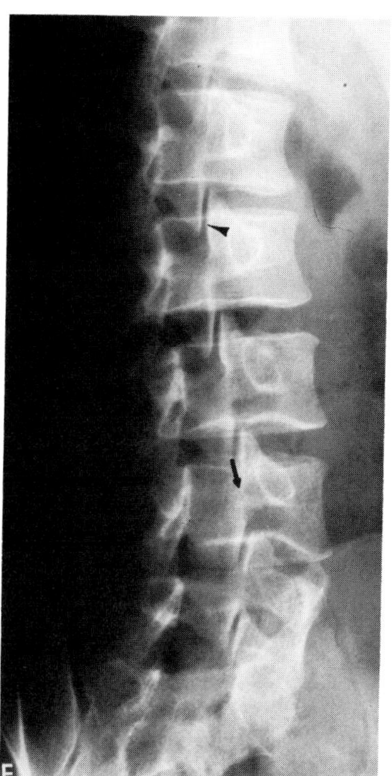

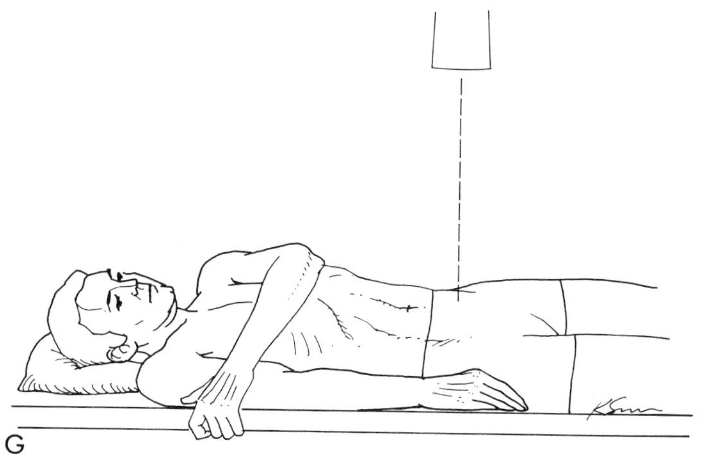

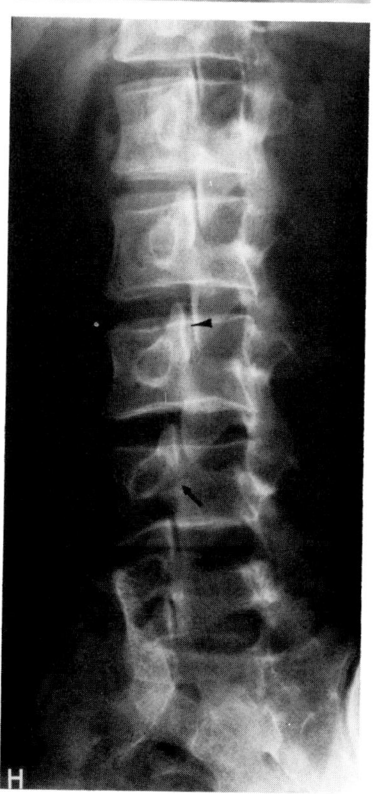

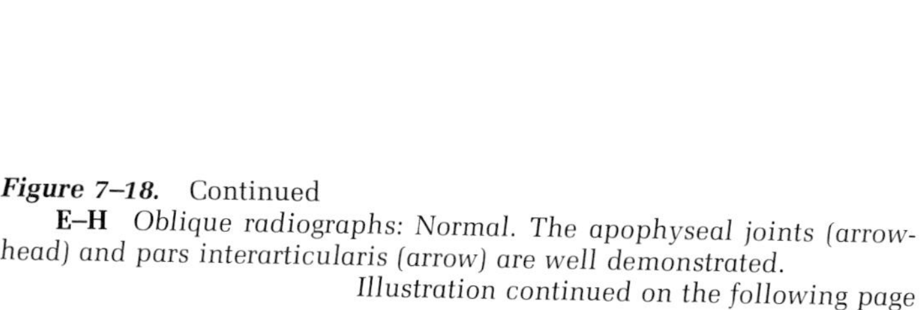

Figure 7–18. Continued

E–H *Oblique radiographs: Normal. The apophyseal joints (arrowhead) and pars interarticularis (arrow) are well demonstrated.*

Illustration continued on the following page

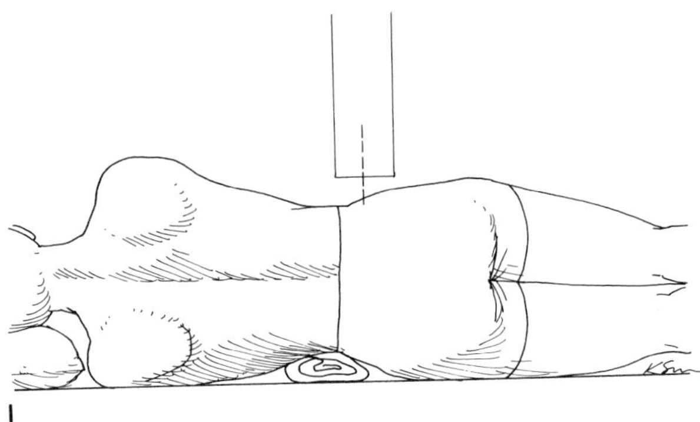
I

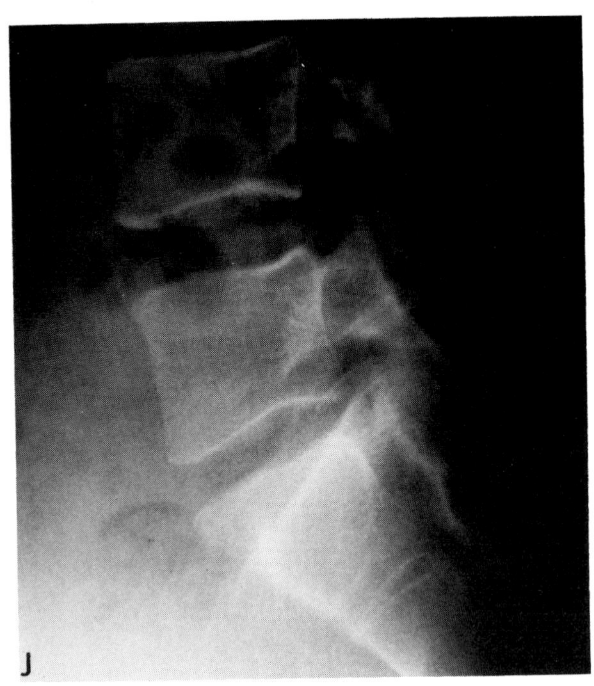
J

Figure 7–18. Continued
I, J *Coned-down lateral radiograph: Normal. The lumbosacral junction can be evaluated. Note that the intervertebral disc between the fifth lumbar vertebral body and top of the sacrum normally may appear narrow compared to the other lumbar intervertebral discs.*

patient supine (Fig. 7–19). The feet are placed in approximately 15 degrees of internal rotation. This is done to overcome the normal anteversion of the femoral necks and place their longitudinal axes parallel to the film. To evaluate the pubis, a posteroanterior radiograph is probably superior to an anteroposterior roentgenogram and may be supplemented with axial projections obtained by angulating the beam or torso.

Various methods have been utilized to examine the sacroiliac joints (Fig. 7–20); none is ideal, as the normal undulating articular surfaces make evaluation of these joints extremely difficult. Oblique views of this articulation can be obtained in either the supine or the prone position.[61, 62] In either instance, the side of the body is elevated approximately 25 degrees, and the beam can be directed perpendicular to the film or angulated to the feet or head. Radiographs of both right and left sacroiliac joints are obtained.

A more ideal method for radiography of the sacroiliac joints utilizes frontal projections (Fig. 7–20). An anteroposterior radiograph can be taken with the tube angulated 25 to 30 degrees in a cephalad direction or a posteroanterior radiograph can be taken with 25 to 30 degrees caudal angulation of the tube. In either case, both sacroiliac joints are exposed on a single film, facilitating comparison of the two articulations. Although we favor the anteroposterior projection, proponents of the posteroanterior

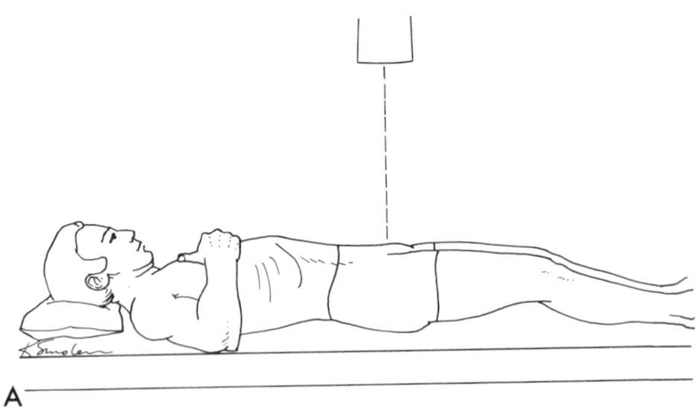
A

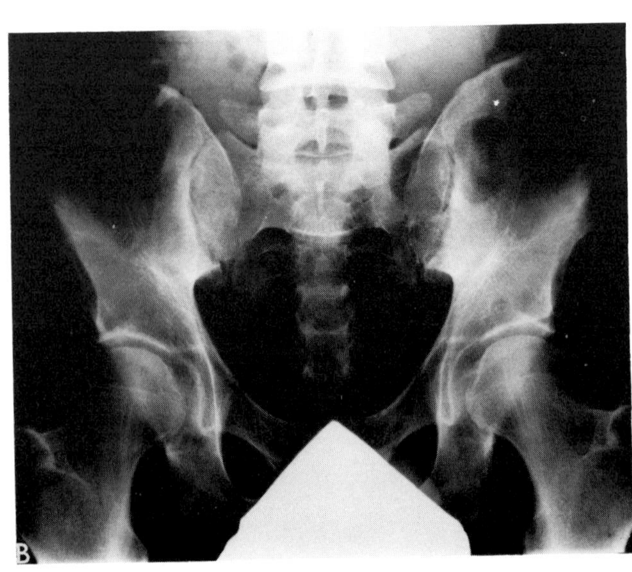
B

Figure 7–19. *Pelvis: Routine radiographs. Anteroposterior radiograph of pelvis: Normal. Internal rotation of the lower legs allows elongation of the femoral necks.*

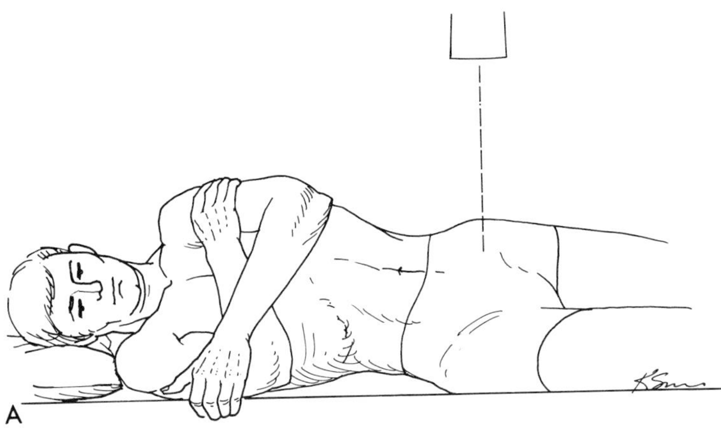

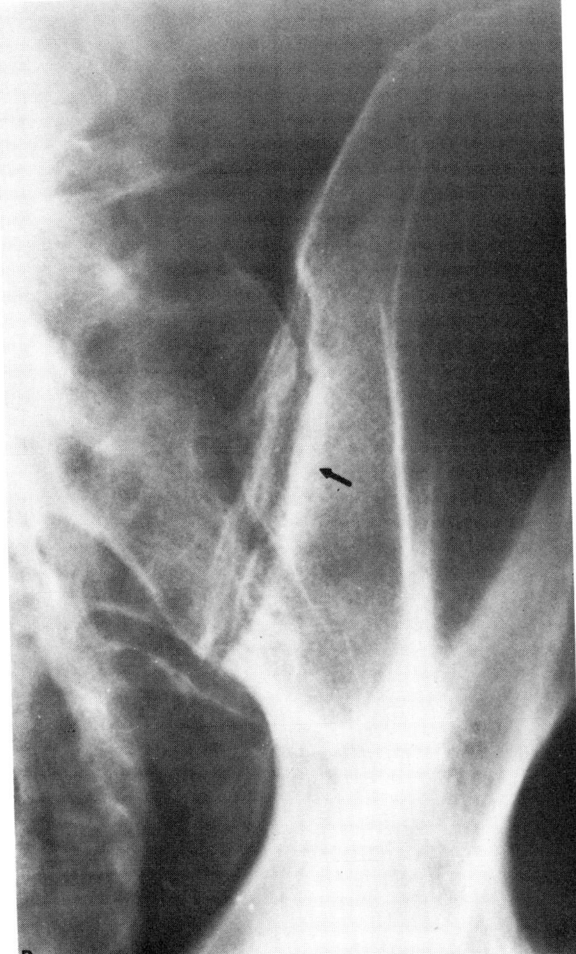

Figure 7–20. *Sacroiliac joints: Routine radiographs.*

A, B *Oblique radiograph: Normal. The side of the body which is being examined is elevated approximately 25 degrees. The sacroiliac joint is demonstrated* **(B)** *and mild sclerosis on the ilial aspect of the articulation (arrow) represents minimal degenerative joint disease.*

Illustration continued on the following page

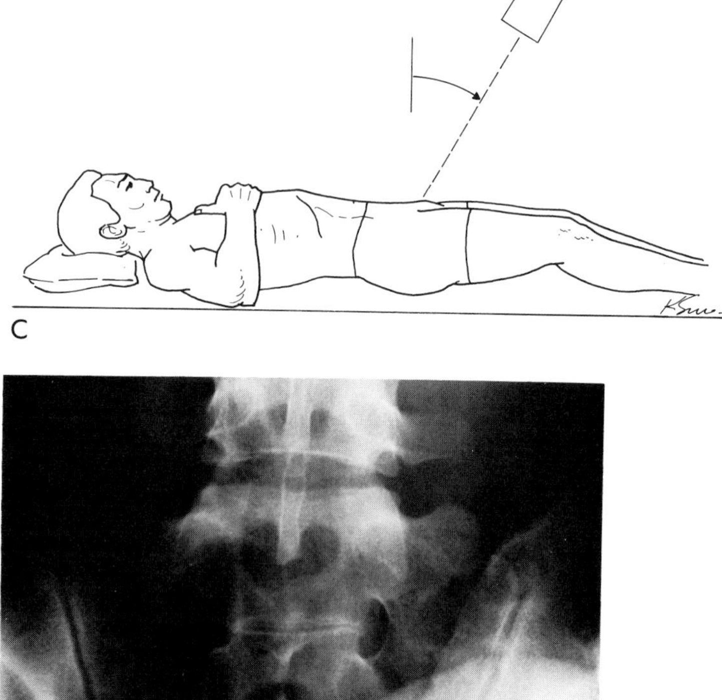

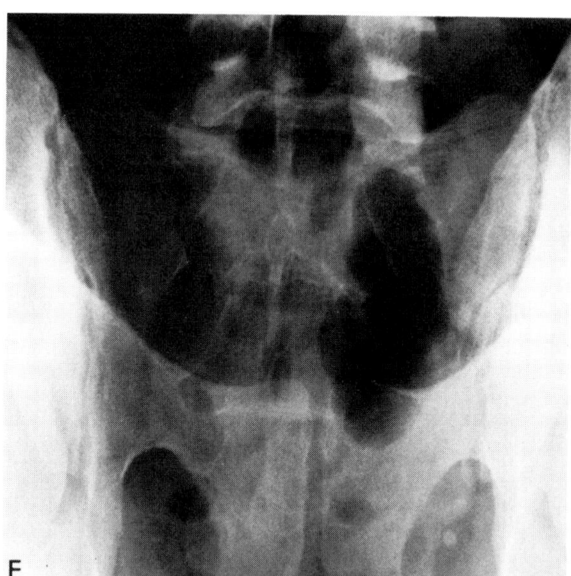

Figure 7–20. Continued

C, D *Anteroposterior radiograph with cephalad angulation: Normal. The tube is angled 25 to 30 degrees in a cephalad direction. Both sacroiliac articulations are projected on a single film.*

E *Posteroanterior radiograph with caudal angulation: Normal. The central ray is angled 25 to 30 degrees in a caudal direction.*

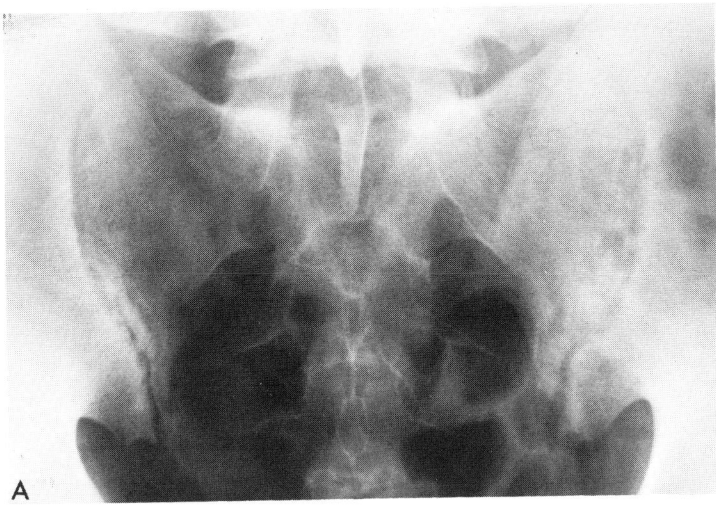

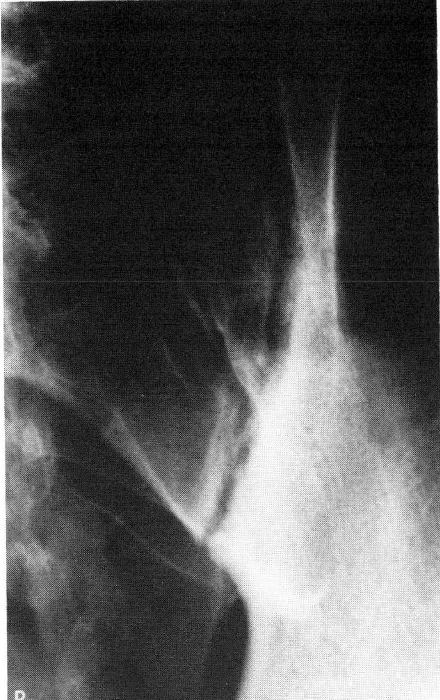

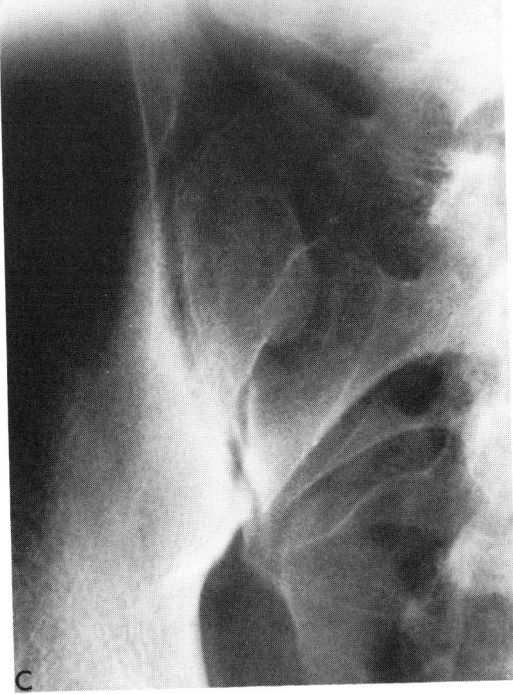

Figure 7–21. *Sacroiliac joint: Sacroiliitis.*

A–C *Anteroposterior and oblique radiographs demonstrate bilateral sacroiliac joint abnormalities consisting of ill-defined osseous surfaces, erosions, and bony eburnation.*

projection claim its superiority because of the normal inclination of the articulation (Fig. 7–21).

A craniocaudal axial view of the sacroiliac joint may better delineate abnormalities along the anterior aspect of the joint[63] (Fig. 7–22). In this view, the patient sits on the x-ray table with slight forward flexion of the trunk. The tube is angled approximately 10 to 20 degrees along the craniocaudal axis of the articulation. This view may be modified by increasing or decreasing the degree of trunk flexion and by not angulating the x-ray tube.[2] Other modifications have also been suggested.[108]

Obtaining anteroposterior views with the patient erect, with the weight borne first on one leg and then on the other, may provide information about motion at the sacroiliac joint and symphysis pubis.[2, 64] This examination can also be accomplished under fluoroscopy[65] or with stereophotogrammetry.[109] The sacroiliac joints and symphysis pubis are part of a single functional unit. Any increase in mobility of the sacroiliac joint is transferred to the symphysis pubis and appears as abnormal motion at this latter site. A 1 mm displacement of the symphyseal part of the pubic bone is probably within normal limits[64] and a permanent displacement of the symphysis pubis may occasionally be noted in certain patients, particularly multiparous women. True instability of the symphysis pubis and

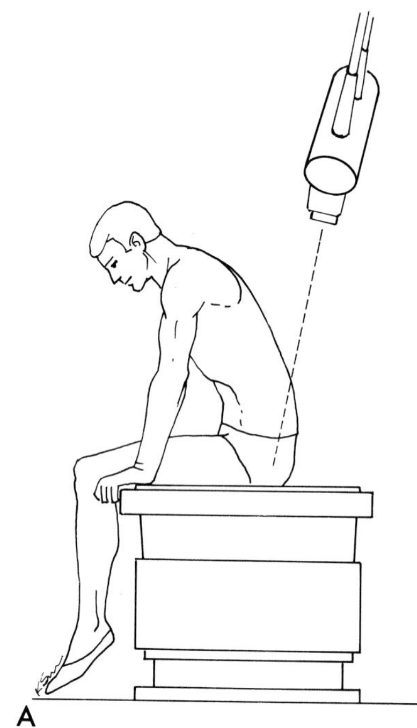

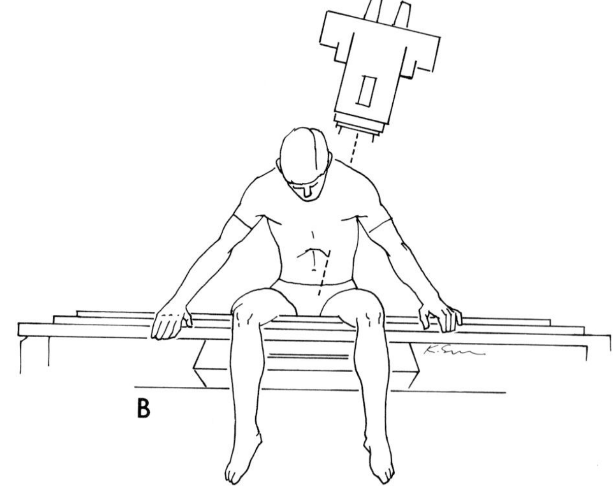

Figure 7–22. *Sacroiliac joint: Additional radiographs.*

A, B *A craniocaudal axial view is obtained with the patient sitting on the x-ray table. The tube is angled 10 to 20 degrees in a lateral to medial direction. Anterior angulation may also be utilized.*

sacroiliac joint is indicated by abnormal widening of either articulation or rotation of one pubic bone in relation to the other on these specialized views.

Basic Examination: Sacroiliac Joint
Anteroposterior with 30 Degree Cephalad Angulation

SACRUM AND COCCYX

The radiographic examination of the sacrum and coccyx includes frontal and lateral projections (Fig. 7–23). To visualize the upper sacrum, an anteroposterior radiograph is obtained with 15 degrees of cephalad angulation of the tube. To visualize the lower sacrum, an anteroposterior radiograph without beam angulation is useful. To visualize the coccyx, an anteroposterior radiograph with 10 degrees of caudal angulation of the tube is required. Any of these films can be done in a prone rather than supine position; in the prone position, the direction of beam angulation is reversed. A lateral projection of sacrum or coccyx is the second required view.

Basic Examination: Sacrum, Coccyx
Anteroposterior with 30 Degrees of Cephalad Angulation (Sacrum) or 10 Degrees of Caudal Angulation (Coccyx)
Lateral

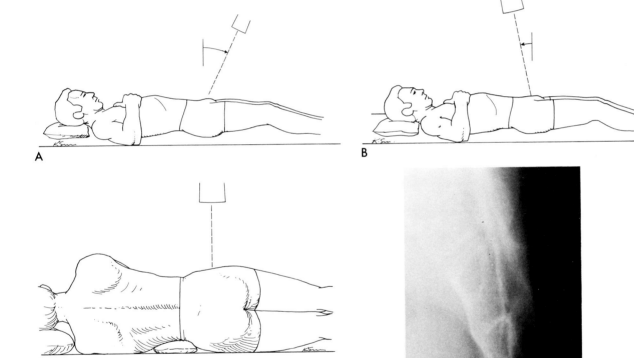

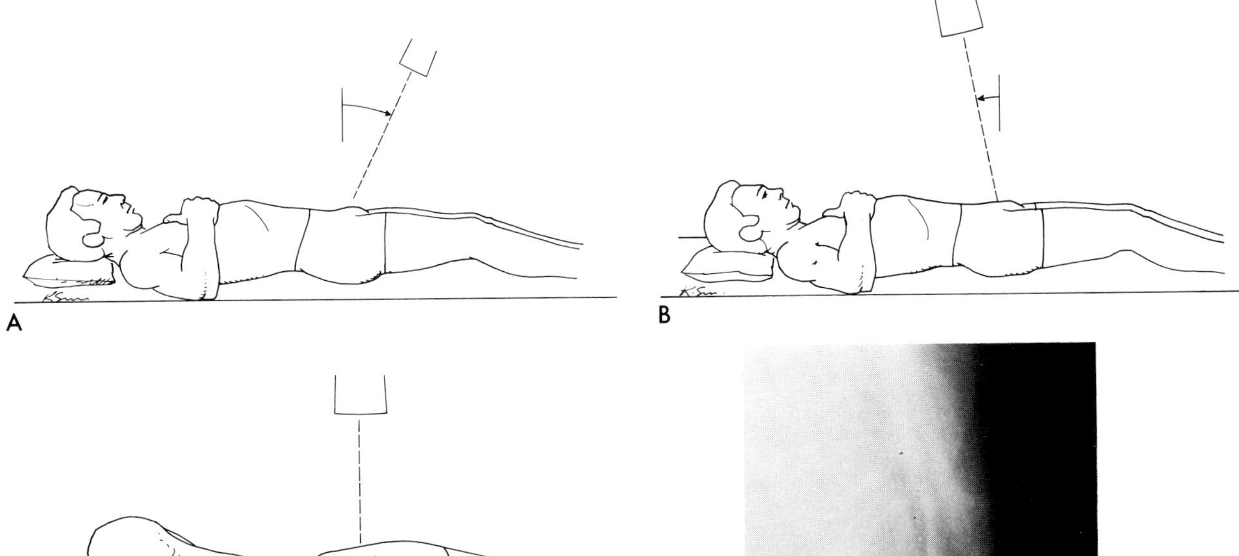

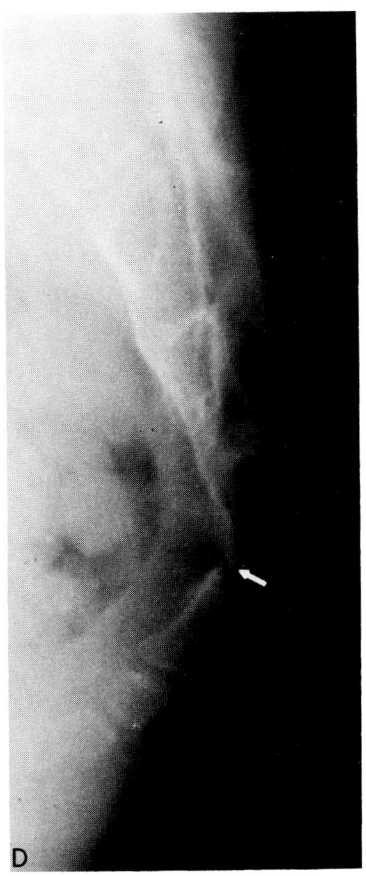

Figure 7–23. *Sacrum and coccyx: Routine radiographs.*
A–C *Frontal radiographs of the sacrum* **(A)** *utilize 15 degrees of cephalad angulation; frontal radiographs of the coccyx* **(B)** *require 10 degrees of caudal angulation. The lateral radiograph* **(C)** *is also obtained.*
D *Lateral radiograph of sacrum: Fracture. The displaced fracture can be observed (arrow).*

HIP

The most common method of examining the hip joint includes an anteroposterior radiograph of the pelvis and a coned-down anteroposterior radiograph of the hip, both obtained with internal rotation of the foot to elongate the femoral neck, and a "frog" view obtained with the hip abducted (Fig. 7–24). Supplementary views are suggested under certain clinical situations. These views include a semiaxial projection, the Chassard-Lapine position, obtained with the patient sitting on the table and the central ray directed vertically through the lumbosacral region,[66, 67] an axial lateral projection, obtained in an inferosuperior direction, and an angulated lateral projection.[68] (Fig. 7–25).

In the evaluation of the hip joint and acetabulum following trauma, 45 degree anterior and posterior oblique projections have been recommended to visualize the anterior and posterior acetabular rims and important bony columns of the pelvis.[69] Our investigation has indicated that shallower oblique projections may be more useful.[70] (Fig. 7–25). A lateral acetabular view has also been recommended.[71]

Roentgenograms of the hip obtained during traction of 14 to 23 kg (30 to 50 lb) have been

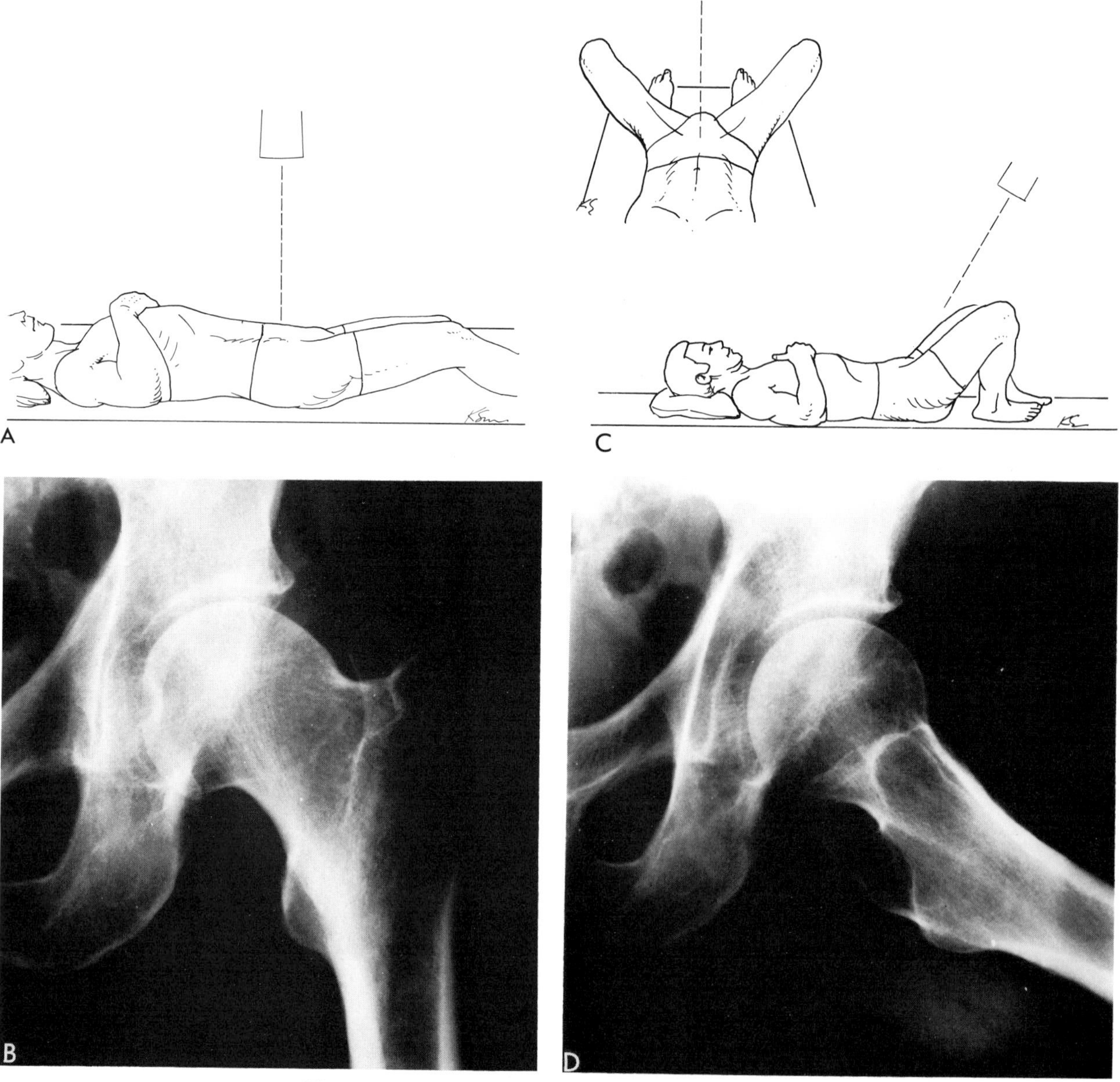

Figure 7–24. *Hip: Routine radiographs.*
A, B *Anteroposterior radiograph: Normal.*
C, D *"Frog-leg" view: Normal. The hip is abducted.*

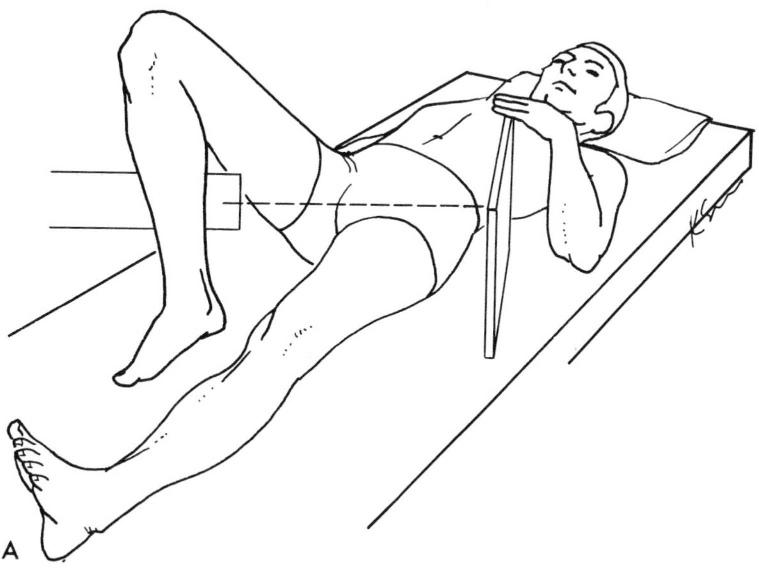

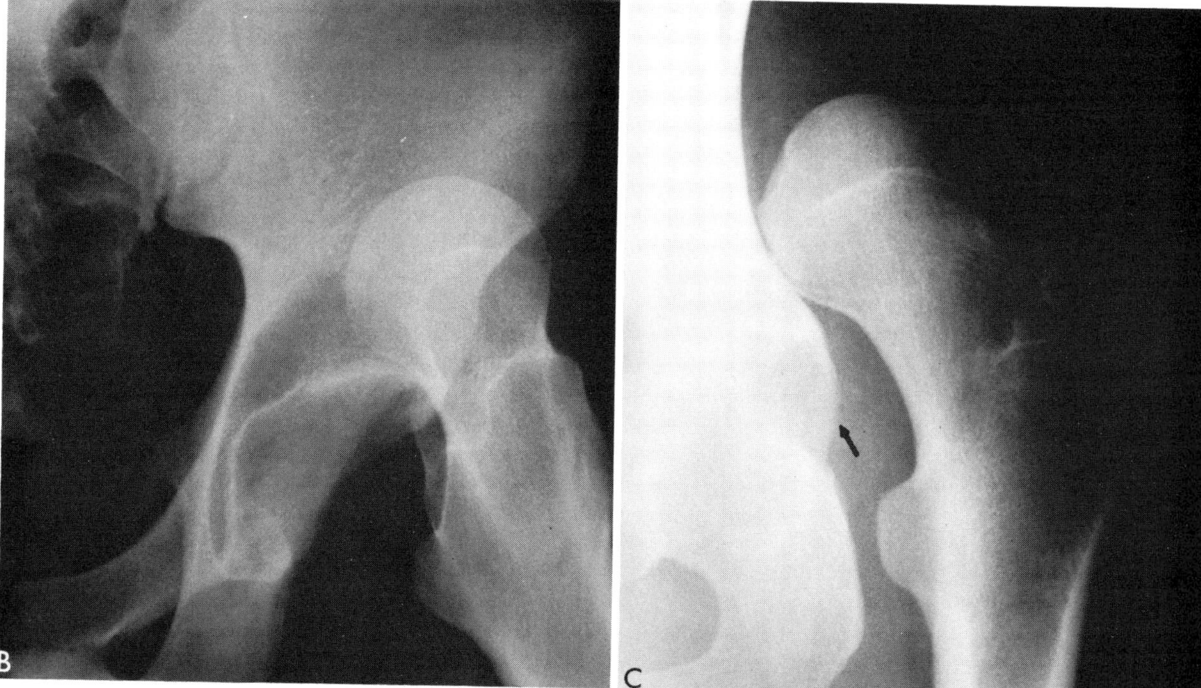

Figure 7–25. Hip: Additional radiographs.

A Inferosuperior radiograph. This technique provides a lateral view of the hip. The tube is placed beneath the flexed knee and the central ray is angled in a superior direction.

B, C Anteroposterior and oblique radiographs: Posterior dislocation of the hip. Although the frontal radiograph **(B)** demonstrates that the femoral head is displaced superiorly, the oblique radiograph **(C)** reveals its posterior displacement and provides information regarding the posterior acetabular rim (arrow).

Illustration continued on the following page

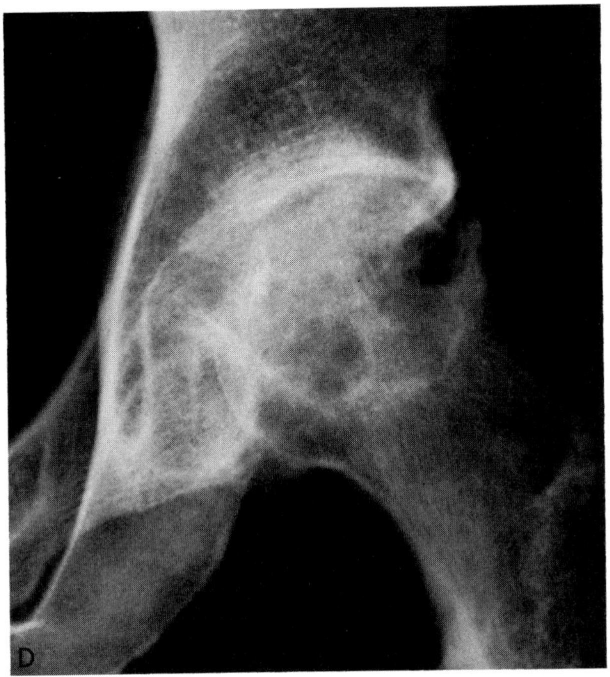

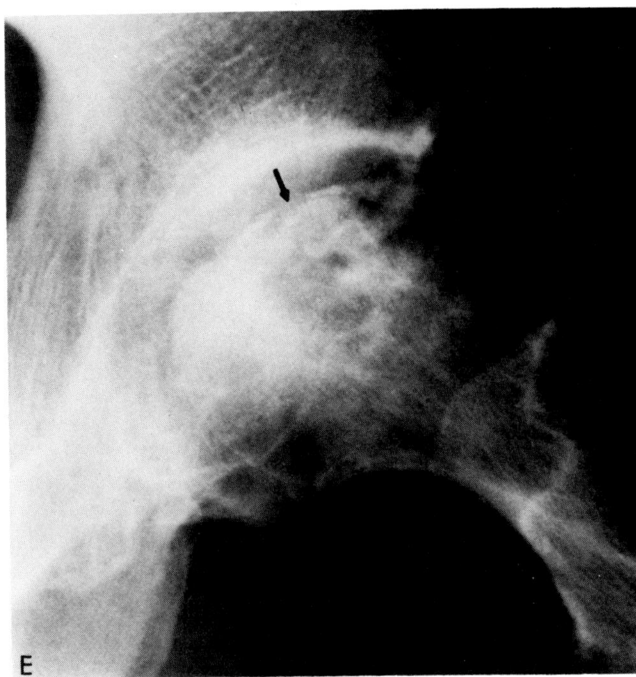

Figure 7–25. Continued
D, E *Traction radiograph: Osteonecrosis. On the initial anteroposterior radiograph* **(D)**, *cystic abnormalities are apparent in the femoral head. With traction and abduction* **(E)**, *osseous collapse and subchondral fractures (arrow) are seen.*

recommended as a useful technique in a variety of articular disorders.[72] This maneuver produces spontaneous intra-articular release of gas, the "vacuum" phenomenon, outlining the integrity of the articular cartilage. The pneumoarthrogram is not obtained if the patient has a hip effusion. In the presence of osteonecrosis, gas may be released into the separated fragment of subchondral bone, allowing earlier diagnosis of this condition[73] (Fig. 7–25).

Basic Examination: Hip
Anteroposterior View of Pelvis
Anteroposterior View of Hip
"Frog" View of Hip

KNEE

An anteroposterior radiograph of the knee is obtained with the beam directed 5 to 7 degrees toward the head, and a lateral radiograph is obtained with the knee flexed 20 to 35 degrees (Fig. 7–26). Forty-five degree oblique projections are necessary in a patient who has experienced knee trauma and in an individual whose problems relate to the proximal tibiofibular articulation. An angulated frontal view with the knee flexed 40 to 50 degrees, the "tunnel" view, is utilized to visualize the intercondylar notch.[74] This can be obtained in an anteroposterior or posteroanterior projection. Some investigators have suggested that radiographs should be obtained in a greater degree of knee flexion to provide better visualization of the articular space and intercondylar area.[75] In patients with knee trauma, a cross-table lateral projection should be added to the examination allowing demonstration of fat-fluid levels, indicative of fractures with release of medullary fat into the articular cavity. (Fig. 7–27).

Various techniques have been described for adequate evaluation of the patellofemoral joint (Fig. 7–28). Original descriptions suggested utilization of the prone position with acute knee flexion, the "sunrise" view.[76] This degree of knee flexion results in the patella becoming deeply situated within the intercondylar fossa. As most cases of subluxation of the patella occur in lesser degrees of knee flexion, this view is not ideal. Hughston[77] suggested that a view obtained with the patient prone and the knee flexed to 50 or 60 degrees was a more suitable technique for visualization of the patellofemoral articulation, although in this view distortion is created by severe angulation of the incident beam. Subsequently, some investigators described techniques in which the patient was examined supine.[78-80] Recently Merchant and co-workers[81] proposed a technique in which the patient is positioned supine on the table with the leg flexed 45 degrees over the end of the table. The tube is angulated 30 degrees toward the floor. Unfortunately, this method requires a special film-holding apparatus and patellar magnification is apparent. The direction of the beam can be reversed and radiographs can be obtained at various degrees of knee flexion, perhaps providing a more accurate appraisal of the patellofemoral area.[82, 83, 114]

Text continued on page 303

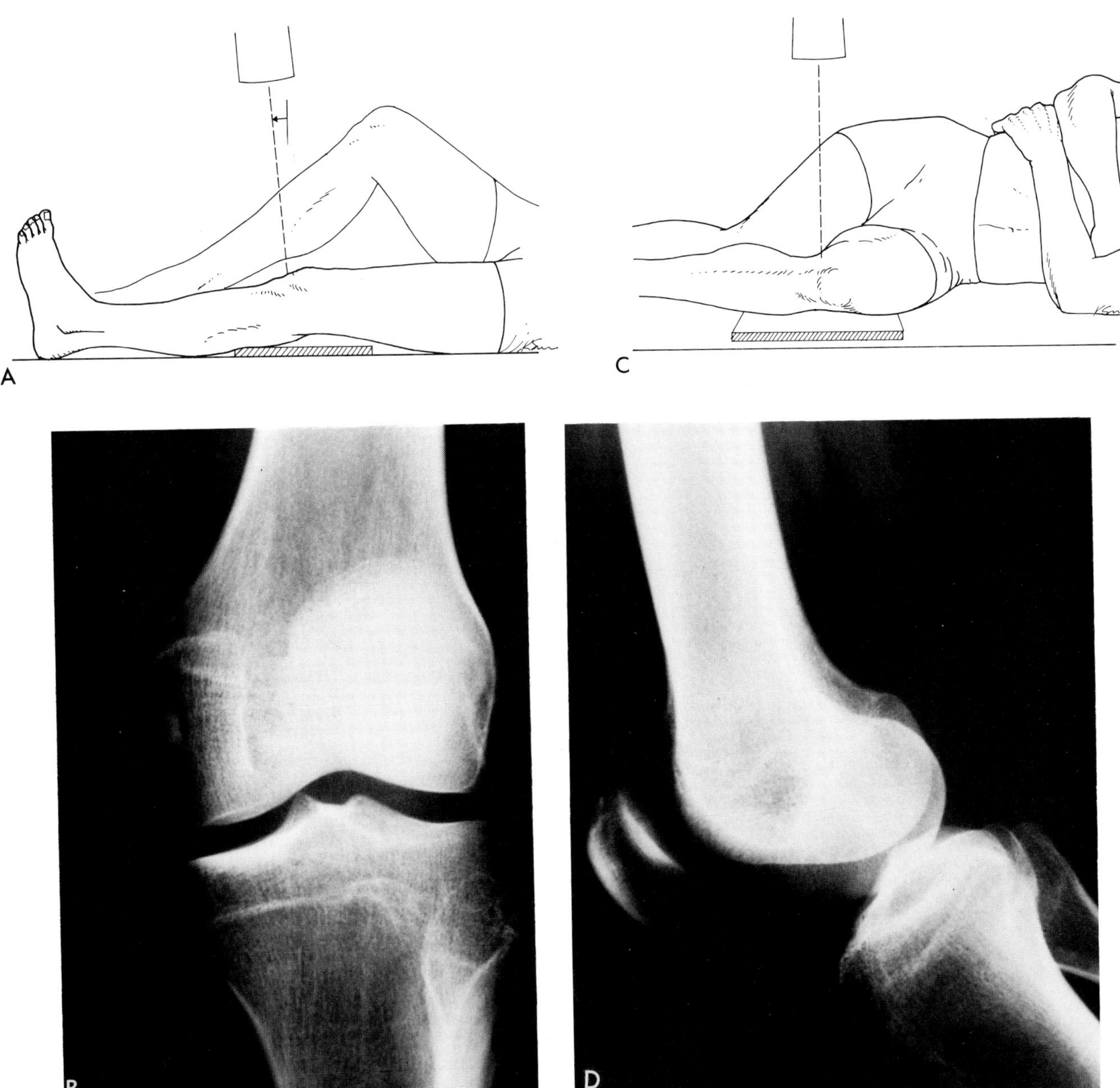

Figure 7–26. Knee: Routine radiographs.

A, B *Anteroposterior radiograph: Normal. Observe that the central ray is directed in a cephalad direction with an angle of 5 to 7 degrees.*

C, D *Lateral radiograph: Normal. The knee is flexed 20 to 35 degrees.*

Illustration continued on the following page

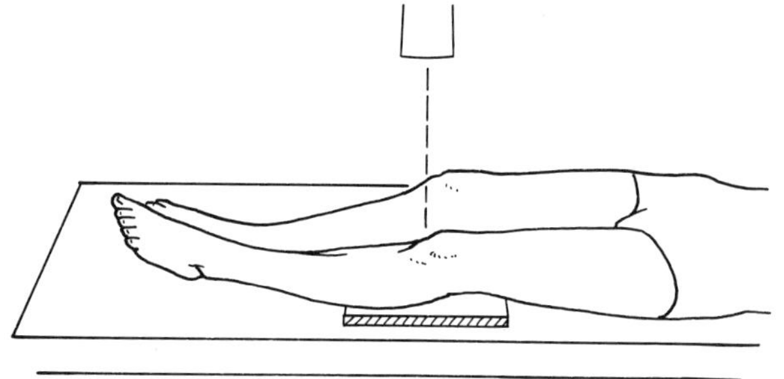

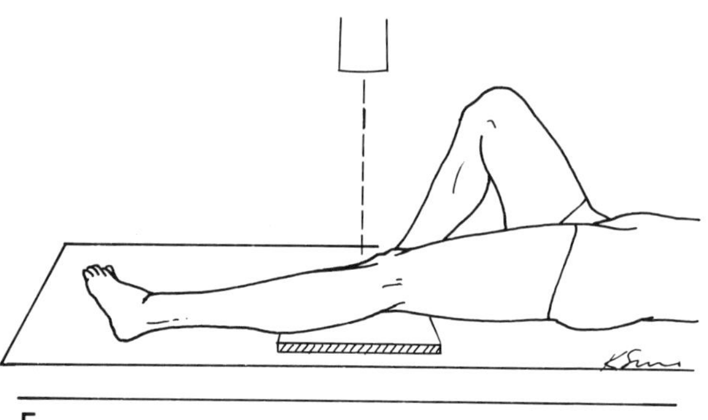

E

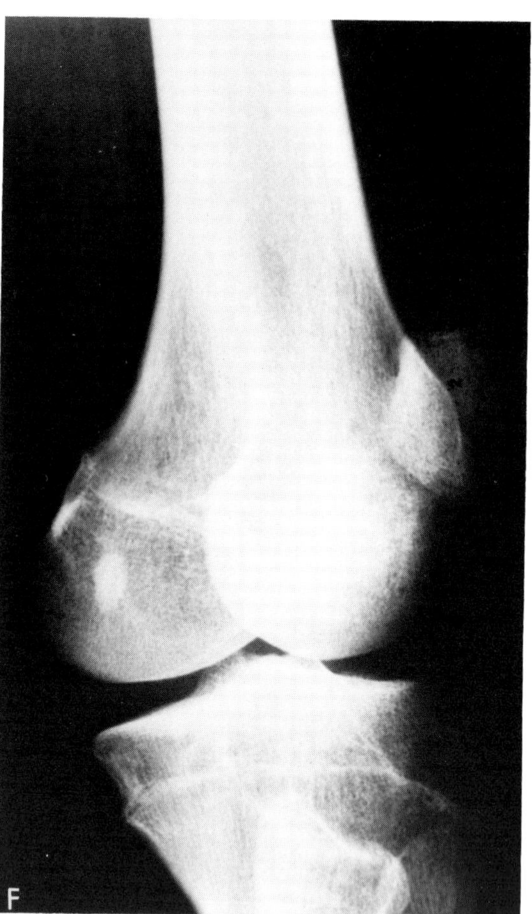

F

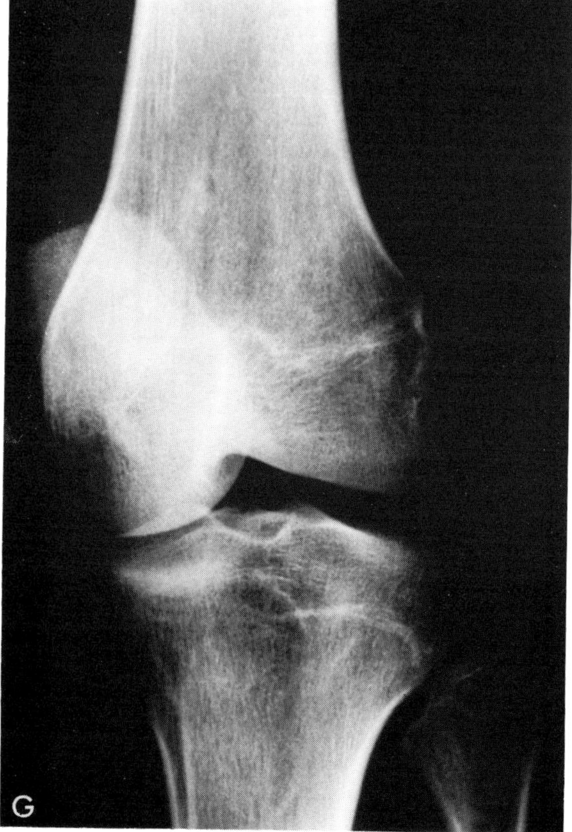

G

Figure 7–26. Continued
E–G *Oblique radiographs: Normal. These films are obtained with the patient turned 45 degrees in either direction.*

Illustration continued on the opposite page

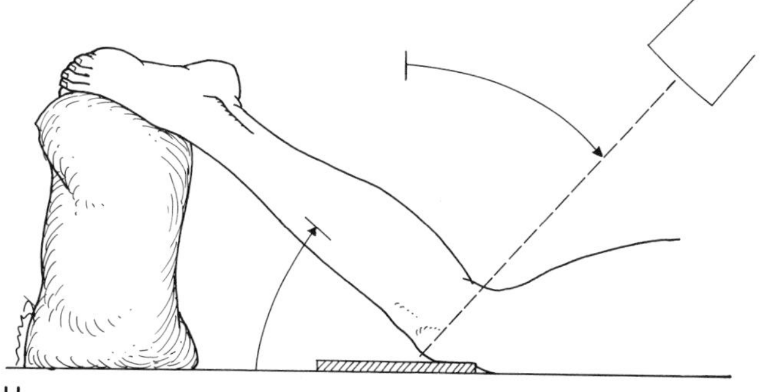

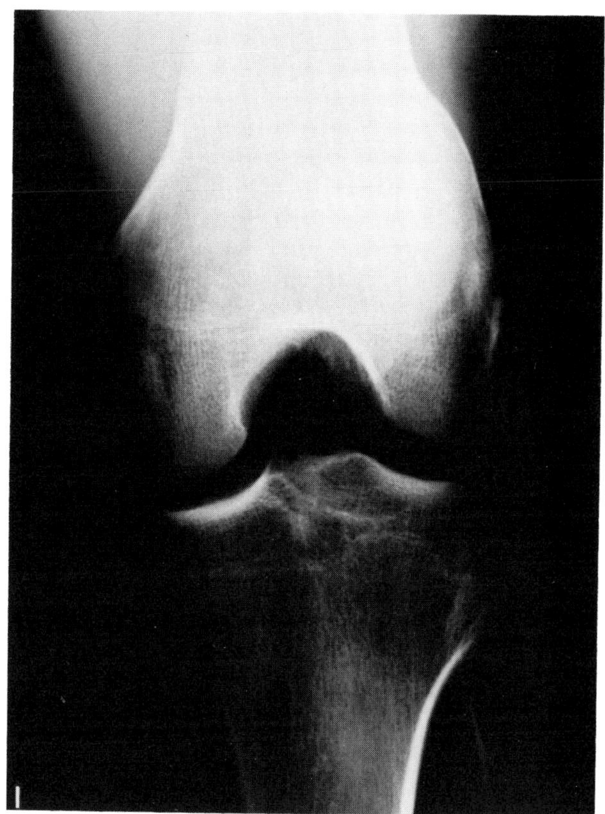

Figure 7–26. Continued

H, I *"Tunnel" view: Normal. The knee is flexed 40 to 50 degrees and rests upon a sandbag. The central ray is angulated 40 to 50 degrees in a caudal direction. The intercondylar notch is well visualized.*

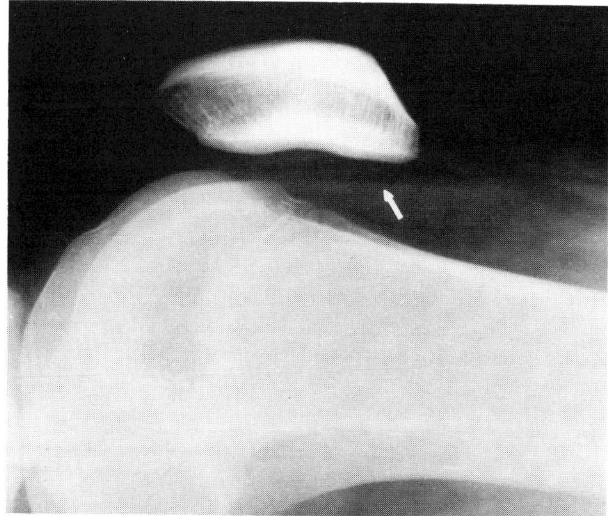

Figure 7–27. Knee: *Additional radiograph. Cross-table lateral projection: fat-fluid level in a patient with a tibial plateau fracture. Note the sharply delineated horizontal radiodense line representing the fat-fluid interface (arrow). The fat originated in the medullary cavity and was released into the joint following the fracture.*

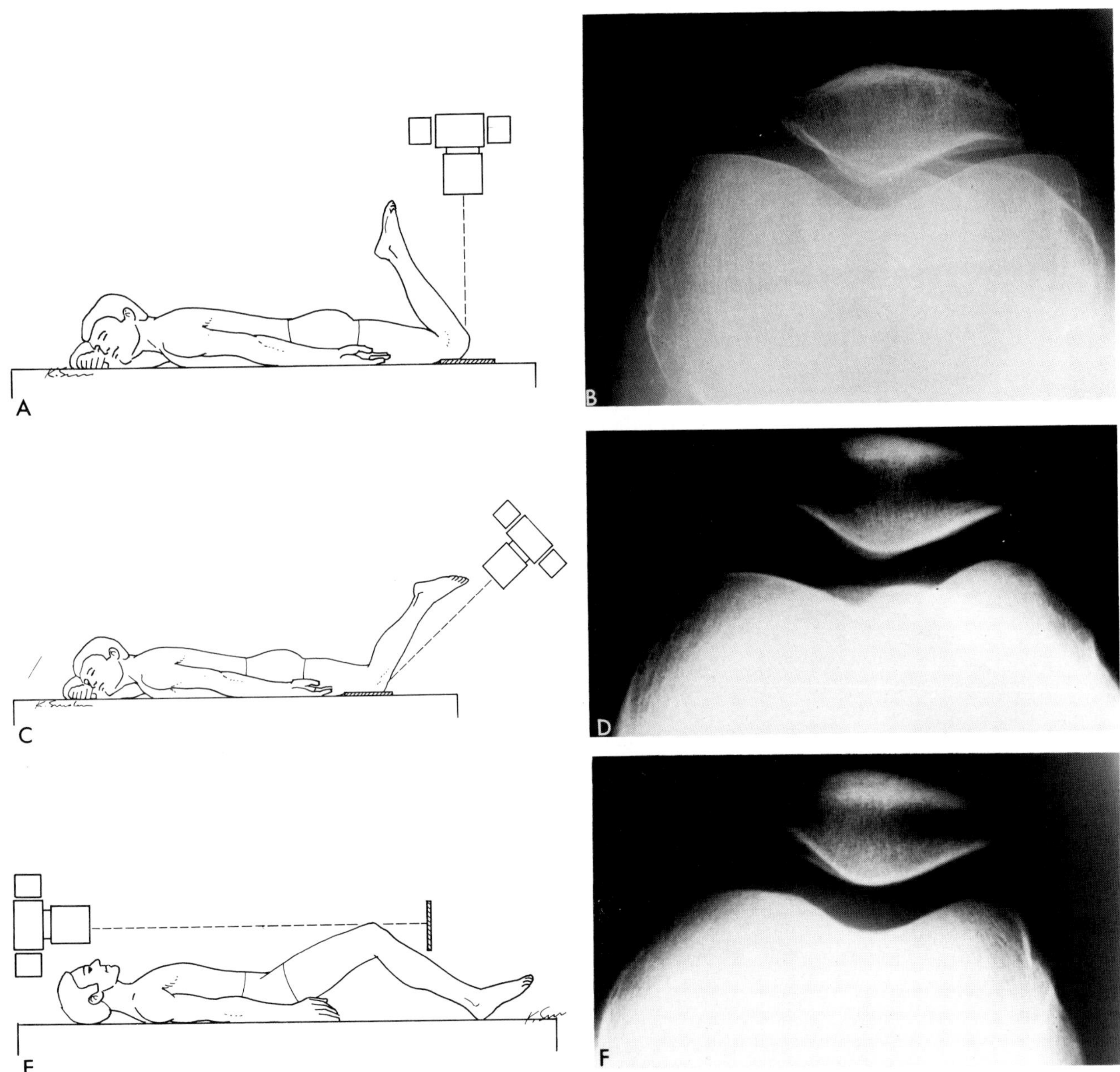

Figure 7–28. *Patellofemoral joint: Routine and specialized radiographs.*

A, B *"Sunrise" view: Normal. This can be obtained with the knee flexed more than 90 degrees. The patella is situated deeply within the intercondylar fossa.*

C, D *Hughston view: Normal. In this projection, the knee is flexed 50 to 60 degrees. The patella is not so closely applied to the femur.*

E, F *Knutsson view: Normal. The patient is supine and the slightly flexed knee rests on the table. A special film holder is necessary.*

Illustration continued on the opposite page

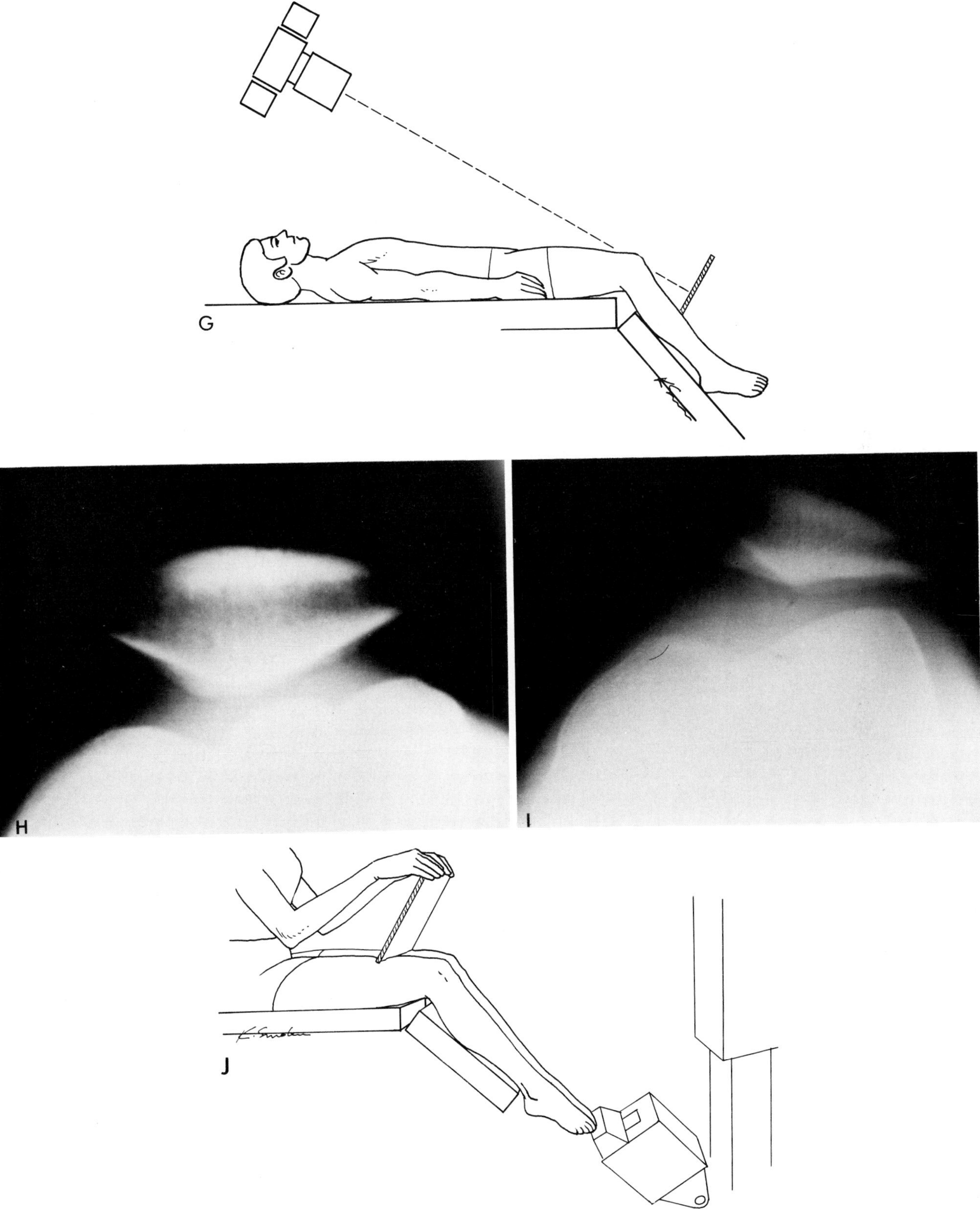

Figure 7–28. Continued

G–I *Merchant view: Normal and abnormal. The patient is placed supine on the table and the knees are flexed 45 degrees over the end of the table* **(G)**. *The central ray is angled 30 degrees from the horizontal in a caudal direction. The normal* **(H)** *and abnormal* **(I)** *appearance is illustrated. In the latter situation, observe the lateral subluxation of the patella.*

J *Inferosuperior view. Direction of the beam has been reversed. There is less distortion of the patella and the patient is able to hold the film.*

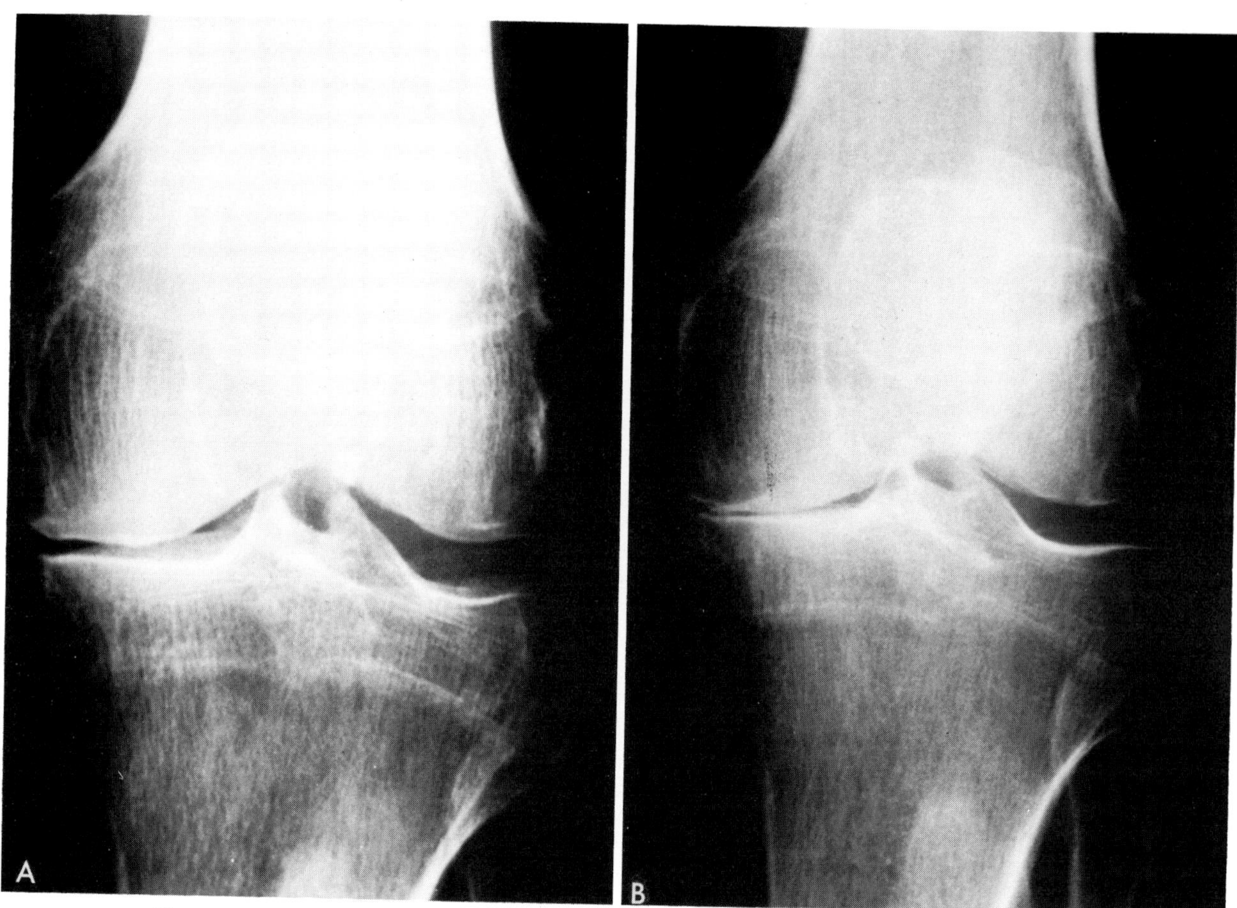

Figure 7–29. *Knee: Weight-bearing radiography.*

A, B *Anteroposterior* **(A)** *and weight-bearing* **(B)** *radiographs in a patient with degenerative joint disease. With weight-bearing, there is further loss of joint space between the medial femoral condyle and tibia, allowing more accurate appraisal of the articular cartilage.*

Weight-bearing radiography of the knee is particularly helpful in the evaluation of degenerative joint disease, providing a more accurate assessment of articular space.[84-86] (Fig. 7–29). In our experience,[87] these views should be obtained on vertically oriented 7 × 17 inch films with the patient standing on the leg being examined. This allows better delineation of the degree of angulation and subluxation at the knee, and serves as a more reliable indication of the extent of joint space loss.

Radiography performed during varus and valgus stress of the knee allows evaluation of ligament instability.[88]

Basic Examination: Knee
Anteroposterior
Lateral
"Tunnel" View
"Sunrise" View

ANKLE

Anteroposterior and lateral radiographs of the ankle are considered routine (Fig. 7–30). To better evaluate the medial articular space, an anteroposterior radiograph with 15 to 20 degrees of internal rotation of the foot — the mortise view — is optimal[89] to compensate for the fact that the ankle is oriented at approximately 15 to 20 degrees of external rotation in reference to the coronal plane of the knee.[90] Forty-five degree medial and lateral oblique roentgenograms are also useful in the patient with a history of trauma to better evaluate the osseous structures, including the malleoli. In this clinical situation, anteroposterior radiographs obtained with varus and valgus stress will document the presence of ligamentous damage, and a "poor" lateral view obtained during slight external rotation of the foot will better delineate the posterior tibial lip[91, 115, 116] (Fig. 7–31).

Basic Examination: Ankle
Anteroposterior
Lateral
Mortise

FOOT

Anteroposterior, medial oblique, and lateral projections are standard views for evaluation of the foot (Fig. 7–32). Of these, the single best view for evaluation of the articulations of the midfoot and forefoot is the medial oblique projection. Similarly, for visualization of the toes, frontal, oblique, and lateral radiographs are necessary.

Adequate radiography of the sesamoid bones

Text continued on page 308

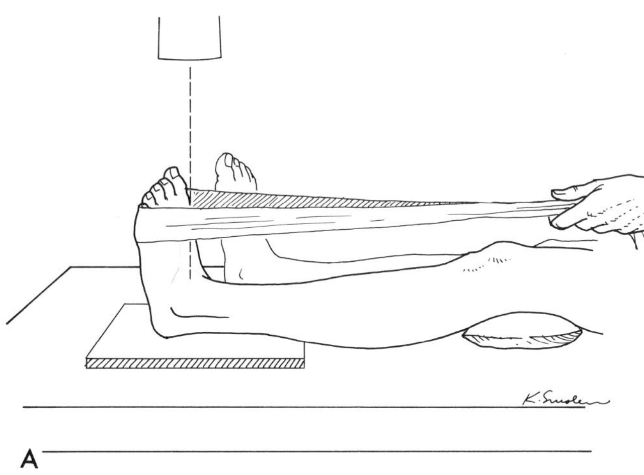

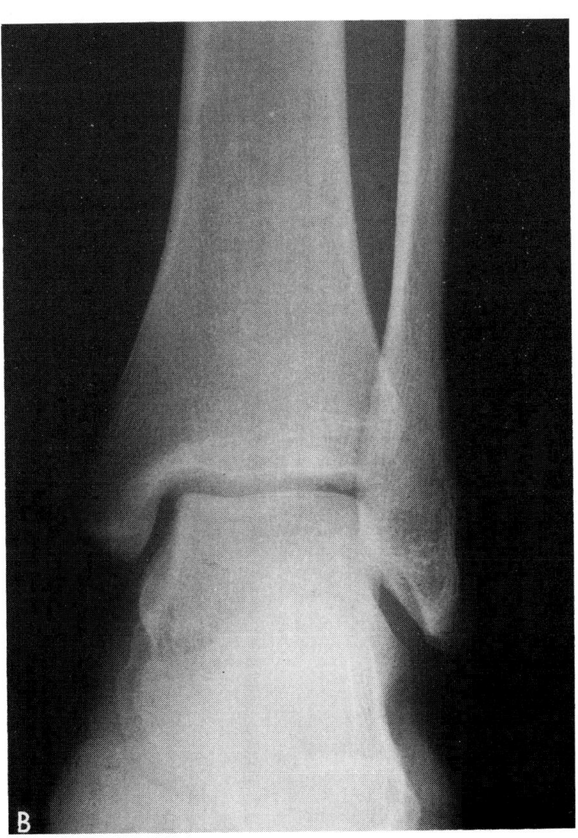

Figure 7–30. *Ankle: Routine radiographs.*
A, B *Anteroposterior radiograph: Normal. A sling may be utilized to provide mild dorsiflexion of the ankle.*

Illustration continued on the following page

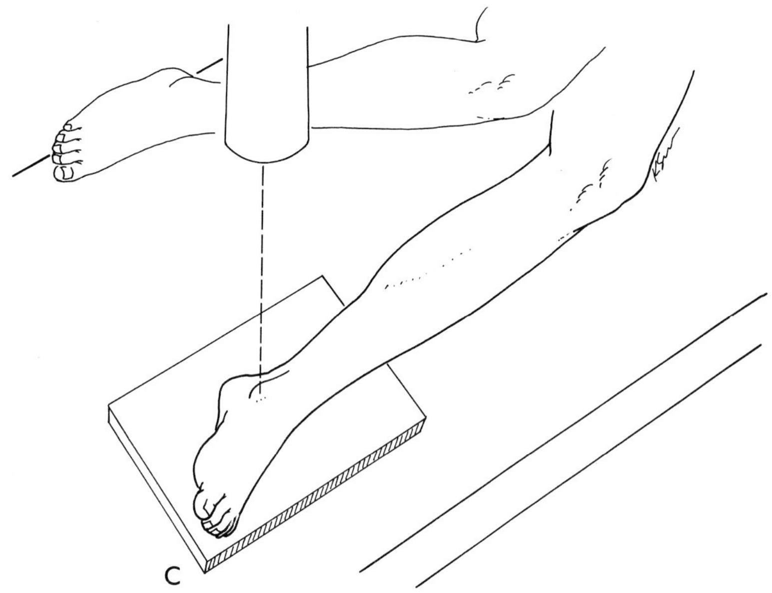

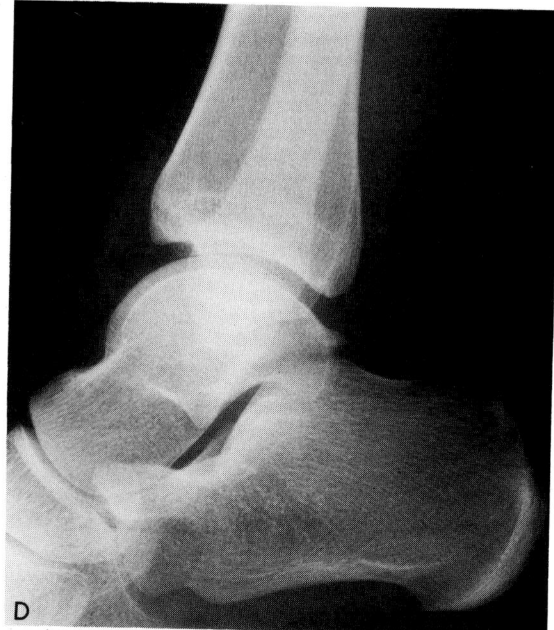

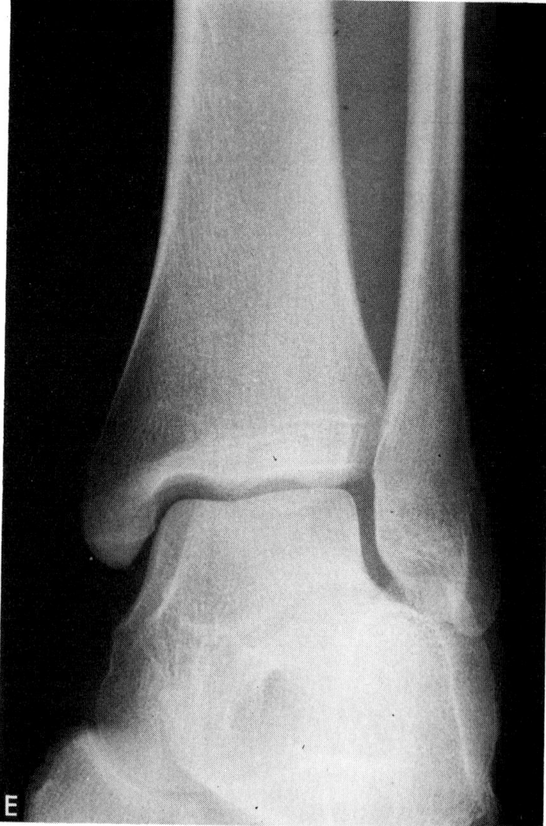

Figure 7–30. Continued

C, D *Lateral radiograph: Normal.*

E *Mortise view: Normal. An anteroposterior radiograph with 15 to 20 degrees of internal rotation allows optimal visualization of the articular cavity.*

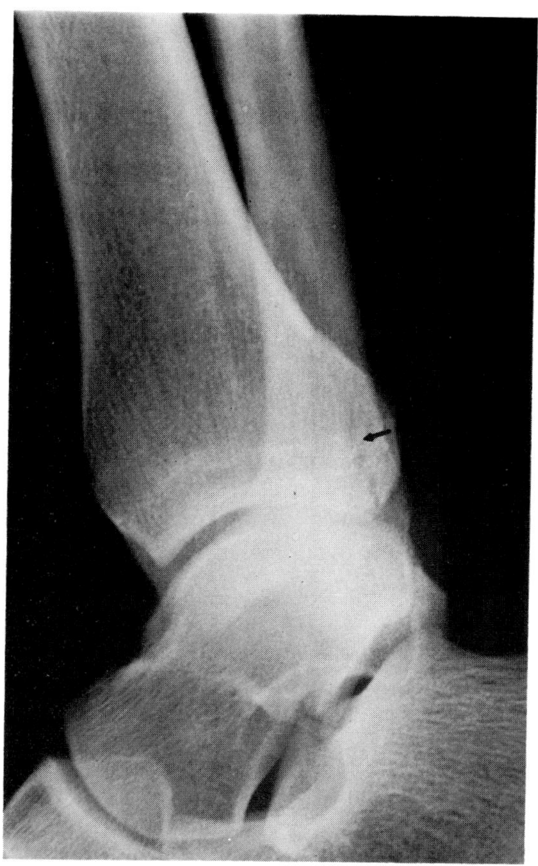

Figure 7–31. *Ankle: "Poor" lateral view in a patient with tibial fracture. The fracture line is apparent (arrow).*

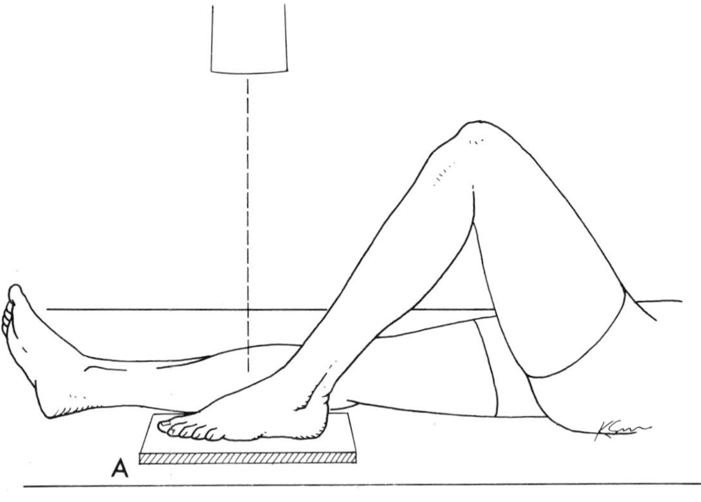

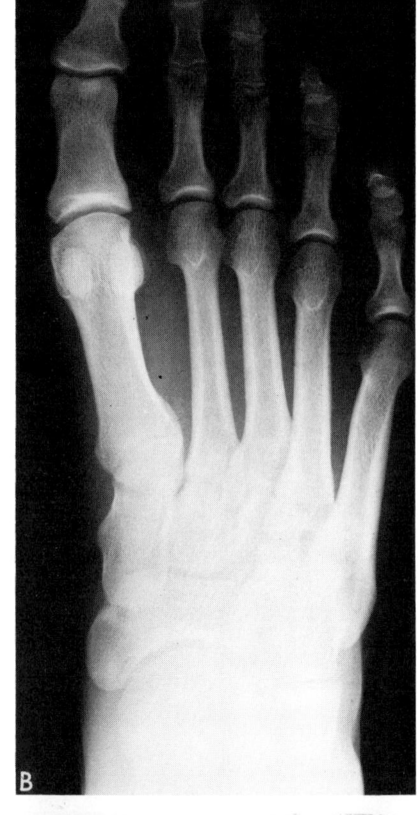

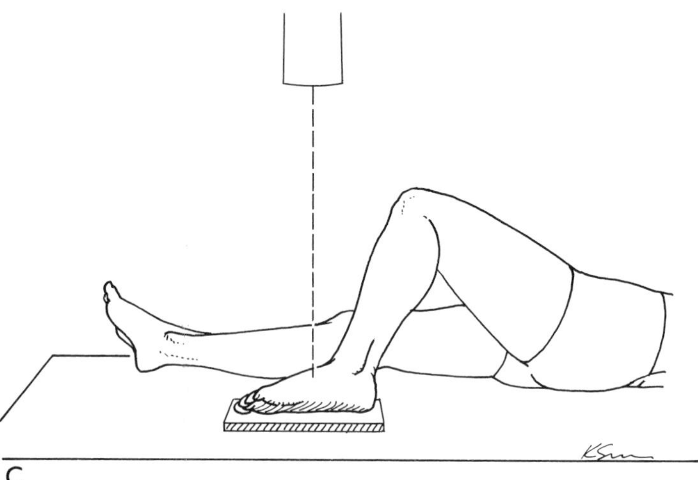

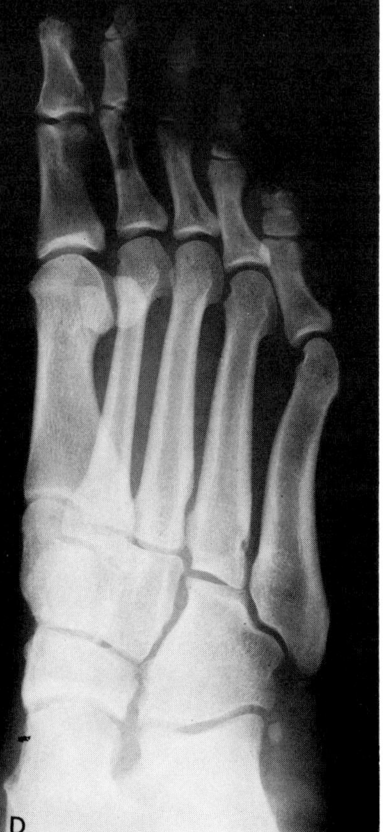

Figure 7–32. *Foot: Routine radiographs.*

A, B *Anteroposterior (dorsoplantar) radiograph: Normal.*

C, D *Medial oblique radiograph: Normal. Observe that the articulations of the forefoot and midfoot are well seen.*

Illustration continued on the opposite page

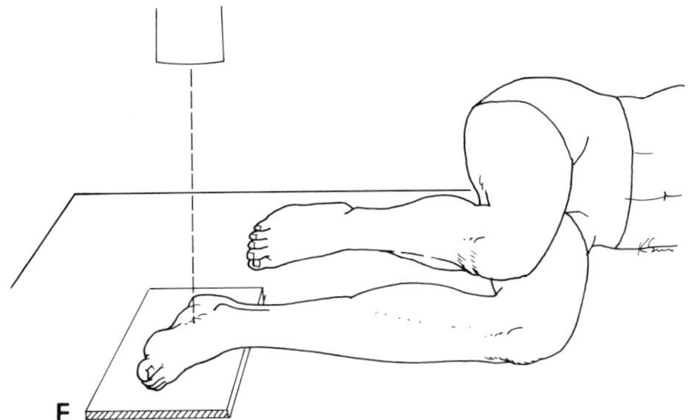
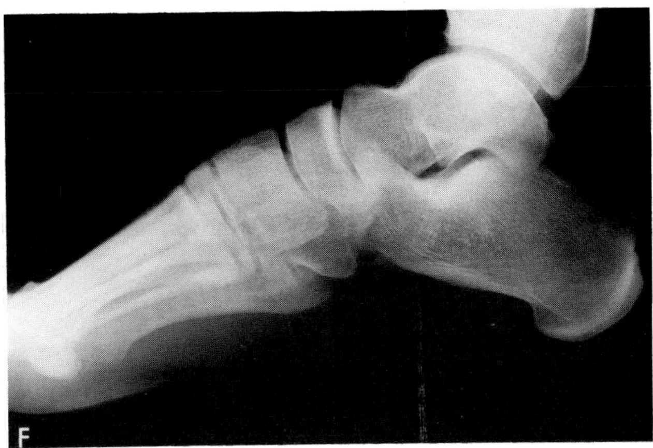

Figure 7–32. Continued
E, F *Lateral radiograph: Normal.*

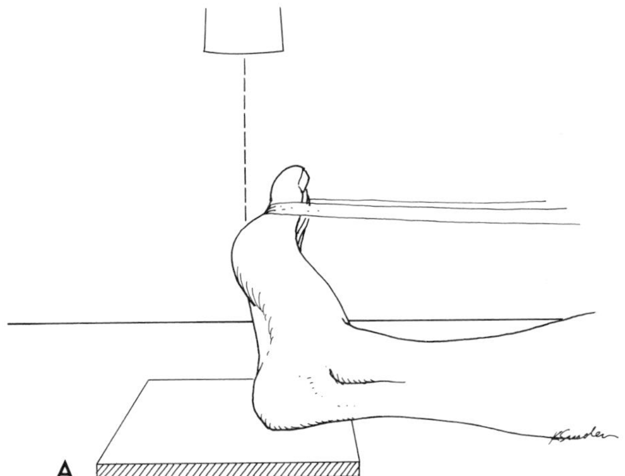
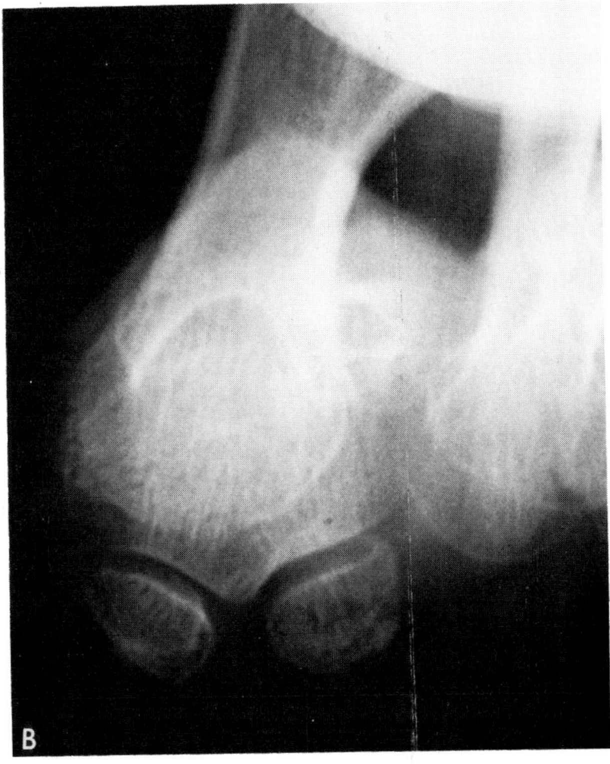

Figure 7–33. Sesamoid bones: Radiography–normal. The patient is supine. The toes are extended and a tangential radiograph demonstrates normal sesamoid bones beneath the first metatarsal head.

beneath the first metatarsal head requires an axial projection[92, 93] and, rarely, an angulated lateral view[94] (Fig. 7–33).

Evaluation of the calcaneus can be accomplished by utilizing a lateral projection, similar to that obtained for evaluation of the ankle, and an angulated frontal view, which can be obtained in an anteroposterior or posteroanterior direction (Fig. 7–34).

The tarsal articulations require special radiographic projections (Fig. 7–35). A penetrated axial view, the Harris-Beath view, is utilized for demonstration of the subtalar joint and that portion of the talocalcaneonavicular joint about the middle facet of the calcaneus.[95] This view, which is similar to the angulated frontal view of the calcaneus, must be obtained with high kilovoltage technique so that the subtalar articulations are identified. In addition, it is advantageous to obtain several axial radiographs with varying degrees of beam angulation, as some variation occurs in the configuration of these articulations.[96] Medial and lateral oblique views are also helpful in visualization of the subtalar and talocalcaneonavicular joints.[97, 98]

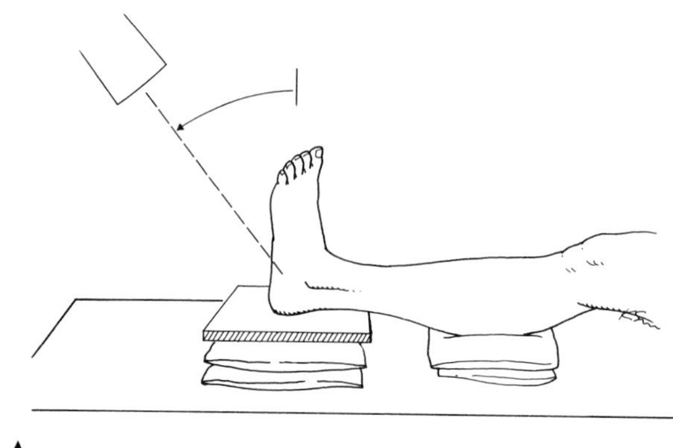

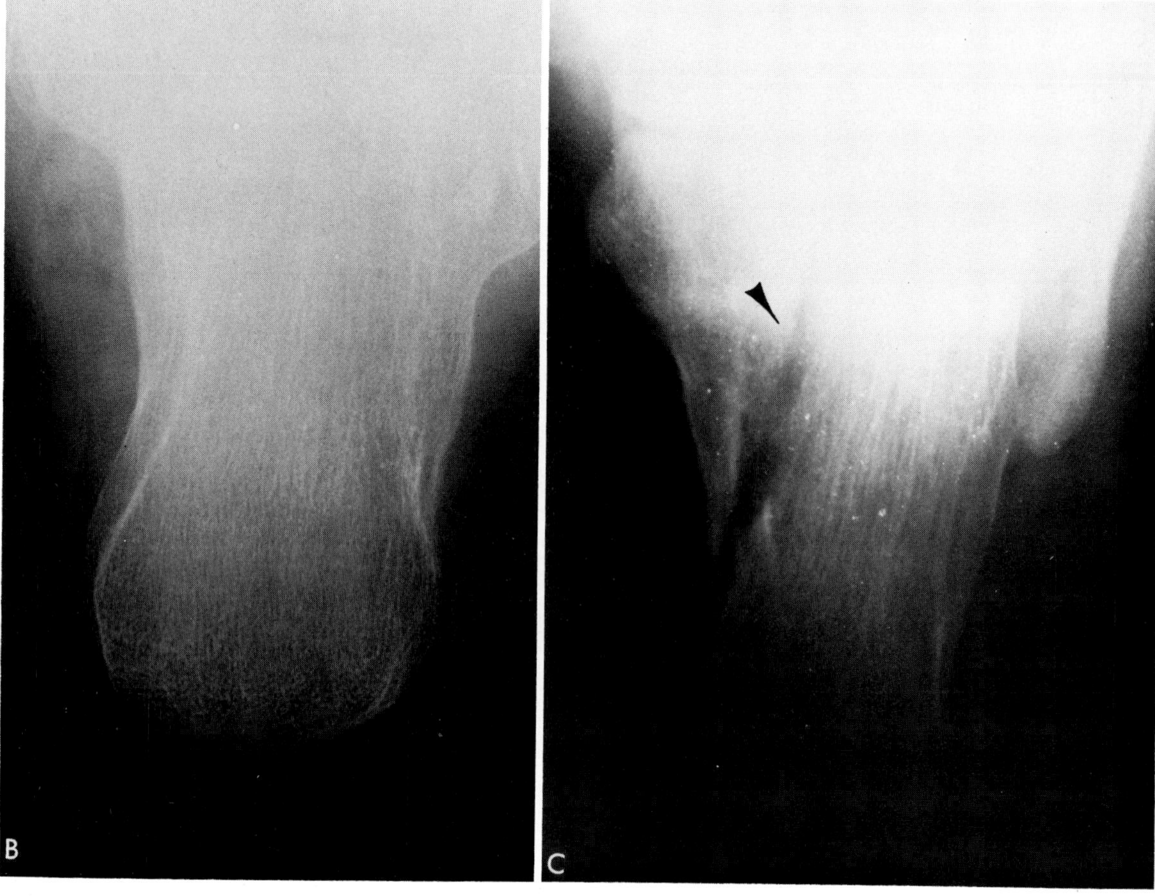

Figure 7–34. *Calcaneus: Angulated frontal radiographs–normal and abnormal. With the patient supine, the central ray is angled at 40 degrees with the long axis of the foot* **(A)**. *The normal* **(B)** *and abnormal* **(C)** *situations are indicated. Observe the calcaneal fracture (arrowhead) extending through the sustentaculum tali.*

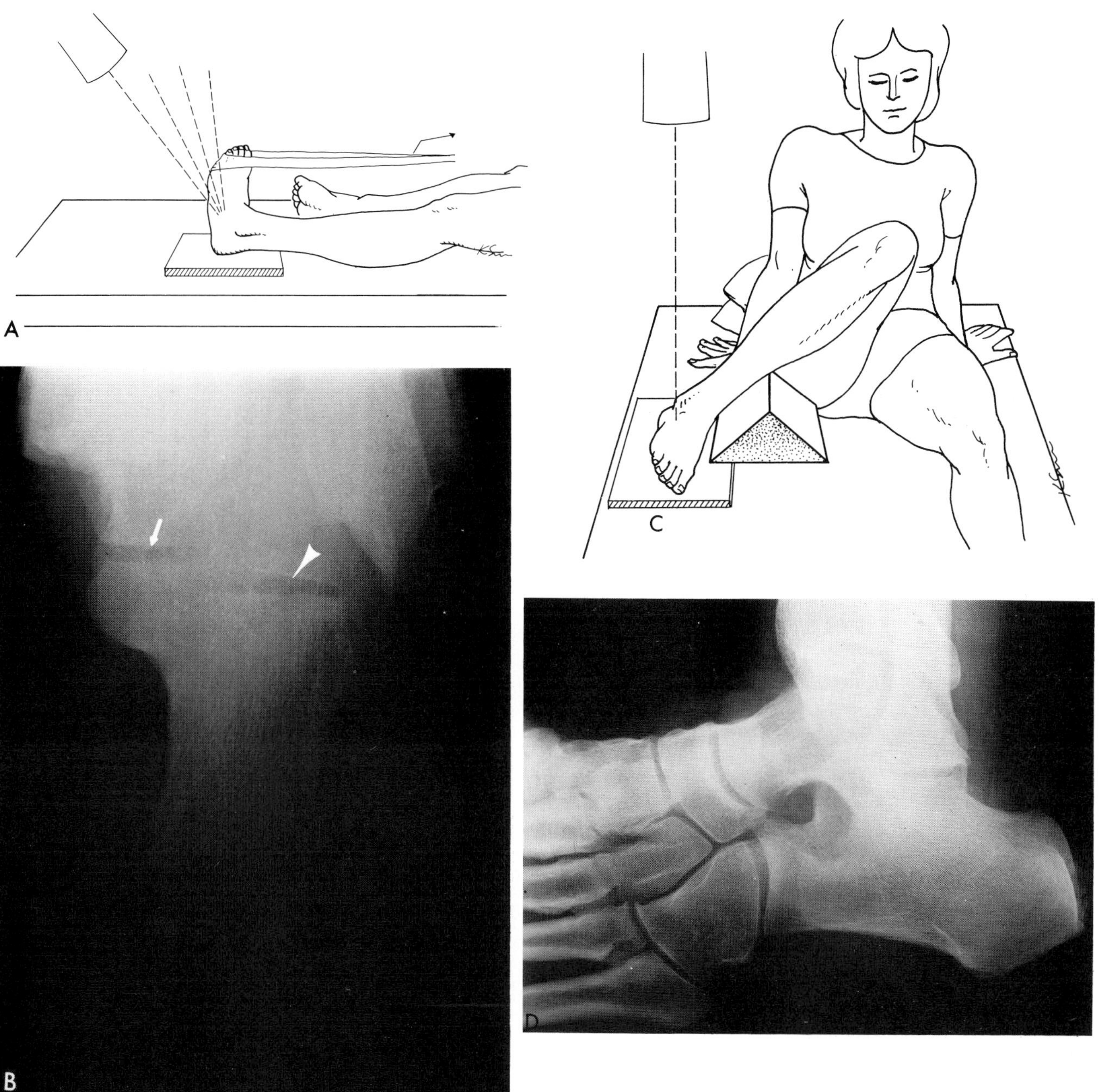

Figure 7–35. *Tarsal articulations: Normal radiography.*

A, B *Axial (Harris-Beath) view. The central ray can be directed at various angles. The subtalar joint (arrowhead) and talocalcaneal portion of the anterior talocalcaneonavicular joint (arrow) are demonstrated.*

C, D *Oblique radiograph. The lateral aspect of the foot is elevated approximately 45 degrees. A vertical beam is utilized. The tarsal bones and articulations are well seen.*

In children or adults with foot deformities, additional roentgenograms are suggested. In general, weight-bearing radiography is necessary utilizing a lateral view of the foot in dorsiflexion and an anteroposterior view with the sagittal plane of the leg perpendicular to the film.[99, 100] Additional roentgenograms are also described.[101-103]

Basic Examination: Foot
Anteroposterior
Oblique
Lateral

SURVEY ROENTGENOGRAMS

"Survey" roentgenograms are obtained in the initial evaluation of patients with polyarticular disorders and at various intervals, during subsequent examinations. The type of radiographs required will depend in large part upon the specific disorder that is suspected clinically and its distribution, as indicated by the patient's symptoms and signs. Thus, survey articular roentgenograms must be "tailored" to each patient and carefully monitored. In this fashion, abnormalities may be detected on initial roentgenograms, and additional views may be obtained for better delineation of these alterations. Despite this necessity for individualizing the survey examination in articular disorders, certain general comments are appropriate.

Initial survey roentgenograms in a patient with polyarticular disease, particularly when the exact diagnosis has not yet been clinically established, must reveal enough information to delineate the type and extent of the disorder without representing an overutilization either of the patient's, technician's, and physician's time or of radiation and expense. This can be accomplished by following a protocol, which includes a minimal number of high-yielding roentgenograms.[104] Our experience has suggested that a protocol relying on the following projections is most useful in these individuals:

Hands:	Posteroanterior
	Semipronated oblique
Wrists:	Posteroanterior
	Lateral
	Semipronated oblique
	Semisupinated oblique
Shoulders:	40 degree posterior oblique
Feet:	Medial oblique
Ankles:	Lateral, to include heel
Knees:	Anteroposterior
	Lateral
Pelvis:	Anteroposterior
Cervical Spine:	Lateral, with neck flexion

It should be emphasized that these guidelines will require modifications depending upon the specific diagnosis that is to be established and the clinical questions that need to be answered. For example, in a patient with ankylosing spondylitis, emphasis must be placed on obtaining radiographs of the axial skeleton, including the sacroiliac joints, whereas in a patient with calcium pyrophosphate crystal deposition disease, a radiographic search for the presence or absence of cartilage calcification should include a coned-down view of the symphysis pubis, posteroanterior radiographs of the wrist, and anteroposterior radiographs of the knees. Furthermore, when a patient with polyarticular disease has more severe symptoms in one or two specific joints, a more detailed radiographic analysis of these joints must be obtained.

Follow-up radiographic examinations in patients with widespread articular disorders need not be so extensive as the initial survey. Attention should be paid to known target areas of the specific disorder and to additional areas that are symptomatic. In this way, radiographs can assess the distribution and extent of disease and its response to therapy.

REFERENCES

1. Clark KC: Positioning in Radiography. 8th Ed. New York, Grune & Stratton, 1964, p 1.
2. Merrill V: Atlas of Roentgenographic Positions. Vol 1. 3rd Ed. St Louis, CV Mosby Co, 1967, p. 3.
3. Meschan I, Farrer-Meschan RMF: Radiographic Positioning and Related Anatomy. Philadelphia, WB Saunders Co, 1968, pp 29, 169.
4. Resnick D, Danzig LA: Arthrographic evaluation of injuries of the first metacarpophalangeal joint: Gamekeeper's thumb. Am J Roentgenol *126*:1046, 1976.
5. Norgaard F: Earliest roentgen changes in polyarthritis of the rheumatoid type. Continued investigations. Radiology *92*:299, 1969.
6. Resnick D: Early abnormalities of pisiform and triquetrum in rheumatoid arthritis. Ann Rheum Dis *35*:46, 1976.
7. Stecher WR: Roentgenography of the carpal navicular bone. Am J Roentgenol *37*:704, 1937.
8. Bridgman CF: Radiography of the carpal navicular bone. Med Radiogr Photogr *25*:104, 1949.
9. Ziter FMH Jr: A modified view of the carpal navicular. Radiology *108*:706, 1973.
10. Templeton AW, Zim ID: The carpal tunnel view. Missouri Med *61*:443, 1964.
11. Nisenfeld FG, Neviaser RJ: Fracture of the hook of the hamate: A diagnosis easily missed. J Trauma *14*:612, 1974.
12. Carter PR, Eaton RG, Littler JR: Ununited fracture of the hook of the hamate. J Bone Joint Surg *59A*:583, 1977.
13. Stark HH, Jobe FW, Boyes JH, Ashworth CR: Fracture of the hook of the hamate in athletes. J Bone Joint Surg *59A*:575, 1977.
14. Lentino W, Lubetsky HW, Jacobson HG, Poppel MH: The carpal bridge view. J Bone Joint Surg *39A*:88, 1957.
15. Burman M: Anteroposterior projection of the carpometacarpal joint of the thumb by radial shift of the carpal tunnel view. J Bone Joint Surg *40A*:1156, 1958.
16. Schmitt H: Die röntgenologische Darstellung des Radiusköpfchens. Roentgenpraxis *11*:33, 1939.
17. Laquerrière, Pierquin: De la nécessité d'employer une technique speciale pour obtenir certains détails squelettiques. J Radiol Electrol Med Nucl *3*:145, 1918.
18. Viehweger G: Zum problem der Deutung der Knoöchernen Gebilde distal

des Epikondylus medialis humeri. Fortschr Geb Rontgenstr Nuklearmed *86*:643, 1957.
19. Berens DL, Lockie LM: Ossification of the coraco-acromial ligament. Radiology *74*:802, 1960.
20. Slivka J, Resnick D: An improved radiographic view of the glenohumeral joint. J Can Assoc Radiol *30*:83, 1979.
21. Cleaves EN: A new film holder for roentgen examination of the shoulder. Am J Roentgenol *45*:288, 1941.
22. Rubin SA, Gray, RL, Green WR: The scapular "Y": A diagnostic aid in shoulder trauma. Radiology *110*:725, 1974.
23. Neer CS II: Displaced proximal humeral fractures. J Bone Joint Surg *52A*:1077, 1970.
24. Neer CS II, Rockwood CA Jr: Fractures and dislocations of the shoulder. *In* CA Rockwood Jr, DP Green (Eds): Fractures. Philadelphia, JB Lippincott, 1975, p. 585.
25. Hill HA, Sachs MD: The grooved defect of the humeral head. A frequently unrecognized complication of dislocations of the shoulder joint. Radiology *35*:690, 1940.
26. Hermodsson I.: Röntgenologische Studien über die traumatischen und habituellen Schultergelenkverrenkungen nach vorn und nach unten. Acta Radiol Suppl *20*:1, 1934.
27. Adams, JC: The humeral head defect in recurrent anterior dislocations of the shoulder. Br J Radiol *23*:151, 1950.
28. Hall RH, Isacc F, Booth CR: Dislocation of the shoulder with special reference to accompanying small fractures. J Bone Joint Surg *41A*:489, 1959.
29. Didiee J: Le radiodiagnostic dans la luxation récidivante de l'épaule. J Radiol Electrol Med Nucl *14*:209, 1930.
30. Bloom MH, Obata WG: Diagnosis of posterior dislocation of the shoulder with use of Velpeau axillary and angle-up roentgenographic views. J Bone Joint Surg *49A*:943, 1967.
31. Fisk C: Adaptation of the technique for radiography of the bicipital groove. Radiol Technol *37*:47, 1965.
32. Zanca P: Shoulder pain: Involvement of the acromioclavicular joint. Analysis of 1000 cases. Am J Roentgenol *112*:493, 1971.
33. Alexander OM: Radiography of the acromioclavicular articulation. Med Radiogr Photogr *30*:34, 1954.
34. Bearden JM, Hughston JC, Whatley GS: Acromioclavicular dislocation: Method of treatment. J Sports Med *1*:5, 1973.
35. Alexander OM: Dislocation of the acromio-clavicular joint. Radiography *15*:260, 1949.
36. Tarrant RM: The axial view of the clavicle. X-ray Techn *21*:358, 1950.
37. Quesada F: Technique for the roentgen diagnosis of fractures of the clavicle. Surg Gynecol Obstet *42*:424, 1926.
38. Kattan KR: Modified view for use in roentgen examination of the sternoclavicular joints. Radiology *108*:8, 1973.
39. Ritvo M, Ritvo M: Roentgen study of the sternoclavicular region. Am J. Roentgenol *58*:644, 1947.
40. Kurzbauer R: The lateral projection in roentgenography of the sternoclavicular articulation. Am J Roentgenol *56*:104, 1946.
41. Hobbs DW: Sternoclavicular joint: A new axial radiographic view. Radiology *90*:801, 1968.
42. Heinig CF: Retrosternal dislocation of the clavicle: Early recognition, x-ray diagnosis and management. J Bone Joint Surg *50A*:830, 1968.
43. Lee FA, Gwinn JL: Retrosternal dislocation of the clavicle. Radiology *110*:631, 1974.
44. Christenson PC: The radiologic study of the normal spine. Cervical, thoracic, lumbar and sacral. Radiol Clin North Am *15*:133, 1977.
45. Weir DC: Roentgenographic signs of cervical injury. Clin Orthop *109*:9, 1975.
46. Miller MD, Gehweiler, JA, Martinez S, Charlton OP, Daffner RH: Significant new observations on cervical spine trauma. Am J Roentgenol *130*:659, 1978.
47. Scher A, Vambeck V: An approach to the radiological examination of the cervicodorsal junction following injury. Clin Radiol *28*:243, 1977.
48. Smith GR, Abel MS, Cone L: Visualization of the posterolateral elements of the upper cervical vertebrae in the anteroposterior projection. Radiology *115*:219, 1975.
49. Jacobs LG: Roentgenography of the second cervical vertebra by Ottonello's method. Radiology *31*:412, 1938.
50. George AW: Method for more accurate study of injuries to the atlas and axis. Boston Med Surg J *181*:395, 1919.
51. Dorland P, Frémont J, Parer, Perez J: Techniques d'examen radiologique de l'arc postérieur des vertèbres cervicodorsales. J Radiol Electrol Med Nucl *39*:509, 1958.
52. Buetti C: Zur Darstellung der Atlanto-epistropheal-gelenke. bzw. der Procc. transversi atlantis und epistrophei. Radiol Clin *20*:168, 1951.
53. McCall I, Park W, McSweeney T: The radiological demonstration of acute lower cervical injury. Clin Radiol *24*:235, 1973.
54. Wortzman G, Dewar FP: Rotary fixation of the atlantoaxial joint: rotational atlantoaxial subluxation. Radiology *90*:479, 1968.
55. Fuchs AW: Thoracic vertebrae. Radiogr Clin Photogr *17*:2, 1941.
56. Oppenheimer A: The apophyseal intervertebral articulations roentgenologically considered. Radiology *30*:724, 1938.
57. Fuchs AW: Thoracic vertebrae. II. Radiogr Clin Photogr *17*:42, 1941.
58. Abel MS, Smith GR: Visualization of the posterolateral elements of the lumbar vertebrae in the anteroposterior projection. Radiology *122*:824, 1977.
59. Kovacs A: X-ray examination of the exit of the lowermost lumbar root. Radiol Clin *19*:6, 1950.
60. Gianturco C: A roentgen analysis of the motion of the lower lumbar vertebrae in normal individuals and in patients with low back pain. Am J Roentgenol *52*:261, 1944.
61. Resink JEJ: Zur Röntgenologie der sacroiliakalen Gelenke. Acta Radiol *38*:313, 1952.
62. Jaeger E: Zur Aufnahmetechnik der Sacroiliocalgelenke. Fortschr Geb. Roentgenstr Nuklearmed *71*:630, 1949.
63. Dory MA, Francois RJ: Craniocaudal axial view of the sacroiliac joint. Am J Roentgenol *130*:1125, 1978.
64. Chamberlain WE: The symphysis pubis in the roentgen examination of the sacroiliac joint. Am J Roentgenol *24*:621, 1930.
65. Kamieth H, Reinhardt K: Der ungleiche Symphysenstand; ein wichtiges Symptom der Beckenringlockerung. Fortschr Geb Roentgenstr Nuklearmed *83*:530, 1955.
66. Chassard, Lapine: Étude radiographique de l'arcade pubienne chez la femme enceinte: une nouvelle méthode d'appréciation du diamètre bi-ischiatique. J Radiol Electrol Med Nucl *7*:113, 1923.
67. Broderick TF: Complementary roentgenographic view of the hip. J Bone Joint Surg *37A*:295, 1955.
68. Johnson CR: A new method for roentgenographic examination of the upper end of the femur. J Bone Joint Surg *14*:859, 1932.
69. Judet R, Judet J, Letournal E: Fractures of the acetabulum: Classification and surgical approaches for open reduction — preliminary report. J Bone Joint Surg *46A*:1615, 1964.
70. Armbuster TG, Guerra J Jr, Resnick D, Goergen TG, Feingold ML, Niwayama G, Danzig LA: The adult hip: An anatomic study. I. The bony landmarks. Radiology *128*:1, 1978.
71. Dunlap K, Swanson AB, Penner RS: Studies of the hip joint by means of lateral acetabular roentgenograms. J Bone Joint Surg *38A*:1218, 1956.
72. Martel W, Poznanski AK: The value of traction during roentgenography of the hip. Radiology *94*:497, 1970.
73. Martel W, Poznanski AK: The effect of traction on the hip in osteonecrosis. A comment on the "radiolucent crescent line." Radiology *94*:505, 1970.
74. Camp JD, Coventry MB: Use of special views in roentgenography of the knee joint. US Naval Med Bull *42*:56, 1944.
75. Holmblad EC: Postero-anterior x-ray view of the knee in flexion. JAMA *109*:1196, 1937.
76. Settegast: Typische Roentgenbilder von normalen Menschen. Lehmanns Med Atlanten *5*:211, 1921.
77. Hughston JC: Subluxation of the patella. J Bone Joint Surg *50A*:1003, 1968.
78. Wiberg G: Roentgenographic and anatomic studies on the femoropatellar joint. Acta Orthop Scand *12*:319, 1941.
79. Knutsson F: Über die Röntgenologie des Femoropatellargelenks sowie eine gute Projektion für das Kniegelenk. Acta Radiol *22*:371, 1941.
80. Furmaier A, Breit A: Uber die Roentgenologie des Femoropatellargelenks. Arch Orthop Unfall-Chir *45*:126, 1952.
81. Merchant AC, Mercer RL, Jacobsen RH, Cool CR: Roentgenographic analysis of patellofemoral congruence. J Bone Joint Surg *56A*:1391, 1974.
82. Ficat P, Phillipe J, Bizour H: Le défilé fémoro-patellaire. Rev Méd Toulouse *6*:241, 1970.
83. Ficat RP, Hungerfor DS: Disorders of the Patello-Femoral Joint. Baltimore, Williams & Wilkins Co, 1977, p. 40.
84. Leach RE, Gregg T, Ferris JS: Weight-bearing radiography in osteoarthritis of the knee. Radiology *97*:265, 1970.
85. Arlbäck S: Osteoarthrosis of the knee. A radiographic investigation. Acta Radiol Suppl *277*:7, 1968.
86. Leonard LM: The importance of weight-bearing x-rays in knee problems. J Maine Med Assoc *62*:101, 1971.
87. Thomas R, Resnick D, Alazraki N, Daniel D, Greenfield R: Compartmental evaluation of osteoarthritis of the knee: A comparative study of available diagnostic modalities. Radiology *116*:585, 1975.
88. Jacobsen K: Radiologic technique for measuring instability in the knee joint. Acta Radiol (Diagn)*18*:113, 1977.
89. Goergen TG, Danzig, LA, Resnick D, Owen CA: Roentgenographic evaluation of the tibiotalar joint. J Bone Joint Surg *59A*:874, 1977.
90. Hutter CG Jr, Scott W: Tibial torsion. J Bone Joint Surg *31A*:511, 1949.
91. Mandell J: Isolated fracture of the posterior tibial lip at the ankle as demonstrated by an additional projection, the "poor" lateral view. Radiology *101*:319, 1971.

92. Holly EW: Radiography of the tarsal sesamoid bones. Med Radiogr Photogr *31*:73, 1955.
93. Lewis RW: Non-routine views in roentgen examination of the extremities. Surg Gynecol Obstet *67*:38, 1938.
94. Causton J: Projection of sesamoid bones in the region of the first metatarsophalangeal joint. Radiography *9*:39, 1943.
95. Harris RI, Beath T: Etiology of peroneal spastic flat foot. J Bone Joint Surg *30B*:624, 1948.
96. Brodén B: Roentgen examination of the subtaloid joint in fractures of the calcaneus. Acta Radiol *31*:85, 1949.
97. Isherwood I: A radiological approach to the subtalar joint. J Bone Joint Surg *43B*:566, 1961.
98. Feist JH, Mankin HJ: The tarsus: Basic relationships and motions in the adult and definition of optimal recumbent oblique projection. Radiology *79*:250, 1962.
99. Freiberger RH, Hersh A, Harrison MO: Roentgen examination of the deformed foot. Semin Roentgenol *5*:341, 1970.
100. Ritchie GW, Keim HA: A radiographic analysis of major foot deformities. Can Med Assoc J *91*:840, 1964.
101. Cobey JC: Posterior roentgenogram of the foot. Clin Orthop *118*:202, 1976.
102. Kandel B: Suroplantar projection in congenital club foot of the infant. Acta Orthop Scand *22*:161, 1952.
103. Gamble FO: A special approach to foot radiography. Radiogr Clin Photogr *19*:78, 1943.
104. Mink J, Gold R, Bluestone R: Radiographic arthritis survey. Arthritis Rheum *20*:1564, 1977.
105. Yousefzadeh DK: The value of traction during roentgenography of the wrist and metacarpophalangeal joints. Skel Radiol *4*:29, 1979.
106. Abel MS: Symmetrical anteroposterior projections of the sternoclavicular joints with motion studies. Radiology *132*:757, 1979.
107. Shackelford GD, McAlister WH: Axial radiography of the spine: A projection for evaluation of the neural arches in children. Radiology *130*:798, 1979.
108. Chevrot A: Incidence cranio-caudale oblique unilatérale de l'articulation sacro-iliaque. J Radiol *60*:143, 1979.
109. Egund N, Olsson TH, Schmid H, Selvik G: Movements in the sacroiliac joints demonstrated with roentgen stereophotogrammetry. Acta Radiol (Diagn) *19*:833, 1978.
110. Sauser DD, Billimoria PE: Equalization filter for the shoulder. Am J Roentgenol *133*:952, 1979.
111. Rhea JT, DeLuca SA, Llewellyn HJ, Boyd RJ: The oblique view: An unnecessary component of the initial adult lumbar spine examination. Radiology *134*:45, 1980.
112. DeSmet AA: Anterior oblique projection in radiography of the traumatized shoulder. Am J Roentgenol *134*:515, 1980.
113. DeSmet AA: Axillary projection in radiography of the nontraumatized shoulder. Am J Roentgenol *134*:511, 1980.
114. Laurin CA, Dussault R, Levesque HP: The tangential x-ray investigation of the patellofemoral joint: X-ray technique, diagnostic criteria and their interpretation. Clin Orthop Rel Res *144*:16, 1979.
115. Van Moppes FI, Van Engelshoven JMA, Van de Hoogenband CR: Comparison between talar tilt, anterior drawer sign and ankle arthrography in ankle ligament lesions. J Belge Radiol *62*:441, 1979.
116. Seligson D, Gassman J, Pope M: Ankle instability: Evaluation of the lateral ligaments. Am J Sports Med *8*:39, 1980.

8

CONVENTIONAL TOMOGRAPHY

by Donald Resnick, M.D.

This chapter summarizes the role of tomography in evaluating patients with articular disorders. A comprehensive discussion of the physics, techniques, and orthopedic applications of tomography is beyond the scope of this book, and the interested reader should consult other available sources.[1-3]

Most skeletal structures can be readily evaluated with routine radiographs. Specialized views, coned-down projections, and fluoroscopic monitoring are additional methods that may supplement initial films, providing adequate visualization of most skeletal sites. Certain structures, such as the vertebral column, sternum, ribs, and sella turcica, are more difficult to evaluate, because of their size, particular orientation in the body, or surrounding tissues. Likewise, certain articulations may not be adequately visualized during initial radiography, necessitating application of tomography. This is particularly true for the sternoclavicular (Fig. 8–1), temporomandibular (Fig. 8–2), sacroiliac, costovertebral, apophyseal, atlanto-occipital, atlanto-axial, subtalar (Fig. 8–3), and intertarsal (Fig. 8–4) articulations.[4-8]

Tomographic evaluation of articular disorders can be accomplished in several ways. Preliminary films must be studied prior to tomography and should be available during the procedure. These radiographs must also be available when the tomograms are being interpreted. The optimal patient position utilized during tomography can generally be ascertained from the plain films; the patient should be placed in an attitude that most ideally demonstrates the articulation. In general, tomograms in a frontal projection are most helpful in visualizing the sacroiliac and sternoclavicular joints; tomograms in an oblique projection may be beneficial in evaluating the costovertebral and apophyseal joints; tomograms performed in frontal and lateral projections may be required for delineating the temporomandibular, atlanto-occipital, atlanto-axial, and subtalar articulations.

The optimal type of radiographic tube motion and the correct thickness and spacing of the tomographic sections will vary. Hypocycloidal tube motion provides extremely thin tomographic sections and can be very helpful in evaluating patients with vertebral fractures. Zonography produces sections of increased thickness and has been applied to abnormalities of the sacroiliac and sternoclavicular joints. The increased thickness of the tomographic projections obtained with zonography allows more contrast on the exposures. We most commonly employ hypocycloidal motion to obtain tomographic images in the evaluation of joint disorders. Although we usually obtain a tomographic section every 5 mm, the studies are carefully monitored, and additional tomograms may be obtained at selected intervals or in another projection to supplement the initial tomographic images.

Text continued on page 319

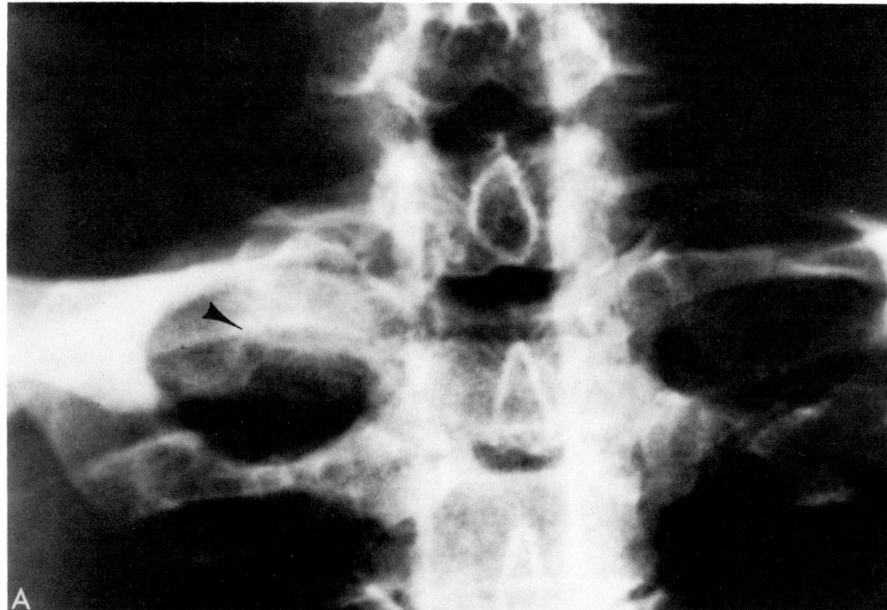

Figure 8–1. Sternoclavicular joint: Osteomyelitis and septic arthritis.

A The initial radiograph outlines erosion and eburnation (arrowhead) of the medial aspect of the right clavicle. Sternal alterations are not well delineated.

B Hypocycloidal tomography reveals considerable osseous erosion of both clavicle (arrowhead) and sternum (arrow). The extensive bony sclerosis, loss of articular space, and superior subluxation of the clavicle are readily apparent.

C Joint aspiration followed by arthrography documented the presence of staphylococci and outlined synovial irregularity, capsular rupture, and soft tissue abscesses (arrows).

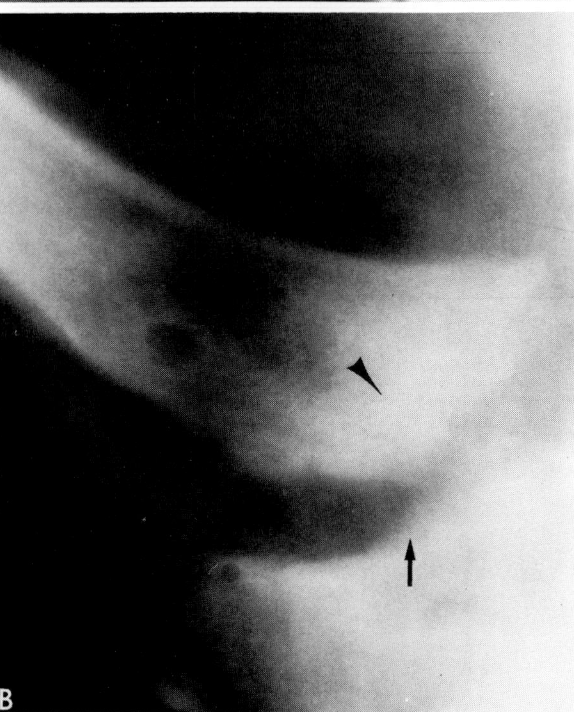

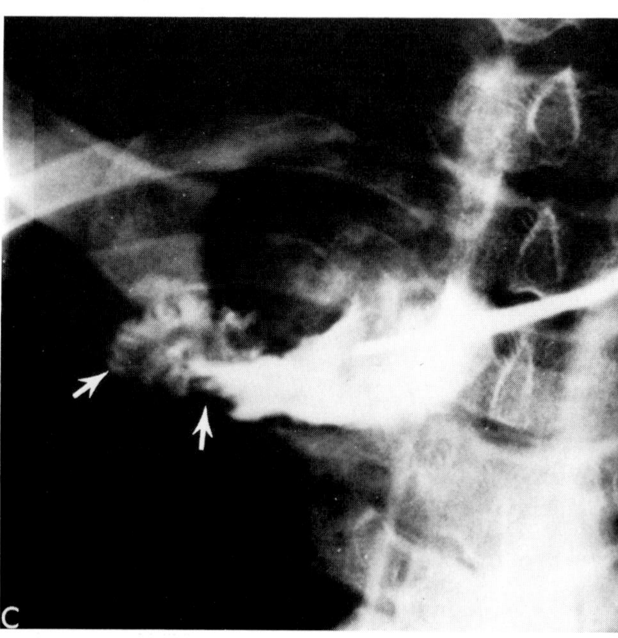

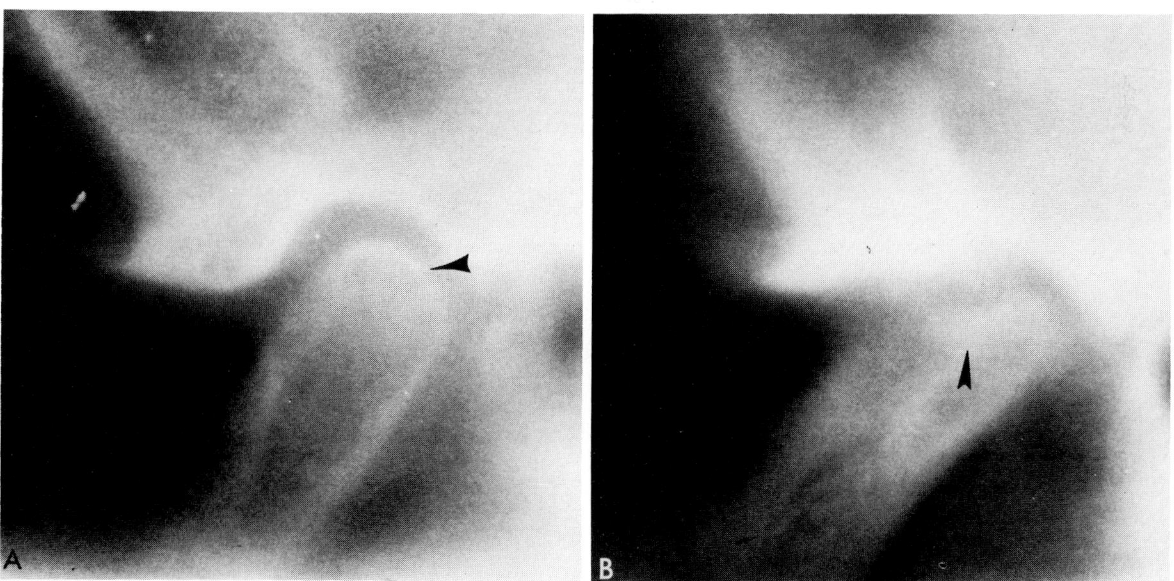

Figure 8–2. *Temporomandibular joint: Normal and abnormal.*

A *Normal situation. Tomogram reveals a smooth condylar head (arrowhead) and temporal fossa and normal joint space.*

B *Posttraumatic degenerative joint disease. Tomography delineates flattening of the condylar head with bony eburnation (arrowhead) and loss of articular space.*

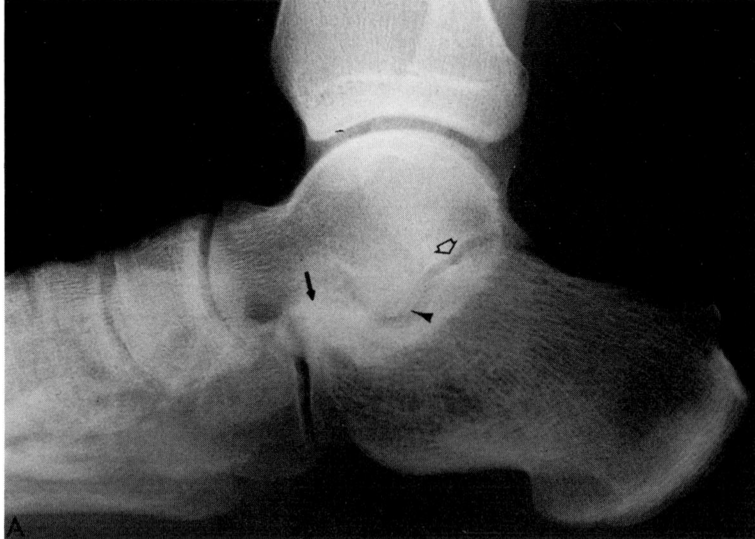

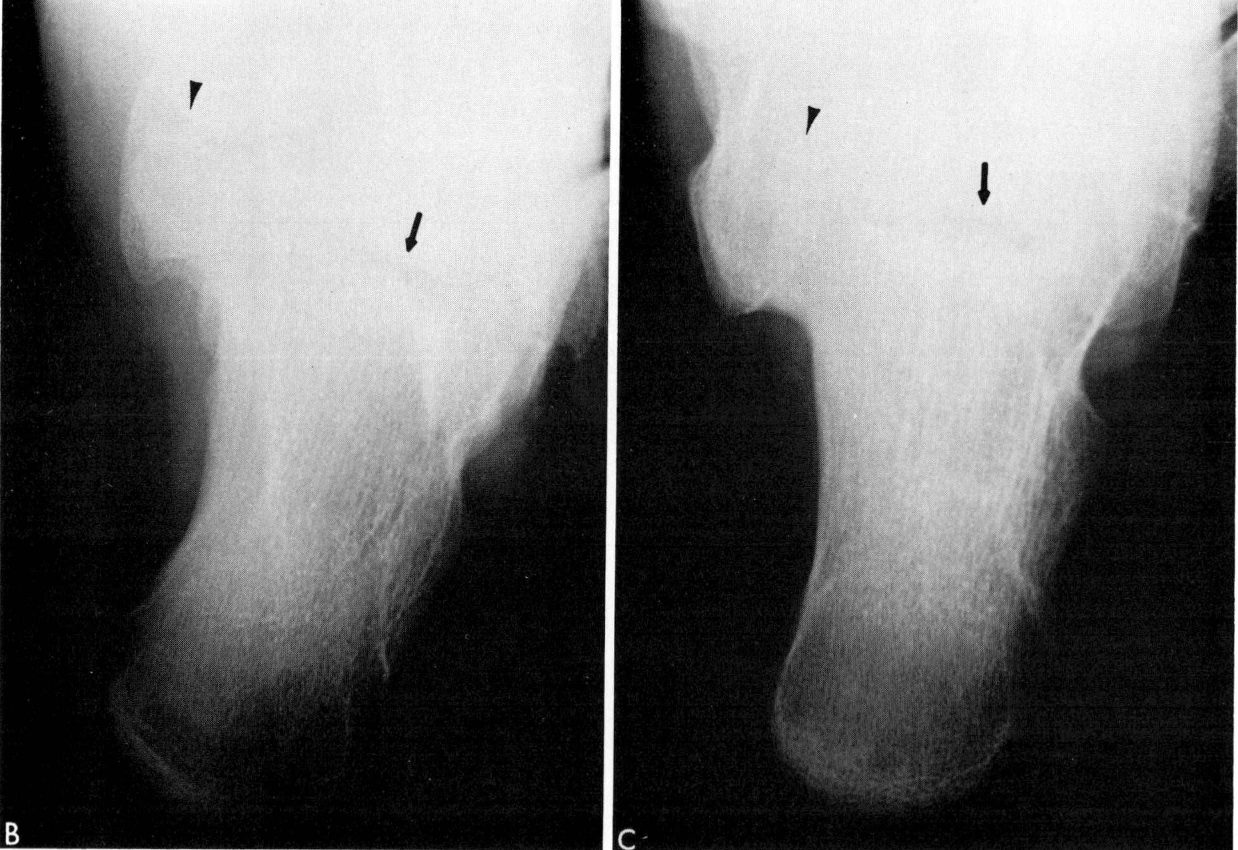

Figure 8–3. *Talocalcaneal articulations: Tarsal coalition.*

A *An initial lateral radiograph of the ankle and foot reveals narrowing of the subtalar joint (open arrow), enlargement of the lateral process of the talus (arrowhead), and poor definition of the anterosuperior aspect of the calcaneus (arrow).*

B *Axial radiograph (Harris-Beath view) of the normal side delineates the subtalar (arrow) and anterior talocalcaneonavicular (arrowhead) articulations, the latter being located above the sustentaculum tali.*

C *Axial radiograph (Harris-Beath view) of the abnormal side demonstrates a relatively normal subtalar joint (arrow) and apparent osseous bridging or coalition (arrowhead) between the sustentaculum tali and talus.*

Illustration continued on the opposite page

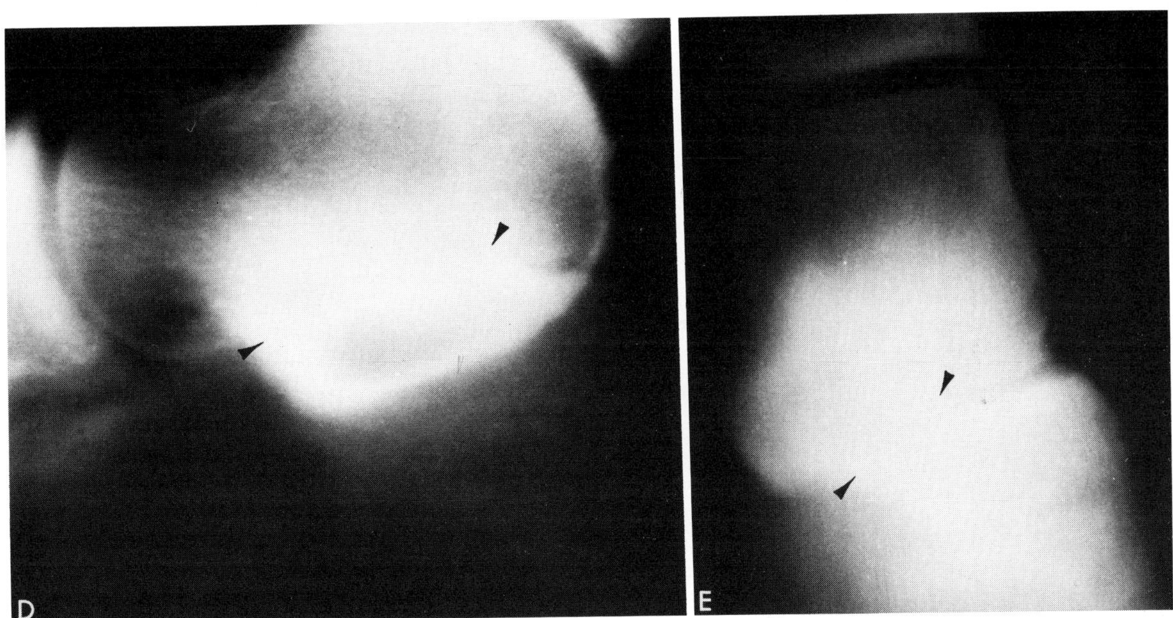

Figure 8–3. Continued
D, E *Tomography in lateral* **(D)** *and frontal* **(E)** *projections confirms the osseous coalition (arrowheads) between the sustentaculum tali and inferior surface of the talus.*

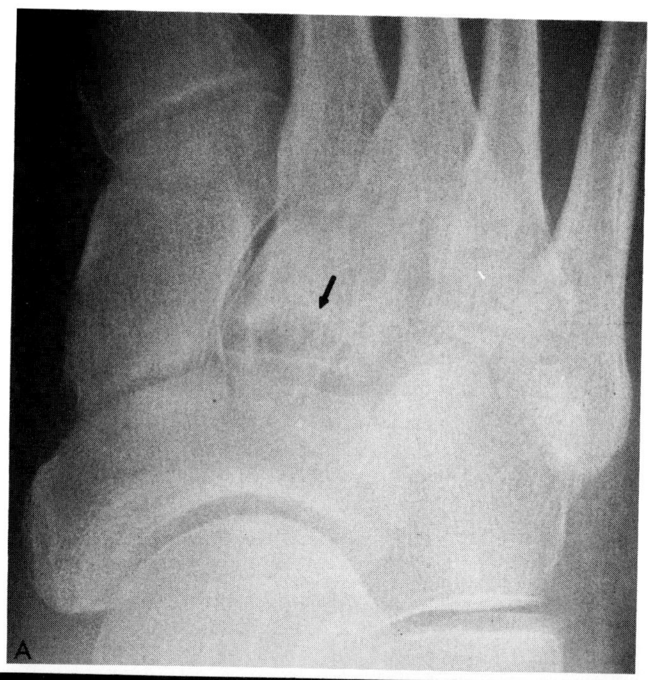

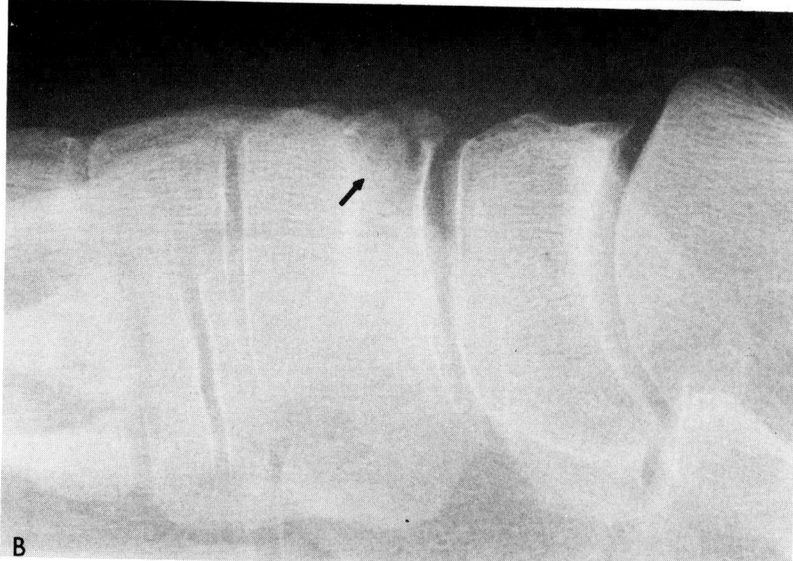

Figure 8–4. *Cuneonavicular joint: Posttraumatic osteonecrosis.*

A, B *Frontal* **(A)** *and lateral* **(B)** *radiographs demonstrate soft tissue swelling, bony fragmentation, and a radiolucent lesion of the intermediate cuneiform bone (arrow).*

Illustration continued on the opposite page

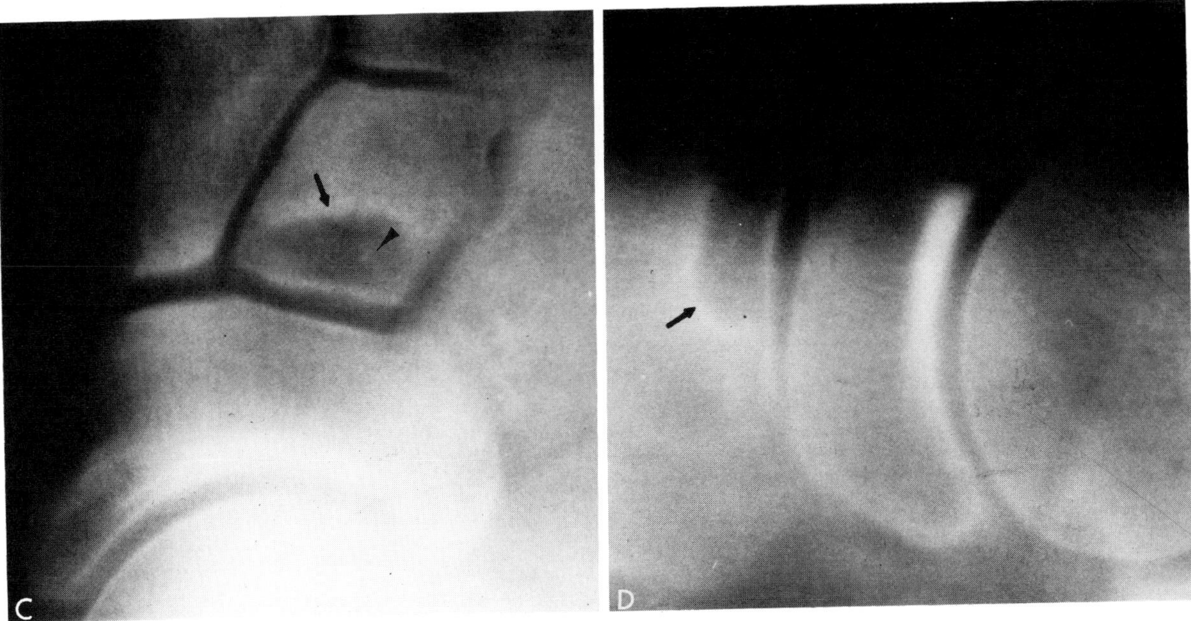

Figure 8–4. Continued
C, D *Frontal* **(C)** *and lateral* **(D)** *tomograms better delineate the size of the lesion (arrow), a central sequestrum (arrowhead), surrounding bony eburnation, and normal articular space. A subsequent biopsy documented posttraumatic osteonecrosis of this bone.*

The clinical situations that may be evaluated with tomography are countless. Only a few such situations will be mentioned here; others are indicated elsewhere in the book. Tomography may be applied to skeletal trauma to detect and delineate vertebral column and hip fractures, to identify osteochondral defects, and to evaluate fracture healing. Intra-articular osseous bodies can be outlined with tomography; intra-articular cartilaginous bodies may require arthrotomography. The early detection of osteonecrosis, particularly of the femoral head, may rely upon tomography. Correct differentiation between severe osteoporosis and infection necessitates scrutiny of subchondral bone to detect early osseous destruction. In this situation, tomography allows evaluation of the articular bone. Tomography can also be beneficial in evaluating patients with chronic osteomyelitis by identifying areas of cortical disruption and sequestrae, findings that imply active disease. Tomographic evaluation of bone neoplasms may identify a nidus of an osteoid osteoma, matrix calcification in cartilaginous tumors, and soft tissue extension of malignant disease.

It is apparent that tomography is a useful adjunct to plain film radiography and should be utilized when standard and specialized views fail to provide needed information for correct diagnosis and adequate treatment.

REFERENCES

1. Christensen, EE, Curry TS, Nunnally J: Introduction to Physics of Diagnostic Radiology. Philadelphia, Lea & Febiger, 1972.
2. Andrews JR: Planigraphy. I. Introduction and history. Am J Roentgenol *36*:575, 1936.
3. Littleton JT, Crosby EH, Durizch ML: Adjustable versus fixed fulcrum tomographic systems. A microdensitometric examination of two tomographic systems. Am J Roentgenol *117*:910, 1973.
4. Wilkinson M, Meikle JAK: Tomography of the sacro-iliac joint. Ann Rheum Dis *25*:433, 1966.
5. Morag B, Shahin N: The value of tomography of the sterno-clavicular region. Clin Radiol *26*:57–62, 1975.
6. Hazan H, Labrune M, Massias P, Segond P: Etude tomographique de la charnière cervico-occipitale au cours des polyarthrites rheumatoides. A propos de 50 observations. Ann Radiol *19*:743, 1976.
7. Reichmann S: Tomography of the lumbar intervertebral joints. Acta Radiol *12*:641, 1972.
8. Elhabali M, Scherak O, Seidl G, Kolarz G: Tomographic examinations of sacroiliac joints in adult patients with rheumatoid arthritis. J Rheumatol *6*:417, 1979.

9

MAGNIFICATION RADIOGRAPHY

by Harry K. Genant, M.D.

The quality of a radiographic image is important for accurate and detailed assessment of subtle skeletal abnormalities. To maximize diagnostic information, high-resolution radiographic techniques have been developed. The purpose of this chapter is to examine quantitatively the fundamental imaging properties and qualitatively the clinical applications of conventional and high-resolution magnification techniques.

Magnification techniques have received increased attention for skeletal radiography, and in recent years have been widely applied.[8, 17-19, 26, 27, 31, 35, 38, 46, 49, 52] The expanded application of magnification has resulted from three factors: (a) advances in radiologic sciences; (b) optimization of physical parameters and exposing factors; and (c) delineation of the meaningful areas for clinical use. High-resolution magnification is achieved by two different techniques.[8, 17, 26] The first is optical magnification of fine-grain films, and the second is direct radiographic magnification (Fig. 9–1).

The *optical magnification* technique consists of contact exposures obtained with conventional x-ray equipment and fine-grain industrial films, such as Kodak Type M. The resultant image is viewed with optical enlargement. Clinical studies with this technique are not new. In the early 1950s, Fletcher and

OPTICAL MAGNIFICATION
1.2 mm FOCAL SPOT
50 KVP
500 MA
0.5 SEC
100 cm FFD
(M=1.02)
20 mm
INDUSTRIAL FILM

RADIOGRAPHIC MAGNIFICATION
100 μm FOCAL SPOT
25 cm
50 KVP
5 MA
1.0 SEC
75 cm FFD
(M = 3)
RARE - EARTH SCREEN - FILM

Figure 9–1. *Comparison of optical and radiographic magnification.*

Rowley[15] reported their experience with fine-grain films and photographic enlargement in the study of peripheral skeletal abnormalities. In a monograph published in 1969, Berens and Lin[2] reported their observations in rheumatoid arthritis with the use of industrial films and optical magnification. More recently, Meema and associates,[38, 39] Weiss,[52] Genant and co-workers,[17, 18, 20, 21] Mall and co-workers,[35, 36] and Jensen and Kliger[32] have reported extensive experience with this technique in various metabolic and arthritic skeletal disorders. Thus, the clinical importance of the optical magnification technique appears established for selected skeletal examinations.

Direct radiographic magnification for skeletal radiography[17, 19, 22, 26, 27, 31, 46, 49, 51] has received less attention than has optical magnification. Only with the recent development of x-ray tubes having small focal spots (100 to 150 μm) and adequate output for clinical examination has this technique become available. Limited clinical experience with direct radiographic magnification of the skeleton has been reported by Gordon and associates,[27] Sundaram and co-workers,[51] Ishigaki,[31] Doi and colleagues,[8] and Genant and co-workers.[17, 19, 26] The initial results have been promising and applications for both thin and thick body parts are being established.

RADIOGRAPHIC TECHNIQUES

Optical Magnification

The standard technique[17] for optical magnification employs Kodak industrial Type M film, which is exposed with approximately 50 to 60 kVp, 500 mA, and 0.5 sec at 100 cm focus-film distance. A conventional x-ray tube with a 1.2 mm focal spot is used for these contact exposures and the inherent magnification for thin parts is low (approximately 1.01 to 1.04 times).[8, 12] Thus, for the peripheral skeleton, exposure times are kept relatively short, and geometric unsharpness is minimal because of the low degree of inherent magnification. The industrial film must be developed manually or by means of an industrial processor. A rapid-process fine-grain film such as Kodak RP/M may be substituted for ease of X-omat processing at a modest loss of image quality. The completed industrial radiograph is surveyed with-

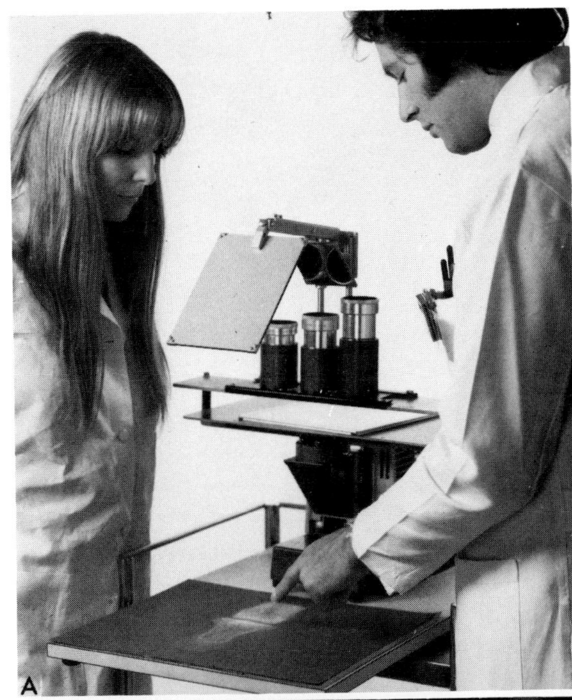

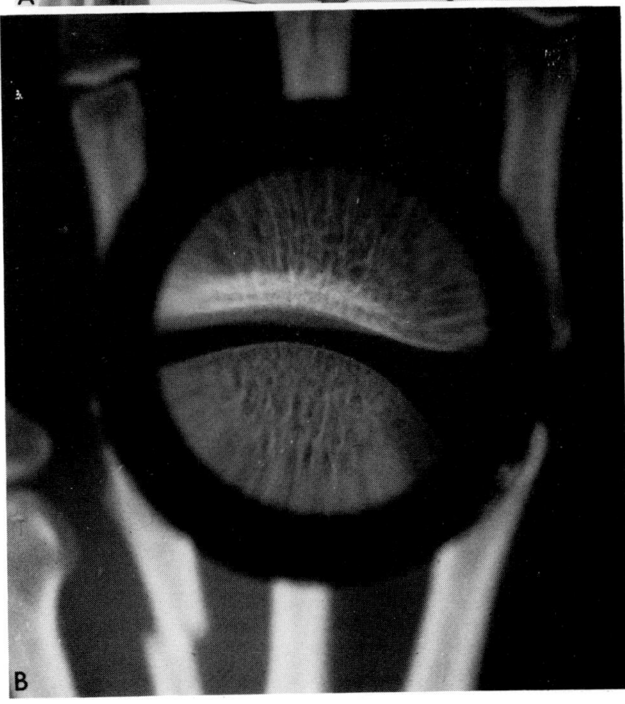

Figure 9–2. *Optical magnification achieved by two methods.* **A,** *For group viewing, a projector, such as the Leitz Macro Promar, is used.* **B,** *For individual viewing, a loupe or hand lens is placed in direct contact with the fine-grained industrial film and the image is viewed at close range.*

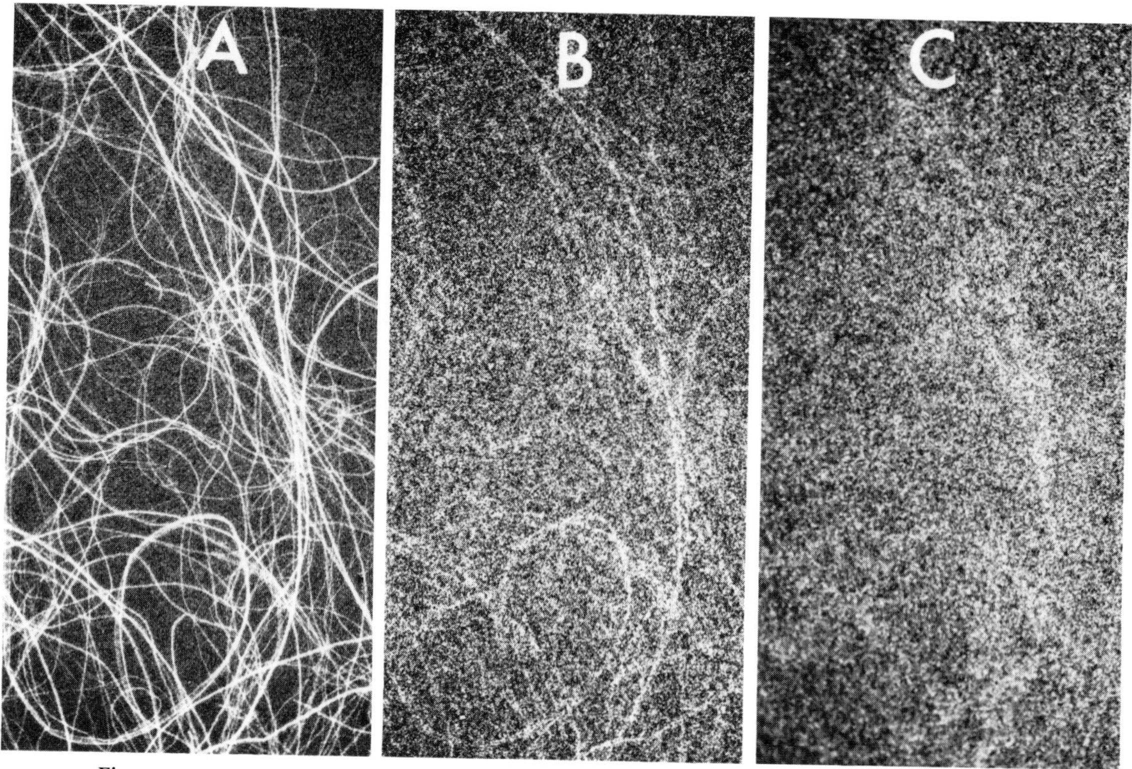

Figure 9–3. *For qualitative comparison, fine steel wool has been radiographed with Type M technique* **(A)**, *nonscreen cardboard technique with medical RP film* **(B)**, *and fine screen-film system, RP-Detail* **(C)**. *Type M technique affords higher resolution, greater contrast, and lower noise compared with the other two standard techniques. Images in* **B** *and* **C** *are fairly comparable. (From Genant HK, et al: Invest Radiol 11:486, 1976.)*

out magnification initially, then viewed with a hand lens or a projector for optical magnification. Such magnification is important to take full advantage of the Type M film, since fine bone structure may not be visible to the unaided eye. For individual viewing, a loupe or hand lens[17, 38] is most convenient, whereas for demonstration or for group viewing, a projector[36] is most convenient (Fig. 9–2).

Inherent in the optical magnification technique is obtaining a contact radiograph of high quality. A comparison[18] of the imaging properties of the Type M film technique and two widely used conventional techniques for peripheral skeletal radiography is given in Figure 9–3. The Type M technique is compared with (1) a standard, nonscreen cardboard technique using RP medical film and (2) a fine screen-film system using detail screens and RP medical film. The small wire structures are best imaged with the Type M technique because of its higher resolution, lower noise, and greater contrast. These

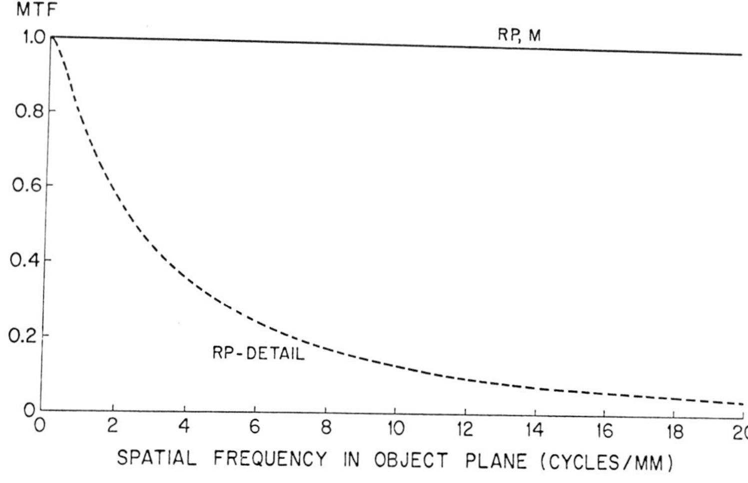

Figure 9–4. *The modular transfer functions (MTFs) of recording systems. The MTFs for direct exposure of RP and Type M film show only 1 per cent decline in the demonstrated range of spatial frequency. The MTF for RP-Detail is quite poor by comparison. (From Genant HK, et al: Invest Radiol 11:486, 1976.)*

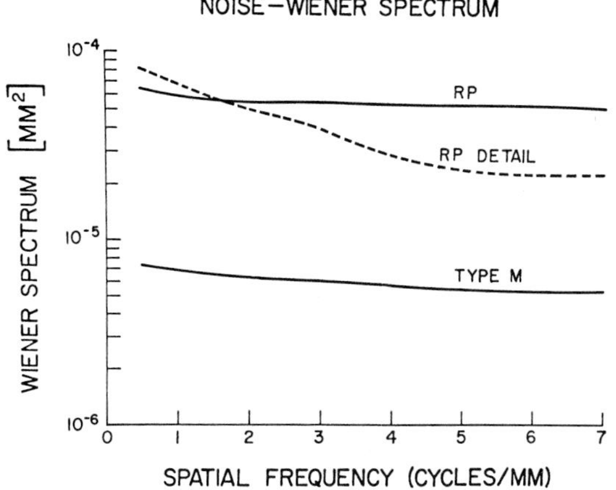

Figure 9–5. *The Wiener spectrum values for Type M, medical RP, and RP-Detail techniques are shown. The noise with Type M is appreciably lower than with either of the other two techniques. (From Genant HK, et al: Invest Radiol 11:486, 1976.)*

imaging properties — i.e., resolution, noise, and contrast — are compared quantitatively by means of the modulation transfer functions (MTF), Wiener spectral analyses, and gradient curves, respectively (Figs. 9–4 to 9–6).

The MTF is a measure of sharpness and describes the signal-transmitting capability of the imaging system in the spatial frequency domain, which may be compared to the frequency response of a "hi-fi" system.[44, 45] The MTF is defined as the ratio of the amplitude of the image to the amplitude of the sinusoidal object, expressed as a function of the spatial frequency. The higher the MTF value, the better the imaging system, i.e., the more closely the image obtained resembles the object. An ideal imaging system with regard to resolution is one that contains a flat MTF curve such as that derived for Type M film (Fig. 9–4). The MTF for imaging components may be measured by a number of methods[10, 11]—for example, the Fourier transformation of slit images was used for these experimental data.[18]

The Wiener spectral value of noise is plotted against the spatial frequency in Figure 9–5. For Wiener spectra of similar shape, the higher the spectral value, the greater the noise level. The noise at high frequencies corresponds to the fine noise pattern, whereas the low frequency component corresponds to the coarse pattern. The Wiener spectra are determined by an electronic Fourier analysis method,[10] in which the film is scanned circularly by a light spot and the fluctuating noise signal in a photomultiplier that corresponds to the radiographic noise is analyzed by an electronic wave analyzer.

The characteristic or "H&D" curve of a screen-film system may be derived by several methods[29] and reflects the relative speed, latitude, and contrast of the recording system. The gradient curve is a plot of gradient or contrast as a function of film density. The H&D and gradient curves for the three comparison techniques are shown in Figure 9–6.

Of the two conventional techniques displayed in Figure 9–3 and quantified in Figures 9–4 to 9–6, the cardboard technique has higher resolution and lower contrast than the detail screen-film system, and the noise is comparable. The overall image quality for the cardboard and detail screen-film techniques is comparable, and is far inferior to that obtained with the Type M technique. Thus, the superior imaging properties of the Type M technique permit optical magnification of up to 10 times for improved detection of subtle abnormalities. Radiation exposure is high,[18] however, resulting in approximately 1 rad to the hand or foot, three times the dose given with the cardboard technique, and 70 times the dose for detail screens. For this reason, the industrial film with optical magnification should be used selectively in those instances in which delineation of subtle abnormalities in the peripheral skeleton is important.

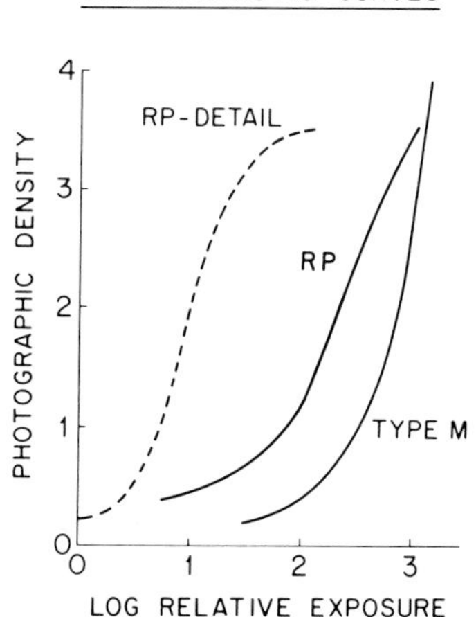

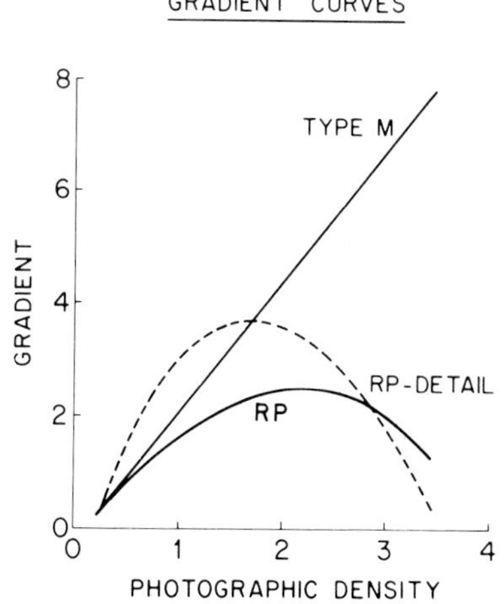

Figure 9–6. *The characteristic and gradient curves for Type M and RP medical film techniques, as well as RP-Detail screen-film technique, are shown. The contrast or gradient with RP medical film technique is quite low compared with that of the other two techniques. (From Genant HK, et al: Invest Radiol 11:486, 1976.)*

Radiographic Magnification

More proximal to the peripheral skeleton, where body parts become thicker, the optical magnification technique with Type M film becomes less feasible. The limitations are attributed to the high radiation exposure that is required and the degradation of image quality related to increased geometric unsharpness, blurring by motion, and scattered radiation. Direct radiographic magnification with a microfocus x-ray tube provides a reasonable alternative.

In radiographic magnification, a screen-film system and geometric enlargement of two to four times are employed in conjunction with a microfocus x-ray tube having a nominal focal spot size of 100 μm (Fig. 9–7*A*, *B*). This technique may overcome some of the limitations of optical magnification, including the high radiation dose to the patient and the special viewing procedure required.[26]

The magnification technique affects the quality of the radiographic image in a complex way.[26] The technical *advantages* of radiographic magnification are based on the following: (1) the sharpness effect, (2) the noise effect, (3) the air-gap effect, and (4) the visual effect.[1, 8, 13, 19, 28, 40, 47, 49] The potential *disadvantages* of radiographic magnification result from the following: (1) the size of the body part examined is limited to small areas compared to those able to be examined with contact exposure; (2) the proper positioning of the area with the lesion may be difficult; and (3) the skin dose is high compared to that with the conventional screen-film technique, although it is low compared to that with Type M film and optical magnification.[17]

Sharpness Effect. The most widely recognized advantage of the magnification technique may be called the sharpness effect. When the x-ray pattern is enlarged, the relative or effective unsharpness of the recording system, which is the unsharpness relative to the input x-ray pattern, is reduced. Therefore, the resolution of the recording system can be improved linearly by the magnification factor. Thus, at 4× magnification, the resolution at the recording system is better by a factor of 4. Similarly, the transfer characteristic of the imaging system — namely, the MTF of the recording system — at four times magnification is derived from the conventional MTF at contact exposure by shifting of the spatial frequency by a factor of four (Fig. 9–7*C*).

Noise Effect. The reason for the noise effect in magnification radiography is similar to that for the sharpness effect. The inherent noise of the recording system does not change, regardless of the magnification. When the x-ray pattern is enlarged, however, the "effective noise," which is the noise relative to the magnified object, is reduced by the square of the magnification factor.[13]

Theoretical study[13] indicates that the effect of radiographic magnification on the Wiener spectrum of the effective noise in the recording system is twofold: (1) the Wiener spectral value decreases by a factor equal to the square of the magnification and (2) the spatial frequency increases by a factor equal to the magnification (Figure 9–7*D*). Thus, the general result is that the higher the magnification, the more drastic the reduction of effective noise by the radiographic magnification technique.

Air-Gap Effect. The air-gap effect has been known for many years to be a technical advantage of magnification radiography.[3, 40, 49] The air-gap usually reduces the scattered radiation relative to contact exposure and thus enhances the contrast of the x-ray pattern used as input to the recording system. The contrast gained, however, may not be as high as that obtained by contact exposure using a grid technique.

Visual Effect. The advantage of magnified radiographs to the observer is called the visual effect. Enlargement of the image is usually helpful for either visual detection or recognition of fine details in the radiograph. It is not helpful, however, for large, low-contrast images because the MTF of the visual system decreases at low spatial frequencies. In practice, therefore, large, low-contrast images are viewed at a greater distance from the radiographs or by a minification lens. These viewing methods are advantageous because noise is suppressed as well. The MTF of the human visual system has been measured,[6, 34] and numerous reported experimental results are now available. These results vary considerably; however, one common point is that the MTF of the visual system peaks at an intermediate spatial frequency and drops on both the high and low frequency sides. The approximate peak position is near the spatial frequency of 1 cycle per mm (an object 1 mm in diameter) at the normal viewing distance of 30 cm, but varies with the brightness of the scene. Enlargement of the image detail is equivalent to shifting the frequency of this detail to the lower side (to the left) in the MTF curve. Therefore, when the image is very large, the enlargement may cause a decrease in the MTF of the visual system unless optical minification is employed.

Effect of Focal Spot Size on Magnification. The selection of the size of the focal spot in magnification radiography affects the resolution of the imaging system, but does not affect contrast or noise. Inherent in achieving the sharpness effect in the direct geometric magnification technique is minimizing the adverse effect of focal spot unsharpness. The potential effect of geometric unsharpness is shown dramatically in Figure 9–8*A*, where fine steel wire has been radiographed at contact as well as elevated 4 cm and 8 cm from a fine-grain film.[21] A standard 1.2 mm focal spot was used at 100 cm focus-film distance. It can be seen that with such a large focal

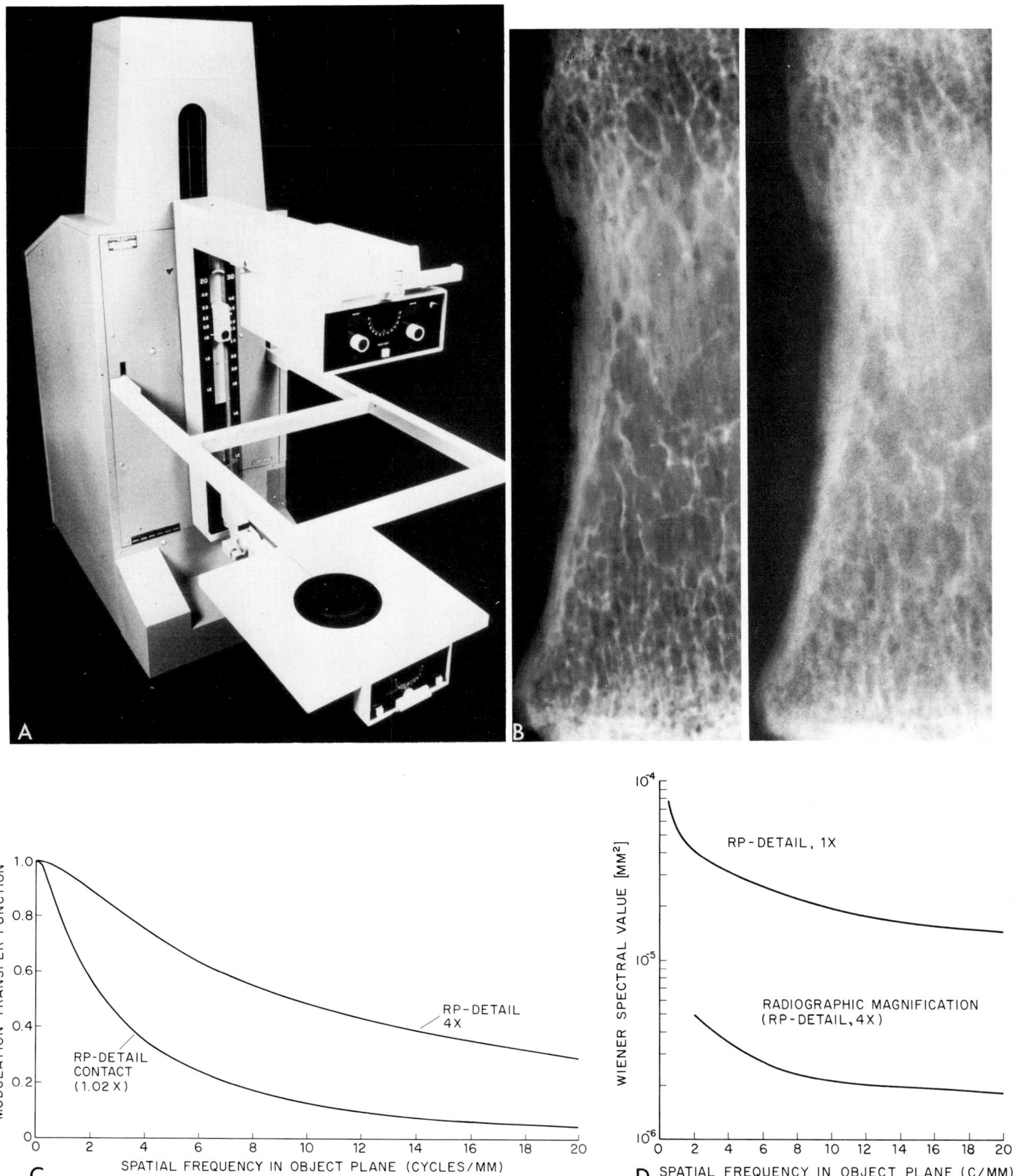

Figure 9–7. **A,** *The most widely used magnification system, the RSI Mag. II.* **B,** *Comparison images of a phalanx at 4× magnification (left) and contact exposure (1.02×), both using RP film and detail screens.* **C,** *The MTF of RP-Detail system at 1.02× (contact exposure) and 4× magnification.* **D,** *Noise Wiener spectra for RP-Detail system for contact exposure (1×) and 4× magnification.* (**C, D,** *Reproduced with permission from Genant HK, Doi K: High-resolution skeletal radiography: Image quality and clinical applications. In RD Moseley Jr, et al [Eds]: Current Problems in Diagnostic Radiology. Copyright © 1978 by Year Book Medical Publishers, Inc, Chicago.)*

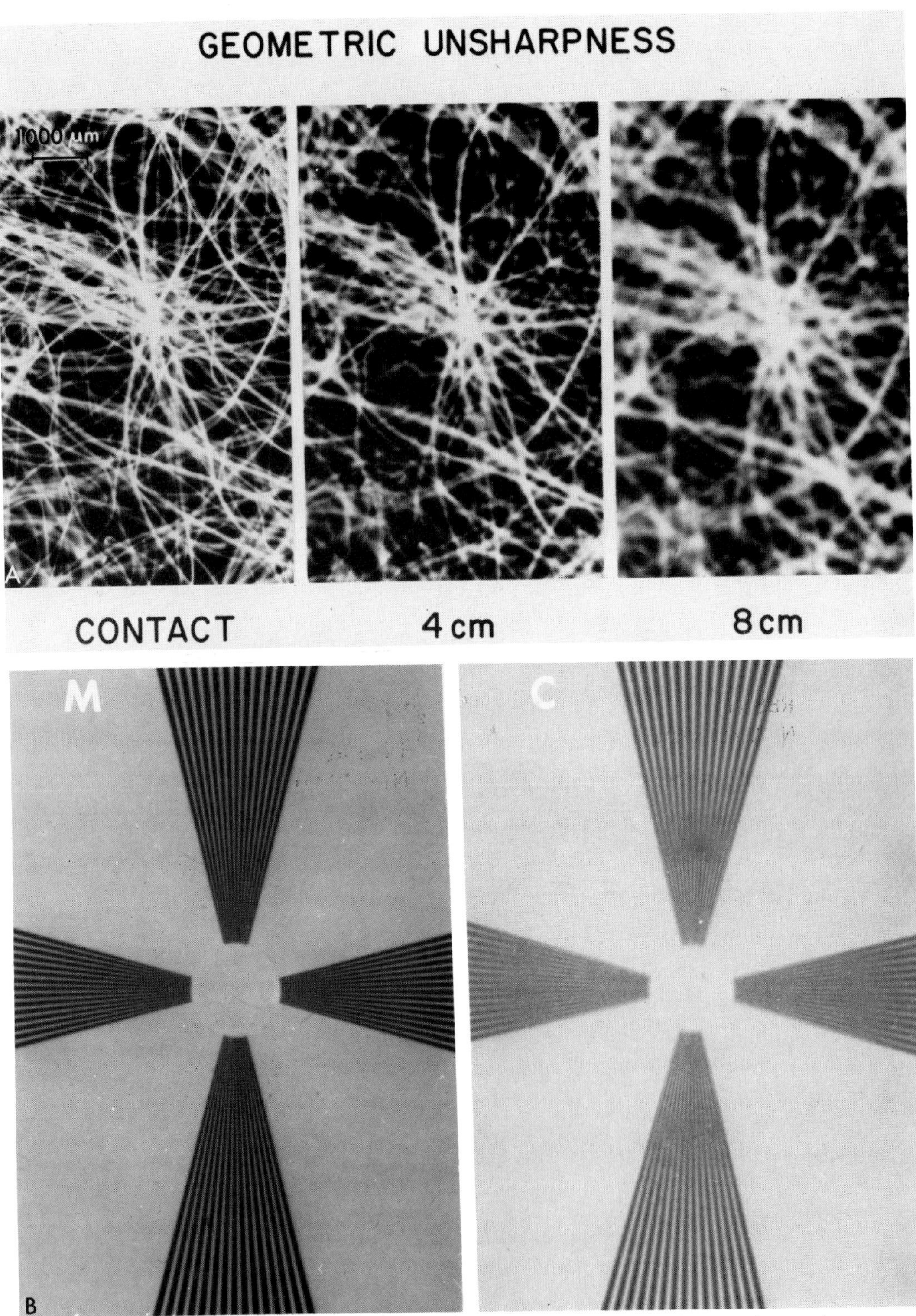

Figure 9–8. **A,** *Fine steel wire radiographed at contact and elevated 4 cm and 8 cm from a fine-grained film using a standard 1.2 mm focal spot at 100 cm focus-film distance (FFD).* **B,** *Star test pattern radiographed at 4× direct magnification using the RSI microfocal spot tube* (M) *(nominal, 0.1 mm) and a rotating anode, small focal spot tube* (C) *(nominal, 0.3 mm).*

spot, even small degrees of magnification introduce considerable geometric unsharpness due to the focal spot penumbra.

A Siemen's star test pattern, which is used to examine focal spot performance, is shown in Figure 9–8*B*. The star test pattern was radiographed at 4× direct magnification, using a microfocal spot tube nominal, 0.1 mm)* and a rotating anode, small focal spot tube (nominal, 0.3 mm). The measured performance of the "small" focal spot is close to 0.5 mm, and is too large for the two to four times geometric magnification used for skeletal examination.[17] The considerably superior image of the Siemen's star pattern with the microfocal spot can be readily appreciated.

Image Comparison and Dosimetry. Insight into the value of direct radiographic magnification compared with a widely used conventional technique is provided by Figure 9–9, which was obtained by (1) direct magnification using a rare-earth screen-film system (3M Trimax Alpha 4-XD) and (2) contact exposure using a midspeed screen-film (Par-RP) with Bucky technique. This qualitative comparison shows the superiority of direct magnification over conventional technique. These results are further supported by the quantitative analysis of resolution and noise given in Figures 9–10 and 9–11.

Despite its excellent imaging characteristics, direct radiographic magnification, like optical magnification, should be used selectively because of its potentially high radiation exposure. Magnification results in an approximately fourfold increase in exposure per surface area (skin dose) compared to conventional techniques when recording-system speeds, air-gap, and grid are considered.[4] The size of the field with magnification is significantly reduced, however, which helps lower the total-body radiation to a level nearly equivalent to that of conventional techniques.

A variety of experimental and, now, commercially available screen-film systems have been used for direct magnification to help reduce radiation exposure. Most of these consist of rare-earth screen-film systems that have high photon-absorption effi-

*Approximate size as specified by the manufacturer.

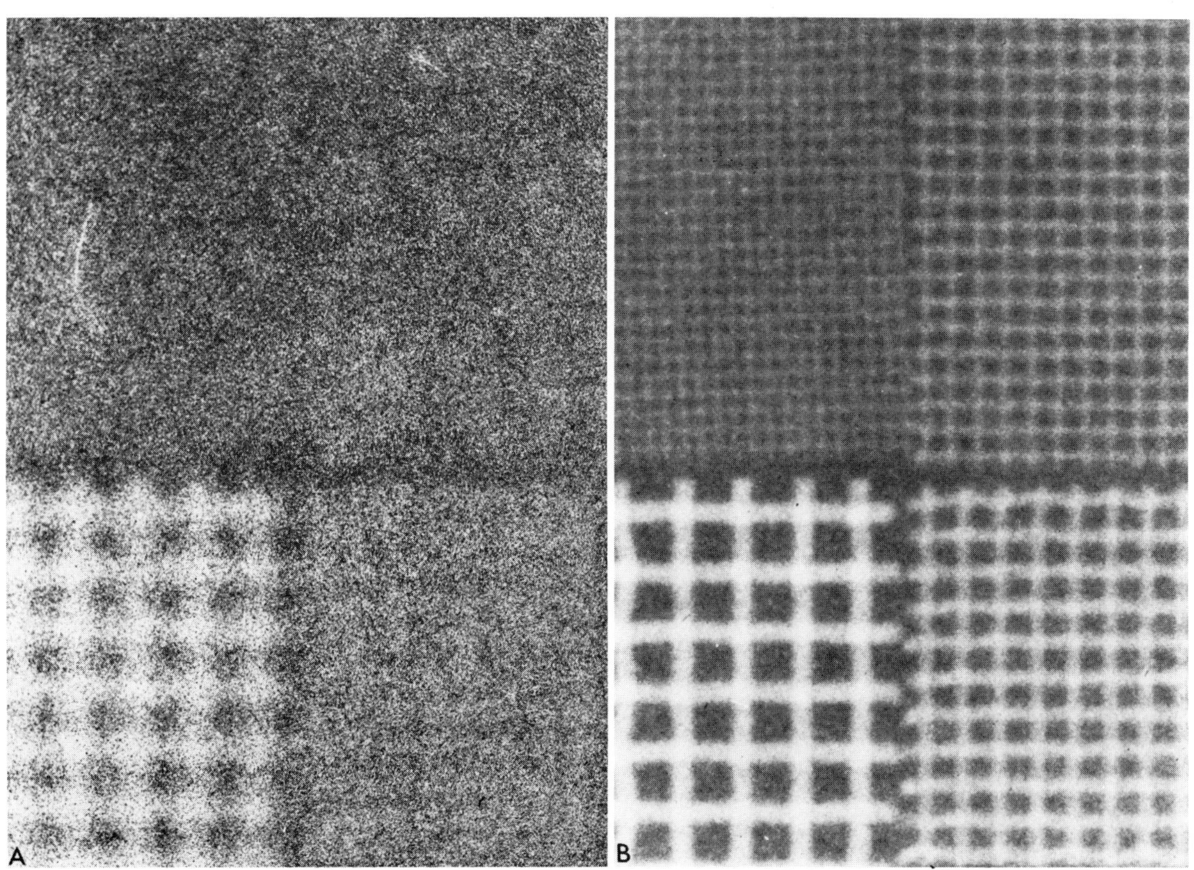

Figure 9–9. *Wire mesh test object that contains cyclic fine structures ranging from one to four line pairs per mm has been radiographed in appropriate thicknesses of lucite to simulate clinical conditions for a thick part such as the hip.* ***A,*** *With conventional technique, two wire meshes are seen.* ***B,*** *With magnification technique, all wire meshes, including four line pairs per mm, can be seen. The effect of lower noise level and higher resolution of magnification relative to conventional technique can be appreciated. Images are made equal in size photographically. (From Genant HK, et al: Radiology 123:47, 1977.)*

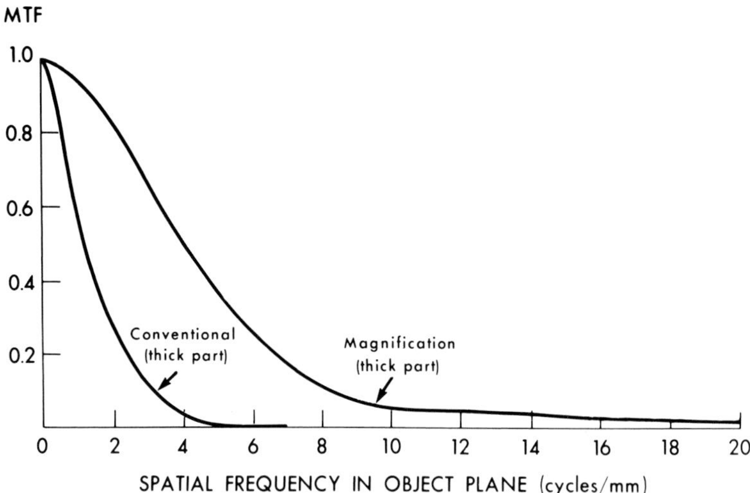

Figure 9–10. *Total MTF (corresponding to test conditions in Figure 9–9) is derived from the product of components, namely, the recording system and the geometric unsharpness. For thick parts, total MTF of radiographic magnification technique is considerably higher than that of conventional contact technique. (From Genant HK, et al: Radiology 123:47, 1977.)*

ciency and high light-conversion efficiency, thus providing an approximately 50 per cent reduction in exposure compared to conventional calcium-tungstate screens.[5] For thin anatomic parts, single-emulsion/single-screen systems are often used, whereas for thicker anatomic parts, double-screen/double-emulsion systems are used.

CLINICAL APPLICATIONS OF MAGNIFICATION RADIOGRAPHY

Based upon this background in physical principles and technical factors, the clinical applications of magnification radiography will be considered. The following general categories of disorders have been studied, which encompass the majority of skeletal examinations: articular, metabolic, infectious, neoplastic, and traumatic disorders and dysplasias.

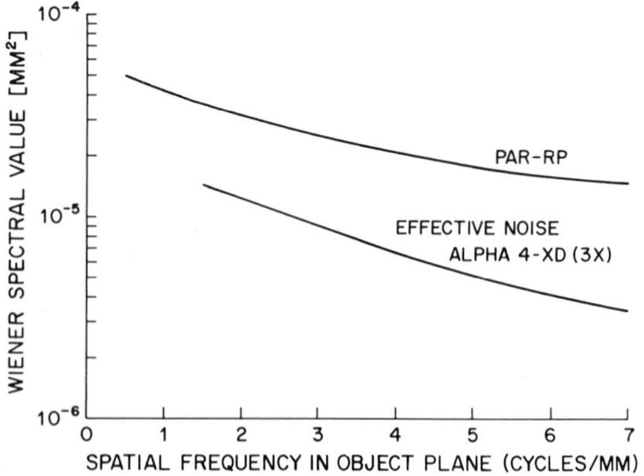

Figure 9–11. *Noise Wiener spectra (corresponding to test conditions in Figure 9–9) for conventional contact and radiographic magnification techniques for thick parts. Magnification technique (Alpha 4-XD system at 3× yields approximately one half to one fourth the effective noise of the conventional contact technique (Par-RP). (From Genant HK et al: Radiology 123:47, 1977.)*

Articular Disorders

Rheumatoid Arthritis. The largest area of clinical application for high-resolution skeletal radiography has been the assessment of rheumatoid arthritis. High resolution radiography using industrial film and *photographic* enlargement was first used in investigations by Fletcher and Rowley[15] in rheumatoid arthritis patients in the 1950s. Berens and Lin[2] later employed fine-detail radiography routinely in the clinical evaluation of patients with various arthritides, including rheumatoid arthritis. An objective analysis of the relative merit of this technique, however, had not been undertaken. To determine objectively whether fine-detail radiography afforded significant advantage over conventional radiography in the clinical evaluation of proved or suspected rheumatoid arthritis, the following study[35] was undertaken.

Twenty-five patients with proved but early rheumatoid arthritis[43] and 20 controls who were normal or had osteoarthritis were studied. The hands of all patients were imaged using a detail screen-film combination and a fine-grain industrial film, and the radiographs were viewed with optical magnification. The sets of radiographs for each patient were read independently by two radiologists without reference to clinical information. A diagnosis was recorded, and erosions and soft tissue swelling were graded as 0 (none), 1 (questionable), 2 (definite), or 3 (severe) according to the most advanced change that was present.

The results demonstrated conclusively that fine-detail radiography was more sensitive than conventional radiography for the detection and evaluation of erosive disease in early rheumatoid arthritis (Fig. 9–12). Further analysis indicated that severe erosions (grade 3) were observed in about the same number of patients with each technique, but minimal erosions (grade 2) were usually detectable only

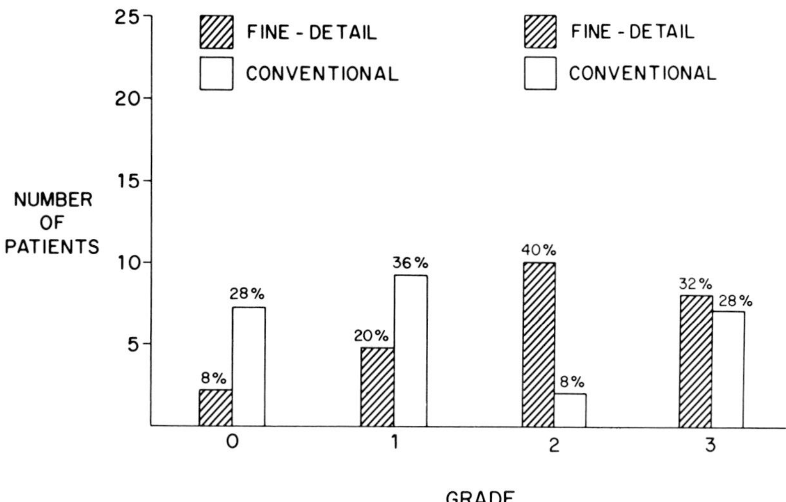

Figure 9–12. *Difference in the detection and grading of erosions with fine-detail and conventional radiography. The difference in the detection rate results almost entirely because of improved detection of subtle (grade 2) erosions. (From Mall JC, et al: Radiology 112:37, 1974.)*

with fine-detail radiography because of its increased sensitivity. These subtle erosive changes were most easily identified as a sawtooth or a "dot-dash" appearance in the metacarpal head (Fig. 9–13) or ulnar styloid (Fig. 9–14) but were also noted in other locations, described by Martel as "bare areas."[2] Detection of surface erosions of this type permitted the identification of subtle progression of disease in some patients. These observations are of particular prognostic significance, since the detection of erosive disease may be an indication for more aggressive therapeutic measures.

The detection of soft tissue swelling was also improved by the high contrast of fine-detail radiography (Fig. 9–15), primarily because of enhanced visualization of subtle changes (grade 2) such as

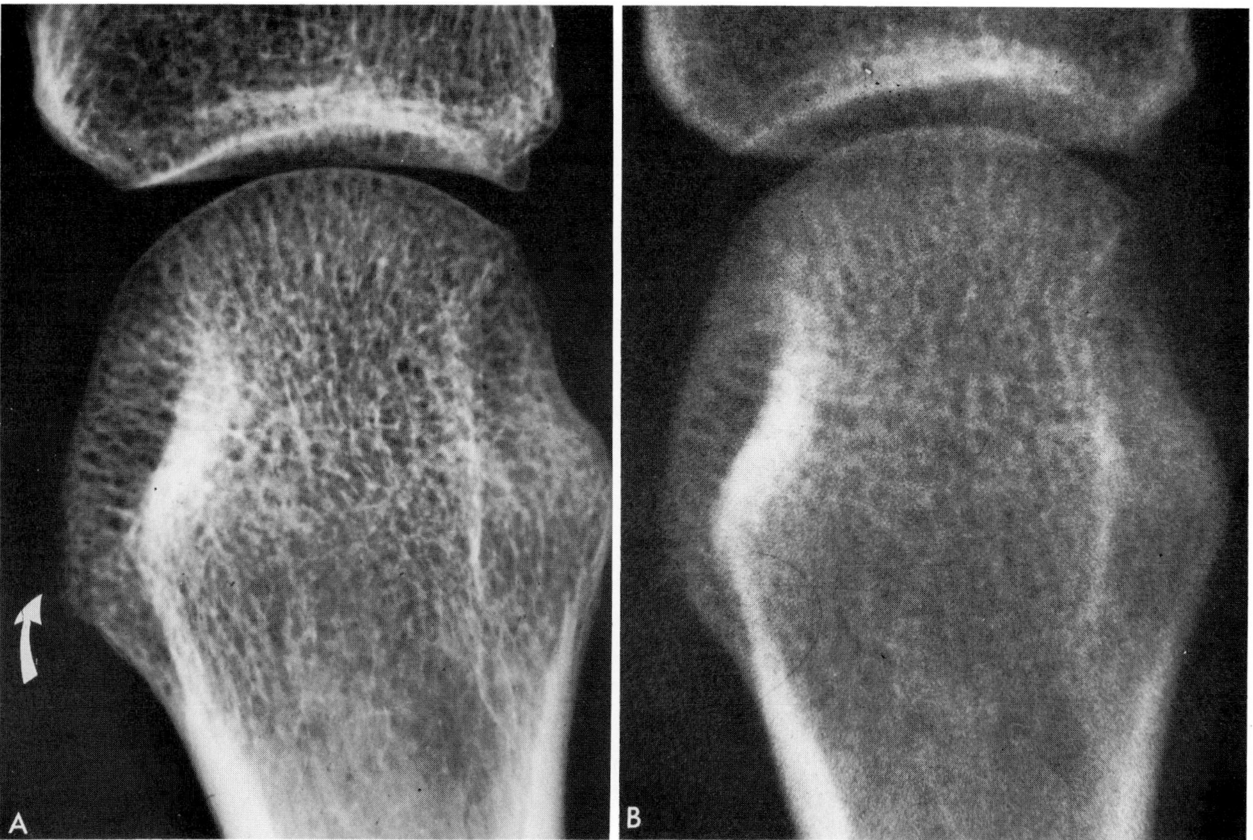

Figure 9–13. *The "dot-dash" appearance of subtle surface erosion (arrow) is clearly identified with fine-detail radiography* **(A)**, *but not with conventional radiography* **(B)**.

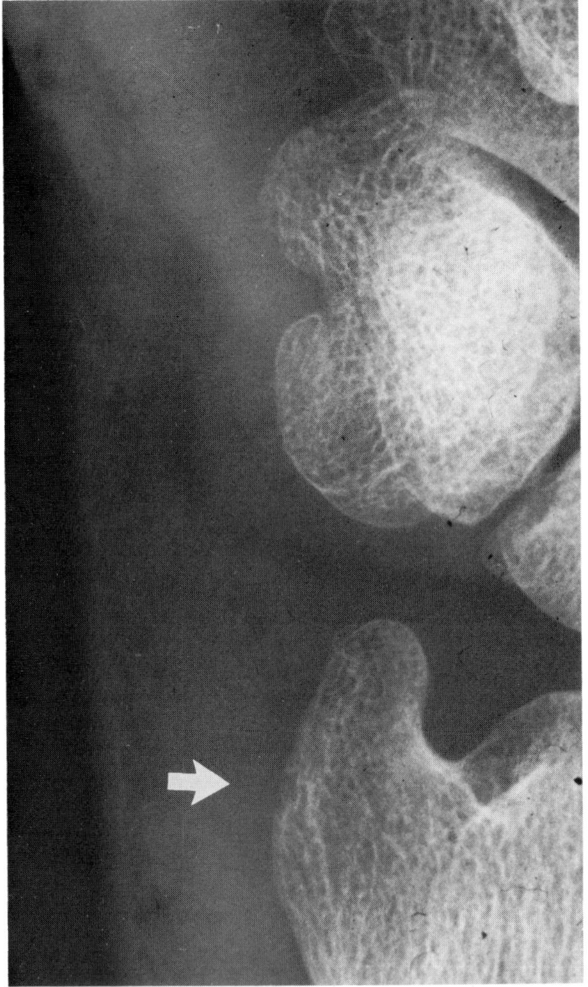

Figure 9–14. Subtle surface erosion (arrow) of ulnar styloid illustrated by magnification radiography.

capsular distention and obliteration of normal fat planes. Such changes were most easily identified at the proximal interphalangeal joints, the first metacarpophalangeal joint and over the ulnar styloid. The detection of soft tissue swelling is important because it is nearly always present at an inflamed joint and occasionally is the only manifestation of disease.

It may be concluded from this study[35] that fine-detail radiography in rheumatoid arthritis has several advantages over conventional radiography: (1) greater sensitivity in detecting erosive disease and joint swelling, (2) improved evaluation of subtle disease progression, and (3) possibly improved diagnostic potential.

Other Arthritides. Magnification radiography may be helpful not only in detecting erosive disease but also in characterizing and differentiating the appearances of various joint afflictions. For example, the erosions seen in psoriatic arthritis, Reiter's syndrome, and the other HLA B27–associated arthritides are characterized by bony proliferation producing a fluffy appearance in juxta-articular regions as well as a linear periosteal new bone response in the adjacent shafts of bones (Fig. 9–16). This appearance is distinct from the typical erosions seen in rheumatoid arthritis. Another form of arthritis, calcium pyrophosphate crystal deposition disease, is characterized radiographically by chondrocalcinosis, which corresponds to intra-articular deposition of calcium pyrophosphate dihydrate crystals. When subtle, the fine linear and punctate calcifications in the hyaline cartilage and fibrocartilage may be detected only with high resolution magnification techniques (Fig. 9–17). Advanced articular calcification (Fig. 9–18) will easily be recognized with conventional radiographic techniques.

Metabolic Disorders

Hyperparathyroidism. The radiographic assessment of osseous changes in hyperparathyroidism has undergone substantial modifications in recent

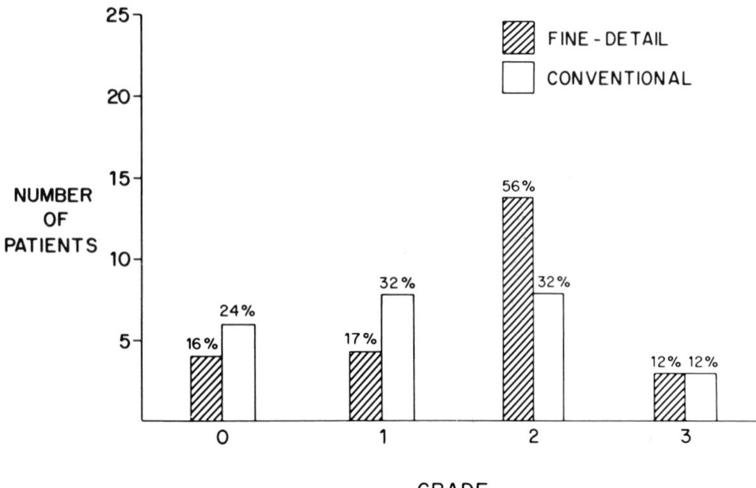

Figure 9–15. Difference in the detection and grading of soft tissue swelling with fine-detail and conventional radiography. (From Mall JC, et al: Radiology 112:37, 1974.)

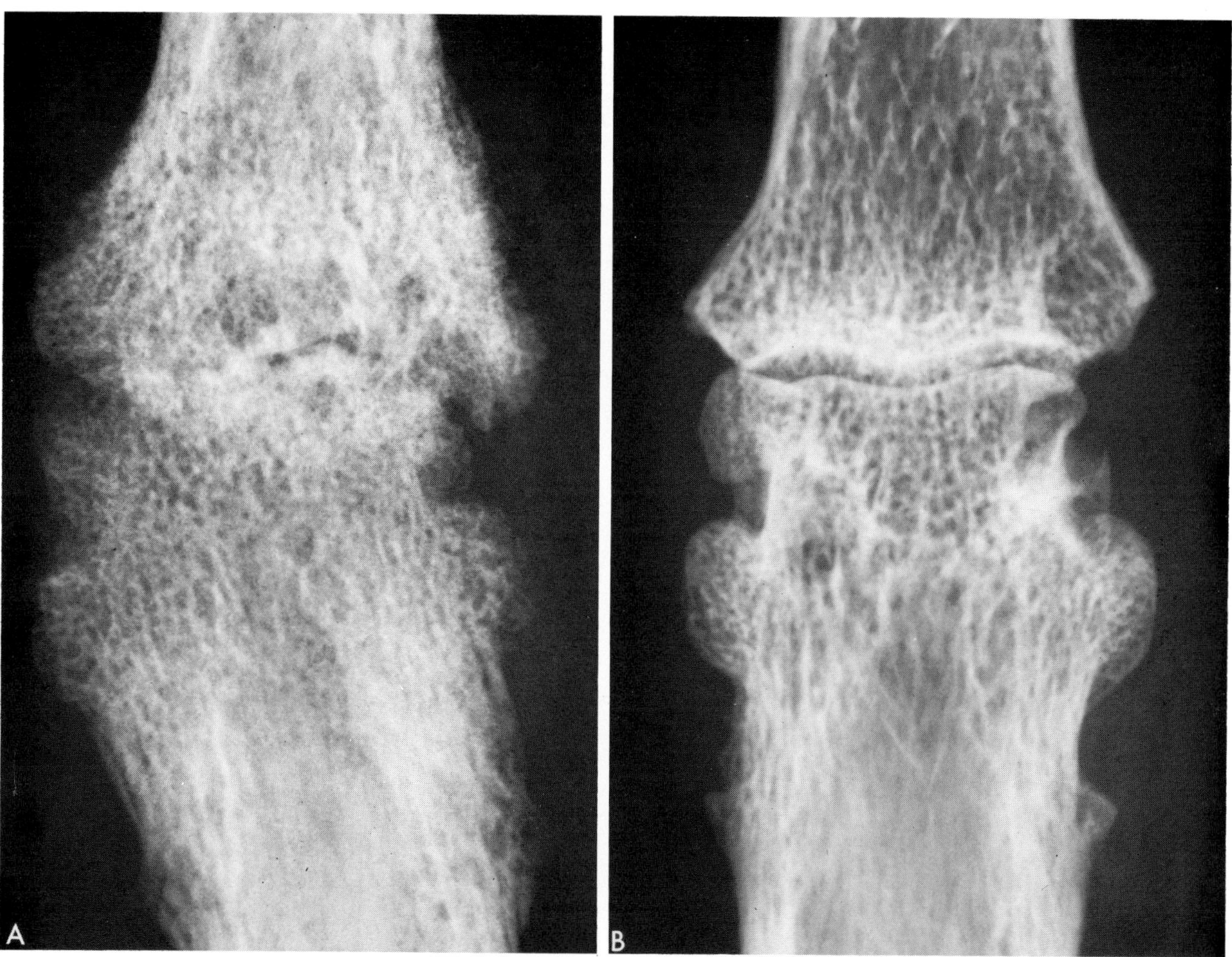

Figure 9–6. *Proliferative erosions and periostitis of psoriatic arthritis* **(A)** *differ in appearance from the well-defined erosions and reactive bone formation of gouty arthritis* **(B)**.

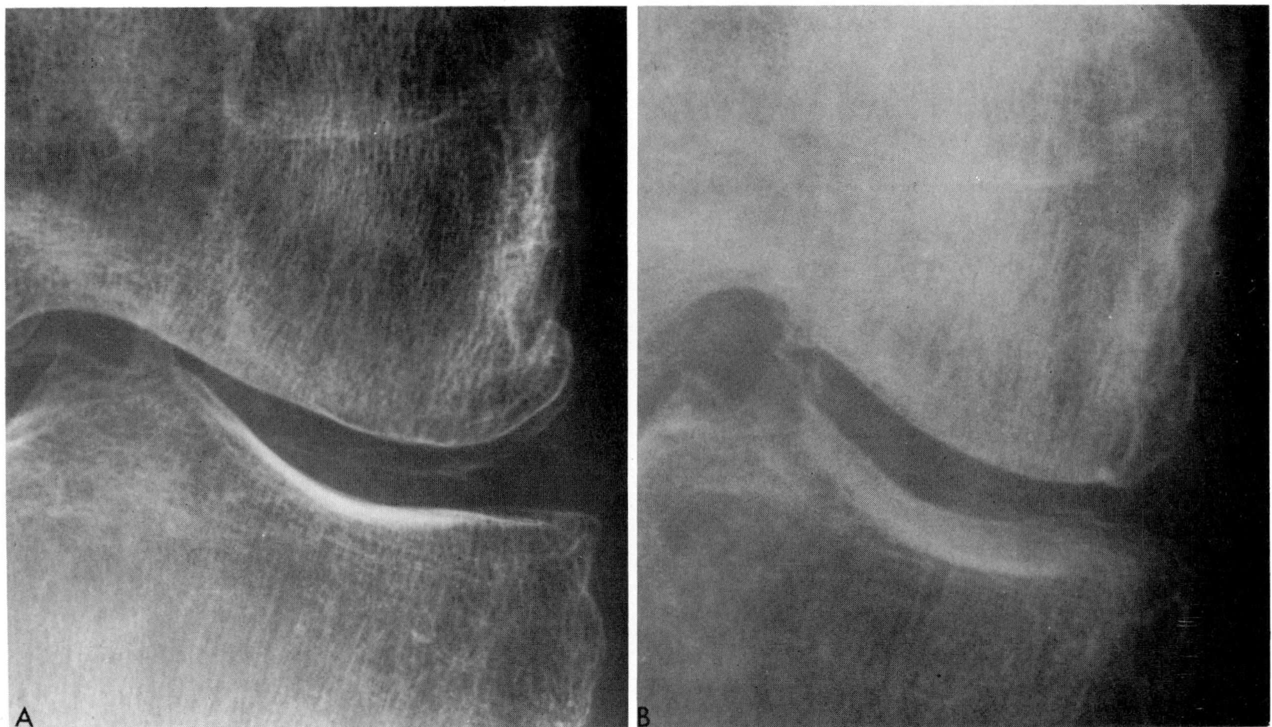

Figure 9–17. *Magnification* **(A)** *and conventional* **(B)** *views of the knee in a patient with pseudogout. Magnification view clearly shows fine linear calcification of the hyaline cartilage and fibrocartilage, diagnostic of calcium pyrophosphate crystal deposition disease. The conventional radiograph fails to reveal definite chondrocalcinosis.*

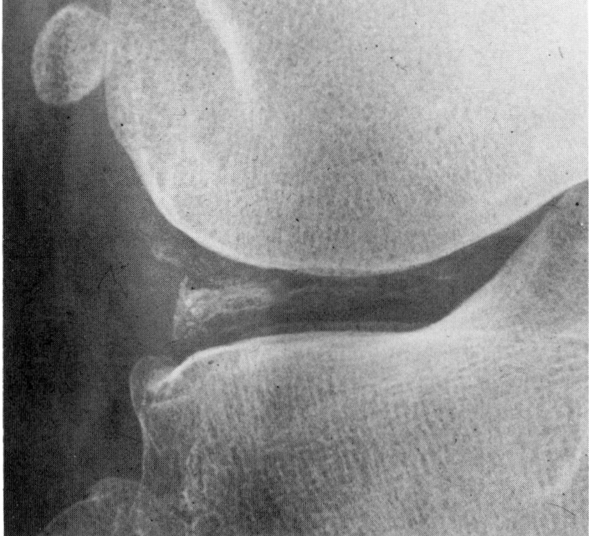

Figure 9–18. *Magnification radiograph of knee shows fine linear and punctate calcifications characteristic of calcium pyrophosphate dihydrate crystal deposition disease.*

years. The classic findings of advanced hyperparathyroid skeletal disease, with striking cortical erosions and cystic brown tumors, are rarely seen today.[16, 20, 46] This change probably reflects the earlier stage of detection[4] and the greater preponderance of benign chemical hyperparathyroidism.[23, 42] In a recent large study[20] of primary hyperparathyroidism, subperiosteal bone resorption limited to the phalanges was revealed by conventional radiography in only 7 of 87 patients (8 per cent). This experience contrasts with the incidence (and severity) of bony abnormalities in hyperparathyroid patients cited in the earlier classic roentgenologic reviews of Pugh,[41] who reported a 33 per cent incidence in 1951, and of Steinbach and co-workers,[48] who reported an incidence of 23 per cent in 1961. For this reason, high resolution radiographic techniques were introduced to detect subtle resorptive changes in the peripheral skeleton.[20, 21, 38, 39, 52]

In a recent study[23] of 20 hyperparathyroid patients imaged by conventional radiography (detail screens) and industrial-film radiography with optical magnification, both subperiosteal and intracortical bone resorption was assessed.

With fine-detail radiography, diagnostic *subperiosteal bone resorption* was observed in 6 of 20 patients (30 per cent), all of whom appeared normal or showed only nonspecific osteopenia with conventional radiographs. Figure 9–19 shows a phalanx of a hyperparathyroid patient radiographed with fine-detail and conventional techniques. The fine-detail radiograph shows the minute skeletal structure and demonstrates clearly the irregular resorption of the outer cortical margins that is pathognomonic of hyperparathyroidism.[24, 41, 48]

Even with high resolution techniques, such subperiosteal bone resorption is being detected uncommonly in primary hyperparathyroidism while being encountered frequently in secondary hyperparathyroidism accompanying renal osteodystrophy. Figure 9–20 shows the magnification radiograph of a knee of a child with chronic renal disease and suspected hyperparathyroid bone disease. The conventional radiograph was nondiagnostic, but the direct magnification film with superior image quality demonstrates definite subperiosteal resorption of the proximal medial metaphysis of the tibia as well as mild osteosclerosis of trabecular bone. The combination of findings is nearly pathognomonic of renal osteodystrophy.

When subperiosteal bone resorption becomes advanced, high resolution radiographic techniques are not necessary for detection. However, for monitoring the course of the disease or the response to therapy, magnification may be helpful. Figure 9–21 shows advanced subperiosteal bone resorption accompanying chronic renal disease. These radiographic findings as well as clinical and biochemical

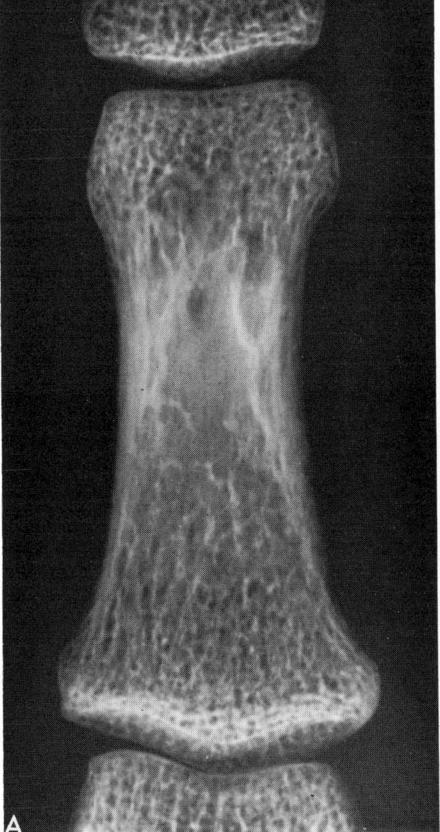

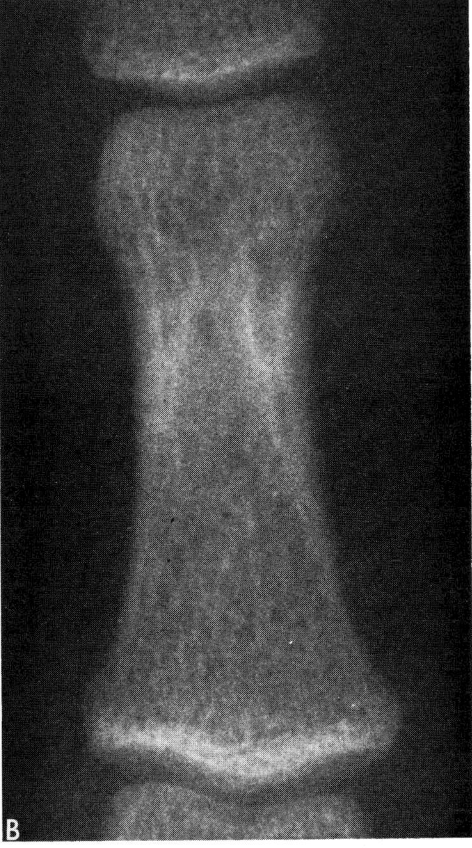

Figure 9–19. *Radiograph of a phalanx of a hyperparathyroid patient. Type M film* **(A)** *shows the irregular resorption of the outer cortical margin not detected in the detail screen-film system* **(B)**. *(From Genant HK, et al: Radiology 109:513, 1973.)*

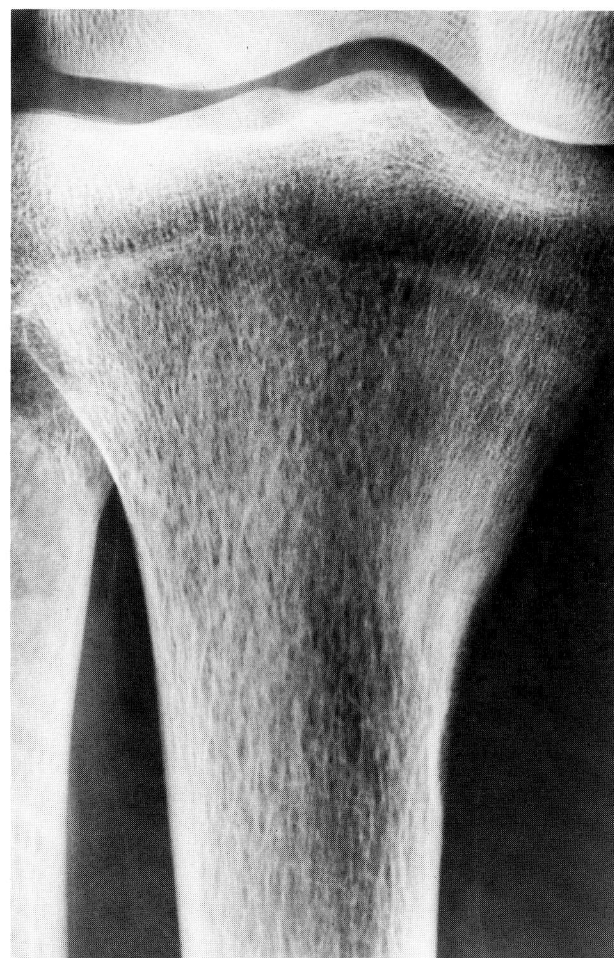

Figure 9–20. *Magnification radiograph of a knee of a child with chronic renal disease demonstrates definite subperiosteal resorption of the proximal medial metaphysis of the tibia, as well as mild osteosclerosis of trabecular bone, nearly pathognomonic of renal osteodystrophy.*

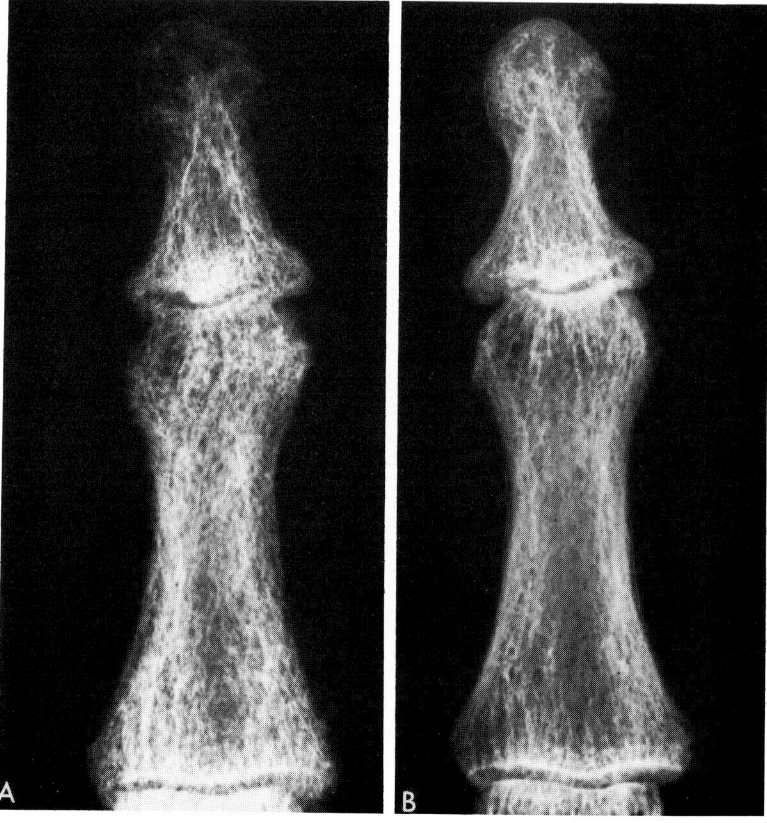

Figure 9–21. *Advanced subperiosteal bone resorption accompanying chronic renal disease* **(A)**. *Following parathyroidectomy, there was remarkable reconstitution of the cortex and healing of the subperiosteal bone resorption* **(B)**.

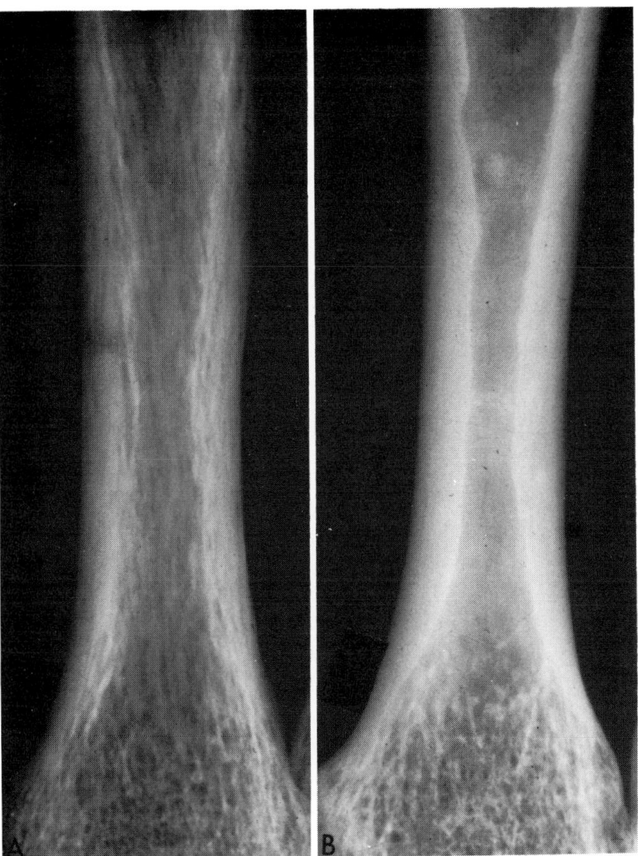

Figure 9–22. Radiographs of metacarpals of a hyperparathyroid (**A**) and of a normal (**B**) patient. Intracortical striation is excessive (grade 3) in **A**, compared with solid cortex (grade 0) in **B**. (From Genant HK, et al: Radiology 109:513, 1973.)

data may indicate the need for subtotal parathyroidectomy. Six months following this surgery, there was remarkable reconstitution of the cortex and healing of the subperiosteal bone resorption.

The second, more sensitive but less specific, finding in hyperparathyroidism is *cortical striation* or *tunneling* (Fig. 9–22). It corresponds histologically to widened haversian systems and resorptive spaces that result from excessive bone resorption in the hyperparathyroid state[14, 20, 39] and it is detected only on fine-detail radiographs unless extremely advanced. In the 20 hyperparathyroid patients[23] referred to previously, cortical striation was graded as 0 (none) to 3 (excessive), after the method of Meema and associates.[38, 39] A striation index was derived for each patient by averaging the grades for the second and third metacarpals of both hands.[23] The striation indices for the 20 hyperparathyroid patients and 50 controls are shown in Figure 9–23. The mean striation index of 1.81 for hyperparathyroid patients is significantly higher than the mean value of 0.49 for controls ($p<0.01$). The values for 15 of the 20 hyperparathyroid patients are more than 1 standard deviation (SD) above the normal mean.

Excessive cortical striation on fine-detail radiographs may be considered the most helpful manifestation in the detection of hyperparathyroidism. It is not a specific change, however, occurring in a variety of conditions with high-bone-turnover states, such as renal osteodystrophy, thyrotoxicosis, immobilization, reflex sympathetic dystrophy, osteomalacia, and rheumatoid arthritis.[53]

Additionally, the changes of increased intracortical tunneling are not limited to the small tubular bones of the hands but may be seen in the long bones as well. For example, Figure 9–24 shows radiographs of the left hip and femoral shaft in a patient who had sustained a fracture of the left hip 3 months earlier. The magnification view of the femur demonstrates the increased intracortical tunneling as well as aggressive resorption of the endosteal surface, findings indicative of an aggressive disuse osteoporosis.[14, 24, 30]

Infectious Disorders

The diagnosis of osteomyelitis or septic arthritis is generally made on the basis of clinical symptoms and findings since conventional radiography demonstrates characteristic features only later in the course. Occasionally, however, magnification radiography may be helpful in delineating subtle cortical destruction or periosteal new bone prior to its demonstration on conventional films. For example, a problem is frequently encountered in an elderly, osteoporotic patient who has ulceration of the soft

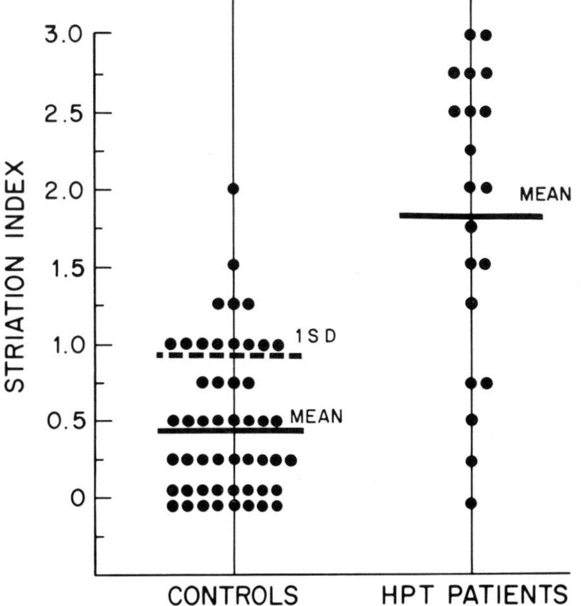

Figure 9–23. Striation indices for 50 controls (mean age, 47 years) and 20 hyperparathyroid (HPT) patients (mean age, 50 years). (From Genant HK, et al: In RB Mazess [Ed]: Proceedings of the International Conference on Bone Mineral Measurement. Chicago, October 12–13, 1973.)

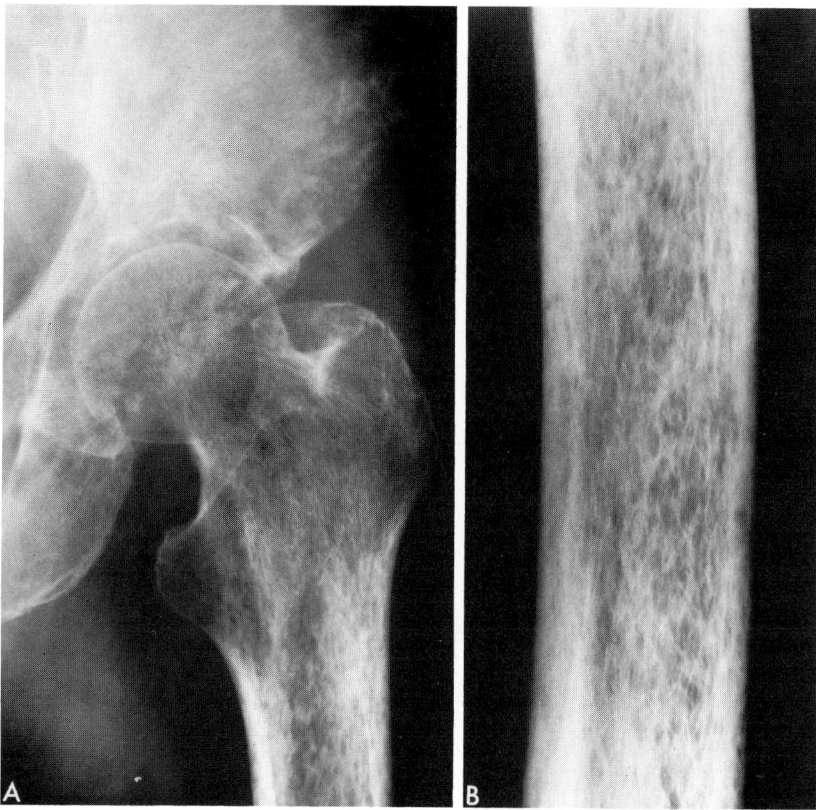

Figure 9–24. *Radiograph of the left hip and femoral shaft* **(A)** *in a patient who had sustained a pathologic fracture of the acetabulum 3 months earlier. The magnification view* **(B)** *of the femur demonstrates the increased intracortical tunneling as well as the extensive resorption of the endosteal surface, all indicative of an aggressive disuse osteoporosis.*

tissues of the foot related to diabetes or arterial insufficiency (Fig. 9–25). The diagnostic problem is to determine whether or not there is underlying osteomyelitis. In this setting, conventional radiography often fails to adequately visualize the bone margins due to the low inherent subject contrast of osteopenic bone. Magnification radiography, however, may clearly delineate the cortical margins and reveal irregular destruction of the outer cortical surfaces, thus permitting a specific diagnosis.

Similarly, Figure 9–26 demonstrates radiographs of the distal leg of an elderly patient with chronic venous stasis, skin ulcerations, and suspected active osteomyelitis. Both the magnification radiograph and the conventional contact radiograph demonstrate nonspecific solid periosteal new bone. With magnification, additional irregular, lacy new bone extending into the adjacent soft tissues can be seen, which supports the diagnosis of active osteomyelitis.

Finally, Figure 9–27 demonstrates radiographs from an elderly man who has had pain in the region of the symphysis for 2 months following a suprapubic prostatectomy. Both the magnification and the conventional radiographs demonstrate a widened symphysis pubis. Additionally, magnification shows an irregular lysis of the subchondral bone, which indicates the aggressive nature of this process and supports a diagnosis of infectious osteitis pubis. The superior visualization of the coccyx is also well demonstrated.

Neoplastic Disorders

Both primary and metastatic neoplasms of bone have been examined with magnification techniques.[22] These examinations are largely of the thick skeletal parts, such as ribs, pelvis, hips, spine, and femora and, therefore, direct radiographic magnification is employed. In some applications, conventional radiographs appear normal or equivocal, and magnification serves to delineate permeative, lytic destruction or subtle periosteal reaction. In other instances, conventional radiography readily demonstrates the presence of the lesion; however, the character or pattern of host response or aggressiveness is best determined by magnification. Frequently, direct magnification is initiated after a positive bone scan and conventional radiographs provide inconclusive results. Serial assessment of the progression of the neoplasm or the response to therapy is also improved by magnification.

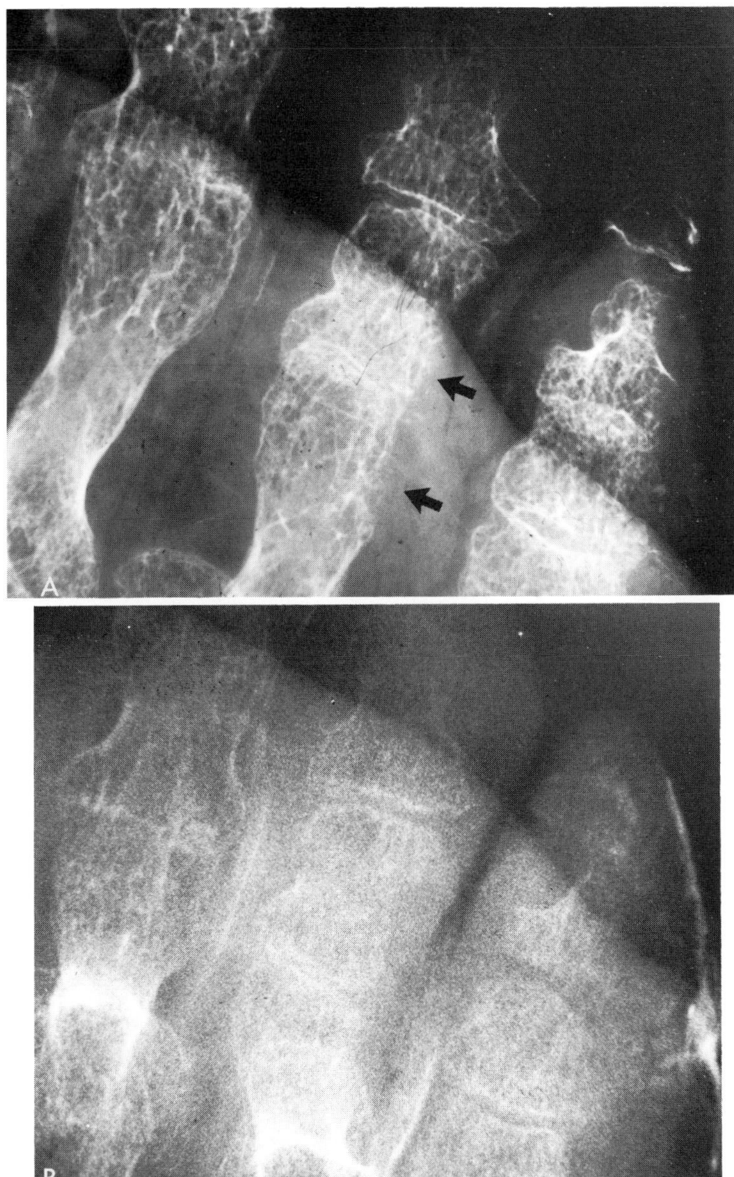

Figure 9–25. *Distal aspect of foot of diabetic patient with suspected osteomyelitis.* **A,** *Cortical destruction of the lateral aspects of the middle and proximal phalanges of the fourth digit (arrows) is readily detected with the Type M technique.* **B,** *The cortical outlines are inadequately delineated for accurate interpretation with the cardboard technique.*

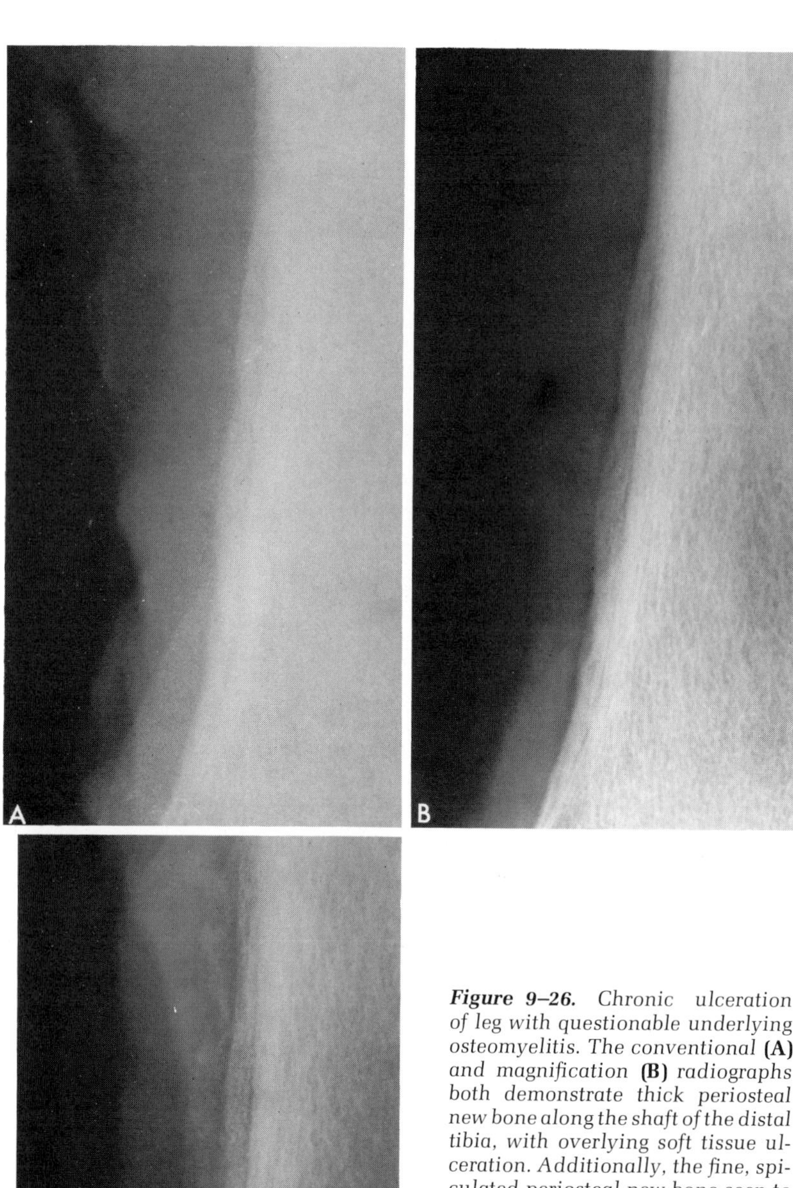

Figure 9–26. *Chronic ulceration of leg with questionable underlying osteomyelitis. The conventional* **(A)** *and magnification* **(B)** *radiographs both demonstrate thick periosteal new bone along the shaft of the distal tibia, with overlying soft tissue ulceration. Additionally, the fine, spiculated periosteal new bone seen to extend into the adjacent soft tissues in the magnification film indicates an evolving process and supports a diagnosis of active osteomyelitis. Serial magnification view* **(C)** *1 month later shows further progression of periosteal new bone, confirming the dynamic nature of the process. Such serial assessment is enhanced by magnification. (From Genant HK, et al: Radiology 123:47, 1977.)*

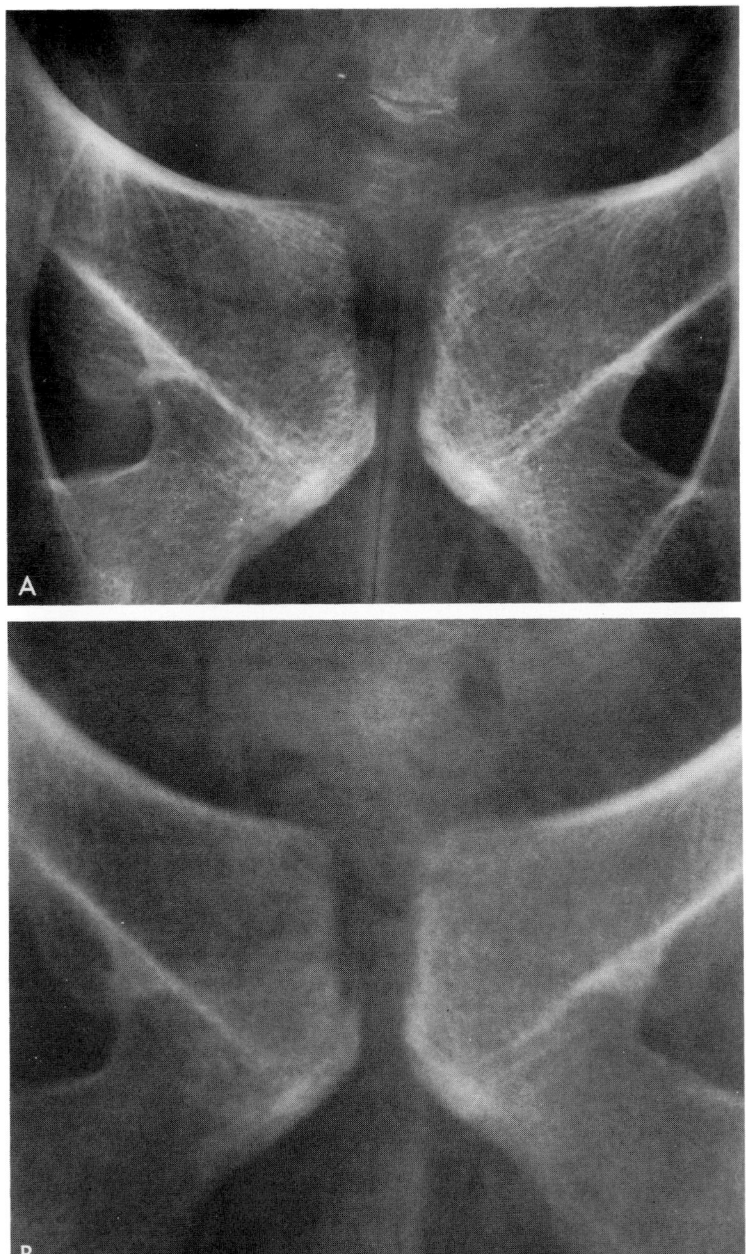

Figure 9–27. *The magnification* **(A)** *and the conventional radiographs* **(B)** *demonstrate widening of symphysis pubis. The magnification study, in addition, shows irregular destruction of the subchondral cortical line, producing a ragged, lace-like appearance. These features indicate an aggressive, evolving process and support the diagnosis of infectious osteitis pubis. (From Genant HK, et al: Radiology 123:47, 1977.)*

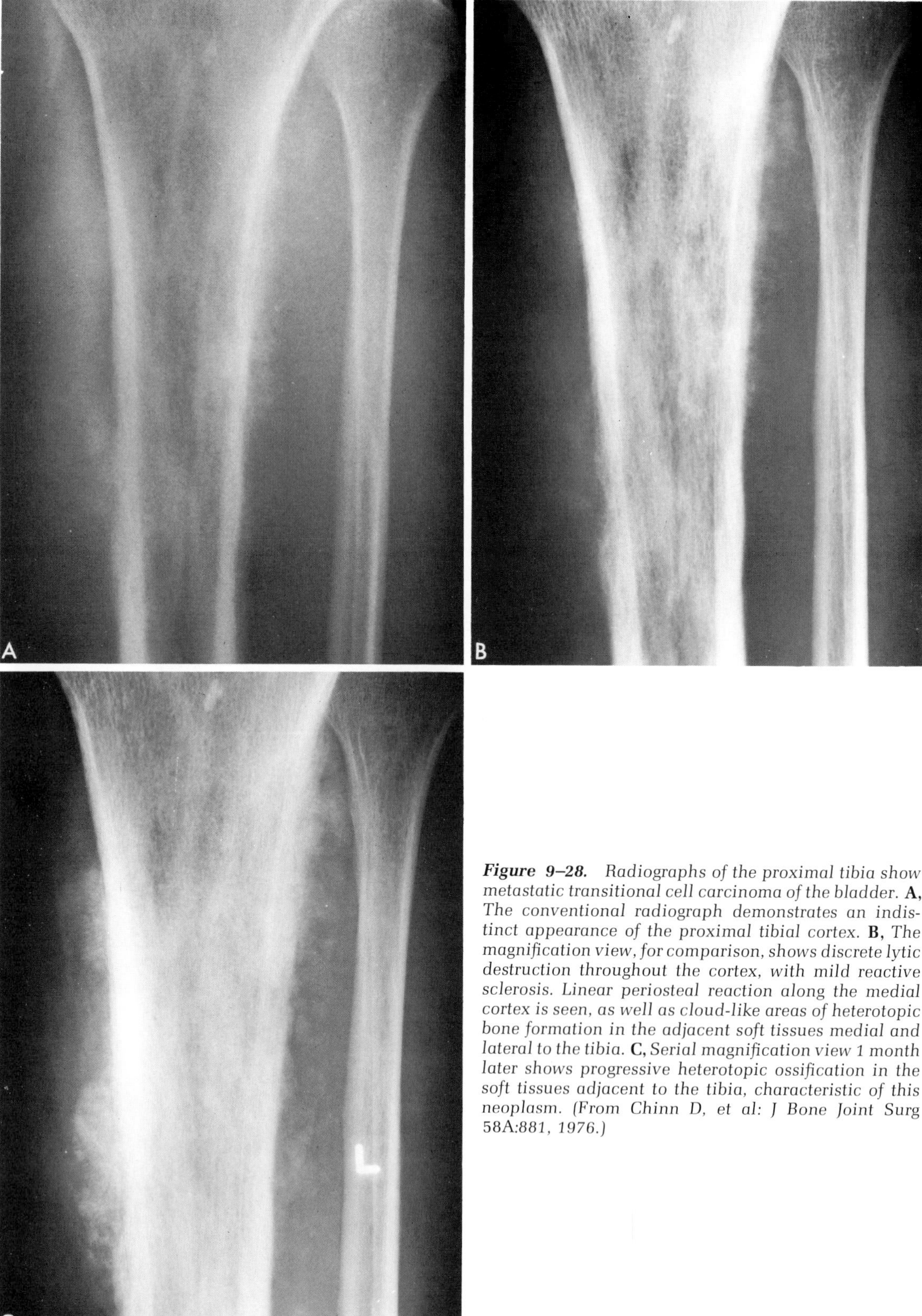

Figure 9–28. *Radiographs of the proximal tibia show metastatic transitional cell carcinoma of the bladder.* **A,** *The conventional radiograph demonstrates an indistinct appearance of the proximal tibial cortex.* **B,** *The magnification view, for comparison, shows discrete lytic destruction throughout the cortex, with mild reactive sclerosis. Linear periosteal reaction along the medial cortex is seen, as well as cloud-like areas of heterotopic bone formation in the adjacent soft tissues medial and lateral to the tibia.* **C,** *Serial magnification view 1 month later shows progressive heterotopic ossification in the soft tissues adjacent to the tibia, characteristic of this neoplasm. (From Chinn D, et al: J Bone Joint Surg 58A:881, 1976.)*

In Figure 9–28, the radiographs of the proximal tibia of a patient with metastatic transitional cell carcinoma of the bladder are shown. The conventional radiograph suggests destruction in the proximal tibia; however, the nature of the lesion is not clearly defined. The comparison magnification radiograph shows permeative destruction extending through both medial and lateral cortices associated with mild reactive sclerosis in the medullary space and considerable periosteal new bone. Additionally, there is ossification in the soft tissues adjacent to the tibia, which represents a rare feature of metastatic transitional cell carcinoma — namely, induction of heterotopic ossification.[7] These important features are difficult to define with conventional radiography. Also, a serial magnification radiograph taken one month later clearly demonstrates advancing heterotopic ossification in the soft tissues. Similar clarification by magnification of the pattern of bony destruction in cystic hemangiomatosis of the shoulder girdle is illustrated in Figure 9–29.

Figure 9–30 demonstrates radiographs of the forearm of a 4 year old child who presented with pain and swelling of the extremity. Permeative destruction of cortical bone, sclerosis of cancellous bone, and fine, laminated periosteal new bone are all depicted in the ulna. Only the gross features of this Ewing's sarcoma can be seen with the conventional contact radiograph. Additionally, a comparison of the industrial film technique and the direct magnification technique is shown, each radiograph displayed at equal size for visual comparison.. The two images are relatively comparable in quality; however, the direct magnification resulted in one fourth the radiation exposure required for the industrial film technique.[17]

The largest application of magnification for assessing metastatic disease has been in imaging the ribs. Figure 9–31 demonstrates radiographs from a woman who underwent a left mastectomy for breast carcinoma, and subsequently presented with pain and swelling of the lateral chest wall. The conventional chest radiograph demonstrates a soft tissue mass and rib destruction. The magnification radiograph shows to greater advantage the lytic destruction with expansion of a rib, the complete destruction of an adjacent rib, and the mixed lysis and sclerosis of a third rib. Although aiding in demon-

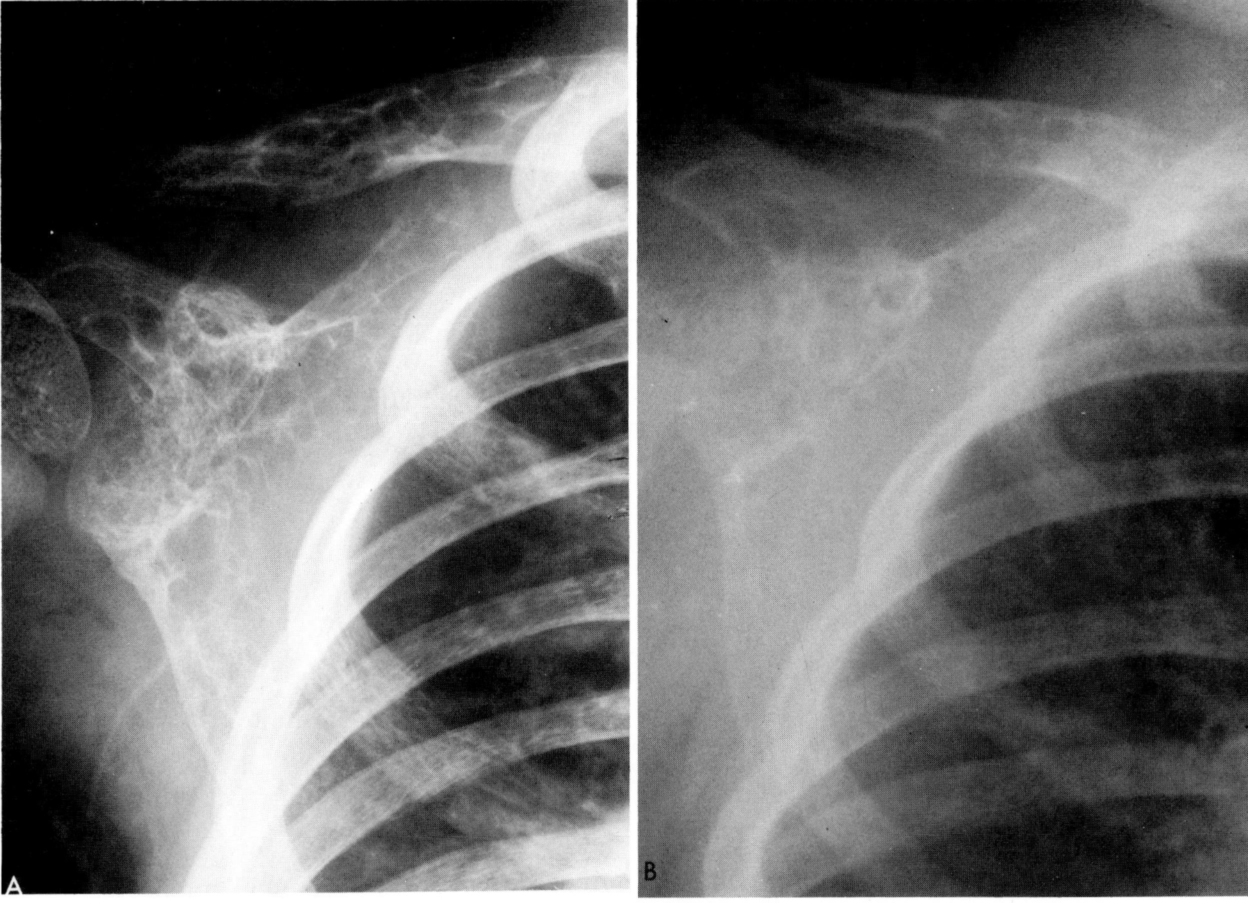

Figure 9–29. *Multiple well-defined cystic and lytic destructive lesions in the scapula and clavicle in a patient with hemangiomatosis of bone. Although large lesions are seen with both magnification and conventional techniques, evaluation of extent of involvement is far superior in the magnification view* **(A)**.

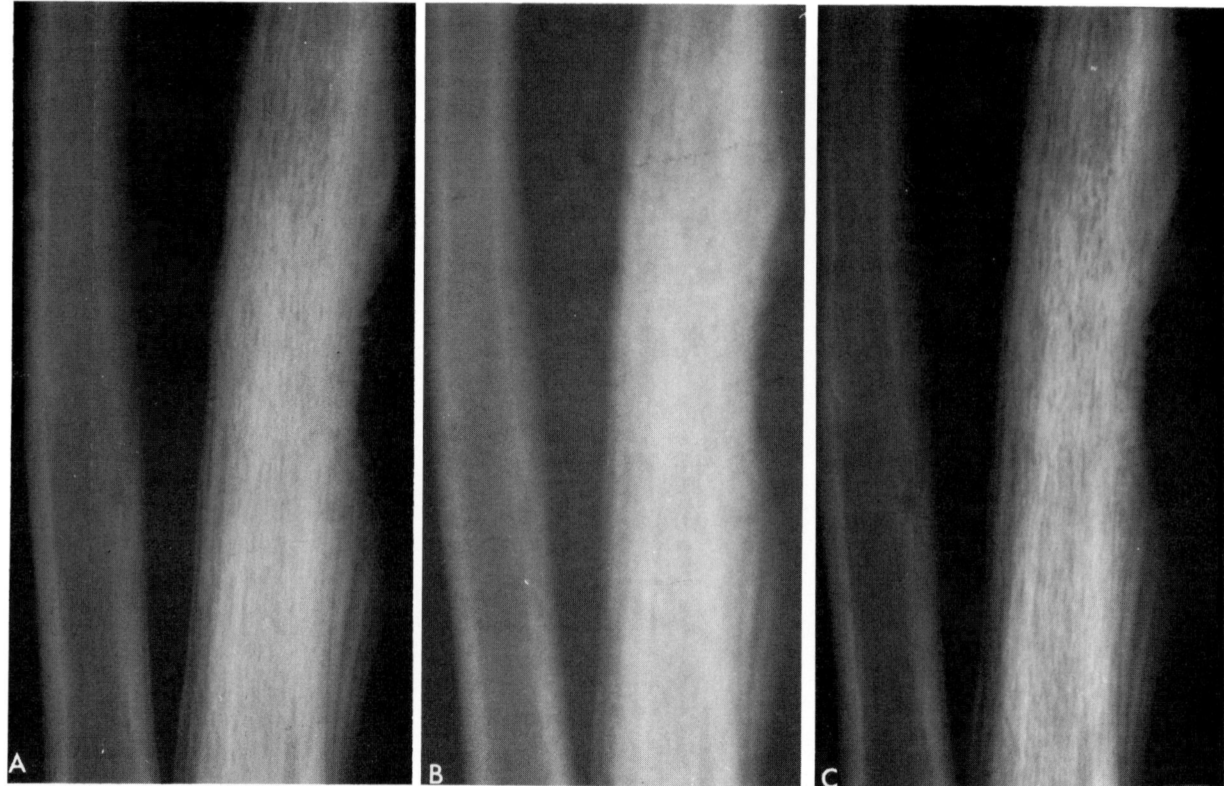

Figure 9–30. *The forearm of a child with Ewing's sarcoma has been radiographed with Type M* **(A)**, *contact RP-Detail* **(B)**, *and 4 × magnification* **(C)** *techniques. The superior imaging performances in* **A** *and* **C** *may permit improved assessment of the aggressiveness of a neoplasm and better delineation of its geographic extent. Type M and 4 × magnification techniques demonstrate similar resolution, contrast, and noise, yet the latter required approximately one fourth the amount of radiation exposure to the patient.*

strating these varied features of metastatic disease, magnification does not provide any new, essential information in this case.

Traumatic Disorders

Magnification radiography has had more limited application in the evaluation of trauma, since the detection of fractures by conventional radiography is generally adequate. Figure 9–32 demonstrates magnification and conventional radiographs of a patient with an oblique fracture of the proximal phalanx of the fifth toe. The fracture can be seen with both techniques, although more clearly with magnification. In this instance, magnification does not provide additional useful information. Occasionally, however, it may be helpful in delineating and defining subtle fractures.

Dysplasias

Magnification techniques have not been found useful in the majority of patients with bone dysplasias. The radiographic findings in these cases are generally advanced and encompass multiple foci and broad anatomic regions. Although high-resolution radiography favorably displays the altered osseous structures, it does not provide new or essential information.

SUMMARY

In Table 9–1, the relative clinical value of magnification compared with conventional radiography for skeletal applications is presented qualitatively. It is based upon our experience with over 25,000 cases in which magnification has been used. For most areas in which magnification (optical or geometric) proves useful, subtle abnormalities of clinical importance are present at bone surfaces or at host-lesion interfaces. This is particularly true for arthritis and metabolic and infectious disorders of bone. In additional instances, serial assessment of the progression of disease or response to therapy is enhanced by magnification. When gross abnormalities are present, as in most instances of trauma and bone dysplasia, the

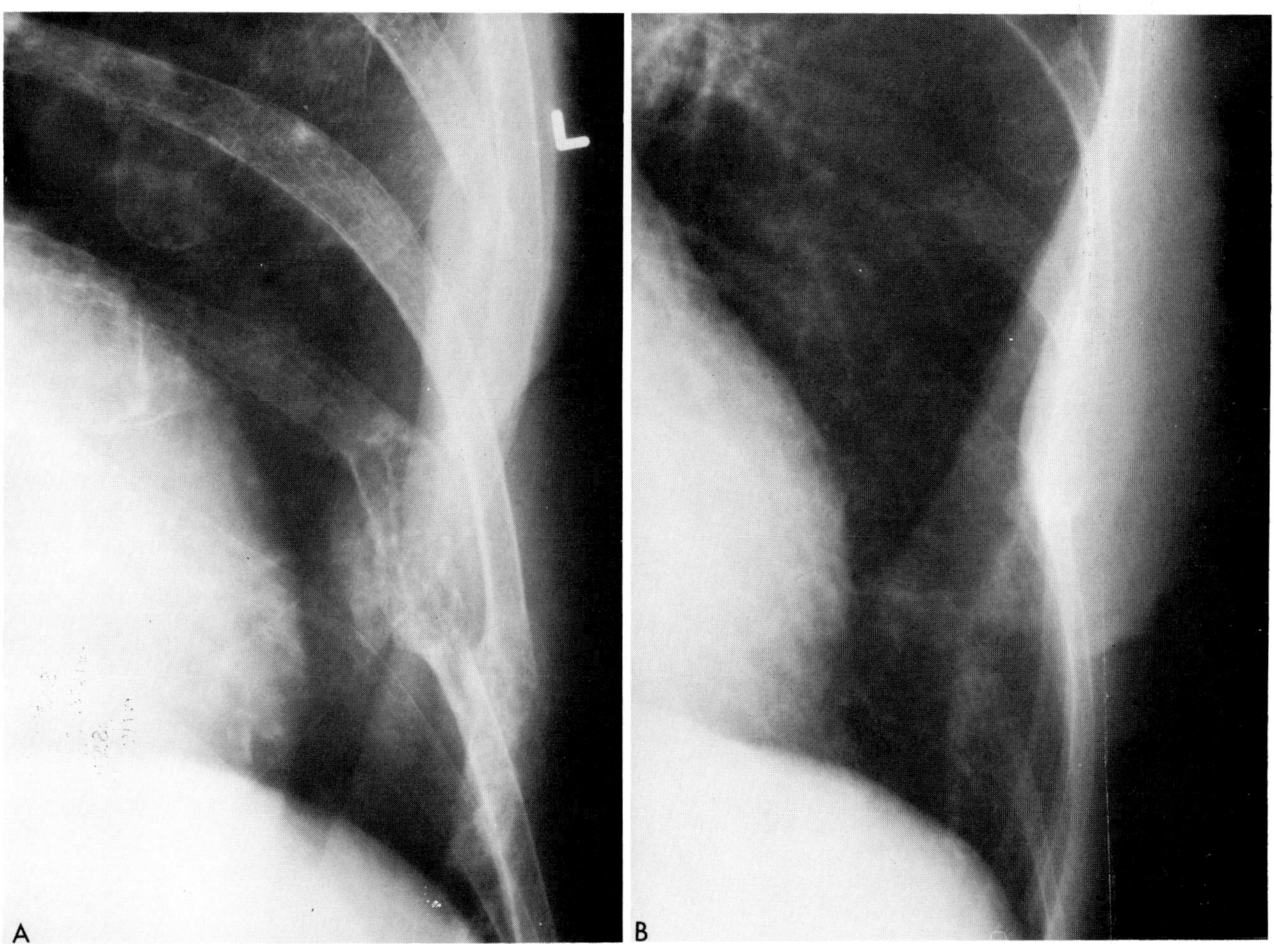

Figure 9–31. *Metastatic carcinoma of breast producing mixed lytic and sclerotic osseous destruction, as well as expansion of bone. Direct magnification technique* **(A)** *is used frequently when rib lesions are suspected on conventional radiography of chest. Conventional radiograph of chest* **(B)** *shows lateral soft tissue mass and rib destruction; however, the extent of involvement is not well defined.*

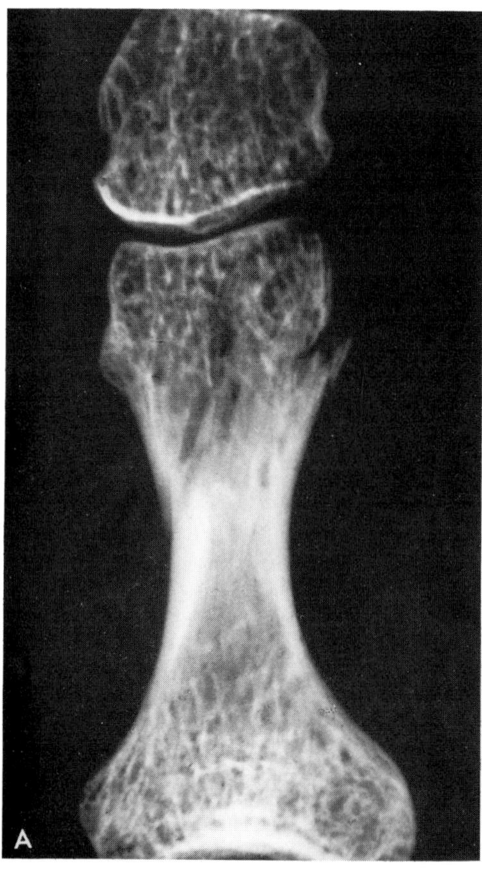

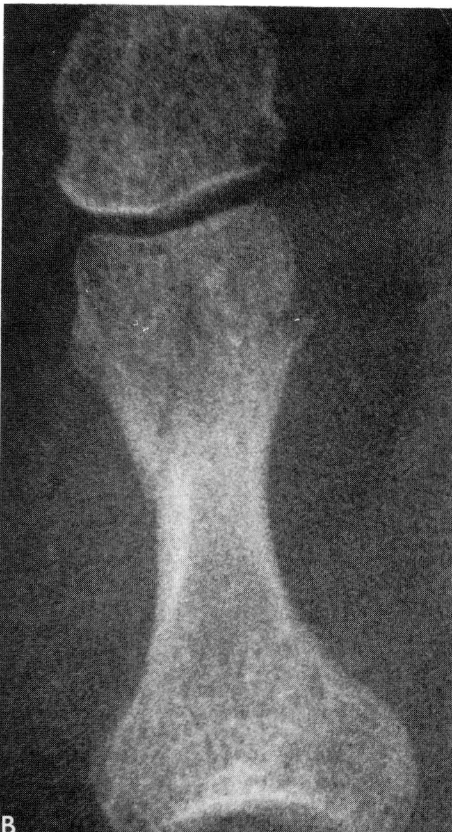

Figure 9–32. *Oblique fracture of the proximal phalanx of the left foot. Although the Type M technique* **(A)** *demonstrates the fracture more clearly, it does not provide additional useful information over that of the cardboard technique* **(B)**.

findings are obvious on conventional radiography, and magnification is not necessary. Thus, the magnification techniques appear to provide important diagnostic information, depending upon the anatomic part that is studied and the clinical question that is posed. It is also apparent that the demonstration of subtle skeletal abnormalities to clinical colleagues for educational purposes is greatly enhanced by magnification radiography. The important and characteristic features of specific skeletal disorders can be clearly delineated and correlated with known clinical, biochemical, and pathologic data. Similarly, the increased sensitivity of magnification may be useful for clinical investigation, in which careful serial assessment of disease and therapeutic response is monitored and recorded.

From dosimetry measurements, it is apparent that relatively high radiation doses result from magnification techniques. For this reason and because of the somewhat greater technical difficulty of performing the examination, magnification is recommended as a selective procedure. Such selection may be based upon analysis of the clinical history and suspected diagnosis, or may be in response to the inadequacies of conventional radiography. When employed in this manner, magnification radiography may be an important tool in the diagnostic study of skeletal diseases.

Table 9–1
RELATIVE VALUE OF MAGNIFICATION

Disorder	Not Helpful	Helpful	Essential
Trauma	X	X	
Dysplasia	X		
Arthritis		X	X
Metabolic Disorders		X	X
Infection		X	X
Neoplasm	X	X	

REFERENCES

1. Ayakawa, Y.: Optimal magnification ratio of direct macroradiography in high magnification. Modulation transfer function study on system combined with intensifying screen-film and object. Nagoya J Med Sci *34*:227, 1972.
2. Berens DL, Lin RK: Roentgen Diagnosis of Rheumatoid Arthritis. Springfield, Ill, Charles C Thomas, Publisher, 1969.
3. Bookstein JJ, Powell TJ: Short-target-film rotating-grid magnification. Comparison with air-gap magnification. Radiology *104*:399, 1972.
4. Boonstra CE, Jackson CE: Hyperparathyroidism detected by routine serum calcium analysis: Prevalence in a clinic population. Ann Intern Med *63*:468, 1964.
5. Buchanan RA, Finkelstein SI, Wickersheim KA: X-ray exposure reduc-

tion using rare-earth oxysulfide intensifying screens. Radiology *105*:185, 1972.

6. Campbell FW, Kulikowski JJ, Levinson J: The effect of orientation on the visual resolution of gratings. J Physiol (Lond) *187*:427, 1966.
7. Chinn D, Genant HK, Quivey J, Carlsson AM: Heterotopic bone formation in metastatic tumor from transitional cell carcinoma of the urinary bladder: A case report. J Bone Joint Surg *58A*:881, 1976.
8. Doi K, Genant HK, Rossmann K: Comparison of image quality obtained with optical and radiographic magnification techniques in fine-detail skeletal radiography: Effect of object thickness. Radiology *118*:189, 1976.
9. Doi K, Genant HK, Rossmann K: Effect of geometric unsharpness upon image quality in fine-detail skeletal radiography. Radiology *113*:723, 1974.
10. Doi K, Rossmann K: Measurements of optical and noise properties of screen-film systems in radiography. *In* Proceedings of the Symposium on Application of Optical Instrumentation in Medicine. Vol 56. Bellingham, Washington, Society of Photo-Optical Instrumentation Engineers, 1975, p. 45.
11. Doi K, Fromes B, Rossmann L: A new device for accurate measurement of the x-ray intensity distribution of x-ray tube focal spots. Med Phys *2*:268, 1975.
12. Doi K, Genant HK, Rossmann K: Effect of film graininess and geometric unsharpness on image quality in fine-detail skeletal radiography. Invest Radiol *10*:35, 1975.
13. Doi K, Imhof H: Noise reduction by radiographic magnification. Radiology *122*:479, 1977.
14. Duncan H: Cortical porosis: A morphological evaluation. *In* Z Jaworski (Ed): Proceedings of the First Workshop on Bone Morphometry. Ottawa, Ontario, University of Ottawa Press, 1976, p. 78.
15. Fletcher DE, Rowley KA: Radiographic enlargements in diagnostic radiology. Br J Radiol *24*:598, 1951.
16. Forland M, Strandjord NM, Paloyan E, Cox A: Bone density studies in primary hyperparathyroidism. Arch Intern Med *122*:236, 1968.
17. Genant HK, Doi K, Mall JC: Optical versus radiographic magnification for fine-detail skeletal radiography. Invest Radiol *10*:160, 1975.
18. Genant HK, Doi K, Mall JC: Comparison of non-screen techniques (medical vs. industrial film) for fine-detail skeletal radiography. Invest Radiol *11*:486, 1976.
19. Genant HK, Doi K, Mall JC, Sickles EA: Direct radiographic magnification for skeletal radiology. An assessment of image quality and clinical application. Radiology *123*:47, 1977.
20. Genant HK, Heck LL, Lanzl LH, Rossmann K, Vander Horst J, Paloyan E: Primary hyperparathyroidism: Comprehensive study of clinical, biochemical and radiographic manifestations. Radiology *109*:513, 1973.
21. Genant HK, Doi K, Rossmann K, Williams JR: Fine-detail radiography — theoretical and practical considerations. *In* Z Jaworski (Ed): Proceedings of the First International Workshop on Bone Morphometry. Ottawa, Ontario, University of Ottawa Press, 1976, p. 63.
22. Genant HK, Doi K: High-resolution radiographic techniques for the detection and study of skeletal neoplasms. *In* Encyclopedia of Medical Radiology. Vol 6, Bone Tumors. New York, Springer-Verlag, 1977, p. 677.
23. Genant HK, Vander Horst J, Lanzl LH, Mall JC, Doi K: Skeletal demineralization in primary hyperparathyroidism. *In* RB Mazess (Ed): Proceedings of the International Conference on Bone Mineral Measurement. Washington, D.C., National Institute of Arthritis, Metabolism, and Digestive Diseases, 1973, p. 177.
24. Genant HK, Kozin F, Bekerman C, McCarty DJ, Sims J: Reflex sympathetic dystrophy syndrome: A comprehensive analysis using fine-detail radiography, photon absorptiometry, and bone and joint scintigraphy. Radiology *117*:21, 1975.
25. Genant HK: Roentgenographic aspects of calcium pyrophosphate dihydrate crystal deposition disease (pseudogout). Arthritis Rheum *19*(Suppl 3):307, 1976.
26. Genant HK, Doi K: High-resolution skeletal radiography: Image quality and clinical applications. Curr Prob Diagn Radiol *7*:3, 1978.
27. Gordon SI, Greer RB, Weidner WA: Magnification roentgenographic technic in orthopedics. Clin. Orthop *91*:169, 1973.
28. Greenspan RH, Simon AL, Ricketts HJ, Rojas RH, Watson JC: In vivo magnification angiography. Invest Radiol *2*:419, 1967.
29. Haus AG, Rossmann K: X-ray sensitometer for screen-film combinations used in medical radiology. Radiology *94*:673, 1970.
30. Herrmann LG, Reineke HG, Caldwell JA: Post-traumatic painful osteoporosis: Clinical and roentgenological entity. Am J Roentgenol *47*:353, 1942.
31. Ishigaki T: First metatarsal-phalangeal joint of gout — macroroentgenographic examination in 6 times magnification. Nippon Acta Radiol *33*:839, 1973.
32. Jensen PS, Kliger AS: Early radiographic manifestations of secondary hyperparathyroidism associated with chronic renal disease. Radiology *125*:645, 1977.
33. Keating FR: The clinical problem of primary hyperparathyroidism. Med Clin North Am *54*:511, 1970.
34. Lowry EM, DePalma JJ: Sine-wave response of the visual system. The Mach phenomenon. J Opt Soc Am *51*:740, 1961.
35. Mall JC, Genant HK, Silcox DC, McCarty DJ: The efficacy of fine-detail radiography in the evaluation of patients with rheumatoid arthritis. Radiology *112*:37, 1974.
36. Mall JC, Genant HK, Rossmann K: Improved optical magnification for fine-detail radiography. Radiology *108*:707, 1973.
37. Martel W: The pattern of rheumatoid arthritis in the hand and wrist. Radiol Clin North Am *2*:221, 1964.
38. Meema HE, Schatz DL: Simple radiologic demonstration of cortical bone loss in thyrotoxicosis. Radiology *97*:9, 1970.
39. Meema HE, Meema S: Comparison of microradioscopic and morphometric findings in the hand bones with densitometric findings in the proximal radius in thyrotoxicosis and in renal osteodystrophy. Invest Radiol *7*:88, 1972.
40. Moore R, Krause D, Amplatz K: A flexible grid–air gap magnification technique. Radiology *104*:403, 1972.
41. Pugh DG: Subperiosteal resorption of bone: Roentgenologic manifestation of primary hyperparathyroidism and renal osteodystrophy. Am J Roentgenol *66*:577, 1951.
42. Purnell DC, Smith LH, Scholz DA, Elveback LR, Arnaud CD: Primary hyperparathyroidism: A prospective clinical study. Am J Med *50*:670, 1971.
43. Ropes MW, Bennett GA, Cobb S, Jacox R, Jessar RA: 1958 revision of diagnostic criteria for rheumatoid arthritis. Bull Rheum Dis *9*:175, 1958.
44. Rossmann K: Point spread function, line spread function and modulation transfer function. Radiology *93*:257, 1969.
45. Rossmann K: Image quality and patient exposure. Curr Probl Diagn Radiol *2*(2):3, 1972.
46. Sakuma S, Ayakawa Y, Fujita T: Macroroentgenography in twenty-fold magnification taken by means of 50μ focal spot x-ray tube and evaluation of its reduced image. Nippon Acta Radiol *30*:205, 1971.
47. Stargardt A, Angerstein W: Der optimale Abbildungsmassstab bei der direkten Röntgenvergrösserung. Fortschr Geb Roentgenstr Nuklearmed *123*:73, 1975.
48. Steinbach HL, Gordan GS, Eisenberg E, Crane JT, Silverman S, Goldman L: Primary hyperparathyroidism: A correlation of roentgen, clinical and pathologic features. Am J Roentgenol *86*:329, 1961.
49. Takahashi S, Sakuma S: Magnification Radiography. New York, Springer-Verlag, 1975.
50. Takahashi S, Sakuma S, Ayakawa Y, Maekoshi H, Ohara K: Radiation levels of macroradiography: Radiation exposure and image quality. Radiology *112*:709, 1974.
51. Sundaram MB, Brodeur AE, Burdge RE, Joyce PF, Riaz MA, Poling ER: The clinical value of direct magnification radiography in orthopedics. Skel Radiol *3*:85, 1978.
52. Weiss A: A technique for demonstrating fine detail in bones of the hands. Clin Radiol *23*:185, 1972.
53. Wilson JS, Genant HK: In vivo assessment of bone metabolism using the cortical striation index. Invest Radiol *14*:131, 1979.

LOW KILOVOLT RADIOGRAPHY

by Erich Fischer, M.D.

10

PHYSICAL PRINCIPLES

Soft tissue radiography of the extremities is based upon the same physical and technical principles as mammography. For the extremities as well, the usable voltage range is from 25 to 35 kilovolts (KV), since it is only this radiation range that will result in large differences in film blackening and greater contrast between bone (calcium), water-equivalent tissue, and fat.[1] Differences in tissue densities are prerequisites for detailed differentiation of bones, calcifications, and soft tissues. The transition from 30 KV to 20 KV almost doubles the contrast,[2] although at 20 KV the transmittance of most tissue layers is markedly reduced; for example, the transmittance for a 5 cm water layer is 2.7 per cent at 30 KV and is 0.17 per cent at 20 KV, and for a 5 cm thick lipid layer is 7.5 per cent and 1.2 per cent respectively.[3]

This low energy x-ray spectrum necessary for contrast enhancement can be favorably selected for the range of 18 to 20 KV by using a molybdenum target and molybdenum filter because of the K-alpha edge produced by molybdenum at 17.5 KV.[4] Contrast differences obtainable with this spectrum are greater than those with a tungsten target and aluminum filter.[2, 5, 6]

The energy spectrum of a tungsten anode with aluminum or molybdenum filters is more suitable for penetrating the bones of the hands and feet, but contrast between fatty tissue and water-equivalent tissue is reduced to such a point that, for visual perception, important details are substantially lost — e.g., signs of incipient or moderate edema.[7]

The radiation obtained by selective molybdenum filtration is polychromatic and has particular spectral ranges, each with distinctive contrast and characteristic patient exposure. For clarity in clinical usage, contrast and exposure have been calculated relative to each other for each of these spectral ranges, and the integrated value is listed as a "quality factor."[3] Accordingly, the optimum for both contrast and radiation exposure of a water layer of 2.5 cm would be expected to be in the range of 28 to 30 KV, which coincides with clinical experience in soft tissue radiography of the extremities.

For low KV radiation to be released at all, the exit window of tubes used in soft tissue radiography must be made of ultrathin glass or of beryllium to keep intrinsic filtration to a minimum.

HISTORY

The principal goal in using low kilovoltage for radiography of the extremities is to improve the diagnostic evaluation of soft tissues. However, soft tissue radiography has been done with conventional techniques for a long time with quite remarkable results. The descriptions of the soft tissue components were first published as follows: subcutaneous vessels, 1913[8]; periarticular soft tissue analysis of large joints, 1936[9, 10]; edema in skin and subcutaneous tissue, 1944[11]; engorgement of the capsule of the ankle joint, 1952[12]; and engorgement of the capsule of the elbow joint, 1954.[13]

Low KV radiography, in the strict sense of the term (employing voltages below 35 KV), was introduced in 1951 with radiographs done with an apparatus designed for dermatologic therapy, mainly in cases of dermatologic interest.[14] In 1957, using 32.5 KV radiation, small capsular distentions in the finger joints in patients with rheumatoid arthritis were first demonstrated.[15] However, only when mammography machines, equipped with molybdenum targets and molybdenum filters, were used for the examination of the extremities was a further improvement in low KV diagnostic capability possible. The very first publication describing this technique in the investigation of the extremities demonstrated numerous applications.[16] A further refinement was achieved by devising more useful views to demonstrate the hand[17, 18] and the ankle[19] for soft tissue detail of the retrocalcaneal bursa. With these improvements, small foreign bodies of low opacity[20] and minute calcifications were initially demonstrated in 1973.[16, 21]

Low KV radiography has contributed to the improved evaluation not only of soft tissues but also of thin bones. Since the early 1970s, low KV radiographs have been used to monitor skeletal changes in patients on chronic hemodialysis[16, 22] or on anticonvulsive chemotherapy.[23] Discrete osseous changes in rheumatoid arthritis and its variants have been demonstrated best with multiple views of the hands and feet.[16, 18]

METHODS AND TECHNIQUES

Low KV radiographs are produced by x-ray tubes with an ultrathin exit window and a tungsten anode,[24] by normal mammography machines with a molybdenum anode and molybdenum filter,[16, 23, 25] or by mammography machines modified to suit the needs of extremity radiography.[18]

"Immersion technique" refers to low KV radiography of the entire hand immersed in a 2.5 cm deep layer of a 1:1 water-ethanol solution. Compared with "dry" low KV radiography, this technique improves the recognizable detail of the skin and some subcutaneous structures.[26] Since the uniformly deep liquid layer equalizes the differences in thickness of the normally tapering fingers, all the small joints of the fingers can be penetrated properly in a single radiograph. But when the thickness of the part to be examined exceeds 2.5 cm, as in the case of the wrist, these differences in object thickness are no longer compensated for and the modulation transfer function (MTF) deteriorates, with loss of detail. A further disadvantage of the immersion technique is that the oblique views of the hand and wrist necessary in the early evaluation of rheumatoid arthritis, osteoarthritis, and tenosynovitis cannot be performed in a bath of only 2.5 cm.

In contrast, "dry" technique low KV radiography of the hands and feet in three views offers the most comprehensive visualization of the changes in the soft tissues as well as in the bones.[18, 27] For low KV films of the extremities, precise and reproducible positioning is mandatory. The exposure must be adjusted individually, according to the clinical problem and to the variations in patient size. Therefore, a separate exposure will have to be obtained for the digits of the hand to include the metacarpophalangeal (MCP) joints and a second exposure for the joints of the wrist to include the metacarpals. For comparison, views of the contralateral extremity must be taken in exactly the same positions. The following rules for positioning for low KV radiographs have proved useful.

Three-View Examination of the Hand and Foot

Fingers. The extended fingers are spread moderately so that in the oblique projections the soft tissues and bones will show the least possible overlap. The area to be radiographed extends from the fingertips to the midshaft of the metacarpals. One film is obtained in a true posteroanterior (PA) (orthogonal) position; two oblique films are taken in PA projection with the radial or ulnar aspects of the fingers elevated 25 degrees relative to the direction of the central beam of the x-ray.

Because the radiation tube and film support assembly are rigidly interconnected by a C-arm in commercially available low KV machines, the two oblique views are obtained by using a wedge or an adjustable angular support device to hold the film and support the hand. The C-arm is then rotated so that the film and the hand are in a horizontal position, resulting in an oblique tube angulation. An additional benefit of this technique is that the hand is resting in a comfortable position during exposure.

For the fingers, the 25 degree oblique projection is the most advantageous compromise, combining a minimum of overlap with a maximum of information gained from the osseous structures, joint capsules, extensor tendons, tendon sheaths, and skin and subcutaneous tissues. This is especially true for the proximal phalanges and the MCP joints. The thumb is included to the extent permitted by film size and the necessary slight abduction. Depending on the clinical findings, additional films of the thumb in the true PA and lateral views may be necessary. For the fingers, a film size of 13 × 18 cm or 8 × 10 in usually suffices.

Wrist. The three projections used in examining the wrist provide a quite comprehensive visualization of the bones and soft tissues of the wrist, despite the complex anatomy. In the first view, the hand and wrist are in true PA projection, with the hand in slight ulnar deviation, so that the radius and second metacarpal align in a straight line. Even slight radial deviation may produce apparent thickening of the tendon sheaths and joint capsules on the radial side owing to their relaxation and thus may mimic pathologic engorgement. The second view is in the anteroposterior (AP) projection, with the radial aspect of the hand elevated 25 degrees. The third view is a straight, true lateral, radioulnar projection.

Because of the common and very early involvement of the pisiform-triquetral joint in rheumatoid arthritis and the frequently encountered painful calcifications on the volar aspect of the pisiform, an additional AP oblique view with the radial aspect of the hand angulated as much as 50 degrees may be necessary. The area to be taken is the direct extension of that for the fingers. Frequently, additional information can be gained due to the fact that the MCP region is included in both sets of films. Proximally, the proximal end of the tendon sheaths and the proximal extension of the adipose layer anterior to the pronator quadratus must be included.

Generally, a 13 × 18 cm or 8 × 10 in film size is adequate.

Forefoot. The forefeet radiographs are taken in three views, corresponding to those of the fingers. The area to be included extends proximally to the distal third of the fifth metatarsal.

Horizontal Beam Lateral View of the Ankle

For the tibiofibular lateral view, the foot is in midposition and rotated slightly inward so that the fibula is projected on the middle third of the tibia. This slight inward rotation is necessary for the anterior surface of the Achilles tendon to be seen exactly in profile. Radiographs not precisely positioned will produce an unsharpness of the anterior margin of the Achilles tendon that mimics a pathologic finding and prohibits measuring of the thickness of the tendon.

In addition, this lateral view shows the capsule of the tibiotalar joint, the tendons and sheaths of the extensor muscles anteriorly, and the tendon sheaths of the fibular and tibial flexor muscles dorsal to the tibia. By changing the degrees of foot rotation, the tendon sheaths described above can be separated and delineated as they move in relation to each other.

Slight enlargements of the retrocalcaneal bursa are demonstrable on a lateral view in maximal plantar flexion.[19] Normally, in this position the fatty tissue between the flexor muscles and the Achilles tendon will extend as a narrow pointed wedge between the calcaneal tubercle and the Achilles tendon to the insertion of the latter. Slight enlargements of the bursa prohibit the extension or widening of this fatty wedge.

The Achilles tendon remains smoothly curved in active flexion; however, in passive flexion it becomes undulate. This normal undulation is reduced in local rigidity of the tendon from various causes or in slight thickening due to edema, even though this may be within normal range.

An 18 × 24 cm or an 8 × 10 in film is adequate.

Horizontal Beam Lateral View of the Knee

Because the knee is quite thick, only the anterior soft tissues — i.e. the patellar ligament, the infrapatellar fat pad, and the quadriceps tendon can be evaluated.

The patellar ligament radiograph is taken in tibiofibular lateral projection with slight inward rotation to render the ligament's anterior and posterior surfaces perpendicular to the film. This view is similar to that for the Achilles tendon. The quadriceps tendon appears as a straight soft tissue stripe of about the same width as the patellar ligament.

In the regions of the ankle and the knee joint, only soft tissue structures can be evaluated; the bones will not be penetrated adequately for diagnostic evaluation.

Other Regions

Low KV radiographs can be taken of any other region that can be sufficiently penetrated and positioned close to the film; however, this is seldom possible.

Correctly exposed films of the fingers, wrist, and forefoot will optimally depict all soft tissue structures and the thinner portions of the bones to show the important marginal osseous structures. Thicker and denser portions of the bones will not be sufficiently penetrated. However, for a precise evaluation of the bones, proper penetration can be achieved by increasing the milliampere-second (mas) value, by increasing KV, or by using a tungsten spectrum instead of the molybdenum spectrum. All of these measures will necessarily greatly impair or totally eliminate the possibility of distinguishing the soft tissues adequately.

SYNOPSIS OF SOFT TISSUE CHANGES

Soft Tissues of Water Density

On radiographs certain soft tissues are "of water density" and may be difficult to identify at times. The following changes are mainly to be found in the soft tissues of water density such as skin, tendon or ligament, tendon sheath, joint capsule, or muscle.

Thickened Soft Tissues. Normal dimensions for the listed soft tissues are given later in this chapter (see *Clinical Examples of Low KV Radiography*, page 351). The reasons for thickening are manifold. In the context of joint diseases the main causes are as follows:

1. *Skin:* Edema, scleroderma, acromegaly, myxedema.
2. *Tendons/ligaments:* Rheumatoid arthritis and its variants; damage due to stress; inclusions of cholesterol, urates, calcifications, or amyloid.
3. *Tendon sheaths and joint capsules:* Mechanical and inflammatory synovial irritation, synovial deposits, proliferation of certain cellular elements, such as reticulohistiocytes, and unknown causes, as in multiple epiphyseal dysplasia.

Narrowed Soft Tissues. Narrowing due to atrophy can be demonstrated only in the skin and muscles. Even slight degrees of atrophy are recognizable, particularly in the interosseous muscles and in the muscles of the calf because lipid structures between single muscles or muscle fibers become visible or increase in thickness before a measurable reduction in muscle mass is noted clinically.

Hazy Soft Tissue Margins. Normally, most soft tissues of water density have distinct contours if adjacent to a fat layer of adequate thickness. Such a layer may be physiologically absent or thin and divided by numerous fibers of connective tissue between the skin and periarticular soft tissues. On both sides of the finger joints, on the radial side of the proximal interphalangeal (PIP) and MCP joints of the index finger, and on the medial side of the metatarsophalangeal (MTP) and interphalangeal (IP) joints of the great toe, this may lead to a physiologic blurring of the marginal contour, rendering any precise measurement of thickness impossible.[18] Another cause of haziness of the exterior margin of the joint capsules is an increase in connective tissue in sites of unusual mechanical wear — e.g., the medial side of the joints of the great toe and the lateral side of the MTP joint of the small toe.[28]

Unsharpness of contours adjacent to fatty tissues not due to these causes or to hematomas is usually the result of a localized edema originating in water-equivalent tissue. This minimal unsharpness due to early edema is not appreciated in xeroradiography because of the effect of edge enhancement, which obscures this earliest of signs. Edema due to general disturbances of venous or lymphatic drainage causes alterations restricted mainly to areolar tissue, whereas the contours of water-equivalent tissues remain precise.

Embedded Calcifications, Other Opaque Foreign Bodies, and Fat Deposition. Due to the great contrast and increased resolution with low KV technique, even very small calcifications and opaque foreign bodies are easily recognizable. Minute calcifications are frequent, diverse, and, in many cases, reversible; these must not be overestimated as signs of generalized disturbances of mineral metabolism or generalized connective tissue diseases.

Fine, single, dust-like intracutaneous calcifications similar to comedo calcifications of the skin are to be found in all regions of the skin and have no pathologic meaning. Beginning in the third decade, stripe-like calcifications not related to any specific disease are frequently found within many periarticular soft tissues, especially those of the fingers. In the hands and feet tiny glass chips, metal dust, and particles of sand embedded by minor abrasions may commonly be encountered. If the bare foot touches the floor when preparing for the radiograph, minute grains of grit or sand may adhere to the skin and simulate a peculiar pattern of "soft tissue calcifications."

The replacement of muscle by fatty tissue has already been mentioned (see *Narrowed Soft Tissues*).

Areolar Tissue

In areolar tissue alterations occur in the vasculature, fine connective tissue, and fatty tissue. Masses, calcifications, and opaque foreign bodies can be encountered.

Increase in the Number and Thickness of Vessels. The vessels recognizable in areolar tissue are, for the most part, veins. There is a marked symmetry in width and number of normal subcutaneous veins. In fingers with abundant adipose tissue, an ample network of venous vessels is commonly found.[18] Among the changes due to increased localized circulation secondary to inflammation,[29] only those pertaining to the veins can be observed. Venous dilatation is caused by increased circulation as well as inflammatory damage to venous walls.[30]

If the venous pattern of single fingers is augmented, one should look for subtle changes of synovitis of the corresponding joints and tendon sheaths of that finger. In rheumatoid arthritis, normalization of the vascular pattern documents a decrease in acuity of local inflammatory lesions.

Haziness of Vessel Contours. Like all contours, those of vessels also may be obscured by edema or hematoma.

Changes in Structure of Fine Connective Tissue. Normal areolar tissue contains a variously shaped fine pattern of connective tissue,[31, 32] which shows numerous manifestations typical of various particular regions, with alterations depending upon function and mechanical wear. The texture of normal areolar tissue in the fingers depends upon the particular finger and aspect of the finger; and it is most marked on the radial side of the second and third digit.[18]

Edema leads to widening and an increase in the number of the normally thin strands of connective tissue. Structures not normally visible (e.g., fascial layers) will become visible when enlarged due to edema. Edematous fatty tissue increases the distance between fascial layers and muscles. In scleroderma, however, there is a pathologic increase in the texture of areolar tissue of the fingers that is not due to edema.[33]

Increased Density of Fatty Tissue. Augmentation and persistence of edema produce a diffuse increase in the density of fatty tissues, which eventually may approach water density.

Local Growth of Soft Tissue Masses. In the context of joint disease, gouty tophi and rheumatoid nodules must be considered in the interpretation of such growths.[18, 34]

Calcifications and Opaque Foreign Bodies. As a consequence of the technical improvement in low KV radiography, minimal calcifications have become demonstrable. Judged by the experience with mammography, it is presumed that even more calcifications will become visible in the extremities as well. Thus, the traditional rules concerning the significance and prevalence of soft tissue calcifications in the extremities will have to be modified. Only those that surpass a certain minimal size and number may be taken as signs of generalized mineral or connective tissue disorders. Likewise, the criteria applicable to calcifications of peripheral arteries must be modified. The ankle region is especially useful for demonstrating incipient stages in the calcification of peripheral arteries.

Owing to their contrast with fatty tissues, embedded foreign bodies like glass or wood chips, thorns, and plastic particles are easily recognizable.

INDICATIONS FOR LOW KV RADIOGRAPHY

The following list of disorders are indications for low KV radiographic evaluation:

Rheumatoid arthritis
Seronegative spondyloarthropathies or rheumatoid "variants" (psoriatic arthritis, Reiter's disease, ankylosing spondylitis)
Scleroderma
Arthralgia in Whipple's disease, regional enteritis, and ulcerative colitis
Detritus-synovitis, especially in osteoarthritis of the fingers
Synovial involvement in reflex sympathetic dystrophy syndrome (Sudeck's atrophy)
Stress damage to tendons, tendon sheaths, and ligaments:
  a. Tendons of the abductor longus and extensor brevis of the thumb
  b. Achilles tendon
  c. Tendon of the quadriceps femoris
  d. Patellar ligament
Bursitis, especially of the retrocalcaneal bursa
Hyperparathyroidism
Osteomalacia
Gout
Calcium pyrophosphate crystal deposition disease (chondrocalcinosis)
Hemochromatosis
Hyperlipoproteinemia type II with xanthomatosis of tendons
Synovial involvement in amyloidosis
Synovial changes in multiple epiphyseal dysplasia
Multicentric reticulohistiocytosis
Minute soft tissue calcifications
Nonmetallic foreign bodies composed of glass, wood, or plastic

CLINICAL EXAMPLES OF LOW KV RADIOGRAPHY

This chapter offers an introduction to the clinical usage of low KV radiography. Examples of pertinent diseases are arranged according to anatomic regions in the following sequence: hand (fingers, wrist), forefoot, ankle, knee. Localized and generalized synovial changes such as distention and thickening of joint capsules, tendons, or tendon sheaths and subcutaneous edema must always be viewed and interpreted with respect to other manifestations of a particular disease.

In spite of electronic contrast harmonization and enhancement, the limited range of photographic material permits only a portion of the original gray scale to be reproduced. On the original films of thin objects (e.g., fingers), both soft tissues and bony structures can be evaluated well. However, reproductions of soft tissues show the bones as if not penetrated and reproductions of bones imply a loss of soft tissue detail.

Fingers and Wrist

Normal Radiographic Anatomy of Soft Tissues of Water Density. The normal radiographic anatomy of water-equivalent soft tissues of the fingers is shown in Figure 10–1 for PA views, in Figure 10–2 for cross sections of fingers, and in Figure 10–3 (*A–C*) for the three standard views of the wrist.

The *skin* of the fingers, especially of the second and third fingers, is much thicker on the radial aspect than on the ulnar aspect, which must be considered when evaluating skin thickness.

The *extensor tendon*, being part of the U-shaped dorsal aponeurosis (Fig. 10–2), can commonly be seen in PA views as thin stripes on both sides of the proximal phalanx and occasionally on one side of the middle phalanx. In oblique views it appears as stripes dorsolateral to the phalanges. These stripes blend with the mass formed by periarticular soft tissues.

The *periarticular soft tissues* of the *fingers* are composed of joint capsules and their contents and collateral ligaments in the distal (DIP) and proximal (PIP) interphalangeal joints with the addition of the adjacent interosseous and lumbrical muscles in the metacarpophalangeal (MCP) joints. The thickness of periarticular soft tissues is measured by taking the

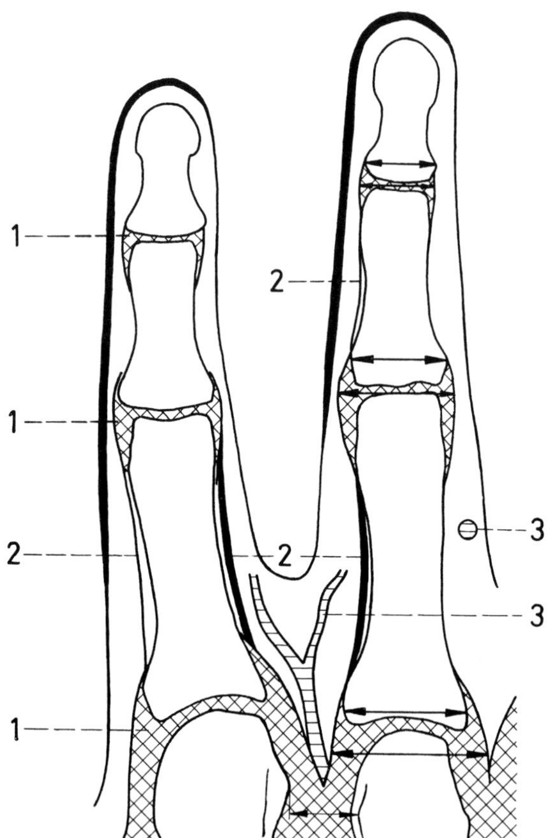

Figure 10–1. Schematic representation of the posteroanterior (PA) view of the right second and third fingers, showing outlines of normal soft tissues and bones. 1, Total periarticular soft tissues (cross-hatched area). 2, Disproportionately thick lateral portion of extensor tendon. 3, Subcutaneous vessels (horizontally shaded area). Note variations in thickness as indicated. The method of measuring the relative widths of periarticular soft tissues and intermetacarpal distance is shown for the third finger. (From Fischer E: Radiologe 19:119, 1979.)

maximum transverse diameter of the periarticular soft tissues as described above minus the maximum transverse diameter of the base of the corresponding phalanx (Fig. 10–1); this measurement is called "relative width of periarticular soft tissues." Mean values for the PIP joints in three views and for the MCP joints in the PA view at a 60 cm focus-film distance (FFD) taken from adults with no known joint disease are listed in Table 10–1. Normal periarticular soft tissues regularly show the same thickness on either side, with differences rarely being of more than 1 mm.[18] By dividing the relative width of periarticular soft tissues by the width of the adjacent phalangeal base, an index has been calculated.[35] Because the absolute dimensions are small and errors in measuring are inevitable, this index gives a false sense of precision. Instead, it is more important to take into account soft tissue dimensions in oblique views, as these show an increase in thickness in incipient capsular distention earlier than is seen in the lateral views. It is also important to be aware of the spectrum of normal variations (see Fig. 10–10).

The periarticular soft tissues of the DIP joints may measure up to 1 mm more than the width of the distal phalangeal base.

In the *wrist*, soft tissue opacities of the joint capsules are imperceptible between the bases of the metacarpals, whereas a maximum width of 2 mm is normal for the intercarpal joints, the radial aspect of the radiocarpal joint, and the inferior radioulnar joint in the true PA view and in the 25 degree oblique AP views (Fig. 10–3*A*, *B*). In the lateral view the soft tissues of the joints and tendon sheaths blend unless they are separated by slender strands of fatty tissue (Fig. 10–3*C*).

The *tendon sheaths* and bones of the second, third, fourth, and fifth fingers overlap completely in the true PA projection and in the 25 degree oblique PA views (Fig. 10–2, *A*) if the transverse axis of the phalanx is parallel to the film. Since the radial side of the hand is thicker than the ulnar side, the fourth and especially the fifth finger are moderately supinated relative to the second and third fingers. Varying degrees of this supination may allow even normal tendon sheaths to be seen in PA views as soft tissue ridges adjacent to the bone (Fig. 10–2, *G*). Therefore, one must take into account the varying positions of individual fingers when evaluating the thickness of tendon sheaths.

Individual tendon sheaths on the radial and ulnar aspects of the wrist are approximately 3 to 4 mm in diameter (Fig. 10–3*A*, *B*). Surprisingly, however, they are not always visible, especially if the areolar tissue is thick and rich in connective tissue fibers. Tendon sheaths will then become visible only if they are slightly enlarged. The tendon sheaths on the ulnar side of the palm that are projected between the ulna and the proximal row of carpal bones in the true PA and in the 25 degree oblique views are frequently separated by a thin fat plane (Fig. 10–3*A*,

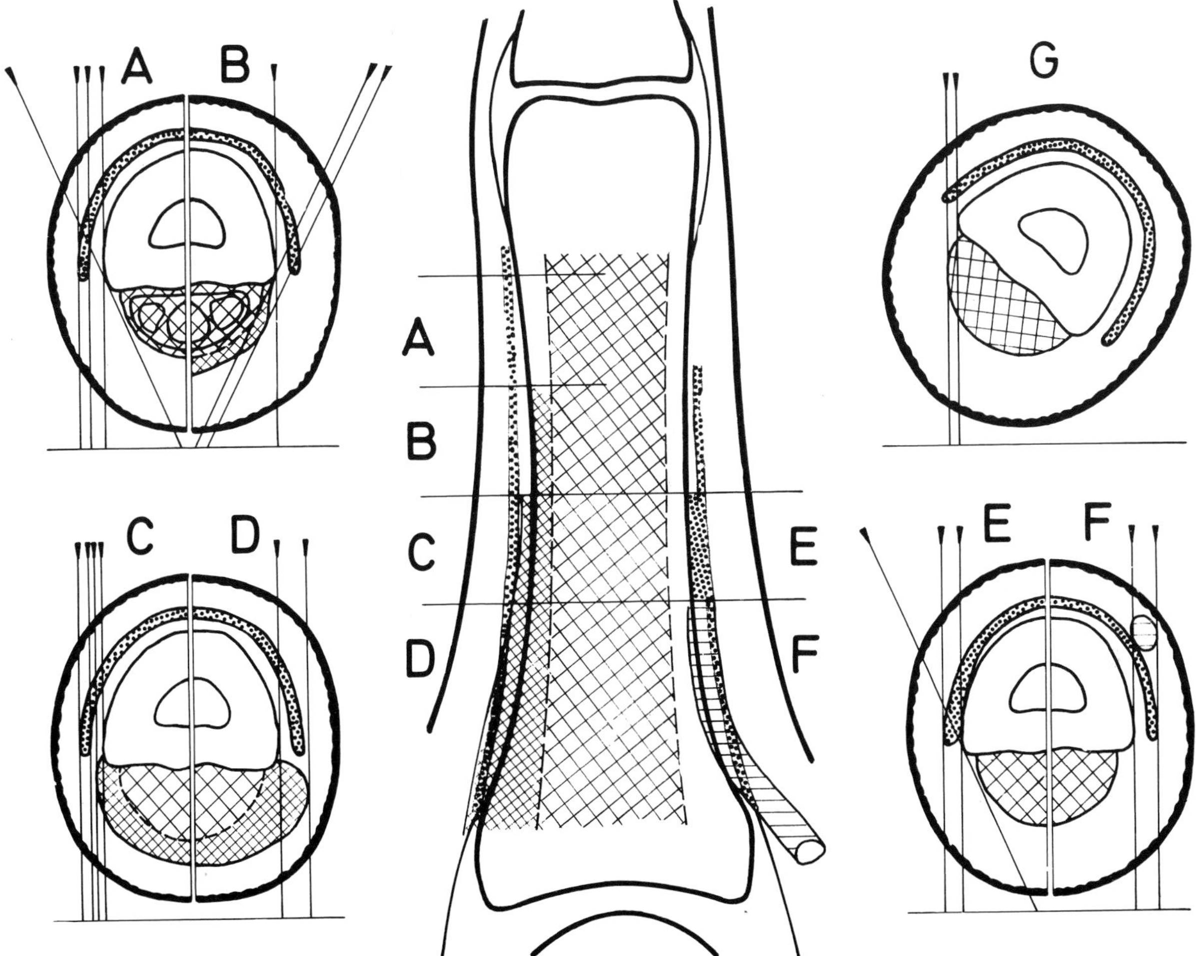

Figure 10–2. Extensor tendons and tendon sheath of a phalanx of a finger, schematically, as seen from above and in cross section. In cross sections A through F, the transverse axis of the phalanx is parallel to the film; posteroanterior (PA) and 25 degree PA oblique projections are shown. In cross section G, the finger is oblique relative to the film. Normal tendon sheath, coarse cross-hatched area; pathologic thickening of tendon sheath, fine cross-hatched area; extensor tendon, dotted area; subcutaneous vein, horizontally lined area. (From Fischer E: Radiologe 19:119, 1979.)

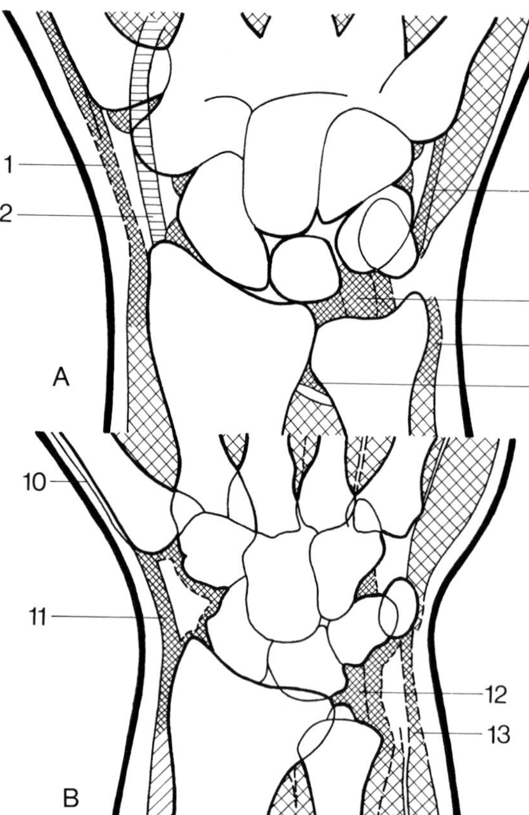

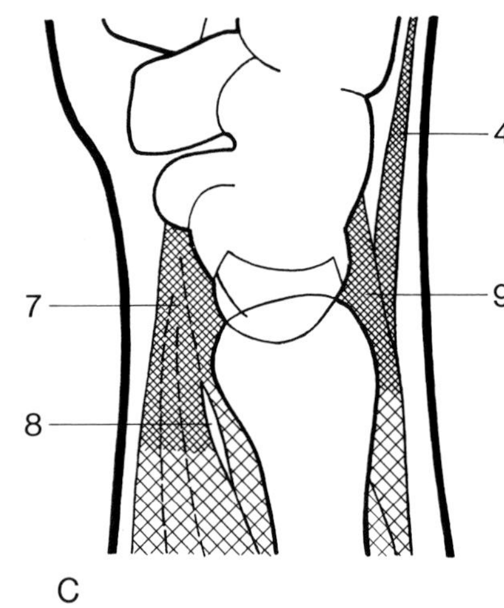

Figure 10–3. *Schematic outlines of soft tissues and bones of the wrist. Tendon sheaths and joint capsule, fine cross-hatched area; muscles, coarse cross-hatched area; vein, horizontally lined area.*

A *Posteroanterior view. 1, Tendon sheath of abductor longus and extensor brevis of the thumb. 2, Vein commonly encountered; overlapping the adjacent tendon sheath or periarticular tissue, this vein may simulate thickening of these structures. 3, Distal portion of the tendon sheath of the extensor carpi ulnaris. 4, Palmar tendon sheaths. 5, Proximal portion of the sheath of extensor carpi ulnaris. 6, Part of the saccular recess of the distal (inferior) radioulnar joint bordered proximally by the fat layer that delineates the distal margin of the pronator quadratus.*

B *25 Degree anteroposterior (AP) oblique view, radial elevation. 10, Fascial stripe; 11, sheath of extensor pollicis longus; 12, palmar tendon sheaths; 13, tendon of flexor carpi ulnaris.*

C *Lateral view. 7, Tendon sheaths of flexors of fingers; 8, fat layer volar to the pronator quadratus; 4, tendons and tendon sheaths of the extensors of the fingers; 9, posterior periarticular soft tissues.*

4; 3*B*, 12). On the radial side, the tendon sheaths of the abductor longus and extensor brevis of the thumb are commonly visible as a single opaque stripe in the PA view, whereas in the 25 degree oblique AP views the tendon sheath of the extensor longus is delineated. Overlapping veins may simulate distention of joint capsules and tendon sheaths (Fig. 10–3*A*, 2).

Special Nonspecific Soft Tissue Calcifications of the Distal Phalanx. Two kinds of soft tissue calcification not related to generalized disease have been recently observed in the distal phalanges of fingers examined for other reasons.[35, 36] Beginning at the age of 20 years, small, round calcifications near the sides of ungual tufts are found appearing and disappearing without symptoms (Fig. 10–4). These occur most frequently in the second and third fingers. Since the tips of the same fingers suffer the heaviest wear, it has been suggested that the strain

Table 10–1

MEAN VALUES IN MILLIMETERS OF THE RELATIVE WIDTHS OF THE PERIARTICULAR SOFT TISSUES OF ADULTS WITH NORMAL FINGER JOINTS

		Finger							
		FEMALES				*MALES*			
Joint	**View**	*2nd*	*3rd*	*4th*	*5th*	*2nd*	*3rd*	*4th*	*5th*
PIP	PA	2.2	2.1	1.8	1.9	2.5	2.6	2.3	2.0
	25°u.e.*	3.1	2.9	2.2	1.5	3.9	3.5	2.7	1.6
	25°r.e.*	2.9	3.1	2.8	3.0	3.0	3.4	3.7	3.5
MCP	PA	3.9	4.2	2.6	2.6	4.6	4.2	3.1	2.6

u.e. = Ulnar aspect elevated; r.e. = radial aspect elevated; PIP, proximal interphalangeal joint; MCP, metacarpophalangeal joint.

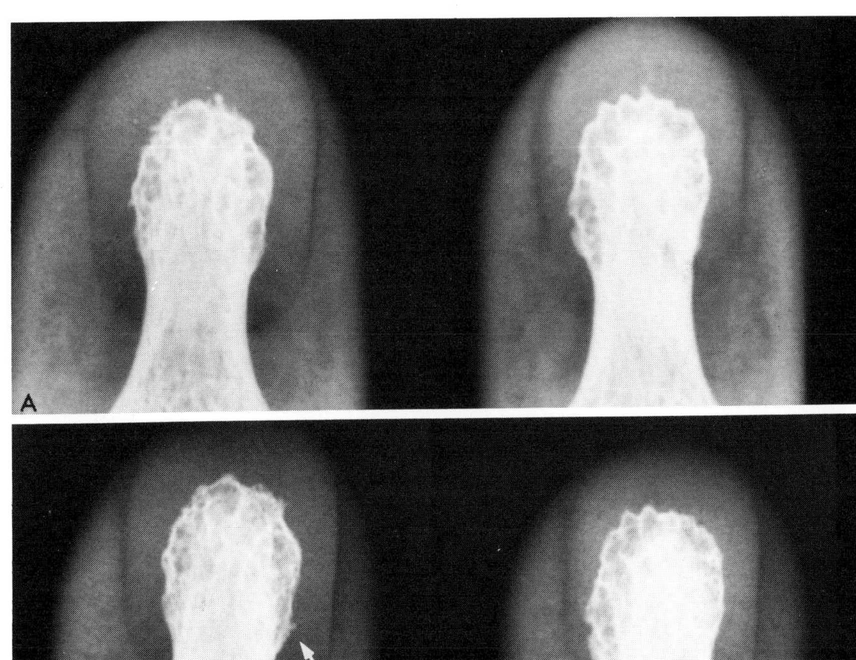

Figure 10–4. *Distal phalanx of the third and fourth fingers; 39 year old female with rheumatoid arthritis.*

A *Several small calcifications in close proximity to the ungual tuft are present.*

B *Two years later, calcifications are no longer visible, and there is new calcification at the junction of the ungual tuft and the shaft of the distal phalanx of the third finger (arrow).*

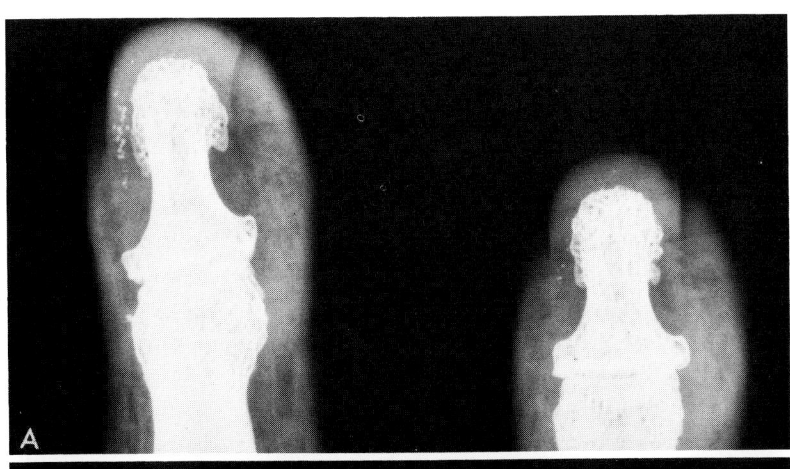

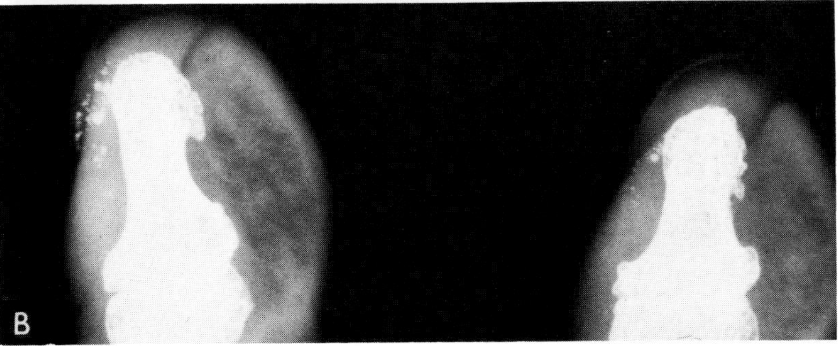

Figure 10–5. *Left second and third fingers; 77 year old woman, nails clinically normal. Radiographs show multiple subungual calcifications.*

A *Posteroanterior (PA) view.*

B *25 Degree PA oblique view, ulna elevation.*

of excessive bending of connective tissue fibers close to their osseous attachments may lead to local damage and subsequent calcifications analogous to the well-known changes at the insertions of certain tendons.[21] Some 10 per cent of patients examined for joint disorders show these calcifications. It is remarkable that such calcifications were not found in disproportionate frequency in numerous patients on chronic hemodialysis under prolonged observation.

Very rarely, in some 0.7 per cent of cases, small, round subungual calcifications are found underlying normal nails in fingers with no history of trauma. These may occur as a single calcification in a single finger or as innumerable calcifications in almost every finger (Fig. 10–5). At present middle-aged adult women appear to be most frequently affected.

Osseous Turnover in Distal Phalanges. The thinnest bones with the least soft tissue coverage are the distal phalanges, which contain the fewest trabeculae, and which therefore offer the most promising circumstances for studying changes in a single trabecula.

The margins of the ungual tufts are the site of two *normal* processes persisting throughout adult life: a slow and rather early inhomogeneous appositional growth subsequently replaced by cancellous bone; and, occasionally, apposition and resorption occurring alternately in zones that are just perceptible (0.2 mm wide) or clearly perceptible (up to 1 mm wide). Such turnover occurs even within a span of 3 to 6 months.

Another region where small changes can occur in rather short intervals is the attachment of tendon sheaths to the shafts of the proximal and middle phalanges. At these sites, osseous apposition may be found and the osteoporosis in association with long-standing rheumatoid tenosynovitis becomes noticeable with ease.

Increased turnover as in *hyperparathyroidism* is clearly evident at the margins of the ungual tufts. In contrast to the changes just described, this occurs simultaneously in several fingers. Small areas of endosteal and periosteal resorption can be observed here prior to the appearance of definite subperiosteal resorption at the lateral aspects of phalangeal shafts. This fact is worth mentioning because at both sides of the shaft of a phalanx near the junction with its base, along ligamentous attachments, there may be normal irregularities of cortical bone that are indistinguishable from subperiosteal resorption. Additionally, there is no clear-cut limit at which incipient stages of augmented streaky intracortical resorption can be called pathologic. Therefore, since even slight osseous turnover can be seen by meticulously comparing the cancellous structure at the sides of the ungual tufts (Fig. 10–6), a PA view of the second and third fingers is helpful in monitoring the skeleton in patients on chronic hemodialysis or anticonvulsive chemotherapy.

Osteoarthritis (Degenerative Joint Disease). One of the earliest radiographic signs of osteoarthritis is the presence of small, predominantly dorsolaterally oriented osteophytes that may be found as early as the middle of the third decade in a non–manually working population. Symptoms of osteoarthritis frequently are reported at the start of the fifth decade. Even grave changes are missed if only PA views are taken of the fingers. More advanced osteoarthritic lesions evident at the volar aspects of the heads of the phalanges and visible only in oblique views are budlike condensations at the osseous margins (Fig. 10–7) or erosions of varying size (Fig. 10–8).

The prevalence of osteoarthritic lesions in middle and advanced age will have to be considered in the evaluation of marginal erosions in late-onset rheumatoid arthritis.

Debris from marginal erosions in osteoarthritis elicits joint pain and causes acute or chronic distention of joint capsules and a corresponding increase in thickness of periarticular soft tissues.

Shallow or angular notches up to 2 mm in length and depth occasionally found on the volar aspect of the heads of the metacarpals and phalanges constitute normal variants and must not be mistaken for degenerative or inflammatory lesions. As a rule, they occur symmetrically in corresponding fingers.

Rheumatoid Arthritis and Its "Variants" (Seronegative Spondyloarthropathies). These diseases can affect any tissue that can be evaluated radiographically.

Edema of the skin (Fig. 10–9) at the level of an inflamed joint has been observed as marked thickening of the skin in 2 per cent of a large population.[18] Edema in rheumatoid arthritis is not always merely a perifocal reaction but can also be due to altered lymph drainage[37] since the disease is known to often affect the lymph nodes.[38]

In *edema of the subcutaneous soft tissues* the texture of the areolar tissue is accentuated and coarse; fatty tissue appears turbid; and the contours of vessels, periarticular soft tissue, tendons, and tendon sheaths become hazy (Figs. 10–9, and 10–10).

An engorgement of *periarticular soft tissues* subsequent to inflammatory irritation can be shown in all finger joints. In comparison with the PIP and MCP joints, the DIP joints are much less distensible. Thus, swellings there are difficult to demonstrate. However, such periarticular swellings have been found in one of two patients with proved arthritis of the PIP and MCP joints.[18] Engorgement of periarticular soft tissues may be homogeneous (Fig. 10–10) or inhomogeneous (Fig. 10–11).

The distention of periarticular soft tissues of the MCP joints can be assessed indirectly by observing changes in the form and size of the fatty wedge in the interdigital web space that usually reaches the level

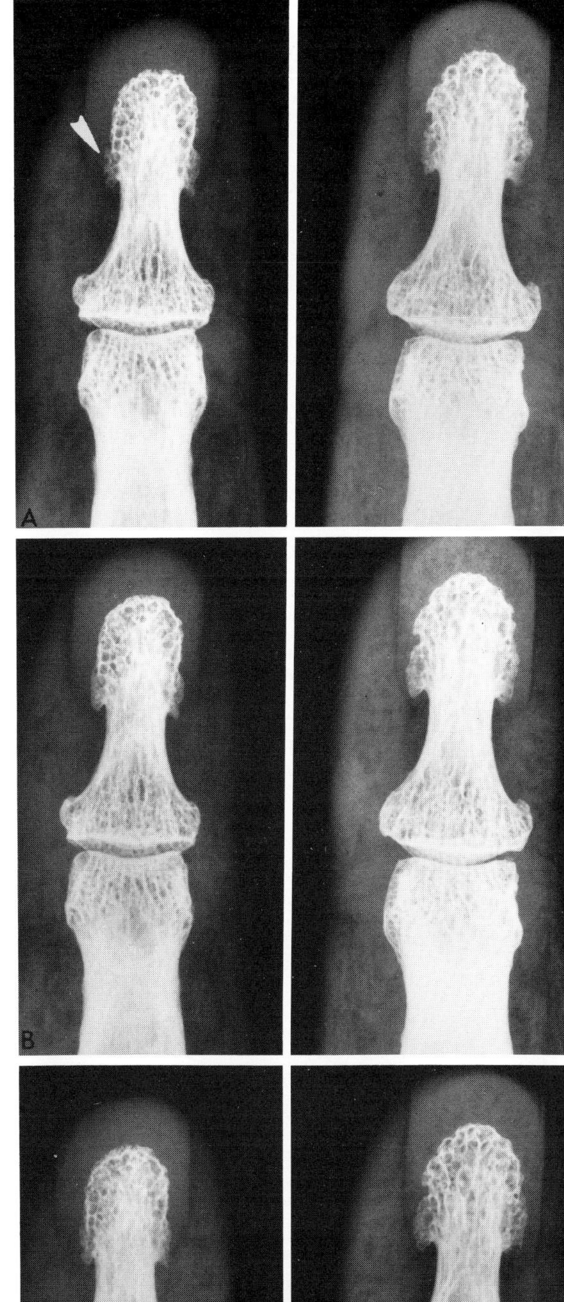

Figure 10–6. *Distal phalanx of the second (on left) and third (on right) fingers; secondary hyperparathyroidism in chronic renal failure.*

A *Minute subperiosteal resorption only at the margin of the ungual tuft of the second finger at the onset of chronic hemodialysis (arrowhead).*

B *12 months later; remineralization of the lesion in* **A** *has occurred.*

C *42 months later; once again fine subperiosteal resorption has taken place at the margin of the ungual tuft of the second finger; there is a large defect near the proximal lateral margin of the ungual tuft of the third finger.*

At no time was subperiosteal resorption seen at the lateral margins of the diaphyses of the phalanges of the fingers.

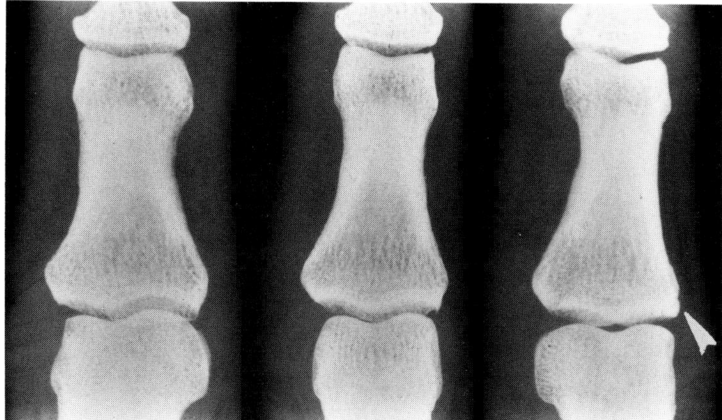

Figure 10–7. Three views of the distal (DIP) and proximal (PIP) interphalangeal joints of the right index finger; 41 year old woman. Shallow sclerotic apposition at the margins of the heads of the phalanx is visible only in oblique views (arrowhead). True posteroanterior (PA) view is shown in the center.

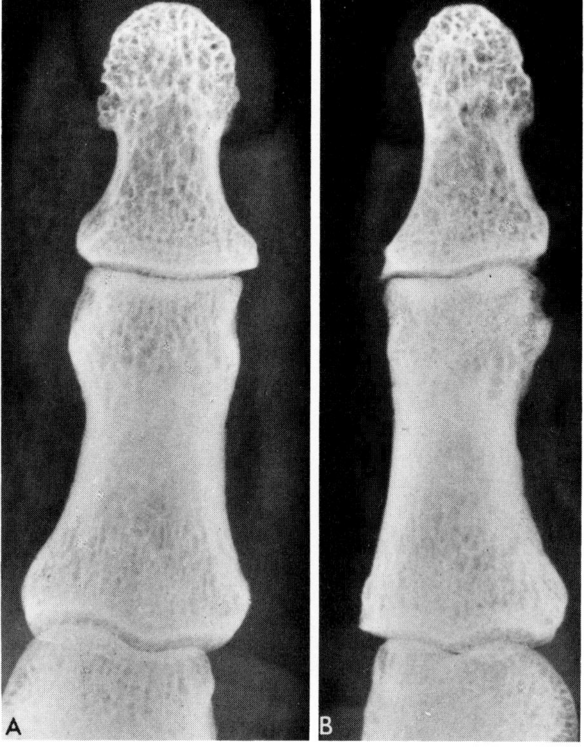

Figure 10–8. Left index finger including distal (DIP) and proximal (PIP) interphalangeal joints; 46 year old diabetic man, obese.

A Posteroanterior view.

B Oblique view. Degenerative erosion at the palmar aspect of the head of the middle phalanx, visible only in the oblique view. Similar changes are found at the DIP and PIP joints.

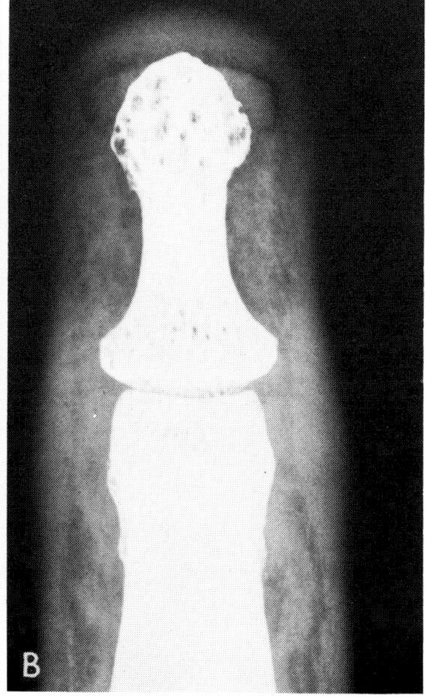

Figure 10–9. Edema of the skin in an inflamed joint.

A Normal right third finger.

B Right fourth finger; inflammation of small joints of this finger in psoriatic arthritis. Note edema of the skin at the level of the thickened periarticular soft tissues of the distal interphalangeal (DIP) joint, subcutaneous edema, and thickened veins.

(From Fischer E: Radiologe 19:119, 1979.)

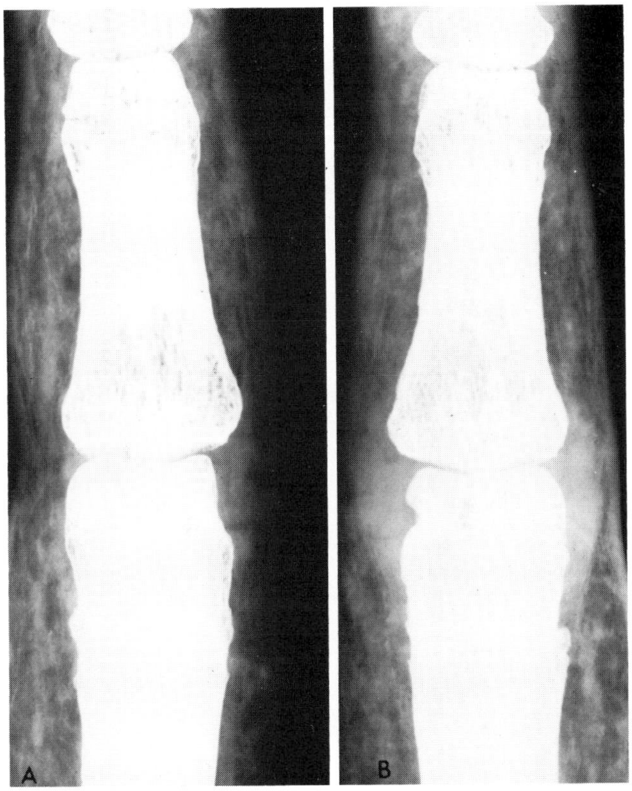

Figure 10–10. *Edema of subcutaneous soft tissues.*

A *Normal left index finger; very narrow periarticular soft tissues at the proximal interphalangeal (PIP) joint; accentuated subcutaneous venous texture.*

B *Right index finger; moderate homogeneous distention of the capsule of the PIP joint; moderate thickening of the veins.*

(From Fischer E: Radiologe 19:119, 1979.)

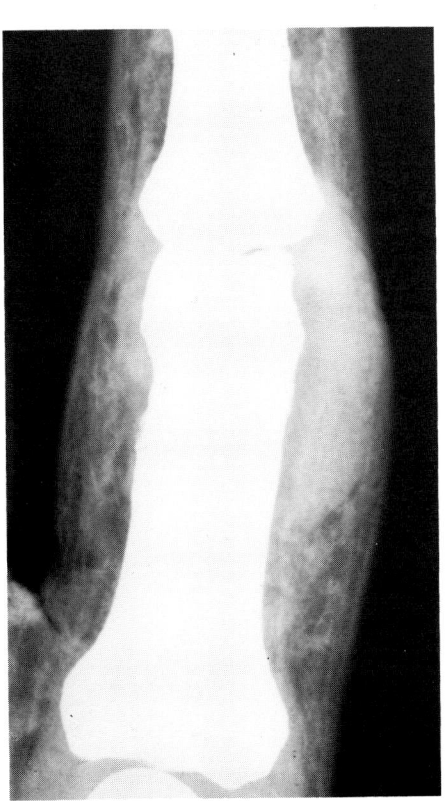

Figure 10–11. *Left index finger, 25 degree posteroanterior (PA) oblique view with ulnar elevation. Enormous engorgement of the capsule of the proximal interphalangeal (PIP) joint is present at the radial aspect only. (From Fischer E: Radiologe 19:119, 1979.)*

of the heads of the metacarpals (Fig. 10–12).[39] Only in significant degrees of distention of adjacent MCP joints will the transverse distance between the heads of the respective metacarpals be increased.

As a rule, this capsular distention initially points in a dorsomedial or dorsolateral direction. Therefore, minor degrees of distention can be seen only in the oblique projections (Fig. 10–12). If *tendon sheaths* of the *fingers* are involved, they will be enlarged also. Minor degrees of this enlargement will be visible only in oblique views, whereas marked degrees are likewise evident in the PA view, presenting as stripes of water density directly adjacent to the volar or lateral aspects of the shafts of the phalanges, as explained schematically in Figure 10–2, (*B*, *C*, *D*). In general, thickening of tendon sheaths in rheumatoid arthritis has been found with this technique about half as frequently as distentions of the PIP and MCP joints.[18] Initial stages as well as exacerbations of rheumatoid arthritis may present solely as tenosynovitis[40] (personal observation). Depending upon the pressure in a tendon sheath and its distensibility, and upon the arrangement and stability of the reinforcing ligaments (anular and cruciform portions of the fibrous sheath), the engorgement will be homogeneous (see Fig. 10–21) or the tendon sheath will herniate between these ligaments (Figs. 10–13 and 10–14).

Capsular distention of the *radiocarpal joint* is directed first dorsolaterally toward the anatomic snuffbox. In this stage it is discernible only in the 25 degree oblique AP views (Fig. 10–15). An enlarged soft tissue mass between the radial styloid and the scaphoid is visible in the PA view only in advanced degrees of distention. At the *radial aspect of the wrist*, fatty tissue of normally triangular shape is delineated by the tendon sheaths of the abductor longus and extensor brevis of the thumb and the soft tissue adjacent to the scaphoid and multangular bones (trapezium, trapezoid) (Fig. 10–3*B*). This triangle is deformed by the distended capsule of the radiocarpal joint. Likewise, hematomas in this joint secondary to fractures of the radial styloid or the scaphoid lead to similar distention of the capsule and deformity of this fat pad; the condition is called a positive "navicular fat stripe sign."[41]

One of the most common soft tissue changes is an enlargement of the *saccular recess* of the inferior radioulnar joint (Fig. 10–3*A*).[17] Since a communication between the inferior radioulnar and the radiocarpal joints is frequently found, especially in rheumatoid arthritis, added synovial contents can

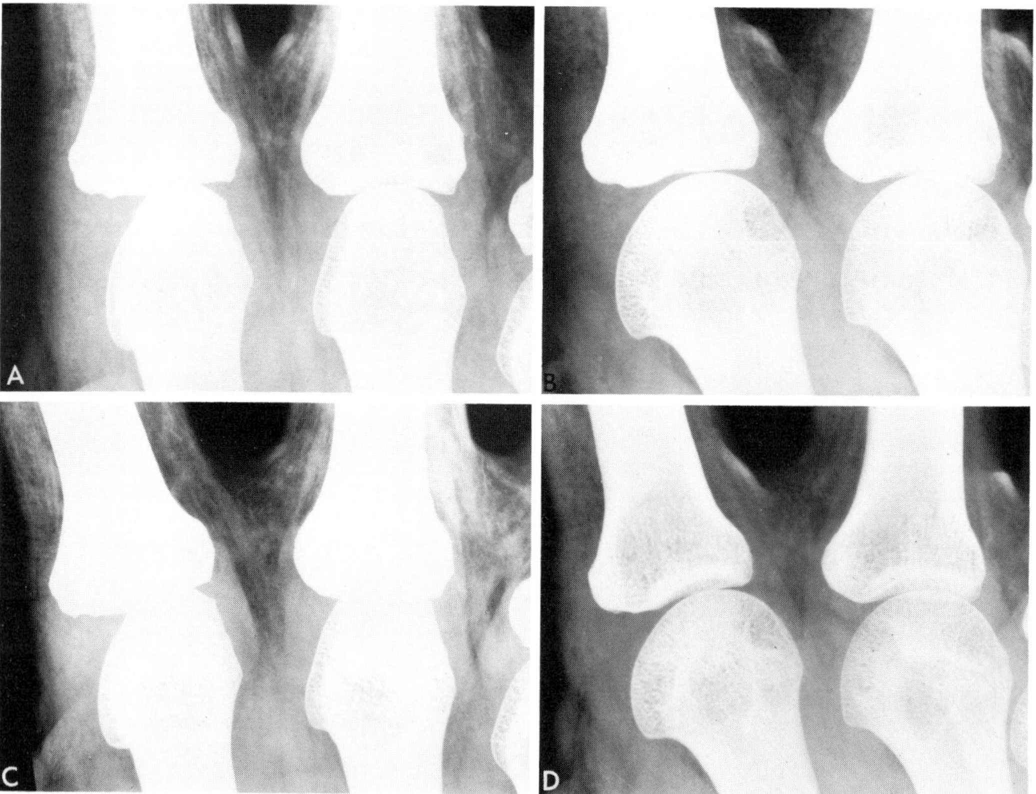

Figure 10–12. *Second and third right metacarpophalangeal (MCP) joints.* **A, C,** *True posteroanterior (PA) views;* **B, D,** *25 degree PA oblique views with radial elevation.* **A, B,** *Minor thickening of the periarticular soft tissues and dorsoulnar distention of the capsule of the second MCP joint are visible, especially in the oblique view.* **C, D,** *Eighteen months later. Normalization of the interdigital fatty wedge secondary to reversal of engorgement of adjacent joint capsules is seen. (From Fischer E: Radiologe 19:119, 1979.)*

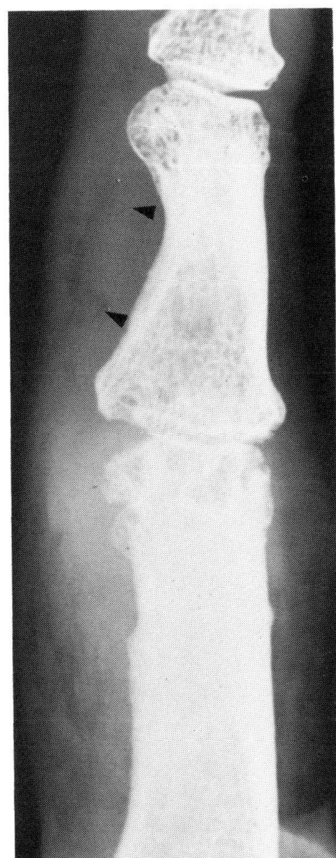

Figure 10–13. *Right third finger, 25 degree posteroanterior (PA) oblique view with radial elevation. Advanced rheumatoid arthritis with destruction of the proximal interphalangeal (PIP) joint. Note the huge engorgement of the tendon sheath, which herniates through reinforcing ligaments of the middle phalanx (arrowheads). Similar engorgement and prolapse were present in the other fingers. In no case could herniation of the tendon sheath be diagnosed clinically. (From Fischer E: Radiologe 19:119, 1979.)*

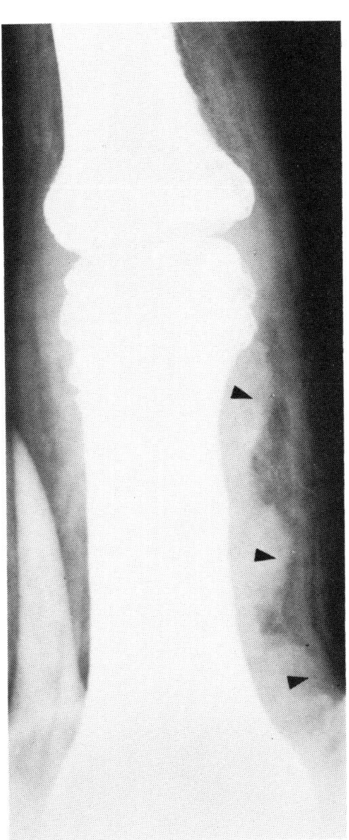

Figure 10–14. *Left third finger, 25 degree PA oblique view with radial elevation. Threefold herniation of the tendon sheaths at the MCP joint with only minor engorgement of the sheaths (arrowheads). The herniations were not palpable.*

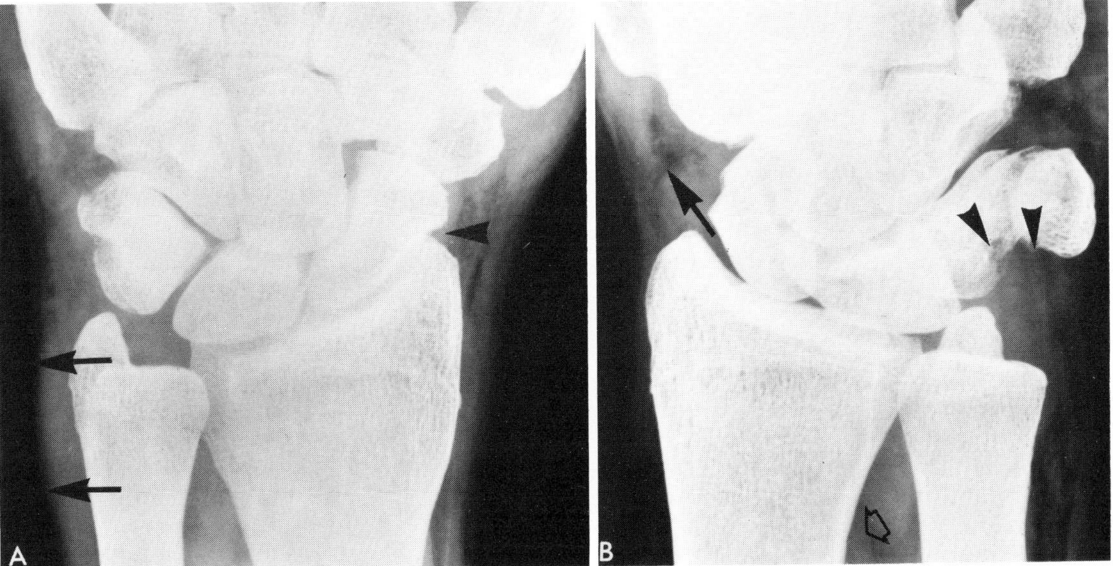

Figure 10–15. *Distention of the ulnar bursa and the capsule of the radiocarpal joint.*

A *Posteroanterior (PA) view of the wrist. There is no discernible radial enlargement of the capsule of the radiocarpal joint (arrowhead). Moderate thickening of the proximal portion of the tendon sheath of the extensor carpi ulnaris is present (arrows). Diffuse opacification between the distal radius and ulna is due to distention of the ulnar bursa.*

B *Same joint, 25 degree anteroposterior (AP) oblique view with radial elevation. Note ballooning of the capsule of the radiocarpal joint directed toward the anatomic snuffbox (solid arrow), distention of the ulnar bursa (open arrow), and erosions of the triquetrum and pisiform bones (arrowheads).*

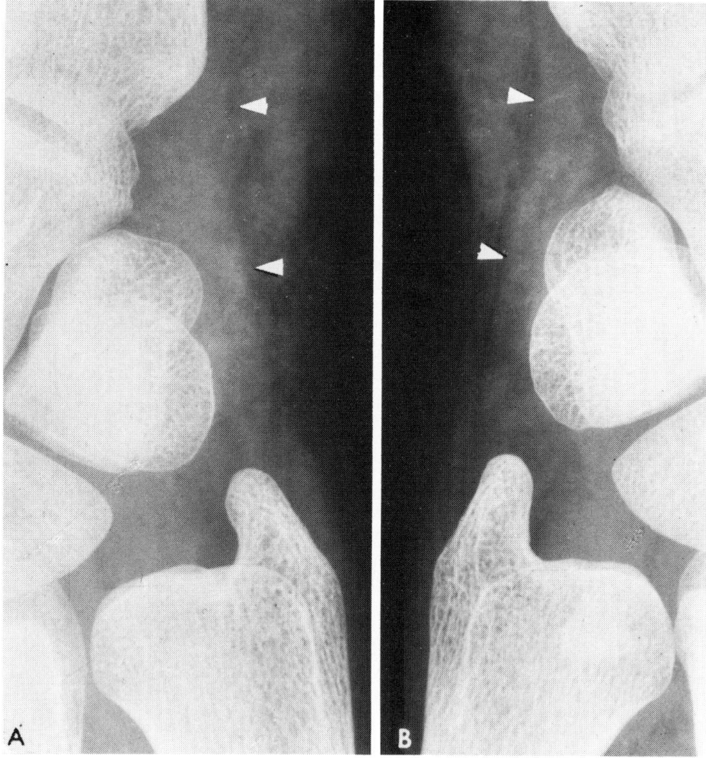

Figure 10–16. Extensor carpi ulnaris tendon sheath in rheumatoid arthritis.

A Ulnar aspect of the right wrist.

B Ulnar aspect of the left wrist. Note minor thickening of the distal portion of the tendon sheath of the extensor carpi ulnaris, discernible only in the right wrist (arrowheads).

quickly enlarge this easily distensible pouch.[42] Severe distention of the *ulnar bursa* may opacify the soft tissues homogeneously between the distal radius and ulna and be indistinguishable from perifocal edema secondary to an enlarged saccular recess. In the lateral or 25 degree oblique AP views, the enlarged ulnar bursa is easily recognized (Fig. 10–15).

Another *tendon sheath* frequently involved in rheumatoid arthritis is that of the *extensor carpi ulnaris,*[17] which may be distended totally or partially (Figs. 10–15*A*, 10–16 and 10–17).

Joint capsules and tendon sheaths may communicate in rheumatoid arthritis more frequently than normal and may produce significant cyst-like extensions.[38] Large synovial masses may thus be formed, the anatomy of which can only be understood correctly by performing an arthrogram.

Three-view low KV radiographs offer a comprehensive demonstration not only of most soft tissues but also of most osseous structures. Prevailing areas of early changes in bones, the so-called "bare areas,"[43] can thus be adequately studied. The charactersitic lesion of the proximal medial margin of the triquetrum[44] is depicted without overlapping structures in the 25 degree AP oblique view (Fig. 10–15*B*).

Ganglion of Tendon Sheath. This nodule presents as a smooth, circular mass adjacent to the normal or slightly thickened tendon sheath, with the radiographic findings corresponding well

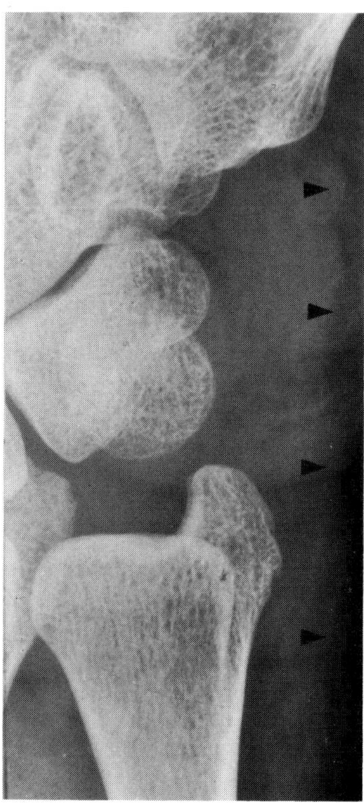

Figure 10–17. Ulnar aspect of the right wrist. Substantial thickening of the entire tendon sheath of the extensor carpi ulnaris with globular distention of its distal portion (arrowheads).

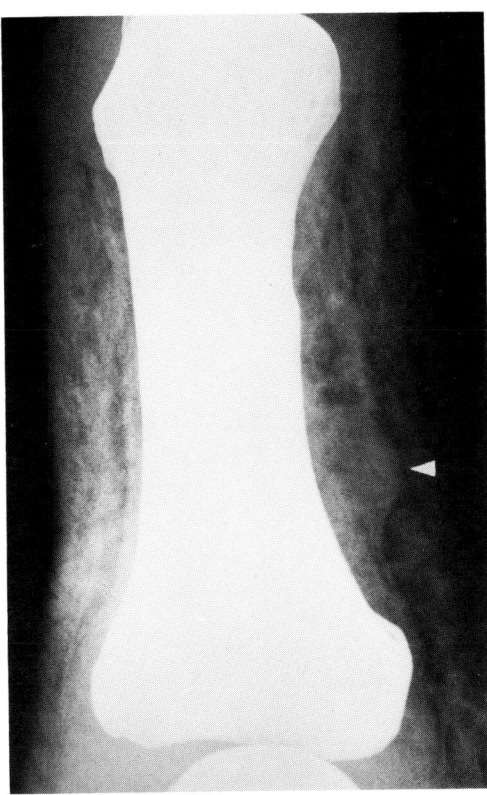

Figure 10–18. Right second finger, posteroanterior (PA) oblique view with 35 degree ulnar elevation. Normal tendon sheath with ganglion (arrowhead) – compare with Figure 10–14. Clinically, a hard nodule was felt. Spontaneous normalization occurred within 1 year. (From Fischer E: Radiologe 19:119, 1979.)

with the physical examination (Fig. 10–18). It is surprising how easily nodules even smaller than the one that is illustrated are palpable. In contrast, rheumatoid enlargement of tendon sheaths, although often more extensive, may not be felt or may be perceived as a diffuse increase in resistance.[18]

De Quervain's Disease. Stress damage of the tendon sheaths of the abductor longus and extensor brevis muscles of the thumb at the radial aspect of the radial styloid is called de Quervain's disease. Only those forms with distended tendon sheaths can be recognized radiographically (Fig. 10–19). If pain occurs in the radial side of the wrist, it is advisable to take a 25 degree AP oblique view because disorders of the sheath of the extensor longus tendon of the thumb occur both in de Quervain's disease and as a separate lesion.

Reflex Sympathetic Dystrophy Syndrome (Sudeck's Atrophy). This syndrome[45] affects all tissues, including the synovial membrane, but radiographically visible synovial changes have not been extensively described. In 1975, the first report of distention of joint capsules and of erosions was published.[46] An involvement of the tendon sheaths is to be expected in this disease, and, indeed, by use of appropriate techniques, tendon sheaths are found to be engorged (Fig. 10–20).

Synovial Involvement in Multiple Epiphyseal Dysplasia. This congenital disease can produce contractures of the extremities beginning in adolescence and progressing thereafter.[47] Performed for the exclusion of a variant of juvenile chronic arthritis, the fortuitous examination of one such case at a stage when contractures were beginning revealed marked thickening of all synovial compartments of the joints, tendons, and tendon sheaths of the hands (Fig. 10–21). The causes of these generalized synovial changes are unknown.

Synovial Involvement in Amyloidosis. In multiple myeloma occasionally even large amounts of amyloid are deposited in synovial tissues. Initially, exercise produces pain in the involved regions; later, joint capsules and tendon sheaths are engorged, thus possibly simulating rheumatoid arthritis.[48, 49] Six year follow-up studies of a case of generalized synovial amyloidosis in multiple myeloma are presented

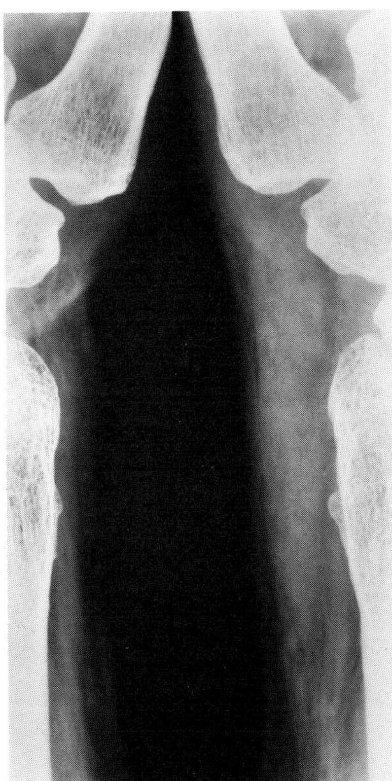

Figure 10–19. de Quervain's disease. Radial aspect of the left and right wrists, posteroanterior (PA) view. There is substantial thickening of the entire tendon sheath of the abductor longus and extensor brevis of the right thumb.

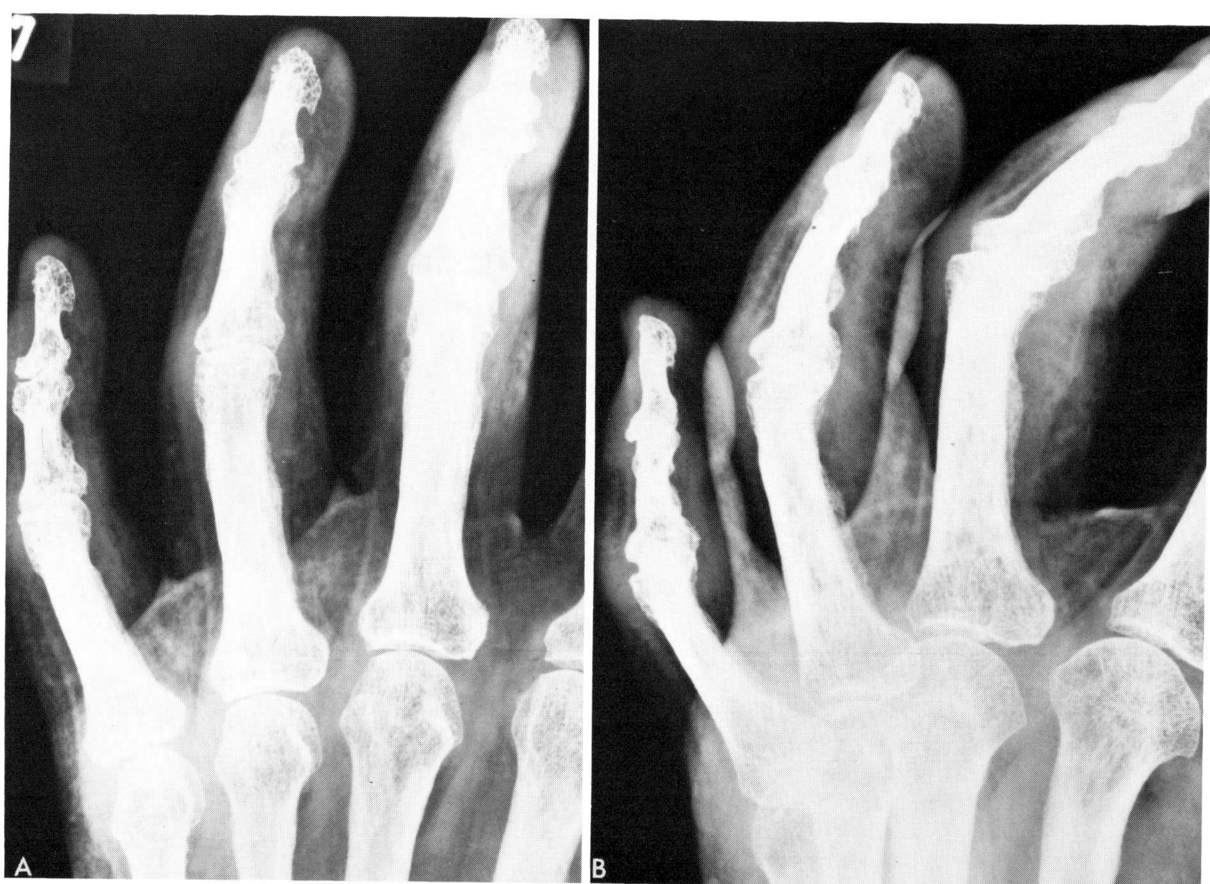

Figure 10–20. *Reflex sympathetic dystrophy syndrome (Sudeck's atrophy).*
A *Left fingers, posteroanterior (PA) view.*
B *Left fingers, PA oblique view, with 25 degree radial elevation. Engorgement of all tendon sheaths and all capsules of the small joints of the fingers is seen.*

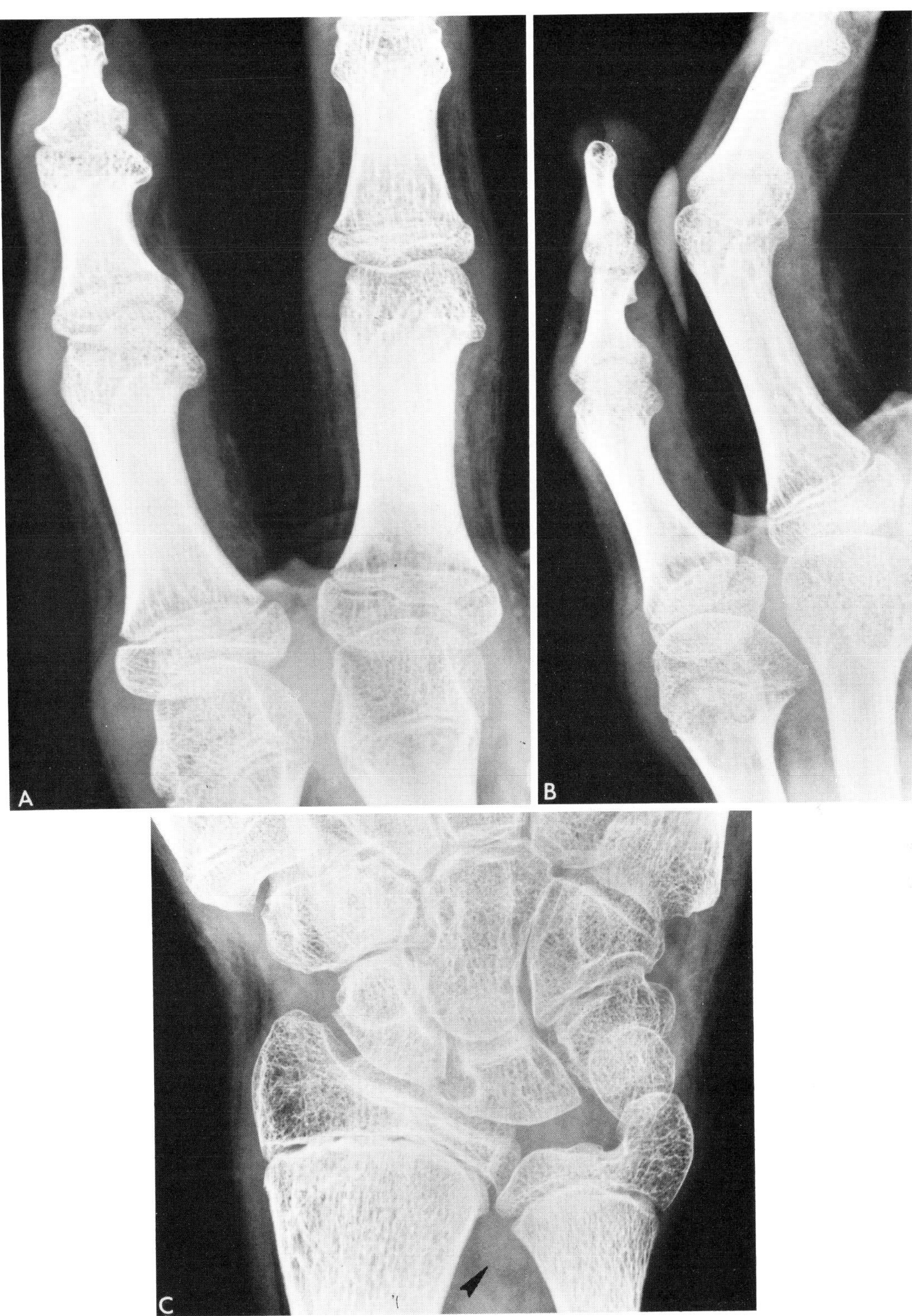

Figure 10–21. Multiple epiphyseal dysplasia; 15 year old girl with retarded growth. There has been progressive thickening and flexion of the finger joints for 8 years.

A Moderate thickening of the periarticular soft tissue of all the small joints.

B Substantial homogeneous thickening of the tendon sheaths of all fingers.

C Ballooning of the saccular recess of the inferior radioulnar joint (arrowhead).

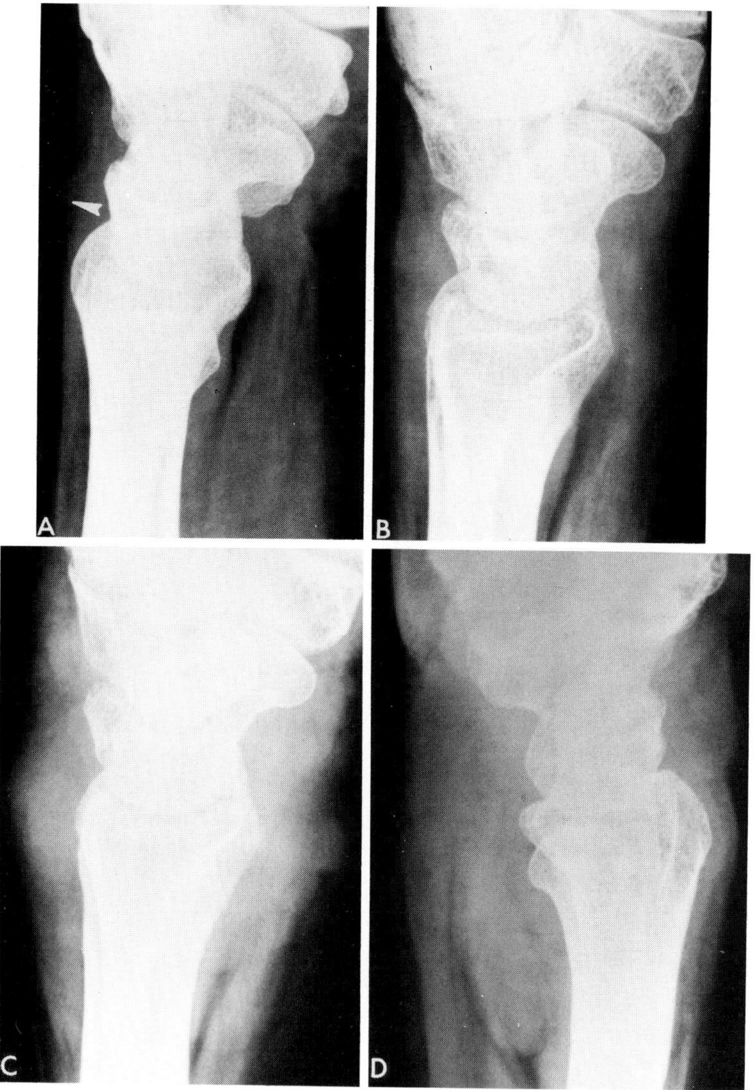

Figure 10–22. *Generalized synovial amyloidosis in multiple myeloma.*

A *Left wrist joint, lateral view. There is bulbous thickening of a short segment of a posterior tendon sheath (arrowhead); otherwise there are normal posterior and palmar soft tissues and normal fat lines separating the anterior tendon sheaths. Patient had pain with exercise.*

B *Four years later. Homogeneous thickening of the posterior and palmar tendon sheaths. Substantial increase in discomfort.*

C *Six years later. Enormous thickening of all tendon sheaths and all joint capsules.*

D *Lateral view of right wrist 6 years after onset of joint discomfort. Note gigantic enlargement of the ulnar bursa and displacement of the fat layer anterior to the pronator quadratus. Predominantly homogeneous thickening of the palmar and posterior tendon sheaths and of posterior joint capsules.*

as illustrations of synovial alterations at the dorsal and palmar aspects of the wrist (Fig. 10–22).

Forefoot

Tendons, tendon sheaths, and muscles of the joints of the toes correspond to those of the fingers. Nevertheless, normal as well as slightly enlarged and inflamed periosseous soft tissues of the toes are much more difficult to recognize radiographically than those of the fingers. Apparently the thick pad on the soles of the toes, which contains substantial fatty tissue, may abolish many soft tissue contours. If perceptible, normal periarticular soft tissues of the second through fifth MTP joints are not wider than the transverse diameter of the adjacent bases of the respective toes. Large masses of water density are found with regularity at the medial aspect of the first IP and MTP joints and at the lateral aspect of the fifth MTP joint. These masses correspond to the plantar cushions of the foot, which are rich in connective tissue in these regions. Because the toes of adults commonly are curved, it may be impossible to do radiographic studies other than of the MTP joints, the IP joint of the great toe, and the soft tissues surrounding these joints.

Rheumatoid Arthritis and Its "Variants" (Seronegative Spondyloarthropathies). The essential soft tissue signs are thickening of periarticular soft tissues and, most importantly, pericapsular edema. This regional edema surrounding the MTP joints, especially of the second through fifth toes, is much larger and frequently of greater density than that of the MCP joints (Fig. 10–23).

Edematous engorgement of the dorsal aponeurosis and distention of the tendon sheaths of the toes are much more difficult to recognize than similar changes in the fingers.

Gout. An acute attack of gout causes a moderate inflammatory distention of the capsule of the

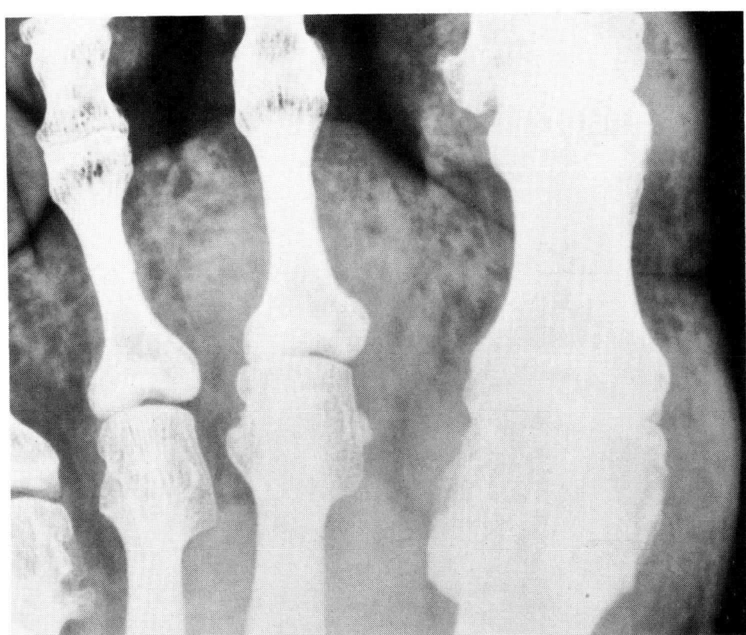

Figure 10–23. Rheumatoid arthritis. Left first through third toes. Note distention of the capsules of the first and second metatarsophalangeal (MTP) joints and of the first interphalangeal (IP) joint. Substantial capsular edema is visible only in the vicinity of the second proximal phalanx. Periarticular soft tissues of the third and fourth MTP joints are normal.

involved joint, as well as periarticular swelling and an augmentation of surrounding veins. The latter may persist for days after the local arthritic attack has subsided.

Ankle Region

Normal Achilles Tendon. The Achilles tendon is normally between 4 and 9 mm thick. The tendon is thinnest in its distal third and commonly increases in thickness proximally. Its junction with the triceps surae muscle is rather extended; terminal fascicles of the muscle sometimes insert asymmetrically into the very distal portions of the tendon. With proper positioning, the Achilles tendon has well-defined margins anteriorly and, if there is sufficient fatty tissue between it and the skin, posteriorly as well. Nevertheless, there are thin opacities accompanying the anterior margin produced by slender lateral extensions of the tendon. These opacities may be due to the plantaris tendon as well, which frequently courses alongside the medial aspect of the Achilles tendon.[50]

In normal posture, the slightly curved contour of the skin posterior to the Achilles tendon forms an obtuse angle of at least 150 degrees, opening posteriorly (Toygar's angle).[51] Since the skin and tendon are closely parallel, the figure formed by the margin of the skin reflects the tension of the Achilles tendon.

Damage of the Achilles Tendon Due to Strain. Lesions related to overstrain range from irritation of the paratenon to complete rupture, usually secondary to degenerative changes that reduce the strength of the tendon.

The signs of *paratenonitis (crepitans) achillea* are increased thickness and unsharpness of the anterior margin as a result of edema (Fig. 10–24), which may extend considerably into the pre-achilles fatty tissue.

In *incomplete rupture,* the course of the tendon is normal. Local thickening due to edema or hematoma may represent sequelae of incomplete rupture (Fig. 10–25).

Perifocal edema as well as shredding of the severed ends of the Achilles tendon are likely to abolish its outline at the site of *complete rupture.* However, even when its contours are well outlined and its thickness is normal, an increase in the anterior curvature of the tendon reducing Toygar's angle to less than 150 degrees is indicative of complete rupture.

Spontaneous healing of an incomplete rupture presents as tapered thickening, whereas surgically treated ruptures commonly lead to shortening and considerable thickening.

Rheumatoid Paratenonitis Achillea. The entire Achilles tendon may be involved in rheumatoid arthritis and its variants. The edematous paratenon causes the outlines of the tendon to broaden with possible, but not mandatory, blurring of its contours and with edema in the preachilles fatty tissue.[50] The thickness of the tendon may approach that of twice normal. If it is still not certain whether slight unilateral thickening of the Achilles tendon and haziness of its anterior border are due to improper positioning (i.e., insufficient inward rotation of the lower limb) or to true paratenonitis, an additional view in passive flexion will reveal whether there is a normal or diminished undulation (Fig. 10–26).

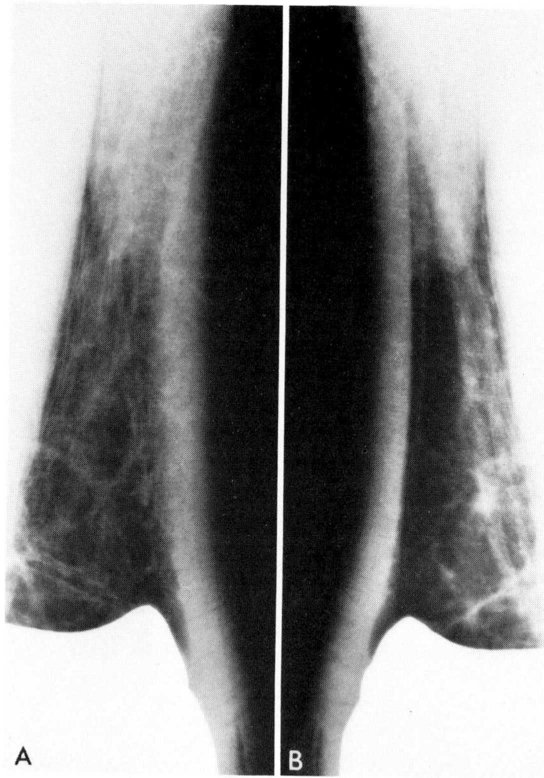

Figure 10–24. *Ankle joint of 31 year old woman with painful right ankle after 4 weeks of strenuous gymnastic exercise.*

A *Right ankle: Paratenonitis achillea due to overstrain. Note moderate thickening and hazy and irregular anterior margin of the Achilles tendon with increased opacity of the pre-achilles fat-pad due to edema.*

B *Normal left ankle of same patient for comparison.*

(From Fischer E: Radiologe 14:457, 1974.)

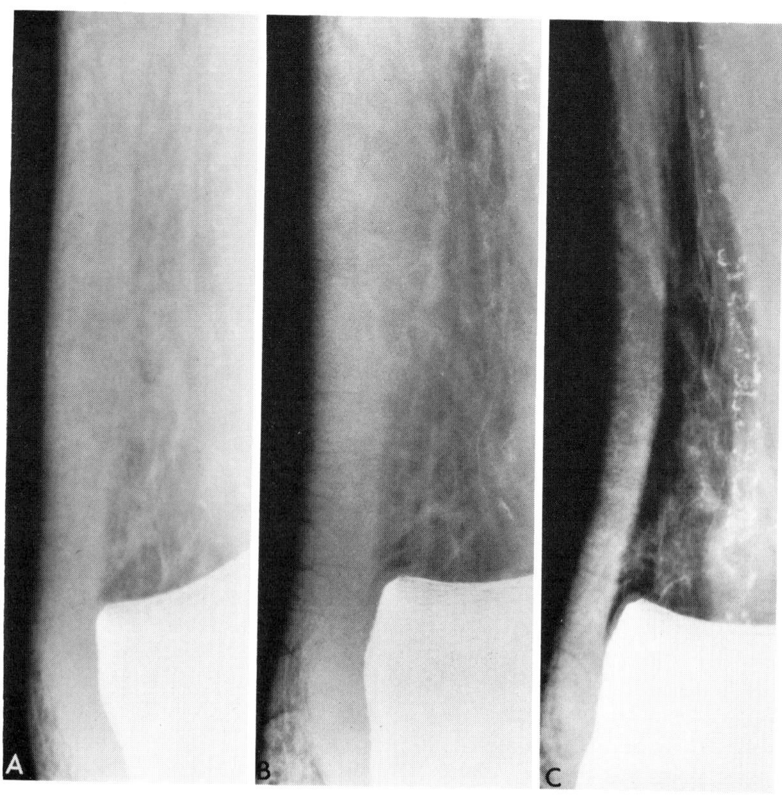

Figure 10–25. *Paratenonitis achillea with subsequent incomplete rupture and later spontaneous healing.*

A *Left Achilles tendon. Note substantial thickening of the tendon and marked edema of the entire ankle following 2 weeks of strenuous digging by this 70 year old unconditioned man.*

B *Two weeks later, while descending from a ladder, the patient experienced sudden excruciating pain in the Achilles tendon with a clearly audible "pop." Note incomplete rupture. This was treated with conservative management and underwent spontaneous healing.*

C *After 3 years the Achilles tendon is almost normal in thickness and shape.*

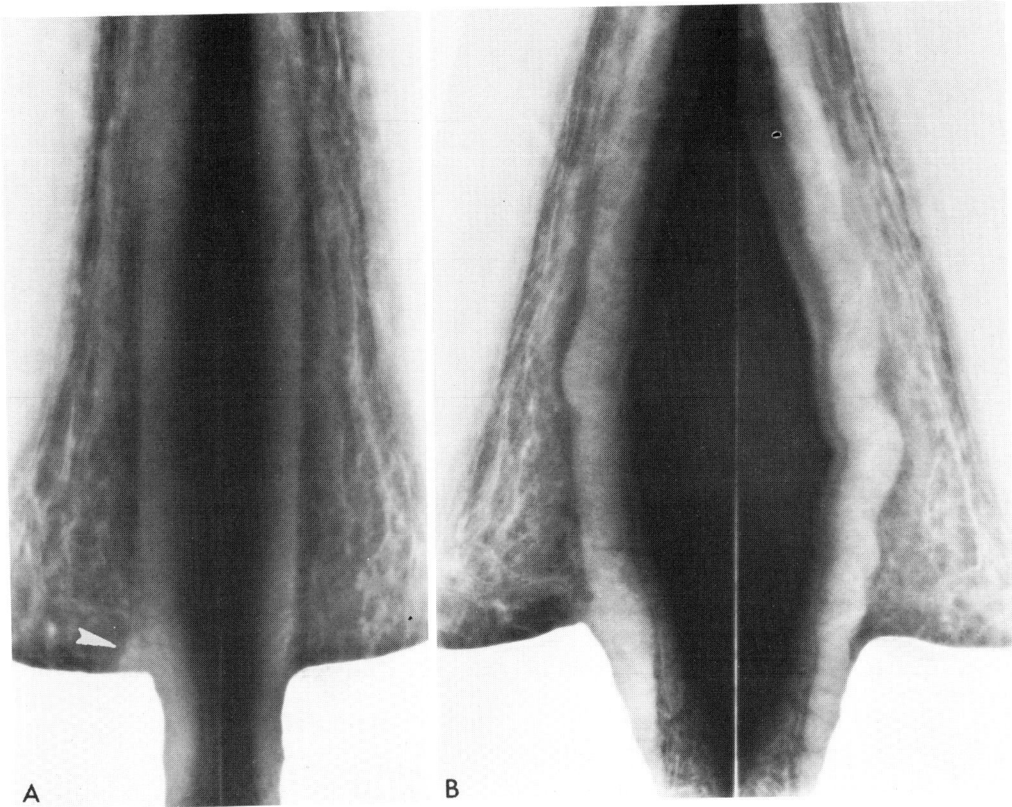

Figure 10–26. *Paratenonitis of the right Achilles tendon with retrocalcaneal bursitis in rheumatoid arthritis.*

A *Both Achilles tendons with both feet in normal midposition. Note moderate thickening of the right tendon and a minor degree of enlargement of the right retrocalcaneal bursa (arrowhead).*

B *Both Achilles tendons in passive relaxation. Note reduced undulation on the right side.*

Retrocalcaneal Bursitis. The retrocalcaneal bursa is frequently involved in rheumatoid arthritis and its variants. The radiographic sign is an opacity of water density of varying size situated between the Achilles tendon and the superior posterior limit of the calcaneal tubercle (Figs. 10–26 and 10–27). When this corner of the calcaneus is prominent (a common finding), the Achilles tendon is in close contact with this bone and an inflammatory expansion of the bursa extends toward the distal posterior margin of the preachilles fatty tissue. Mechanical factors will certainly aggravate the irritation of an already inflamed bursa, as was shown in cases of unilateral Haglund's disease.[50]

The distention in bursitis is often only moderate; the only radiographic sign is a striped edematous texture in the vicinity of the bursa, which may be considerable (Fig. 10–27). Retrocalcaneal bursitis frequently causes a thickening of the adjacent Achilles tendon as evidence of secondary localized rheumatoid paratenonitis.

Xanthomatosis of the Achilles Tendon. Large amounts of cholesterol may be deposited in hyperlipoproteinemia type II in many tendons and ligaments. Such deposits are particularly evident in the Achilles tendon, and in this site the radiographic demonstration of minor degrees of thickening secondary to cholesterol deposition surpasses that of physical examination in reliability (Fig. 10–28).) Therefore, low KV radiography of this tendon is recommended to monitor patients with hyperlipoproteinemia type II.[52]

Thickening of Skin Overlying the Achilles Tendon. Palpation is often inconclusive in deciding whether nodular masses in the vicinity of the Achilles tendon pertain to the skin or to the tendon because there are commonly rather taut interconnections. With low KV radiographs, however, skin and tendon can be clearly distinguished.

Although cutaneous and subcutaneous nodes posterior to the Achilles tendon are a familiar finding in rheumatoid arthritis, it is not as well known that gouty tophi can occur in the same site (Fig. 10–29).

Soft Tissues of the Knee Joint

In the slightly bent, healthy knee, the *patellar ligament* appears as a stripe, 4 to 7 mm in width, that is perpendicular to the joint surface or shows a

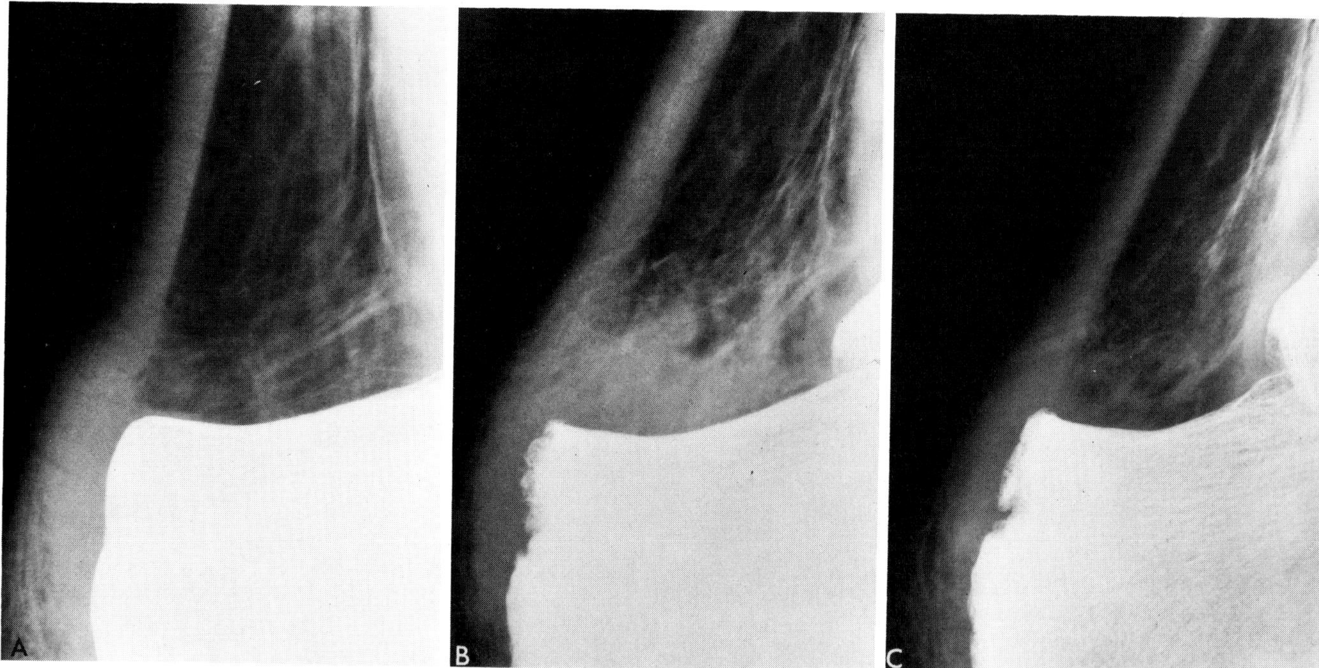

Figure 10–27. *Retrocalcaneal bursitis in ankylosing spondylitis; 22 year old woman.*

A *Note edema in the vicinity of the bursa as the only radiologic sign of bursitis. There is a minor degree of thickening of the adjacent distal Achilles tendon.*

B *Two years later. Substantial destruction has taken place at the posterior margins of the calcaneal tubercle, and there is marked distention of the bursa proximally and substantial streaky edema proximal to the bursa.*

C *Four years later. The erosions show partial restitution. However, the coarse streaky edema proximal to the calcaneal tubercle persists.*

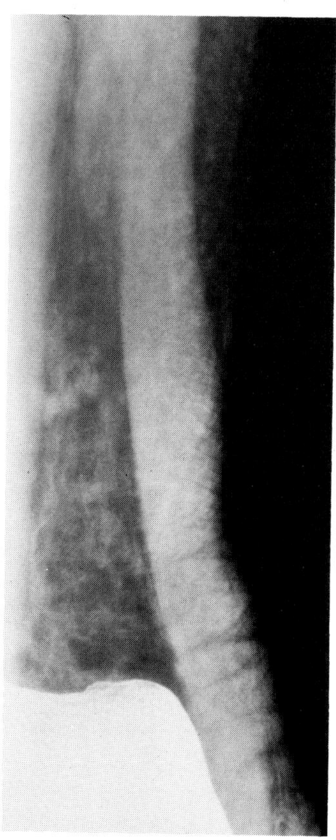

Figure 10–28. *Xanthomatosis of the Achilles tendon in hyperlipoproteinemia type II. Note thickening of the right Achilles tendon. This was barely perceptible on clinical examination.*

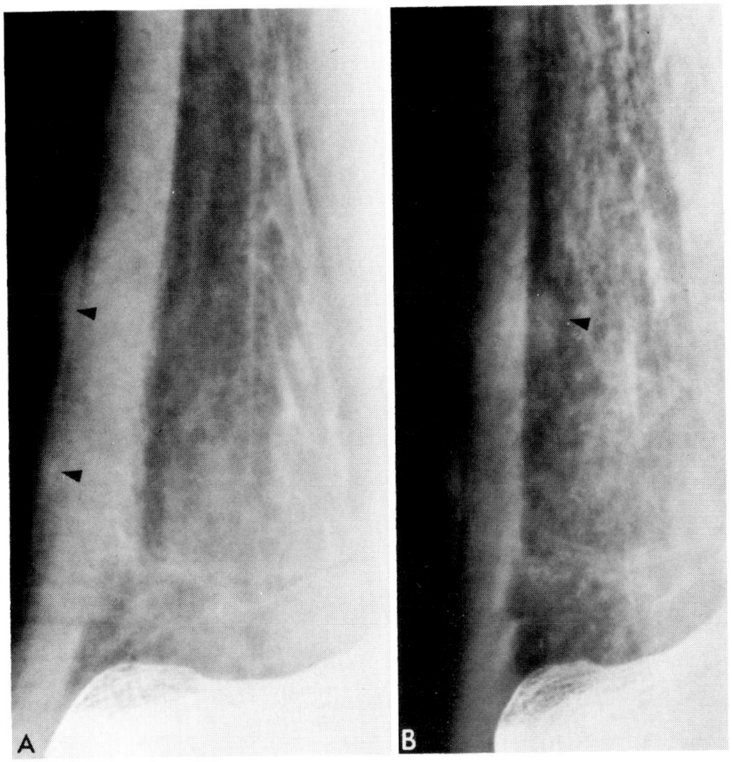

Figure 10–29. Gout.

A Note the thickened Achilles tendon and two cutaneous tophi (arrowheads).

B Three years later. Normal Achilles tendon. There has been an increase in the size of the proximal gouty tophus (arrowhead). (From Fischer E: Radiologe 14:457, 1974.)

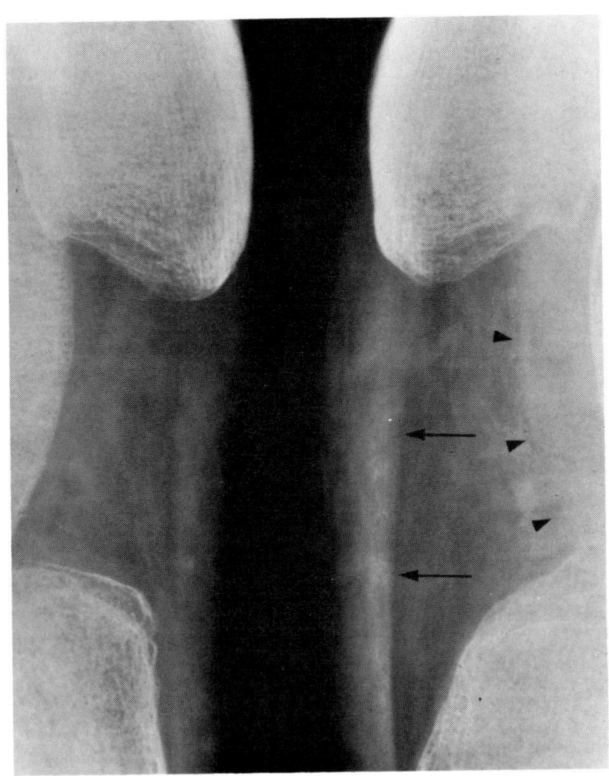

Figure 10–30. Rheumatoid arthritis of the right knee. On a lateral projection, note dorsally open curvature of the patellar ligament (arrows) and widening of the periarticular soft tissues (arrowheads). Soft tissues of the other knee are normal.

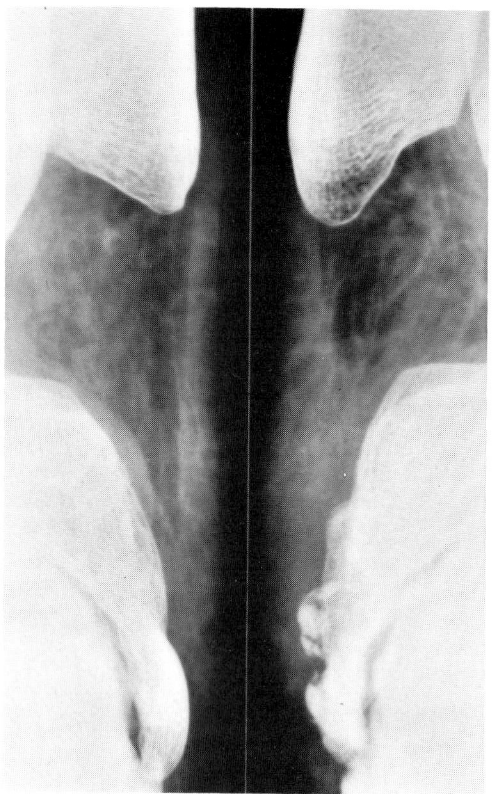

Figure 10–31. Osgood-Schlatter's disease of the right knee. Patient is 13 year old boy with a history of playing soccer, using predominantly his right leg, who developed a painful swelling distal to the patella. Note thickening of the distal two thirds of the patellar ligament and the alteration of the inferior and anterior portions of the infrapatellar fat pad secondary to edema. Normal left knee is shown for comparison.

shallow convexity pointing posteriorly but never anteriorly. A curvature of the patellar ligament directed anteriorly is produced by an augmentation of the *infrapatellar fat pad* (hypertrophy or edema) and by displacement of this fat pad by recurrent effusions in the knee joint (Fig. 10–30). Following trauma or inflammation, low KV radiographs can demonstrate edema in the infrapatellar fat pad in close proximity to the capsule of the knee joint that persists for a long period of time.

Osgood-Schlatter's disease is a lesion not only of the anterior tibial tubercle but also of the patellar ligament as a result of repeated injury.[53] In Osgood-Schlatter's disease, the entire ligament or just its distal portion may be thickened. Additionally, edema of the anterior and inferior portions of the infrapatellar fat pad[54] is frequently found (Fig. 10–31).

FINAL REFLECTIONS ON LOW KV RADIOGRAPHY

Because of the increase in contrast and resolution obtainable with low KV radiography, many minute details of bones and soft tissues are clearly perceptible that would otherwise not be visible. These minute details often pertain to different tissues that are situated very close to each other. The number of structures to be observed is further increased because multiple views are frequently necessary. A magnifying glass is required to analyze the radiographic details in low KV radiography. This limits the field of vision and facilitates a systematic analysis of these detailed radiographic images.

To justify the use of this radiographic technique, which is more laborious than conventional radiography, the radiologist's evaluation must include a detailed examination of all the barely perceptible structures in keeping with the clinical objective. The implication is that minimal and, therefore, very early changes are diagnosed. The patient's diagnosis will be achieved more easily and more accurately if the patient's history and physical examination are specifically recorded for the radiologist.

Presupposing only reasonable indications and diligent evaluation, the patient dose necessary in low KV radiography is tolerable. Depending upon the size of the patient, use of industrial (fine-grain) non-screen films involves a skin dose per exposure between 2 and 10 centigray (cGy)* similar to the skin dose in mammography. Reduction of this dose by means of more sensitive recording media is therefore necessary. The low-dose system is adequate if the soft tissues alone are to be considered, whereas the newer rare-earth screens have not been sufficiently tested.

*The gray is a unit of radiation measurement (a unit of absorbed dose) that replaces the rad. One gray (Gy) = 1 joule/kg = 100 rads.

REFERENCES

1. Ter-Pogossian MM: The Physical Aspects of Diagnostic Radiology. New York, Hoeber Medical Division, Harper and Row, 1969, p 173.
2. Rini JM, Horowitz A, Balter S, Watson RC: A comparison of tungsten and molybdenum as target material for mammographic x-ray tubes. Radiology *106*:657, 1973.
3. Gajewski H, Reiss KH: Physik und Technik der Weichteildiagnostik. Radiologe *14*:438, 1974.
4. Gajewski H.: Aufnahmetechnische Grundlagen der Mammographie. *In* W Hoeffken, M Lanyi: Röntgenuntersuchung der Brust. Stuttgart, Georg Thieme, 1977, p 8.
5. Hach G: Betrachtungen zur optimalen Mammographietechnik. Fortschr Geb Roentgenstr Nuklearmed *117*:298, 1972.
6. Marshall M, Peaple LHJ, Ardran GM, Crooks HE: A comparison of x-ray spectra and outputs from molybdenum and tungsten targets. Br J Radiol *48*:31, 1975.
7. Fischer E: Unpublished data.

8. Révész V: Röntgenbilder normaler peripherischer Blutgefässe. Fortschr Geb Roentgenstr Nuklearmed *20*:39, 1913.
9. Bonola A: Sulla interpretazione radiografica delle ombre normali e pathologiche delle parti molli del ginocchio senza mezzi di contrasto. Chir Organi Mov *23*:39, 1936.
10. Carty JR: Soft tissue roentgenography. Anatomical, technical and pathological considerations. Am J Roentgenol *35*:474, 1936.
11. Frantzell A: Röntgenologische Weichteilsstudien von Cutis and Subcutis. Ein Beitrag zur röntgenologischen Ödemdiagnostik. Acta Radiol (Stockh) *25*:460, 1944.
12. Chiappa S: Studio radiologico sulle parti molli articolari e periarticolari.. Le parti molli dell'articolazione tibiotarsica nel quadro normale e nelle lesioni da trauma. Radio Med (Torino) *38*:621, 1952.
13. Norell HG: Roentgenologic visualization of the extracapsular fat: Its importance in the diagnosis of traumatic injuries to the elbow. Acta Radiol (Stockh) *42*:205, 1954.
14. Bonse G: Anwendungsmöglichkeiten röntgenologischer Weichteildiagnostik ohne Kontrastmittel. Fortschr Geb Roentgenstr Nuklearmed *74*:450, 1951.
15. Soila P: The roentgen demonstration of soft tissue changes in rheumatoid arthritis. Acta Rheum Scand *3*:328, 1957.
16. Fischer, E, Braun J: Neue diagnostische Möglichkeiten an den Extremitäten durch Weichstrahlaufnahmen mit Mammographiegeräten. Electromedica p 90, 1973.
17. Fischer E: Die röntgenologische Weichteildiagnostik der rheumatischen Arthritis (Weichstrahlaufnahmen der Hand). *In* Frommhold-Gerhardt: Klinisch-radiologisches Seminar *3*, p 17. Stuttgart, Georg Thieme, 1974.
18. Fischer E: Die Weichteilveränderungen der Finger bei der rheumatischen Polyarthritis. Ergebnisse nach Weichstrahlaufnahmen in drei Ebenen. Radiologe *19*:119, 1979.
19. Fischer E: Weichteildiagnostik an den peripheren Extremitäten mittels Weichstrahltechnik. Teil III. Der Nachweis diskreter Reizzustände der Bursa subachillea. Radiologe *14*:468, 1974.
20. Fischer E: Der Nachweis von Holz- und kleinen Glassplittern durch die Weichstrahlaufnahme. Fortschr Geb Roentgenstr Nuklearmed *118*:309, 1973.
21. Fischer E: Der Nachweis einer chronischen Insertionstendinopathie am Epicondylus humeri durch Weichstrahlaufnahmen. Fortschr Geb Roentgenstr Nuklearmed *119*:358, 1973.
22. Bosert W, Schulz W: Ausmass, Schweregrad und Verlaufsbeobachtung der renalen Osteopathie mittels. Mikroradioskopie der Handkortikalis. Nieren-Hochdruckkr p 52, 1978.
23. Prager PJ, Krause KH, Ritz E, Schmidt-Gayk, H: Handskelettaufnahmen in Mammographietechnik bei Patienten unter antiepileptischer Behandlung. Fortschr Geb Roentgenstr Nuklearmed *126*:371, 1977.
24. Reichmann S, Deichgräber E Strid KG, Heyman F, Strand T: Soft tissue radiography of finger joints. Acta Radiol. (Diagn) *15*:439, 1974.
25. Mäkelä P, Haataja M: Soft tissue radiography of the hands in rheumatoid arthritis. Scand J Rheumat *5*:113, 1976.
26. Mäkelä P, Haaslahti JO: Immersion technique in soft tissue radiography. Acta Radiol (Diagn) *19*:89, 1977.
27. Fischer E: Unpublished data.
28. Fischer E: Röntgenologische Weichteildiagnostik der rheumatoiden Polyarthritis an Händen und Füssen. Verh Dtsch Ges Rheumatol *4*:176, 1976.
29. Wegelius U: Angiography of the hand. Acta Radiol (Suppl) *315*:86, 1972.
30. Cooper NS: Pathology of rheumatoid arthritis. Med Clin North Am *52*:607, 1968.
31. Bohndorf W: Uber die Röntgendiagnostik der Hautkrankheiten. Radiologe *5*:39, 1965.
32. Schraub S: Radiographie de la peau. *In* T Trial, M Laval-Jeantet, M-C Plainfossé (Eds): Traité de radiodiagnostic. Rhumatologie, articulations, parties molles. Paris, Masson, 1976, p 423.
33. Fischer E: Die progressive Sklerodermie der Finger im Weichstrahlbild. Fortschr Geb Roentgenstr Nuklearmed *119*:372, 1973.
34. Brower AC, NaPombejara C, Stechschulte DJ, Mautz F, Ketchum L: Rheumatoid nodulosis: another cause of juxtaarticular nodules. Radiology *125*:669, 1977.
35. Fischer E: Weichteilverkalkungen am Rande der Tuberositas unguicularis der Finger. (in preparation).
36. Fischer E: Subunguale Verkalkungen (in preparation).
37. Kalliomäki JL, Vastamäki M: Chronic diffuse oedema of the rheumatoid hand. A sign of local lymphatic involvement. Ann Rheum Dis *27*:167, 1968.
38. Weston WJ, Palmer DG: Soft Tissues of the Extremities. A Radiologic Study of Rheumatic Disease. Berlin, Springer Verlag, 1978, pp 13, 14, 60.
39. Mäkelä P, Virtama P: The "pre-erosive" radiologic signs of rheumatoid arthritis in soft tissue radiography of the hands. Skel Radiol *2*:213, 1978.
40. Jacobs JH, Hess EV, Beswick IP: Rheumatoid arthritis presenting as tenosynovitis. J Bone Joint Surg *39B*:288, 1957.
41. Terry DW, Ramin JE: The navicular fat stripe. A useful roentgen feature for evaluating wrist trauma. Am J Roentgenol *124*:25, 1975.
42. Fischer E: Weichstrahldiagnostik des vergrössberten Recessus sacciformis des distalen Radio-ulnargelenks. Radiologe *15*:157, 1975.
43. Martel W, Hayes JT, Duff IF: The pattern of bone erosion in the hand and wrist in rheumatoid arthritis. Radiology *84*:204, 1965.
44. Resnick D: Early abnormalities of pisiform and triquetrum in rheumatoid arthritis. Ann Rheum Dis *35*:46, 1976.
45. Steinbrocker O, Argyros, TG: The shoulder-hand syndrome: Present status as a diagnostic and therapeutic entity. Med Clin North Am *42*:1533, 1958.
46. Genant HK, Kozin F, Bekerman C, McCarty DJ, Sims J: The reflex sympathetic dystrophy syndrome. Radiology *117*:21, 1975.
47. Poznanski AK: The Hand in Radiologic Diagnosis. WB Saunders Co, Philadelphia, 1974, p. 297.
48. Goldberg A, Brodsky I, McCarty D: Multiple myeloma with paramyloidosis presenting as rheumatoid disease. Am J Med *37*:653, 1964.
49. Gordon DA, Pruzanski W, Ogryzlo MA, Little HA: Amyloid arthritis simulating rheumatoid disease in five patients with multiple myeloma. Am J Med *55*:142, 1973.
50. Fischer E: Weichteildiagnostik an den peripheren Extremitäten mittels Weichstrahltechnik. Teil II. Erkrankungen der Achillessehne und ihrer angrenzenden Gewebe. Radiologe *14*:457, 1974.
51. Toygar O: Subkutane Ruptur der Achillessehne (Diagnostik und Behandlungsergebnisse). Helv Chir Acta *14*:209, 1947.
52. Gatterau A, Davignon J, Langelier M, Levesque HP: An improved radiological method for the evaluation of achilles tendon xanthomatosis. Can Med Assoc J *108*:39, 1973.
53. Alexander CJ: Effect of growth rate on the strength of the growth plate-shaft junction. Skel Radiol *1*:67, 1976.
54. Scotti DM, Sadhu VK, Heimberg F, O'Hara AE: Osgood-Schlatter's disease, an emphasis on soft tissue changes in roentgen diagnosis. Skel Radiol *4*:21, 1979.

11 XERORADIOGRAPHY

by Harry K. Genant, M.D.

Xeroradiography is an electrostatic imaging system that utilizes selenium as a photoconductor. It is a radiographic application of the xerographic process first discovered by Carlson in 1937. This methodology initially was applied in the field of graphic arts, where the process was used as a photographic recording medium. McMaster and Schaffert[22] first used the selenium plate with x-rays for the nondestructive testing of metal castings. The initial medical adaptation of xeroradiography was undertaken in the early 1950s by Roach and Hilleboe,[27-29] who explored the system as a means of providing diagnostic x-ray facilities during civilian disasters.

In the past 12 years, considerable investigative effort has been directed by Wolfe[34-37] at the medical applications of xeroradiography. Wolfe has written extensively on xeroradiography as an imaging modality for mammography and has also supported its use in other areas of diagnostic radiography. These applications include skeletal trauma, metabolic bone disease, musculoskeletal neoplasms, and arthritis.

TECHNICAL CONSIDERATIONS

The physical qualities of semiconductors form the basis for the xeroradiographic imaging process.[18, 29, 37] The ability of a semiconductor to change from a material of high electrical resistance in the resting state to one of relatively low resistance when activated by radiant energy is fundamental for capturing a latent image. The xeroradiographic plate upon which the latent image is formed has an aluminum base that is coated with a thin photoconductive layer of vitreous selenium. Although a number of semiconductors are available, selenium has been utilized most extensively.

Image Production

Briefly, the steps in image production are as follows[18, 29, 37]: The metal plate is charged to a high positive potential by coronal discharge; then it is placed in a cassette and used as an image receptor similar to a conventional screen-film system; when the X rays strike the selenium plate, photoconduction occurs, which produces a latent charge image of the object; the latent image is made visible by the use of charged developer particles or toner particles, which are brought in close proximity to the plate; and finally, the resultant powder image is transferred to a paper and fused thermally, providing a permanent opaque image.

Edge Enhancement

One of the unique features of the xeroradiographic imaging process is the phenomenon of edge enhancement. To understand this process, one must examine closely the mechanism of image production in xeroradiography[18, 37, 41] (Fig. 11–1).

Prior to x-ray exposure, the xeroradiographic plate undergoes *relaxation*, a process of heating that removes any residual charge pattern on the plate.[18, 42] This relaxation prevents ghosting or the faint appearance of information from the previous image on the new image. After relaxation, the plate has a uniform level of surface potential.

In order for the image to be captured, the plate must be charged by submitting the plate to a uniform surface charge, thus sensitizing it for x-ray exposure.

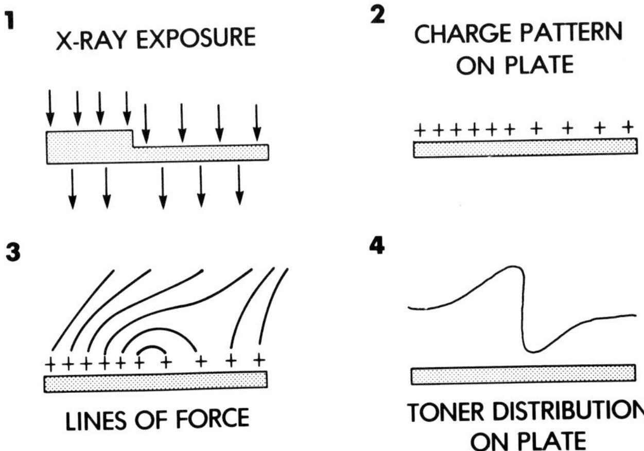

Figure 11–1. *Schematic representation of the steps in production of the xeroradiographic image. (From Xerox corporation: Technical Application Bulletin 3, November 1975.)*

The surface charge is applied by a series of coronal discharge wires that are electromechanically passed close to the selenium plate, depositing a positive electrostatic charge on the surface of the selenium.

During radiographic exposure, X rays are transmitted through the object and are absorbed by the selenium plate, causing a selective *discharge*. The amount of discharge is proportional to the radiation striking the selenium plate. The information in the transmitted x-ray beam is present as a residual charge pattern on the plate, a *latent image*. Although the latent image is not edge enhanced, charge differences in the latent image and the resulting electric fields do cause edge enhancement during later development steps. To make the latent image visible, the selenium plate is processed, during which a cloud of negatively charged fine powder, called toner, is attracted to the charge pattern on the plate. This attraction is related to the amount of residual charge and is controlled by the *electric fields* occurring during development.

Electric fields exist during development as a result of two phenomena. First, a voltage is applied to the back of the plate and the development chamber. This provides a uniform contribution to the electric field and aids in delivering toner near the plate. Second, charge differences in the latent image cause *fringe fields*. These are strong near the plate surface and contribute to the electric field nonuniformly. Fringe fields are strongest at the boundary between areas of different charge and are weakest in areas of uniform charge. The latter phenomenon results in broad area contrast suppression. Wherever there is an abrupt change in charge as shown for the step edge exposure (Fig. 11–1), the fringe field directs more toner to the high charge side of the step edge and less toner to the lower charge side, producing the edge effect.

Thus, following the distribution of the lines of electric force, an edge or boundary is developed with increased toner on one side producing a darker band juxtaposed to a lighter band with less toner deposition. This accentuated toner distribution at contrast interfaces then produces the *edge enhancement* characteristic of xeroradiography.[18, 37]

IMAGE QUALITY AND DOSIMETRY

The recording characteristics of *edge enhancement* and *broad latitude* found with the xeroradiographic system can be appreciated from Figure 11–2, which demonstrates the density tracings of a step-wedge exposure using xeroradiography, a screen-film system, and a nonscreen system.[9, 18] The exaggerated edge effect and the suppressed broad area contrast of the xeroradiographic system can be appreciated from the tracing and are the result of the electric lines of force discussed previously. With the screen-film system, a blurred edge effect can be seen, which represents unsharpness resulting from light

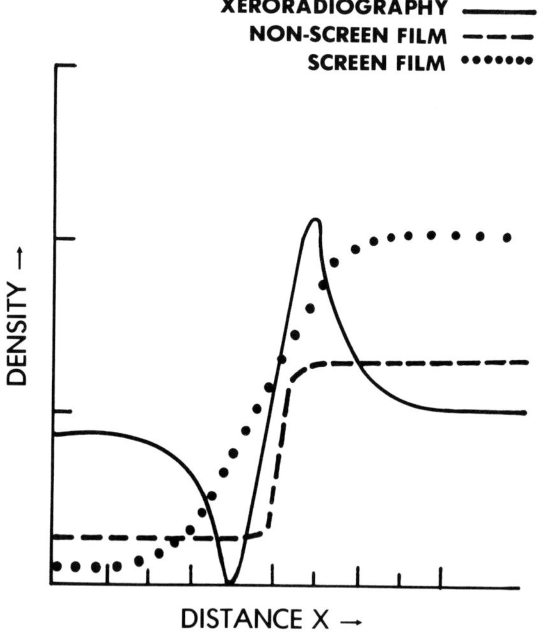

Figure 11–2. Schematic representation of density tracings of a step wedge for three recording systems (adapted from Fender[9]).

diffusion in the phosphor screen. This blurring is characteristic of screen-film systems. The nonscreen-film technique demonstrates a sharp edge interface but no edge enhancement, as with xeroradiography. Additionally, the nonscreen technique has lower contrast than the screen-film system but does not show the broad area contrast suppression of the xeroradiographic system.

It is of importance to note that the amount of edge enhancement and the degree of broad area contrast suppression can be manipulated by appropriate selection of the kilovoltage for exposure, the amount of charge potential initially placed on the plate, and the level of back voltage applied during developing.[18] The latter two steps provide added recording flexibility, which is not achievable with conventional radiography. Generally, a relatively high kilovoltage exposure (~ 120 kVp) is selected for musculoskeletal applications[40] in order to increase the recording latitude and to diminish the excessive edge enhancement, which can produce a halo effect or toner deletion at the high contrast interfaces between bone and soft tissue. It can be inferred from Figure 11–2 that the sharpness or *spatial resolution* of the xeroradiographic system is high relative to conventional screen-film radiography but is less than that of nonscreen techniques using medical or industrial film. The mottle or *noise* of the xeroradiography similarly falls between that of a conventional screen-film system and that of a nonscreen-film technique. As a result of these inherent image characteristics, a xeroradiograph may be optically magnified 1.5 to 2 times using a hand lens, and additional useful information may occasionally be derived. The use of higher degrees of optical magnification, as are commonly employed for industrial film radiography, however, does not provide additional diagnostic information for xeroradiography. Here, the four- to eightfold enlargement simply produces a greater visual awareness of the inherent unsharpness and mottle of the xeroradiographic image.

The *radiation exposure* required for xeroradiography is relatively high compared to that needed for conventional screen-film radiography, but it is lower than that for nonscreen industrial film.[16, 19, 35, 36] Typically skin doses of 0.3 to 2.0 rads are needed for musculoskeletal applications, which generally limits the use of xeroradiography to the thinner body parts.

CLINICAL APPLICATIONS

By far the largest clinical application for xeroradiography has been in the area of *mammography.*[21, 30, 34, 36] In this field the broad latitude of the recording system and the edge enhancement have proved valuable in assessing the breast for benign and malignant neoplasms. In comparison with the nonscreen industrial film technique used earlier by Egan, xeroradiography provides lower radiation exposure and possibly greater ease of interpretation. These factors have contributed to the widespread use of xeroradiography as a mammographic recording system. With the recent advent of the low-dose, high-resolution screen-film systems for mammography,[3, 25, 31, 32] however, the continued use of the higher dose xeromammography is in question.

Xeroradiography has not been widely employed as a recording medium for anatomic parts other than the breast. Although studies have been reported outlining its value in selected applications, a widespread use of xeroradiography in routine clinical practice has not been observed. It appears to have greatest potential in the depiction of *soft tissue masses*[17, 26, 35] in an extremity or limb girdle, in which situations the broad recording latitude and the edge enhancement show the subtle density interfaces of the soft tissue lesions to advantage (Fig. 11–3). Differentiation between benign and malignant soft tissue neoplasms has been observed in some cases. This application, however, is rapidly being supplanted by computed tomography,[2, 4, 14, 15] which has far superior density resolution and the advantage of providing cross-sectional display.

Another area in which xeroradiography has found some success is in the depiction of subtle skeletal abnormalities in patients with early *arthritis* or *metabolic bone disease.*[35, 39, 40] In the former situation the ability to show with a single radiographic

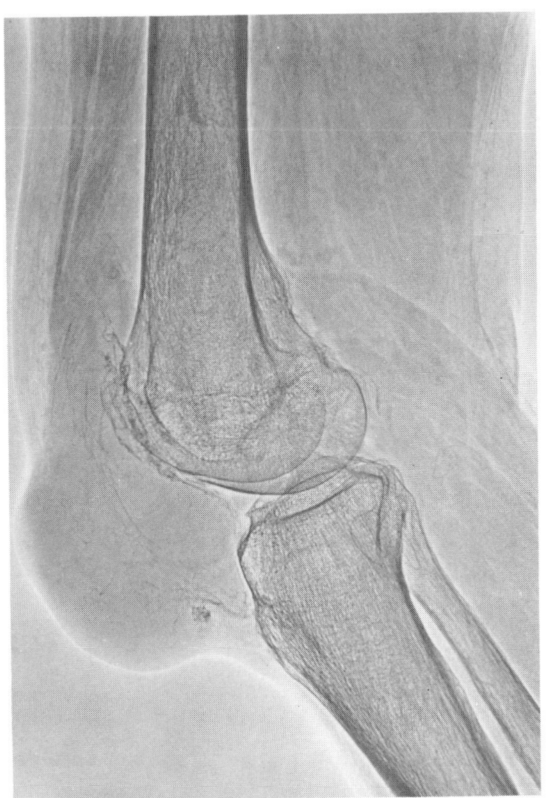

Figure 11–3. *Xeroradiograph of the knee, which demonstrates a lytic destructive process with a large soft tissue component that has replaced the patella. The edge enhancement and broad latitude of the xeroradiographic system can be appreciated.*

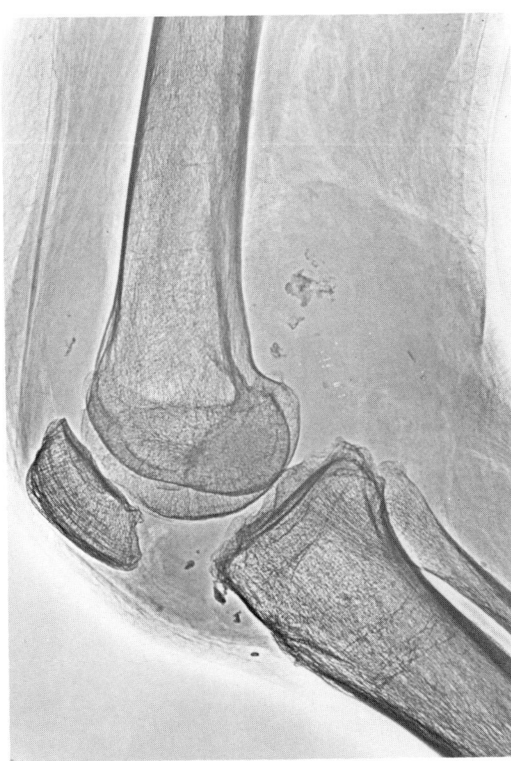

Figure 11–4. *Xeroradiograph of the knee demonstrating moderately advanced degenerative arthropathy complicated by a large joint effusion and a Baker's (popliteal) cyst. The soft tissue planes are particularly well demonstrated by xeroradiography.*

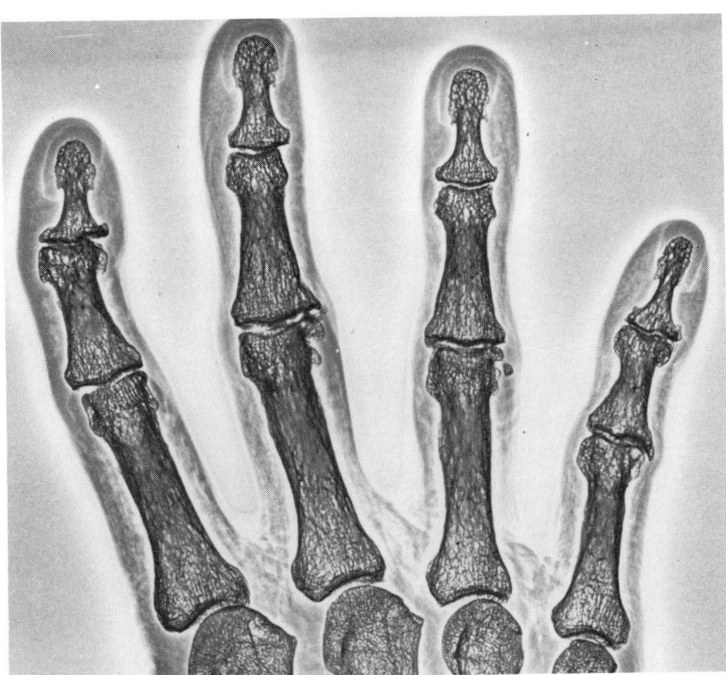

Figure 11–5. *Xeroradiograph of the distal hand of a patient with primary generalized osteoarthritis. Articular and periarticular structures are well shown with the xeroradiographic technique.*

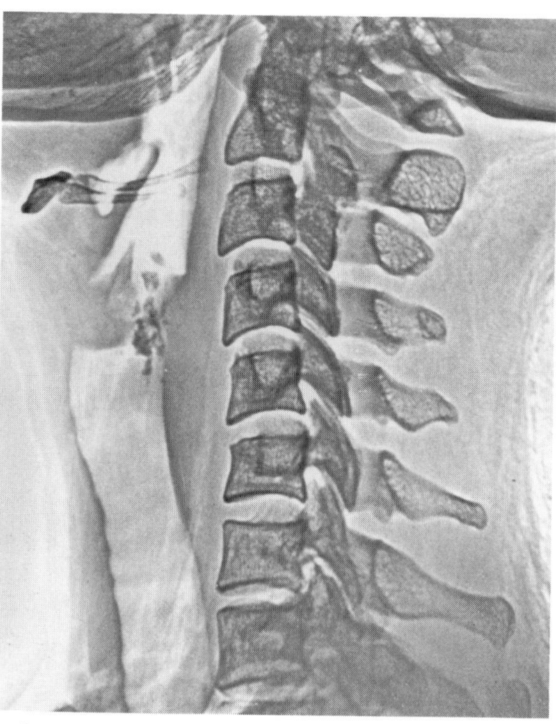

Figure 11–6. Xeroradiographic view of the neck demonstrates the osseous as well as the soft tissue structures to advantage.

exposure the osseous structures of the joint as well as the periarticular soft tissues is a potential advantage (Figs. 11–4 and 11–5). It appears, however, that for this application, the use of magnification techniques, either optical or radiographic, are more widely accepted, since they provide superior images.[1, 5, 11, 12, 13, 20, 31] Similarly, in the assessment of suble structural changes in the hands or feet in metabolic bone disease, xeroradiography, although superior to conventional screen-film radiography, is inferior to the alternative high-resolution magnification techniques.[7, 10, 11, 12, 23, 24, 33]

In selected cases, xeroradiography has been shown to provide high-quality images for viewing the *cervical spine* and *ribs*.[26, 35] Here xeroradiography can record many tissues of different density and thicknesses; for example, bone, fat, air, and muscle are readily delineated on a single image. On a lateral view of the cervical spine, one can easily see the primary areas of interest, the vertebrae, and also the thinner, less dense parts such as the trachea, cartilages, epiglottis, valleculae, and so forth (Fig. 11–6). Thus, when the soft tissues of the neck are of particular importance, xeroradiography may be used.[6] Similarly, the detection of subtle abnormalities in the rib cage may be difficult with conventional radiography due to the broad latitude required, and xeroradiography may be used.

Xeroradiography has had some success in imaging the skeletal structures of an extremity that has been immobilized in a *plaster cast*.[38] In this situation, the superimposition of structures and the broad range of subject density make visualization by conventional radiography difficult. The xeroradiographic process, with the high kilovoltage generally applied, permits the cast to be penetrated readily, whereas the edge enhancement and wide recording latitude permit the edges of bones and fractures to be easily detected.

SUMMARY

In summary, the xeroradiographic imaging process differs considerably from conventional screen-film or nonscreen radiography, having unique imaging characteristics of edge enhancement, subdued broad area response, and large object latitude. These imaging characteristics make this modality useful in selected cases for imaging low-contrast objects that are defined by sharp edges. Nevertheless, the widespread acceptance and usage of xeroradiography for routine musculoskeletal examinations appear unlikely owing to the relatively high radiation exposure required and the comparatively limited availability of the system.

REFERENCES

1. Berens, DL, Lin RK: Roentgen Diagnosis of Rheumatoid Arthritis. Springfield, Ill, Charles C Thomas, 1969.
2. Berger, PE, Kuhn JP: Computed tomography of tumors of the musculoskeletal system in children. Radiology *127*:171, 1978.
3. Chang CHJ, Sibala JL, Martin NL, Riley RC: Film mammography: New low radiation technology. Radiology *121*:215, 1976.
4. DeSantos LA, Goldstein HM, Murray JA, Wallace S: Computed tomography in the evaluation of musculoskeletal neoplasms. Radiology *128*:89, 1978.
5. Doi K, Genant HK, Rossmann K: Comparison of image quality obtained with optical and radiographic magnification techniques in fine-detail skeletal radiography: Effect of object thickness. Radiology *118*:189, 1976.
6. Doust BD, Ting YM: Xeroradiography of the larynx. Radiology *110*:727, 1974.
7. Doyle FH: Radiological patterns of bone disease associated with renal glomerular failure in adults. Br Med Bull *28*:220, 1972.
8. Egan RL: Mammography and breast diseases. *In:* LL Robbins (Ed): Golden's Diagnostic Radiology. Baltimore, Williams & Wilkins, 1970, p. 240.
9. Fender WD: Radiographic image analysis through application of the radiographic modulation transfer function and system phase response. *In*: Quantitative Imagery in the Biomedical Sciences. Proceedings of the Society of Photo-Optical Instrumentation Engineers, Bellingham, Washington, Vol. 26, 1971.
10. Genant HK, Heck, LL, Lanzl LH, et al: Primary hyperparathyroidism. A comprehensive study of clinical, biochemical and radiographic manifestations. Radiology *109*:513, 1973.
11. Genant HK, Doi K, Mall JC: Optical versus radiographic magnification for fine-detail skeletal radiography. Invest Radiol *10*:160, 1975.
12. Genant HK, Doi K, Mall JC, Sickles EA: Direct radiographic magnification for skeletal radiology: An assessment of image quality and clinical application. Radiology *123*:47, 1977.
13. Genant HK, Doi K: High-resolution skeletal radiography: Image quality and clinical applications. Curr Probl Radiol *7*:3, 1978.
14. Genant HK, Wilson JS, Bovill EG, Brunelle FO, Murray WR, Rodrigo JR: Computed tomography of the musculoskeletal system. J Bone Joint Surg (in press).
15. Hunter JC, Johnston WH, Genant HK: Computed tomography evaluation of fatty tumors of the somatic soft tissues: Clinical utility and radiologic pathologic correlation. Skeletal Radiology *4*:79, 1979.
16. Jaeger SS, Cacak RK, Barnes JE, Hendee WR: Optimization of xeroradiographic exposures. Radiology *128*:217, 1978.
17. Jing BS: Xeroradiography of the soft tissues. Cancer Bull *26*:31, 1974.
18. Kearns WJ: Xeroradiography — Principles and Practice. *In*:Quantitative Imagery in the Biomedical Sciences. Proceedings of the Society of Photo-Optical Instrumentation Engineers, Bellingham, Washington, Vol 26, 1971.
19. Lester RG: Risk versus benefit in mammography. Radiology *124*:1, 1977.
20. Mall JC, Genant HK, Silcox DC, McCarty, DJ: The efficacy of fine-detail radiography in the evaluation of patients with rheumatoid arthritis. Radiology *112*:37, 1974.
21. Martin JE: Xeromammography — an improved diagnostic method. A review of 250 biopsied cases. Am J Roentgenol *117*:90, 1973.
22. McMaster RC, Schaffert RM: Xeroradiography — a basic development in x-ray. Nondestructive Testing 9:11, 1950.
23. Meema HE, Schatz DL: Simple radiologic demonstration of cortical bone loss in thyrotoxicosis. Radiology *97*:9, 1970.
24. Meema HE, Meema S: Comparison of microradioscopic and morphometric findings in the hand bones with densitometric findings in the proximal radius in thyrotoxicosis and in renal osteodystrophy. Invest Radiol *7*:88, 1972.
25. Ostrum BJ, Becker W, Isard HJ: Low-dose mammography. Radiology *109*:323, 1973.
26. Otto RC, Pouliadis GP, Kumpe DA: The evaluation of pathologic alterations of juxtaosseous soft tissue by xeroradiography. Radiology *120*:297, 1976.
27. Roach JF, Hilleboe HE: Xeroradiography. Arch Surg *69*:594, 1954.
28. Roach JF, Hilleboe HE: Xeroradiography. Am J Roentgenol *73*:5, 1955.
29. Roach JF: Xeroradiography. Radiol Clin North Am *8*:271, 1970.
30. Rothenberg LN, Kirch RLA, Snyder RE: Patient exposure from film and xeroradiographic mammographic techniques. Radiology *117*:701, 1975.
31. Sickles EA, Doi K, Genant HK: Magnification film mammography: Image quality and clinical studies. Radiology *125*:69, 1977.
32. Sickles EA, Genant HK: Controlled single-blind clinical evaluation of low-dose mammographic screen-film systems. Radiology *130*:347, 1979.
33. Weiss A: A technique for demonstrating fine detail in bones of the hands. Clin Radiol *23*:185, 1972.
34. Wolfe JN: Xerography of the breast. Radiology *91*:231, 1968.
35. Wolfe JN: Xeroradiography of the bones, joints and soft tissues. Radiology *93*:583, 1969.
36. Wolfe JN, Dooley R, Harkins LE: Xeroradiography of the breast: A comparative study with conventional film mammography. Cancer *28*:1569, 1971.
37. Wolfe JN: Xeroradiography: Image content and comparison with film roentgenograms. Am J Roentgenol *117*:690, 1973.
38. Xerox Corporation: Xeroradiography for casted extremities. Pasadena, California, Xerox Medical Application Bulletin 105, June 1973.
39. Xerox Corporation: Xeroradiography for detection of hyperparathyroidism. Pasadena, California, Xerox Medical Application Bulletin 108, June 1973.
40. Xerox Corporation: Xeroradiography for extremities. Pasadena, California, Xerox Medical Application Bulletin 117, December 1973.
41. Xerox Corporation: What is edge enhancement and how does it affect the mammographic image? Pasadena, California, Technical Application Bulletin 1, November 1974.
42. Xerox Corporation: What are the most common xeroradiographic terms and what do they mean? Pasadena, California, Technical Application Bulletin 3, November 1975.

12

COMPUTED TOMOGRAPHY

by Harry K. Genant, M.D.

In less than a decade since its introduction, computed tomography (CT) has revolutionized neurologic diagnosis and now is having impact on many other medical disciplines, including orthopedic surgery and rheumatology. It has been properly observed that no advancement comparable to CT has been made in radiologic sciences since Roentgen discovered the X ray in 1896. Following the development of the first scanner and the subsequent recognition of its diagnostic capability, the entire field of CT technology rapidly evolved.[3-5, 7] In the United States today, there are over 1400 brain and body scanners in operation. The impact of this technology is extending far beyond medicine per se and is currently a focal point of broader social, economic, and political discussion.[2, 14, 22] These matters, however, are beyond the scope of this chapter, which will focus on the technology of CT and its potential applications in orthopedics and rheumatology.

TECHNOLOGY

What then is the origin of this new technology? Reconstruction from projection profiles dates back to 1917 and the mathematical investigations of

Radon.[50] This method was subsequently studied by many investigators using mathematical and photographic models. The first medical applications were carried out independently by Oldendorf,[45] Cormack,[13] and Kuhl and Edwards[32] in the early 1960s, but it was Godfried Hounsfield[28] of England who developed the first clinically useful brain scanner in 1970.

The essential components of a CT system consist of a scanning gantry frame with patient table, x-ray generator, and a data processing system. The total cost for such a system ranges from several hundred thousand to eight hundred thousand dollars.

To provide insight into the method of image reconstruction and display, it is useful to review the chronologic development of commercial scanners.[7, 30] First generation brain scanners (Fig. 12–1*A*) utilize an x-ray source with a tightly collimated pencil beam that is interfaced with a single sodium iodide detector by means of a gantry frame. The gantry frame translates or moves in a linear fashion, causing the x-ray beam to traverse the head. Multiple readings of x-ray intensities are made across the path. At the completion of the first transverse scan, the entire gantry frame rotates through a small angle, typically 1 degree, and the linear scan is repeated. The entire translate-rotate process is continued through 180 degrees, and a total of several hundred thousand measurements are recorded and transmitted to the computer for processing. The first generation scanners are extremely slow, requiring 5 to 10 minutes per scan.

Second generation scanners (Fig. 12–1*B*) are capable of imaging the body and greatly shorten the scanning time, to between 20 and 120 seconds per scan. This is accomplished by incorporating a narrow fan-beam technology and multiple, rather than single, detectors. A translate-rotate motion is still used but multiple readings are obtained simultaneously; and larger increments of rotation are employed. These scanners are widely used today.

Third generation scanners employ a continuous 360 degree rotary motion rather than the complex translate-rotation motion. This is accomplished by the use of a broad fan-beam, which exposes the entire cross section of the body with one pulse, eliminating the linear translation. The fan-beam is interfaced with a large array of detectors, up to 600 in number (Fig. 12–1C). The resulting scan time for one complete sweep is shortened to 5 to 10 seconds,

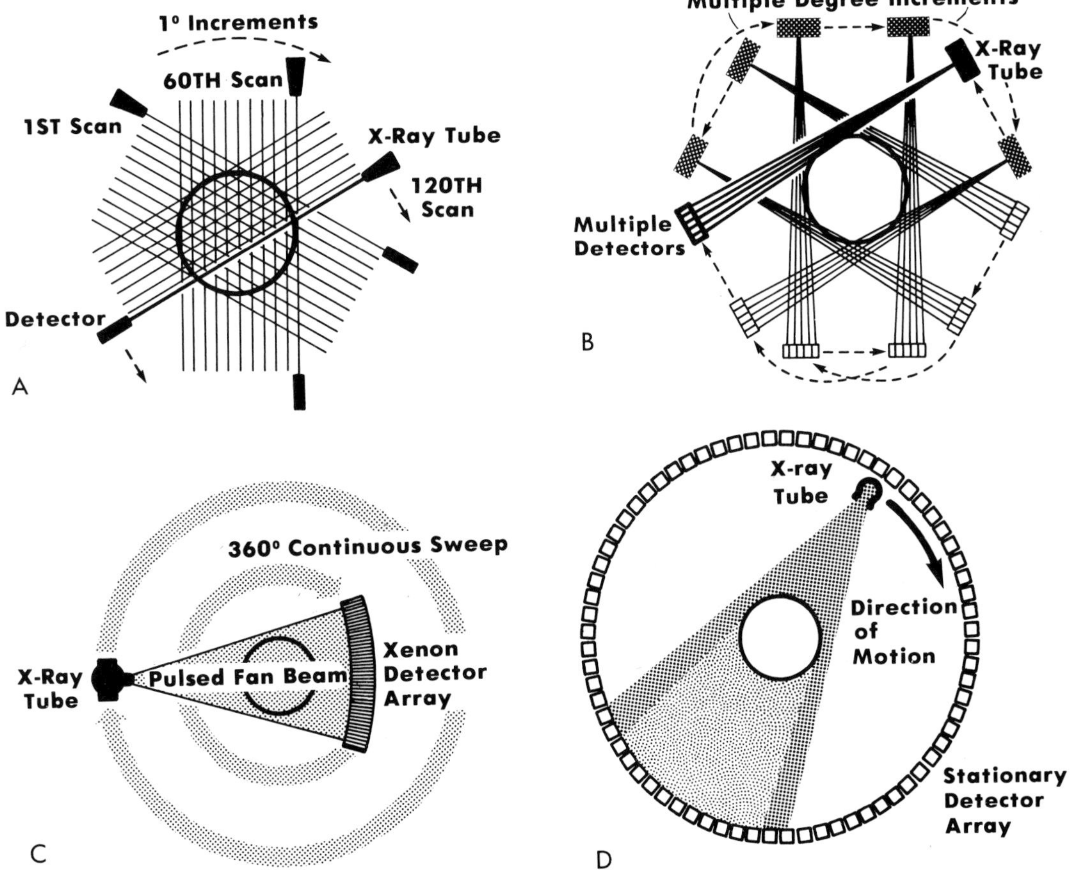

Figure 12–1. *Schematic representation of first generation* **(A)**, *second generation* **(B)**, *third generation* **(C)**, *and fourth generation* **(D)** *CT scanners.*

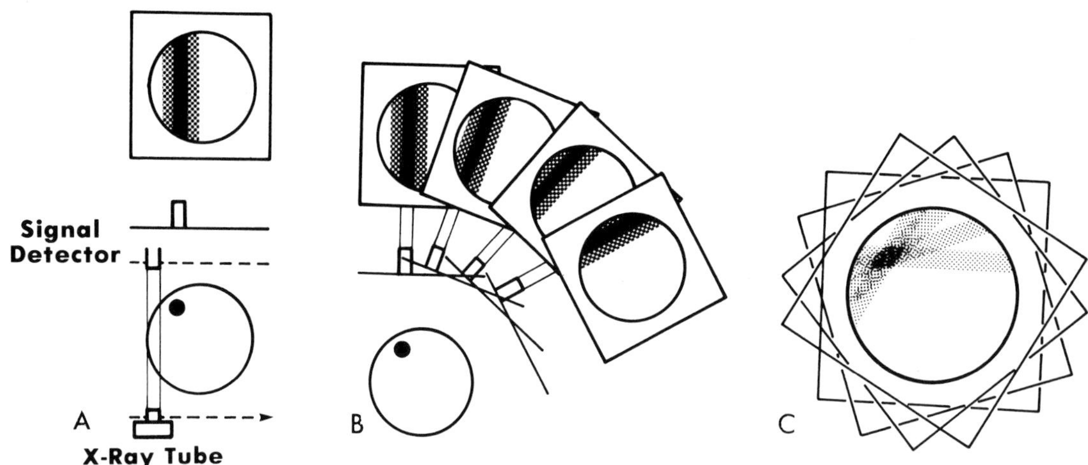

Figure 12–2. *Reconstruction of an image from profiles is shown schematically.*[30] *First, a single scan ray* **(A)** *is generated, followed by multiple scan rays* **(B)**, *and finally a composite of scan rays* **(C)**.

and image reconstruction time is approximately 90 seconds.

Fourth generation scanners (Fig. 12–1*D*) similarly utilize a rotary fan-beam, but in these the detection configuration is a fixed stationary ring. This scanning geometry offers some advantages and disadvantages over third generation scanners.

Reconstruction of an image from profiles is shown graphically in Figure 12–2, in which a brain lesion is simulated and a single scan or array is demonstrated. The computer stores and analyzes multiple arrays and generates an image based upon a mathematical calculation called an algorithm.[9, 26, 30] With appropriate programming, the computer-synthesized image may be nearly artifact-free.

The manner of image computation and presentation by CT scanners is shown schematically in Figure 12–3. The cross-sectional slice, typically 0.5 to 1.3 cm thick, is divided into numerous small volume elements by a coarse grid. Specific x-ray attenuation values are determined for each volume element based upon the density and anatomic number of the tissue within the element.[38, 47, 51] The attenuation values are expressed as CT numbers, shown here on a scale of −1000 for air, 0 for water, and +1000 for dense bone. Typical values[3] computed for various organ tissues are represented in Figure 12–4. The distinction between subtle tissue and organ densities is a unique capability of computed tomography.

For display purposes, the reconstructed slice is regarded as a two dimensional matrix of picture elements called pixels. The computer displays the array of pixels on a video monitor using a color scale or more commonly varying shades of gray to represent the computed CT numbers. The range of CT numbers displayed by the gray scale can be altered by adjusting the window width and level on the video monitor (Fig. 12–5).

Representative technical parameters[7, 8, 25, 30] of

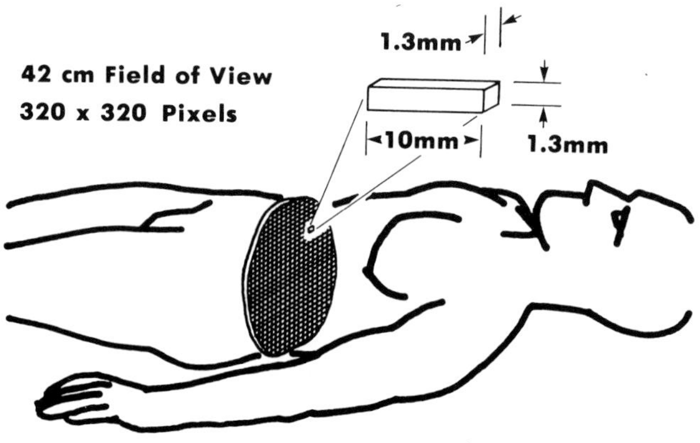

Figure 12–3. *The manner of image computation and presentation by a typical scanner is shown schematically.*

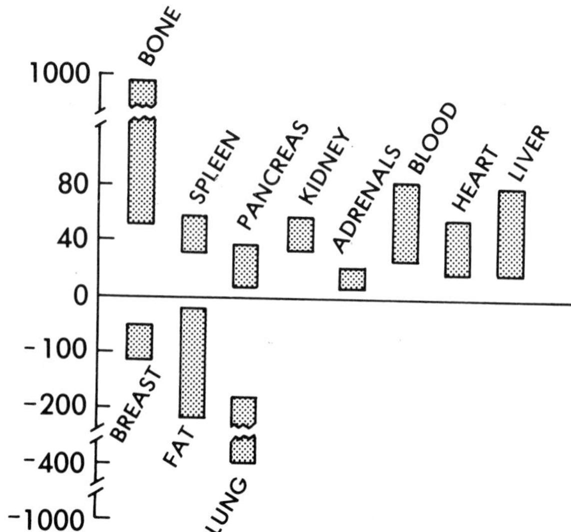

Figure 12–4. *Typical CT values computed for various organ tissues are represented graphically. (From Alfidi RJ, et al: Am J Roentgenol 124:199, 1973.)*

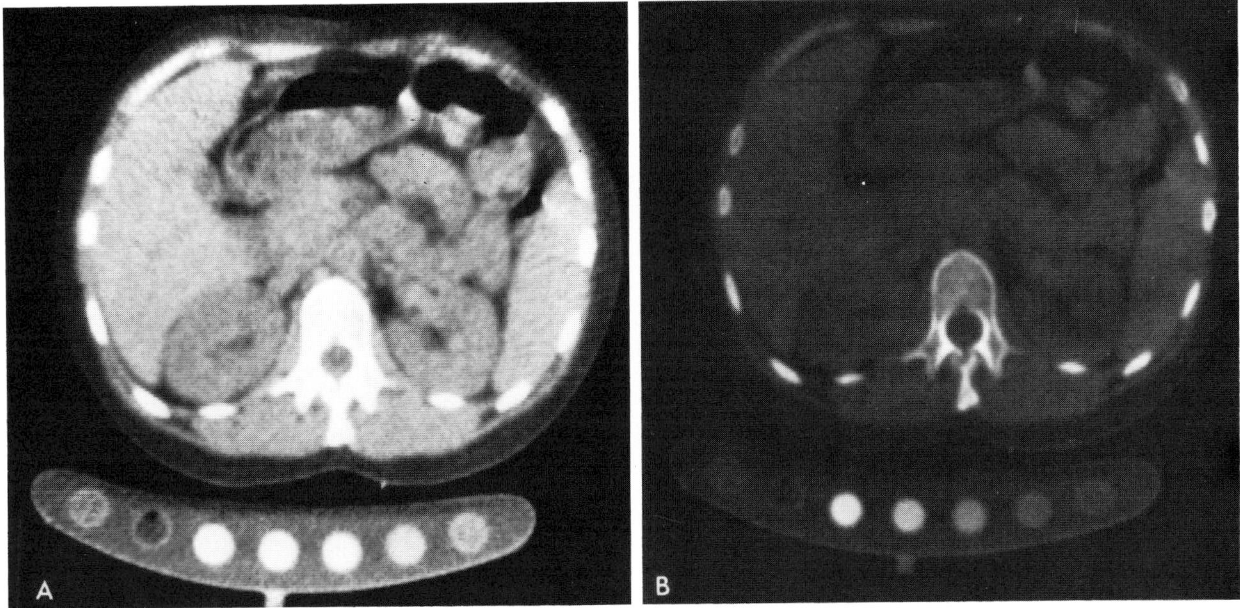

Figure 12–5. *The range of CT numbers displayed by the gray scale can be altered by adjusting the window width and level on the video monitor. A window setting optimal for viewing abdominal viscera* **(A)** *and a window setting optimal for viewing a vertebra* **(B)** *are shown.*

CT scanners are given in Table 12–1. The spatial resolution which is a measure of sharpness, is about 1.5 mm, slightly less than that for conventional radiography. The density resolution, which is a measure of ability to differentiate subtle tissue densities, is about 0.5 per cent, an order of magnitude greater than that for conventional radiography. The radiation exposure for a series of images is in the acceptable range of 1 to 3 rads for the entire examination.[8, 39]

The potential advantages, then, of CT relative to conventional radiography are the cross-sectional display, the excellent density resolution, and the accurate measurement of attenuation coefficient. The manner in which these potential advantages may be specifically applied to examinations of the musculoskeletal system will be illustrated.

TECHNICAL FACTORS

The technical requirements for optimal examination of disorders of the musculoskeletal system differ from those for examinations of the brain and abdomen. Although each study must be tailored to the specific needs of the patient, general principles can be outlined.[21, 40, 41, 55] A preliminary radiograph is obtained with external radiopaque markers to facilitate localization. The patient is positioned to maintain anatomic symmetry of the skeleton, a measure that aids in detecting subtle differences in osseous or muscular tissues. Intravenous contrast is administered if the precontrast scan fails to identify a suspected mass (isodense lesion) or if major vessel encroachment is suspected. Additionally, if the degree of vascularity of a soft tissue mass is of diagnostic or therapeutic importance, intravenous contrast may be utilized to answer this question. The CT study is performed using contiguous scans through the lesion to the nearest joint. Slices 0.5 cm thick for bony lesions and 1.0 cm thick for soft tissue lesions are used. The video display and hard copy images should utilize a maximum, or near-maximum, window width (~1000 Hounsfield units) and a relatively high window level (~200 Hounsfield units) in order to visualize the broad range of subject contrast and the highest density of musculoskeletal structures. In order to distinguish and confirm subtle differences in marrow and soft tissue densities, the measure mode should be employed for quantification. Careful attention to these technical details will improve the interpretation of CT scans of the musculoskeletal system and enhance their diagnostic and therapeutic utility.

Table 12–1

COMPUTED TOMOGRAPHY – TECHNICAL PARAMETERS

Spatial Resolution	~1.5 mm
Density Resolution	~ 0.5%
Radiation Exposure	~1–3 rads

CLINICAL APPLICATIONS

A broad experience using computed tomography has been gained at the University of California,

Table 12–2
CLASSIFICATION OF 200 CASES

	Number
Neoplastic Disorders	78
Primary	
Metastatic	
Non-neoplastic Disorders	62
Anatomic variant	
Infection	
Trauma	
Spinal stenosis	
Bone stock deficiency	
Quantitative Bone Mineral Analyses	60

San Francisco (UCSF), during the past 5 years.[1, 10, 20, 22, 23, 51, 52, 55] During this period, over 200 examinations for musculoskeletal disorders have been performed. An analysis of these cases and a review of pertinent literature[6, 15, 16, 37, 40, 41, 44, 46, 54] provide the basis for this discussion.

The major categories (Table 12–2) to be considered are neoplastic (78 cases) and non-neoplastic (62 cases) disorders and quantitative bone mineral analyses (60 cases). Our largest experience has been with *neoplastic disorders.* As experience is gained and technology advances, however, it is likely that CT applications for *non-neoplastic disorders* will have greater impact on orthopedics and rheumatology. Finally, the potential of CT for *quantitative bone mineral analysis* will be briefly addressed (see also Chapter 18).

Neoplastic Disorders

An analysis of the role of CT in the evaluation of neoplasms of the musculoskeletal system will be considered first. For *primary bone tumors*[15, 16, 17, 21, 50, 55], CT scanning is useful in (1) localizing the lesion by cross-sectional display; (2) determining its intramedullary and extra-osseous extent; and (3) defining the relationship between tumor and vital structures. Representative cases illustrating these points are given later in this chapter.

Figure 12–6*A* demonstrates a radiograph of an adolescent boy with leg pain, which shows solid periosteal reaction circumscribing the femur. This appearance is consistent with a diagnosis of osteoid osteoma, Brodie's abscess, or stress fracture. CT scans are shown using two different window settings, one optimal for visualizing soft tissue (Fig.

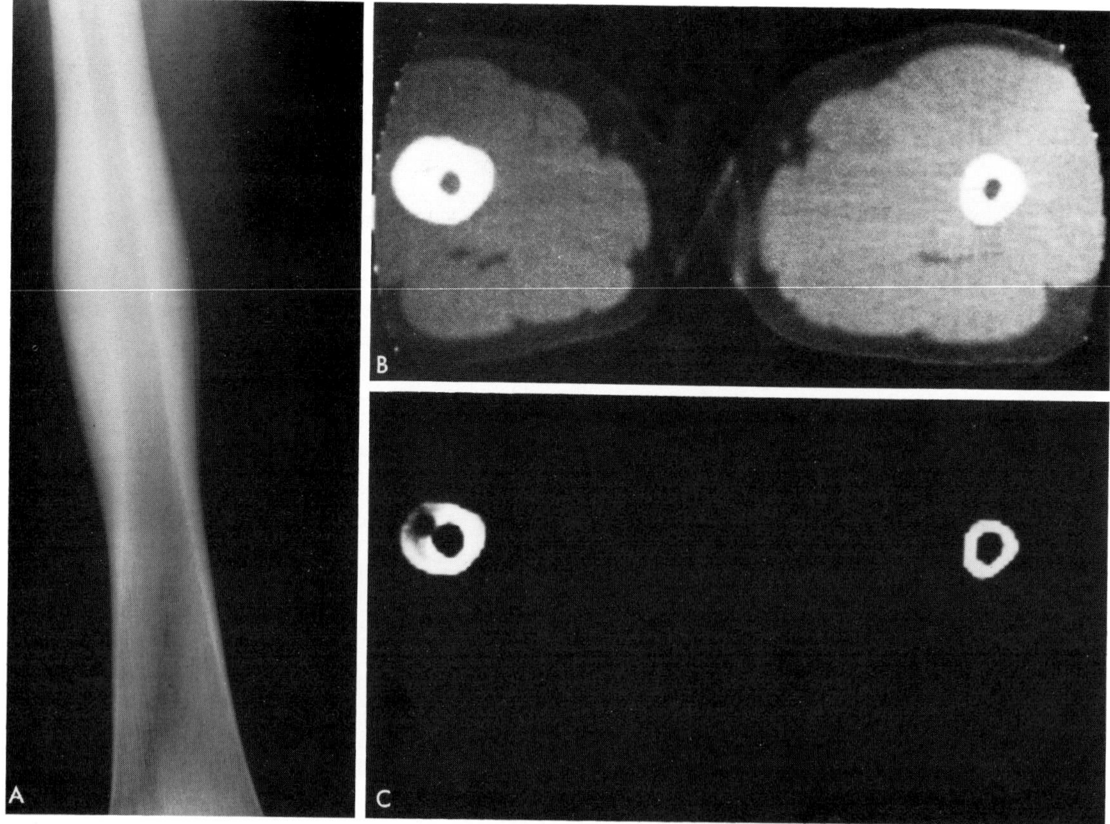

Figure 12–6. *Conventional radiograph* **(A)** *of the femur demostrates solid periosteal reaction circumscribing the femur. CT scans are shown at two different window settings, one optimal for soft tissues* **(B)** *and one optimal for skeletal structures* **(C)**. *The lucent nidus surrounded by dense bone on CT is nearly diagnostic of an osteoid osteoma.*

12–6*B*) and one optimal for visualizing skeletal structure (Fig. 12–6*C*). The lucent nidus surrounded by dense bone shown on CT is virtually diagnostic of an osteoid osteoma. More importantly, this type of precise preoperative localization by cross-sectional display may be helpful for the surgeon when, as in this case, a small focus within dense cortical bone is to be resected.

Figure 12–7*A* shows a radiograph of a young lady presenting with low back pain. A well-defined, lytic, expansile process in the sacroiliac (SI) region is demonstrated. The CT scan (Fig. 12–7*B*) reveals this lesion to be in the ilium, abutting, but not crossing, the SI joint. The CT number or density of this lesion is that of water, not fat or muscle, suggesting the diagnosis of a benign fluid-filled cyst. More importantly, an anterior approach was being considered prior to the study, but CT clearly indicates that the lesion should be unroofed by a posterior approach. This benign bone cyst was subsequently curetted and packed using a posterior approach.

In contrast to this example of a fluid-filled cyst, the following case illustrates a solid intraosseous lesion in a young man presenting with pain in his shoulder. A plain film (Fig. 12–8*A*) shows lytic destruction of the proximal humerus abutting the articular surface, an appearance suggestive of giant cell tumor. The CT (Fig. 12–8*B*) here confirms the solid nature of the mass. Unlike the previous case, this lesion has nearly the same density as the adjacent muscle. More significantly, CT shows that the humeral cortex is entirely intact and that no extraosseous soft tissue mass is present. This assessment may be important in benign but locally aggressive lesions when the surgeon is considering an allograft or a custom prosthesis.[15]

Figure 12–9 reveals images of a patient who presented with a painless mass in the calf. Conventional radiographs (Fig. 12–9*A*,*B*) show an ossifying process in the region of the tibia and fibula. Even with tomograms, the relationship of the mass to the underlying tibia and fibula and the presence of an intramedullary component could not be determined. These features are important in differentiating osteo-

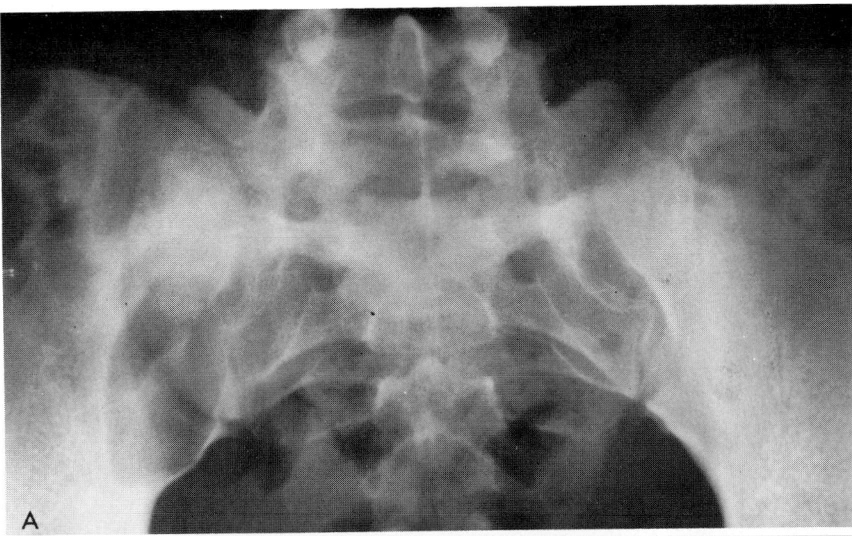

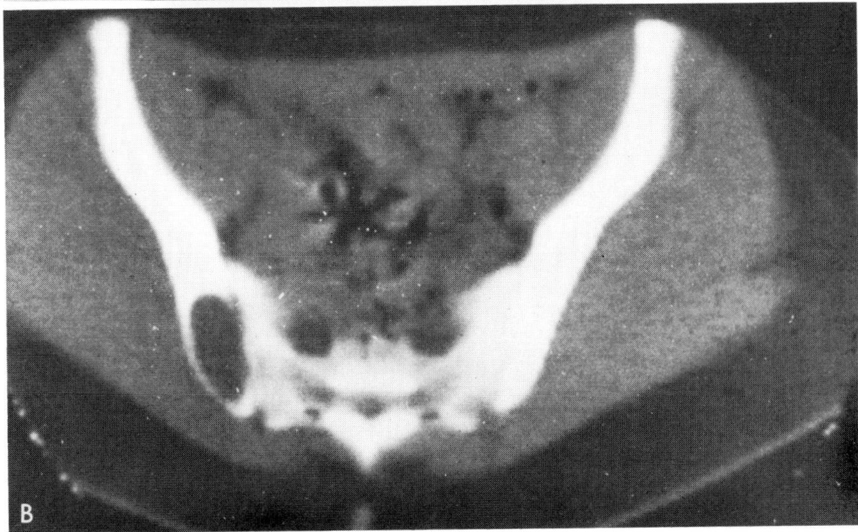

Figure 12–7. *Conventional radiograph* **(A)** *demonstrates a well-defined, lytic, expansile lesion in the right sacroiliac region. CT scan* **(B)** *demonstrates the precise posterior location and fluid nature of the lesion.*

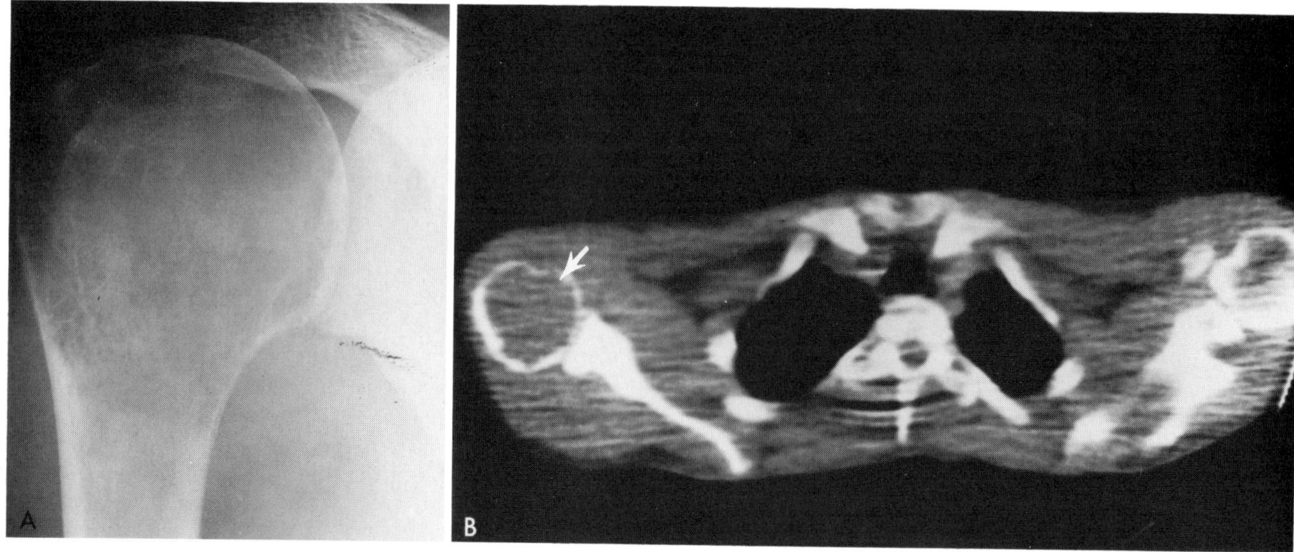

Figure 12–8. *Conventional radiograph* **(A)** *demonstrates a lytic, destructive lesion in the proximal humerus abutting the articular surface. CT scan* **(B)** *confirms the solid nature of this giant cell tumor (arrow) and shows the integrity of the humeral cortex.*

sarcoma from parosteal sarcoma and myositis ossificans. The CT scans (Fig. 12–9*C,D*) are helpful in showing the intimate relationship of this ossifying mass to the underlying tibia and the sparing of the fibula. There is only focal involvement of the medullary canal. This appearance is most consistent with a parosteal sarcoma, and the cross-sectional display is helpful in planning surgical management.

The next example is that of a young woman with hip pain and restricted range of motion. Radiographically (Fig. 12–10*A*) a large calcified cap is evident, suggesting an osteochondroma. The CT scan (Fig. 12–10*B*) provides information regarding the surgical management. It indicates that if the lesion is resected to the base of the stalk, adequate cortex will remain to provide structural integrity. It also shows there is no soft tissue mass outside of the calcified portion, which lends support to its benign nature. Additionally, following the administration of intravenous contrast material to this patient, it can be seen that the femoral artery and vein are not entrapped within the lesion, an important surgical consideration.

In contrast to this case of benign cartilage neoplasm, Figure 12–11 depicts a patient who presented with a mass in the shoulder and whose plain chest film showed only a faint density in the axillary region. On a magnification radiograph (Fig. 12–11*A*), discrete, speckled calcification characteristic of a cartilage tumor can be seen. The CT scan (Figure 12–11*B*) reveals the precise posterior relationship of the stalk attaching to the scapula. Additionally, a large soft tissue component is seen that suggests this is not simply an osteochondroma but more likely a chondrosarcoma. This was confirmed at surgery.

The role of CT in assembling soft tissue tumors[15, 29, 41, 54, 55] will be considered next. Here, CT has two functions: it not only determines the extent of the process but also provides a specific diagnosis in many cases. An example is illustrated by a young lady who presented with an increasing girth of the right thigh (Fig. 12–12). The displacement of the normal soft tissue planes can be seen radiographically (Fig. 12–12*A*), but it is difficult to define a mass. CT (Fig. 12–12*B*) clearly demonstrates a homogeneous mass of low density that has a CT number comparable to subcutaneous fat (approximately −100 Hounsfield units). This appearance is diagnostic of a lipoma. There is encapsulation peripherally, but permeation of the musculature centrally indicates an infiltrating lipoma. The complete resection of this type of lipoma is facilitated by preoperative mapping using CT.[29]

Another fatty neoplasm is demonstrated in Figure 12–13. The conventional radiograph documents an extensive, mottled soft tissue mass in the popliteal region. The precontrast CT scan (Figure 12–13*B*) shows a poorly marginated, inhomogeneous mass containing areas of fat density as well as regions of higher density. Following administration of intravenous contrast material (Fig. 12–13*C*), there are areas of enhancement, indicating a vascular component. This appearance, in contrast to that of the previous case, is diagnostic of liposarcoma.[29] CT is largely replacing arteriography as a means of defining the boundaries of soft tissue masses and determining their vascularity.[15, 41, 55]

Not all masses of relatively low density are lipomatous. The CT scan of a patient presenting with mild swelling of the thigh (Fig. 12–14) identifies a sharply marginated, low density mass. On CT, this cylindric lesion extended over 15 cm within the neurovascular bundle of the posterior thigh, an interpretation that was based upon its shape, location and density. A nerve-sheath tumor of the sciatic

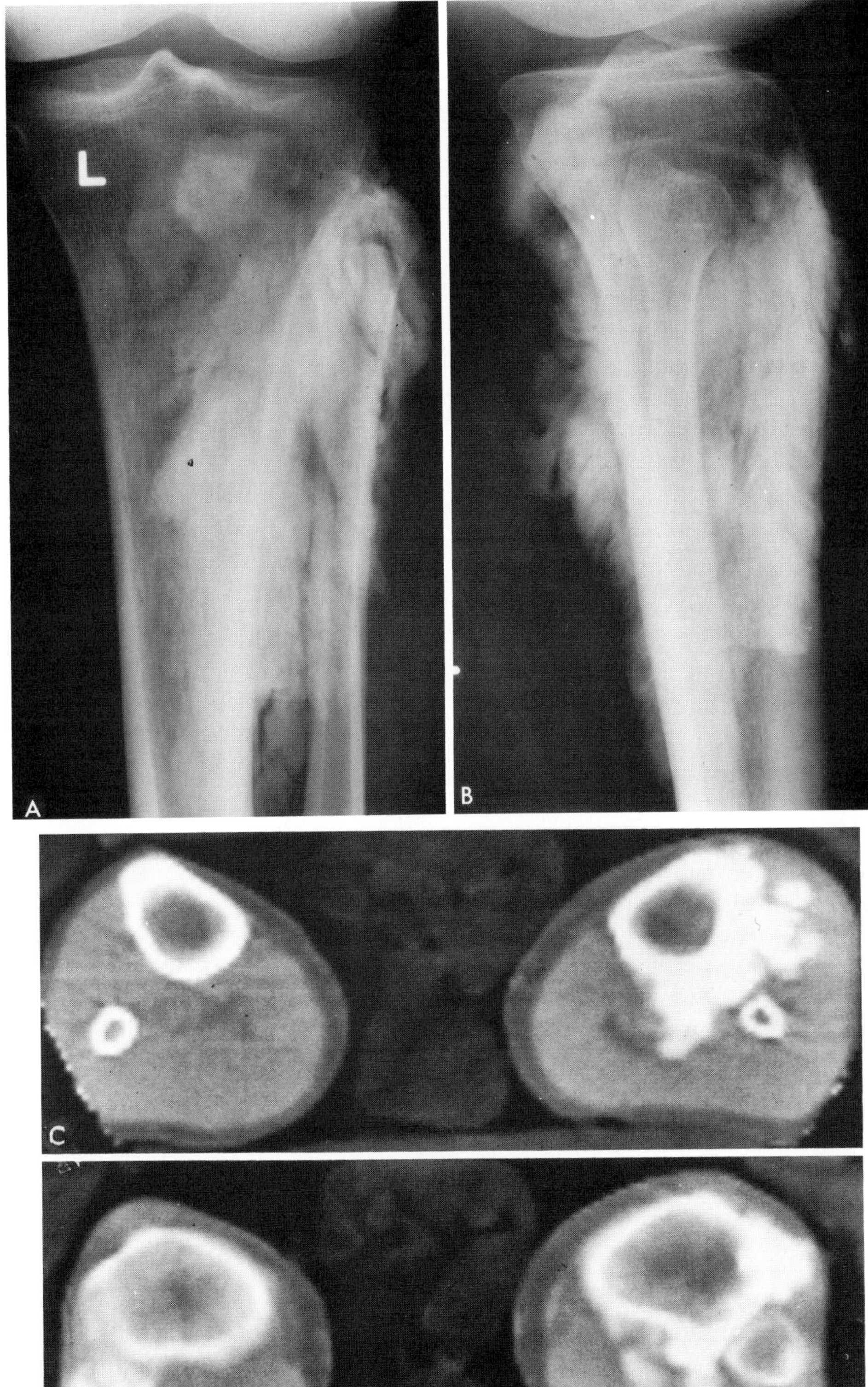

Figure 12–9. *Conventional radiographs* **(A, B)** *show an ossifying process in the region of the tibia and fibula. CT scans* **(C, D)** *demonstrate the intimate relationship of this ossifying mass to the underlying tibia, the sparing of the fibula, and the minimal involvement of the medullary canal. This appearance is nearly diagnostic of parosteal sarcoma.*

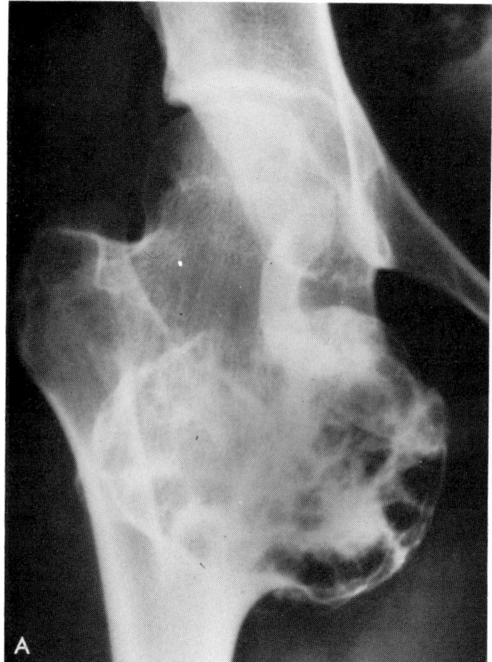

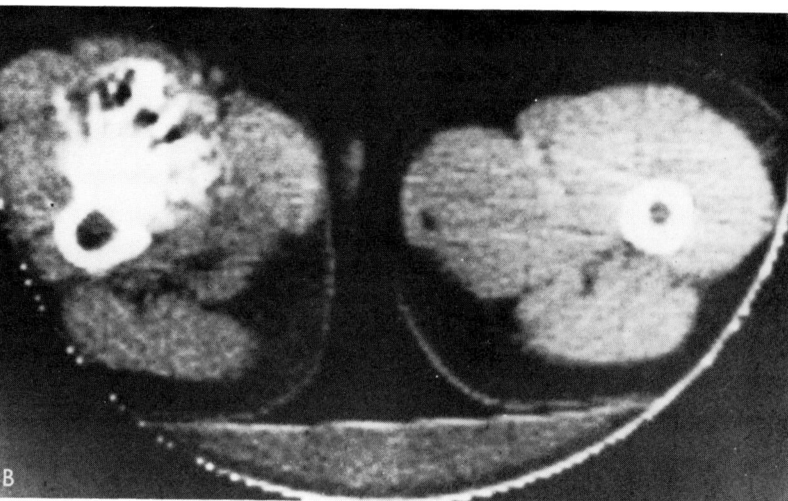

Figure 12–10. *Conventional radiograph* **(A)** *demonstrates a calcified mass projecting from the proximal femur consistent with an osteochondroma. CT scan* **(B)** *demonstrates precise attachment of the stalk to the underlying femur, the absence of a significant soft tissue mass, and the absence of femoral artery and vein entrapment.*

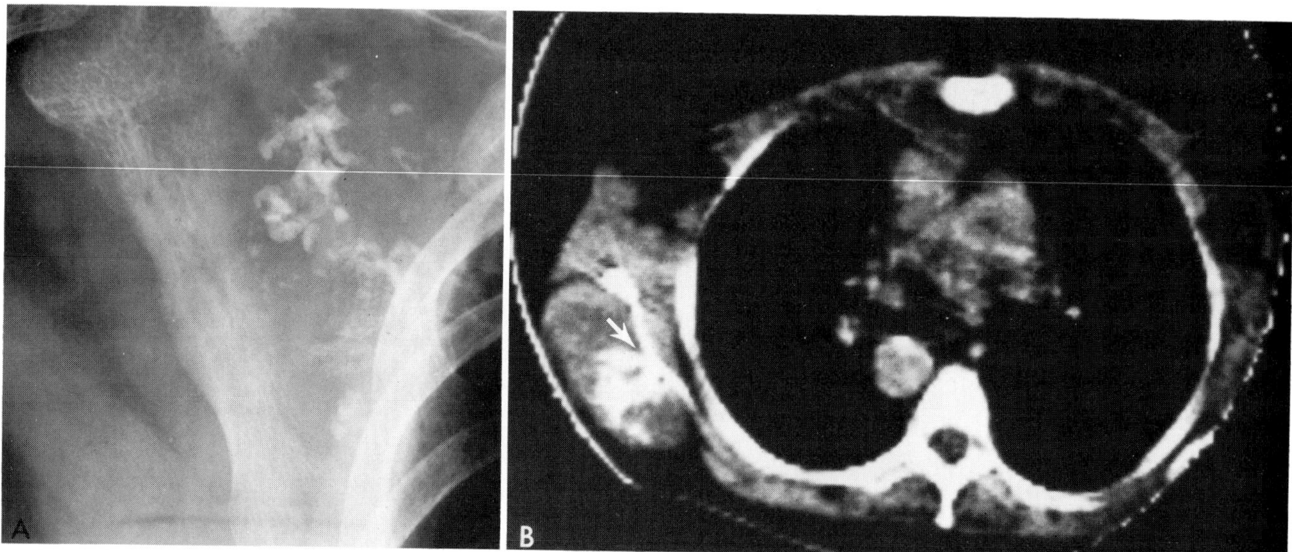

Figure 12–11. *Magnification radiograph* **(A)** *of the shoulder demonstrates a calcified mass in the region of the scapula. CT scan* **(B)** *defines the precise posterior relationship of the stalk to the scapula (arrow) and shows an extensive soft tissue component beyond the calcified portion, suggesting a chondrosarcoma.*

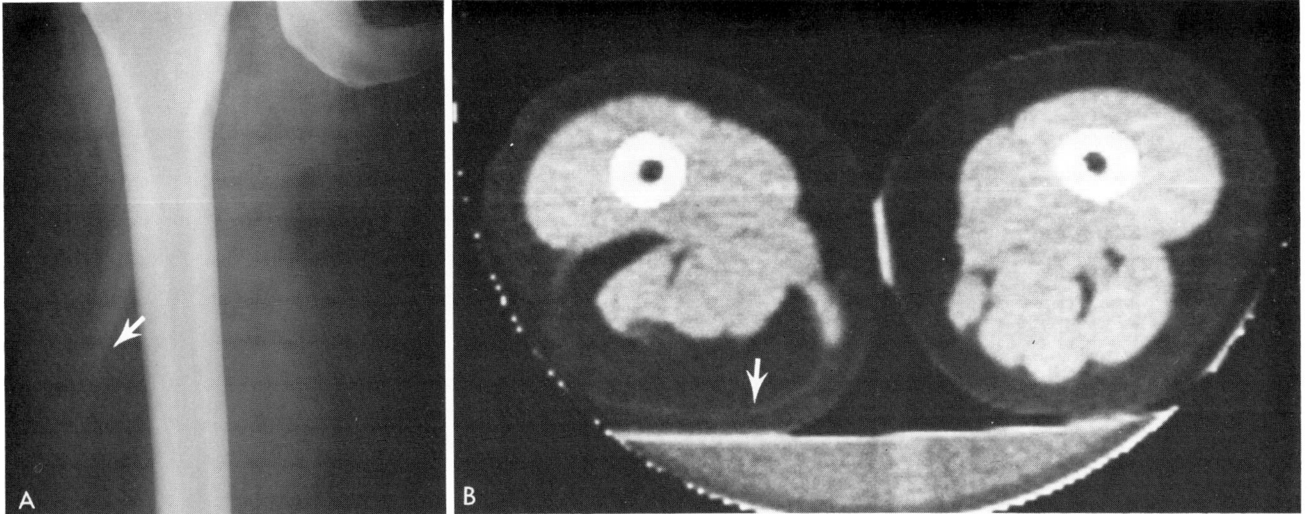

Figure 12–12. Conventional radiograph **(A)** demonstrates displacement of normal soft tissue planes lateral to the femur (arrow). CT scan **(B)** defines a low density, homogeneous mass with a CT number comparable to subcutaneous fat (~ minus 100 Hounsfield units). Encapsulation of the mass is seen peripherally (arrow) and permeation of adjacent musculature is evident centrally, indicating an infiltrating lipoma.

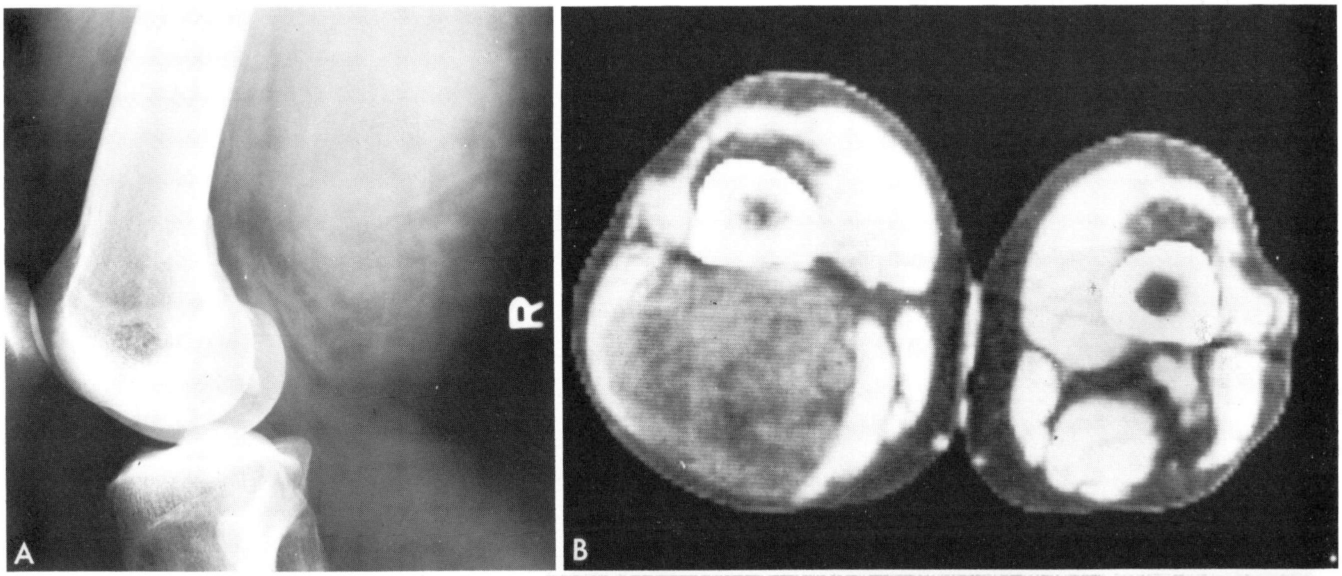

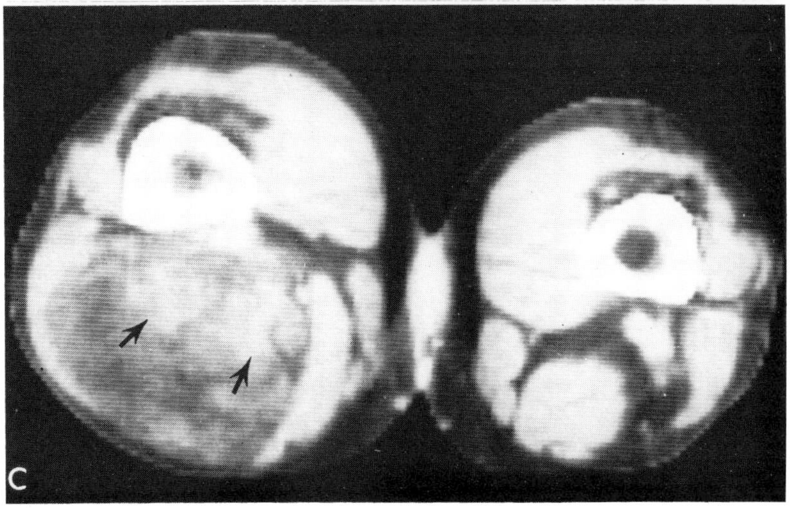

Figure 12–13. Conventional radiograph **(A)** demonstrates a large soft tissue mass in the popliteal region. Precontrast scan **(B)** shows a poorly marginated, nonhomogeneous, low density mass. Postcontrast scan **(C)** reveals areas of enhancement (arrows), indicating the vascular nature of this liposarcoma.

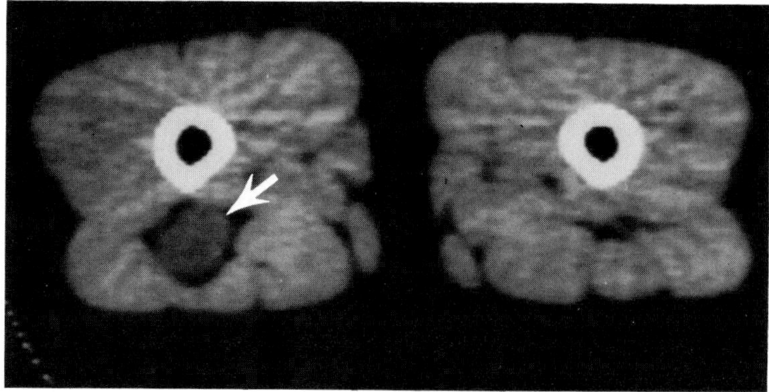

Figure 12–14. *CT scan demonstrates a relatively low density mass within the neurovascular bundle of the posterior thigh (arrow). This cylindric mass was shown by CT to extend over 15 cm, suggesting the correct diagnosis of schwannoma.*

nerve was suspected. A schwannoma was confirmed at surgery.

Many soft tissue masses are of the same density as muscle, as is illustrated in a patient who presented with a faintly palpable mass in the left gluteal region (Fig. 12–15) and who had normal conventional radiographs. The CT scan shows a soft tissue mass of approximately the density of muscle, which is clearly outlined and contrasted by the subcutaneous fat. It is attached by a stalk to the underlying gluteus medius musculature. Surgery confirmed a desmoid tumor, a locally aggressive and frequently recurrent process. Preoperative mapping of the extent of the process by CT may be helpful in this setting.

The role of CT in the evaluation of *metastatic disease to bone*[10, 21, 55] can also be illustrated. Here CT is used to (1) document the presence of metastasis, and (2) evaluate its intramedullary and extraosseous extent.

Figure 12–16 reveals images that were obtained in a patient with bronchogenic carcinoma who had pain in the left hip and a limp for several months. The conventional radiograph (Fig. 12–16*A*) is normal; however, the bone scan (Fig. 12–16*B*) shows increased uptake in the proximal femur, suggesting the presence of metastatic disease. The CT scan (Fig. 12–16*C*) shows increased density of the left femoral head and the greater trochanter relative to that on the right side. Increased medullary density by CT has been found in metastatic processes involving the long bones and it is nearly diagnostic in this setting.[10] In this case, the increased density extended inferiorly to the level of the lesser trochanter, which documents the extent of medullary involvement.

An additional important application for computed tomography in metastatic disease is determining the extent of soft tissue masses in treatment planning, i.e., radiation port selection or surgical debulking procedures. Figure 12–17 demonstrates images of the spine and pelvis of a patient with multiple myeloma and advanced destruction of the vertebrae. The CT scans do not provide additional

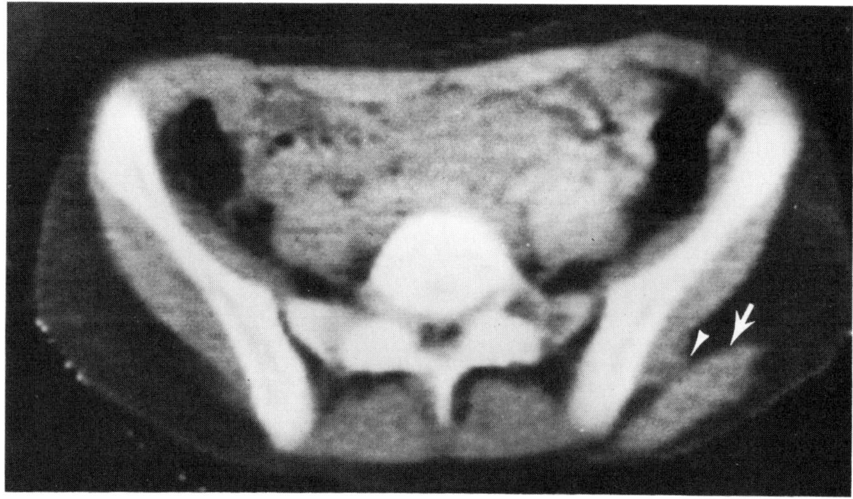

Figure 12–15. *CT scan demonstrates a soft tissue mass having a density approximately equal to that of muscle but clearly outlined and contrasted by the subcutaneous fat of the buttock (arrow). This desmoid tumor was found at surgery to be attached to the underlying gluteus musculature by a stalk (arrowhead).*

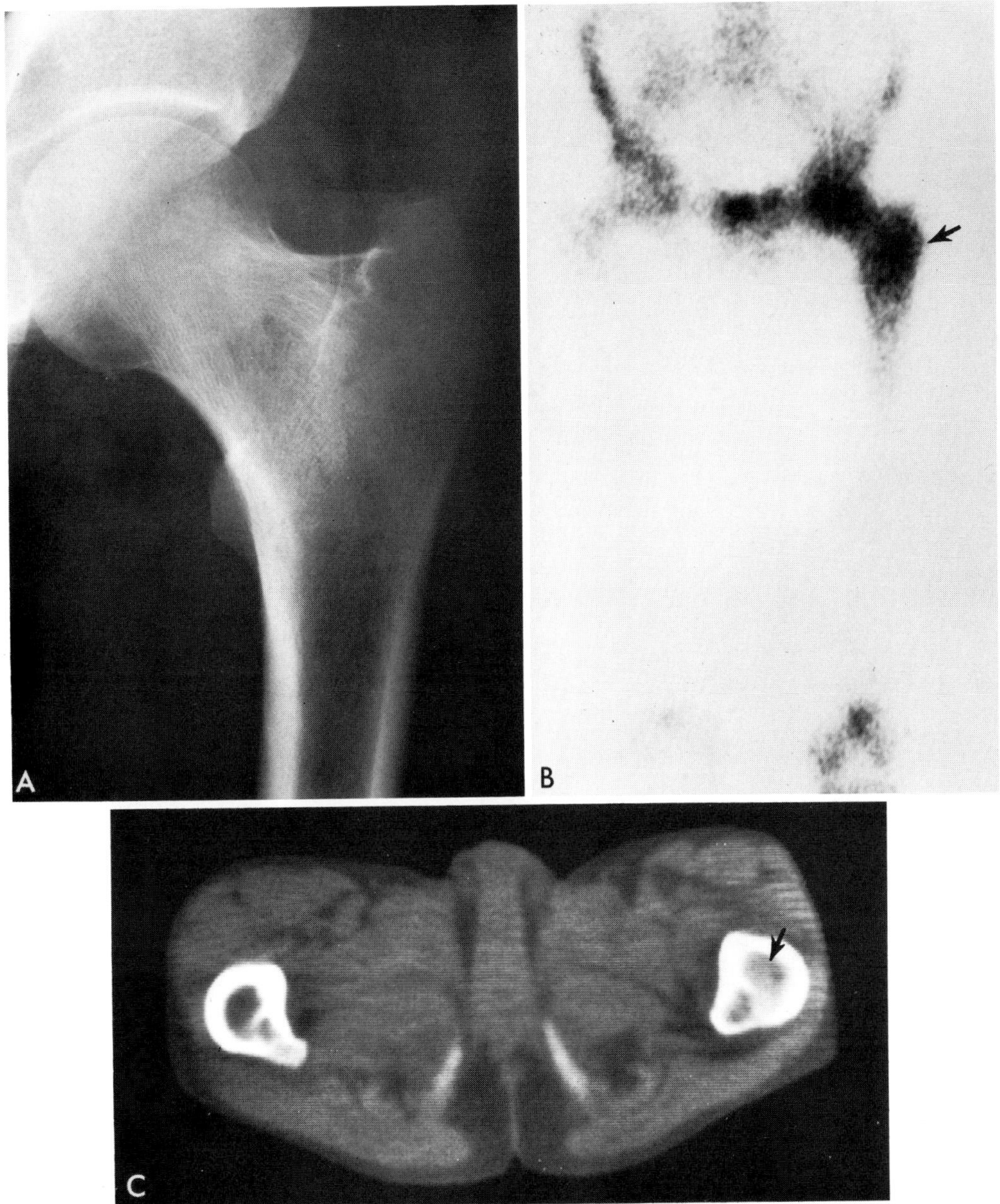

Figure 12–16. *A patient with suspected metastatic disease has normal conventional radiograph of the femur* **(A)** *but focally increased activity on bone scan* **(B)** *in the proximal femur (arrow). CT scan* **(C)** *shows ipsilateral increased density of the medullary canal (arrow), strongly supporting a diagnosis of a metastatic focus.*

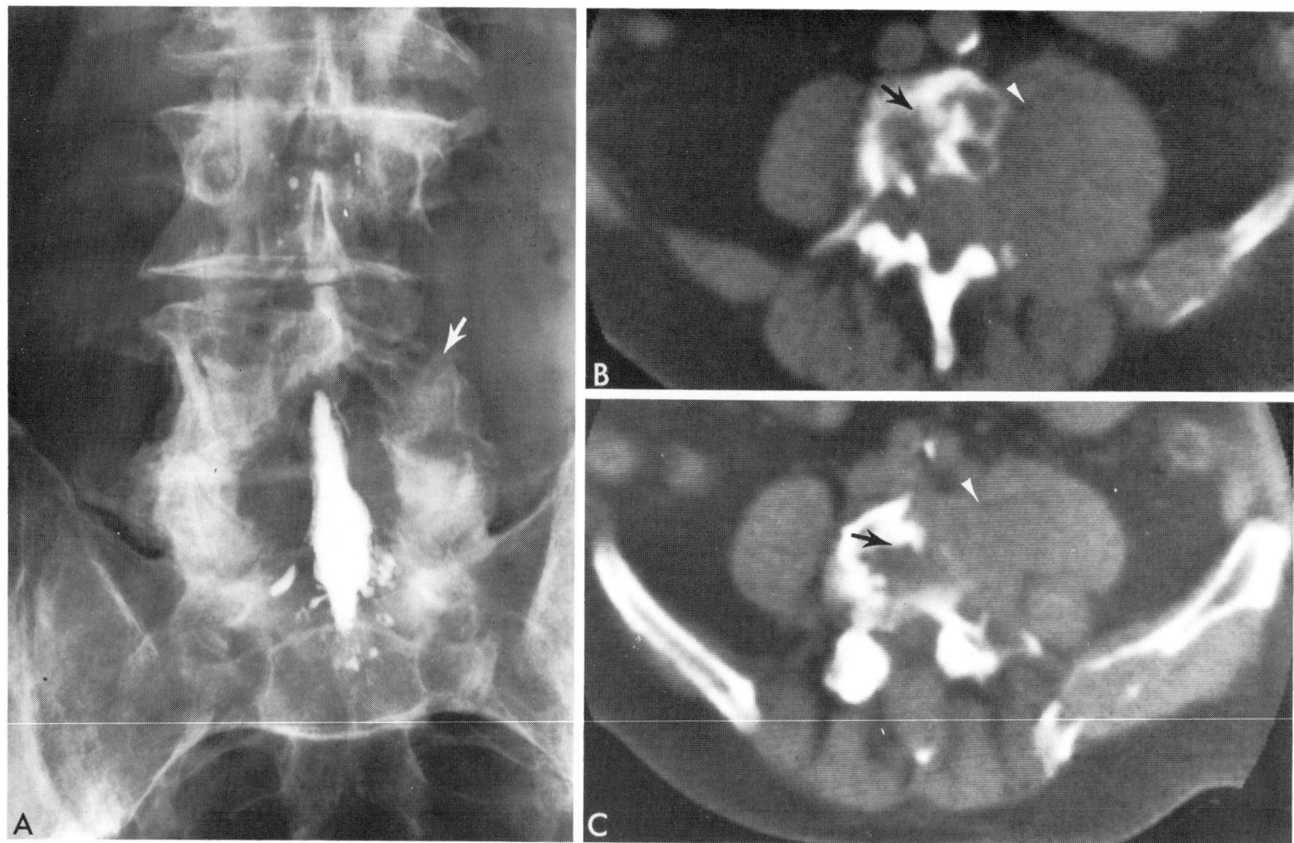

Figure 12–17. *Conventional radiograph* **(A)** *demonstrates marked destruction of lower lumbar vertebrae due to myeloma (arrow). CT scans* **(B, C)** *confirm the advanced bony destruction (arrows) but, more importantly, define the extraosseous extent of the paraspinous and extrapelvic soft tissue masses (arrowheads).*

information regarding the bone destruction but do reveal to advantage the large paraspinal masses as well as the extension beyond the pelvic wall.

Locally recurrent neoplasms[21, 40, 42, 55] may be an indication for CT scanning. Here a baseline CT study may be performed postoperatively when a tumor cannot be completely resected or when the aggressive nature of a tumor makes local recurrence a likely possibility. In this fashion, CT can be used to identify and assess recurrent disease serially.

Figure 12–18*A* shows a patient who, as a child, underwent resection of a desmoplastic fibroma of the ilium. Now, as a young adult (Fig. 12–18*B*) following multiple resections, radiation therapy, and a cup arthroplasty, he was considered to be free of tumor. Serial CT studies were performed in this case. The initial scan (Fig. 12–18*C*) demonstrates only postoperative changes, with no evidence of recurrence. One year later (Fig. 12–18*D*), following administration of intravenous contrast material, an area of enhanced vascularity, which encroaches on the ischiorectal space, is identified, representing recurrent desmoplastic fibroma.

Non-Neoplastic Disorders

This analysis of the role of CT in the evaluation of non-neoplastic disorders is based upon a fairly broad exposure but not an in-depth experience[22, 52, 55] in the categories of disorders listed in Table 12–2. Selected examples of potential CT applications will be illustrated, but the preliminary nature of this assessment must be emphasized.

A number of patients with suspected masses have been studied by CT, in whom the "abnormalities" were found, in reality, to be *anatomic variants*, such as prominent muscle groups or skeletal asymmetry; as a result, exploratory surgery was avoided.

CT may be useful in evaluating *infections of bone or joint.*[33, 40, 46, 55] In this setting, CT may con-

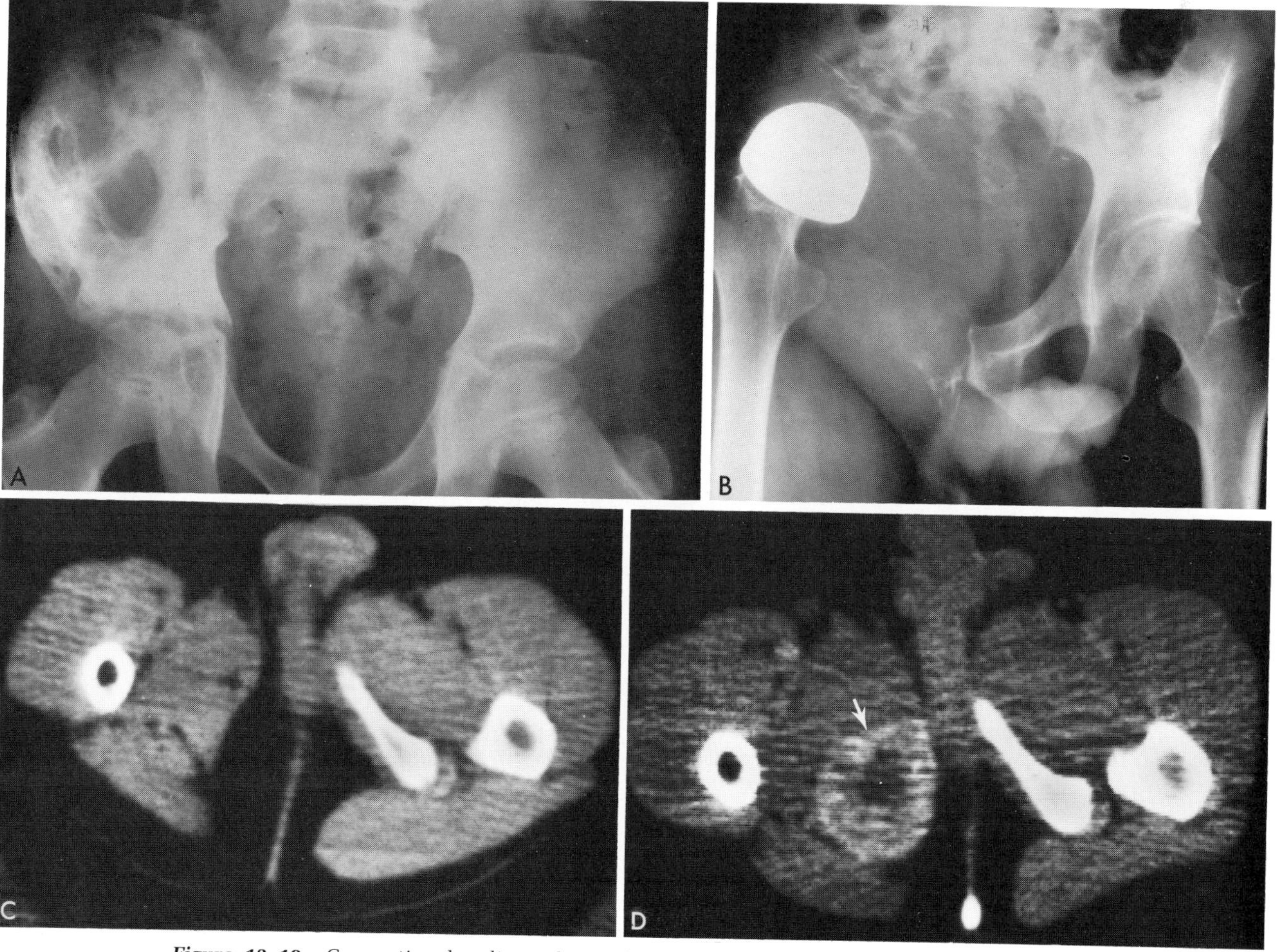

Figure 12–18. *Conventional radiograph* **(A)** *demonstrates advanced destruction of the right ilium due to desmoplastic fibroma. Ten years later, conventional radiograph* **(B)** *shows extensive post-surgical alterations. CT scan* **(C)** *at the same time similarly shows these changes. One year later, however, post-contrast CT scan* **(D)** *shows a doughnut-shaped vascular mass (arrow) and encroachment on the ischiorectal space, representing recurrent desmoplastic fibroma.*

firm increased intramedullary density in an area of suspected osteomyelitis or may provide information of therapeutic significance regarding the appropriate approach for aspiration or debridement. For example, in Figure 12–19, images of an adolescent boy with left hip pain reveal a lytic, expansile process, which appears to involve the region of the lesser trochanter. Periosteal reaction can be seen extending from the lesion. The differential diagnosis includes Brodie's abscess, osteoid osteoma, and primary bone malignancy, and a posterior approach for open biopsy of the lesser trochanter was considered by the surgeon. The frog-leg view, however, demonstrates a relatively normal appearance of the lesser trochanteric apophysis and suggests an abnormality deep in the medullary space. The cross-sectional capability of CT clarifies this matter by demonstrating precisely the anteromedial location of this abscess, indicating the advisability of an anterior rather than a posterior approach. Additionally, the increased density of the

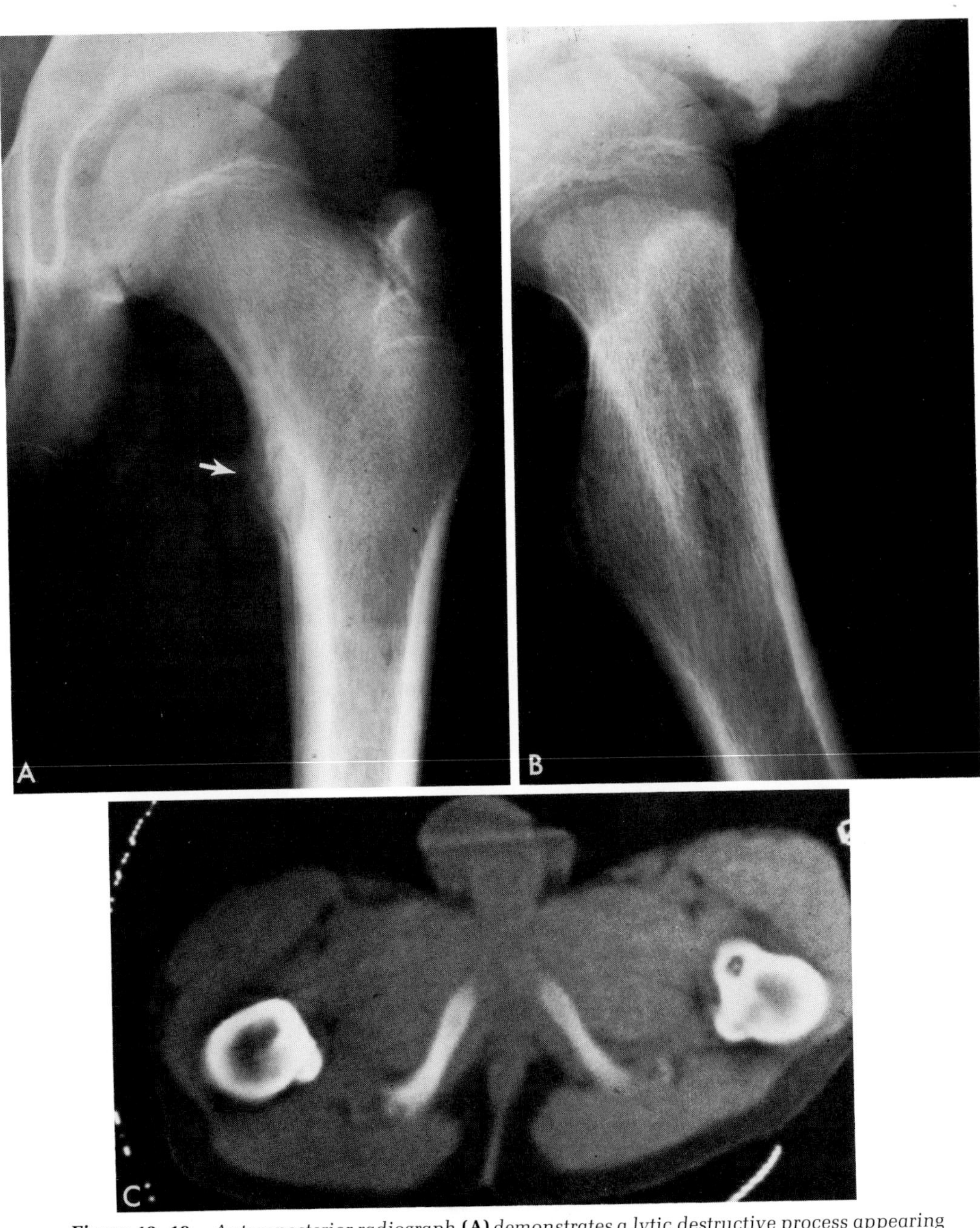

Figure 12–19. *Anteroposterior radiograph* **(A)** *demonstrates a lytic destructive process appearing to involve the lesser trochanter and associated with periosteal reaction (arrow). Lateral radiograph* **(B)** *fails to confirm destruction of the lesser trochanteric apophysis but suggests altered trabecular architecture of the medullary shaft. CT scan* **(C)** *demonstrates a normal lesser trochanteric apophysis and shows focal expansion of the anteromedial femoral cortex. Additionally, ipsilateral increased density of the medullary canal is seen in this case of Brodie's abscess.*

ipsilateral medullary space as shown here on CT may be a useful sign of early osteomyelitis, although it may also be encountered in intramedullary neoplasms.

Figure 12–20 concerns a patient who underwent discectomy several months prior to the time the radiograph was obtained and who presented with increasing back pain. Obvious destruction of the vertebral end plates at the L4-5 level can be seen on the conventional radiograph (Fig. 12–20*A*) consistent with an intervertebral disc infection. The CT scan (Fig. 12–20*B*), obtained at the same time, demonstrates a large prevertebral abscess, suggesting the necessity of surgical drainage and debridement. Following drainage, the patient was rescanned (Fig. 12–20*C*), and the resolution of the abscess was confirmed by CT.

Similarly, Figure 12–21 illustrates the case of a woman with low back pain who demonstrates destruction of the L5-S1 disc space, reactive sclerosis, and erosion of the right sacroiliac joint. An infectious process, possibly tuberculous in origin, was suspected. CT was performed to determine whether there was a presacral abscess and to provide localization for needle biopsy. There is no evidence of anterior extension of an abscess. Furthermore, the

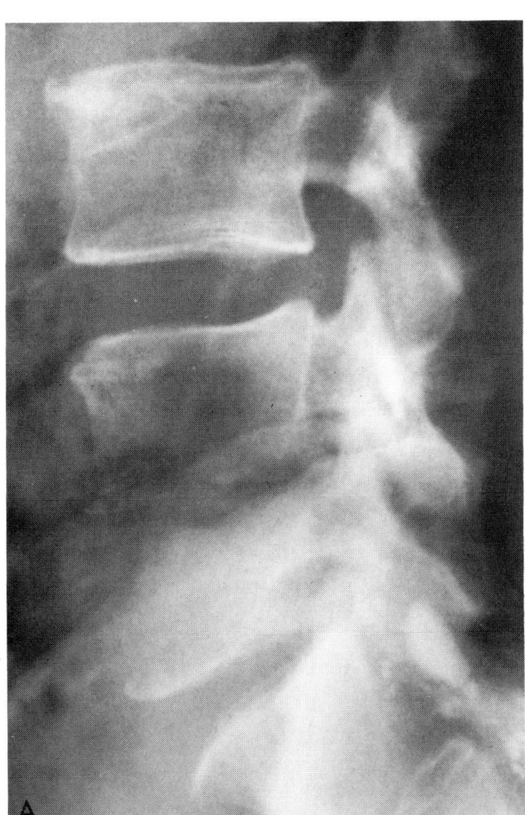

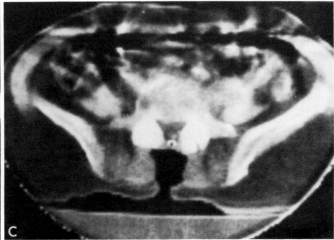

Figure 12–20. *Conventional radiograph* **(A)** *demonstrates extensive destruction of disc and end-plates at L4–5 consistent with infection. CT scan* **(B)** *demonstrates vertebral destruction, and additionally shows a large prevertebral abscess. CT scan* **(C)** *following surgical debridement demonstrates resolution of the abscess.*

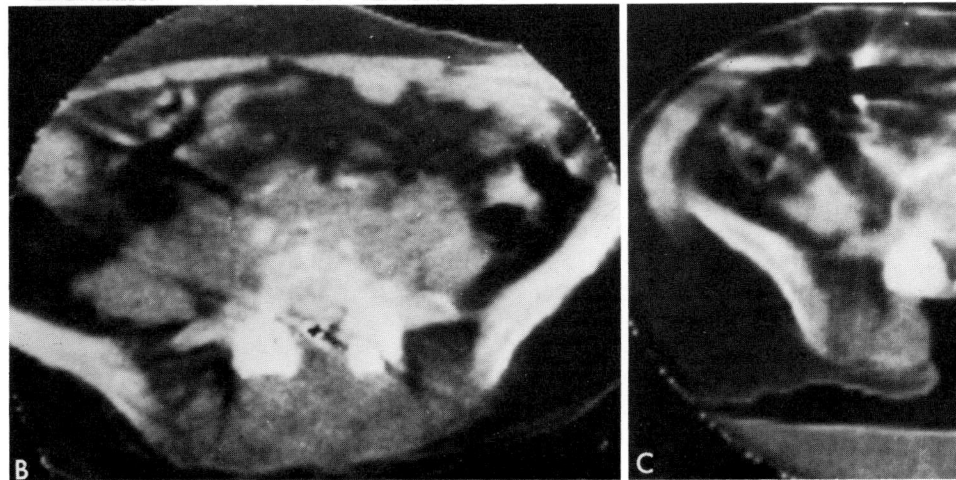

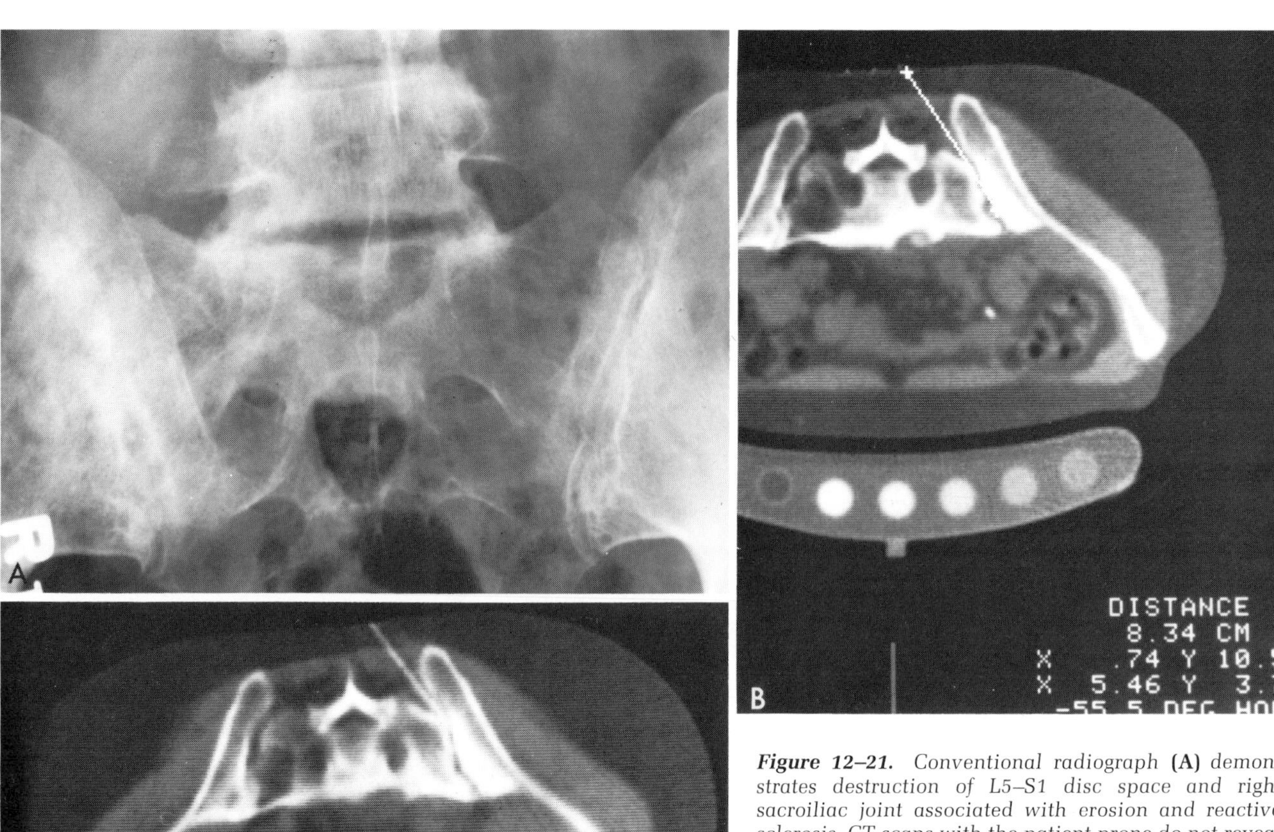

Figure 12–21. *Conventional radiograph* **(A)** *demonstrates destruction of L5–S1 disc space and right sacroiliac joint associated with erosion and reactive sclerosis. CT scans with the patient prone do not reveal a presacral abscess. The proposed approach for needle aspiration has been designated by a straight line connecting two points marked on the video monitor, and the distance and angle for insertion of the needle are given. Subsequent CT scan* **(C)** *confirms the position of the needle.*

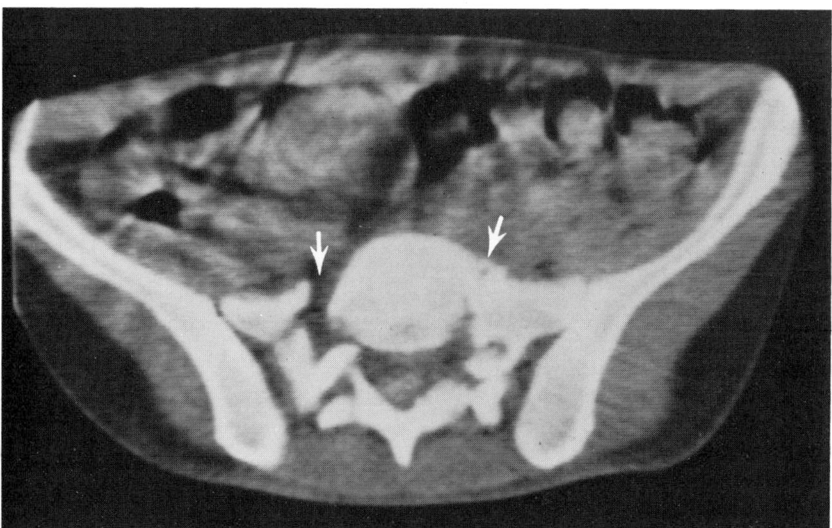

Figure 12–22. *Extensive comminuted fracture of the sacrum is well seen by CT (arrows). (Courtesy of Dr. William O'Shea.)*

extent of involvement of the sacroiliac joint can be seen (Fig. 12–21*B*,*C*). With the patient prone, an aspiration biopsy was performed in the scanner room using new developments in software and hardware. An X can be indicated on the video monitor at the proposed point of entrance of the needle and at the point where the tip is to be placed. The computer connects the two points with a straight line (Fig. 12–21*B*) and determines the distance needed to insert the needle, 8 cm in this case. It also recalculates the angle at which the needle should enter the skin, 55 degrees to the horizontal. In subsequent scans, the hub of the needle can be seen, and the shaft has been inserted into the sacroiliac joint (Fig. 12–21*C*). This case illustrates the capability of computed tomography for needle biopsy localization of relatively inaccessible sites.[19, 22]

To date, there has been only limited experience regarding the role of computed tomography in the evaluation of fractures or dislocations.[12, 36, 41, 46, 55] However, CT may indeed be important in this regard, particularly in anatomically complex regions, such as the spine and pelvis. Figure 12–22 shows an extensive comminuted fracture of the sacrum, an

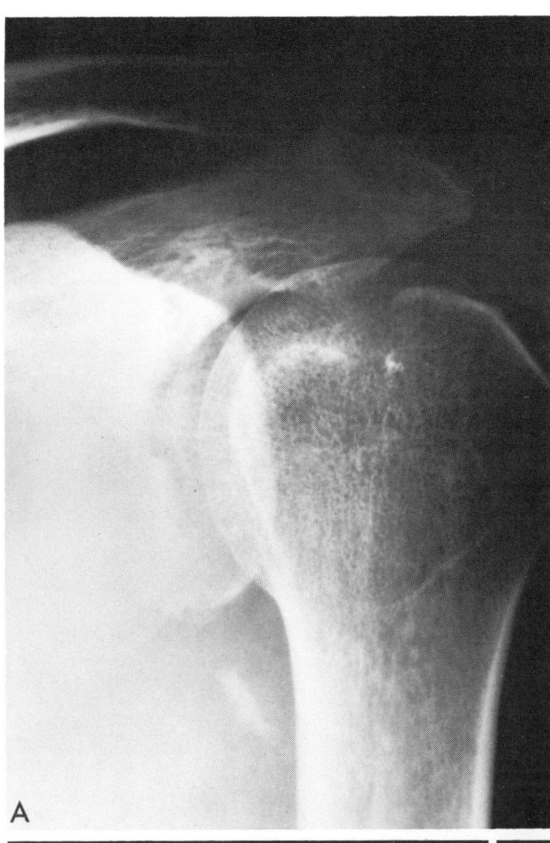

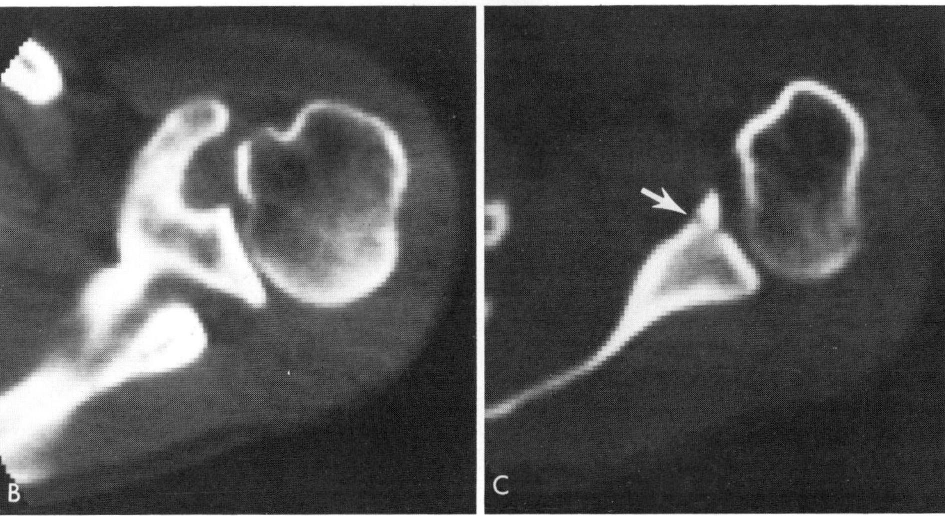

Figure 12–23. *Post-reduction radiograph* **(A)** *following an anterior shoulder dislocation demonstrates a displaced bony fragment and a fracture involving the glenoid. Serial CT scans demonstrate that the major portion of the glenoid surface is intact* **(B)** *and only the inferior anterior margin is fractured* **(C)** *(arrow).*

anatomically complex region. At this site, the cross-sectional display of CT can allow evaluation of the spatial relationships of these fractures.

Figure 12–23 illustrates a patient who sustained a fracture-dislocation of the shoulder. The postreduction view (Fig. 12–23*A*) reveals a displaced bony fragment, and a fracture involving the glenoid base. In such a case, the integrity of the glenoid and the need for open reduction may be in question. A CT scan with contiguous 0.5 cm cuts shows that the major extent of the glenoid surface is completely intact (Fig. 12–23*B*). Only at the inferoanterior margin of the glenoid can a small, nondisplaced fracture be seen (Fig. 12–23*C*). Conservative management was employed.

A small number of patients with complicated spinal fractures have been scanned. In Figure 12–24, anteroposterior and lateral radiographs (*A*,*B*) dem-

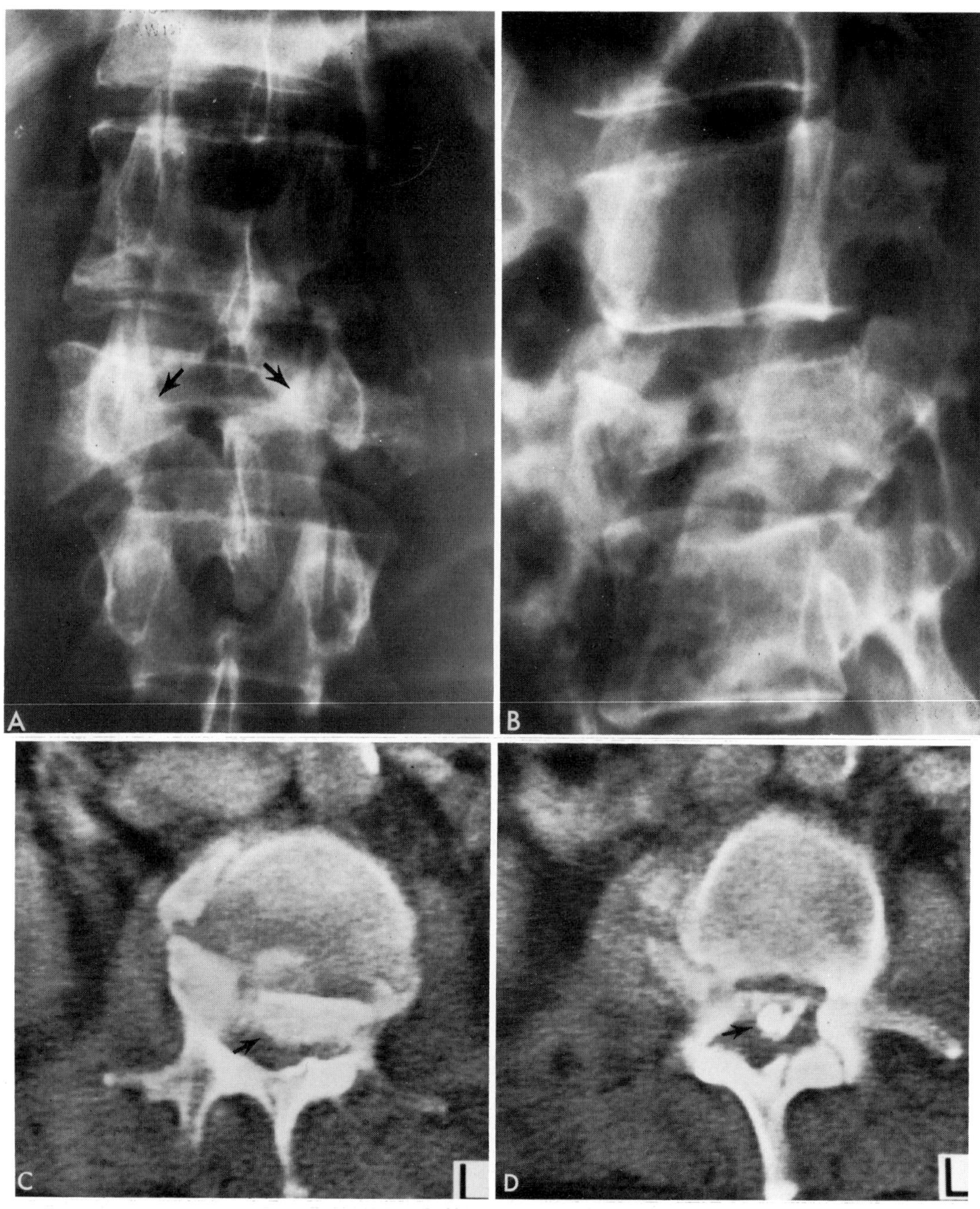

Figure 12–24. *Conventional radiographs* **(A, B)** *demonstrate a "burst" fracture of the body of L2 and associated splaying of the posterior elements (arrows). CT scans* **(C, D)** *optimally display the relationship of the fractured elements to the cord (arrows) and the extent of posterior column involvement.*

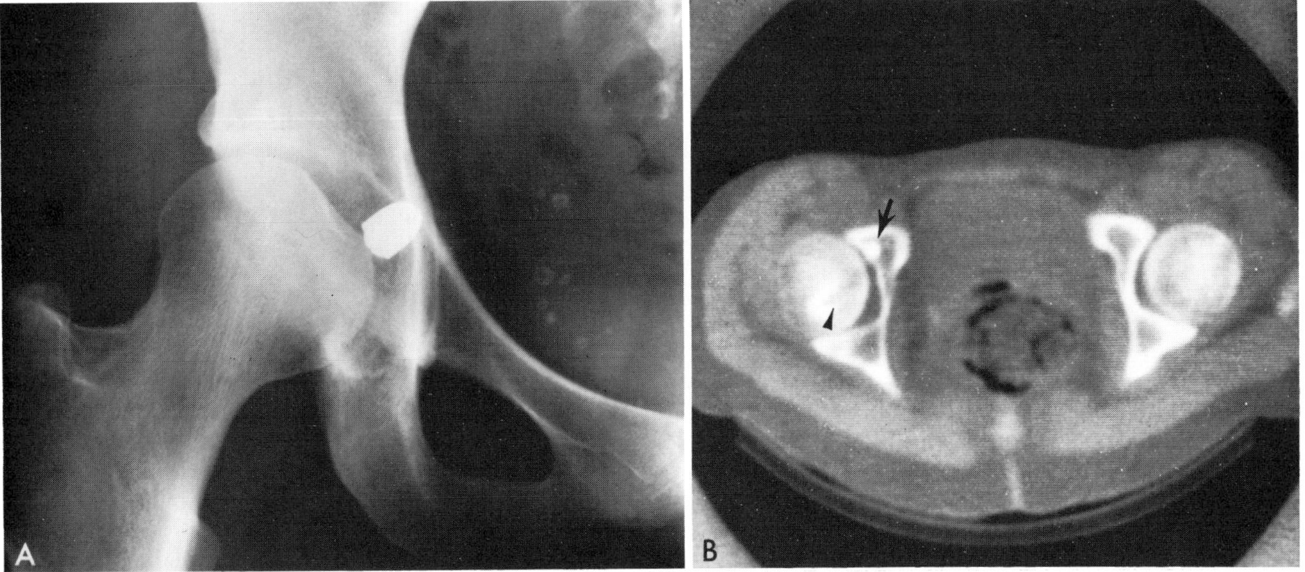

Figure 12–25. *Conventional radiograph* **(A)** *demonstrates a bullet in the region of the right hip. CT scan* **(B)** *demonstrates the precise location of the bullet, which is lodged in the subchondral bone of the acetabulum (arrow), and also shows the bullet track where it had traversed the femoral head (arrowhead).*

onstrate a burst fracture involving the second lumbar veterbral body as well as its posterior elements. In this setting, the CT scan can optimally display the relationship of fractured elements to the spinal cord and the extent of posterior column involvement (Fig. 12–24*C,D*). As computed tomographic procedures become faster and more accessible, this manner of studying complicated fractures may partially replace conventional tomography, which is more time-consuming and difficult to perform.[22, 42]

Figure 12–25 illustrates the case of a young women who presented with progressive right hip pain several months following a gunshot wound to the right buttock. A plain radiograph (Fig. 12–25*A*)

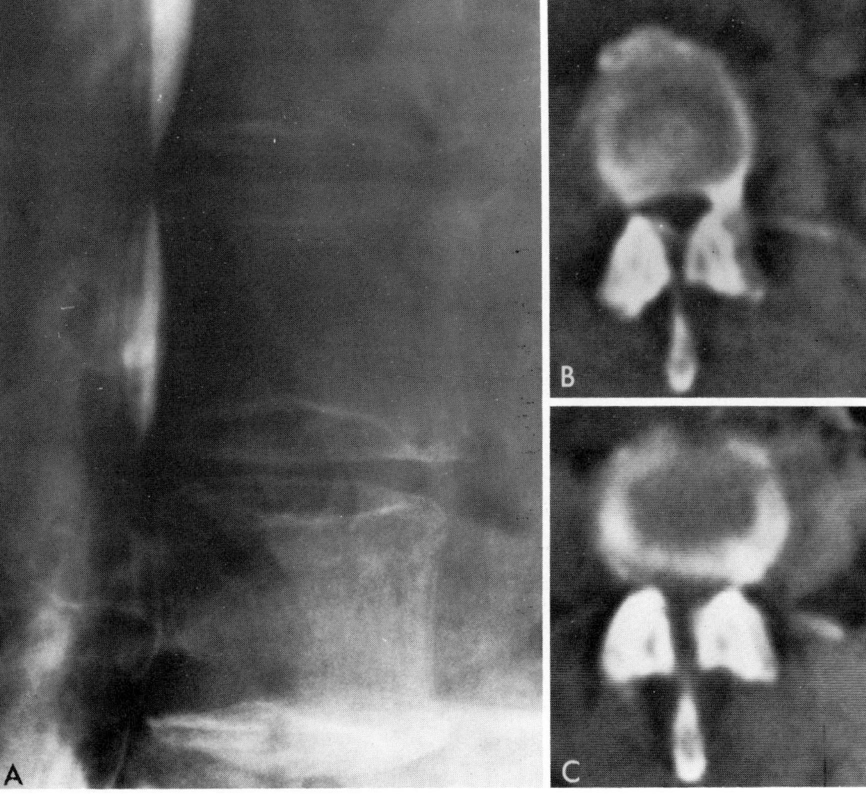

Figure 12–26. *Metrizamide myelogram* **(A)** *demonstrates typical, multilevel incomplete obstruction due to spinal stenosis. CT scans* **(B, C)** *show an abnormally small spinal canal with a trefoil configuration. Additionally, encroachment on the neural foramina is visualized.*

reveals a bullet in the region of the right hip, but its precise intra- or extra-articular location is unclear. The cross-sectional and tomographic display of CT shows curvilinear surfaces such as the acetabulum to advantage.[35] Here the CT scan (Fig. 12–25*B*) indicates that the bullet is lodged in subchondral bone of the acetabulum and that the bullet track traverses the femoral head and presumably violates the femoral articular cartilage.

The evaluation of *spinal stenosis* and other congenital and acquired disorders that compromise the spinal cord and nerve roots[18, 27, 34, 36, 43, 48, 49, 53] is an important potential application of computed tomography. Here the cross-sectional display of CT permits precise definition of the critically important transverse configuration and size of the spinal canal. Computed tomography is superior to transaxial tomography (TAT) because of its higher spatial and density resolution and its lower radiation exposure.[22, 48]

Figure 12–26*A* demonstrates typical stenotic changes and multilevel incomplete obstruction on a metrizamide myelogram in a middle-aged man whose symptoms suggested spinal claudication. A noninvasive CT scan (Fig. 12–26*B*,*C*) provides similar information regarding the stenotic canal. By analysis of multiple consecutive 0.5 cm thick slices, the cause and level of maximum stenosis can be determined. Additionally, narrowing of the neural foramina and lateral recesses can be visualized. To what extent CT may supplement or replace myelography in this setting has not yet been determined.[18]

CT may be useful in the pre-operative assessment of the adequacy of bone stock in special problem cases.[22] Figure 12–27*A* shows a pelvic radiograph of a patient with cerebral palsy and a left hip dislocation who is being evaluated for total hip arthroplasty. The CT scan (Fig. 12–27*B*,*C*) demonstrates the shape and cross-sectional dimensions of the iliac bone stock. In this instance, the stock appears adequate, although the bone is osteoporotic compared to that on the right side.

Similarly, Figure 12–28*A* demonstrates a patient who has undergone several previous hip

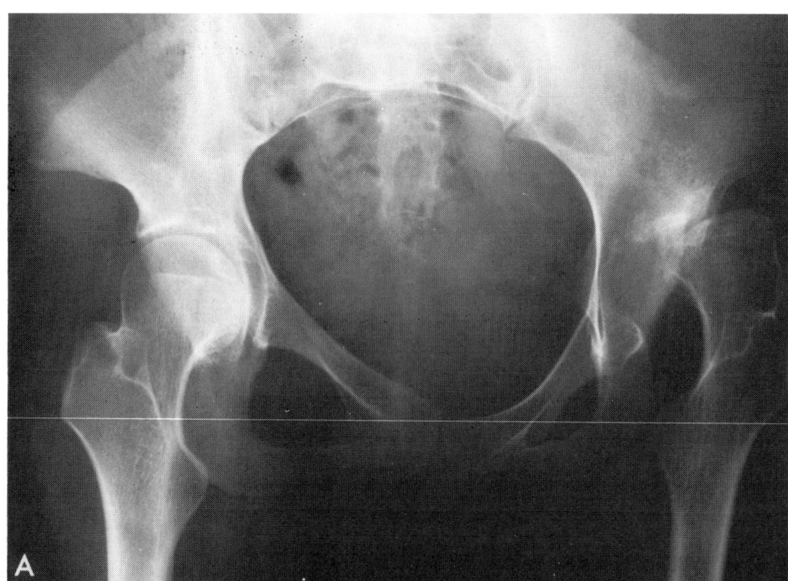

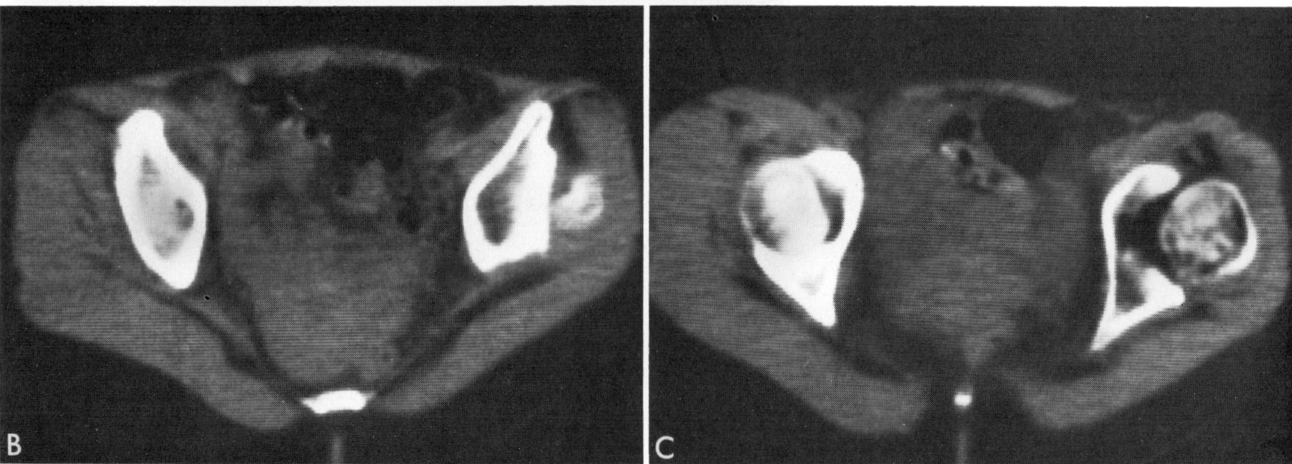

Figure 12–27. *Conventional radiograph* **(A)** *demonstrates deformity and dislocation of the left hip. CT scans* **(B, C)** *demonstrate the shape and cross-sectional dimensions of the iliac bone stock, which in this case appears adequate although osteoporotic relative to the contralateral side.*

arthroplasties and is now having pain. The physician, who suspected loosening of the prosthesis, anticipated a complicated revision. In this clinical setting, a CT scan can define the spatial relationship of the acetabular component to the underlying innominate bone and determine the adequacy of bone stock. In this case (Fig. 12–28*B*), there is minimal iliac bone stock remaining. The femoral component, and the saturn ring of the acetabular component, can be seen projecting far into the pelvis. A tomographic cut (Fig. 12–28*C*), which is slightly below that in Figure 12–28*B*, reveals streak artifacts, which are frequently encountered at metal-bone interfaces. In this case, these artifacts do not interfere significantly with interpretation.

Quantitative Bone Mineral Analysis

Because of its ability to clearly define a specific volume and to accurately measure the density of that volume, CT offers promise for *quantitative bone mineral analysis*. It also provides the unique capability for measuring cancellous bone of the axial skeleton, a site sensitive to metabolic stimuli. Thus, CT may be used to diagnose osteoporosis or to assess

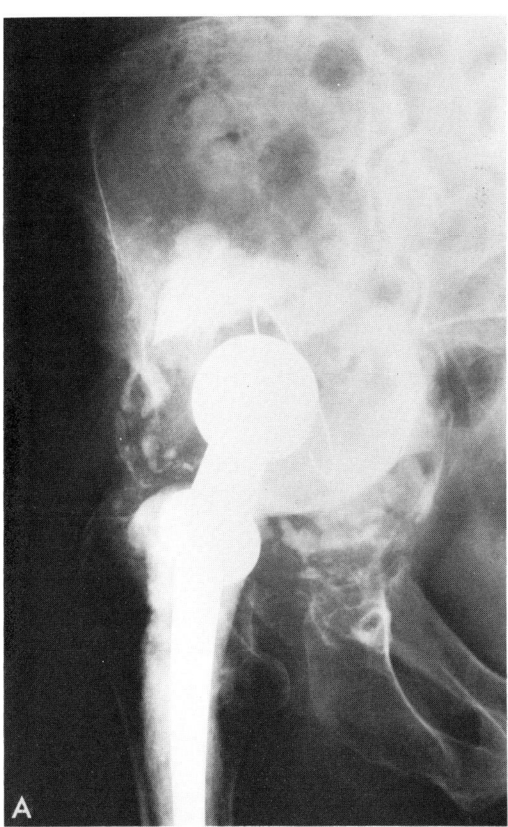

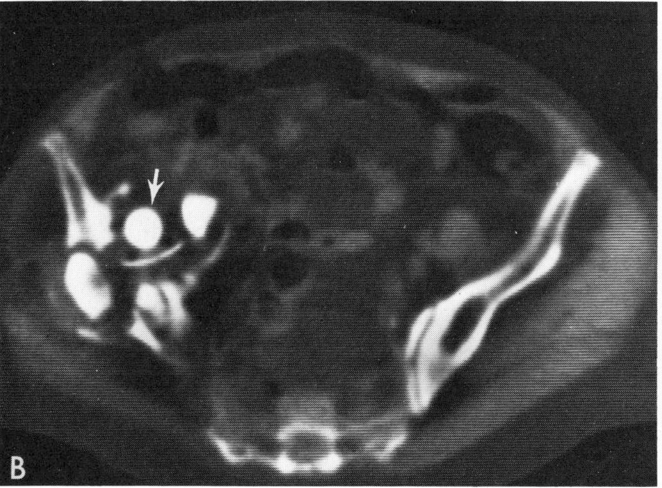

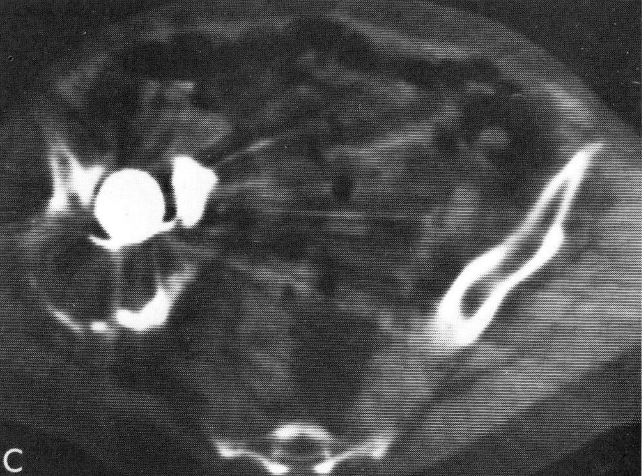

Figure 12–28. *Conventional radiograph* **(A)** *demonstrates a right total hip arthroplasty with superior and medial migration of the acetabular component and subluxation of the femoral head. CT scan* **(B)** *demonstrates the femoral head and the saturn ring of the acetabular component projecting far into the pelvis (arrow). Minimal iliac bone stock remains. CT scan* **(C)** *inferior to this shows streak artifacts that are frequently encountered at metal-bone interfaces, but which do not interfere with interpretation in this case.*

bone mineralization serially in a variety of metabolic bone disorders. At UCSF, computed tomography for spinal bone mineral quantitation has been applied in over 60 patients having metabolic bone disease. The initial results[1, 20, 51] are encouraging, and are discussed in detail in Chapter 18.

EFFICACY

In order to provide insight into the utility of CT, it is useful to analyze the 140 clinical cases represented in this series.

The pre-CT workup was not prospectively planned but rather reflected the usual plan undertaken at UCSF. Primary bone tumors were examined by conventional or magnification[23] radiography and, in most cases, polytomography. Metastatic tumors were examined by conventional radiography and, commonly, by radionuclide imaging of the entire skeleton. Soft tissue masses were examined with routine and xeroradiographic filming. Occasionally a patient had only standard radiographic projections prior to CT.

Each individual in the total group of 140 patients was evaluated in the following manner.[55] First, the results of conventional imaging procedures, including standard radiography, tomography, and xeroradiography, were reviewed and validated. Second, the results of each CT scan were reviewed and compared with the information obtained by the conventional procedures. Finally, after a critical review of each patient's medical record and personal interviews with referring physicians, an estimate of the clinical utility of each CT examination was made.

The CT examination was judged useful if it contributed uniquely in (1) establishing a correct diagnosis; (2) demonstrating the extent of a disease process; or (3) planning the medical or surgical management. CT was not considered useful if it only confirmed information gained by the other imaging modalities. Accordingly, CT was considered useful for diagnosis if it correctly established the presence or absence of a suspected lesion, or if it correctly suggested the specific histologic nature of a lesion. CT was judged useful for treatment planning when it helped determine the optimal mode of therapy (surgery, radiation, chemotherapy, or no therapy), or when it provided information about the extent of disease and its relation to specific bones, muscle bundles, or large nerves and blood vessels that affected the size of incision and the degree of dissection, thus reducing the duration of surgery and the amount of tissue destruction. In most cases, the ability of CT to offer additional and useful information in the categories of diagnosis, extent of disease, and treatment planning was assessed in consultation with the referring clinician.

Table 12–3
OVERALL UTILITY OF CT IN 140 CASES

Diagnosis	61(44%)
Extent	100(71%)
Treatment	96(69%)

Using these criteria, CT provided unique diagnostic information in 61 of 140 patients (44 per cent) (Table 12–3). The ability of CT to depict precisely the anatomy of a lesion and its relation to surrounding vital structures was considered useful in 100 patients (71 per cent). CT proved efficacious in planning surgical or nonsurgical management in the majority of patients (69 per cent).

Applied specifically to disorders in the *neoplastic* category, CT was useful diagnostically in a small percentage of cases (29 per cent) but was helpful in determining the extent of disease in 88 per cent and in optimizing treatment planning in 68 per cent. In contrast, in the *non-neoplastic* category CT was quite helpful in establishing a diagnosis (61 per cent) but was slightly less useful for defining the extent of the process (50 per cent) than it was in neoplastic conditions. CT was efficacious in treatment planning in 69 per cent of non-neoplastic cases, a result that is similar to that noted with regard to neoplasms.

FUTURE CONSIDERATIONS

What then is the anticipated role for CT in the near future? The rapid advancement in CT brain scanning that has taken place over the past 7 years is dramatically represented in Figure 12–29. Similarly, in 5 years, CT technology applied to body scanning has improved tremendously. This explosive technologic development defies long-range predictions, but short-range speculation is possible.[22]

The continued development of computer hardware and software will permit greater facility of patient studies. Faster scanning time (on the order of 1 second per slice) and nearly instantaneous image reconstruction will be commonplace. There will be a greater application of multiplanar reconstruction[24]; thus, from a single series of cross-sectional scans, coronal and sagittal planes as well as those in any desired projection may be reconstructed, allowing a broad spectrum of spatial orientations without additional patient time or radiation exposure. Any number of planes and slice thicknesses can be selected and, in the movie mode, a rapid consecutive display of images can be observed on the monitor. Static images reflecting this capability are shown in Figure 12–30.

Options are now available on prototype scanners[14] that provide for extremely high spatial and

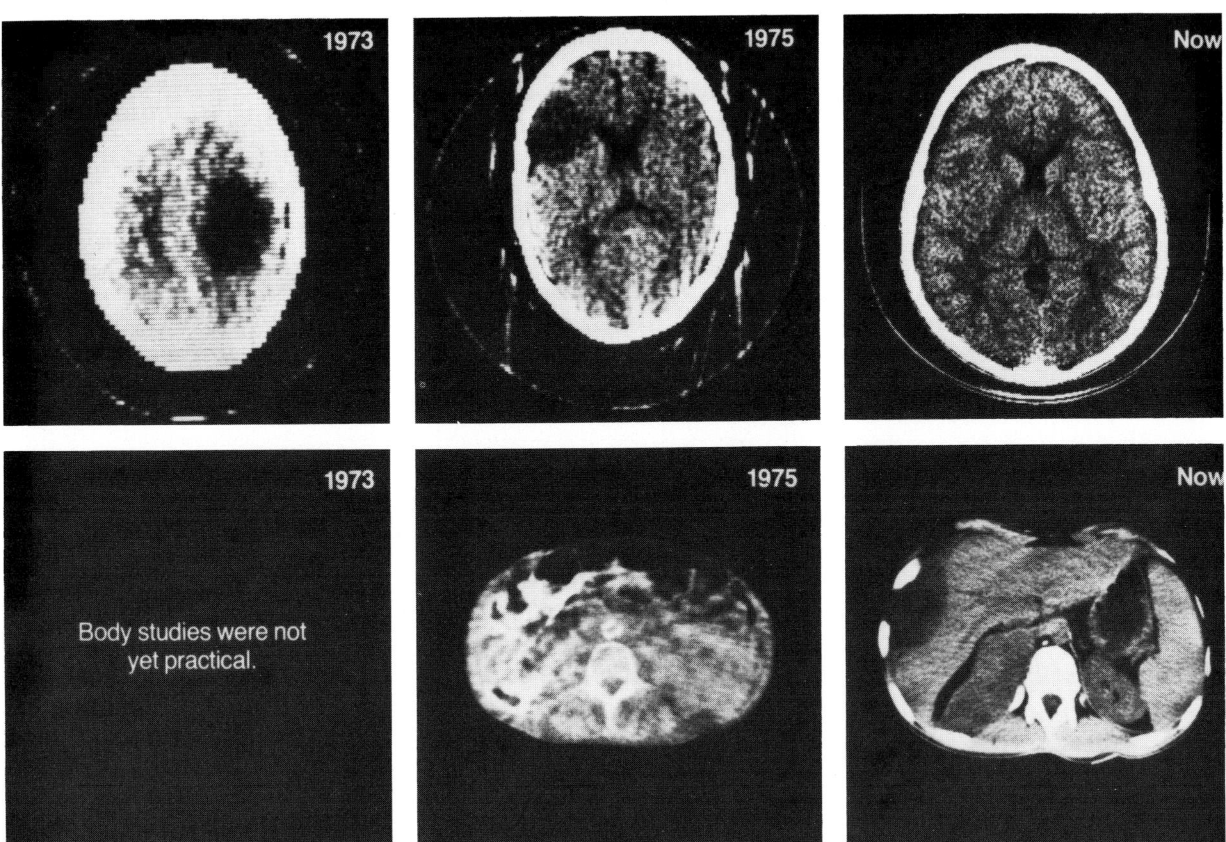

Figure 12–29. *The evolution of CT imaging capability*[14] *for the head (top) and the body (bottom) are shown dramatically.*

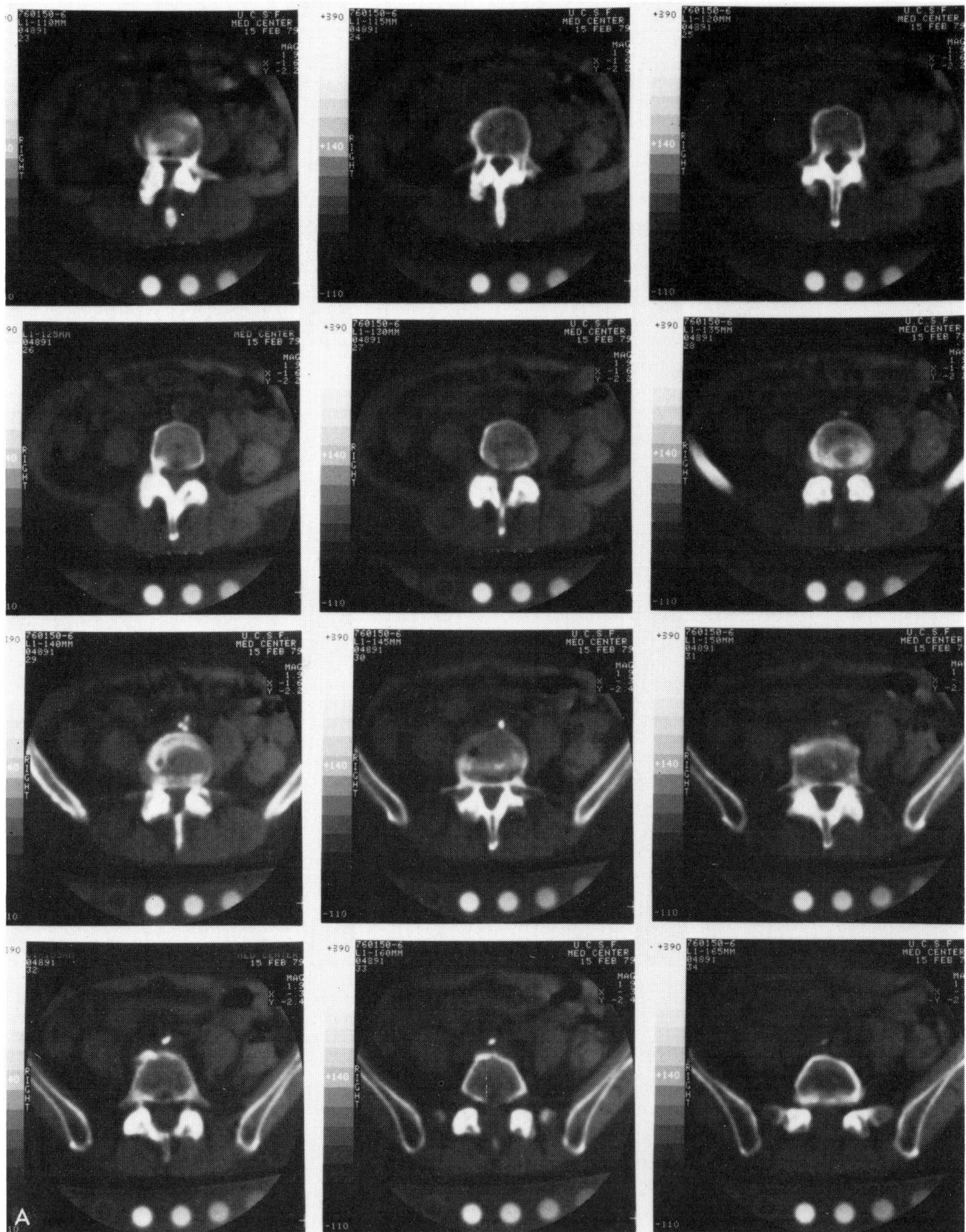

Figure 12–30. *Static images reflecting the "movie mode" capability for viewing cross sectional* **(A)**, *coronal* **(B)**, *or sagittal* **(C)** *images of the lumbar spine.*

Illustration continued on the opposite page

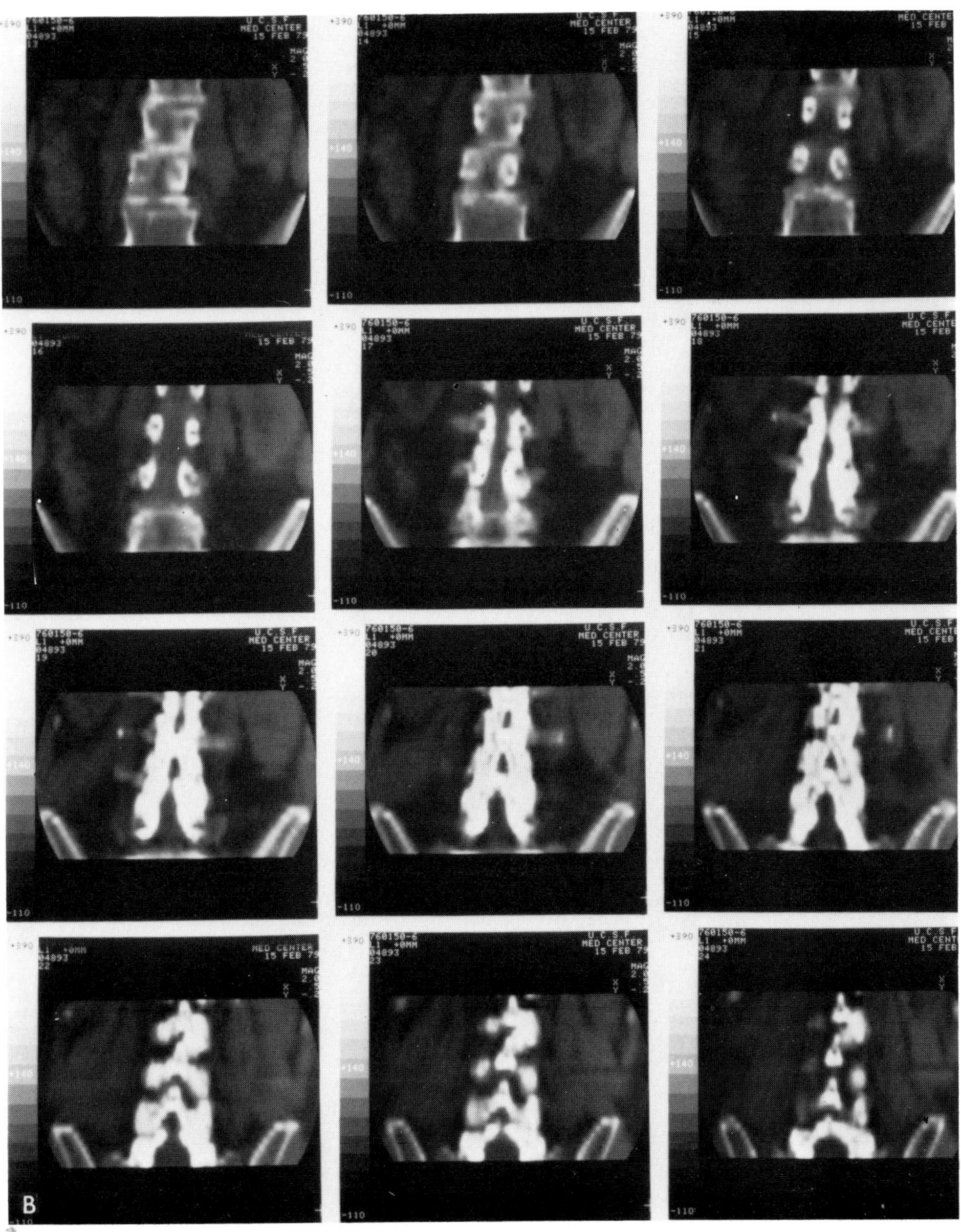

Figure 12–30. Continued

Illustration continued on the following page

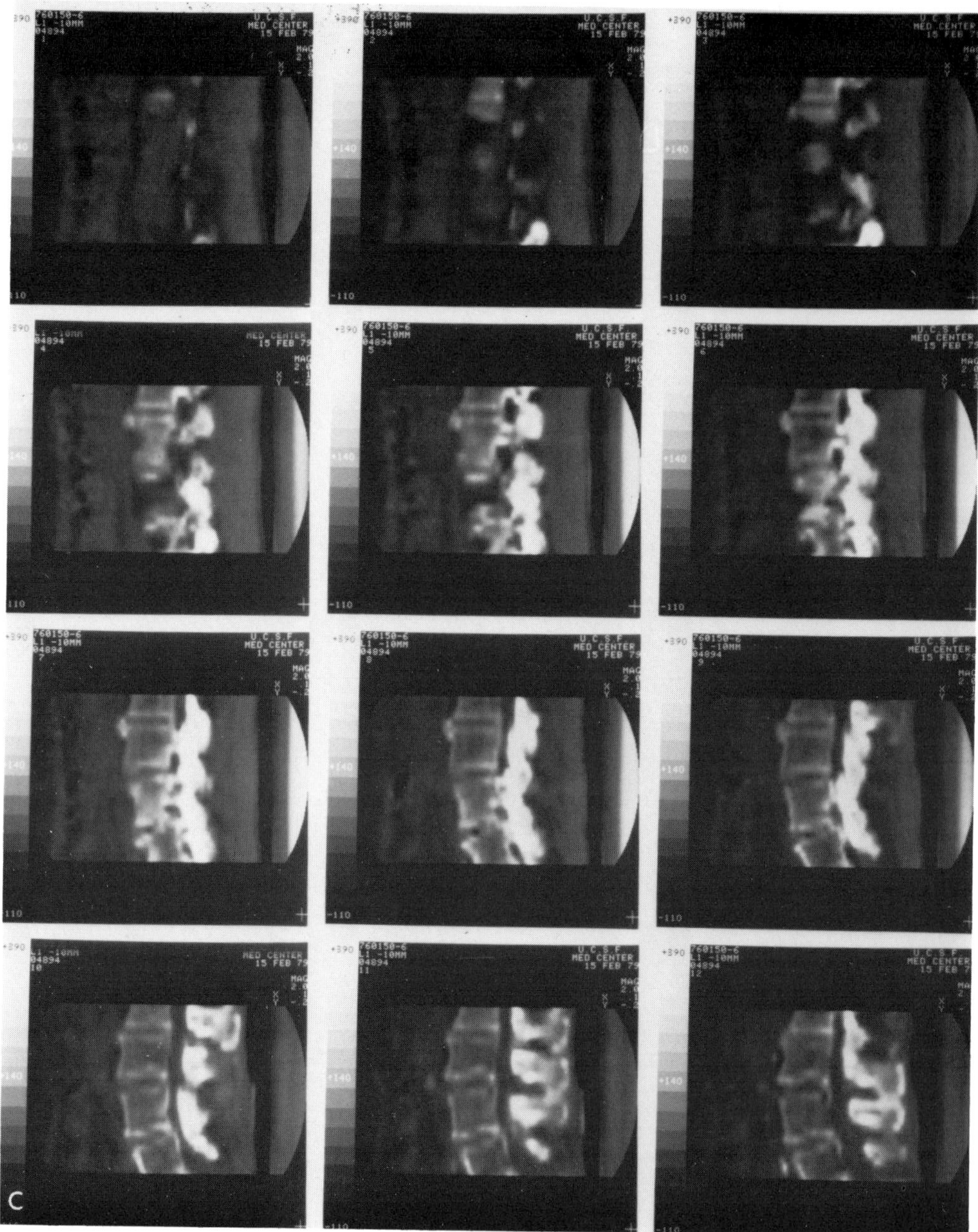

Figure 12–30. Continued

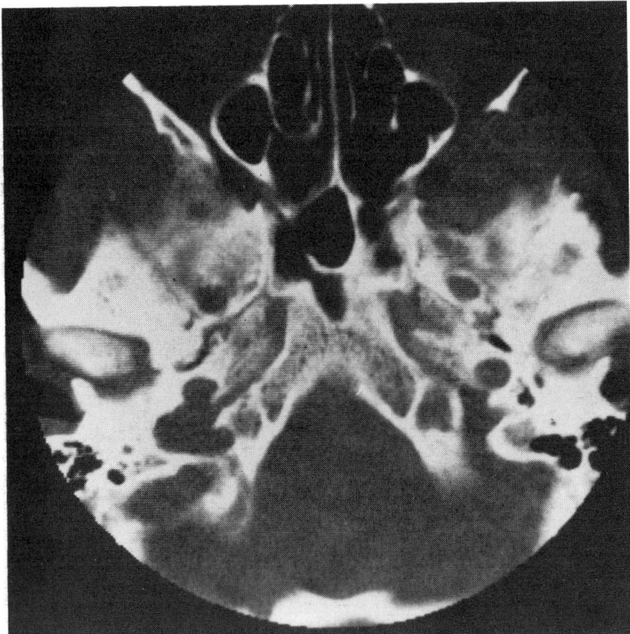

Figure 12–31. High resolution CT scan of the base of the skull performed with the Elscint Exel-905.

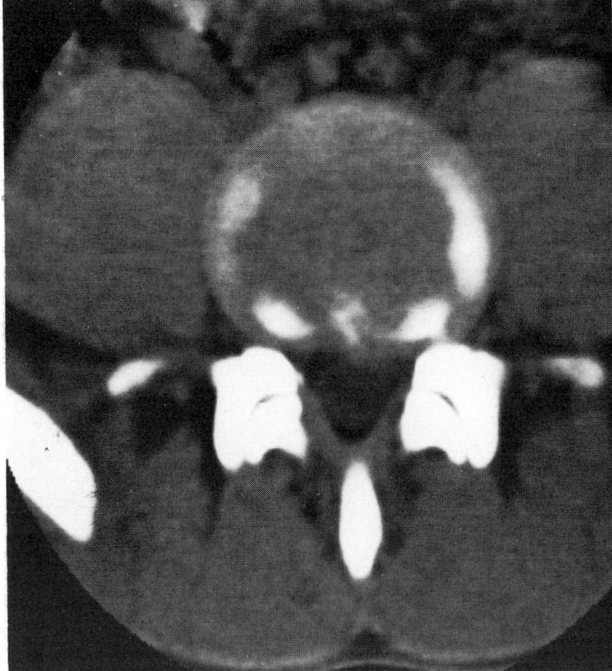

Figure 12–32. High resolution CT scan of the lumbar spine using the GE 8800 body scanner. Posterior disc protrusion and displacement of the thecal sac are readily identified without the use of contrast.

density resolution. This improved spatial resolution or sharpness combined with an ability to obtain thinner slices will permit visualization of small bony structures as seen in the base of the skull (Fig. 12–31) and the spine. The improved density resolution will result in direct visualization of structures such as the spinal cord, nerve roots, and intervertebral discs (Fig. 12–32).

Another advancement in technology that is currently available is termed scout film or computed radiography. Here the scanning equipment itself is used to generate a projection radiograph similar in configuration to a conventional radiograph. The patient is scanned longitudinally on a motor-driven table. The projection image on the video monitor is indexed to the table position, providing precise anatomic localization for subsequent transverse scanning. In addition, lateral scout films may be obtained to facilitate localization or to show the need for angulation of the gantry frame to maintain a true transverse orientation (Fig. 12–33).

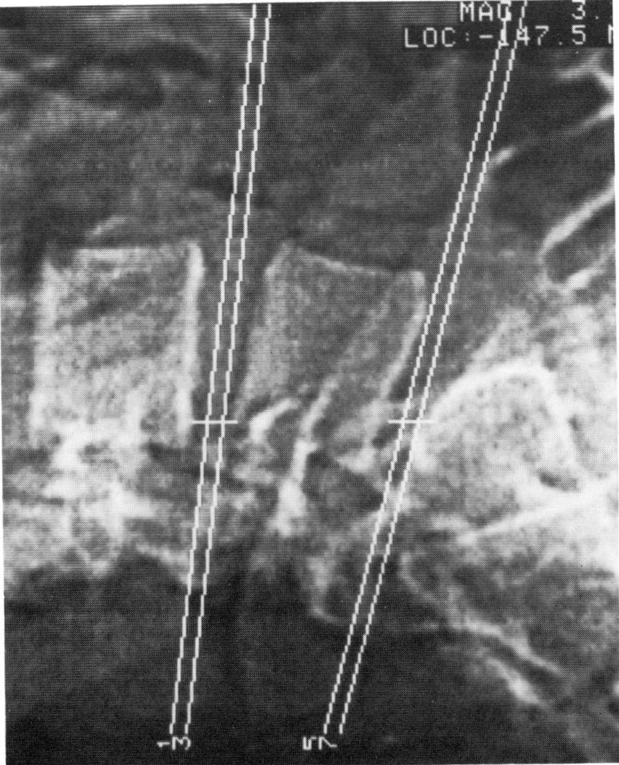

Figure 12–33. Lateral scout film shows the capability for selecting appropriate angulation for the gantry frame when scanning the lower spine.

SUMMARY

The remarkable technology of computed tomography has been reviewed. A spectrum of important potential applications of this technique to the musculoskeletal system has been defined, and the new developments that appear on the horizon have been discussed. The future of computed tomography in orthopedic and rheumatologic diagnosis and management appears promising; however, its ultimate impact clearly awaits further investigation and delineation.

REFERENCES

1. Abols Y, Rosenfeld D, Genant HK: Spinal bone mineral determination using computed tomography in patients, controls, and phantom. *In* RB Mazess (Ed): Proceedings of 4th International Conference of Bone Measurements. Washington DC, US Government Printing Office, 1979.
2. Abrams HS, McNeil BJ: Computed tomography: Cost and efficacy implications. Am J Roentgenol *131*:81, 1978.
3. Alfidi RJ, MacIntyre WJ, Meany TF. Chernack ES, Janicki R, Tarar R, Levin HL: Experimental studies to determine application of CAT scanning to the human body. Am J Roentgenol *124*:199, 1973.
4. Ambrose J: Computerized transverse axial scanning (tomography). II. Clinical application. Br J Radiol *46*:1023, 1973.
5. Baker HL Jr, Campbell JK, Houser OW, Reese DF, Sheedy PF, Holman CB, Kurland RL: Computer assisted tomography of the head; early evaluation. Mayo Clin Proc *49*:17, 1974.
6. Berger PE, Kuhn JP: Computed tomography of tumors of the musculoskeletal system in children. Radiology *127*:171, 1978.
7. Boyd, DP, Korobkin MT, Moss A: Engineering status of computerized tomographic scanning. Optical Eng *16*:37, 1977.
8. Brasch RC, Boyd DP, Gooding CA: Computed tomographic scanning in children: Comparison of radiation dose and resolving power of commercial CT scanners. Am J Roentgenol *131*:95, 1978.
9. Brooks RA, DiChiro G: Theory of image reconstruction in computed tomography. Radiology *117*:561, 1975.
10. Brunelle FO, Genant HK, Cann CE, Helms C, Gilula LA: Detection of subtle foci of metastatic disease in the skeleton using computed tomography (in preparation).
11. Coin CG, Chan YS, Keranen V, Pennink M: Computed assisted myelography in disc disease. J Comp Assist Tomogr *1*:398, 1977.
12. Colley DP, Dunsker SB: Traumatic narrowing of the dorsolumbar spinal canal demonstrated by computed tomography. Radiology *129*:95, 1978.
13. Cormack AM: Representation of a function by its line integrals with some radiological applications. J Appl Physics *34*:2722, 1963.
14. Computed Tomography — Continuum. Milwaukee, Wisconsin, General Electric Company, Medical Systems Division, 1978.
15. DeSantos LA, Murray JA: Evaluation of giant cell tumor by computerized tomography. Skel Radiol *2*:205, 1978.
16. DeSantos LA, Goldstein HM, Murray JA, Wallace S: Computed tomography in the evaluation of musculoskeletal neoplasms. Radiology *128*:89, 1978.
17. Destouet JM, Gilula LA, Murphy WA: Computed tomography of long bone osteosarcoma. Radiology *131*:439, 1979.
18. DiChiro G, Schellinger D: Computed tomography of spinal cord after lumbar intrathecal introduction of metrizamide (computer assisted myelography). Radiology *120*:101, 1976.
19. Ferrucci JT, Wittenberg J: CT biopsy of abdominal tumors: Aids for lesion localization. Radiology *129*:739, 1978.
20. Genant HK, Boyd DP: Quantitative bone mineral analysis using dual energy computed tomography. Invest Radiol *12*:545, 1977.
21. Genant HK: Musculoskeletal applications of computerized tomography. *In* F Feldman (ed): Radiology, Pathology, and Immunology of Bones and Joints. A Review of Current Concepts. New York, Appleton-Century-Crofts, 1978, p 253.
22. Genant HK: Advances in orthopedic diagnosis: The emergence of computed tomography. President's Guest Lecture presented at the Annual Assembly of the American Academy of Orthopedic Surgeons, San Francisco, February 24, 1979.
23. Genant, HK, Doi K, Mall JC, Sickles EA: Direct radiographic magnification for skeletal radiology. An assessment of image quality and clinical application. Radiology *123*:47, 1977.
24. Glenn WV, Johnston RJ, Morton PE, Dwyer SJ: Image generation and display techniques for CT scan data: Thin transverse and reconstructed coronal and sagittal planes. Invest Radiol *10*:403, 1975.
25. Goodenough DJ, Weaver KE, Davis DO: Potential artefacts associated with the scanning patterns of the EMI. Radiology *117*:615, 1975.
26. Gordon R, Herman GT, Johnson SA: Image reconstruction from projections. Sci Am *233*:56, 1975.
27. Hammerschlag SB, Wolpert SM, Carter BL: Computed tomography of the spinal canal. Radiology *121*:361, 1976.
28. Hounsfield GN: Computerized transverse axial scanning (tomography). I. Description of a system. Br J Rad *46*:1016, 1973.
29. Hunter JC, Johnston WH, Genant HK: Computed tomography evaluation of fatty tumors of the somatic soft tissues. Clinical utility and radiologic pathologic correlation. Skel Radiol *4*:79, 1979.
30. Introduction to Computed Tomography. Milwaukee, Wisconsin, General Electric Company, Medical Systems Division, 1976.
31. Kirkpatrick RH, Wittenberg J, Schaffer DL, Black EB, Hall DA, Braitman BS, Ferrucci JT Jr: Scanning techniques in computed body tomography. Am J Roentgenol *130*:1069, 1978.
32. Kuhl DE, Edwards RQ: Reorganizing data from transverse section scans of brain using digital processing. Radiology *91*:975, 1978.
33. Kuhn JP, Berger PE: Computed tomographic diagnosis of osteomyelitis. Radiology *130*:503, 1979.
34. Lancourt JE, Glenn WV, Wiltse LL: Multiplanar computerized tomography in the normal spine and in the diagnosis of spinal stenosis. A gross anatomic-computerized tomographic correlation. Spine *4*(4):379, July/Aug, 1979.
35. Lasda NA, Levinsohn EM, Yuan HA, Bunnell WP: Computerized tomography in disorders of the hip. J. Bone Joint Surg *60A*:1099, 1978.
36. Lee BCP, Kazam E, Newman AD: Computed tomography of the spine and spinal cord. Radiology *128*:95, 1978.
37. Levitt RG, Sagel SS, Stanley RJ, Evens RG: Computed tomography of the pelvis. Semin Roentgenol *13*:193, 1978.
38. McCullough EC: Photon attenuation in computed tomography. Med Physics *2*:307, 1975.
39. McCullough EC, Payne JT: Patient dosage in computed tomography. Radiology *129*:457, 1978.
40. McLeod RA, Stephen DH, Beabout JW, Sheedy PF, Hattery RR: Computed tomography of the skeletal system. Semin Roentgenol *13*:235, 1978.
41. McLeod RA, Gisvold JJ, Stephens DH, Beabout JW, Sheedy PF: Computed tomography of soft tissues and breast. Semin Roentgenol *13*:267, 1978.
42. Naidich TP, Pudlowski RM, Moran CH, Gilula LA, Murphy W, Naidich J: Computed tomography of spinal fractures. *In* R Thompson, JR Green (eds): Advances in Neurology. Vol 22. New York, Raven Press, 1979, p 207.
43. Nakagawa H, Huang YP, Malis LI, Wolf BS: Computed tomography of intraspinal and paraspinal neoplasms. J Comp Assist Tomogr *1*:377, 1977.
44. O'Connor JF, Cohen J: Computerized tomography (CAT Scan, CT Scan) in orthopedic surgery. J Bone Joint Surg *60A*:1096, 1978.
45. Oldendorf WH: Isolated flying spot detection of radiodensity discontinuities displaying the internal structural pattern of a complex object. IRE Trans Bio-Med Elect BME *8*:68, 1961.
46. Paul D, Morrey BF, Helms C: Computerized tomography in orthopedic surgery. Clin Orthop *139*:142, 1979.
47. Phelps ME, Hoffman EJ, Ter-Pogossian MM: Attenuation coefficients of various body tissues, fluids, and lesion at photon energies of 18 to 136 keV. Radiology *117*:573, 1975.
48. Post MJ, Gargano FP, Vining DQ, Rosomoff HL: A comparison of radiographic methods of diagnosing constrictive lesion of the spinal canal. J Neurosurg *48*:360, 1978.
49. Quencer RM, Murtagh FR, Post MJD, Rosomoff HL, Stokes NA: Postoperative bony stenosis of the lumbar spinal canal: Evaluation of 164 sympatomatic patients with axial radiography. Am J Roentgenol *131*:1059, 1978.
50. Radon J: On the determination of functions from their integrals along certain manifolds. Ber Saech Akad Wiss Leipzig Math Phys Kl *69*:262, 1917.
51. Rosenfeld D, Abols Y, Genant HK: Analysis of multiple energy computed tomography techniques for the measurement of bone mineral content. *In* RB Mazess (Ed): Proceedings of the 4th International Conference of Bone Measurement. Washington DC, US Government Printing Office, 1979.
52. Schumacher TM, Genant HK, Korobkin MT, Bovill EG: Computed tomography; its use in space-occupying lesions of the musculoskeletal system. J Bone Joint Surg *60A*:600, 1978.
53. Sheldon JJ, Sersland T, Leborgne J: Computed tomography of the lower lumbar vertebral column. Radiology *124*:113, 1977.
54. Weinberger G, Levinsohn EM: Computed tomography in the evaluation of sarcomatous tumors of the thigh. Am J Roentgenol *130*:115, 1978.
55. Wilson JS, Korobkin MT, Genant HK, Bovill EG: Computed tomography of musculoskeletal disorders. Am J Roentgenol *131*:55, 1978.

13

DIAGNOSTIC ULTRASOUND

by William Scheible, M.D.

Diagnostic ultrasound has achieved a central role in the evaluation of numerous clinical problems in obstetrics, medicine, and surgery. Ultrasonography is frequently utilized in abdominal and pelvic disease as a correlative modality to other imaging procedures, and many times it functions as a primary diagnostic study. The advent of gray scale signal processing and the routine utilization of higher frequency transducers have broadened the applicability of the technique to encompass assessment of smaller lesions as well as organ parenchymal texture. Although the role of diagnostic ultrasound in problems related to bone, joint, and soft tissue is limited in scope, there are situations in which the technique offers significant information, usually with less discomfort, risk, cost, and time expenditure than alternative radiographic or isotopic procedures.

FUNDAMENTAL PHYSICS OF DIAGNOSTIC ULTRASOUND

No chapter on diagnostic ultrasonography is complete without a requisite review of pertinent physical principles and applications. This contribution will be brief and serve only to emphasize fundamental points.

The heart of ultrasonographic imaging technology is the transducer. A transducer converts one form of energy into another, and in this setting the transformation is from electrical energy to sound energy and back again. A crystalline material such as barium titanate can be physically deformed by an electric current, with the resultant production of sound waves. Sound waves returning from the body then deform the transducer crystal in a similar fashion and produce an electric current. This property of some crystals is called the piezoelectric effect, and it forms the cornerstone for the clinical applications of ultrasound. The transducer acts as a receiver for approximately 999/1000 of any time period, having been only instantaneously operative as a sender of sound waves.

In clinical use, the emitted sound waves have a frequency of 2.25 to 10 megahertz (MHz); 1 MHz is one million cycles per second. These frequencies are far above the range of human hearing, which has an upper limit of approximately 20,000 cycles per second. Frequency is inversely related to wave length and to the depth of penetration into a given material. A higher frequency transducer (10 MHz, for example) is capable of penetrating only a few centimeters into soft tissue. Conversely, the higher the frequency, the better the resolution capability. The superficial location of most musculoskeletal problems is better imaged with higher frequency instrumentation.

The transducer is either placed directly on the surface of the patient or housed in a water bath. A suitable coupling agent, such as mineral oil or aqueous gel, is applied to the skin surface. Scanning is normally undertaken in planes at 90° to one another, although the flexibility of most scanning assemblies allows unlimited positional changes.

The interaction of propagated sound waves with tissue interfaces in the body is a second key consideration in sonographic imaging. Whenever the sound beam encounters an interface between tissues of different acoustic impedance, reflection or refraction occurs. It is the waves reflected back to the transducer crystal and converted into electric input that are recorded and displayed as ultrasonographic images. Early imaging with ultrasound was termed "bistable" display because it was essentially an all-or-none phenomenon. When the transducer face was placed on the surface of the body perpendicularly to a tissue interface, a strong reverberation was recorded. However, this technique practically limited useful information to boundaries or margins of organs or lesions and to characterization of fluid and solid structures. Bistable imaging has been supplanted by gray scale technology. Simply stated, it is now possible to record the diffuse reflections that previously would have been subthreshold. Consequently, much more information about organ parenchyma is now retrievable. Additionally, less technical expertise is required to produce a study of diagnostic quality. Gray scale refers to the fact that all intensities of returning echoes are assigned proportional shades of gray for display on an oscilloscope screen or television monitor. A permanent record can be obtained by photographing this image, either on x-ray film, Polaroid film, or heat-sensitive paper.

Real time ultrasonography is a newer technology that promises to play an important role in clinical diagnosis. One can consider real time as the sonographic equivalent of radiographic fluoroscopy because it entails the recording of dynamic events. If a single transducer is employed, it is made to vibrate or oscillate at high frequency. Alternatively, an array of transducer elements can be sequentially fired to produce the same effect. In addition to static images of the oscilloscope display, videotape recording of real time examinations can be performed.

PRINCIPLES OF CLINICAL ULTRASONOGRAPHY

Descriptive terminology in diagnostic ultrasonography is relatively straightforward. Lesions are characterized as either cystic, solid, or complex. Cystic structures are typified by any fluid-filled mass, such as a renal cyst, a pancreatic pseudocyst, or a normal organ such as the distended urinary bladder. Cystic organs or masses are echo-free. Because their fluid nature does not impede the transmission of the sound beam, a strong build-up of echoes is seen deep to the area. Solid masses and the parenchyma of most organs exhibit a variable pattern of middle-amplitude gray tones. The liver parenchyma, the nongravid uterus, and the thyroid gland are examples. Many neoplasms and inflammatory masses show a complex echographic appearance, containing both solid and fluid elements.

Deterrents to successful ultrasonography are air and bone, since the sound beam is not transmitted through either. For this reason, much of the thorax is blind to ultrasonography. Likewise, intestinal bowel gas sometimes hinders examinations of the abdomen.

The earliest use of diagnostic ultrasound was primarily for differentiation of cystic from solid mass lesions that had generally been detected by clinical or radiographic examinations. While still an important task for sonography, cyst/solid distinction is no longer the only use for ultrasound, which is now employed as a primary imaging study in many clinical situations. Several unique properties of ultrasound make the technique particularly useful. It is noninvasive and painless to the patient. It is generally less expensive and more rapidly performed than alternative studies. The risks of reaction to iodinated contrast material are eliminated. No ionizing radiation is employed. So far as is known, pulsed ultrasound in clinically useful frequency ranges has no deleterious effect on somatic or genetic cells.[1] Sonography is well suited to sequential follow-up studies to determine response to a particular therapeutic regimen. Because it allows localization of lesions in three dimensions, sonography is a useful technique for guiding percutaneous aspiration or biopsy, and for mapping radiation portals.

CLINICAL USE OF DIAGNOSTIC ULTRASOUND IN BONE, JOINT, AND SOFT TISSUE DISEASES

The Popliteal Space

The use of ultrasonography in clinical diagnosis for evaluation of various swellings in the popliteal space gained early acceptance. Because fluid/solid distinction was easily accomplished even by early instruments, and since popliteal cysts and popliteal artery aneurysms constitute the majority of masses in this area, sonography has frequently been utilized for this problem.

Popliteal cysts (Baker's cysts) are thought to arise in abnormal knee joints and to be dependent upon two factors, one anatomic, the other pathologic.[2-5] There must be a communication between the knee joint and the gastrocnemio-semimembranosus bursa. Second, an intra-articular abnormality must be present to produce an effusion capable of distending the joint.

The gastrocnemio-semimembranosus bursa is situated between the medial head of the gastrocnemius muscle and the semimembranosus more laterally.[6, 7] Anatomic connection between the bursa and the knee joint probably is present in about 50 per cent of people. The bursa is lined with synovium continuous with that in the joint space. In many instances, it is thought that a check valve mechanism limits flow of synovial fluid to one direction.[4] As a result, contrast arthrography and intra-articular radionuclide studies might fail to detect some popliteal cysts.[2] It has also been noted that flexion of the knee can collapse the suprapatellar bursa, forcing fluid into the gastrocnemio-semimembranosus bursa.[6] In this circumstance, arthrographic filling of the distended bursa can lead to a false diagnosis of popliteal cyst.

Joint effusion is a response to a number of abnormalities of the knee. As a component in the genesis of popliteal cysts, effusions are most often related to the synovial proliferation of rheumatoid arthritis or to traumatic internal derangements of the knee joint. Popliteal cysts have also been described in patients with osteoarthritis, gout, Reiter's syndrome, pigmented villonodular synovitis, and osteochondritis dissecans.[3]

Sometimes synovial membrane may herniate through a weakened posterior capsule of the knee joint.[5] This probably occurs in those patients who lack anatomic communication between the joint space and the gastrocnemio-semimembranosus bursa, and when rupture occurs, a pseudocapsule forms to contain fluid.[7] These collections are most often located between the gastrocnemius and the soleus muscles.

Arthrographic success rates for detecting popliteal cysts are variable, with cited figures ranging from 7 to 42 per cent.[2] Direct comparisons of sonography with contrast arthrography have generally shown rather close correlation, with no distinct advantage for either technique in terms of overall accuracy.[5, 8-10] Certain circumstances offer potential sources of error for each method. Lack of anatomic continuity between the knee joint and the gastrocnemio-semimembranosus bursa prevents arthrographic or isotopic demonstration of a significant number of cysts. Also, the contrast agent may not fill the entire cyst because of fibrin clots, adhesions, and loculations. Sonography circumvents both of these problems. On the other hand, sonography may fail to detect some ruptured cysts that have decompressed and may miss small cysts. The size threshold for sonographic identification of popliteal cysts should be less than 1 cm, particularly with the use of higher frequency transducers. The sonographic features of a cyst are readily determined, and a popliteal cyst should meet these criteria. Variable amounts of septation, debris, or pannus may be seen within the cyst (Figs. 13–1 and 13–2).

Ultrasonography has been recommended as a screening procedure for patients with rheumatoid arthritis who present with swelling, painful or asymptomatic, of the popliteal space.[4, 9] Since structural integrity of the knee joint is not an issue in these patients, the risks, discomfort, and costs of arthrography can be obviated. Moreover, ultrasonography is a particularly attractive means of performing serial noninvasive studies to monitor response to various therapeutic endeavors.[4, 11] Popliteal cysts are probably best treated by anterior synovectomy, since recurrences and fistula formation are not rare following attempts at cyst removal only.[4, 8] Synovial ablation with radioisotopes has also been advocated, with ultrasonography used in an effort to diagnose synovial thickening prior to the onset of radiographic bony changes.[11]

Rupture of a popliteal cyst or hemorrhage into the cyst can present with a clinical picture that closely mimics deep venous thrombophlebitis.[7, 12, 13] Compression of the popliteal vein by the cyst can also produce physical signs resembling thrombophlebitis.[14] The distinction between a popliteal cyst and thrombophlebitis is an important one to make, since anticoagulant therapy is required in the latter

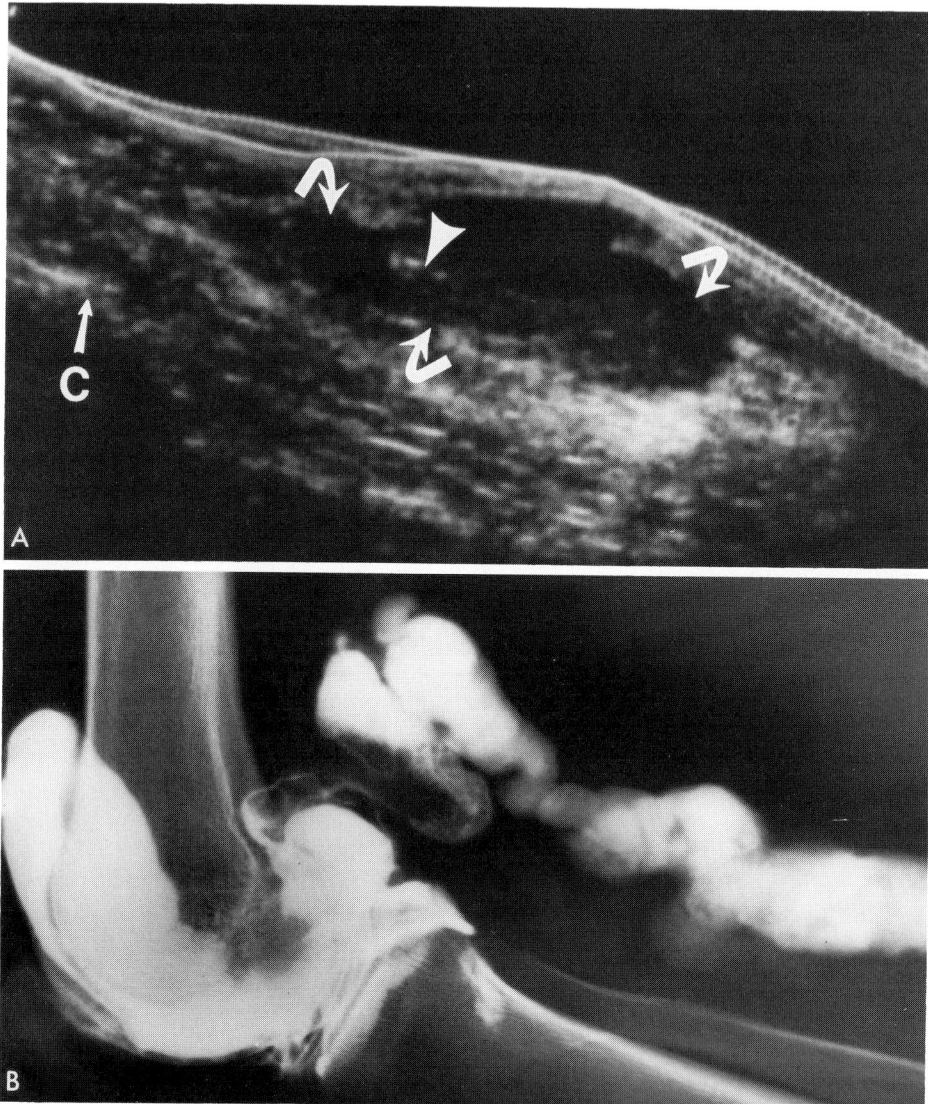

Figure 13–1. *Popliteal cyst.*

A *Longitudinal scan of the popliteal fossa shows a primarily fluid-filled mass (curved arrows) in the proximal calf. Fine internal echoes (arrowhead) represent either synovial proliferation or fibrin strands. The patient is prone, with the head to viewer's left. C, Femoral condyle.*

B *Contrast arthrography confirms an elongated popliteal cyst with numerous soft tissue excrescences.*

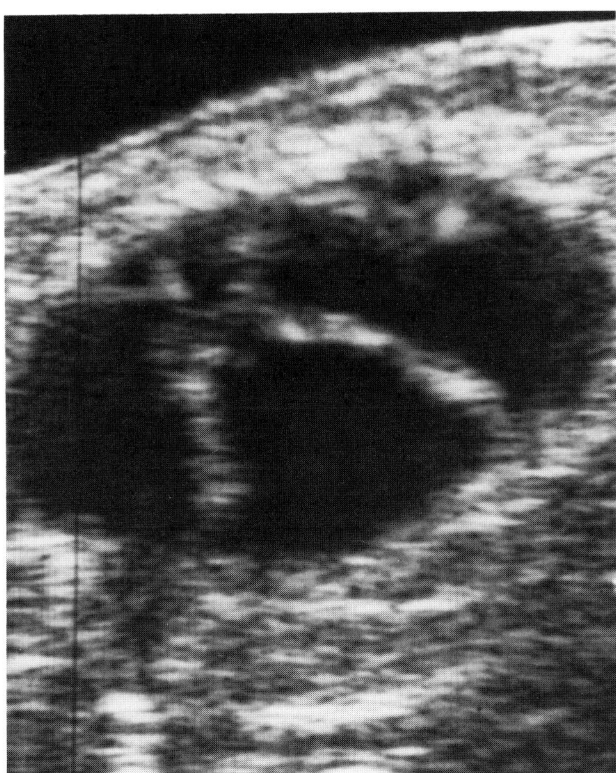

Figure 13–2. *Popliteal cyst. High resolution scan utilizing 10 MHz transducer shows a well demarcated popliteal cyst with internal septation. Frame size is 3 × 4 cm.*

instance and is not without hazard. Ultrasonography has been a valuable aid in this clinical setting.[3, 5, 10, 15, 16] Radioisotope methods have also been employed, but require intra-articular injection and are more time consuming and expensive than sonography.[13, 17]

The role of diagnostic ultrasound is thus relatively well established in conditions involving the popliteal space in patients with rheumatoid arthritis. It is important to remember that not every swelling in this area is secondary to a Baker's cyst, and sonography can conveniently exclude other causes, such as a popliteal artery aneurysm or a soft tissue tumor or abscess.[4, 5, 10] If desired, percutaneous aspiration of popliteal cysts can be guided by sonography.[4] Response of the cyst to therapy is easily monitored by the technique. In those knees in which trauma with internal derangement is the likely cause, contrast arthrography is the preferred method of evaluation, since sonography provides no information about structural integrity of the knee joint.

Ultrasonography is capable of detecting effusions in the knee joint, although the sensitivity of the method is not established.[11, 16] Very small amounts of fluid in the suprapatellar bursa should in theory be identifiable, especially with newer high-resolution transducers. Other joints have been examined with standard transducers, and some success has been claimed for the detection of small effusions of the hip, shoulder, and elbow.[79, 80] Para-articular fluid collections can also be distinguished. Although of doubtful clinical impact, sonography can sometimes identify intra-articular loose bodies, perhaps an aid in diagnosing those that are radiographically nonopaque.[80]

Aneurysms of the popliteal artery represent the most frequent of the peripheral arterial aneurysms.[18] Atheromatous disease is causative in the vast majority of cases, and a significant number of patients have coexisting cardiovascular disease, including abdominal aortic aneurysm.[18-20] The lesions are bilateral in up to 59 per cent of cases, although only one side may be clinically evident.[18, 20, 21] Popliteal artery aneurysms have a high incidence of thromboembolic complications, including thrombosis, venous occlusion, ulceration and gangrene, and peripheral embolization.[18, 21-23, 81] A 3 per cent incidence of limb loss has been cited for untreated popliteal artery aneurysms.[18] Up to 15 per cent of patients may have associated popliteal vein thrombosis, thus being at risk for pulmonary embolism.[24]

Angiography has been the traditional method for diagnosing and evaluating popliteal artery aneurysms. While required to determine the extent of disease and to assess the state of proximal and distal circulation, arteriography is not necessary to establish the diagnosis.[18, 20] In addition, arteriography suffers from several limitations that are overcome by ultrasonography.[21, 22, 25, 26] Many patients with popliteal artery aneurysms have diffuse vascular disease, and compromised proximal inflow may preclude visualization of the popliteal artery. Thrombus within an aneurysm, easily documented by sonography, is not seen with arteriography, which opacifies only the patent lumen carrying flowing blood. Thrombus is considered by some to be an indication for surgery.[25, 26] Clinical diagnosis is not always straightforward, as in cases in which pulsation is absent because of a thrombosed aneurysm.[10]

Because of the high incidence of complications in untreated popliteal artery aneurysms, elective surgical correction is recommended for most patients.[18, 22, 23] A sensitive, noninvasive screening procedure is necessary, and ultrasonography is increasingly utilized in this context, as it is thought by some to be more accurate than either clinical or arteriographic evaluation.[22, 23, 25, 26] The size of the normal popliteal artery has been determined in control groups, and ultrasonography yields accurate measurements because there is no magnification distortion.[25, 26] In addition to the ability of sonography to detect aneurysms and thrombus within them, the technique easily accomplishes a survey of the other leg for clinically silent aneurysms. Also, other causes of a mass behind the knee can be excluded by ultrasonography.[22]

The ultrasonographic diagnosis of popliteal artery aneurysm is relatively straightforward so long as continuity of the mass with a proximal and distal vessel can be ascertained.[22] This may occasionally be difficult when the popliteal artery is exceedingly tortuous.[19]

Investigation of other peripheral arterial aneurysms with ultrasonography has been limited.[82] The femoral artery at the level of the groin and the major vessels in the upper extremity are capable of being imaged in most patients.

Tumors of Bone and Soft Tissue

Modest experience has accumulated utilizing ultrasonography as a correlative modality to evaluate tumors of musculoskeletal origin.[27, 28] Lesions arising in the extremities as well as axial skeleton, pelvis, retroperitoneum, trunk, and abdominal wall have been described.[29-31, 83] Although sonography easily catalogues mass lesions into cystic, solid, or complex groupings, little histologic specificity is obtained from sonographic appearances alone.[32, 33] Fatty tissue is often extremely echogenic and lipomatous tumors can appear quite dense on gray scale sonograms.[34] Neoplasms of lymphatic origin typically contain extensive cystic areas.[29, 31] Highly vascular tumors such as hemangioma also can have numerous fluid regions (Fig. 13–3).

Because many of these lesions either arise from bone or involve bone secondarily, and because ultrasonography has negligible success establishing bone–soft tissue relationships, the role of sonography in this setting is questionable. Computed tomography has significant advantage in detailing

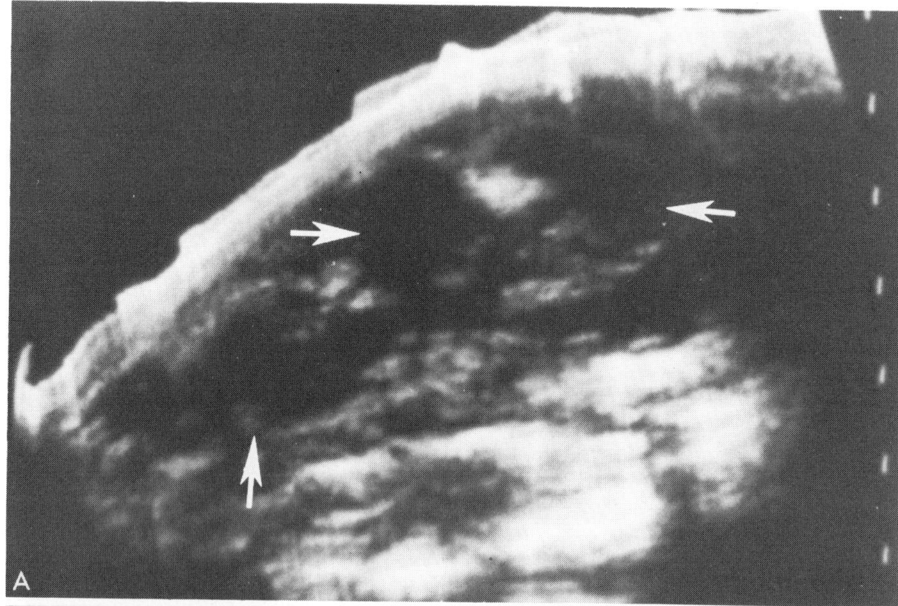

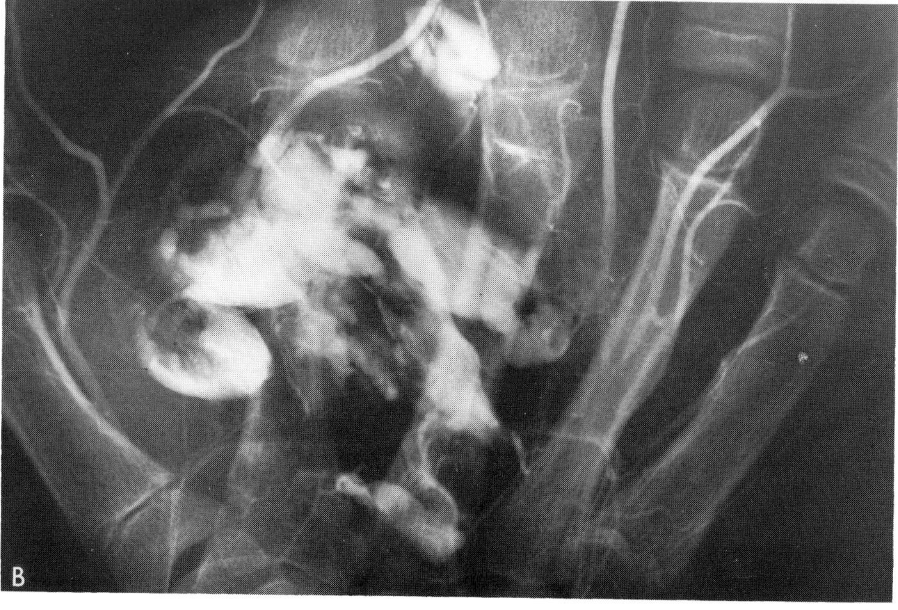

Figure 13–3. Hemangioma.

A *A superficial lesion of the palm contains many fluid-filled spaces representing dilated vascular channels (arrows).*

B *Arteriography shows the extensive vascular pooling within the cavernous hemangioma.*

these problems and is the preferred procedure in most instances.[84]

Once the presence of a lesion is identified, however, sonography can be employed as a means of monitoring the response of any extraosseous tumor bulk to therapeutic regimens.[27, 28, 85] Enlargement of a tumor mass can be the result of hemorrhage or necrosis rather than tumor growth, a distinction sonography can make.[33] The technique is well suited to repeated sequential examinations and is generally reproducible if care is taken to establish reference landmarks. Pretreatment tumor mapping with ultrasonography has been used to guide radiotherapy portals.[28] Finally, sonography offers a rapid and accurate method of localizing a soft tissue mass for percutaneous biopsy.[35] Areas of hemorrhage or necrosis have poor cytologic yield and the needle can be directed to more appropriate regions for sampling.

Infections of Bone and Soft Tissue

Detection of abscesses remains a challenging task for diagnostic imaging. Ultrasonography is frequently called upon in this situation, and when the area of suspicion is superficially located, as in the extremity or abdominal wall, the technique is quite successful. Demonstration of intra-abdominal and retroperitoneal abscesses is also feasible, though often correlative radiographic or isotopic studies are necessary for diagnosis.[36] Ultrasonography is unable to determine bony involvement by infectious proc-

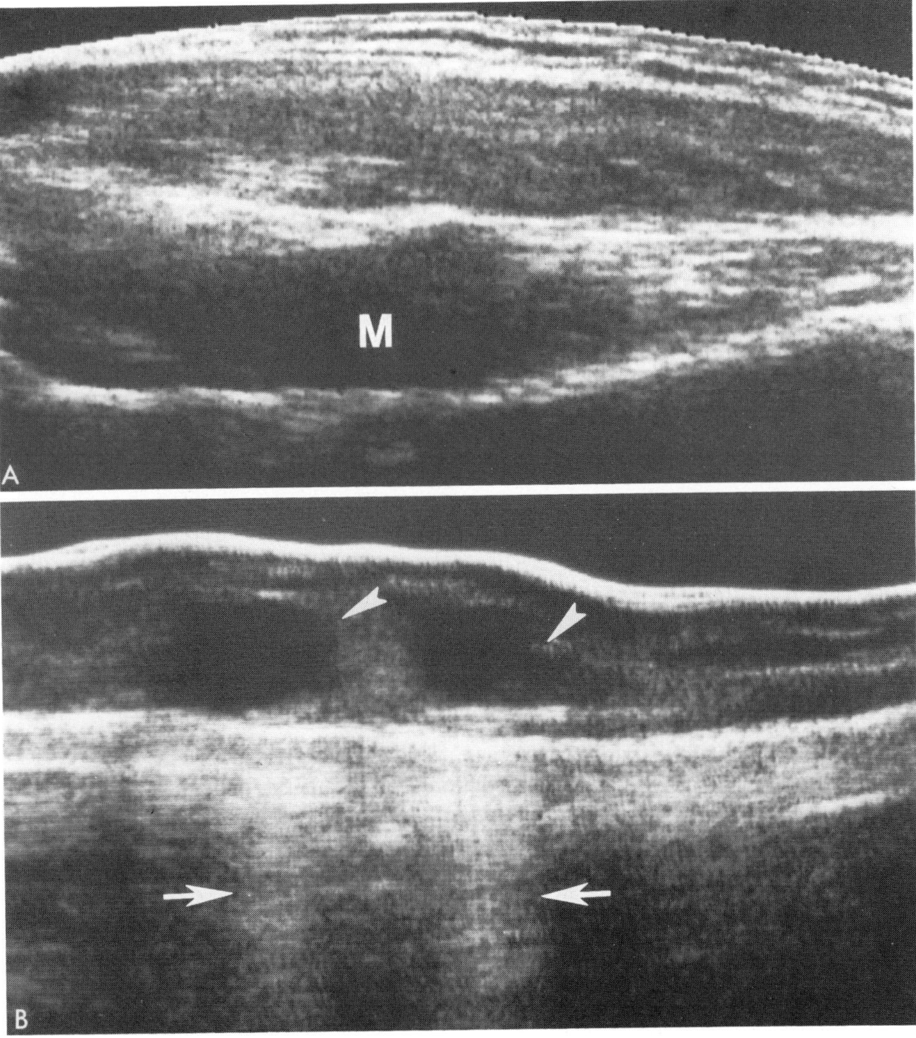

Figure 13–4. *Differentiation of cellulitis from soft tissue abscess.*

A *Cellulitis. Longitudinal scan of the anterior thigh demonstrates diffuse edema of the superficial soft tissues, clearly demaracted from the deeper muscle* **(M).**

B *Soft tissue abscesses. Localized fluid-filled masses (arrowheads) are present within the subcutaneous tissues of the thigh. A build-up of echoes deep to the lesion (arrows) is characteristic of cystic masses.*

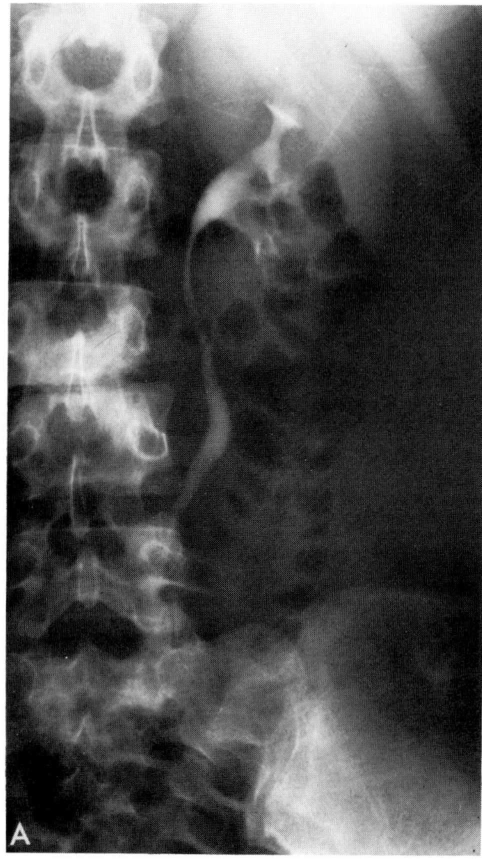

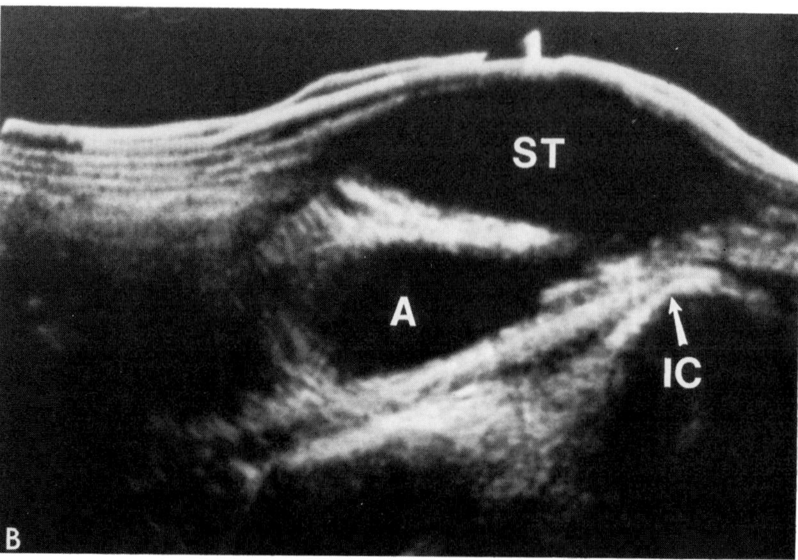

Figure 13–5. Tuberculous psoas abscess.
A Intravenous urogram shows slight lateral deviation of the midureter. The adjacent L3–4 interspace is eroded and narrowed due to tuberculous infection.
B Longitudinal sonogram of the left lower quadrant reveals the psoas abscess **(A)**, which has extended superficially into the subcutaneous tissues **(ST)**. **IC,** Iliac crest.

esses. Delineation of this problem necessitates other examinations.

Sonographic features of abscesses vary considerably.[33, 37-39] A typical abscess contains predominantly fluid but often has debris as well that is manifest as fine, low-level echoes within the cystic mass. This material sometimes accumulates in the dependent portion of the abscess, a phenomenon that can be documented by changing the patient's position. The margins of an abscess are usually indistinct, in contrast to simple cysts. Many abscesses, notably chronic or partially treated lesions, are complex in appearance and can even be difficult to distinguish from surrounding soft tissue. Gas-containing abscesses can be quite dense on sonograms, an appearance thought to be a result of the numerous highly reflective interfaces engendered by "micro bubbles."[39]

Despite the variable sonographic appearance of abscesses and the considerable overlap with other lesions, including hematomas and tumors, sonography is of significant diagnostic aid in this clinical problem. Cellulitis can be treated effectively with antibiotics, but abscesses generally require percutaneous or open surgical drainage. Segregation of abscess from simple cellulitis of the extremity has been accomplished with sonography[10] (Fig. 13–4). This capability can be extended to encompass the abdominal wall, trunk, and neck. Paravertebral abscesses are present in a significant percentage of patients with infections of the spine.[40] The existence of a paraspinous abscess is often difficult to establish with conventional radiography and as a rule ultrasonography is more successful (Fig. 13–5). Apart from detecting the presence of effusion in the knee joint, sonography has no benefit in the evaluation of septic arthritis.

Sonographic guidance for percutaneous needling of various lesions is being undertaken more aggressively. The technique has proved to be quite satisfactory for aspiration or continuous drainage of abscesses.[35, 41-43] This approach can spare a number of patients the risk and expense of surgical intervention. Importantly, sonography is an objective means of monitoring the response of a given inflammatory lesion to appropriate therapy.

Hemophilia and Altered Coagulability States

A significant population is at risk for hemorrhage, either from primary blood dyscrasias or secondary alterations in clotting mechanisms. The latter circumstance is frequently iatrogenic, since many patients are placed on anticoagulant medication. The relative ease with which ultrasonography detects fluid collections such as hematomas makes this an attractive method for evaluating these patients. Sonography has proved efficacious in this clinical problem, both in diagnosing areas of hemorrhage and in following the natural history of the bleeding.[44-46]

Rectus sheath hematoma is a specific clinical entity that is misdiagnosed in as many as 60 per cent of cases.[47, 48] Signs and symptoms often mimic acute abdominal or pelvic conditions, such as intestinal obstruction or hernia, twisted ovarian cyst, or perivesicular inflammatory disease. Factors predisposing to rectus sheath hematoma include violent muscular contraction (cough, sneeze, exercise), trauma (including surgery), pregnancy and labor, tension on the abdominal wall (ascites, obesity), blood dyscrasias, and anticoagulant therapy.[48] Conservative treatment is recommended and entails analgesia, compresses, and rest. Surgery is to be avoided.[47] The sonographic appearance of rectus sheath hematoma is characteristic and consists of an ellipsoid or spindle-shaped fluid collection in the superficial anterior abdominal wall.[49, 50, 86] The tight boundaries of the rectus sheath confine the bleeding, and the process does not cross the midline unless it occurs low, where the posterior portion of the sheath is deficient (Fig. 13–6).

Iliopsoas hematoma is a common complication of hemophilia.[51, 52] A rather typical syndrome of pain and nerve deficit occurs with bleeding isolated to the closed iliacus compartment that contains the femoral nerve. The psoas fascia is looser and allows more extensive hemorrhage to take place. When this occurs on the right side, differentiation from acute appendicitis may be clinically difficult. Sonography is capable of detecting hemorrhage in both of these muscle compartments.[45, 52, 87]

Hemorrhage into the wall of the intestine or into the root of the mesentery is also a complication of altered coagulability. Intramural intestinal hematoma exhibits rather characteristic, albeit nonspecific, echographic features.[53] The diagnosis of occult mesenteric hematoma is often very difficult. Sonography can identify this lesion and establish its origin as being separate from neighboring parenchymal organs.[88]

Intra-articular hemorrhage is not amenable to current ultrasonographic instrumentation, although reference has been made to its potential use in hemophilia to detect fresh blood superimposed upon thickened synovium from previous joint hemorrhage.[11]

Depending on the age and chronicity of the hemorrhage, hematomas display a spectrum of appearances on gray scale sonograms.[44, 46, 54] When fresh and composed of liquid blood, a hematoma is homogeneous and appears virtually echo-free.[44] Internal echoes appear when clot begins to organize and then fragment, resulting in a more complex sonographic appearance. Liquefaction of clot may then lead once again to a variable fluid pattern on sonography. This inconstant pattern causes difficulty in attempting to predict the age of a given collection of blood.[54] Considerable overlap exists with similar features demonstrated by abscesses or tumors, for example. Nonetheless, the appropriate clinical setting generally allows an accurate diagnosis, and the real task of diagnostic ultrasound is to detect an abnormality in this circumstance that often escapes conventional radiographic approaches. By

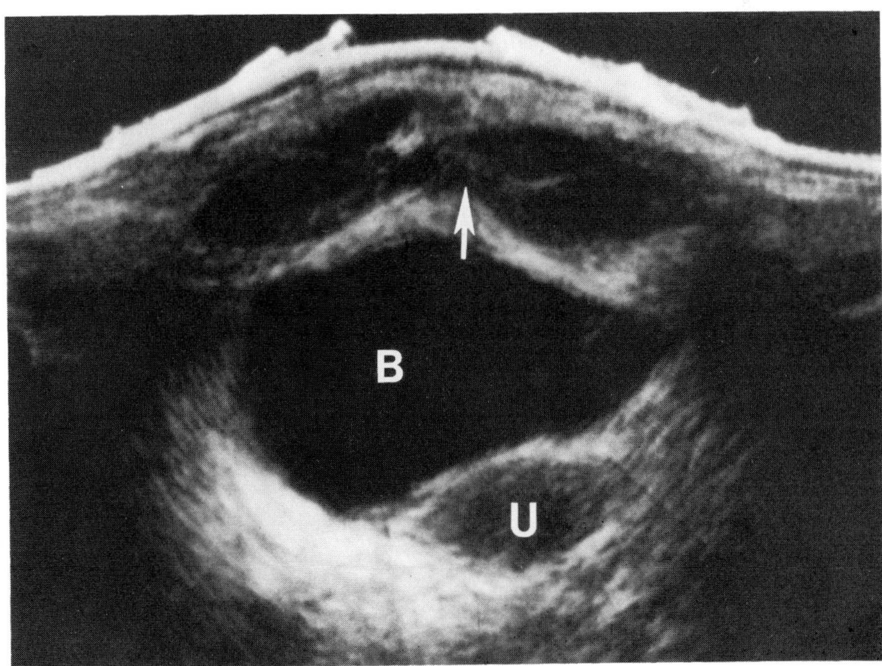

Figure 13–6. *Rectus sheath hematoma. The classic sonographic features of rectus sheath hematoma are demonstrated on this transverse scan through the distended urinary bladder* **(B)**. *The lesions are bilateral, but separated in the midline by the linea alba (arrow).* **U**, *Uterus.*

making the diagnosis, sonography can eliminate the need for a more elaborate and perhaps invasive work-up (Fig. 13–7).

Endocrine Disorders

The parathyroid glands are intimately involved in calcium homeostasis and thus come into the province of diseases involving bone. It is not the osseous changes, but rather the parathyroids themselves, that are of interest to ultrasonographers.

Normal parathyroid glands measure approximately 3 × 4 × 5 mm and have by and large evaded all attempts to image them. It is apparent that sonography does as well, if not better, than alternative methods in depicting enlargement of one or more of these organs. The sonographic findings in both hyperplasia and adenoma have been detailed.[55-57, 89] An overall accuracy rate of 70 per cent has been achieved by diagnosing as abnormal any gland larger than 5 mm in diameter.[58] However, a negative study is unreliable since not all abnormal glands are enlarged.

The goal of ultrasonography should be to reliably identify parathyroid enlargement. Asymptomatic hypercalcemia is identified rather frequently during routine biochemical screening panels. A noninvasive imaging modality such as ultrasonography has potential benefit for this select group of patients. In primary hyperparathyroidism, which is due to an adenoma in 90 per cent of cases, localization of the offending tumor is desirable to shorten an otherwise exhaustive surgical exploration of the

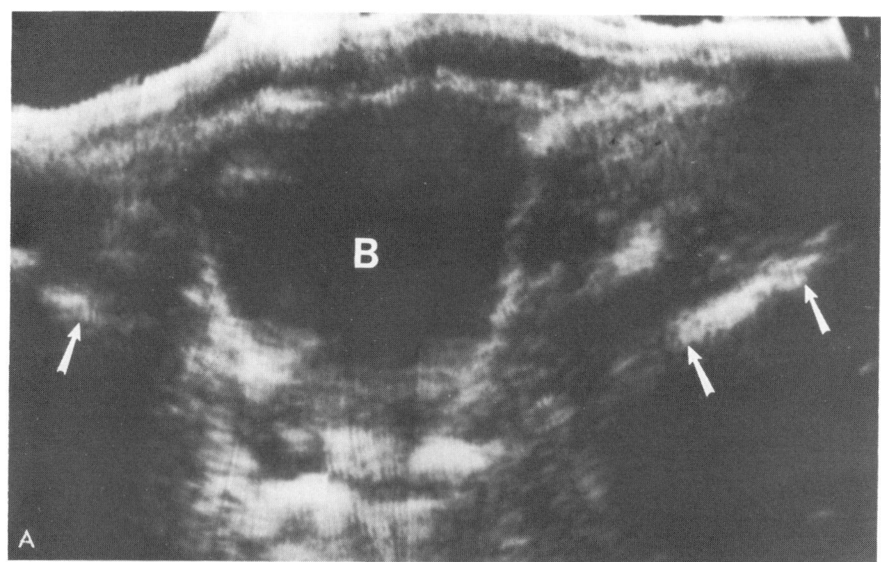

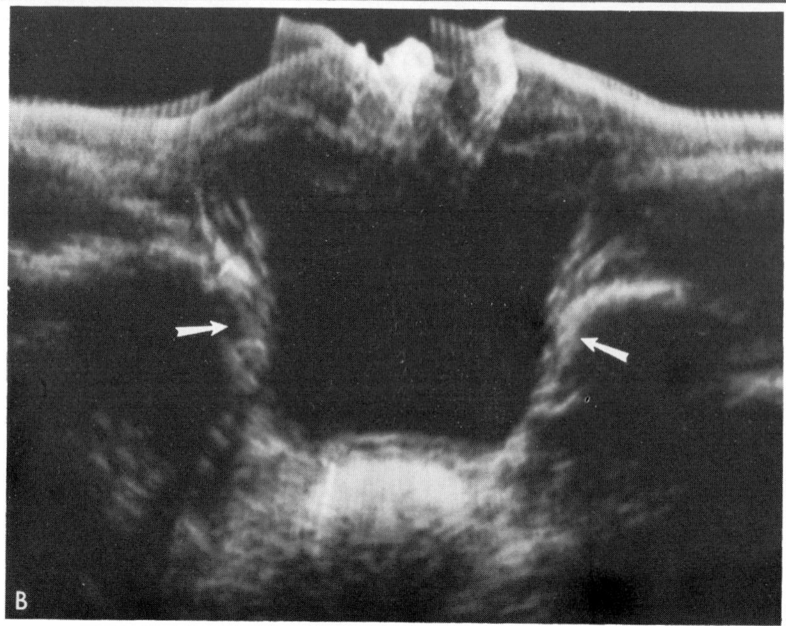

Figure 13–7. *Iliopsoas hematoma.*

A *Transverse sonogram through the urinary bladder* **(B)** *reveals enlargement of the left iliopsoas compartment, with impression upon the lateral wall of the distended bladder. The pelvic sidewall is demarcated by the dense reflection from iliac bone (arrows).*

B *Resolution of iliopsoas hematoma is confirmed by a return to normal anatomic relationships. The posterolateral bladder now abuts upon the pelvic sidewall (arrows).*

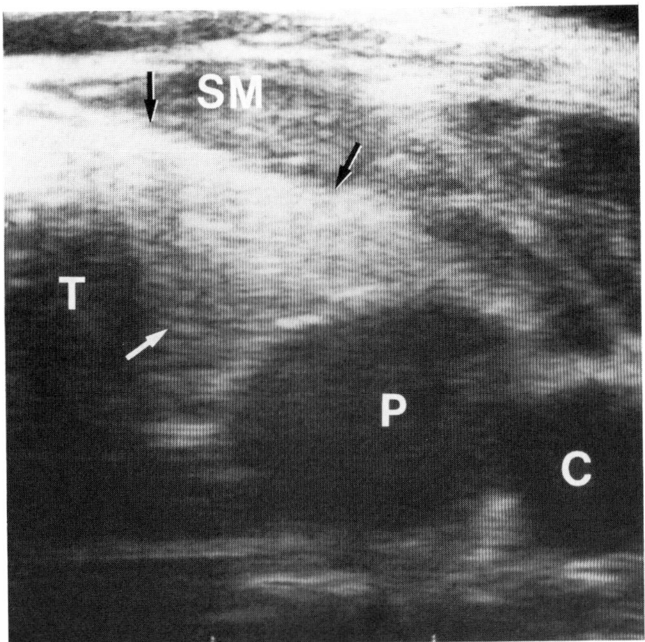

Figure 13–8. *Parathyroid hyperplasia. A high resolution scan transversely through the left lobe of the thyroid (arrows) shows enlargement of the upper parathyroid gland* **(P)**, *measuring 12 mm in diameter.* **C**, *Common carotid artery;* **T**, *trachea;* **SM**, *sternothyroid and sternohyoid muscles.*

neck. Secondary hyperparathyroidism is frequently caused by renal disease and results in hyperplasia of the parathyroid glands, and localization of single glandular enlargement is less important.

Technical advances in high-resolution real time ultrasonography promise to expand the role of diagnostic ultrasound in parathyroid disease. The technique is likely to become the preferred method of parathyroid imaging (Fig. 13–8).

Somewhat related to parathyroid problems is the significant population undergoing chronic hemodialysis for renal failure. Ultrasonography has potential application in these patients, since it is a rapid and noninvasive means of evaluating vascular access grafts and their complications.[59, 60] The superficial placement of dialysis fistulas renders them easily accessible to ultrasound scanning, especially with high resolution transducers.[90] Previously these patients required repeated angiographic studies of their grafts, an expensive and time-consuming procedure not without risk.[61-63]

Complications that confront hemodialysis fistulas include stenosis, thrombosis, aneurysm and pseudoaneurysm, and local infection.[59, 60, 64-66] Each of these can be identified by ultrasonography, and although angiography does quite well, certain situations are better evaluated with diagnostic ultrasound. Partially thrombosed aneurysms may be missed entirely by angiography and the study is precluded altogether in clotted grafts. Early detection of thrombus allows thrombectomy and salvage of the fistula. Graft stenosis may lead to thrombosis, and narrowed segments, if identified early, can be corrected by shunt revision rather than placement of a new fistula. Extrinsic abnormalities such as hematomas and abscesses will not be seen by angiography but should be demonstrable by sonography (Fig. 13–9).

Pleural and Pericardial Disease

Systemic rheumatologic diseases such as rheumatoid arthritis and lupus erythematosus affect the pleural and pericardial surfaces. Detection of fluid in either location is readily accomplished with ultrasonography.

Air and bone, the major constituents of the thorax, both interfere with transmission of sound waves and thereby limit the usefulness of ultrasound in the chest. However, pleural fluid usually accumulates adjacent to the chest wall and displaces the lung away from the transducer. Consequently, sonography can be employed to identify pleural fluid and assist thoracentesis.[67-74] This is especially true for loculated or small collections and in cases in which

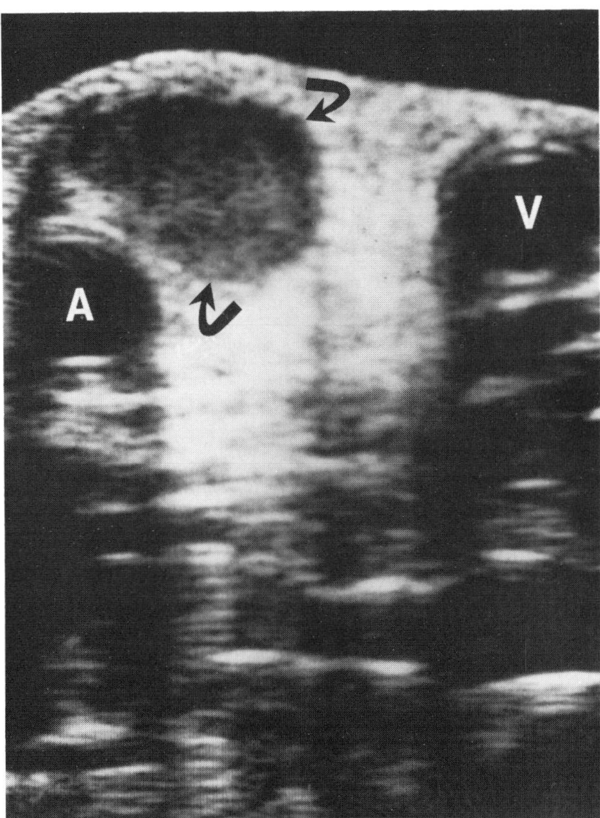

Figure 13–9. *Pseudoaneurysm of hemodialysis graft. A transverse sonogram of the forearm utilizing high resolution real-time instrumentation. The arterial* **(A)** *and venous* **(V)** *limbs of the synthetic graft are seen in cross section. A large pseudoaneurysm (curved arrows) filled with thrombus projects from the arterial limb.*

the position of the hemidiaphragm is crucial information. As little as 5 cc of pleural fluid can be detected.[69, 73] Because the visceral pleural surface can be identified, pneumothorax has been an infrequent complication when sonography is used to guide thoracentesis.[71, 74]

Although in theory a distinction of fluid collections from solid lesions should be easily done with sonography, and in fact usually is, sonographic features alone have poor predictive value regarding the success of fluid retrieval.[68, 71, 73] Organizing effusions may appear echo-free yet defy aspiration. Conversely, many complex-appearing pleural collections yield fluid. The most pertinent finding for documenting free-flowing fluid is the demonstration of a change in position or configuration of the collection when the patient's position is changed.

Any radiographic opacity that abuts upon the chest wall can be investigated by ultrasonography.[73, 75] Some solid lesions such as pulmonary Hodgkin's disease are difficult to distinguish from fluid collections.[76]

Clinically overt rheumatoid heart disease is rare.[91] The echographically determined incidence of pericardial effusion is approximately 15 to 30 per cent.[77, 78] Seldom is the effusion hemodynamically significant. Likewise, indices of left ventricular function may experience mild abnormalities but rarely is there clinical manifestation of left ventricular depression. Echocardiographic abnormalities have been identified in scleroderma and related diseases as well.[92]

SUMMARY

Despite the early clinical application of diagnostic ultrasound to diseases of the musculoskeletal system, the technique has not become widespread. Usually this is because alternative imaging procedures provide more complete information. There are special circumstances wherein ultrasonography is clearly of use, however. Further improvements in and experience with high resolution transducers promise to broaden the potential applicability of sonography to diseases of bone, joint, and soft tissue.

REFERENCES

1. Baker ML, Dalrymple GV: Biological effects of diagnostic ultrasound: A review. Radiology *126*:479, 1978.
2. Wolfe RD, Colloff B: Popliteal cysts: An arthrographic study and review of the literature. J Bone Joint Surg *54A*:1057, 1972.
3. McDonald DG, Leopold GR: Ultrasound B-scanning in the differentiation of Baker's cyst and thrombophlebitis. Br J Radiol *45*:729, 1972.
4. Moore CP, Sarti DA, Louie JS: Ultrasonographic demonstration of popliteal cysts in rheumatoid arthritis: A non-invasive technique. Arthritis Rheum *18*:577, 1975.
5. Carpenter JR, Hattery RR, Hunder GG, Bryan RS, McLeod RA: Ultrasound evaluation of the popliteal space: Comparison with arthrography and physical examination. Mayo Clin Proc *51*:498, 1976.
6. Doppman JL: Baker's cyst and the normal gastrocnemio-semimembranosus bursa. Am J Roentgenol *94*:646, 1965.
7. Pastershank SP, Mitchell DM: Knee joint bursal abnormalities in rheumatoid arthritis. J Can Assoc Radiol *28*:199, 1977.
8. Meire HB, Lindsay DJ, Swinson DR, Hamilton EBD: Comparison of ultrasound and positive contrast arthrography in the diagnosis of popliteal and calf swellings. Ann Rheum Dis *33*:221, 1974.
9. Baumann D, Kremer H: Arthrography and sonography in the diagnosis of Baker's cysts. ROEFO *127*:463, 1977.
10. Lawson TL, Mittler S: Ultrasonic evaluation of extremity soft-tissue lesions with arthrographic correlation. J Can Assoc Radiol *29*:58, 1978.
11. Cooperberg PL, Tsang I, Truelove L, Knickerbocker WJ: Gray scale ultrasound in the evaluation of rheumatoid arthritis of the knee. Radiology *126*:759, 1978.
12. Good AE: Rheumatoid arthritis, Baker's cyst, and thrombophlebitis. Arthritis Rheum *7*:56, 1964.
13. Schmidt MC, Workman JB, Barth WF: Dissection or rupture of a popliteal cyst: A syndrome mimicking thrombophlebitis in rheumatic diseases. Arch Intern Med *134*:694, 1974.
14. Swett HA, Jaffe RB, McIff EB: Popliteal cysts: Presentation as thrombophlebitis. Radiology *115*:613, 1975.
15. Rudikoff JC, Lynch JJ, Philipps E, Clapp PR: Ultrasound diagnosis of Baker cyst. JAMA *235*:1054, 1976.
16. Ambanelli U, Manganelli P, Nervetti A, Ugolotti V: Demonstration of articular effusions and popliteal cysts with ultrasound. J Rheumatol *3*:134, 1976.
17. Levin MH, Nordyke RA, Ball JJ: Demonstration of dissecting popliteal cysts by joint scans after intra-articular isotope injections. Arthritis Rheum *14*:591, 1971.
18. Wychulis AR, Spittell JA, Wallace RB: Popliteal aneurysms. Surgery *68*:942, 1970.
19. Sarti DA, Louie JS, Lindstrom RR, Nies K, London J: Ultrasonic diagnosis of a popliteal artery aneurysm. Radiology *121*:707, 1976.
20. Chitwood WR, Stocks LH, Wolfe WG: Popliteal artery aneurysms: Past and present. Arch Surg *113*:1078, 1978.
21. Silver TM, Washburn RL, Stanley JC, Gross WS: Gray scale ultrasound evaluation of popliteal artery aneurysms. Am J Roentgenol *129*:1003, 1977.
22. Scott WW, Scott PP, Sanders RC: B-scan ultrasound in the diagnosis of popliteal aneurysms. Surgery *81*:436, 1977.
23. Collins GJ, Rich NM, Phillips J, Hobson RW, Andersen CA: Ultrasound diagnosis of popliteal arterial aneurysms. Am Surg *42*:853, 1976.
24. Giustra PE, Root JA, Mason SE, Killoran PJ: Popliteal vein thrombosis secondary to popliteal artery aneurysm. Am J Roentgenol *130*:25, 1978.
25. Davis RP, Neiman HL, Yao JST, Bergan JJ: Ultrasound scan in diagnosis of peripheral aneurysms. Arch Surg *112*:55, 1977.
26. Neiman HL, Yao JST, Silver TM: Gray-scale ultrasound diagnosis of peripheral arterial aneurysms. Radiology *130*:413, 1979.
27. Kobayshi, T, Yoh S, Shinohara N, Fukuma H: Echographic diagnosis of soft tissue tumors in extremity and trunk. Jap J Clin Oncol *5*:97, 1975.
28. deSantos LA, Goldstein HM: Ultrasonography in tumors arising from the spine and bony pelvis. Am J Roentgenol *129*:1061, 1977.
29. Gilsanz V, Yeh HC, Baron MG: Multiple lymphangiomas of the neck, axilla, mediastinum, and bones in an adult. Radiology *120*:161, 1976.
30. Miller WB, Melson GL: Abdominal wall endometrioma. Am J Roentgenol *132*:467, 1979.
31. Leonidas JC, Brill PW, Bhan I, Smith TH: Cystic retroperitoneal lymphangioma in infants and children. Radiology *127*:203, 1978.
32. Goldberg BB: Ultrasonic evaluation of superficial masses. J Clin Ultrasound *3*:91, 1975.
33. Gooding GAW, Herzog KA, Laing FC, McDonald EJ: Ultrasonographic assessment of neck masses. J Clin Ultrasound *5*:248, 1977.
34. Behan M, Kazam E: The echographic characteristics of fatty tissues and tumors. Radiology *129*:143, 1978.
35. Holm HH, Pedersen JF, Kristensen JK, Rasmussen SN, Hancke S, Jensen F: Ultrasonically guided percutaneous puncture. Radiol Clin North Am *13*:493, 1975.
36. Korobkin M, Callen PW, Filly RA, Hoffer PB, Shimshak RR, Kressel HY: Comparison of computed tomography, ultrasonography, and gallium-67 scanning in the evaluation of suspected abdominal abscess. Radiology *129*:89, 1978.
37. Weiner CI, Diaconis JN: Primary abdominal wall abscess diagnosed by ultrasound. Arch Surg *110*:341, 1975.

38. Doust BD, Quiroz F, Stewart JM: Ultrasonic distinction of abscesses from other intra-abdominal fluid collections. Radiology *125*:213, 1977.
39. Kressel HY, Filly RA: Ultrasonographic appearance of gas-containing abscesses in the abdomen. Am J Roentgenol *130*:71, 1978.
40. Allen EH, Cosgrove D, Millard FJC: The radiological changes in infections of the spine and their diagnostic value. Clin Radiol *29*:31, 1978.
41. Smith EH, Bartrum RJ: Ultrasonically guided percutaneous aspiration of abscesses. Am J Roentgenol *122*:308, 1974.
42. Conrad MR, Sanders RC, Mascardo AD: Perinephric abscess aspiration using ultrasound guidance. Am J Roentgenol *128*:459, 1977.
43. Grønvall J, Grønvall S, Hegedüs V: Ultrasound-guided drainage of fluid-containing masses using angiographic catheterization techniques. Am J Roentgenol *129*:997, 1977.
44. Kaplan GN, Sanders RC: B-scan ultrasound in the management of patients with occult abdominal hematomas. J Clin Ultrasound *1*:5, 1973.
45. Nowotny C, Niessner H, Thaler E, Lechner K: Sonography: A method for localization of hematomas in hemophiliacs. Haemostasis *5*:129, 1976.
46. Thomas JL, Cunningham JJ: Echographic detection and characterization of abdominal hemorrhages in patients with altered coagulation states. Arch Intern Med *138*:1392, 1978.
47. Titone C, Lipsius M, Krakauer JS: "Spontaneous" hematoma of the rectus abdominis muscle: Critical review of 50 cases with emphasis on early diagnosis and treatment. Surgery *72*:568, 1972.
48. Spitz HB, Wyatt GM: Rectus sheath hematoma. J Clin Ultrasound *5*:413, 1977.
49. Hamilton JV, Flinn G, Haynie CC, Cefalo RC: Diagnosis of rectus sheath hematoma by B-mode ultrasound: A case report. Am J Obstet Gynecol *125*:562, 1976.
50. Kaftori JK, Rosenberger A, Pollack S, Fish JH: Rectus sheath hematoma: Ultrasonographic diagnosis. Am J Roentgenol *128*:283, 1977.
51. Goodfellow J, Fearn CBD, Matthews JM: Iliacus haematoma: A common complication of haemophilia. J Bone Joint Surg *49B*:748, 1967.
52. Forbes CD, Moule B, Grant M, Greig WR, Prentice CRM: Bilateral pseudotumors of the pelvis in a patient with Christmas disease. Am J Roentgenol *121*:173, 1974.
53. Lee TG, Brickman FE, Avecilla LS: Ultrasound diagnosis of intramural intestinal hematoma. J Clin Ultrasound *5*:423, 1977.
54. Wicks JD, Silver TM, Bree RL: Gray scale features of hematomas: An ultrasonic spectrum. Am J Roentgenol *131*:977, 1978.
55. Seltzer SE, Balikian JP, Birnholz JC, Hargreaves H, Cartier P, Herman PG: Giant hyperplastic parathyroid gland in the mediastinum — partially cystic and calcified. Radiology *127*:43, 1978.
56. Crocker EF, Bautovich GJ, Jellins J: Gray-scale echographic visualization of a parathyroid adenoma. Radiology *126*:233, 1978.
57. Karo JJ, Maas LC, Kaine H, Gelzayd EA: Ultrasonography and parathyroid adenoma. JAMA *239*:2163, 1978.
58. Sample WF, Mitchell SP, Bledsoe RC: Parathyroid ultrasonography. Radiology *127*:485, 1978.
59. Fellner SK, Gonzalez AC, Kottle SP: Ultrasonography: A noninvasive alternative to arteriography for evaluation of vascular grafts. Dial Transplant *7*:680, 1978.
60. Kottle SP, Gonzalez AC, Macon EJ, Fellner SK: Ultrasonographic evaluation of vascular access complications. Radiology *129*:751, 1978.
61. Gilula LA, Staple TW, Anderson CB, Anderson LS: Venous angiography of hemodialysis fistulas. Radiology *115*:555, 1975.
62. Anderson CB, Gilula LA, Harter HR, Etheredge EE: Venous angiography and the surgical management of subcutaneous hemodialysis fistulas. Ann Surg *187*:194, 1978.
63. O'Reilly RJ, Hansen CC, Rosental JJ: Angiography of chronic hemodialysis arteriovenous grafts. Am J Roentgenol *130*:1105, 1978.
64. Rohr MS, Browder W, Frentz GD, McDonald JC: Arteriovenous fistulas for long-term dialysis. Arch Surg *113*:153, 1978.
65. Mennes PA, Gilula LA, Anderson CB, Etheredge EE, Weerts C, Harter HR: Complications associated with arteriovenous fistulas in patients undergoing chronic hemodialysis. Arch Intern Med *138*:1117, 1978.
66. Lemaitre P, O'Regan S, Herba M, Kaye M: Complications in expanded polytetrafluoroethylene arteriovenous grafts: An angiographic study. Am J Roentgenol *131*:817, 1978.
67. Sandweiss DA, Hanson JC, Gosink BB, Moser KM: Ultrasound in diagnosis, localization, and treatment of loculated pleural empyema. Ann Intern Med *82*:50, 1975.
68. Doust BD, Baum JK, Maklad NF, Doust VL: Ultrasonic evaluation of pleural opacities. Radiology *114*:135, 1975.
69. Gryminski J, Krakowka P, Lypacewicz G: The diagnosis of pleural effusion by ultrasonic and radiologic techniques. Chest *70*:33, 1976.
70. Ravin CE: Thoracocentesis of loculated pleural effusions using grey scale ultrasonic guidance. Chest *71*:666, 1977.
71. Laing FC, Filly RA: Problems in the application of ultrasonography for the evaluation of pleural opacities. Radiology *126*:211, 1978.
72. Adams FV, Galati V: M-mode ultrasonic localization of pleural effusion. JAMA *239*:1761, 1978.
73. Hirsch JH, Carter SJ, Chikos PM, Colacurcio C: Ultrasonic evaluation of radiographic opacities of the chest. Am J Roentgenol *130*:1153, 1978.
74. Edell SL: Pleural effusion aspiration with ultrasound. Clin Radiol *29*:377, 1978.
75. Wolson AH: Ultrasonic evaluation of intrathoracic masses. J Clin Ultrasound *4*:269, 1976.
76. Shin MS, Gray PW: Pitfalls in ultrasonic detection of pleural fluid. J Clin Ultrasound *6*:421, 1978.
77. Hernandez-Lopez E, Chahine RA, Anastassiades P, Raizner AE, Lidsky MD: Echocardiographic study of the cardiac involvement in rheumatoid arthritis. Chest *72*:52, 1977.
78. MacDonald WJ, Crawford MH, Klippel JH, Zvaifler NJ, O'Rourke RA: Echocardiographic assessment of cardiac structure and function in patients with rheumatoid arthritis. Am J Med *63*:890, 1977.
79. Seltzer SE, Finberg HJ, Weissman BN, Kido DK, Collier BD: Arthrosonography: Gray-scale ultrasound evaluation of the shoulder. Radiology *132*:467, 1979.
80. Seltzer SE, Finberg HJ, Weissman BN: Arthrosonography: Technique, sonographic anatomy, and pathology. Invest Radiol *15*:19, 1980.
81. Sprayregen S: Popliteal vein displacement by popliteal artery aneurysms: Report of two cases. Am J Roentgenol *132*:838, 1979.
82. Yeh HC, Mitty HA, Wolf BS, Jacobson JH: Ultrasonography of the brachiocephalic arteries. Radiology *132*:403, 1979.
83. El-Khoury GY, Bassett GS: Symptomatic bursa formation with osteochondromas. Am J Roentgenol *133*:895, 1979.
84. Heelan RT, Watson RC, Smith J: Computed tomography of lower extremity tumors. Am J Roentgenol *132*:933, 1979.
85. Levine E, Lee KR, Neff JR, Maklad NF, Robinson RG, Preston DF: Comparison of computed tomography and other imaging modalities in the evaluation of musculoskeletal tumors. Radiology *131*:431, 1979.
86. Wyatt GM, Spitz HB: Ultrasound in the diagnosis of rectus sheath hematoma. JAMA *241*:1499, 1979.
87. Kumari S, Fulco JD, Karayalcin G, Lipton R: Gray scale ultrasound: Evaluation of iliopsoas hematomas in hemophiliacs. Am J Roentgenol *133*:103, 1979.
88. Fon GT, Hunter TB, Haber K: Utility of ultrasound for diagnosis of mesenteric hematoma. Am J Roentgenol *134*:381, 1980.
89. Bambach CP, Riley JW, Picker RH, Reeve TS, Middleton WRJ: Preoperative parathyroid identification by ultrasonic scan. Med J Aust *2*:227, 1978.
90. Scheible W, Skram C, Leopold GR: High resolution real time ultrasonography of hemodialysis vascular access complications. Am J Roentgenol (in press).
91. Burney DP, Martin CE, Thomas CS, Fisher RD, Bender HW: Rheumatoid pericarditis: Clinical significance and operative management. J Thorac Cardiovasc Surg *77*:511, 1979.
92. Gottdiener JS, Moutsopoulos HM, Decker JL: Echocardiographic identification of cardiac abnormality in scleroderma and related disorders. Am J Med *66*:391, 1979.

IMAGING MODALITIES IN INTRASPINAL DISORDERS

by Marc N. Coel, M.D.

14

Radiographic examination for intraspinal pathology dates back to the earliest days of radiology. Initially used to diagnose tumors affecting the spine, myelography developed as the primary examination for all neurologic dysfunctions involving the spinal nerves and the spinal cord. Low back pain is among the most common medical and medicolegal problems encountered in the modern practice of medicine. Many patients with this problem require chronic care and limitation of their previous lifestyles. The orthopedic and neurologic evaluation is of utmost importance in determining both the etiology and the extent of the abnormality. A careful physical examination prior to any radiologic work-up is a necessity. Then, with due consideration to subsequent therapy, the radiologic work-up is initiated.

The roentgenographic evaluation of patients with a spinal abnormality should begin with a complete plain film examination of the region of interest, including anteroposterior, lateral, oblique, and coned-down films. Occasionally, tomography may also be necessary. At this point, several additional examinations are available for more detailed diagnosis. Selection of a specific modality depends upon the clinical situation and on the training and expertise of the examiner. Although myelography is still regarded as the mainstay of these available radiographic techniques, lumbar venography has become a screening procedure for intervertebral disc disease and, on occasion, for other epidural abnormalities. On the other hand, the role of discography in the diagnosis of intervertebral disc disease has diminished. In the past few years, there has been increasing enthusiasm and support for utilization of computed tomography (CT) with its ability to evaluate the bony spinal column, the spinal cord, and the space surrounding the cord, as well as the extraspinal tissues. In the newborn, especially the premature infant, ultrasonic examination can be performed for evaluation of congenital abnormalities of the spinal cord (Fig. 14–1). Lastly, spinal arteriography is indicated for diagnosis and treatment of vascular malformations of the spinal cord.

In any particular case, full consultation between the clinician and the radiologist is mandatory so that the examination that will be of most benefit to the patient is performed. As the examination must evaluate all possible sites that might contain the offending lesion, the myelographer must be cognizant of the neurologic findings and the possible levels at which the pathologic lesion may be located. This will prevent an inappropriately limited examination, one that emphasizes only the first and perhaps insignificant abnormality detected.

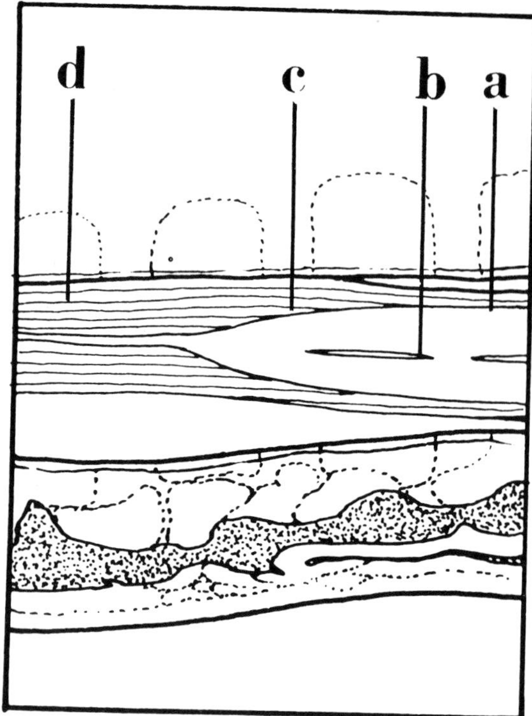

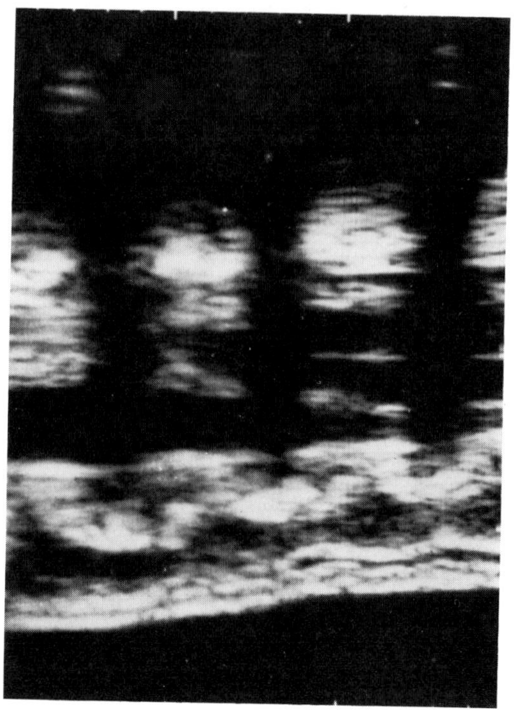

Figure 14–1. Gray scale ultrasound image of spine of a newborn. This examination can be accomplished because of the lack of surrounding bone structure. Demonstrated here are the spinal cord (a), the central canal (b), the conus medullaris (c), and the nerve roots making up the cauda equina (d). (Courtesy of Dr. George Leopold, University Hospital, San Diego, California.)

DIAGNOSTIC MODALITIES

Myelography

HISTORICAL ASPECTS. Myelography developed in the 1920s in the United States and in Europe. Initial studies utilized air,[1,2] a negative contrast medium that appeared radiolucent on the x-ray film. In later years, positive contrast media were developed, which appeared radiodense on the film owing to their absorption of the x-ray beam. Iodinized poppy seed oil was first used as a positive contrast agent, but its high viscosity and immiscibility combined with its irritating effect on the arachnoid and nerve roots reduced its usefulness. In 1931, Arnell and Lidström[3] introduced Skiodan, a water-soluble myelographic contrast medium. This material was the forerunner of the improved water-soluble contrast media that are now well accepted in Europe, particularly in the Scandinavian countries. Currently, there are basically three varieties of contrast media utilized: iophendylate (Pantopaque),* water-soluble contrast medium (Amipaque†, metrizamide), and gas (air, oxygen). There are ongoing investigations to develop cheaper and less toxic water-soluble contrast media for intrathecal injection.

*Lafayette Pharmacal, 522 North Earl Avenue, Lafayette, Indiana 47902.

†Winthrop Laboratories, 90 Park Avenue, New York, New York 10016.

CONTRAST MEDIA

Oily Contrast Media. Iophendylate was introduced by Strain and co-workers[4] in 1946. It contains 30.5 per cent iodine in an oily ester. Although iophendylate has greater viscosity than cerebrospinal fluid and is immiscible with it, it flows smoothly to the dependent portions of the subarachnoid space. Severe reactions to this agent can occur, but they are fortunately extremely infrequent. Modest lymphocytosis and elevation of cerebrospinal fluid protein and gamma globulin levels may be apparent.[5] Iophendylate myelography may be followed by arachnoiditis with encystment,[6-8] although Praestholm and co-workers[9] found a limited reaction of the normal meninges and normal brain to the presence of this substance. In this latter study, there was accumulation of iophendylate in macrophages in the inner lining of the ventricles, suggesting that it is these cellular elements that are important in the removal of residual oily contrast medium from the subarachnoid space and its dispersal into the systemic circulation. It is estimated that such removal occurs at the rate of approximately 0.5 ml per year.

Absolute contraindications to the utilization of

iophendylate are a previous reaction to this drug or, possibly, to other iodinated contrast media, and the presence of an inflammatory disease of the meninges or neural tissue. If introduction of this or other iodinated contrast media is necessary in a patient with an allergic history, pretreatment should include administration of steroids, antihistamines, and heparin. A bloody tap also precludes use of iophendylate as a contrast medium; experiments in monkeys have shown that the combination of bloody cerebrospinal fluid and iophendylate increases the incidence and severity of arachnoiditis. In this situation, either metrizamide or gas should be used, or the study should be delayed 10 to 14 days to permit the resorption of the blood. One further, albeit minor, contraindication to the use of iophendylate is in the patient who may later require diagnostic radioiodine (RAI) uptake studies. The slow, continuous resorption of any residual iodinized oil from the subarachnoid space into the systemic circulation provides a source of iodine for the thyroid and can give a false impression of suppressed RAI uptake.

Although there has recently been great enthusiasm for metrizamide as an appropriate contrast material for myelography, many radiologists are once again utilizing iophendylate for cervical and thoracic spinal examination. This medium is extremely safe and easy to visualize fluoroscopically; it remains visible and in position while the films are being checked.

Water-Soluble Contrast Media. For many years, attempts have been made to develop a water-soluble myelographic contrast medium with low toxicity. There are several potential advantages to this type of contrast medium: It can be placed within the subarachnoid space using a fine, narrow-gauge spinal needle; the needle need not be inserted in the midline nor must it remain in place following injection; the material is not totally miscible with the cerebrospinal fluid, so it can diffuse through smaller spaces, allowing better visualization of the nerve root sleeves (sheaths); and it will be resorbed rapidly from the subarachnoid space, without requiring manual removal. Recently, metrizamide[10-12] has been introduced as such a low-toxicity water-soluble myelographic contrast medium.

Metrizamide is a nonionic substance with a lower incidence of side effects compared with that of previously used water-soluble compounds, which were complicated benzene rings, ionic in nature. Arachnoiditis is infrequent[13] when metrizamide is used in relatively low concentrations; however, other troublesome symptoms and signs may appear. Baker and co-workers[14] detected a 62 per cent incidence of headache, a 38 per cent incidence of nausea or vomiting, and a 26 per cent incidence of new or exacerbated leg or back pain with metrizamide myelography, although none of these manifestations persisted beyond 48 hours following the procedure. Furthermore, mild febrile reactions were encountered in children. The incidence of the reactions that were noted in the study by Baker and associates is higher than that observed in certain Scandinavian reports.[10-12] This may be related to the greater concentration of metrizamide that was used in the American investigation. Nickel and Salem[41] also recorded more adverse reactions than the earlier studies; these two investigators found a 0.4 per cent incidence of major motor seizure activity.

The popularity of water-soluble contrast media, specifically nonionic metrizamide, is based upon the relative ease in performing the examination and the potential for increased diagnostic accuracy compared with iophendylate myelography.[15] Nerve root sleeves are identifiable as far distally as the neural foramina when low-viscosity metrizamide is utilized, allowing detection of minor deviations of these root sleeves by laterally herniated intervertebral discs. Small tumors may also be detected by the less dense water-soluble contrast medium. However, in certain situations, iophendylate is particularly useful; lesions producing tight partial blocks are better delineated with this contrast agent, as both sides of the obstructing lesion can be well visualized. Because of the seizure activity and headaches, many centers now reserve the use of metrizamide for lumbar myelograms and subarachnoid space opacification for CT scanning.

In many institutions steroids are placed in the lumbar subarachnoid space following myelography with water-soluble contrast media in an attempt to decrease postprocedural arachnoiditis. However, Dullerud and Morland[16] detected a marked increase in postmyelographic adhesive arachnoiditis in those patients treated with steroids. Thus, it seems that at this time, no patient should be given subarachnoid steroids as an adjunctive measure in water-soluble contrast myelography.[17]

Simultaneously with the advancements in available contrast media, there have been technical improvements to reduce the complications of this invasive procedure. Needles with short bevels, nontraumatic cannulas for the removal of the oily contrast media, and increasing sophistication of x-ray equipment have combined to make myelography an extremely safe and highly diagnostic procedure.

INDICATIONS. Myelography is used to detect the effects of a pathologic process on the subarachnoid space and its content. This is also its limitation, in that it cannot detect the extraspinal extent of the pathologic process, nor can it detect concomitant disease in other organ systems. The choice of myelography implies that surgery, radiation therapy, or chemotherapy is seriously being considered as an appropriate mode of treatment. In the patient with degenerative disease of the spine in whom symptoms and signs are mild in nature, a trial of rest and special exercises is warranted prior to performing a myelogram. Once myelography is chosen as the appropriate diagnostic modality, the examination should be used to pinpoint the location of a pathologic process and to provide accurate information concerning the likely histologic characteristics of the lesion. It is with this analysis that appropriate therapy can then be applied.

Techniques

Pantopaque Myelography. Myelography should always be performed on a tilting radiographic table, preferably one with a 90 degree to 90 degree tilt. This allows the patient to be positioned vertically, either erect or head down. The table should be equipped with a Bucky filming device as well as image intensification. Fluoroscopy is mandatory and should be utilized for all positioning prior to obtaining overhead or spot films. Shoulder supports or leg-boot harnesses should be available for use in thoracic and cervical examinations, during which the patient must be tipped head down (Trendelenburg position). Preliminary films should be obtained to establish proper technique prior to the introduction of the subarachnoid contrast medium. This is most critical if the new water-soluble contrast media are being used for the study; proper film density must be obtained initially, as the contrast medium dissipates rapidly.

Prior to the insertion of the spinal needle, the patient should be fully informed concerning the side effects and complications of the procedure. Any spinal puncture may be followed by headaches, which are exacerbated by upright positioning. Since headaches are caused by continued leaking of cerebrospinal fluid through the puncture site after withdrawal of the needle, the frequency of this complication is directly related to the size of the needle. Headaches are worse in young females.[18-20] "Allergic reactions" to positive contrast media and arachnoiditis, a sterile inflammatory reaction of the arachnoid lining which can cause pain, are unusual complications about which the patient should be informed. The patient should be well hydrated and should not have eaten solid food for at least 4 hours prior to myelography. As a precautionary measure, the legs should be wrapped with either Jobst stockings or Ace bandages to help prevent blood pooling and exacerbation of symptoms and signs should a hypotensive crisis develop.

The preferred puncture site depends upon the level of the suspected abnormality. The needle should never be placed at the level where the abnormality might exist. For example, since most herniated discs occur at the L4-L5 or L5-S1 disc interspace, the lumbar puncture should be performed at the L3-L4 or L2-L3 intervertebral levels. In addition, if there is suspected infection or an extensive lesion of the lumbar canal, cisternal (suboccipital) or lateral C1-C2 needle puncture should be utilized.[19] No puncture should be performed at levels above the L2-L3 interspace so as to prevent the advancing needle from coming into contact with the conus medullaris. When oily contrast medium is utilized, it must be removed following the procedure. In this situation, the ideal level for puncture is the L3-L4 interspace, which is at the apex of the lumbar lordosis and is thus at the lowest point when the patient is prone. The heavy oily contrast medium, which has a higher specific gravity than the cerebrospinal fluid, pools at this level and can thus be easily removed.

For lumbar puncture, the patient is placed prone with a large cushion beneath his epigastrium in order to reduce the normal lumbar lordosis. This has the effect of spreading the spinous processes, facilitating the introduction of the needle. In addition, the cushion remains under the patient when the contrast medium is moved cephalad. This maintains the contrast medium in a single collection, allowing it to be moved to the appropriate cervical or thoracic region with ease.

Only the skin need be anesthetized, using 1 per cent lidocaine without epinephrine. The choice of needle size depends upon which of the contrast media is selected for the procedure. Bigger needles (18 or 20 gauge) are used for oily contrast media, and the narrower needles (22 gauge) for air and water-soluble agents. Fluoroscopy during performance of the puncture is necessary only for those patients who are receiving oily contrast media. In this case, the needle must be inserted in the midline, into the deepest part of the spinal canal. This placement will facilitate the removal of the contrast medium at the end of the procedure. The needle should be advanced toward the vertebral body rather than directed at the intervertebral disc interspace; this prevents a needle artifact, which might be misinterpreted as an unsuspected disc herniation. When the dural click is felt as the needle enters the subarachnoid space, the pointed stylet is removed, and a blunt aspiration cannula is inserted and locked into the needle hub.[21] This cannula then extends approximately 5 mm beyond the tip of the needle. Both the needle and the cannula may then be advanced until the blunt tip of the cannula touches the vertebral body. The blunt tip prevents rupture of an epidural vein. If the cannula touches the vertebral body before the needle-cannula interlock can be engaged, the needle is withdrawn until it locks onto the hub of the aspiration cannula. This technique permits perfect positioning of the spinal needle within the subarachnoid space, preventing injection of the contrast medium into the subdural or epidural spaces. Cerebrospinal fluid is then removed for laboratory examination.

The amount of contrast medium that should be injected depends upon the type, severity, and location of the suspected lesion. If a complete block is anticipated, smaller amounts are injected in order to determine the affected level and the nature of the obstruction. Otherwise, the examination is modified according to the level of interest in the vertebral column. For examination of the lumbar region, enough contrast material should be present to extend up to the midportion of the third lumbar vertebra when the patient is in an upright position. The examination of the lumbar spine should then be performed with the patient in a semi-upright position (60 degree upright), an attitude that allows full distention of the subarachnoid space owing to the weight of the contrast medium and the entire column of cerebrospinal fluid. Such distention improves the filling of the caudally directed lumbar root sleeves and the degree of contact between the contrast medium and any extradural mass. The upper lumbar canal can subsequently be examined with the patient in the prone position.

For evaluation of the thoracic spine, larger amounts of contrast medium are necessary. Because of the normal thoracic kyphosis, the contrast medium has a tendency to divide into two or more collections and move in a craniad or caudad direction; sufficient contrast material must be injected to provide a single column of contrast medium and to outline both the proximal and the distal contours of any lesion. In general, enough contrast agent is injected to fill the thoracic subarachnoid space to its midpoint while the patient is in the lateral decubitus position (Fig. 14–2). Radiographs are obtained in

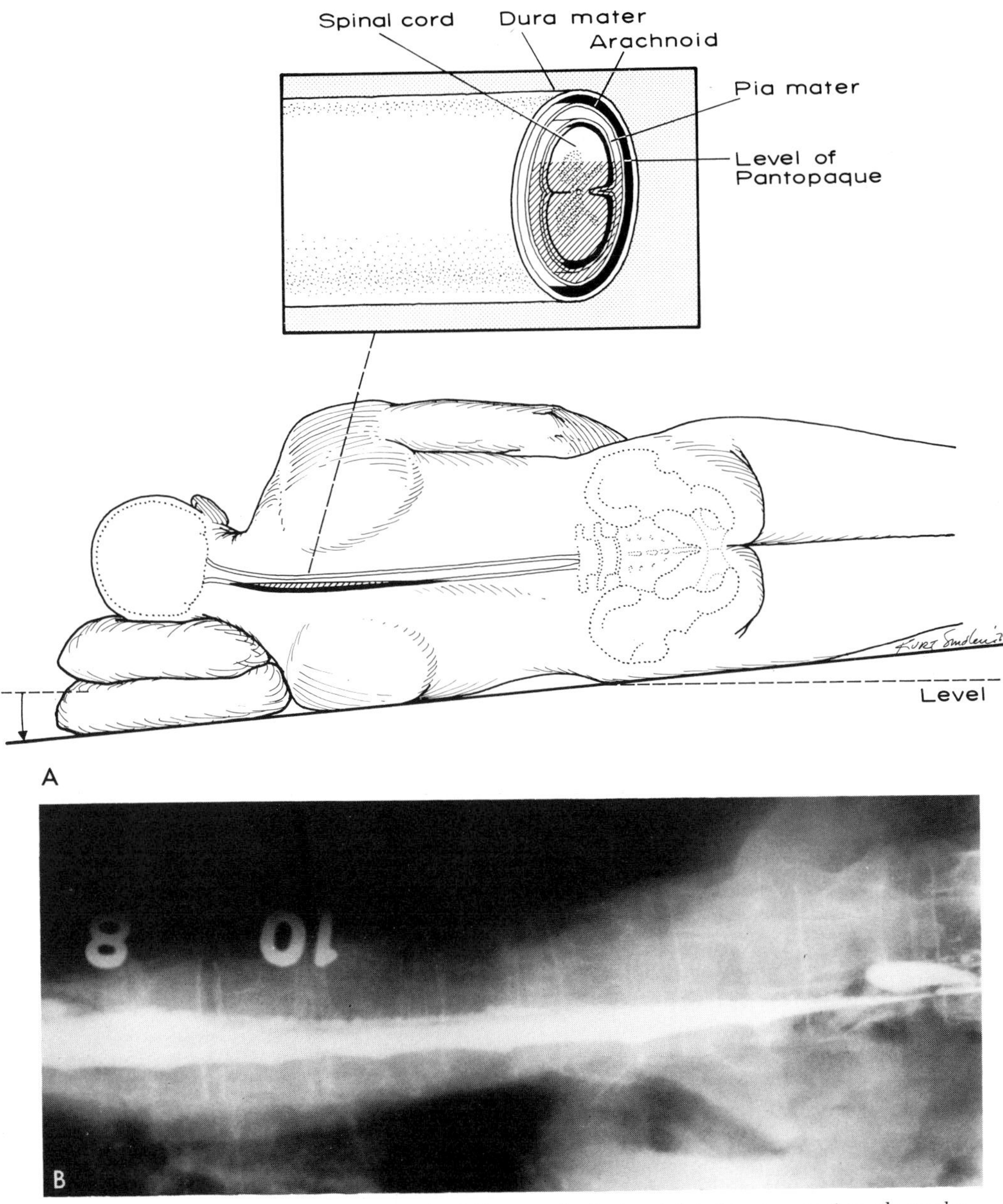

Figure 14–2. The decubitus position should be used for iophendylate (Pantopaque) myelography in the examination of the thoracic spine. A slight Trendelenburg position usually is necessary. Enough iophendylate should be used to fill the spinal canal in the region of interest to about one half of its width.

cross-table anteroposterior and posteroanterior projections and supplemented with lateral spot films exposed during fluoroscopy.

The cervical myelogram can be obtained following the introduction of contrast medium into either the cervical or the lumbar region. In either situation, it is of extreme importance to have the patient's head in such a position as to prevent the contrast medium from extending into the subarachnoid cisterns of the cranium. If positive contrast medium is utilized, the head is maintained in extension. The contrast medium should extend from the clivus to the upper thoracic vertebrae. Radiographs are then obtained in multiple projections. An anteroposterior spot film is employed first. The remaining projections are obtained with the overhead tube, without moving the patient's head. Oblique films are required, which should be obtained by the technique described by Rice and Coyle.[22]

Metrizamide Myelography. Prior to performing a metrizamide myelogram, neuroleptic drugs, including phenothiazines, must be discontinued for at least 48 hours; if it is necessary to maintain patients with seizure disorders on anticonvulsant medication, consideration should be given to changing the diagnostic regimen (i.e., iophendylate). Premedication frequently is necessary, and agents should be used that possess both sedative and anticonvulsant properties (e.g., barbiturates). Complications of this technique are those related to lumbar puncture and to the contrast medium itself: nausea and vomiting, 25 to 35 per cent; backache, 10 per cent; leg pain, 10 per cent; seizures, 0.4 per cent.[41]

The amount of metrizamide that is necessary for myelography depends on the region to be evaluated. A lumbar myelogram requires 170 to 190 mg of iodine per milliliter (mgI/ml) in a volume of 10 to 15 ml diluent; a thoracic myelogram requires 220 mgI/ml in a 10 ml volume; and a cervical myelogram performed from the lumbar route requires 240 to 300 mgI/ml in a 10 ml volume. The cervical myelogram obtained via suboccipital (cisternal) or lateral C1-C2 puncture can be accomplished utilizing a lower concentration of iodine, approximately 220 mg/ml in a 10 ml volume.

These studies should be performed under fluoroscopy. Due to the hypertonicity of the metrizamide, the region of interest must be in a dependent position. This positioning should be done expeditiously to prevent the dilution of the metrizamide by the cerebrospinal fluid; filming, which is accomplished with lower kilovolt peak (kVp) technique (60 to 75 kVp), must be completed within 20 to 30 minutes after the introduction of the contrast medium into the subarachnoid space. Some investigators have recommended that initial filming in the lumbar region be obtained with the patient in the lateral decubitus position, utilizing horizontal beam technique. This method facilitates the filling of the dependent root sleeves with the hypertonic contrast medium. The patient can subsequently be rolled to the opposite decubitus position for additional radiographs. Prone and upright films in the oblique and lateral projections can then be obtained utilizing fluoroscopic spot films.

Thoracic myelography with metrizamide should be accomplished in a room possessing equipment with tomographic capabilities. Initially, with the patient on his back, tomograms are obtained in the anteroposterior projection.

Gas Myelography. Gas myelography has been utilized extensively in Europe, particularly in the Scandinavian countries, where iophendylate was not available.[23, 24] It is the optimal myelographic technique for examination of the thoracic spine, and is especially useful in evaluating lesions around the foramen magnum and posterior fossa cisterns. However, this technique can be used to examine other areas of the spinal canal and to detect most types of lesions, with the exception of those that press solely on the nerve root sleeves.[25]

Although severe complications are unusual,[24] side effects are frequent. Analgesics and sedatives that are helpful prior to the procedure are imperative following the study. Low-grade fever and headaches are frequent following myelography and must be treated. Nausea and muscular cramps occur occasionally. Simon and associates[26] have reported intraocular hemorrhage in 7 of 21 patients undergoing gas myelography; two of these patients had symptoms. Our patients have had no similar symptomatic episodes in over 200 gas myelograms.

Gas myelography can be performed from either the lumbar or the cervical route utilizing a 22 gauge spinal needle. In either case, the study should be accomplished on a tomographic table, preferably a polydirectional unit (e.g., the Philips polytome). Following the puncture, as a normal precaution, a limited injection of approximately 5 ml of gas should be administered with the part of the spine that is most distant from the injection site in a semiupright position. After this small injection, a film is obtained of the uppermost portion of the spine to exclude the presence of a total block somewhere along the subarachnoid space. For example, the head should be elevated during the initial 5 ml aliquot injection when a lumbar injection site is utilized; the sacral sac should be uppermost when a cervical puncture is performed. If a block exists, it should be documented on radiographs. The study is then terminated. If the gas does reach the other end of the subarachnoid space, the patient is positioned for cerebrospinal fluid drainage.

The needle site is placed in a dependent position so that as much spinal fluid as possible can be removed from the subarachnoid space without the use of suction. Following this drainage, the patient is placed in a Trendelenburg position, and oxygen or air is injected into the subarachnoid space until the pressure within the spinal canal reaches 30 to 40 mm of mercury. This measurement can be obtained by having a sphygmomanometer interposed in the tubing that connects the spinal needle and the injecting syringe. Repeated injection of gas is necessary in order to maintain full distention of the subarachnoid space. This distention is as necessary with gas myelography as with positive contrast myelography.

Tomograms should be obtained initially in the lateral projection with the area of interest well distended with gas. These should be 3 to 5 millimeters in thickness, utilizing high kVp technique. Either linear, elliptic, tri-spiral, or hypocycloidal tomography is adequate.

Lumbar Venography

Historical Aspects. Although sixteenth and seventeenth century anatomists described the veins of the vertebral column and canal, it was not until Batson[27] reviewed the spinal venous anatomy and its role in the spread of tumor that modern medicine placed some importance on the presence of these vascular channels. It later became apparent that these same veins could be used for the diagnosis of diseases affecting the epidural space.[28-30]

Contrast Media. For ascending lumbar venography, any of the triiodinated water-soluble contrast media can be utilized. Intravenous utilization of these substances produces serious reactions in approximately 1 in 12,000 injections.[31] These reactions include anaphylaxis, bronchospasm, and renal failure. Less serious reactions such as urticaria, nausea, and vomiting are more frequent. The incidence of death due to utilization of intravenous contrast media has been estimated to be about 1 in 40,000 studies.[31] Persons who have serious allergies or who have had previous contrast medium reactions should either have gas myelography or be pretreated prior to the use of any iodinated contrast medium with high dosages of steroids and antihistamines for 3 days and, possibly, with heparin anticoagulation.[31]

Indications. Epidural venography, accomplished by an intraosseous or catheter method, has a wide range of indications, including the evaluation of the following: space-occupying lesions of the epidural or subdural space; spinal angiomata; destructive lesions of the vertebral bodies that invade the epidural space; degenerative disease; trauma; and inflammatory disease. Epidural venography causes no intrathecal irritation or changes in intraspinal pressure. It is the examination of choice in patients suspected of having lumbar stenosis at multiple levels. This method is frequently used in the patient in whom myelography is either nondiagnostic or contraindicated. It is particularly helpful in evaluating the L5-S1 intervertebral disc space, at which site the thecal sac, owing to its posterior location, may not be deformed from an adjacent herniated disc. As of this time, epidural venography has not been utilized extensively for thoracic or cervical pathology.[32-34]

Techniques. The lumbar venogram is performed most frequently by the Seldinger technique of catheterizing the femoral veins[35] (Fig. 14–3). The intraosseous method is infrequently used, owing to the marked discomfort that it causes to the patient. The left femoral vein is the vessel of choice as the left ascending lumbar vein, arising from the common iliac vein, normally is larger than the one on the right. Injection of the presacral veins is optimal for L5-S1 disc disease. Bilateral filling of the epidural veins is usually obtained, although Guistra and co-workers[36] reported a need for multiple injections in 65 per cent of their patients. At times, catheterization of both femoral veins may be necessary, with simultaneous injection of the ascending lumbar, the presacral, and/or the internal iliac veins. Of marked importance is the use of compression of the inferior vena cava and a strong Valsalva maneuver by the patient; these techniques promote retrograde filling of the valveless epidural veins. Any water-soluble contrast medium is suitable, the concentration of the agent being dependent upon the breadth of the patient. Meglumine iothalamate (Conray 60)* is the

*Squibb & Sons, P. O. Box 4000, Princeton, New Jersey 08540.

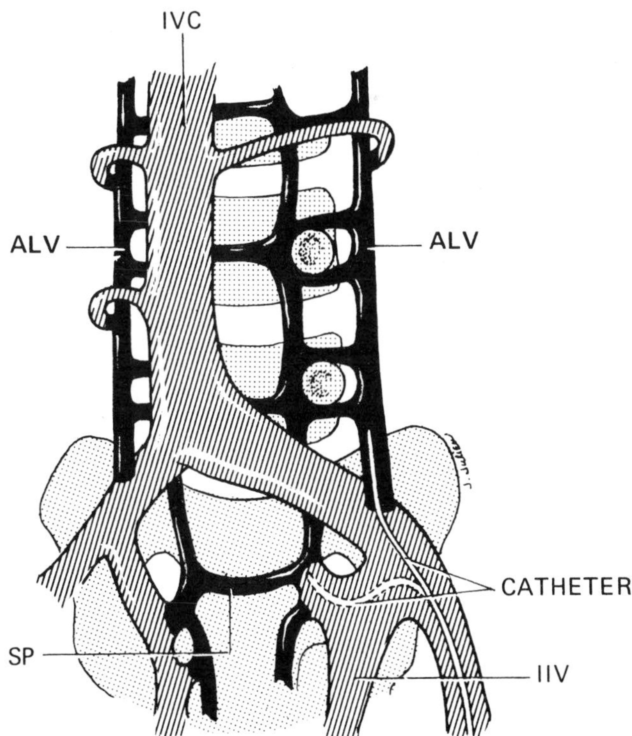

Figure 14–3. The epidural veins of the lumbar spinal canal run within the canal, along the posterior border of the vertebral bodies. The veins can be filled with contrast medium injected in the ascending lumbar vein (ALV) or the presacral vein of the sacral plexus (SP). IVC, Inferior vena cava; IIV, internal iliac vein.

contrast medium we have used most frequently. Thirty milliliters (2 to 5 ml/sec) is injected, and a single film is obtained each second for 10 seconds.

The reported accuracy of epidural venography is quite high (approximately 90 per cent).[30, 37, 38] Its only risk is that attendant on intravenous injections of contrast media.

Computed Tomography

Indications. With the recent advent of computed tomography, there has been tremendous interest in its application in the evaluation of spinal pathology.[39, 40] This modality possesses definite advantages over other available techniques. Two such advantages are its noninvasive nature and lack of intrinsic toxicity except for the radiation exposure. The radiation dosage to the patient has been diminished with improved technology and is approximately 1 to 3 rads per examination. A third advantage of computed tomography is its ability to examine many tissues at the same time, e.g., the vertebral bodies, the neural arches, the spinal cord, and the subarachnoid space. In addition, the paraspinal areas and the other organs within the transverse plane can also be evaluated. A major shortcoming of computed tomography is the lack of detail that exists in differentiating the spinal cord from the subarachnoid and extradural spaces. Furthermore, it is impractical to examine the entire length of the spinal cord when clinical localization of a lesion is not possible.

Computed tomography measures the differential absorption of the x-ray beam traversing the body, and a computer reconstructs the image from the data collected. The x-ray beam is measured as it enters and exits the body; the difference in the measurements indicates the amount of x-ray absorption that has occurred. Similar measurements following x-ray tube rotation through small angles determine the exact radiation absorption of each volume in the scan slice. The computer is then able to reconstruct images in the transverse, coronal, and sagittal plane (Fig. 14–4).

Techniques. The technique for scanning the vertebral column does not differ from that of any other part of the body (see Chapter 12). Scans are obtained along a length of the vertebral column above, through, and below the suspicious area. Following these initial scans, contrast media can be introduced intrathecally, and additional scans can be obtained. The intrathecal contrast medium should not be quite dilute (metrizamide, 170 mgI/ml) because of the modality's exquisite sensitivity to differences in density. Contrast-enhanced scans are particularly valuable in investigating the spinal cord and subarachnoid space, as well as the brain. Intravenous contrast medium (i.e., meglumine iothalamate, 300 MgI) may also be utilized; a bolus or an infusion of contrast material is helpful in evaluating the spinal cord in cases of suspected tumor or vascular malformation.

Complications of this technique are those related to lumbar puncture and to the contrast medium itself.

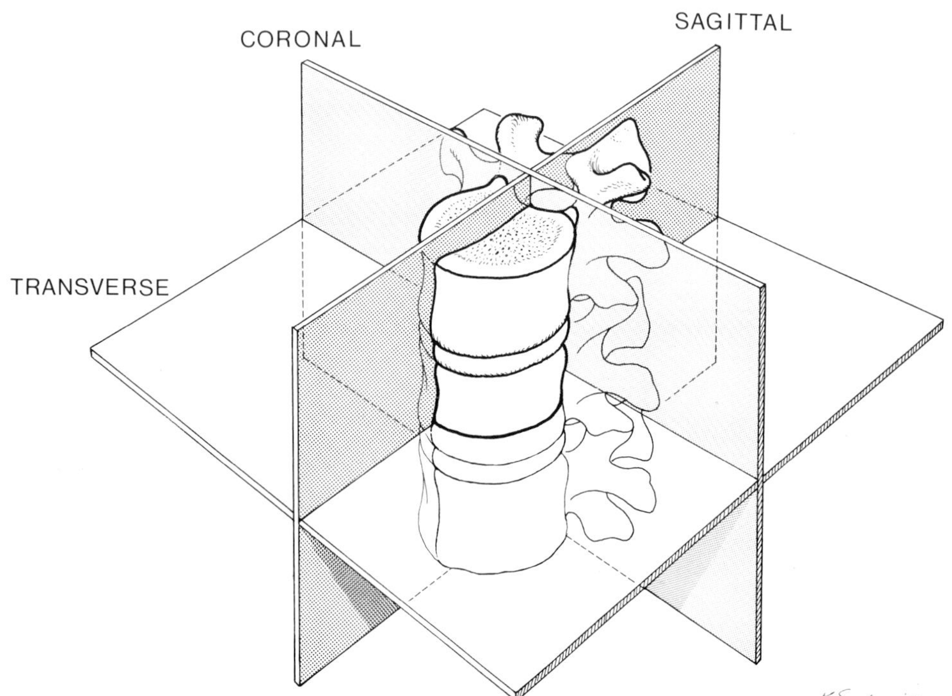

Figure 14–4. *The various planes in which reconstruction of the spinal canal can be obtained by the computed tomography unit are demonstrated here. From the transverse scan initially obtained, the coronal and sagittal planes can be reconstructed by the computer.*

Spinal Arteriography

INDICATIONS. Spinal arteriography was first utilized by Tarlov in 1947[42] in a patient in whom a spinal extradural hemangioblastoma was demonstrated during surgery. From the early 1950s to the present time, the main indication for arteriography of the spinal cord has remained the evaluation of arteriovenous malformations,[43] although this technique has been utilized when investigating other lesions of the vertebral bodies and the spinal cord,[44, 45] including chronic inflammatory processes, hemangiomas, and additional benign and malignant tumors. Furthermore, transcatheter embolization of spinal arteriovenous malformations and tumors has been used to decrease the likelihood and extent of hemorrhagic complications of surgery and to provide symptomatic relief in patients whose conditions are inoperable.[46-48] Spinal arteriography has limited application in the evaluation of traumatic lesions.[49, 50]

TECHNIQUES. The technique is usually performed via the femoral arteries using the Seldinger method. An initial arteriogram defines the precise level of origin of the radicular artery, which supplies the spinal vessels. Subsequently, the small intraspinal vessels are selectively injected utilizing a non–sodium-containing contrast medium (e.g., meglumine iothalamate).[51]

As the arterial supply to the spinal cord is derived from multiple feeding or radicular branches that interconnect along its entire length, multiple arteries may have to be catheterized in order to study the entire cord, including the thyrocervical and costocervical trunks, and the vertebral, intercostal, and lumbar arteries. Any of these vessels can represent the site of origin of a branch that supplies the anterior and posterior spinal arteries. The anterior spinal artery runs the length of the spinal cord, receiving several contributing arteries along the way.

The main complication of this procedure is contrast medium neurotoxicity. Paraplegia, quadriplegia, and seizure disorders have all been recorded following injection into a spinal artery. If a serious complication does occur, it is recommended that immediate lumbar puncture be performed with exchange of 10 ml aliquots of cerebrospinal fluid and isotonic saline solution, a technique that ameliorates the neurologic deficit.[52]

Discography

INDICATIONS. Discography was developed by Lindblom in 1948[53] in studies of normal and pathologic intervertebral discs. This technique provides visual evidence of the integrity of the disc; furthermore, symptoms and signs that develop following intradiscal injection of contrast material provide clinical evidence as to the exact level of involvement. Currently, it is used predominantly in patients in whom a diagnosis of the cause of radicular pain is not clear, and in whom the myelographic findings have not been diagnostic. Discography also allows differentiation of the exact cause of clinical findings in patients who have two coexisting processes, e.g., diabetes mellitus and degenerative intervertebral disc disease. In these instances, reproduction of pain can differentiate between the symptoms of a herniated disc and those of diabetic neuropathy.

TECHNIQUES. The preparation of patients for discography is identical to that for individuals undergoing myelography. The patient should be placed prone on a pillow in order to increase the distance between adjacent spinous processes. The puncture site(s) should correspond to the level(s) of clinical suspicion. A 21 gauge spinal needle is inserted into the intraspinous ligaments in order to establish direction and rigidity for the subsequent insertion of a 26 gauge, 12 cm spinal needle. A sensation of back pain should be felt by the patient as the anterior dura and the anulus fibrosus are entered. If the pain radiates down the legs, a nerve root has been compromised and the needle should be redirected. After the needle is positioned at the midpoint of the intervertebral disc space, a lateral film should be obtained to document precise needle placement. Conray 60 (meglumine iothalamate) is injected manually. A volume of 0.3 to 1.0 ml is sufficient for a normal disc, and a volume of 2 to 3 ml is necessary when the lack of resistance to injection indicates an abnormal disc.

If the differentiation between peripheral neuritis and discogenic disease is the prime reason for the examination, normal saline solution should be employed for injection, as pain related to irritation of the nerves in the anulus fibrosus can be produced by the contrast medium itself. Pain that is experienced during the injection of saline solution is usually related to discogenic disease; if no sensation is experienced, a peripheral neuropathy is the more likely causative process.

Epidurography

Another means of evaluating disease entities involving the spinal canal is epidurography (also called peridurography, canalography).[54, 55] This examination involves catheterization and contrast medium injection in the epidural space. The epidural space surrounds the subarachnoid space with the dura mater of the spinal cord as the central boundary and the periosteum of the vertebral bodies and posterior neural elements as the peripheral margins. This space contains fatty connective tissue, blood vessels, and the exiting nerve root sleeves.

In performing this technique, a curved needle is

placed through the sacral notch into the epidural space. This space has a normal vacuum and will draw in a drop of saline solution held within the needle when the space is entered. A guidewire is then passed through the needle and a catheter is exchanged for the needle. The epidural space is divided posteriorly into two sections by the plica mediana dorsalis, so that separate catheterizations must be performed in order to visualize both sides in most cases. Water-soluble contrast medium is used, preferably metrizamide. The catheter tip is usually left at the L5 vertebral body level, and 15 to 20 ml of contrast medium is injected. Anteroposterior, lateral, and oblique films should be obtained; tomography is only occasionally necessary.

Complications are unusual with this technique, although subarachnoid injection is possible. Spasms of the lower extremities may occur, although they are highly unlikely when a nonionic water-soluble contrast medium is used. Aseptic meningitis has been reported with epidural as well as subarachnoid injection of Conray 60, although it has not been seen to date with metrizamide. Minor complications, such as injection into muscular planes or into the epidural venous plexus, can occur but are of no great significance. Roberson and associates[55] believe that epidurography has several important advantages: The subarachnoid space is not entered, there is no spinal headache produced or risk of arachnoiditis, and immediate ambulation is possible.

The major disadvantage in the use of this technique is the lack of film contrast, particularly in heavy patients, and the inability to visualize the nerve root sleeves. As greater experience is attained, however, the ability to read subtle changes becomes more developed.

NORMAL AND ABNORMAL EXAMINATIONS

Myelography

The normal myelogram allows visualization of the spinal cord (Figs. 14–5, 14–6, 14–10 to 14–13). The nerve root sleeves and neural foramina can be adequately visualized only with positive contrast medium myelography (Figs. 14–5 and 14–7), computed tomography (Fig. 14–8), or epidurography[55] (Fig. 14–9). On positive contrast myelograms, the suspensory ligaments of the spinal cord can be seen; these include the septum posticum posteriorly and the dentate ligaments laterally. Occasionally, the anterior spinal artery may also be evident.

In the cervical region, the spinal cord should be no larger than two thirds the lateral diameter of the bony canal (Fig. 14–10); normally a slight enlargement of the cervical cord occurs at the level where the brachial plexus originates. The sagittal diameter of the cervical cord is optimally identified utilizing gas myelography with lateral tomography (Fig. 14–11). The thoracic cord is smaller than the cervical cord and has an approximate lateral width of 7.5 to 9 mm (Fig. 14–12). At the conus medullaris, the size of the cord increases (Fig. 14–13), terminating at T12 or L1 at the cauda equina. Throughout its course, the spinal cord should possess a smooth contour, with parallel margins. Sleeves containing nerve roots should be apparent at every intervertebral level. In order to fully evaluate these nerve root sleeves, oblique films are mandatory, at least in the cervical and lumbar regions (Fig. 14–10 and 14–14). A dependent position of the root sleeves should be maintained during myelography so that the iophendylate or metrizamide will distend them (Fig. 14–7, 14–10, 14–14).

The normal subarachnoid space surrounding the spinal cord should be applied to the vertebral bodies anteriorly, and to the pedicles laterally (Fig. 14–15). The caudal limit of the subarachnoid space varies in position; it may be located just beyond the L5-S1 disc interspace, or it may extend into the sacrum as far distally as the S3 level. At the L5-S1 interspace, the subarachnoid space may not be intimate with the vertebral bodies because of the presence of epidural fat. This anatomic fact makes it difficult or impossible to diagnose an L5-S1 disc herniation on myelography.

Lesions affecting the spinal nervous system are characterized according to their location as extradural, intradural-extramedullary, and intramedullary (Figs. 14–16 to 14–18). In each of these locations, or compartments, only certain lesions occur, with varying predictability (Table 14–1). Neurologic dysfunction results from compressive effects or by direct involvement of the neural tissue. The findings at myelography include either displacement, compression, or expansion of one of the major elements of the spinal canal.

Extradural lesions will displace and compress the subarachnoid space and secondarily the spinal cord (Fig. 14–19). The degree of abnormality varies with the size and nature of the lesion. Minimal abnormalities such as compression and occlusion ("amputation") of a nerve root and root sleeve are commonly associated with small extradural herniated disc fragments (see Fig. 14–40), whereas extradural total blocks are characterized by a serrated margin ("feathering") as well as displacement of the spinal contents (Fig. 14–20).

Intradural-extramedullary lesions are usually covered by the extremely thin arachnoid but may be considered to lie within the subarachnoid space; thereby, these lesions displace only the spinal cord and nerve roots and not the subarachnoid space (Fig. 14–21). Because of the location of intradural-extramedullary lesions within the subarachnoid space, the contrast medium will abut the lesion and

Text continued on page 445

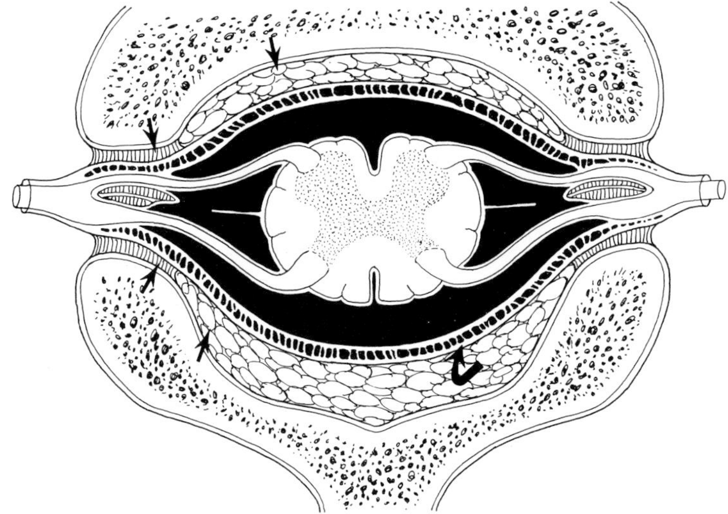

Figure 14–5. The cross section of the spinal canal demonstrates the spinal cord surrounded by the subarachnoid space (in black), the epidural space, containing fat and ligaments (arrows), and the potential subdural space (curved arrow).

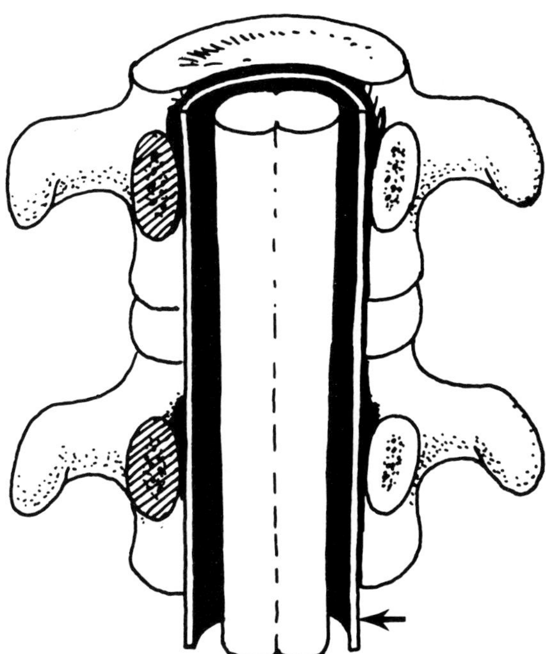

Figure 14–6. A coronal view of the spinal canal with the posterior elements removed demonstrates the spinal cord surrounded by the subarachnoid space (in black) and the epidural space on the other side of the dura mater (arrow).

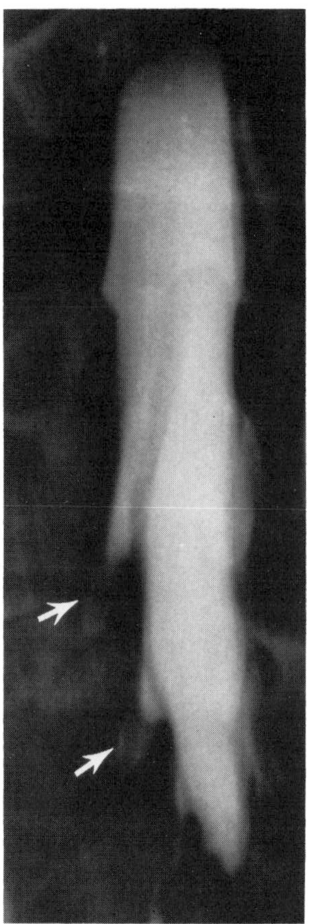

Figure 14–7. *An oblique view obtained during metrizamide myelography demonstrates the nerve root sleeves (sheaths) (arrows) containing the exiting nerve roots (the linear filling defects).*

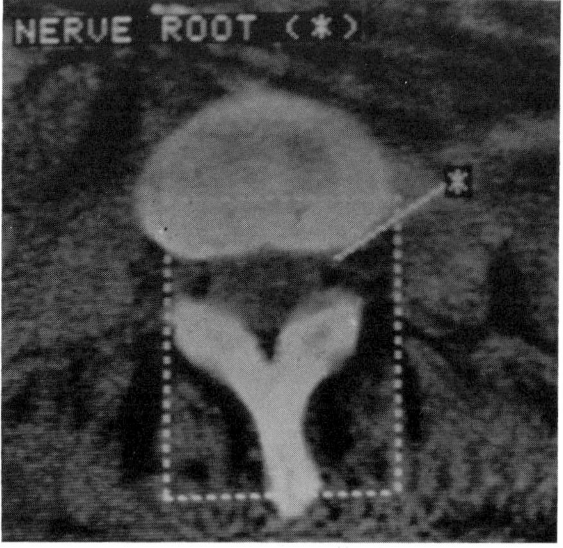

Figure 14–8. *A transverse computed tomography (CT) scan demonstrates an exiting nerve root sleeve (asterisk) within the spinal canal and neural foramen. (Courtesy of Dr. William Glenn, Long Beach Memorial Hospital, Long Beach, California.)*

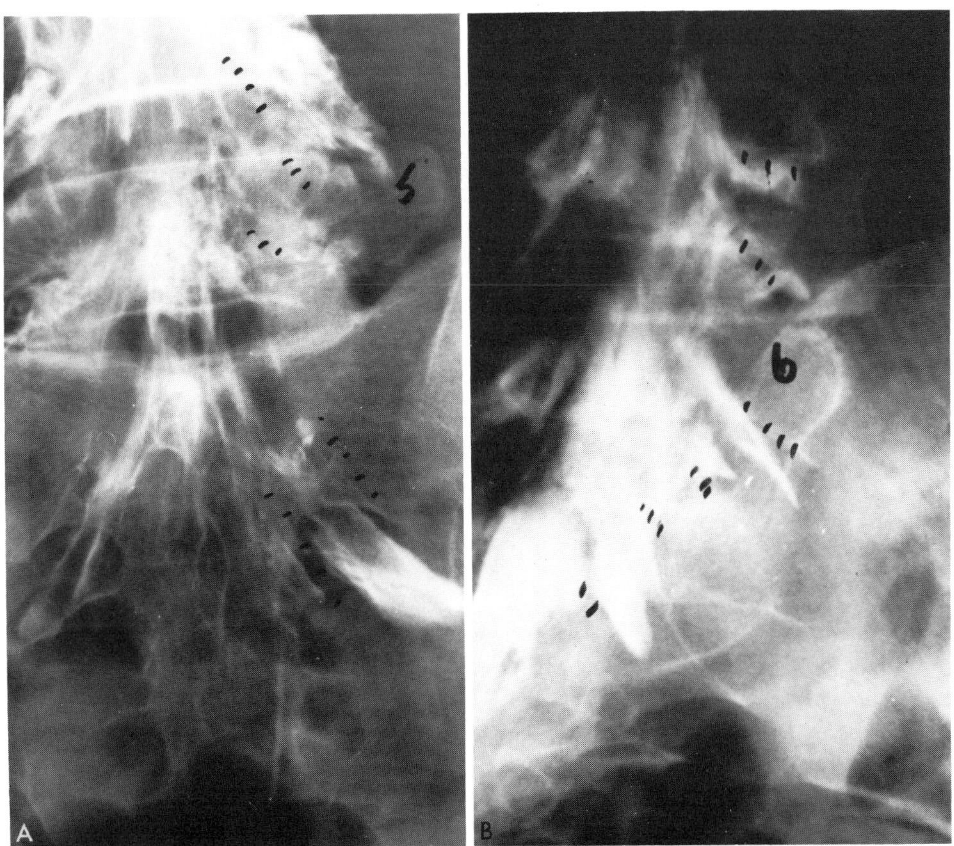

Figure 14–9. *Normal epidurogram. Contrast medium in the epidural space outlines the exiting nerve root sleeves (dotted lines) in the anteroposterior* **(A)** *and oblique* **(B)** *projections. Any mass compressing the nerve root sleeve will also involve the epidural space and will therefore not allow the contrast medium to extend from the spinal canal through the neural foramina. Contrast medium dissipates in the retroperitoneal space and water-soluble types will be totally absorbed in a matter of minutes.*

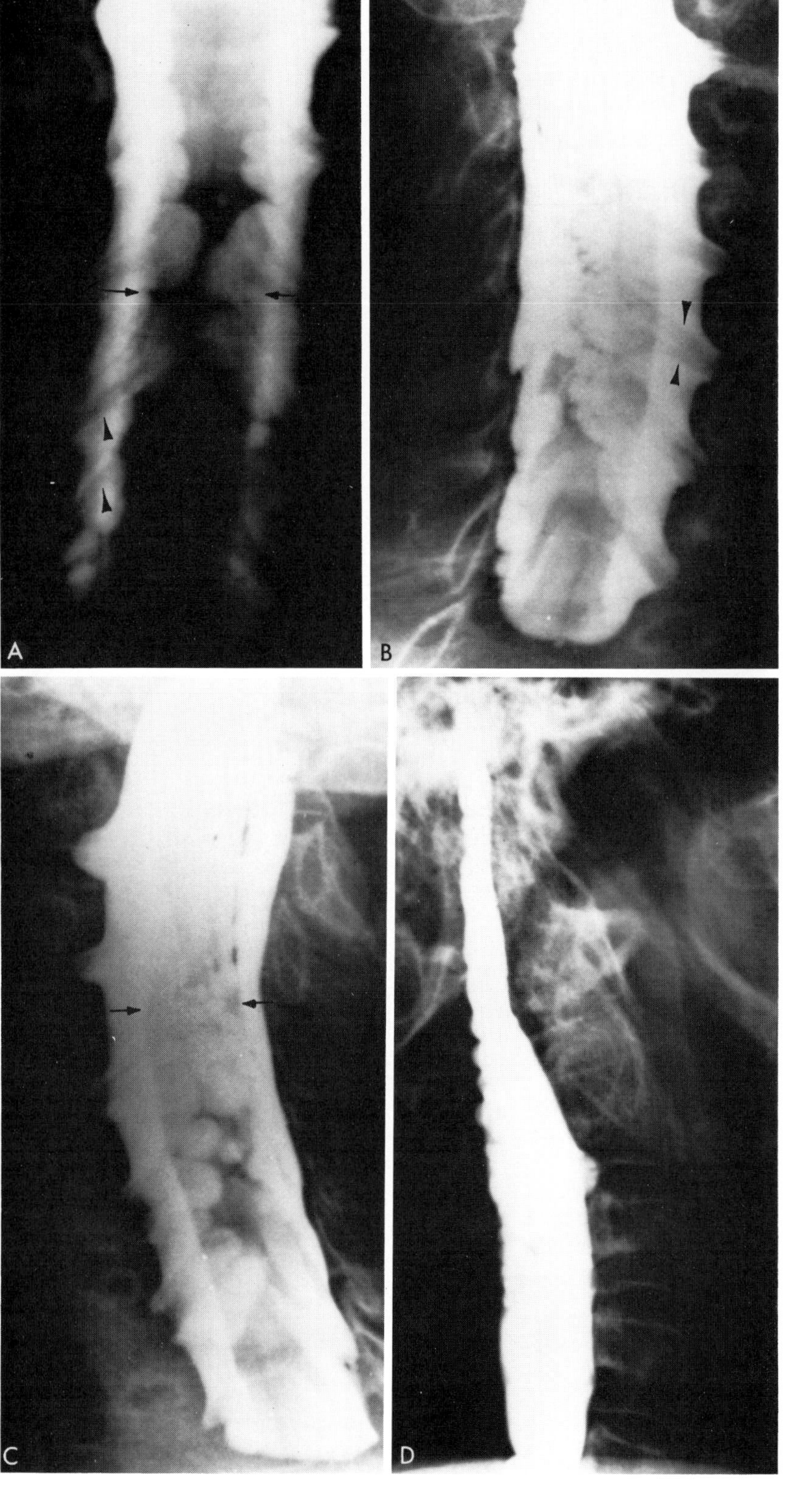

Figure 14–10. *Normal iophendylate (Pantopaque) cervical myelogram. The anteroposterior projection* **(A)** *is important for spinal cord measurements, whereas the oblique films* **(B, C)** *provide the most information concerning the nerve root sleeves. The lateral projection* **(D)** *is critical for exact localization of any mass lesions. Arrows, spinal cord; arrowheads, nerve roots.*

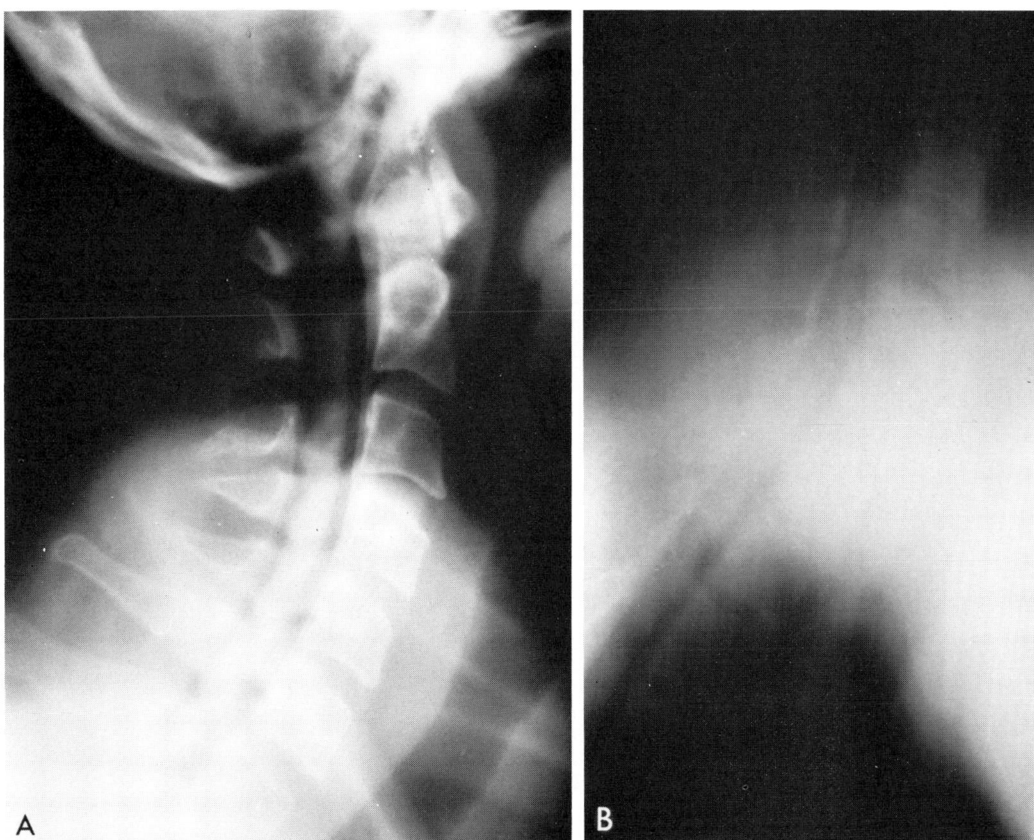

Figure 14–11. **A,** *Normal cervical air myelogram. This demonstrates the normal cervical spinal cord surrounded by the gas (air or oxygen). Compare this with Figures 14–55, 14–97, 14–98, and 14–112.* **B,** *Lower cervical air myelogram. This is more difficult to obtain owing to the thickness of the shoulders; however, with higher kilovoltage technique, good penetration should give films of diagnostic quality.*

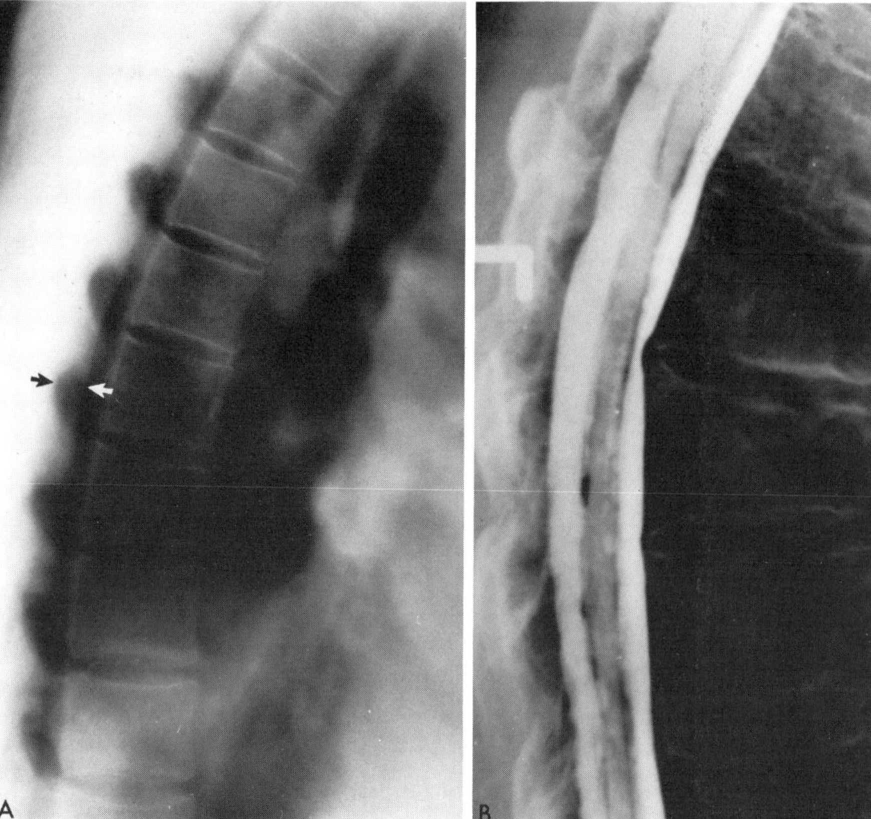

Figure 14–12. A, *Normal thoracic air myelogram. Here the soft tissue density of the spinal cord is seen in the posterior aspect of the thoracic spine. The width of the cord (between arrows) in this region is equal throughout, and the contour is smooth.* **B,** *Iophendylate myelogram usually shows the spinal cord centrally within the spinal canal, surrounded on all sides by the radiopaque (white) iophendylate.*

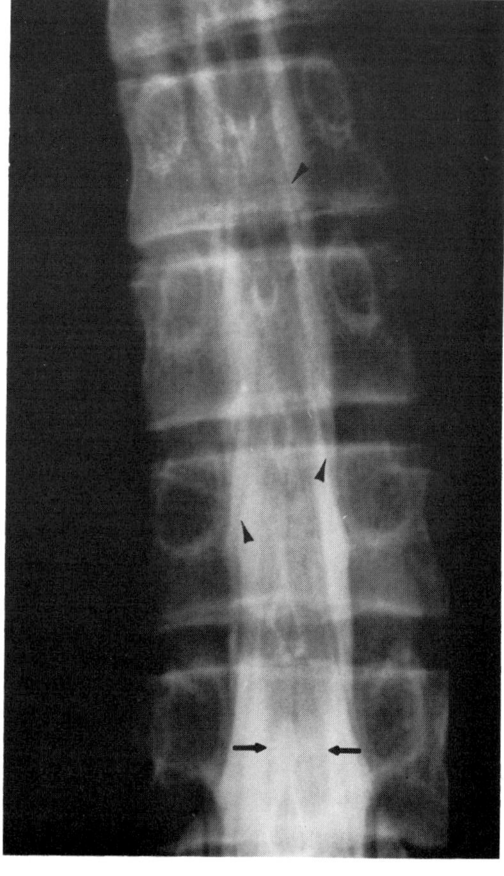

Figure 14–13. *Metrizamide thoracic myelogram. Generally, it is far more difficult to examine the thoracic spinal cord with metrizamide than with air or oily contrast media. At times, tomography is required for full delineation of the spinal cord. This film shows the distal portion of the thoracic spinal cord (between arrows) in the anteroposterior projection. The nerve roots (arrowheads) are also seen.*

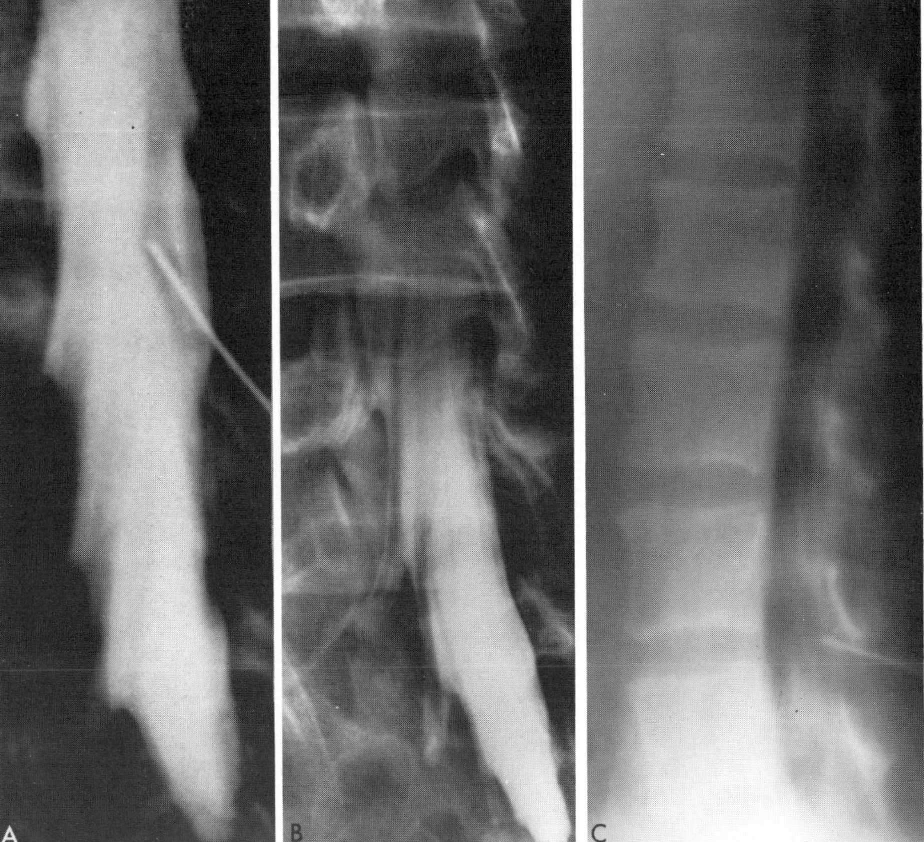

Figure 14–14. *Lumbar myelography is much more frequently performed than any other examination of the spinal canal. A comparison of iophendylate, metrizamide, and gas myelograms demonstrates the value of positive contrast medium and oblique, upright filming.* **A,** *Iophendylate myelogram;* **B,** *metrizamide myelogram;* **C,** *gas myelogram. It has become a standard practice that when only the lower lumbar canal is to be studied, metrizamide is the contrast medium of choice. This is because its low viscosity allows metrizamide to more consistently fill the nerve root sleeves compared with iophendylate.*

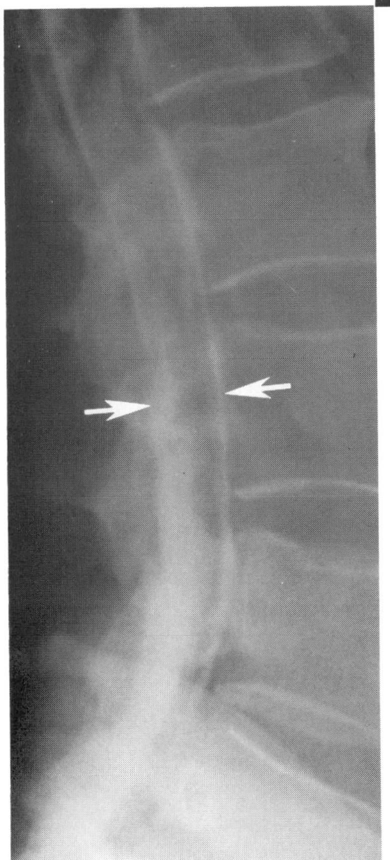

Figure 14–15. *Anteroposterior spinal canal diameter. The subarachnoid space is delineated here by an epidurogram, which outlines the entire lumbar sac in its anteroposterior diameter (arrows). Note the application of the subarachnoid space to the vertebral bodies anteriorly and the neural arches posteriorly. (Courtesy of Dr. Jane Barry, San Diego, California.)*

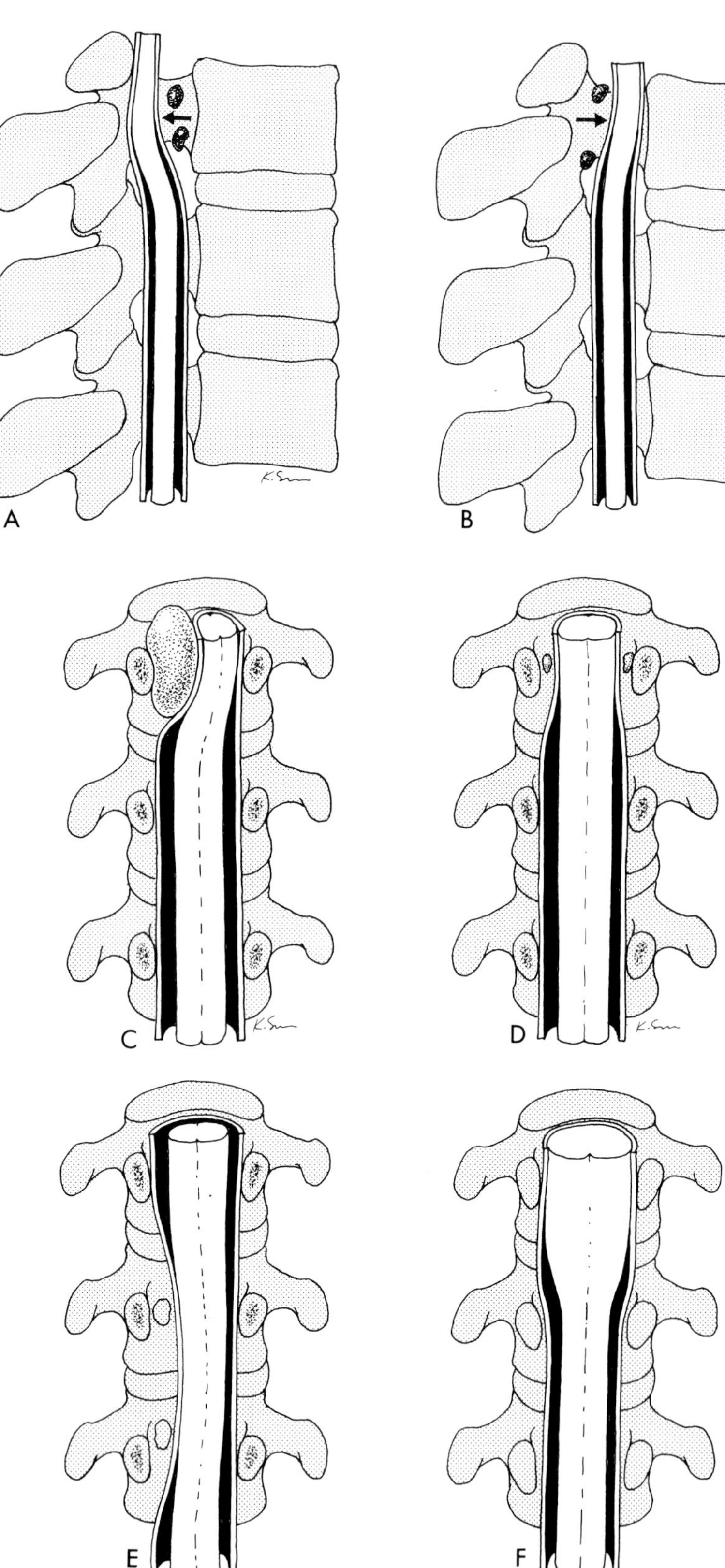

Figure 14–16. *Location of spinal lesions.* **A,** *Anterior extrinsic compression on the dura and subarachnoid space flattens the cord posteriorly. The most frequent anterior extradural masses are nuclear fragments from herniated intervertebral discs, with the extradural impression limited to the intervertebral disc level.* **B,** *Impression on the posterior dura and subarachnoid space from extradural masses occurs most frequently from hypertrophied osteophytes and ligaments in osteoarthritis.* **C,** *A lateral mass will compress the subarachnoid space and spinal cord to one side, separating the subarachnoid space from the pedicle on the affected side and applying it closer to the pedicle on the opposite side.* **D,** *Bilateral or circumferential lesions will compress the subarachnoid space and spinal cord toward the center, away from the pedicles. Epidural tumors, particularly metastatic disease, and peridural fibrosis or arachnoiditis are the most common causes of narrowing and constriction of the subarachnoid space.* **E,** *Long epidural lesions crossing the disc space generally imply tumor or infection.* **F,** *Widening of the spinal cord on one view can occur with any mass in the same plane as the film projection. Epidural, intradural-extramedullary, or intramedullary masses all expand the spinal cord in one projection. With extradural masses, a radiographic projection taken at 90 degrees will demonstrate displacement of the cord and subarachnoid space, with subsequent compression of the cord against the bony elements on the opposite side from the offending mass.*

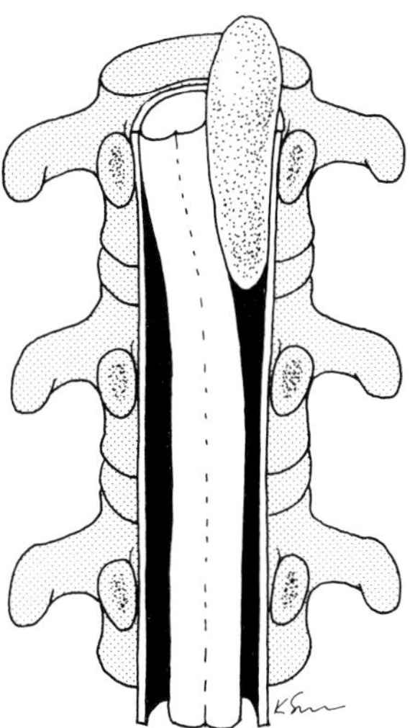

Figure 14–17. *Intradural-extramedullary masses. Such masses separate the spinal cord from the dura. There is narrowing of the subarachnoid space on the opposite side from the offending lesion, and widening of the subarachnoid space along the edges of the mass lesion. In one projection there is displacement of the cord. In the opposite projection, there is apparent widening of the cord, as seen in Figure 14–16***F***.*

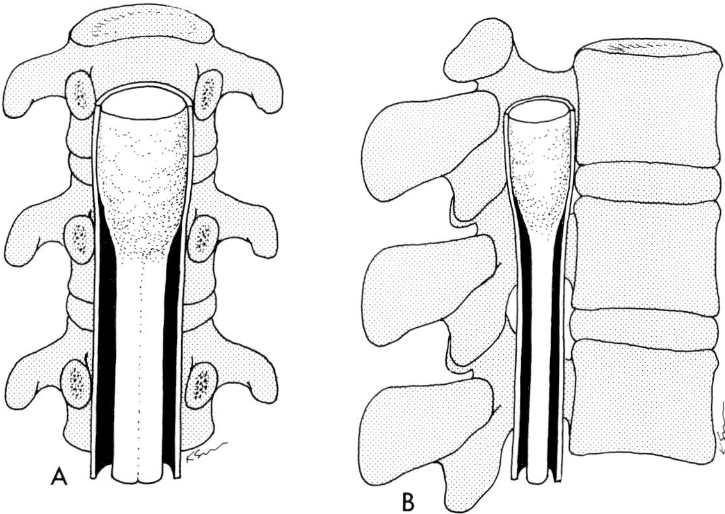

Figure 14–18. *Intramedullary masses. Such masses expand the spinal cord when viewed in any projection.* **A,** *Anteroposterior projection;* **B,** *lateral projection. Note that the subarachnoid space is narrowed symmetrically as the spinal tumor expands the cord.*

Table 14–1

CLASSIFICATION OF SPINAL PATHOLOGY BY COMPARTMENT

EXTRADURAL
- Protruded or herniated intervertebral disc
- Osteophyte; hypertrophic ligament
- Bone fragment
- Tumor (metastatic or primary bone tumor)
- Scar tissue
- Hematoma
- Infection
- Congenital extradural cyst
- Congenital bony abnormality

INTRADURAL-EXTRAMEDULLARY
- Tumor (meningioma or neurofibroma)
- Infection
- Arachnoiditis
- Acquired epidermoid sequestration cyst
- Congenital cyst

INTRAMEDULLARY
- Tumor
- Vascular malformation
- Hydromyelia/syringomyelia
- Hematoma
- Infection
- Radiation and posttraumatic atrophy

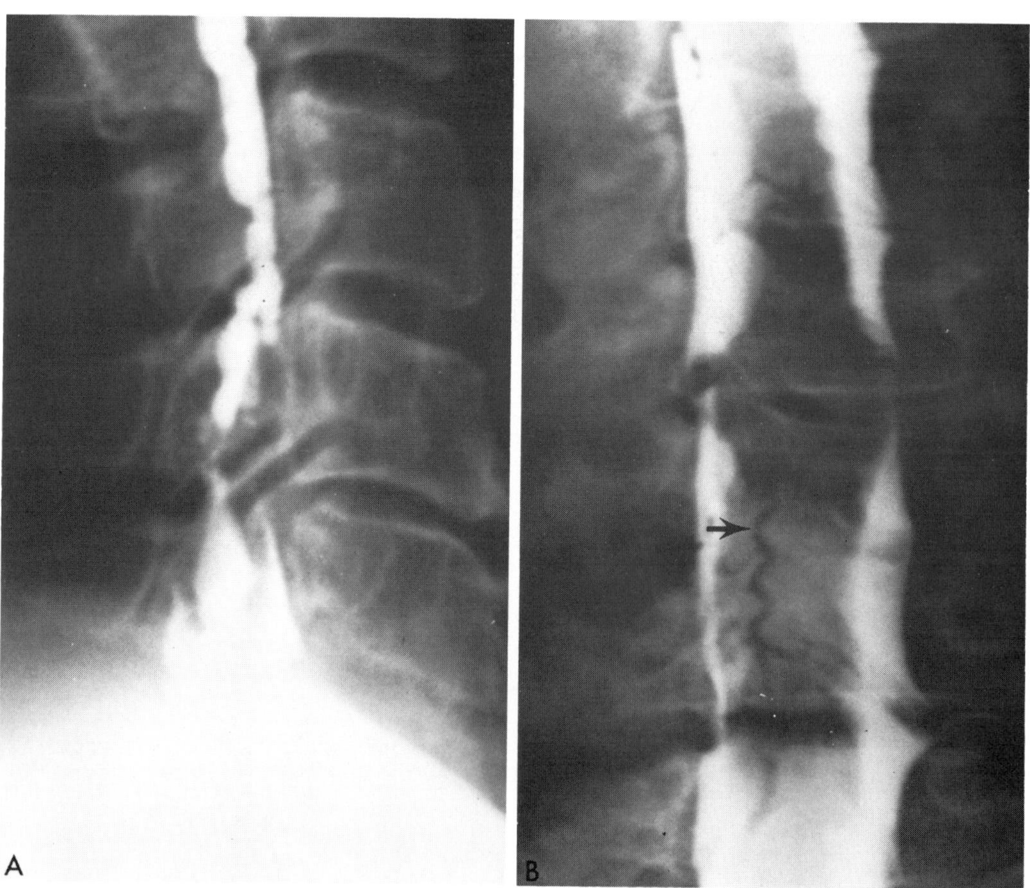

Figure 14–19. *Extradural spinal cord compression.* **A,** *A large osteophyte and herniated cervical disc displace the spinal cord and subarachnoid space posteriorly.* **B,** *Apparent widening of the spinal cord indistinguishable from that accompanying any intramedullary mass is evident on this one projection. Incidentally noted is a large draining vein (arrow) resulting from obstruction of normal venous flow from the cord compression.*

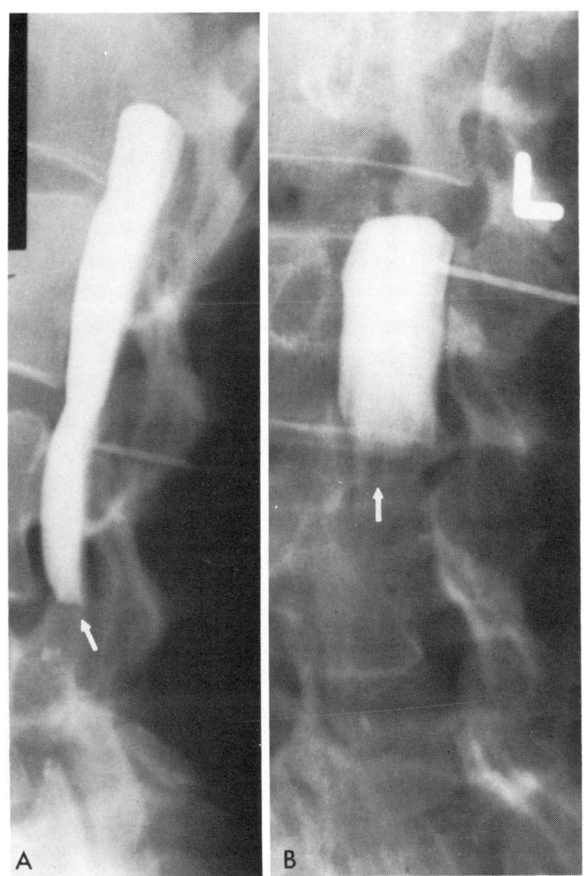

Figure 14–20. *Extradural block.* **A,** *Lateral film of a myelogram demonstrating a total block at the level of L3-L4 from a herniated disc (arrow).* **B,** *The feathering appearance (arrow) seen on this oblique film is most often found with extradural lesions that create a total block.*

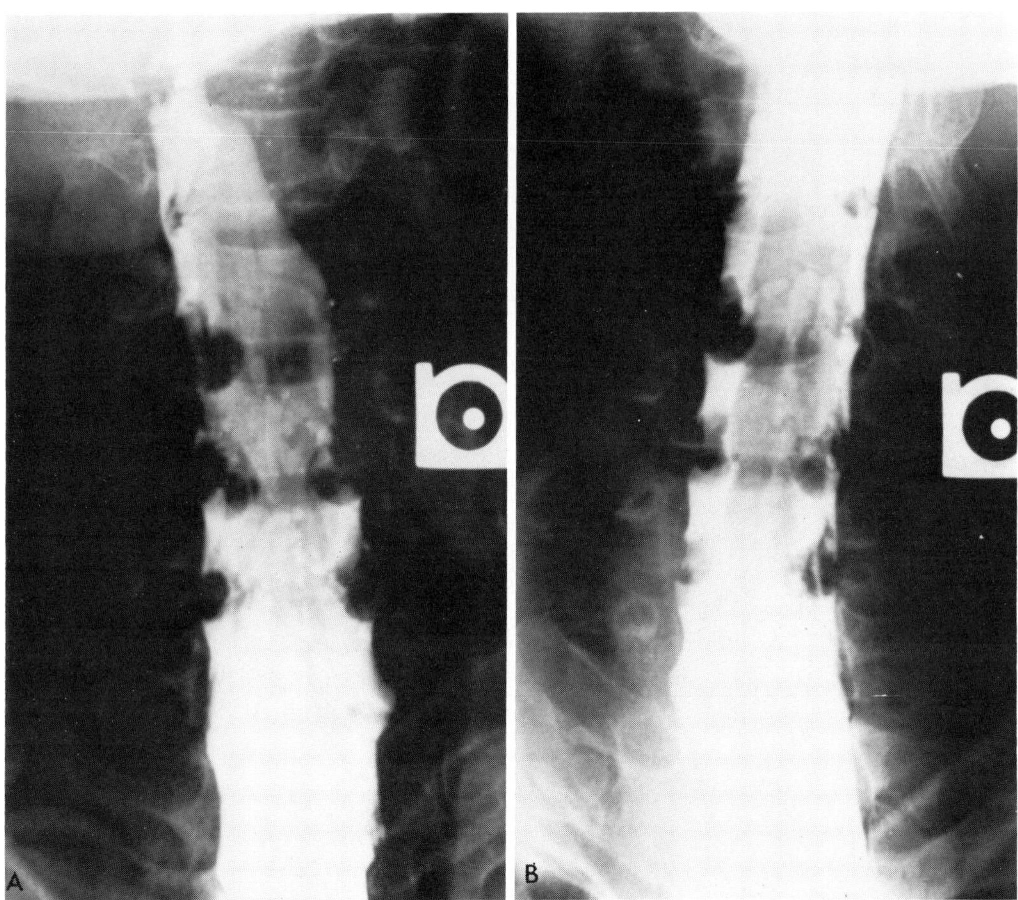

Figure 14–21. *Intradural-extramedullary lesion. Two films demonstrating intradural-extramedullary neurofibromas with minimal displacement of the spinal cord to the left by the larger lesions on the right side. The widening of the subarachnoid space on the right is typical of intradural-extramedullary masses. Cupping of the lesions and sharp borders are other characteristics of masses in this compartment.*

produce a sharp outline. Frequently, there is a rapid transition between the outer margin of the subarachnoid space and the tumor margin. This rapid transition coupled with the "capping" of the mass lesion by the contrast medium differentiates intradural from extradural lesions.

The intramedullary lesions arise within the spinal cord itself. The cord enlarges in a diffuse, fusiform fashion, tapering to either side of the central portion of the lesion (Fig. 14–22). This widening of the spinal cord narrows the subarachnoid space symmetrically so that contrast medium, trapped within the subarachnoid space, tapers from both the cranial and the caudal ends toward the central portion of the lesion. On occasion, there is asymmetric widening of the spinal cord, with narrowing of the subarachnoid space on the involved side and widening of this space on the opposite side.

A widened spinal cord on one roentgenographic projection is not diagnostic of an intramedullary lesion. Any mass displacing one aspect of the cord may flatten its contralateral aspect against the adjacent neural bony elements (Fig. 14–19). It is for this reason that at least two films exposed at 90 degrees to one another be obtained in all cases.

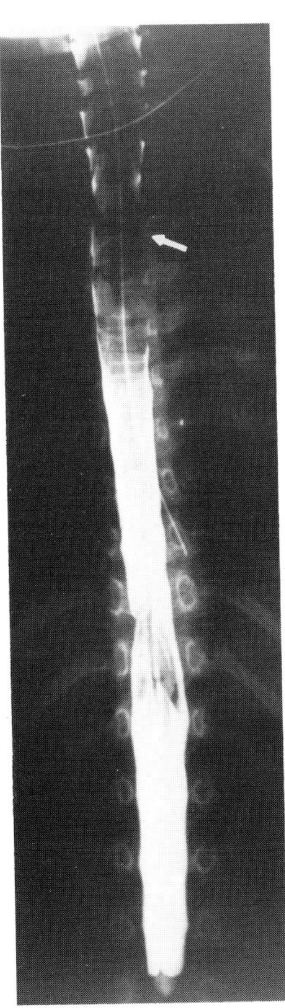

Figure 14–22. *Intramedullary lesion. An intramedullary mass will look the same when viewed from all directions. In this case, a distended syringomyelia enlarges the spinal cord (arrow) from foramen magnum to conus medullaris. It symmetrically narrows the column of contrast medium in the subarachnoid space.*

Table 14–2

CLASSIFICATION OF SPINAL PATHOLOGY BY ETIOLOGY

TRAUMATIC OR DEGENERATIVE
Protruded or herniated intervertebral disc
Osteophyte
Hypertrophied ligament
Spinal stenosis
Hematoma
Posttraumatic intramedullary cyst
Posttraumatic meningocele (posttraumatic root sleeve cyst)
Bone fragment
Cord atrophy
Arachnoiditis (postoperative)
TUMOR
Primary
Metastatic
CONGENITAL
Spinal dysraphism
Syringomyelia, hydromyelia
Vascular malformation
INFLAMMATORY
Infection; abscess
Arachnoiditis (idiopathic or postmyelographic)

Once the precise location of a lesion is determined, a probable tissue type may be suggested, based upon its location, size, and shape. On the basis of an appropriate history, the radiologic findings frequently will provide a single accurate diagnosis (Table 14–2).

Lumbar Venography

Veins draining blood from the spinal cord, the nerve roots, the meninges, the vertebral bodies, and the paravertebral muscles form an intricate network of valveless vessels extending from the presacral plexus to the base of the occiput. There are two communicating venous plexuses: the external vertebral plexus in the lumbar region and the internal vertebral venous system (the epidural veins). Depending upon pressure gradients, blood will flow in a cephalad direction in either of these two systems. The intermediary external system exists between the systemic veins, the inferior vena cava, and the retroperitoneal veins. The internal spinal vertebral veins drain the spinal cord and vertebral bodies. The epidural veins lie between the vertebral bodies and the dura mater. The veins lying against the vertebral bodies and the intervertebral discs are termed the anterior internal vertebral veins (AIVV). These channels have a "rope-ladder" appearance as they extend cephalad (Fig. 14–23). In the normal state, there should be symmetry in the appearance of the two ascending venous groups. In the anteroposterior projection, the AIVV are concave laterally at the level of the pedicles, at which site they receive the

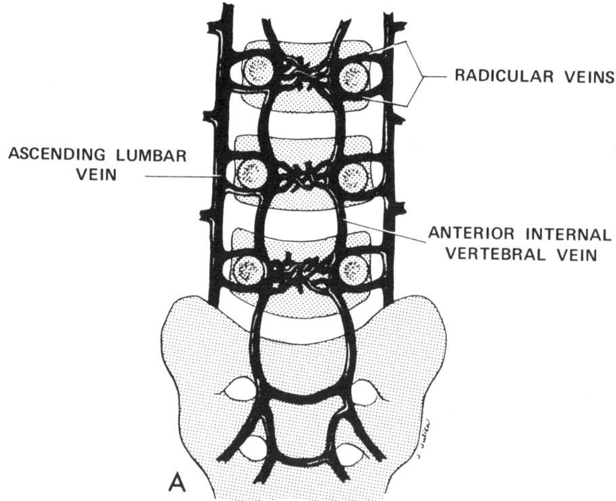

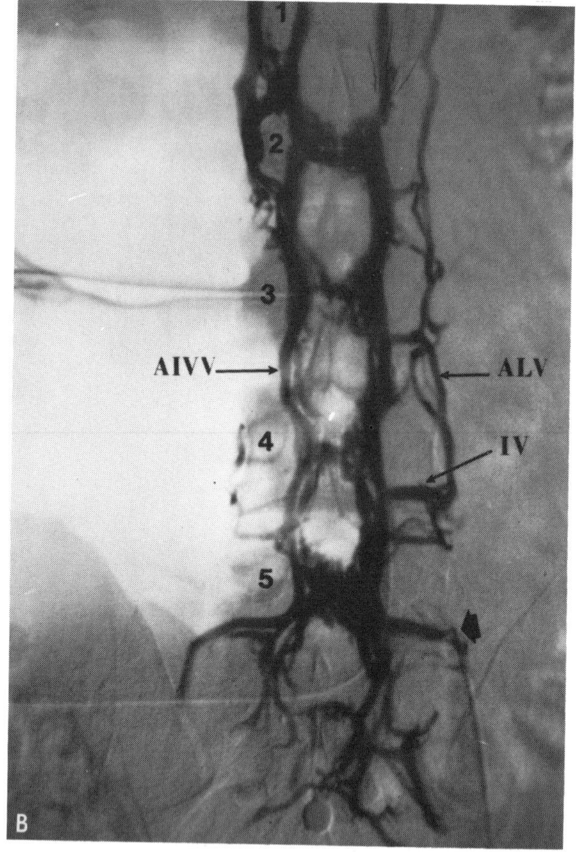

Figure 14–23. Lumbar phlebography. **A,** Diagram demonstrating the spinal venous plexus as viewed on a spinal phlebogram. The ascending lumbar veins are extravertebral, with the radicular veins (also called pedicular or intervertebral veins) carrying the blood to the intravertebral plexus running behind the vertebral bodies in the extradural space. **B,** Subtraction venogram demonstrating the epidural veins. ALV, Ascending lumbar vein; IV, intervertebral veins or radicular veins; AIVV, anterior internal vertebral veins; arrow, catheter tip. (From O'Dell CW, Jr, et al.: J Bone Joint Surg 59A:159, 1977.)

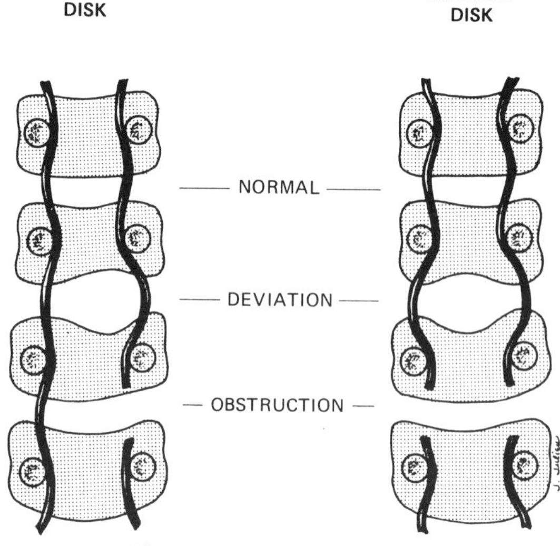

Figure 14–24. Abnormal epidural venous patterns. Diagram demonstrating the various configurations of the ascending internal vertebral veins when a pathologic process affects them. An extreme lateral disc may deviate the veins medially. (From O'Dell CW Jr, et al.: J Bone Joint Surg 59A:159, 1977.)

communicating veins from the external vertebral plexus. At the intervertebral disc level, the AIVV reverse their curvature, becoming concave medially. Asymmetry, thinning, and occlusion of these veins are abnormal findings (Fig. 14–24).

Spinal Arteriography

The normal spinal arteriogram shows a very small, nonbranching single anterior spinal artery, and, on occasion, two posterior spinal arteries (Fig. 14–25). The course of these vessels is longitudinal and nondeviating. The anterior spinal artery extends along the ventral surface of the spinal cord from the upper cervical region to the caudal end of the spinal cord at L1. Any deviation in the course of these vessels or any vascular enlargement indicates abnormality.

Discography

Following the injection of contrast medium into the center of a normal intervertebral disc of a young patient, the nucleus pulposus should appear as a single transverse, homogeneous density. In older individuals, the nucleus bifurcates and will appear on discography as two parallel dense areas with an intervening radiolucent band; the horizontal radiodense regions are usually connected posteriorly, although they may be joined anteriorly. In both young and old patients, the nucleus should be well contained by a radiolucent anulus fibrosus (Figs. 14–26 and 14–36).

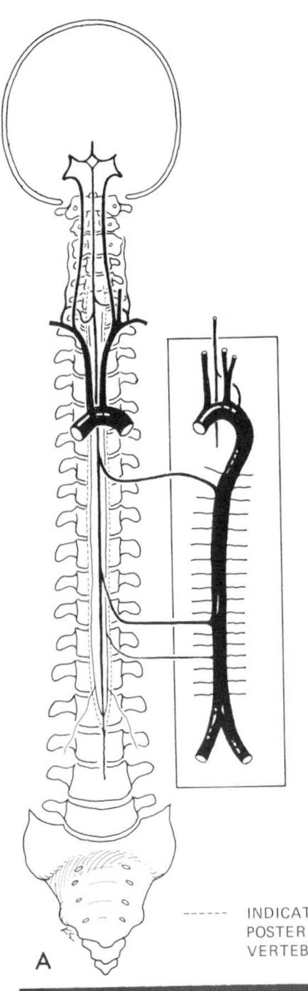

Figure 14–25. Anterior spinal artery. **A**, Diagram demonstrates the multiple contributing arteries that form the anterior spinal arterial chain. The anterior spinal artery is single and runs along the ventral surface of the spinal cord, in the midline. **B, C**, Anteroposterior and lateral vertebral arteriograms (with subtraction technique) demonstrate filling of the anterior spinal artery (arrows). **D**, Injecting an intercostal artery fills the lowest of the contributing arteries to the anterior spinal artery, also known as the artery of Adamkiewicz (arrows). Note the characteristic loop (arrowheads).

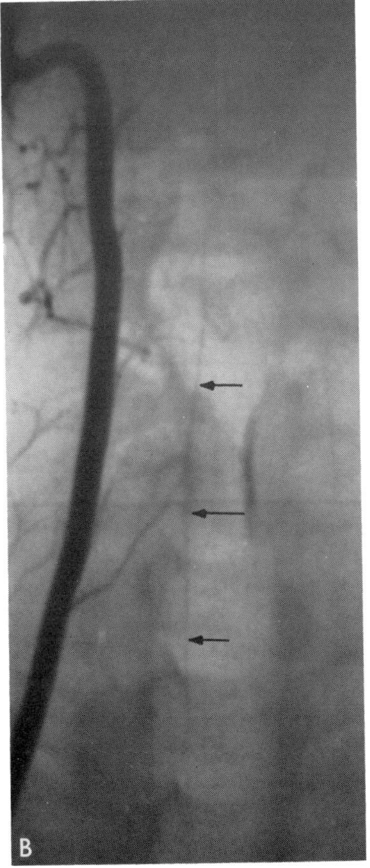

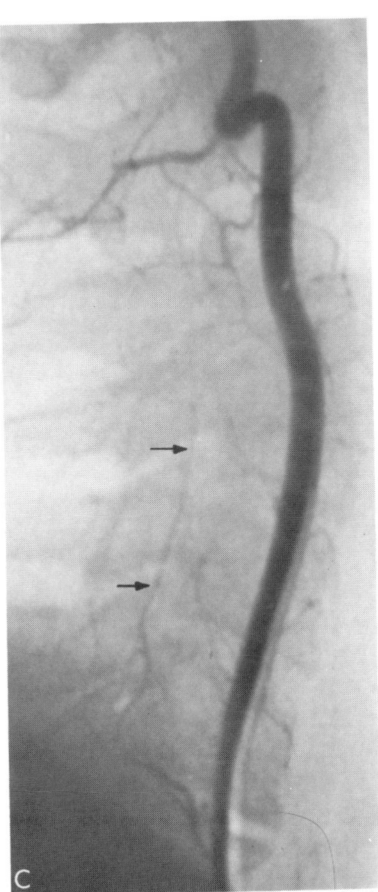

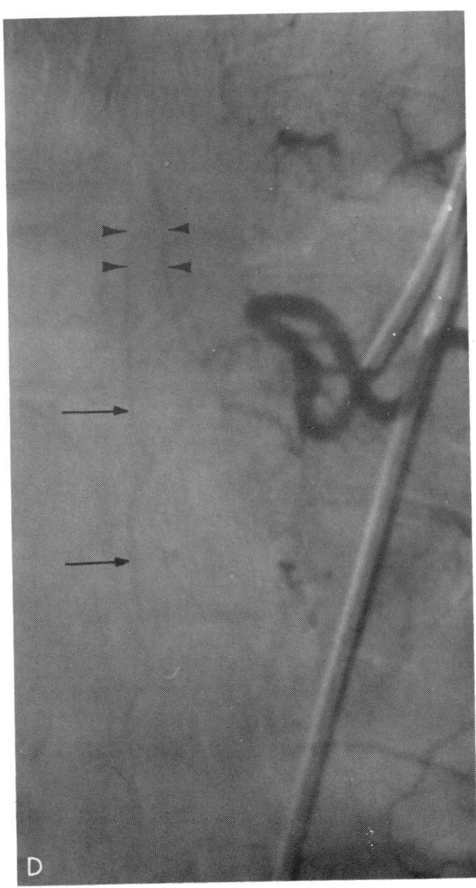

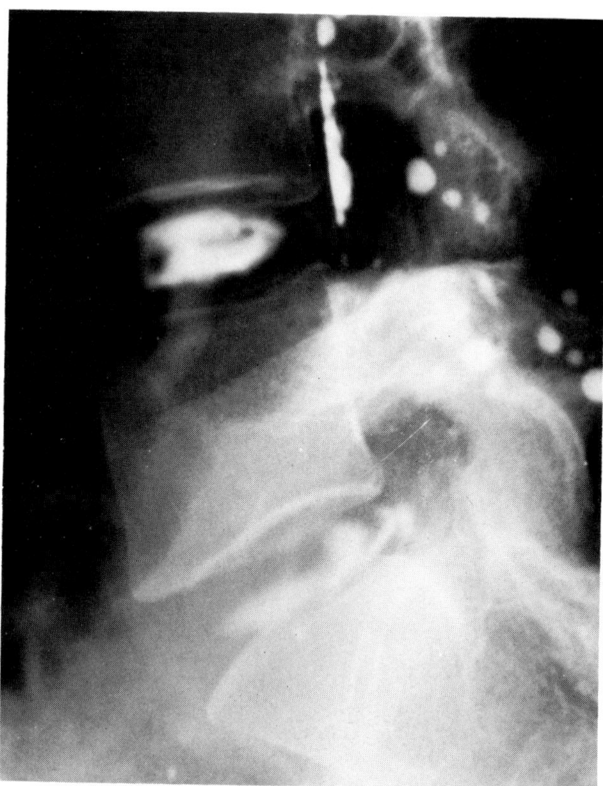

Figure 14–26. Normal findings on a discogram are evident with contrast medium seen in the L4-L5 disc interspace, centrally and without extravasation. The L5-S1 interspace shows abnormal findings, with extravasation of the contrast medium posteriorly. (Courtesy of Dr. Bernard Ghelman, New York, New York.)

Epidurography

In the normal epidurogram contrast material outlines the dural sac (Figs. 14–9 and 14–15). The contrast medium diffuses along the dura mater within the spinal canal and extends into the neural foramina, to eventually become dispersed and resorbed in the retroperitoneal space. Within the contrast column are the nerve root sleeves and exiting nerve roots. Any extrinsic mass, whether it is a disc fragment or bony overgrowth, will be seen as a block to the flow of contrast medium into the neural foramina or as deviation of the epidural space. This technique has been limited to evaluation of lumbar disease, especially degenerative disc processes and spinal stenosis.

Computed Tomography

The normal computed tomogram without intrathecal contrast media can demonstrate the spinal cord and exiting nerve roots (Fig. 14–8). With intrathecal contrast media, the nerve roots are usually not visualized, but the outline of the spinal cord is well demarcated (Fig. 14–50*B*). Intravenous contrast medium usually enhances only pathologic processes — e.g., tumors, arteriovenous malformations.

DISEASE PROCESSES

Degenerative Disorders

The most common spinal problems encountered in humans may be attributed to erect posture. Degenerative lesions of the vertebral column are among the most frequent causes of lost productivity in modern society, and can lead to significant clinical abnormalities. There are several factors that contribute to low back and neck pain and radiculopathies: herniated intervertebral disc material; osteophytosis; hypertrophy of ligaments; and narrowing of the spinal canal.

Comprehension of the mechanism and the appearance of prolapsed disc material requires an understanding of discal anatomy. The intervertebral disc consists of two main components: the anulus fibrosus and the nucleus pulposus. The former is composed predominantly of fibrous and elastic elements, which surround and retain the nuclear material. The anulus fibrosus forms the anterior, the posterior, and the lateral support of the nucleus pulposus, whereas the cartilaginous end-plates contain the nucleus superiorly and inferiorly. If there is weakening of either of these barriers, the nuclear material may prolapse, taking the "path of least resistance." With aging, the posterior anular fibers may develop fissures and cracks, allowing herniation of the nuclear material through the weakened area. If the fissures in the anulus fibrosus are not complete, simple bulging or protrusion of the nucleus occurs; when the nuclear fragment breaks through the confines of the anulus fibrosus, the process is termed discal herniation. The majority of symptomatic lesions due to discal herniation occur in the lumbar and cervical regions.

Neurologic symptoms and signs result from compression of the neural elements (spinal cord or nerve roots) by the protruding or herniated nuclear fragments and by any associated osseous degenerative abnormalities (osteophytes) or hypertrophied ligaments. Additionally, neurologic abnormalities may result from compromised blood supply to either the nerve roots or the spinal cord. Finally, the protruded nuclear material may incite an inflammatory response (arachnoiditis and peridural fibrosis), leading to further compromise of the spinal canal.

Trauma may play an important role in posterior herniation of the nucleus pulposus. Single and acute or repeated and chronic traumatic events place additional stress on the anulus fibrosus. Compression, hyperextension, or hyperflexion of the spinal column and iatrogenic injuries, including lumbar puncture, discography, and orthopedic and chiropractic manipulation and surgery, can lead to bony and ligamentous hypertrophy as well as protrusion of nuclear fragments.

The degree and direction of the herniation of nuclear fragments determine the patient's symptom complex. As would be expected, lateral protrusions and herniations compress nerve roots as they exit the neural foramina, leading to radicular pain and sensory deficits. Local pain, i.e., neck or low back pain, may also be present. Clinical findings may include abnormal reflexes as well as muscle wasting. Central impressions on the spinal cord occur most frequently in the lower cervical spine (Fig. 14–19). In this location, a complex of symptoms and signs occurs, which may be confused with those associated with an intraspinal tumor or a degenerative process (e.g., lateral sclerosis). Further, a midline discal herniation in combination with osteophytosis and ligamentous hypertrophy may press upon the medial pyramidal spinothalamic tracts. If this ventral impression is not midline, a symptom complex known as the Brown-Séquard syndrome[56] may develop, which consists of ipsilateral motor deficit due to pyramidal tract compression and contralateral sensory deficit due to compression of the anterior and lateral spinothalamic tracts, which have not yet crossed over. In the lumbar region, central defects have been associated with bowel and bladder dysfunction as well as lower extremity neurologic deficits.

Routine roentgenographic examination may confirm the presence of degenerative or traumatic vertebral abnormalities. Narrowed intervertebral disc spaces (Fig. 14–27), hypertrophic spurs (Fig. 14–28), vertebral body compression fractures (Fig. 14–29), and calcified discs (Fig. 14–30) are frequent plain film findings. A "vacuum phenomenon" representing a radiolucent collection of nitrogen located in the area of the nucleus pulposus is associated with intervertebral disc space narrowing and osteophyte formation. It is found most frequently in the lower cervical and lower lumbar intervertebral disc spaces (Fig. 14–31).

Despite these characteristic roentgenographic abnormalities, myelography remains the standard examination in delineating discal prolapse. Although any contrast medium that is utilized will demonstrate most of the lesions, the water-soluble media (e.g., metrizamide) allow more optimal visualization of the nerve root sleeves. Lateral intervertebral disc herniations are also better appreciated with these latter agents compared with either iophendylate or gas myelography.

When the myelogram is inconclusive, lumbar venography can represent a helpful additional procedure, especially in a patient with a lateral discal herniation, or with a suspected L5-S1 discal prolapse (Fig. 14–32). The precise role of computed tomography in evaluating discal disorders is not clear at this time although proper computer programing can allow visualization of bony abnormalities as well as the herniated discal fragments (Figs. 14–33 to 14–35). In addition, epidurography or discography at one or multiple levels may be performed to outline the rent in the anulus fibrosus (Figs. 14–26 and 14–36).

Lumbar Disc Disease. The most frequent level for lumbar discal herniation is L4-L5, followed closely by L5-S1 (Table 14–3). Central or lateral discal herniations can occur. On myelography, central discal protrusion will produce a defect that is best delineated on the lateral film as a posterior displacement with a double area of density or zone of diminished contrast (Fig. 14–37). This phenomenon is related to the thin contrast-filled lateral portions of the anterior subarachnoid space that envelop the central herniated discal fragment. The lateral herniation, which is more frequent than the central herniation, is produced by a nuclear fragment that escapes through a fissure of the anulus fibrosus into the lateral portion of the spinal canal and often into the neural foramina. On myelography or epidurography, amputation of a nerve root sleeve or a lateral impression on the subarachnoid column will be

Text continued on page 457

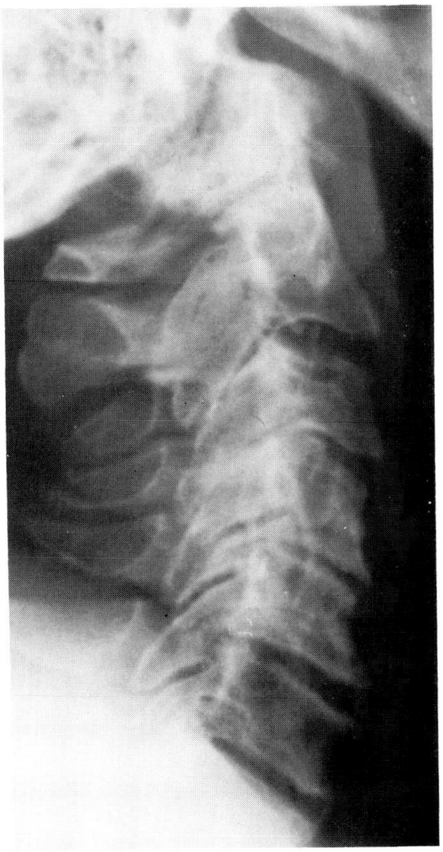

Figure 14–27. *Narrow intervertebral disc spaces with hypertrophic spurs on the anterior and posterior surfaces of the vertebral bodies indicate a marked degree of disc degeneration.*

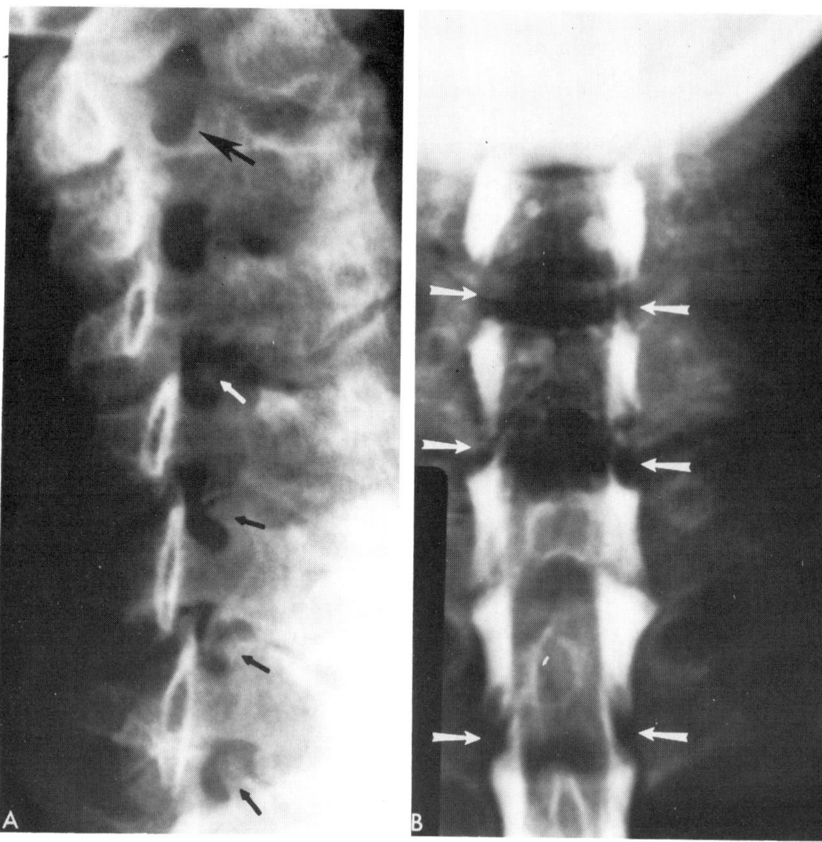

Figure 14–28. Hypertrophic spurs. **A**, The hypertrophic spurs (small arrows) encroach upon neural foramina at multiple levels. The normal foramen is smoothly oval (large arrow). **B**, Anteroposterior projection of iophendylate myelogram demonstrates multiple nerve root amputations by the hypertrophic spurs (arrows).

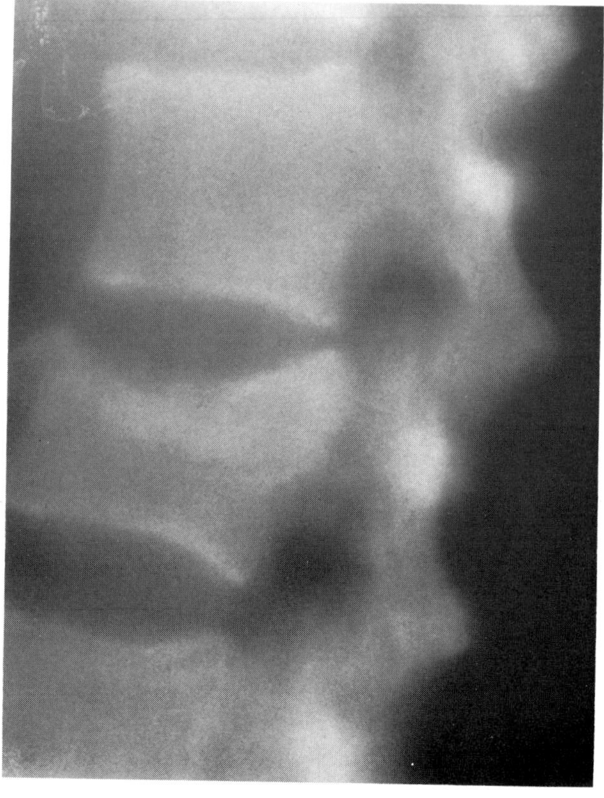

Figure 14–29. Vertebral fracture. This vertebral body compression fracture, demonstrated on tomography, impinges upon the spinal canal. Posttraumatic lesions should be evaluated with computed tomography, myelography, arteriography, or venography when neurologic symptoms and signs are present.

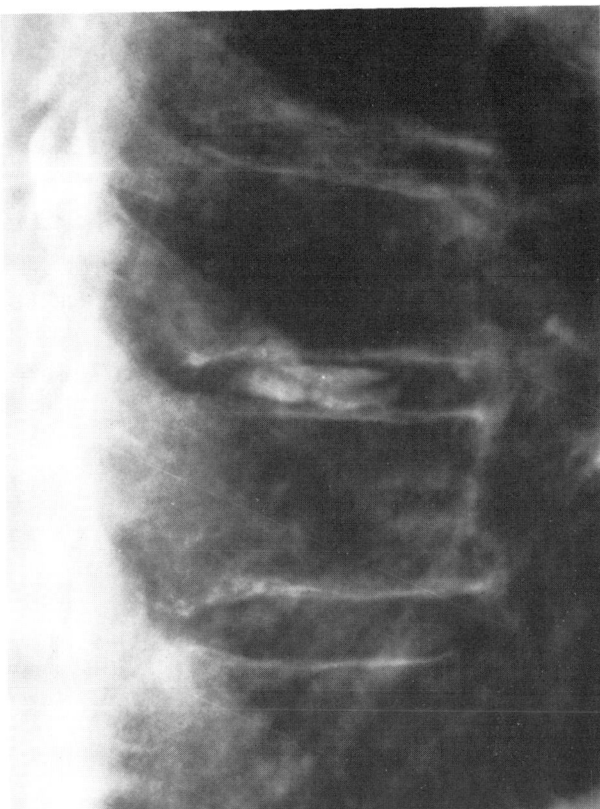

Figure 14–30. *Calcified intervertebral disc. This finding is frequent on plain film examinations of the chest. It is the nucleus pulposus that calcifies. Most cases are asymptomatic.*

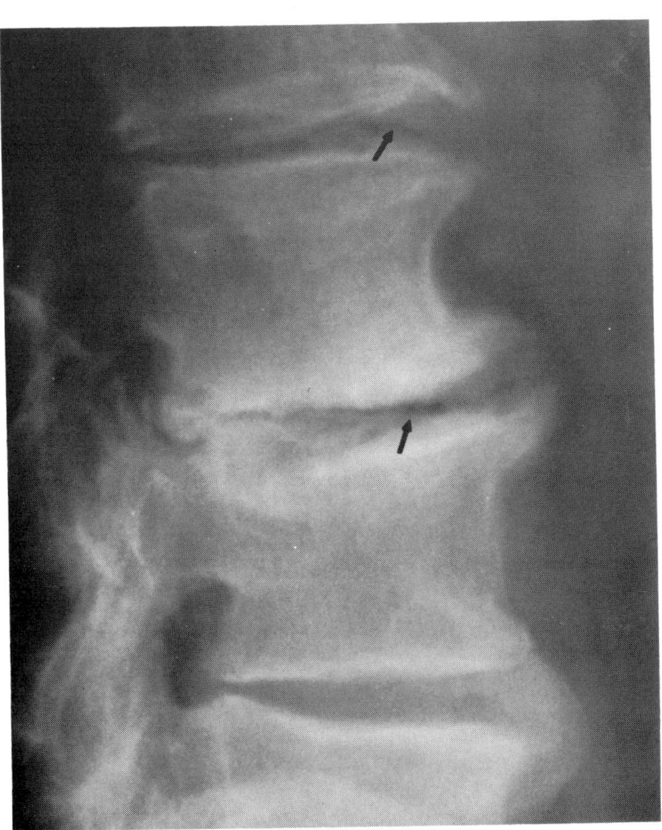

Figure 14–31. *Vacuum phenomenon. Such phenomena are frequent plain film findings and appear as radiolucent streaks between vertebral bodies in narrow intervertebral disc spaces (arrows). They are indicative of degenerative disc disease.*

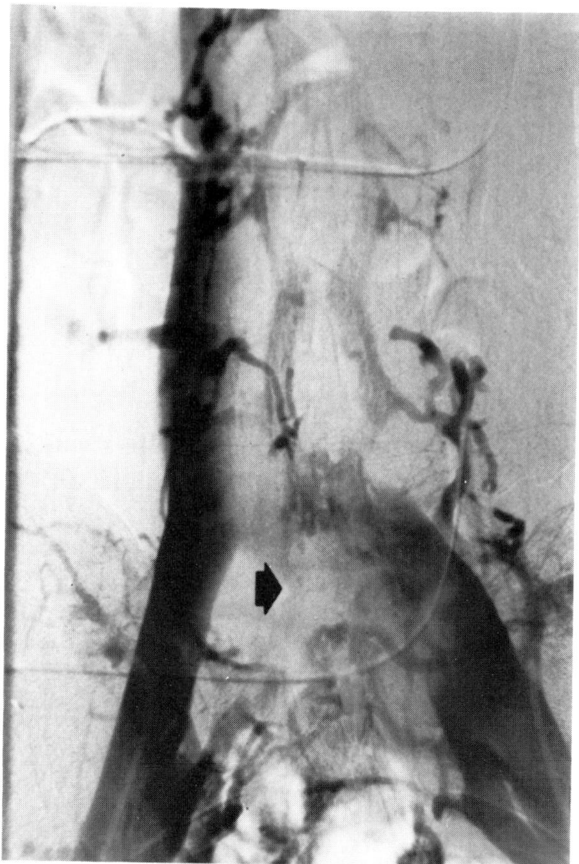

Figure 14–32. Herniated disc. Lumbar venogram demonstrates interruption of the epidural veins at L5-S1 bilaterally (arrow). This is indicative of herniation of nucleus pulposus fragments into both neural foramina. The myelogram failed to document the presence of this herniated disc.

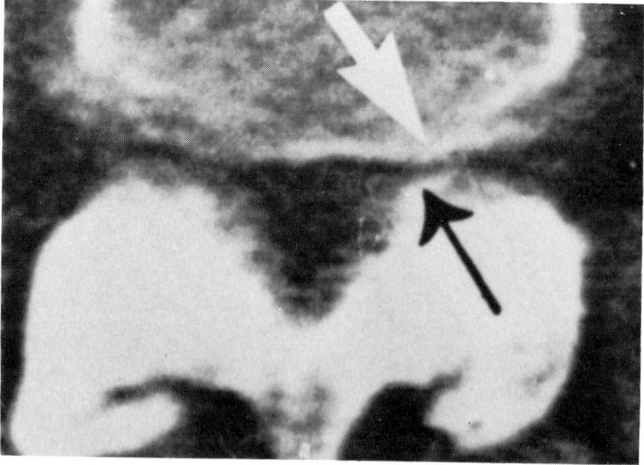

Figure 14–33. Narrow neural foramen. CT scan of the lumbar spine (with the vertebral body at top) demonstrates hypertrophic changes narrowing the neural foramina (arrows), particularly in the superior articular facets. These changes are very difficult to demonstrate on plain film examination. (Courtesy of Dr. William Glenn, Long Beach Memorial Hospital, Long Beach, California.)

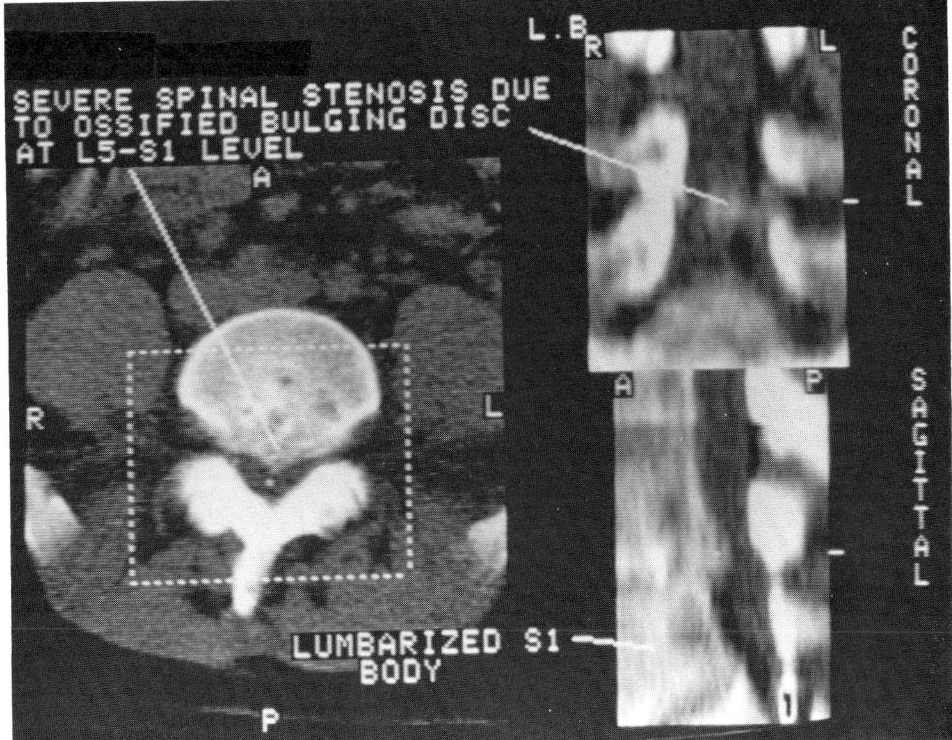

Figure 14–34. *Centrally herniated disc. CT scan demonstrates herniated disc material from the L5-S1 disc space. (Courtesy of Dr. William Glenn, Long Beach Memorial Hospital, Long Beach, California.)*

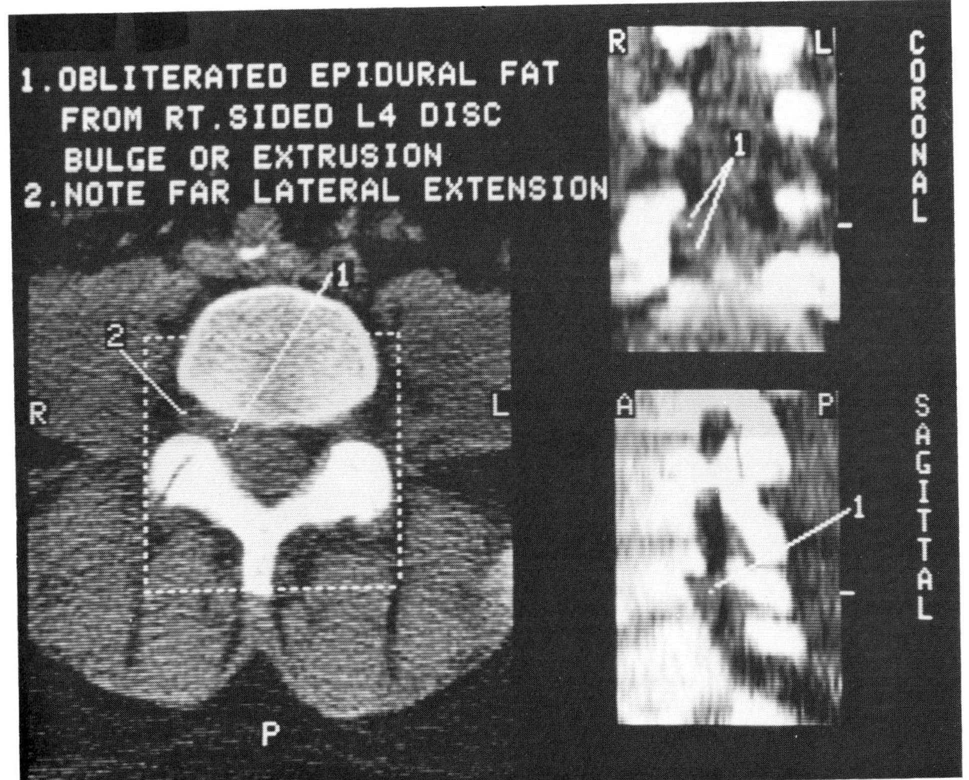

Figure 14–35. *Laterally herniated disc. Disc material herniating into the right lateral neural foramen is demonstrated on CT examination. Compare the densities in each of the neural foramina. Note the normal appearance of the superior articulating facets, ending smoothly with the inferior articulating facets. (Courtesy of Dr. William Glenn, Long Beach Memorial Hospital, Long Beach, California.)*

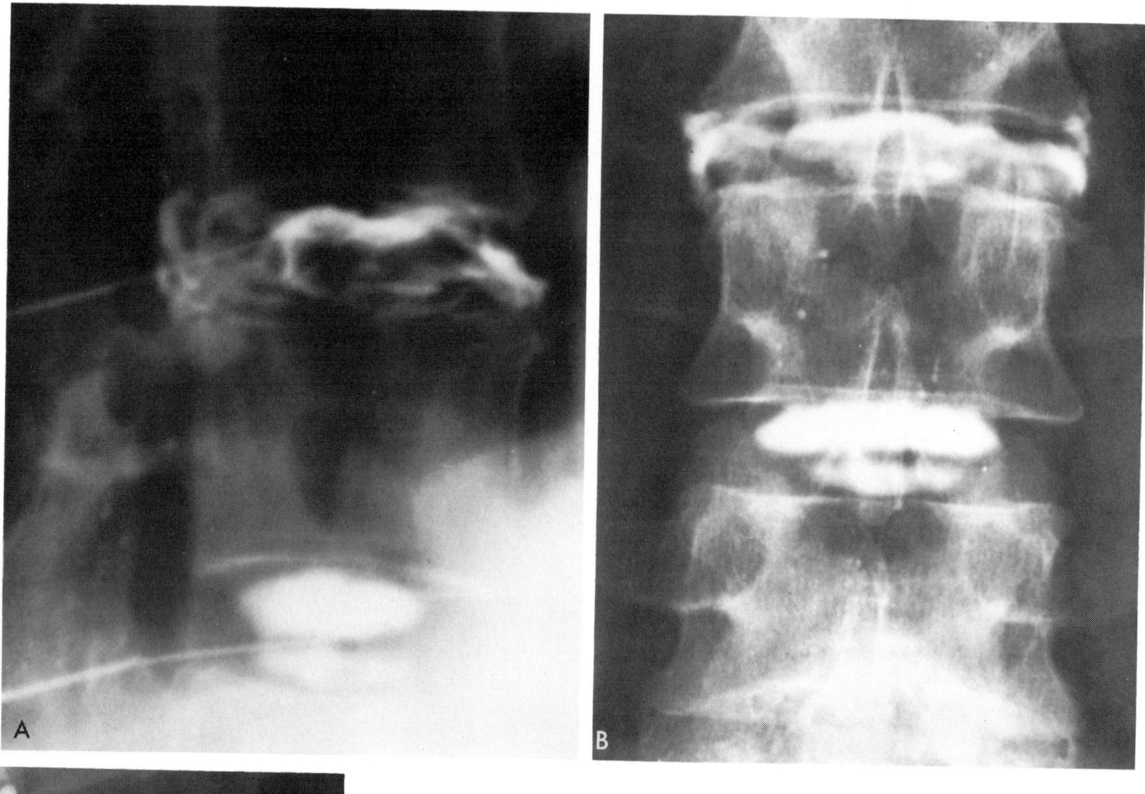

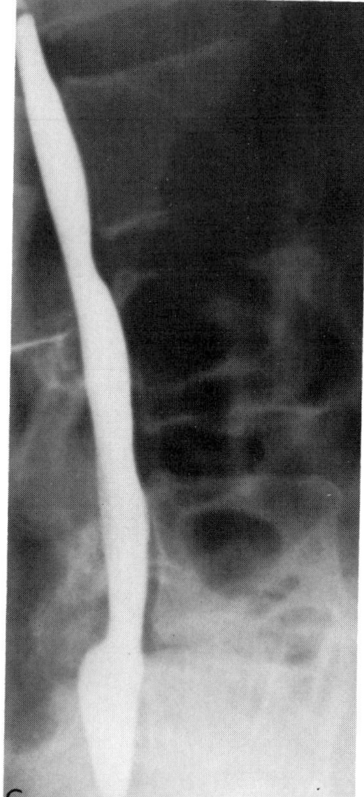

Figure 14–36. **A, B,** *Abnormal discogram. There is extravasation of contrast medium injected at the L3-L4 intervertebral disc level. A simultaneous injection at the L4-L5 disc level is normal.* **C,** *Lateral projection from an iophendylate myelogram showed entirely normal results.*

Table 14–3
LEVELS OF INTERVERTEBRAL DISC HERNIATION

LUMBAR	L4-L5 > L5-S1 >> L3-L4 >>> L2-L3, L1-L2
THORACIC	T4-T5 → T12-L1 all equal T1-T2, T2-T3 rare
CERVICAL	C6-C7 > C5-C6 >>> C7-T1 > C4-C5

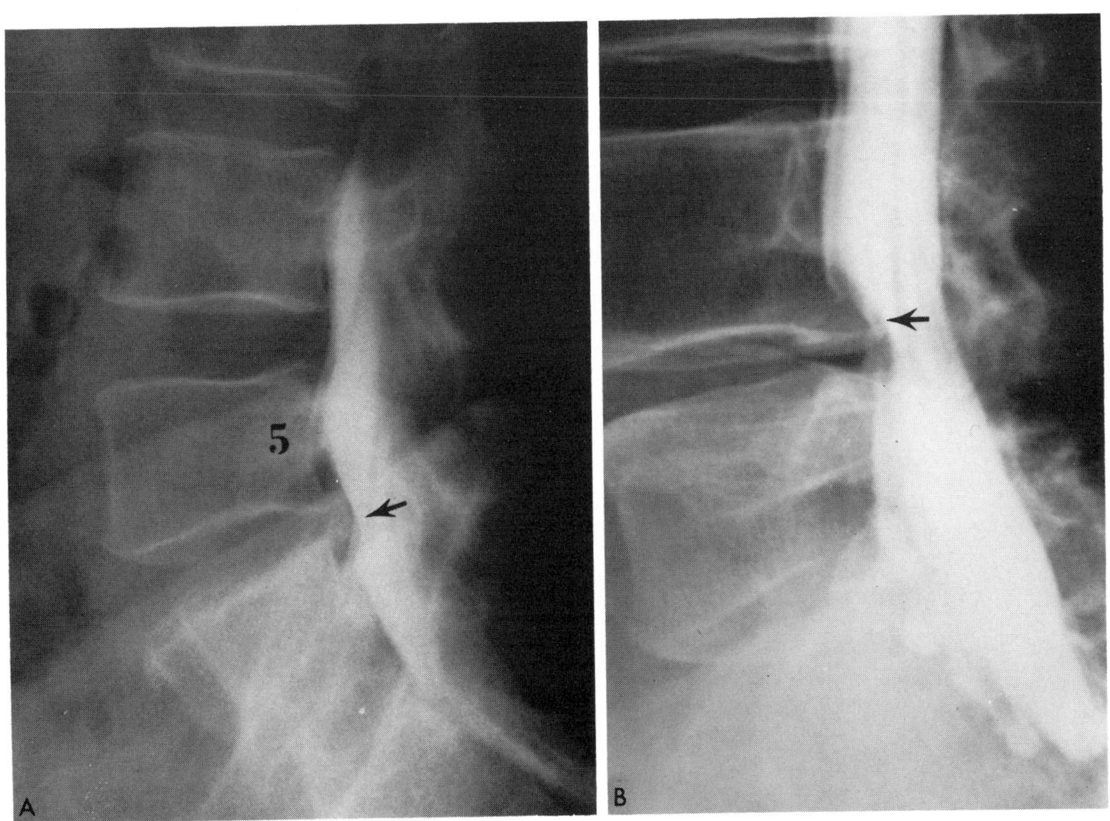

Figure 14–37. *Herniated disc.* **A,** *Posterior displacement at L5-S1 intervertebral disc level is indicative of posterior herniation or protrusion of intervertebral disc material (arrow).* **B,** *At L4-L5, in a different patient, there is the thinning of the contrast column at the level of the intervertebral disc herniation creating a double density appearance (arrow).*

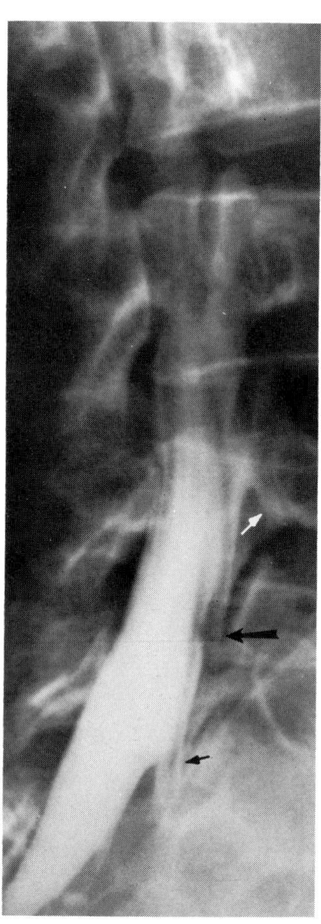

Figure 14–38. Root sleeve amputation. On myelography, nerve root sleeves are seen exiting the neural foramina beneath the pedicles at L4-L5 and S1-S2 (small arrows). There is amputation of the L5-S1 nerve root sleeve with a minimal impression upon the subarachnoid space (large arrow).

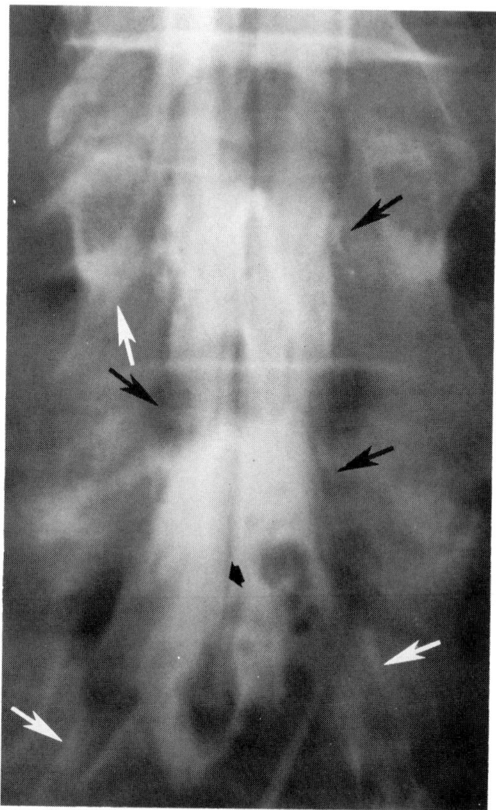

Figure 14–39. Root sleeve amputation. An abnormal epidurogram reveals amputation of the L5-S1 root sleeves bilaterally, as well as at the left L4-L5 level (black arrows). Contrast medium can be seen entering the right L4-L5 foramen and the sacral neural foramina (white arrows). (Courtesy of Dr. Jane Barry, University Hospital, San Diego, California.)

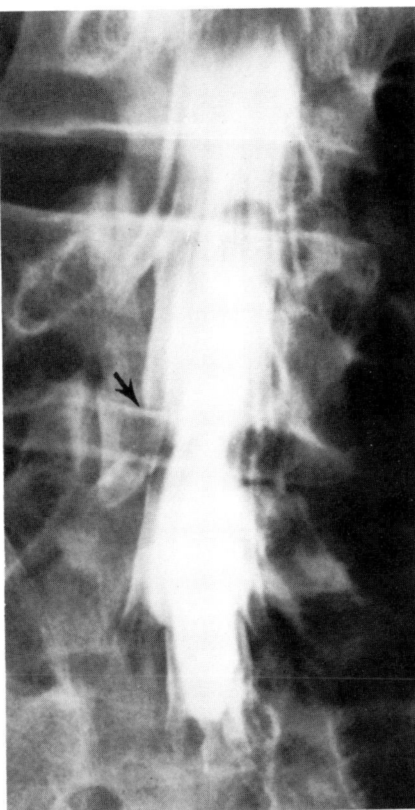

Figure 14–40. Root sleeve deviation. Although the L5-S1 nerve root sleeve fills with contrast medium, there is a superior impression on the nerve root from a laterally herniated disc fragment (arrow).

evident (Figs. 14–38 and 14–39). Minor deviations of nerve root sleeves are also indicative of herniated intervertebral discs (Fig. 14–40).

Other etiologies of extradural defects at the level of an intervertebral disc space are localized arachnoiditis, peridural fibrosis, bony spurs, osteoarthritis (Figs. 14–41 and 14–42), degenerative ligamentous disease, and tumor.

Thoracic Disc Disease. Herniated intervertebral discs are unusual in the thoracic spine, although degenerative changes are frequently evident on films of the dorsal region. Most patients who present with acute symptoms related to a herniated thoracic intervertebral disc detail a history of trauma, although occasionally a patient will be seen with no clear-cut antecedent trauma. Although patients with herniated intervertebral discs in the thoracic region are frequently without significant symptoms (possibly because of the generous subarachnoid space in this region), thoracic discal herniation can occasionally lead to symptoms and signs, even in young patients. In fact, children have been reported with prolapse of calcified nuclear material. Lateral herniation can produce radiculopathy from compression of exiting nerve roots, whereas central discal herniations will impress upon the spinal cord, producing long tract signs (motor and sensory). Impressions upon the conus medullaris and cauda equina may also produce sphincter disturbances, gait abnormalities, and sensory deficits.

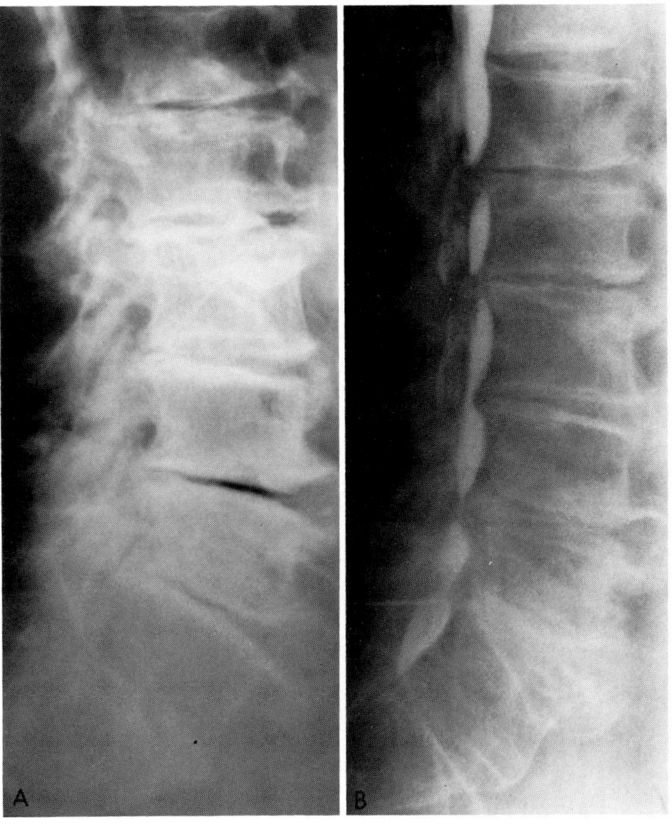

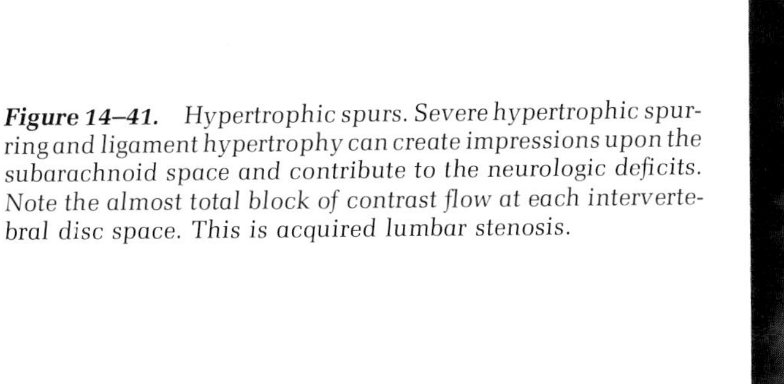

Figure 14–41. Hypertrophic spurs. Severe hypertrophic spurring and ligament hypertrophy can create impressions upon the subarachnoid space and contribute to the neurologic deficits. Note the almost total block of contrast flow at each intervertebral disc space. This is acquired lumbar stenosis.

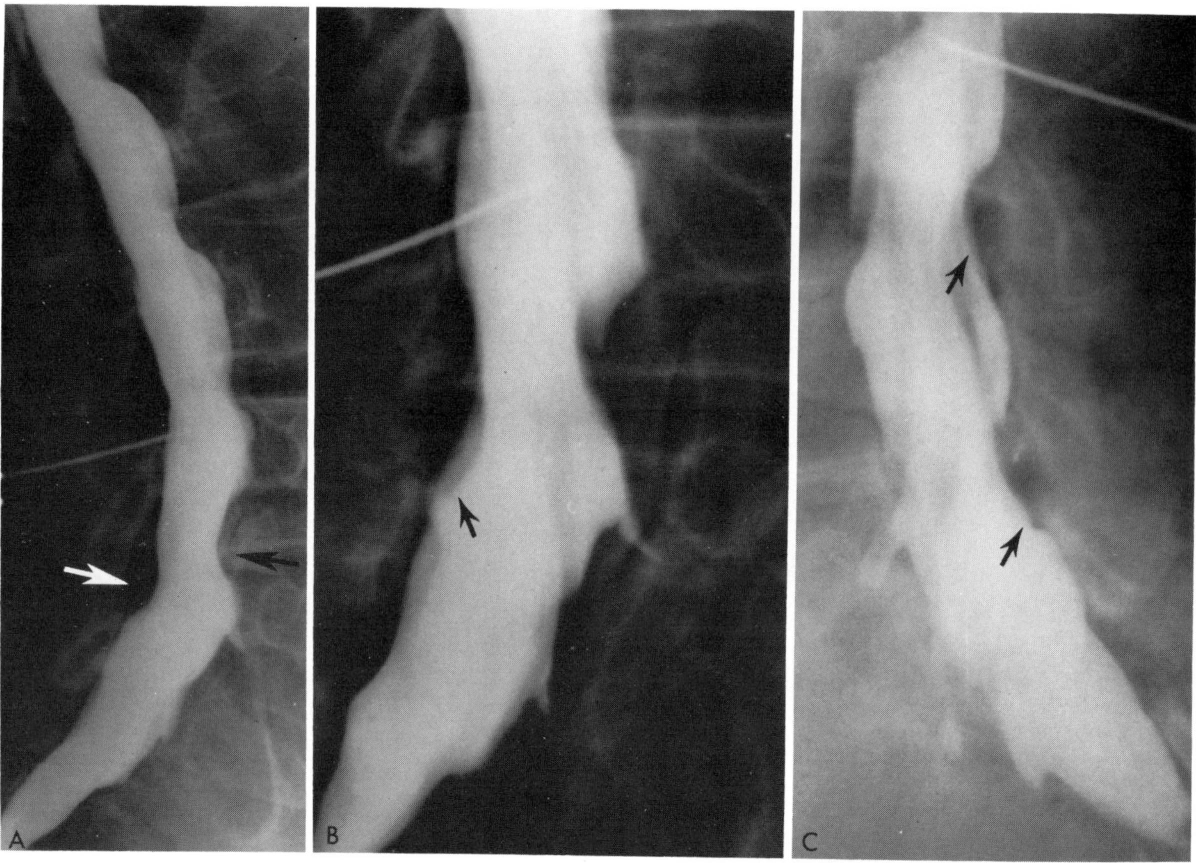

Figure 14–42. Hypertrophic ligaments (ligamentum flavum). **A,** There is marked narrowing of the subarachnoid space caused by herniated intervertebral disc material (black arrow) as well as posterior ligamentous hypertrophy (white arrow). **B,** Oblique projection in same case further delineates the posterior impression by the hypertrophic ligaments (arrow). **C,** In another patient, hypertrophic ligaments and posterior bony elements (arrows) partially narrow the spinal cord.

Routine radiographs of the thoracic spine can reveal intervertebral discal calcification (Fig. 14–30), degenerative spurs (mostly anterior), and disc space narrowing. On myelography, discal prolapse produces a characteristic extradural defect at the level of the involved intervertebral space (Fig. 14–43). The detection of such a lesion should not dissuade the examiner from completing the entire myelogram, as an unsuspected secondary lesion may be responsible for much of the symptom complex. The thoracic spine is a site of predilection for skeletal metastasis, and a careful search for bony erosion and destruction, a paraspinal mass, and elongated extradural defects should be accomplished. This region is also a frequent site for meningiomas, which in most instances are intradural-extramedullary lesions.

Cervical Disc Disease. Extradural compression of the spinal cord and the cervical nerve roots is extremely common. Most cervical discal herniations occur in the lower cervical spine, especially the C5-C6 and C6-C7 levels. Men are more commonly affected than women, and older patients more frequently than younger patients.

Plain film examination may reveal anterior and posterior osteophyte formation and disc space narrowing (Fig. 14–27). On oblique films, the osteophytes often protrude into the neural foramina (Fig. 14–28). Apophyseal joint sclerosis and hypertrophy are also frequent. At myelography, the extradural impression upon the nerve roots and spinal cord usually represents a combination of a herniated nucleus pulposus (Fig. 14–44), osteophytosis (Fig. 14–45), and a hypertrophic ligamentum flavum (Fig. 14–46). Often, multilevel disease is found at myelography, necessitating careful clinical correlation. The major findings include amputation of nerve root sleeves, thinning of the contrast column ("cervical bars") (Fig. 14–45), displacement of the subarachnoid space, and spinal cord compression.

Spinal Stenosis. Spinal stenosis is a condition in which the cross-sectional area of the spinal canal is smaller than normal. It may be developmental or degenerative in etiology.[57] In both of these situations, the anteroposterior diameter is significantly shortened. In developmental stenosis of the lumbar spine, the narrow canal is due to overgrowth of the vertebral laminae and classically involves multiple levels, although a single level may occasionally be affected. Degenerative stenosis may appear in a canal already compromised by develop-

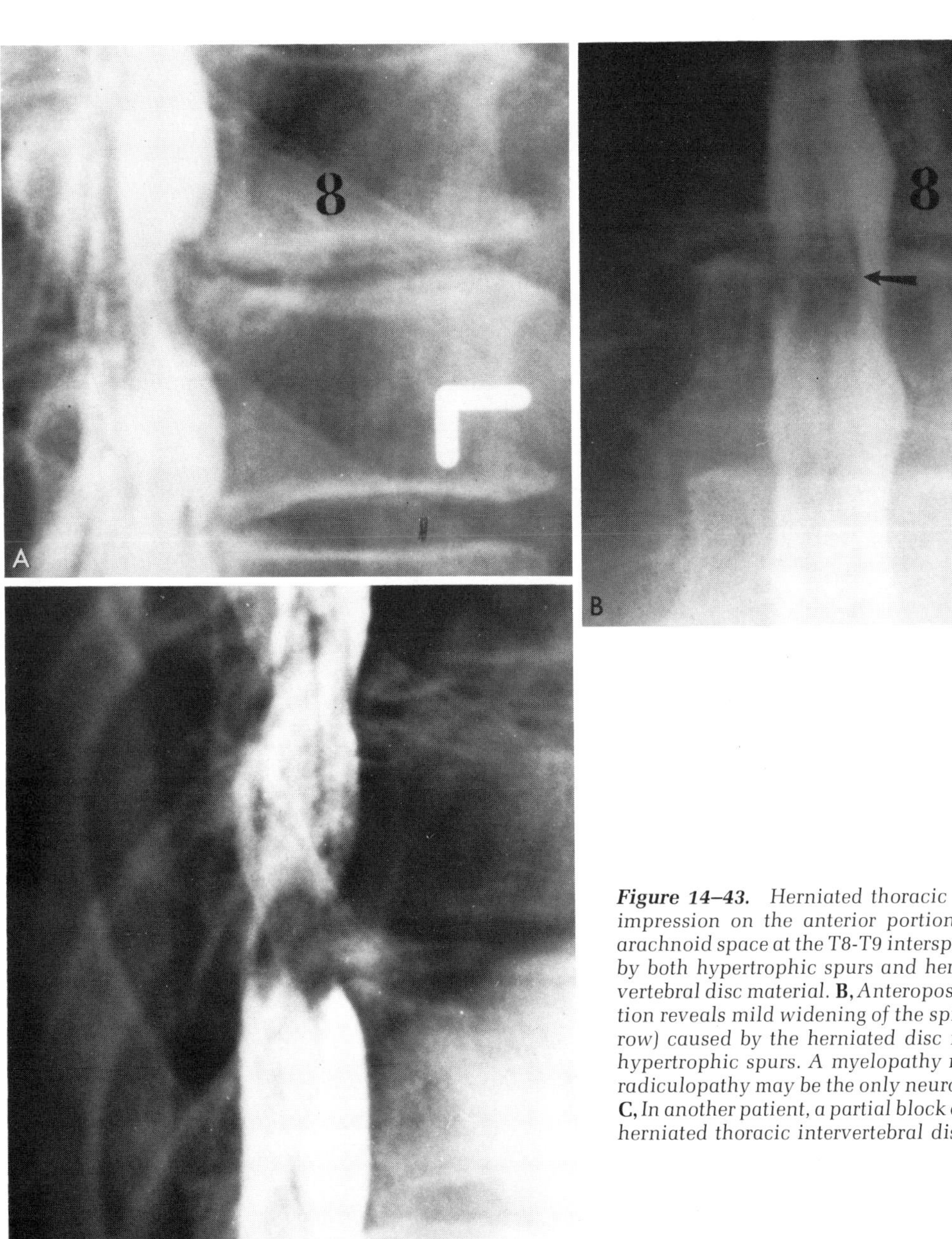

Figure 14–43. *Herniated thoracic disc.* **A,** *The impression on the anterior portion of the subarachnoid space at the T8-T9 interspace is caused by both hypertrophic spurs and herniated intervertebral disc material.* **B,** *Anteroposterior projection reveals mild widening of the spinal cord (arrow) caused by the herniated disc material and hypertrophic spurs. A myelopathy rather than a radiculopathy may be the only neurologic deficit.* **C,** *In another patient, a partial block occurs from a herniated thoracic intervertebral disc.*

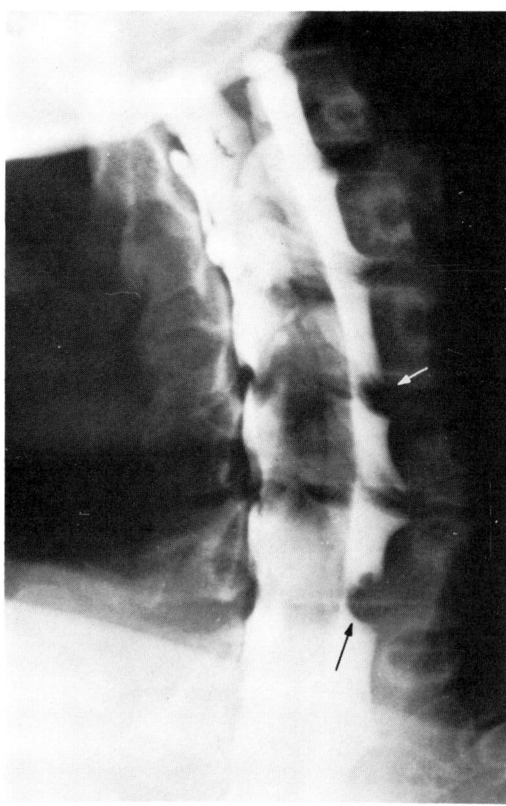

Figure 14–44. Posttraumatic herniated cervical disc. In a patient with a C8 radiculopathy, an amputated nerve root at C7-T1 is found (black arrow). In this patient, no hypertrophic spurs were present at this level. In addition, there is amputation of the C5-C6 nerve root sleeve (white arrow).

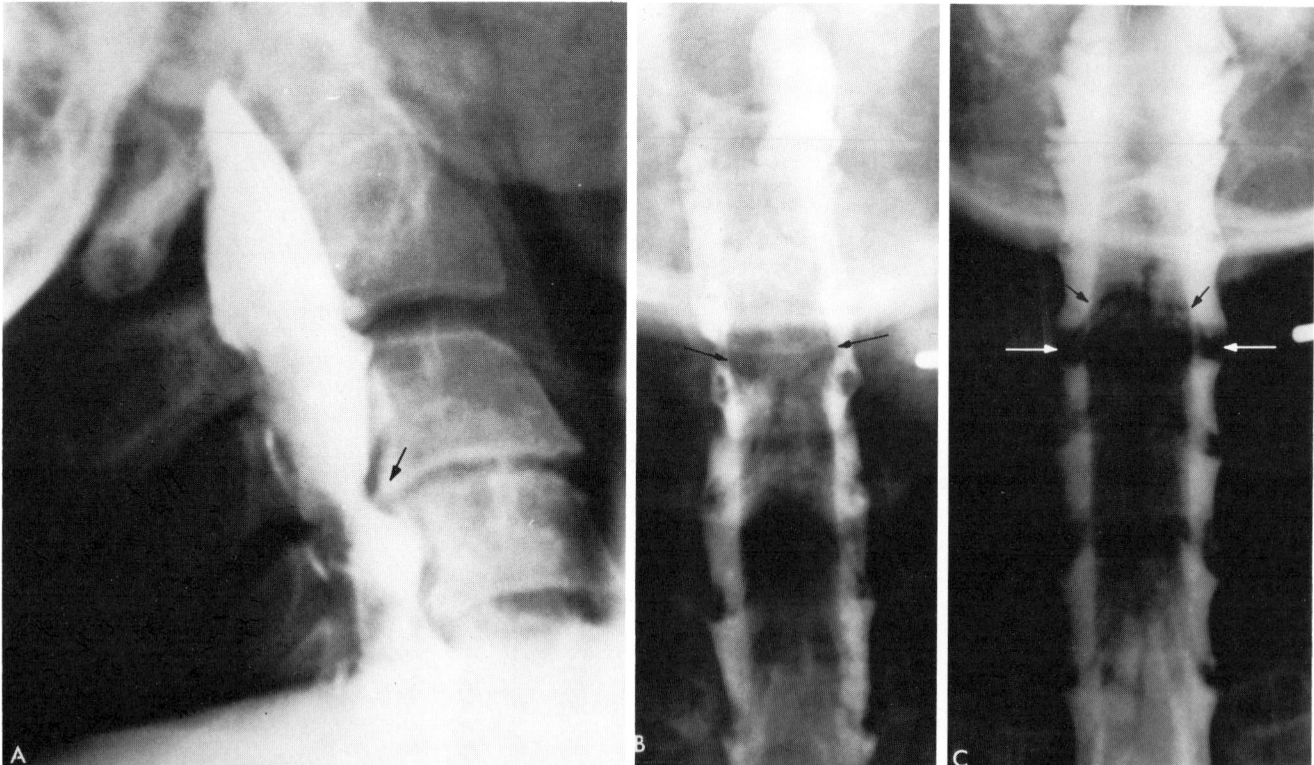

Figure 14–45. Hypertrophic cervical spurs creating myelopathy. **A,** Hypertrophic spurs can be seen impressing upon the subarachnoid space at the C3-C4 intervertebral disc level (arrow). **B,** There is widening of the cervical spinal cord from the anterior spurs compressing the spinal cord in the narrowed canal (arrows). **C,** In another patient, localized widening of the cervical spinal cord (black arrows) results from hypertrophic spurs, creating a lucent horizontal "cervical bar" (white arrows).

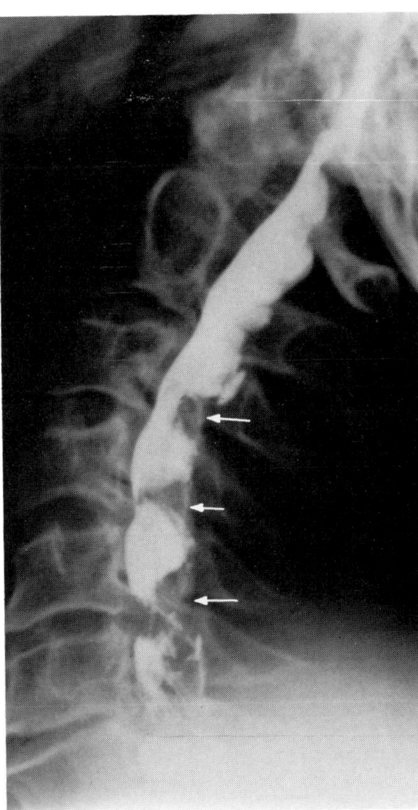

Figure 14–46. Hypertrophic ligamentum flavum. The posterior impressions on the contrast column are due to the elongated and hypertrophied ligamentum flavum (arrows).

mental stenosis or in a normal canal. It relates to hypertrophic ligaments and degenerative changes of the posterior articular processes. In this form of the disease, a single lumbar level is commonly affected, although multiple levels may be altered. In either developmental or degenerative spinal stenosis, a simple bulging of the intervertebral disc may be sufficient to produce symptoms and a herniated intervertebral disc may lead to acute and severe neurologic deficits.

Kirkaldy-Willis and associates[58] refer to an article by Saks and Frankel in 1900 in which the first case of lumbar stenosis is described in the medical literature. In this case, laminectomy revealed a markedly thickened lamina, and the patient's pain was relieved following osseous resection.

Pain is the most frequent complaint in patients with spinal stenosis. This pain, which is exacerbated by walking and relieved by rest, may be confused with intermittent arterial claudication.[59, 60] The character of the pain suggests that with exercise and erect posture, there is protrusion of the intervertebral disc and compression of the arterial or venous blood supply, leading to intermittent claudication of the peripheral nerves to the lower extremity as they exit the neural foramina. Occasionally, the pain may be localized to the back, the buttocks, or the thighs. Sensory deficits and muscle wasting are not prominent.

Radiographic examination of the stenotic lumbar spine may not be rewarding, and subtle alterations require careful evaluation of spinal dimensions. On the lateral roentgenogram, measurements should be made from the posterior border of the vertebral body to the junction of the superior and inferior articular facets (Figs. 14–15 and 14–47). In order to correct the radiographic magnification, the calculated measurements should be multiplied by 0.77 to arrive at the true anteroposterior diameter of the lumbar canal. Eisenstein[61] determined that the lower normal limit of the anteroposterior diameter of the lumbar canal is 15 mm; no significant difference between men and women was detected. This investigator noted that measurements of the transverse diameter of the spinal canal (the interpedicular distance) were not necessary.

In the patient with lumbar stenosis, myelography can be quite difficult. Because of the narrowness of the subarachnoid space, bloody taps are not infrequent. Furthermore, even with fluoroscopic monitoring, it is commonly difficult to localize the injected contrast medium because of the marked narrowing of the spinal canal, and difficulty in interpretation is further accentuated by the fragmen-

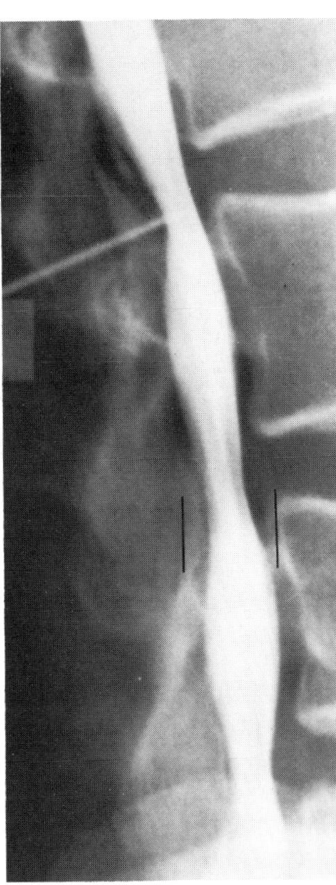

Figure 14–47. Lumbar stenosis. Measurements from a lumbar myelogram corrected for radiographic magnification indicate a narrow anteroposterior diameter of the lumbar canal, 12 mm wide (minimum normal = 15 mm). This is compatible with congenital lumbar spinal stenosis.

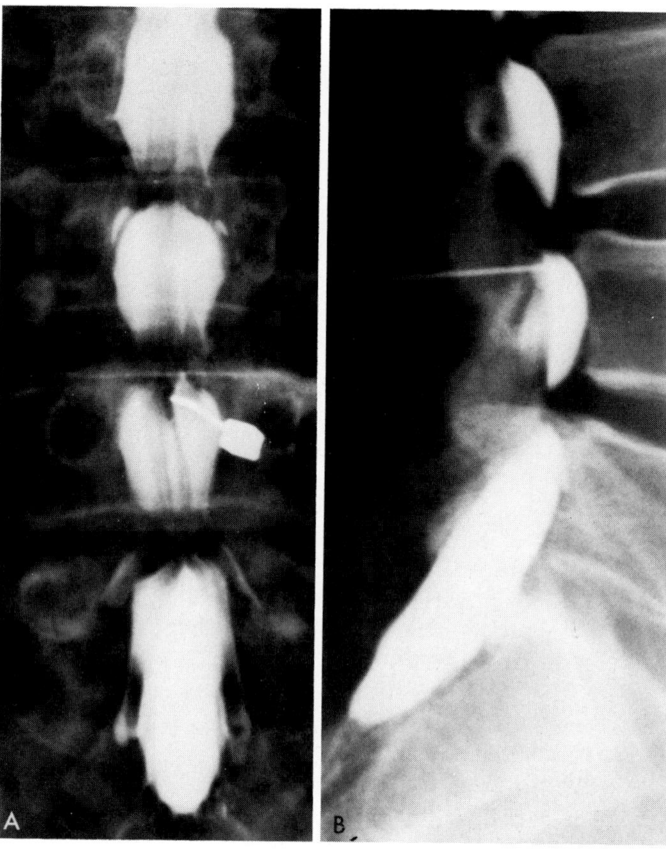

Figure 14–48. Lumbar stenosis. **A,** Anteroposterior film from an iophendylate myelogram shows separation of the contrast column at each intervertebral disc level owing to intervertebral disc protrusion or herniation superimposed upon a narrowed anteroposterior diameter of the lumbar canal. **B,** Lateral film of the same patient demonstrates the separation of the iophendylate column at each of the intervertebral disc levels. Note the lack of hypertrophic osteophytes. This is indicative of the diffuse, congenital form of lumbar spinal stenosis.

tation of the column of contrast material due to the protruding intervertebral discs and hypertrophied bones and ligaments (Figs. 14–41 and 14–48). Crowding of the nerve roots within this narrow canal creates a "streaky" appearance, which may be mistaken for arachnoiditis. Measurements of the anteroposterior diameter of the subarachnoid space should be accomplished with the patient upright, allowing full distention from the hydrostatic pressure of the contrast-filled lumbar thecal sac.

If myelography proves to be inadequate or technically unfeasible, epidural venography may be the next examination of choice. In fact, in our institution, epidural venography is the initial procedure if there is a clinical suspicion of spinal stenosis. In spinal stenosis, the anterior internal vertebral veins are interrupted at multiple intervertebral disc levels (Figs. 14–49 and 14–50). Computed tomography can also be used to delineate the true cross-sectional anatomy of the vertebral canal (Fig. 14–50). With this modality, direct measurement can be made of the anteroposterior distance of the spinal canal, its shape assessed, and the thickened laminae and protruding intervertebral discs visualized. With metrizamide in the subarachnoid space, or with special computer programing, the hypertrophied ligaments can also be seen with this technique[40] (Fig. 14–50).

Lumbar spinal stenosis frequently accompanies certain conditions, such as achondroplasia (Fig. 14–50).

The cervical spine is frequently narrowed in its anteroposterior diameter by various degenerative changes, such as osteophytes and hypertrophic posterior facets and laminae.[62, 63] These changes cause impingement on the cervical spinal cord, leading to a variety of symptoms, including radiculopathies, the Brown-Séquard syndrome, or findings simulating multiple sclerosis or lateral sclerosis.

Traumatic Disorders

Hematoma. Following an acute traumatic event, neurologic deficit may result from spinal cord or nerve root damage. The most serious of the injuries to the spinal cord is transection. This usually occurs with vertebral canal fracture and dislocation. Routine radiography and tomography may demonstrate bony fragments within the spinal canal (Fig. 14–29). Although there may be no demonstrable bony fragments following trauma, neurologic deficits can result from intramedullary or extradural hematoma formation. Spinal cord transection usually occurs with bone and ligament disruption. An intramedullary hematoma is termed a hematomyelia. More commonly, hematomas are located in the

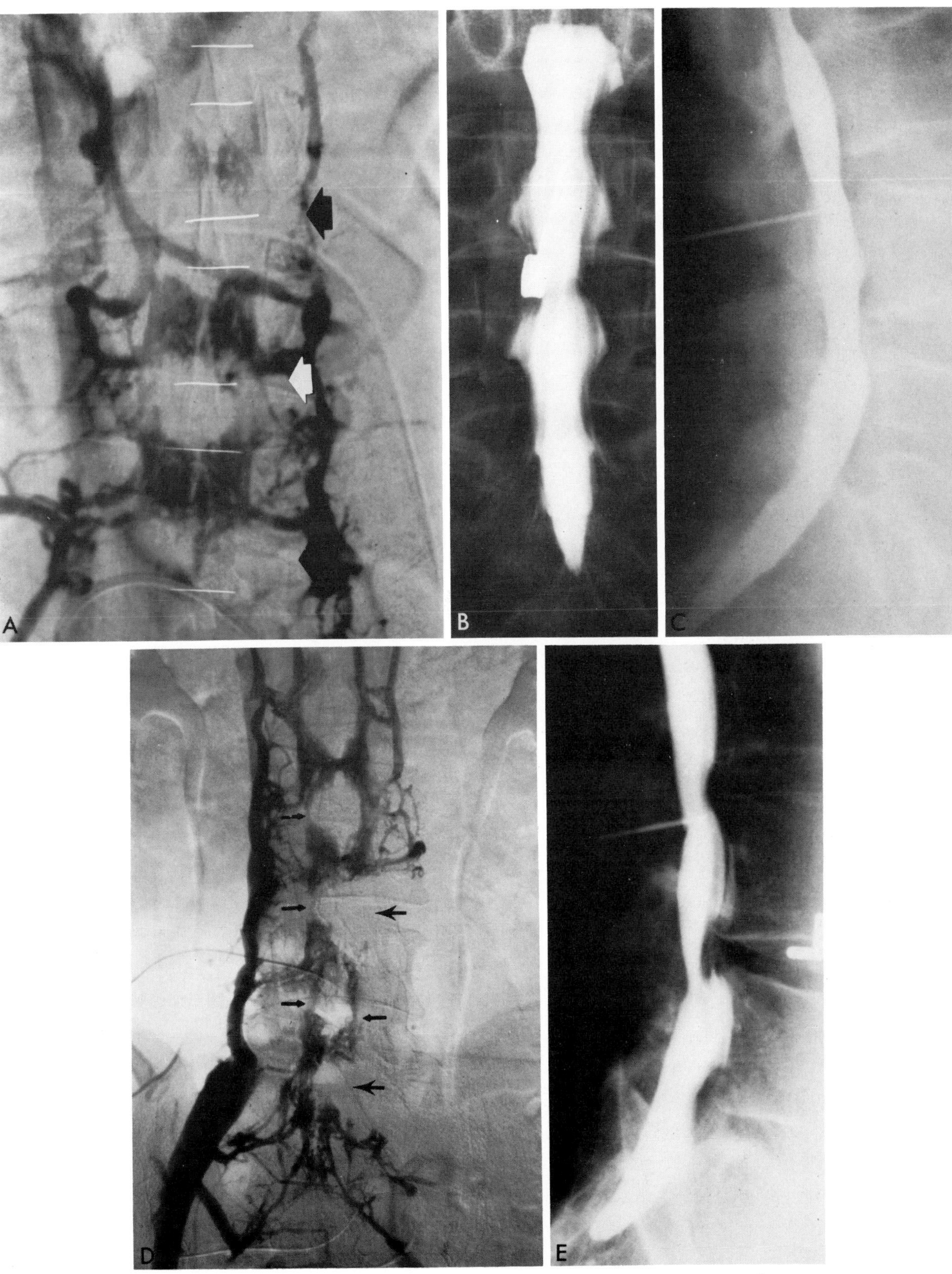

Figure 14–49. *Lumbar stenosis.* **A,** *Subtraction film from a lumbar venogram demonstrates obstruction at all intervertebral disc levels in a patient with lumbar spinal stenosis. The venous plexuses at the vertebral body levels (arrows) not only are present but also are hypertrophic as they act as collateral pathways.* **B,** *Anteroposterior film of the myelogram in the same patient demonstrates bilateral impressions on the subarachnoid space at each of the intervertebral disc levels.* **C,** *The lateral myelographic film does not show anterior discal impressions.* **D,** *In another patient with lumbar spinal stenosis, there is venous obstruction at L3-L4 and L5-S1 on the left (large arrows) with thinning of the veins at L2-L3, L3-L4, L4-L5 on the right and L4-L5 on the left (small arrows).* **E,** *Lumbar myelogram demonstrates at least three of these levels to be abnormal, with marked impressions upon the subarachnoid space. The anteroposterior diameter of the spinal canal is narrowed, indicating lumbar spinal stenosis, a situation that makes the patient extremely sensitive to intervertebral disc protrusion and herniation.*

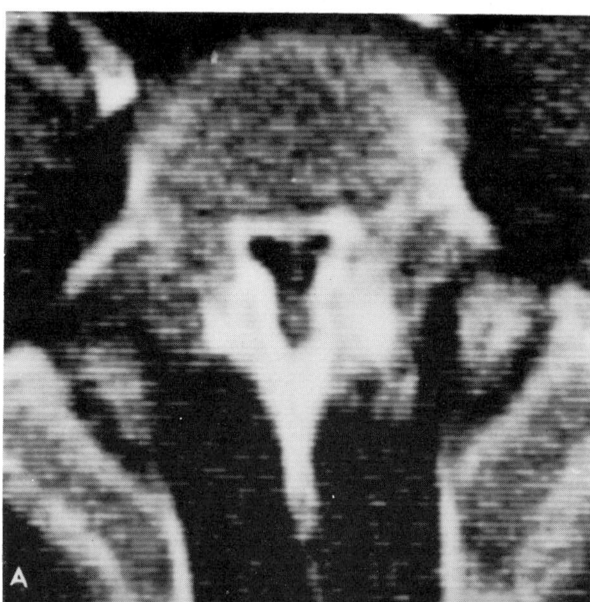

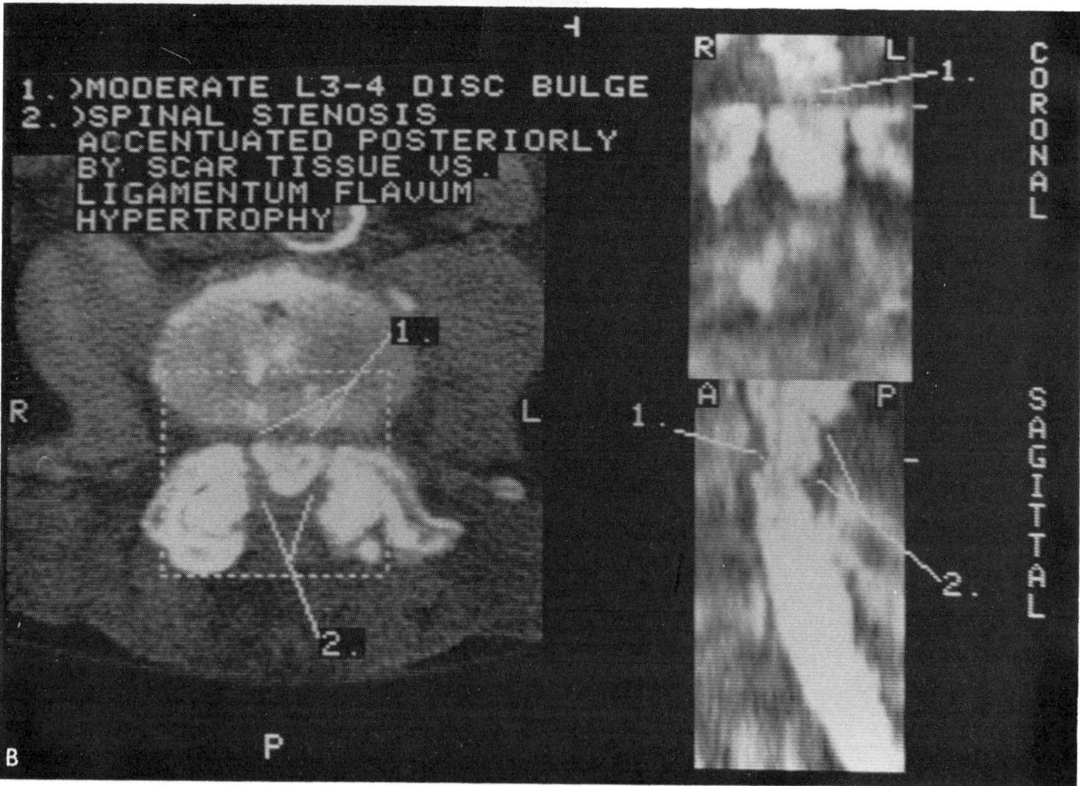

Figure 14–50. *Spinal stenosis.* **A,** *CT scan of a patient with achondroplasia demonstrates a misshapen spinal canal due to shortened pedicles and thickened laminae.* **B,** *A metrizamide CT scan from another patient reveals localized (acquired) spinal stenosis. (Courtesy of Dr. William Glenn, Long Beach Memorial Hospital, Long Beach, California.)*

extradural space, compressing the spinal cord or the nerve roots of the cauda equina[64] (Figs. 14–51 to 14–53). Occasionally, subdural or extradural hematomas may develop from lumbar punctures, particularly in patients with bleeding diatheses, such as leukemia, or in individuals on anticoagulant (even aspirin) therapy.[65] On rare occasions, subdural hematomas may result from falls or other blunt trauma[66] (Figs. 14–54).

Symptoms may be quite dramatic, such as quadriplegia or paraplegia, or more subtle, such as mild motor and sensory deficits. If the cause of the symptoms is not recognized early, the deficits may become permanent despite surgical decompression.

At myelography, hematomas can produce total blocks or mild extrinsic compression. The intramedullary hematoma appears as an intramedullary mass. If it is not evacuated early, the hematoma may become liquefied and cystic in nature.[67] Subsequently, the cord may atrophy[68] (Fig. 14–55). The extradural hematoma usually extends over several vertebral segments, an appearance that is not encountered with herniated intervertebral discs. The resulting myelographic findings must be differentiated from

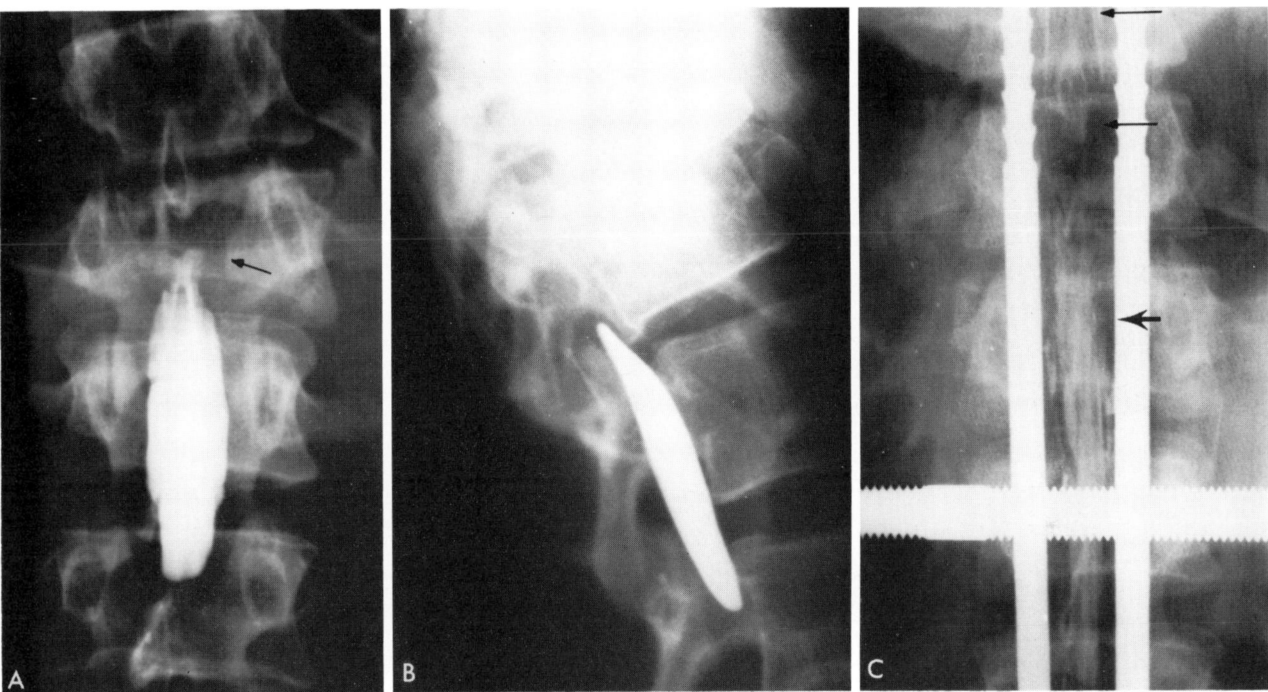

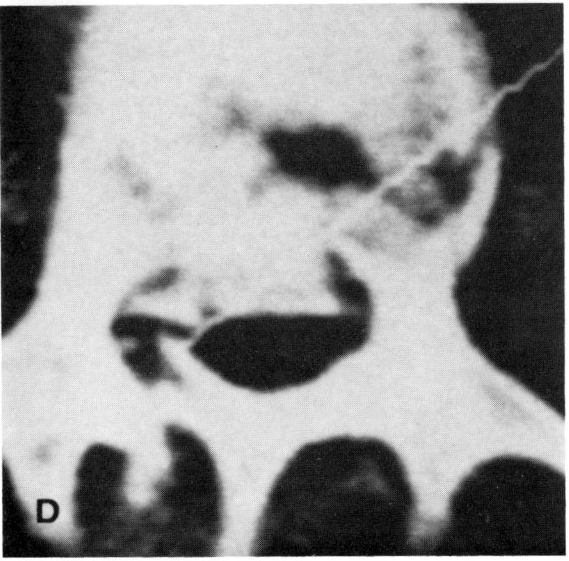

Figure 14–51. *Spinal fracture. A 22 year old man involved in a motor vehicle accident presented with right leg weakness and acute neurologic bladder dysfunction. Myelogram was performed to determine the degree of compromise of the spinal canal.* **A, B,** *There is a total block of the iophendylate column at the inferior margin of the fractured L1 vertebral body. In addition, there is a lamina burst fracture on the left (arrow) with spreading of the pedicles seen on the anteroposterior projection.* **C,** *Postoperative metrizamide myelogram demonstrates contrast medium overlying the fracture at L1 (large arrow). There remains some compromise of the subarachnoid space at T11 and T12 (small arrows), presumably due to residual epidural hematoma. The patient had a total neurologic recovery.* **D,** *A CT scan from another patient demonstrates a burst fracture with a vertebral body fragment displaced posteriorly into the spinal canal. Lamina and pedicle fractures allow for anterior slippage of the posterior neural arch. (Courtesy of Dr. William Glenn, Long Beach Memorial Hospital, Long Beach, California.)*

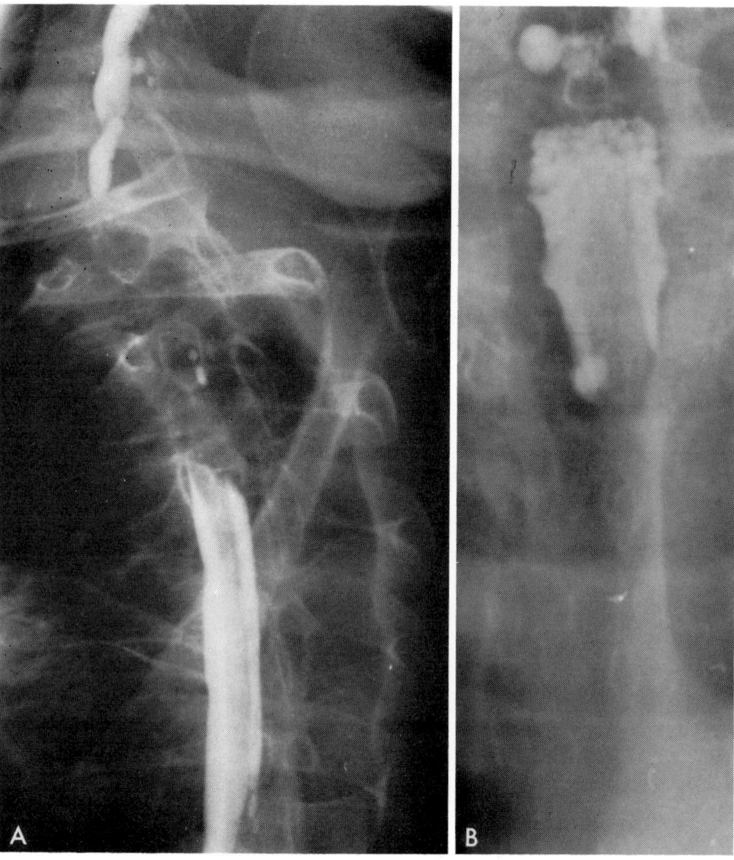

Figure 14–52. Epidural hematoma. *A middle-aged man on anticoagulant therapy sustained a fall, presenting with bilateral lower leg weakness and sensory deficits.* **A,** *Iophendylate introduced from below outlines an incomplete block at the level of T3.* **B,** *In the upright position, the contrast medium stops just above the T3 vertebral body. Also note the deviation of the iophendylate column (subarachnoid space) to the left (away from the right-sided pedicles) by the extensive extradural hematoma.*

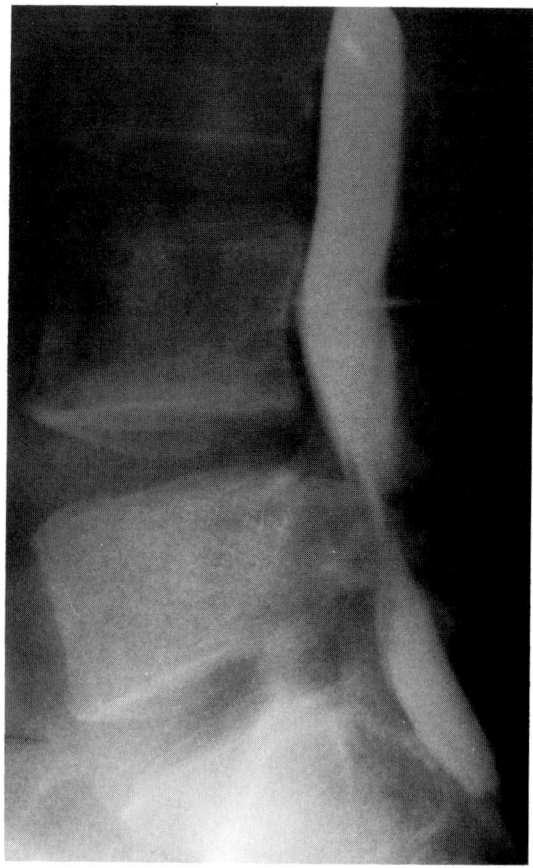

Figure 14–53. Epidural hematoma. *Patient with a bleeding diathesis owing to leukemia had neurologic deficits of the lower extremity following a lumbar puncture. Myelogram demonstrates marked narrowing of the subarachnoid space owing to a large hematoma.*

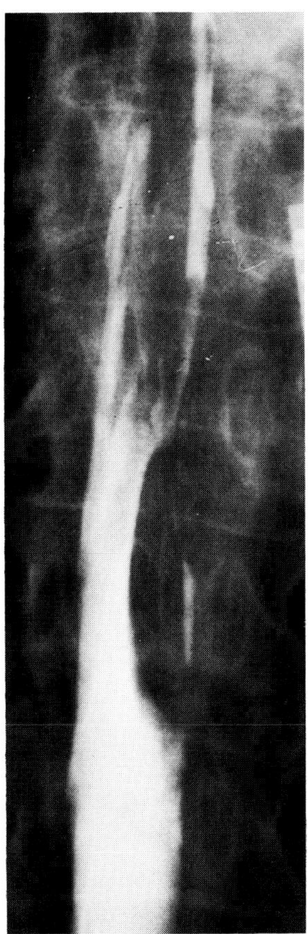

Figure 14–54. *Subdural hematoma. An unusual subdural hematoma resulting from trauma in a patient with ankylosing spondylitis. Note the sharper transition zones of this lesion compared with epidural lesions. (From Sokoloff J, et al: Radiology 120:116, 1976.)*

other extradural masses, e.g., lymphoma and infection.

MENINGOCELE. Traumatic meningoceles (also called pseudomeningoceles) frequently occur in the cervical region. They are the result of a severe force applied to the shoulder and the neck. The position of the arm at the time of injury will determine the type of neurologic deficit that becomes evident. An Erb-Duchenne paralysis, which occurs when the arm is in adduction at the time of trauma, is due to C5-C6 nerve root avulsions. If the injured arm is in a position of abduction, the lower cervical roots (C7-T1) are injured, creating a Klumpke paralysis involving the small muscles of the hand and wrist, as well as an ulnar sensory deficit.[69] After this severance, the nerve roots retract and atrophy. The resultant traumatic meningocele represents an outpouching of the subarachnoid space into the neural foramen, which contains the nerve roots.

Plain film examination may be entirely normal in these instances, although associated fractures of the spinal column can occur. Myelography demonstrates diverticula of the subarachnoid space that do not contain nerve roots (Fig. 14–56). Extensive and irregular outpouching can be evident, and the "traumatic meningocele" may dissect into the neck.[70] Similar injuries may tear the dura and create a fistulous tract extending from the subarachnoid space to the pleura, the extrapleural space, or the mediastinum[71] (Fig. 14–57).

Postsurgical extradural "meningoceles" may result from inadvertent violation of the dura. These may have a complete meningeal covering or a thin fibrous pseudomembrane. These small meningoceles may remain contained within the spinal canal, or, on rare occasions, may enlarge, leading to symptomatic compression of the subarachnoid space and the spinal cord (Fig. 14–58).

EPIDERMOID CYST. Acquired epidermoid sequestration cysts are the result of epidermoid tissue being introduced into the subarachnoid space during lumbar puncture. This complication occurs almost exclusively when open spinal needles, rather than those with occluding obturators, are utilized.

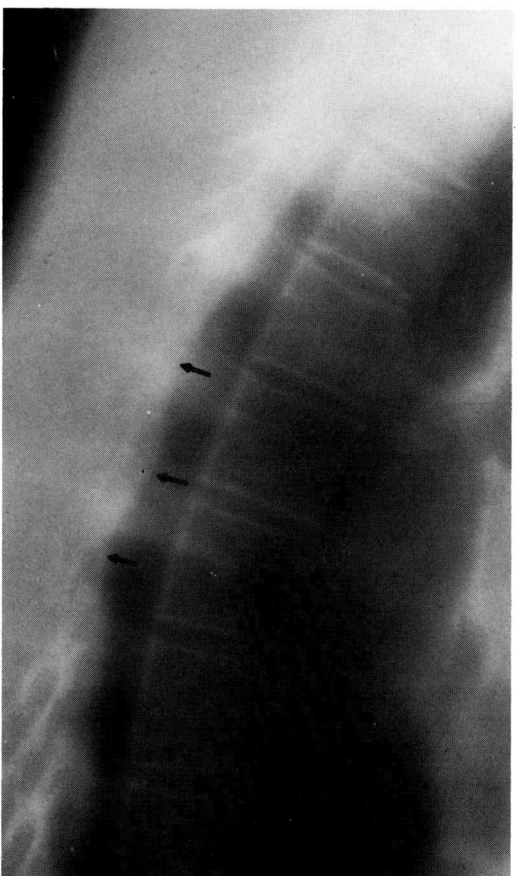

Figure 14–55. *Posttraumatic spinal cord atrophy. A gas myelogram reveals marked atrophy of the thoracic spinal cord in a patient who had sustained extensive trauma 20 years earlier. Lower limb weakness and sensory deficits were present. Note the narrowed and wavy spinal cord shadow (arrows).*

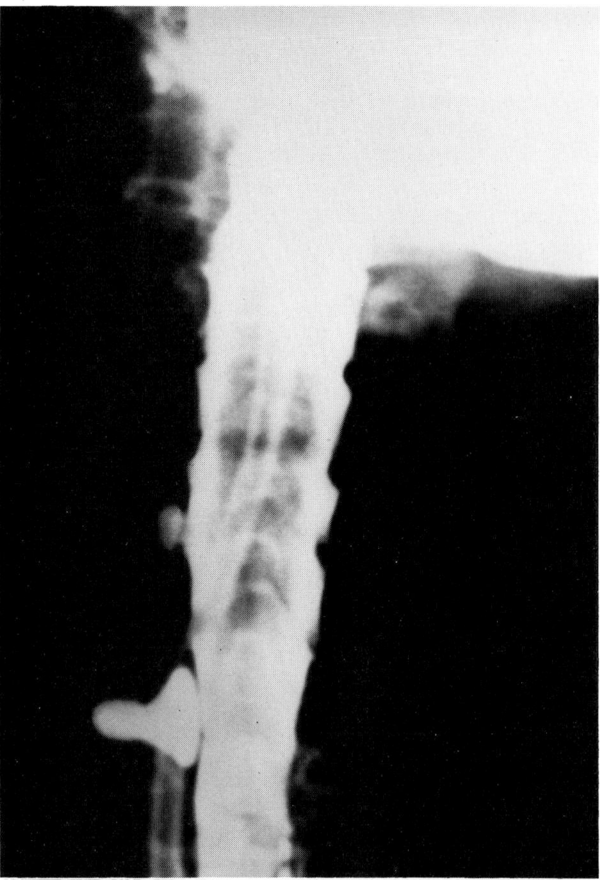

Figure 14–56. Posttraumatic meningoceles. A myelogram in a patient who had had previous neck and shoulder trauma demonstrates extension of the subarachnoid space laterally into the neural foramina, yet no exiting nerve roots are present in these traumatic meningoceles.

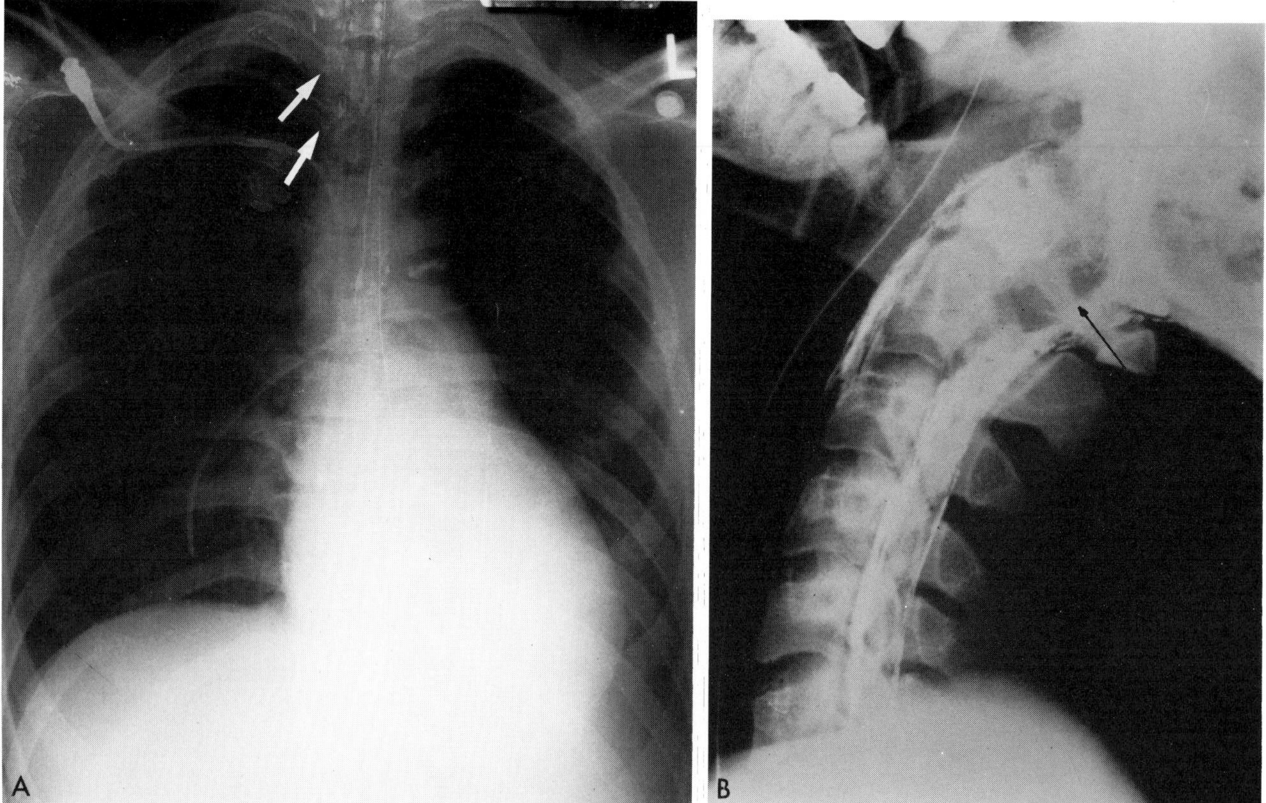

Figure 14–57. Dural tear. **A,** Single anteroposterior chest roentgenogram in a patient who had sustained severe trauma in an automotive accident reveals iophendylate (arrows) dissecting down the soft tissues of the neck. There are bilateral pleural effusions, greater on the left side, proved to be cerebrospinal fluid secondary to a sinus tract originating from the cervical tear of the subarachnoid space and dura. **B,** Lateral film from the iophendylate myelogram demonstrates dissection of the contrast medium from the spinal canal into the soft tissues of the neck, and subsequently through a rent in the pleura. Note the extradural hematoma behind the dens (arrow).

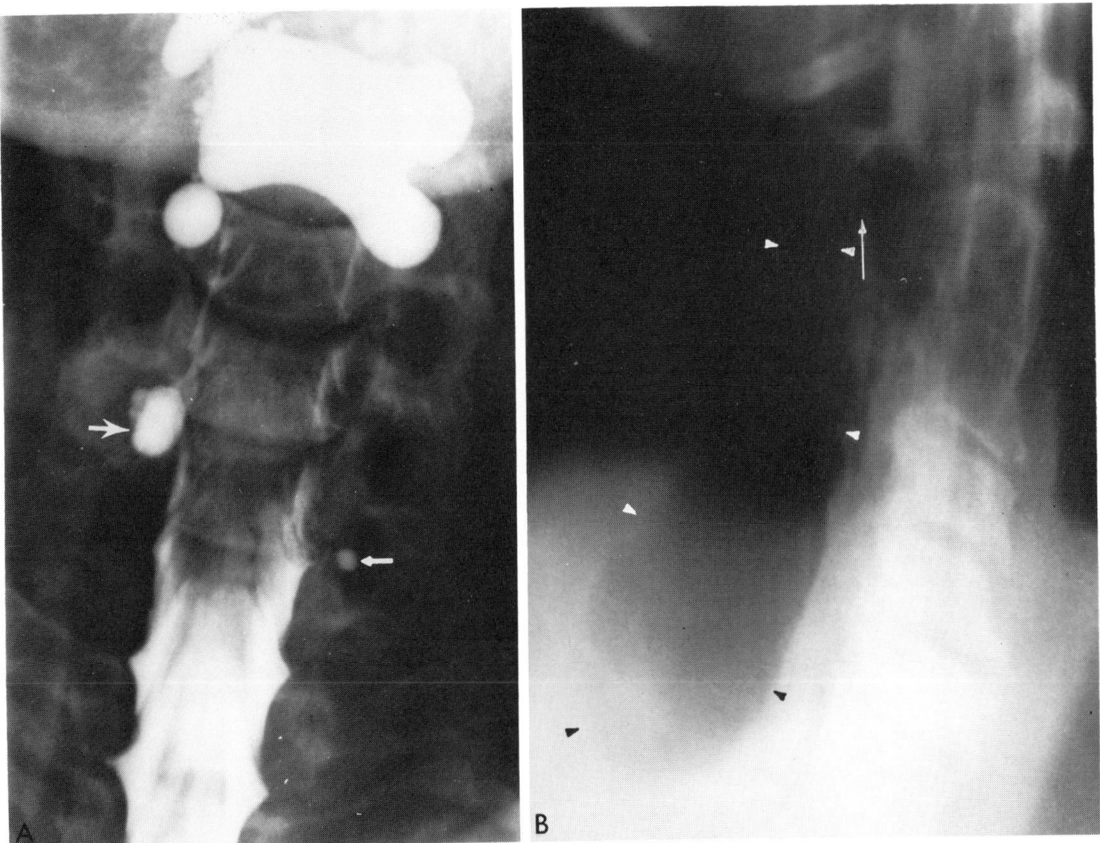

Figure 14–58. Postoperative "meningocele." Several years following extensive laminectomy, this middle-aged man developed myelopathy. **A,** There is apparent expansion of the spinal cord due to its compression by a posterior mass. The irregular collection of iophendylate represents a postoperative meningocele. Incidentally noted are several posttraumatic meningoceles (arrows). **B,** On a gas myelogram, the large posterior meningocele (arrowheads) compressing the subarachnoid space can be seen. Note the complete removal of posterior bony elements. The rent in the dura mater is at C1-C2 (arrow).

Myelography reveals masses that are adherent to the arachnoid and nerve roots at the lumbar puncture site.

Neoplastic Disorders

General Features. All mass lesions involving the spinal cord and canal are categorized as occurring in one of the three anatomic spaces: intramedullary, intradural-extramedullary, and extradural. Intramedullary lesions arise within the spinal cord between the foramen magnum and the conus medullaris. Intradural-extramedullary lesions occur between the outer dura and the neural tissue, and for all intents and purposes can be considered subarachnoid. Extradural lesions occur outside the surrounding dura mater and may extend to the bone and paraspinal tissues. Both primary and secondary benign and malignant neoplasms may involve the spinal cord and canal. Intramedullary lesions account for 10 per cent of tumors, intradural-extramedullary masses for approximately 60 per cent, and extradural tumors for approximately 25 per cent. Metastatic disease is the most common of the neoplastic masses (Table 14–4).

Primary tumors of the spinal cord are considerably less frequent than those of the brain. This may reflect the fact that the neural mass of the cord is one seventh that of the brain. The majority of tumors arising in the spinal canal develop from the meninges or nerve root coverings (meningiomas and neurinoma). Primary tumors of the spinal cord itself account for approximately 10 per cent of all tumors of this region.

The clinical diagnosis of a spinal tumor can be difficult. Symptoms are often nonspecific. Neurologic deficits are more readily apparent in the adult than in the child. Pain, sensory deficits, weakness or sphincter incontinence may bring the adult patient to the physician at an early stage of the disease process. In children, the early signs of intraspinal tumors may not be obvious to the parents nor disruptive to the patient's activities. Rectal and bladder sphincter dysfunction are obscured in infancy and early childhood, and sensory deficits are easily overlooked until quite profound. Abnormally slow de-

Table 14–4
TUMORS AND OTHER MASSES

Intramedullary	Intradural-Extramedullary	Extradural
Glioma	Meningioma*	Metastatic Carcinoma
Ependymoma*	Neurinoma*	Bronchogenic
Astrocytoma*	Neurofibroma*	Prostatic
Oligodendroglioma	Dermoid	Mammary
Spongioblastoma	Epidermoid	Lymphoma
Medulloblastoma	Lipoma	Lymphosarcoma
Vascular Malformation	Metastatic	Sarcoma
Hemangioblastoma	Glioma	Chordoma
Arteriovenous malformation*	Medulloblastoma	Teratoma
Cavernous angioma	Ependymoma	Meningioma
Angioma	Glioblastoma multiforme	Neurinoma
Varices	Pinealoma	Fibroma
Cyst	Metastatic or direct extension of carcinoma	Lipoma
Syringomyelia*		Dermoid
Hydromyelia		Vascular Lesion
Mesenchymal Tumor		
Fibroma		
Lipoma*		
Dermoid		
Teratoma		
Neurinoma		
Metastatic Carcinoma		
Primary and Secondary* Lymphoma		

*Most common.

velopment (e.g., inability to sit or walk) or pain may be the first noticeable manifestation of central nervous system disease. Persistent neck and back pain and stiffness, and progressive scoliosis, should be fully evaluated. An elevated cerebrospinal fluid protein level or cell count mandates a full neurologic and neuroradiologic work-up.

Routine radiologic findings of neoplasm in the child may include expansion of the spinal canal, with widening of the interpedicular and anteroposterior diameters (Figs. 14–22 and 14–59 to 14–61) (Table 14–5). There may be accompanying erosion of the vertebral bodies or the posterior neural elements. Scoliosis (Figs. 14–60 and 14–61) and osteoblastic or osteolytic lesions with or without an associated paraspinal mass are additional plain film findings. Associated spina bifida or tumor calcification can rarely be found.[72]

In the adult, osseous erosion, especially destruction of the vertebral pedicles, is most commonly encountered (Fig. 14–62). On occasion, a paraspinal mass may accompany the destructive process. With slowly growing masses, there may be expansion of the spinal canal or associated scalloping of the posterior surface of the vertebral bodies. Gradually enlarging nerve sheath tumors may widen the neural foramina as they extend from the spinal canal (Fig. 14–63).

The distribution of tumors affecting the spinal cord varies with the age of the patient.[73] Most tumors occur between the ages of 20 and 60 years in both men and women. In childhood, there is an increased incidence of congenital lesions involving the spinal cord, predominantly in the cervical, lumbar, and lumbosacral regions. These lesions include those that are associated with the dysraphic spinal canal: dermoids, epidermoids, lipomas, hamartomas, teratomas, and neurenteric cysts. Syringomyelia, hydromyelia, chordoma, neurofibromatosis, neurofibromas, and arteriovenous malformations are additional developmental lesions that are not associated with dysraphic cords. Gliomas do occur in children, but fortunately are uncommon. Metastases from within and outside the central nervous system, leukemia, or primary sarcoma may occasionally be encountered.

In the adult, over half the tumors affecting the spinal cord occur in the thoracic region. These lesions are most frequently metastatic in nature, although meningiomas, neurilemomas, gliomas, and lymphomas are encountered.

EXTRADURAL LESIONS. The vast majority of extradural tumors are malignant, usually metastatic carcinoma. Lymphosarcoma, Hodgkin's disease, and leukemic infiltrates are the next most frequent tumors, with the rare primary sarcomas accounting for a very small percentage of these lesions. These

Text continued on page 476

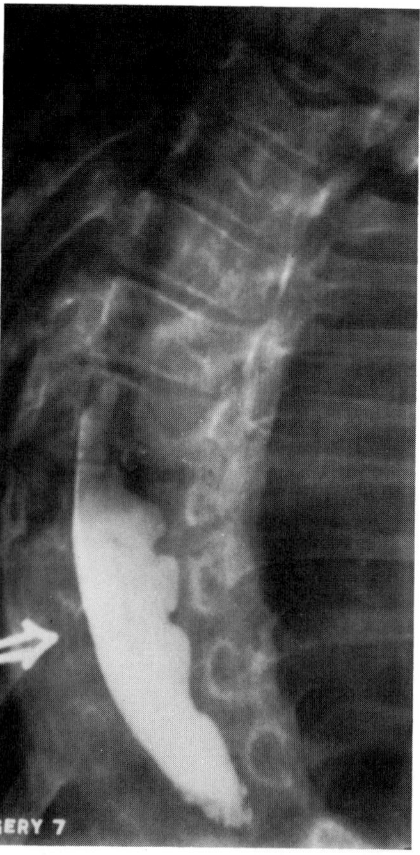

Figure 14–59. *Spinal canal expansion. There is marked widening of the thoracic vertebrae and total obstruction of the iophendylate column due to a large intramedullary spinal glioma. Also note the marked scoliosis.*

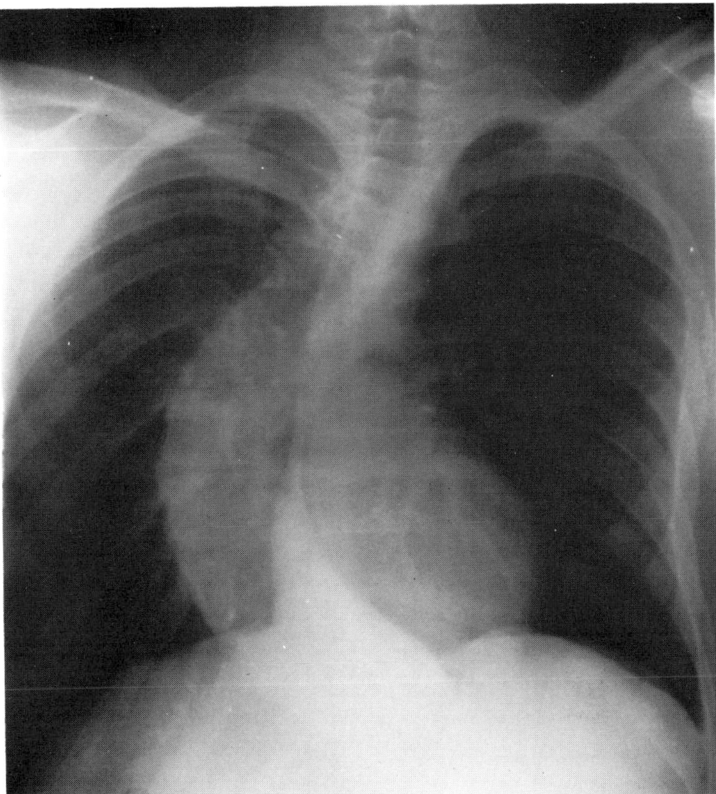

Figure 14–60. Scoliosis. Marked scoliosis and widening of the vertebral canal are noted in a patient with an intramedullary glioma.

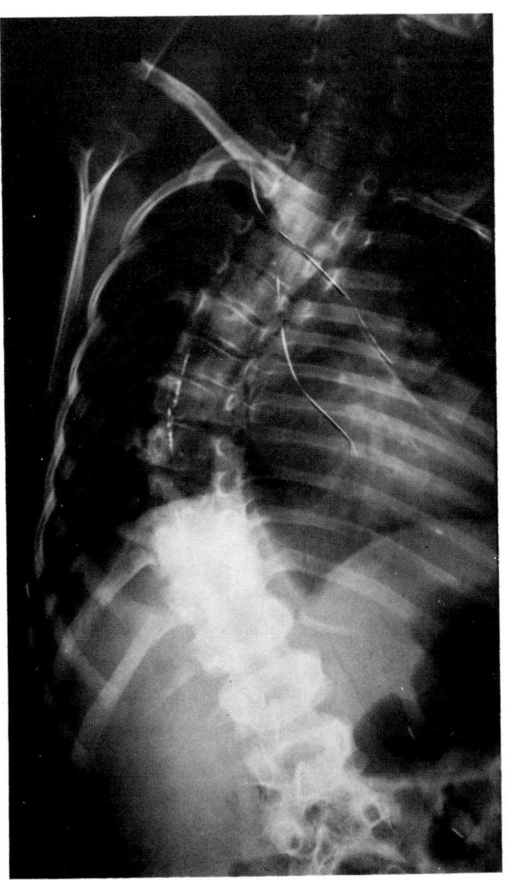

Figure 14–61. Scoliosis and spinal canal expansion. The marked widening and scoliosis of the cervicothoracic spine are due to an intramedullary glioma.

Table 14–5
CAUSES OF WIDE VERTEBRAL CANAL

Syringomyelia-hydromyelia
Meningomyelocele
Diastematomyelia
Neurofibromatosis
Intraspinal tumor
(Aneurysms, nerve sheath tumors, and ectatic vessels may enlarge the neural foramina)

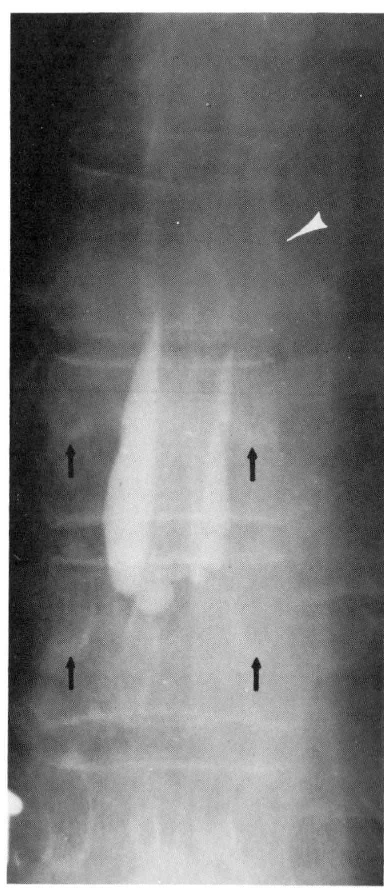

Figure 14–62. *Vertebral destruction. The pedicles and vertebral body of T4 were destroyed by metastatic renal cell carcinoma (arrowhead). (Arrows indicate pedicles present on other vertebral bodies.) The subarachnoid space is deviated by the epidural tumor, indicating an epidural location for the mass.*

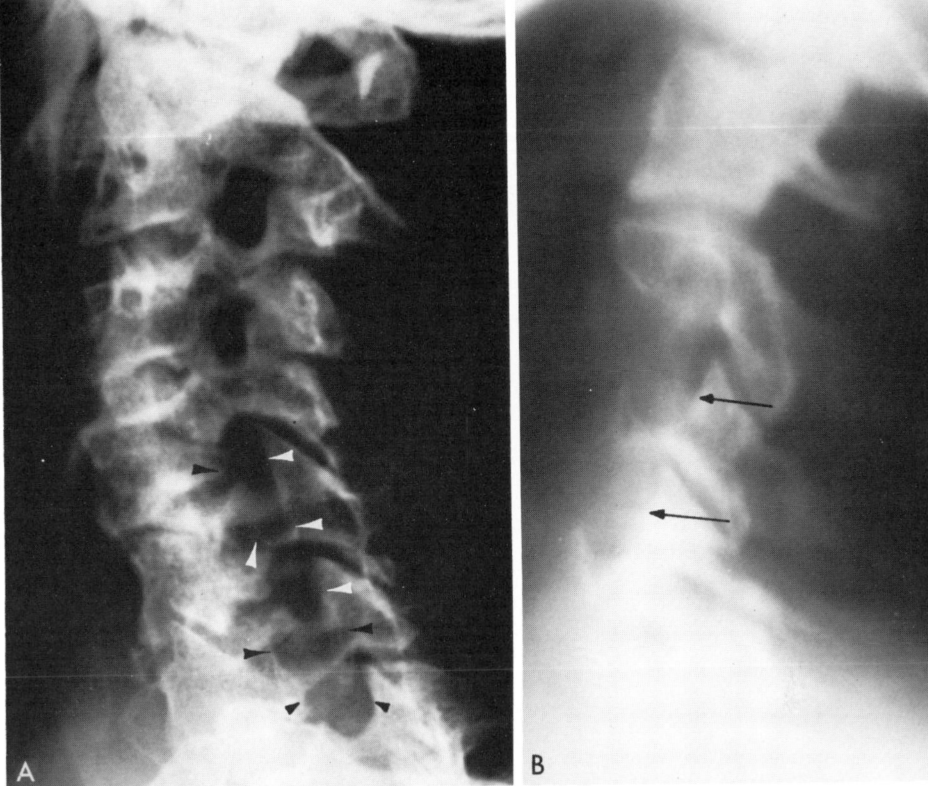

Figure 14–63. *Neural foramina enlargement.* **A,** *Oblique plain film of the cervical spine in a patient with neurofibromatosis reveals enlargement of several neural foramina (arrowheads).* **B,** *Tomography in another patient with the same disease demonstrates the enlargement of the neural foramina (arrows), with complete erosion of some of the bony elements.*

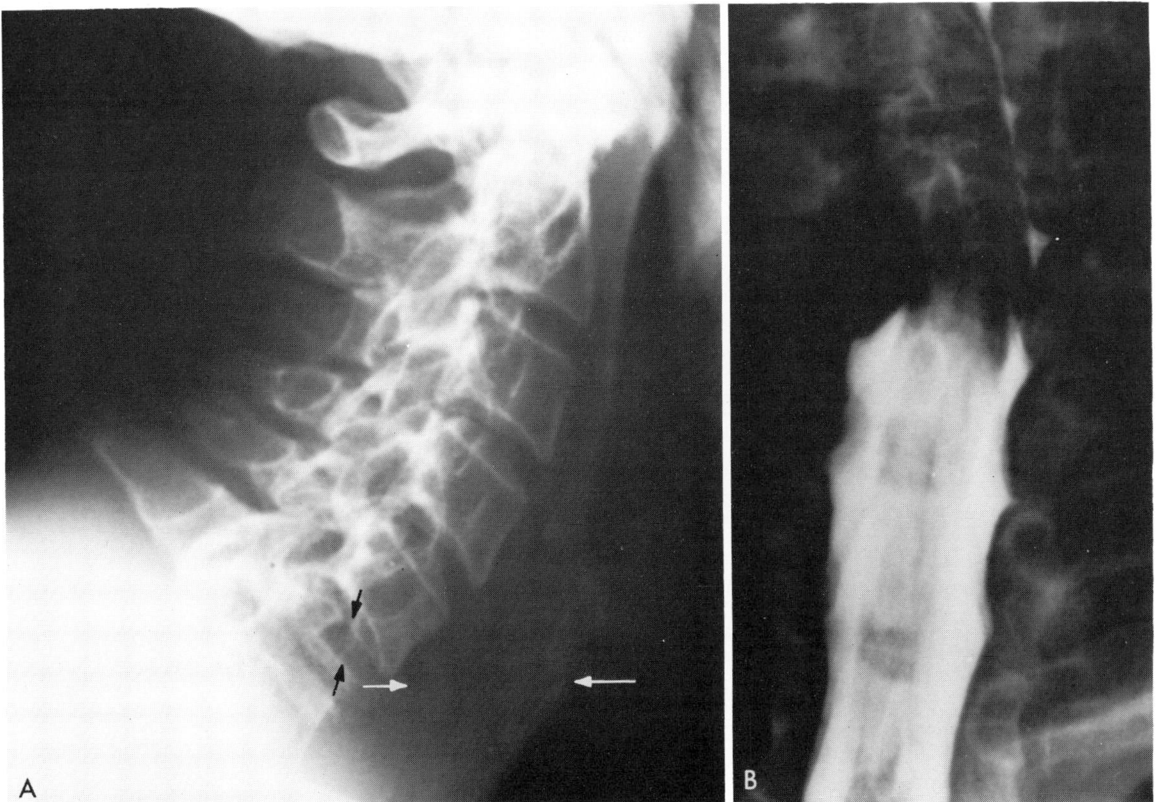

Figure 14–64. *Prevertebral mass.* **A,** *A soft tissue mass (white arrows) is present between the anteriorly displaced trachea and the anterior vertebral borders. Note the bone destruction (black arrows) of the sixth cervical vertebral body.* **B,** *At myelography, there is a partial block owing to invasion by this squamous cell carcinoma originating in the soft tissues of the neck.*

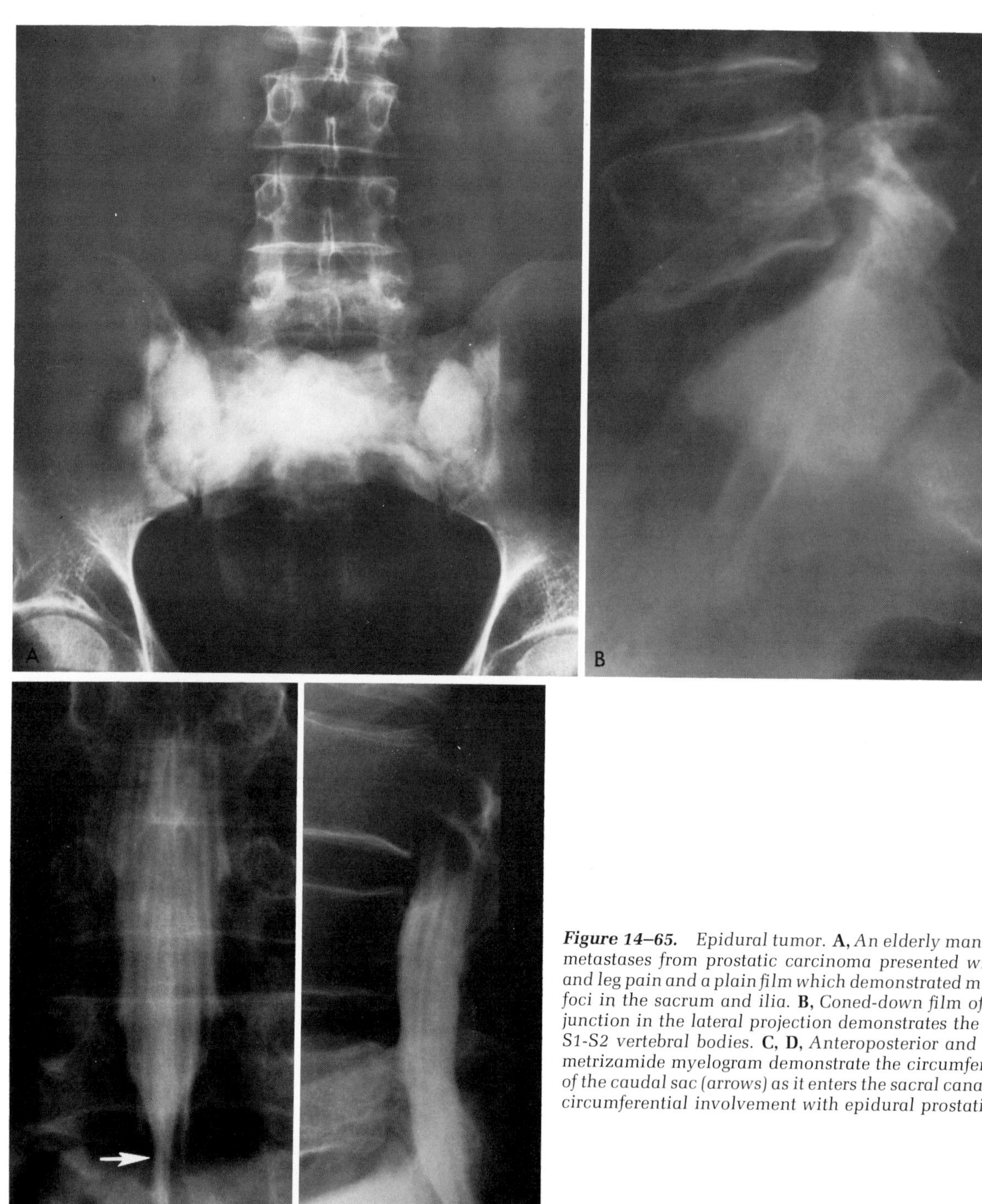

Figure 14–65. Epidural tumor. **A**, *An elderly man with osteoblastic metastases from prostatic carcinoma presented with atypical back and leg pain and a plain film which demonstrated multiple metastatic foci in the sacrum and ilia.* **B**, *Coned-down film of the lumbosacral junction in the lateral projection demonstrates the markedly blastic S1-S2 vertebral bodies.* **C**, **D**, *Anteroposterior and lateral films of a metrizamide myelogram demonstrate the circumferential narrowing of the caudal sac (arrows) as it enters the sacral canal. This was due to circumferential involvement with epidural prostatic carcinoma.*

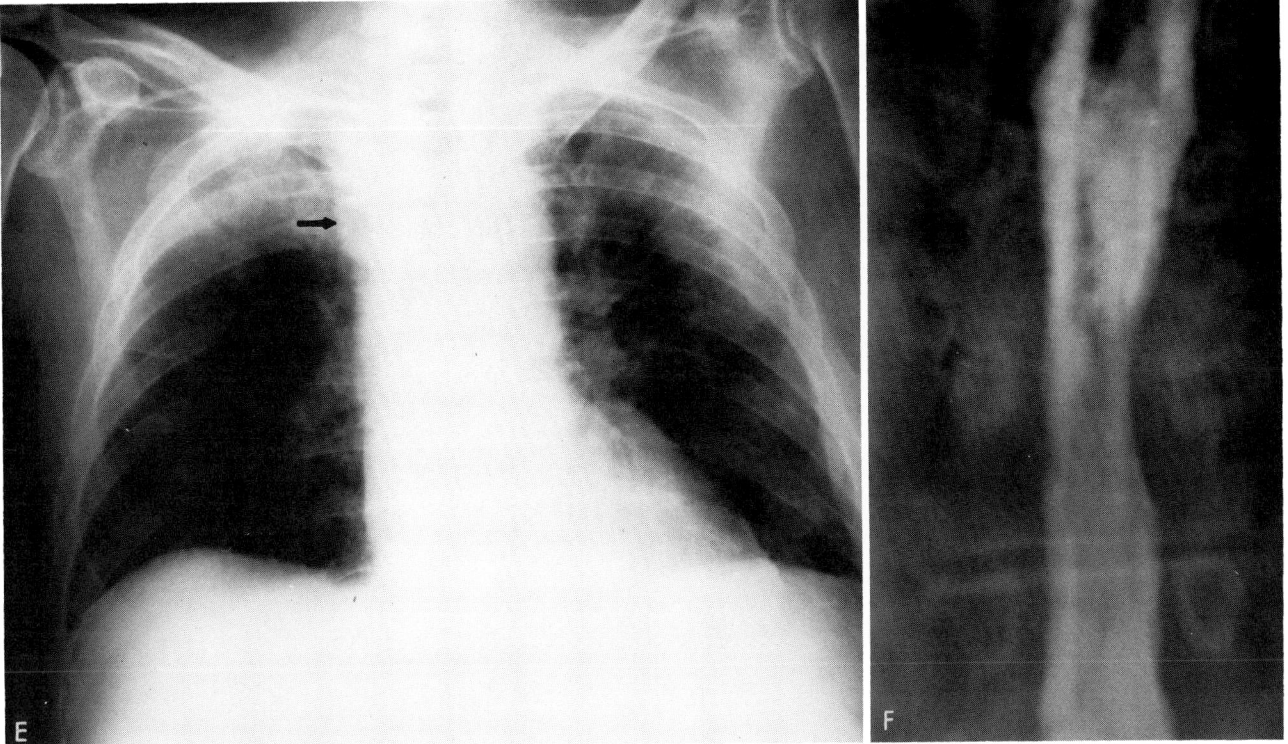

Figure 14–65. Continued

E, F, *Another patient with lymphomatous involvement of the superior mediastinum (arrow). Iophendylate myelogram demonstrates circumferential narrowing of a long segment of upper thoracic vertebral canal secondary to direct invasion by tumor. Note the intact pedicles at the affected levels.*

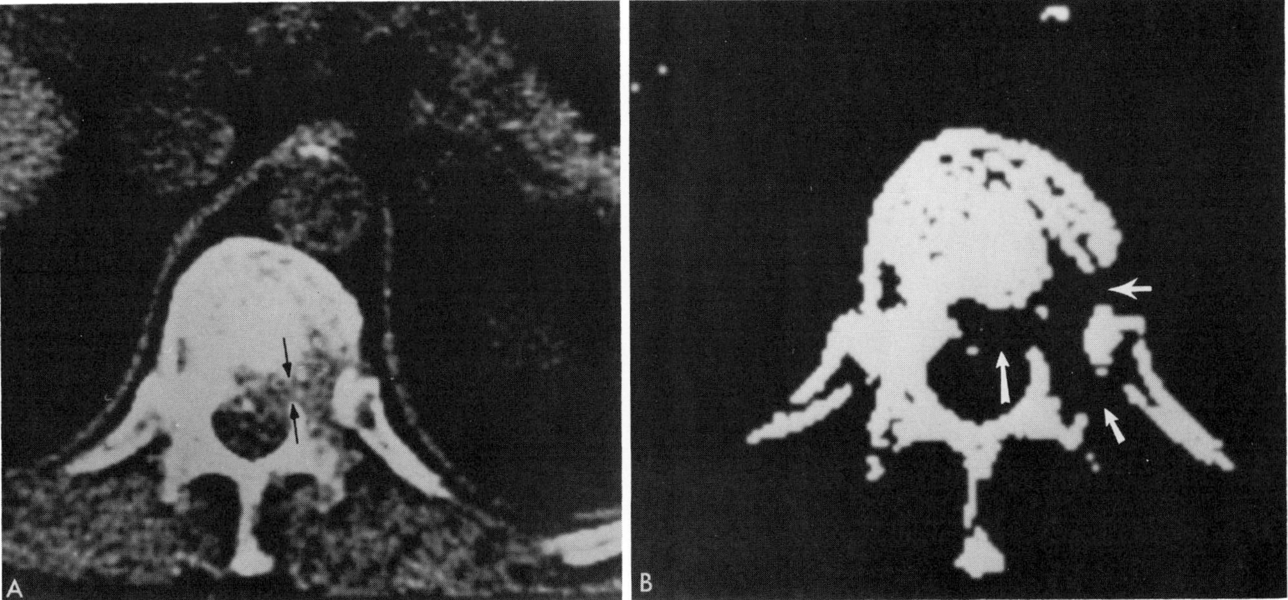

Figure 14–66. *Epidural tumor.* **A,** *The tumor can be seen invading the vertebral body and spinal canal on a computed tomography scan (arrows).* **B,** *At a different setting (for bone), the destruction of the vertebral body and posterior elements as well as the anterior wall of the vertebral canal is better delineated (arrows).*

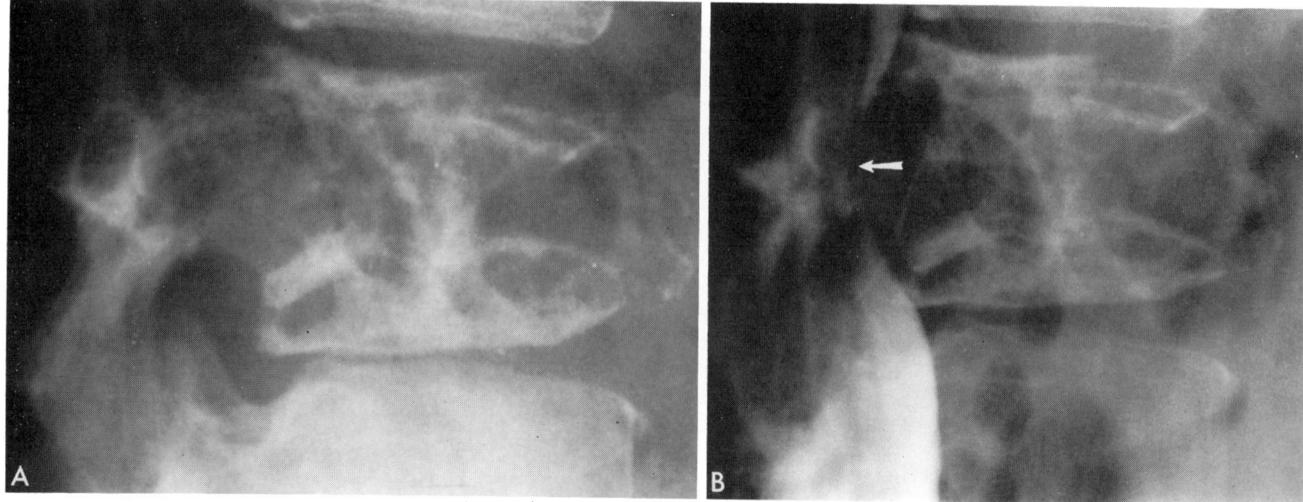

Figure 14–67. *Bone tumor involving spinal canal.* **A,** *This vertebral body was the site of a plasmacytoma.* **B,** *The tumor extends into the spinal canal, compressing the subarachnoid space (arrow).*

neoplasms may involve the spine and the paravertebral tissues as well as the epidural space (Fig. 14–64). It is distinctly unusual, however, for the malignant extradural tumor to invade the dura and involve the subarachnoid space.[74] Rather, these masses compress and deform the subarachnoid space and frequently totally encircle the thecal sac (Fig. 14–65).

The most common neoplasms that metastasize to the spine are carcinomas of the lung, the breast, and the prostate. Most of the symptomatic metastatic lesions reveal some bony involvement. Osteolytic or osteoblastic responses can be detected either with plain film roentgenography (Figs. 14–62 and 14–65) or with the more sensitive modalities, nuclear scan and computed tomography (Fig. 14–66). Any segment of the spine can be affected, although a high proportion of metastases occur in the thoracic region. Metastases to the lumbar spine are seen in approximately 25 per cent of patients, and to the cervical spine in about 7 per cent of patients.[75] Twenty per cent of patients with lymphosarcoma or Hodgkin's disease may have osteolytic or osteoblastic vertebral metastases, although only 5 per cent of these patients will have symptomatic extradural lesions. Primary tumors of the retroperitoneum, pleura, lung, and vertebral bony canal may directly invade the spinal canal[76] (Figs. 14–67 and 14–68).

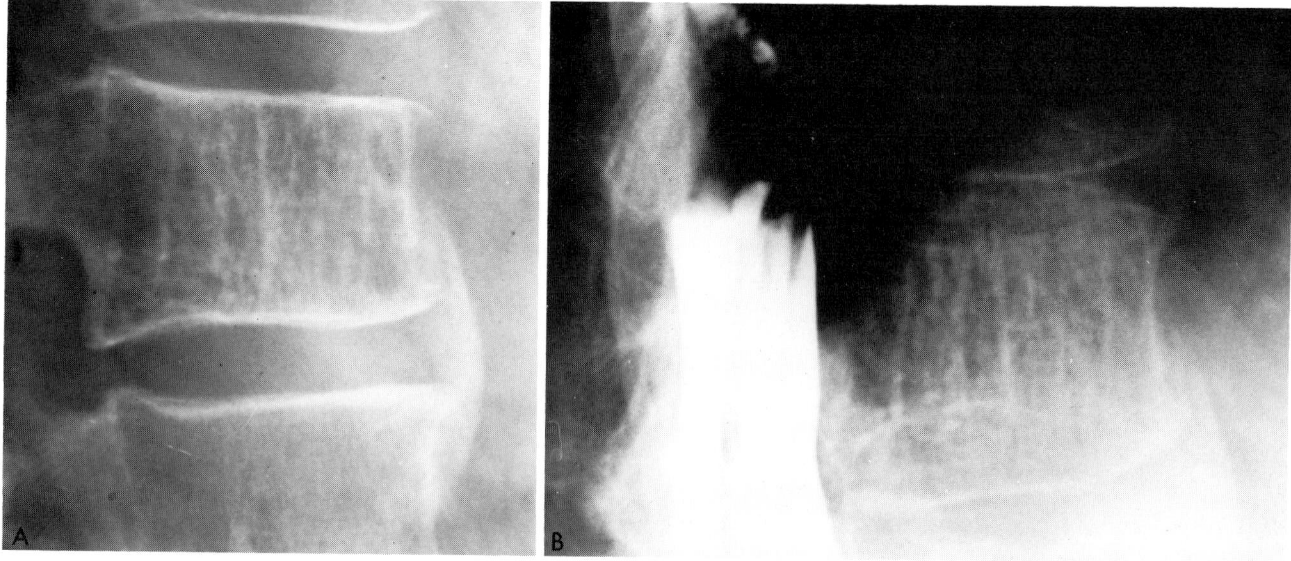

Figure 14–68. *Bone tumor involving spinal canal. The L1 vertebral body is the site of an hemangioma that has extended through the posterior border and obstructed the subarachnoid space* **(B).** *The actual cause of obstruction in these patients may be either direct extension of the vertebral hemangioma or hemorrhage from the lesion.*

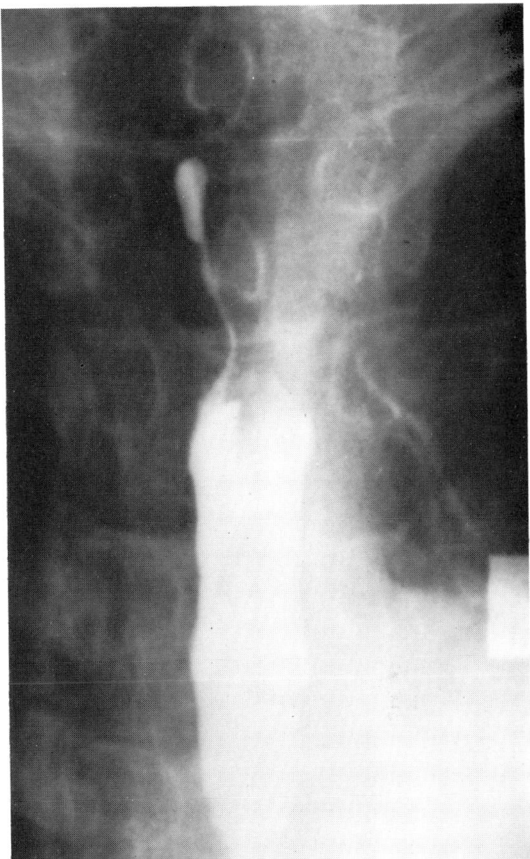

Figure 14–69. Extradural tumor. An extradural mass displaces the subarachnoid space in the upper thoracic region (extradural meningioma).

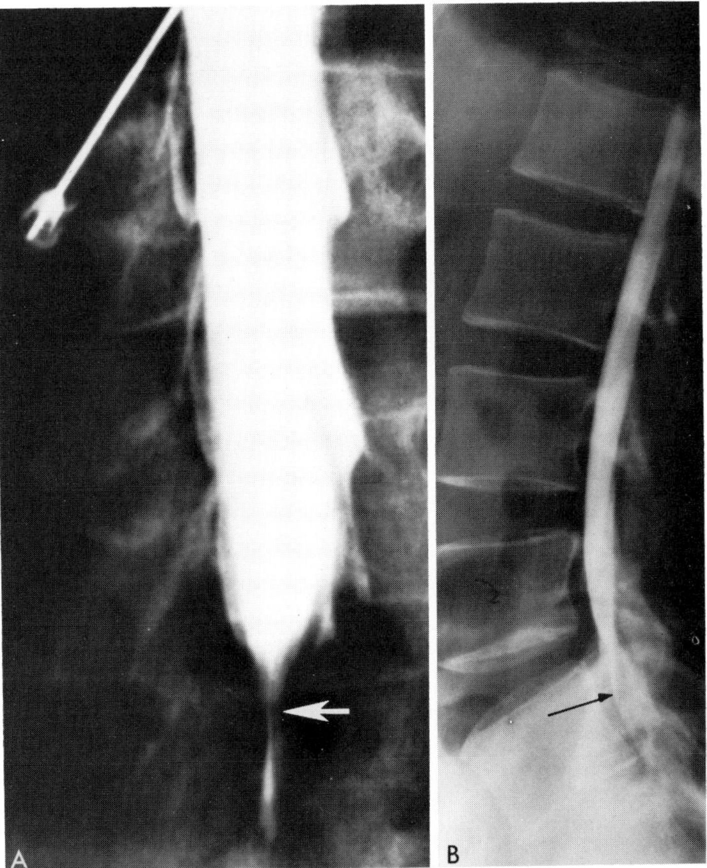

Figure 14–70. Encircling extradural tumor. Metastatic bronchogenic carcinoma in the caudal sac totally surrounds and encases the subarachnoid space, creating a "rat-tail" (arrows).

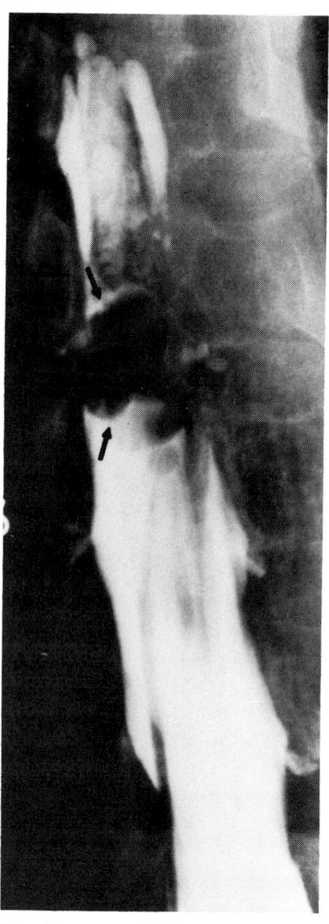

Figure 14–71. Neurilemoma. This tumor mass is multilobulated, involving the conus medullaris and the cauda equina. Note the sharp borders and capping indicative of an intradural-extramedullary lesion (arrows).

Myelography will demonstrate an extradural impression on the subarachnoid space, which may extend from one vertebral body to the next (Fig. 14–69), or over several vertebral segments (Fig. 14–65*F*). The subarachnoid space will be displaced away from the bony elements, especially in the presence of an encircling lesion (Figs. 14–65 and 14–70). These myelographic characteristics pinpoint the extradural nature of the lesion, information that is of fundamental clinical importance. An extradural lesion does not require intradural exploration with possible biopsy of normal neural tissue.[74] If myelography is inconclusive or contraindicated, epidural venography and computed tomography may help in differentiating the extradural nature of the lesion (Fig. 14–66).

Intradural - Extramedullary Lesions. The majority of intradural-extramedullary neoplasms arise from the dura mater or the nerve root sheaths. These tumors consist primarily of meningiomas and neurinomas and constitute approximately 70 per cent of all primary neoplasms of the vertebral canal (Figs. 14–71 to 14–73). They are adherent to the dura and covered by the exeedingly thin arachnoid membrane. Because the tumors involve the meninges and nerve roots, they may grow from the intradural space into the extradural space, forming "dumbbell" lesions (Fig. 14–74). Other neoplasms found in this anatomic space include lipomas, epidermoids, dermoids, and metastatic gliomas. The central nervous system tumors that metastasize to the spinal cord frequently do so after treatment, particularly surgical intervention. Medulloblastoma, ependymoma (Fig. 14–75), and, less commonly, pinealoma and glioblastoma multi-

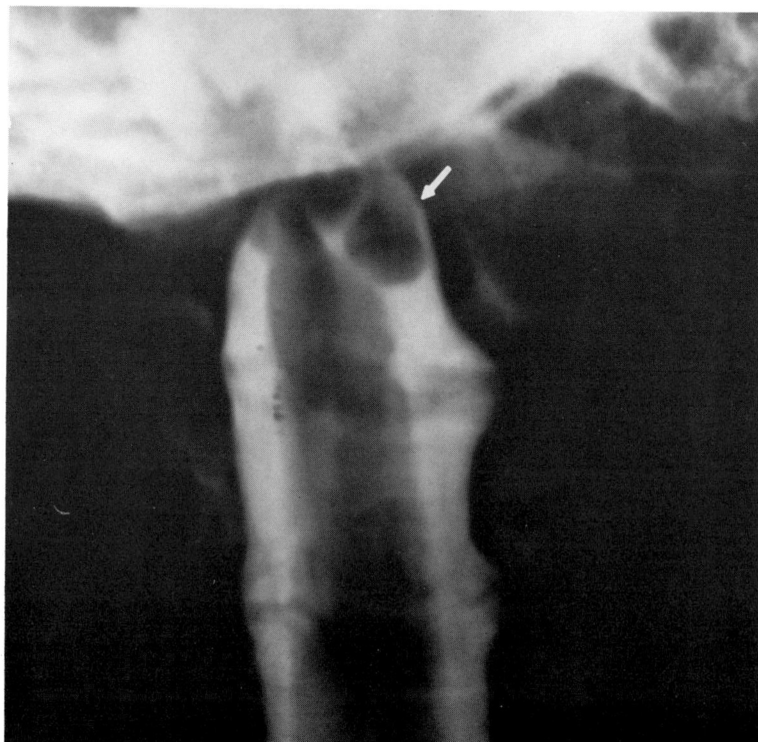

Figure 14–72. Meningioma. This lobulated meningioma (arrow) is quite similar in appearance and spatial location to neurofibromas and neurilemomas.

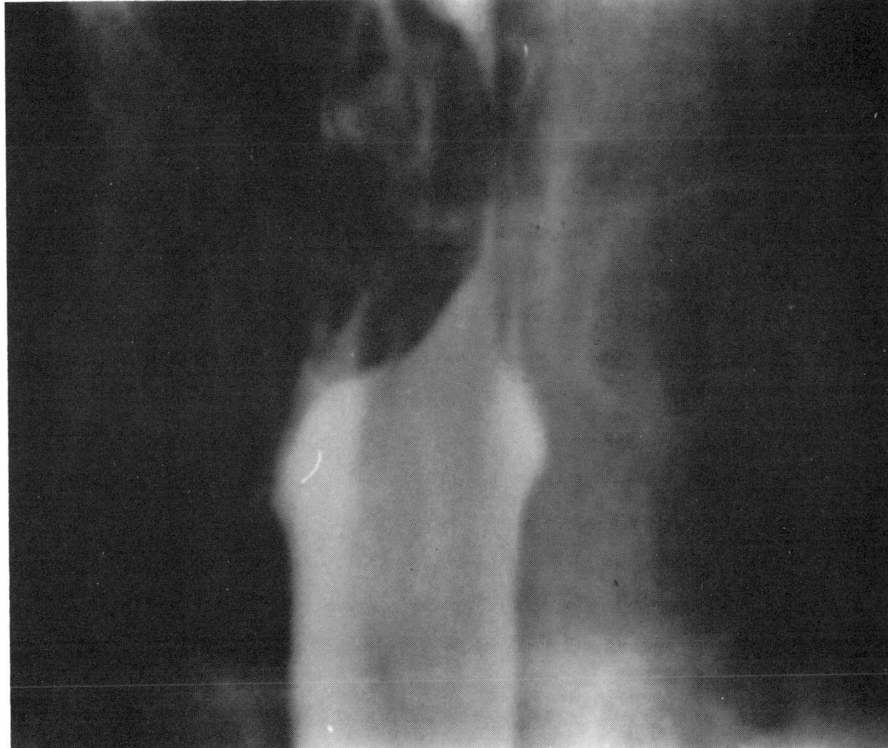

Figure 14–73. Meningioma. This midthoracic meningioma is sharply outlined, as are most intradural-extramedullary lesions. Note the similarity of this lesion to the subdural hematoma in Figure 14–54.

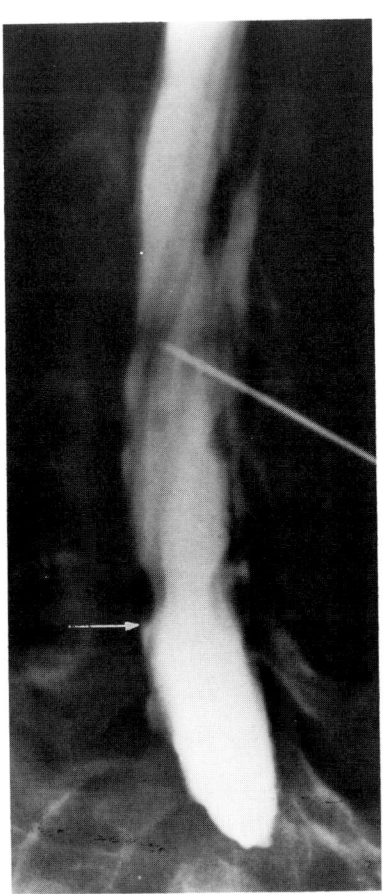

Figure 14–74. Neurofibromas. Multiple neurofibromas are seen arising from lumbar nerve roots. Note the intradural-extramedullary appearance of some of the lesions (arrow), as indicated by the sharp transition zone. These lesions also extend from the normal subarachnoid space along with the nerve root in its passage through the neural foramina ("dumbbell neuromas").

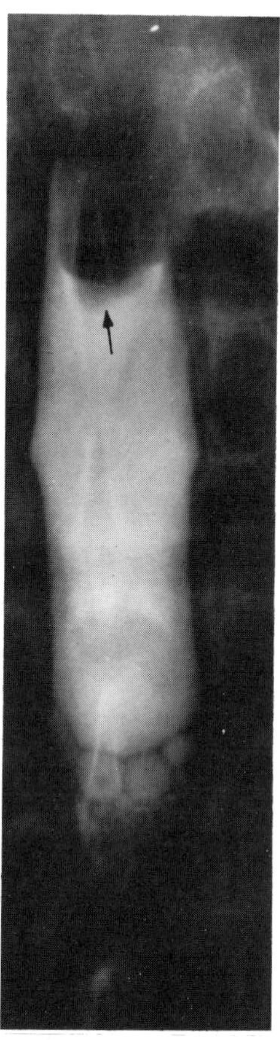

Figure 14–75. *Ependymoma. A lobulated ependymoma (arrow) arises from the cauda equina in a typical location.*

forme seed to the nerve roots. On extremely rare occasions, metastatic carcinoma from sites outside the central nervous system[78] (Figs. 14–76 and 14–77) and adjacent tumors (e.g., bronchogenic carcinoma) with contiguous spread can involve the intradural-extramedullary space.

The routine radiographic findings of neurofibromatosis include expansion of the bony vertebral canal. This is a result of the slow growth of these neoplasms, with widening of the interpedicular space and neural foramina, scalloping of the posterior surface of the vertebral body, and scoliosis (Fig. 14–78). Although such scalloping may be due to direct contact with a neoplastic mass, in patients with neurofibromatosis it occurs at multiple levels and is associated with dural ectasia, not neurofibromas.

Meningiomas rarely produce abnormalities on plain film radiographs. Calcifications within these tumors may be present, but are too faint to be picked up on plain films.

Myelography demonstrates sharply circumscribed filling defects within the contrast-filled subarachnoid space. The spinal cord is displaced away from the offending lesion (Figs. 14–72 and 14–79). Frequently, there is cupping of contrast material around the lesion, identifying its intradural rather than extradural location (Figs. 14–71 to 14–79).

INTRAMEDULLARY LESIONS. Intramedullary tumors of the spinal cord are the least common mass lesions involving the spine. The majority of these tumors are primary gliomas. Of these, ependymomas (Fig. 14–80) account for 65 per cent of lesions, with astrocytomas representing the majority of the remaining tumors (30 per cent) (Figs. 14–81 and 14–82). Ependymomas most frequently originate in the conus medullaris and may extend down the filum terminale into the lumbosacral space. Oligodendrogliomas, spongioblastomas, medulloblastomas, and, rarely, glioblastoma multiforme may arise primarily in the spinal cord. Furthermore, hemangioblastomas may occur as isolated lesions of the spinal cord without indicating the presence of the von Hippel-Lindau disease (hemangioblastoma, retinal angioma, and cystic disease of the pancreas, kidneys, adrenals, and ovaries) (Fig. 14–83). Intramedullary metastatic deposits from primary neoplasms of the brain may also occur. These primarily represent gliomas and, in particular, ependymomas. Intramedullary metastases from carcinomas, most frequently of the breast and the lung, can also be found[77] (Figs. 14–84 to 14–86). Additional unusual intramedullary tumors include neurinomas (Fig. 14–87), dermoids (Fig. 14–88), teratomas, and primary and secondary deposits of lymphoma, sarcoma, and melanoma.

Because of the slow-growing nature of most intramedullary tumors, plain film radiologic examination may reveal widening of the spinal canal with thinning of the pedicles and laminae (Figs. 14–61 and 14–95), scalloping of the posterior margins of the vertebral bodies, and scoliosis (Figs. 14–59 to 14–61). The scoliosis is due to weakness of the paraspinal muscles as a result of involvement of the nerves innervating the musculature. The predominant myelographic finding is fusiform widening of the spinal cord (Figs. 14–18, 14–81, 14–82, and 14–84 to 14–88). Although virtually all intramedullary tumors grow concentrically, hemangioblastoma does demonstrate a tendency to extend onto the surface of the cord into the subarachnoid space (Fig. 14–83). A complete myelogram is necessary to detect all lesions that are affecting the cord or the nerve roots (Fig. 14–89).

Vascular Malformations

Vascular malformations are another commonly encountered lesion of the spinal cord. They represent congenital lesions that usually present before the sixth decade of life, either with acute neurologic signs secondary to subarachnoid hemorrhage (50 per cent) or with slowly progressive signs with clinical remissions[78] (50 per cent). Men are predominantly

Text continued on page 489

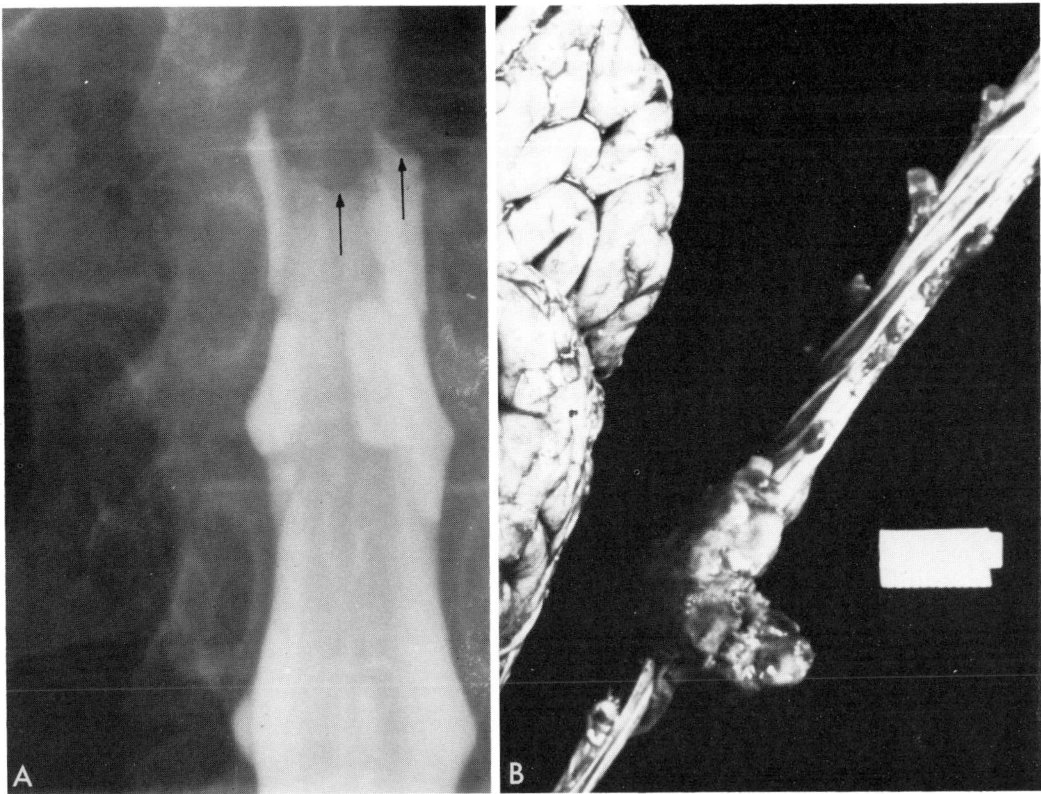

Figure 14–76. *Intradural-extramedullary metastatic tumor.* **A,** *An iophendylate myelogram demonstrates an intradural-extramedullary mass obstructing the flow of contrast medium cephalad (arrows).* **B,** *At autopsy, a metastatic bronchogenic carcinoma was found to envelop the spinal cord and nerve roots, growing within the intradural-extramedullary space.*

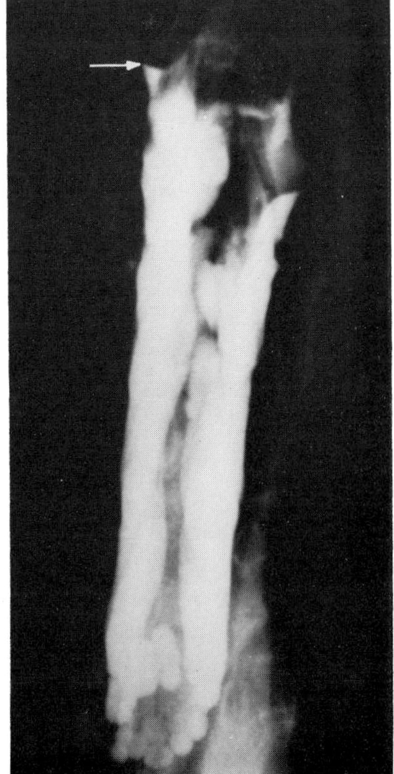

Figure 14–77. *Intradural-extramedullary metastatic tumor. Intradural-extramedullary involvement by bronchogenic carcinoma obstructs the cervical subarachnoid space. The contrast column caps the lesion (arrow), indicating the location of this tumor within the intradural-extramedullary space.*

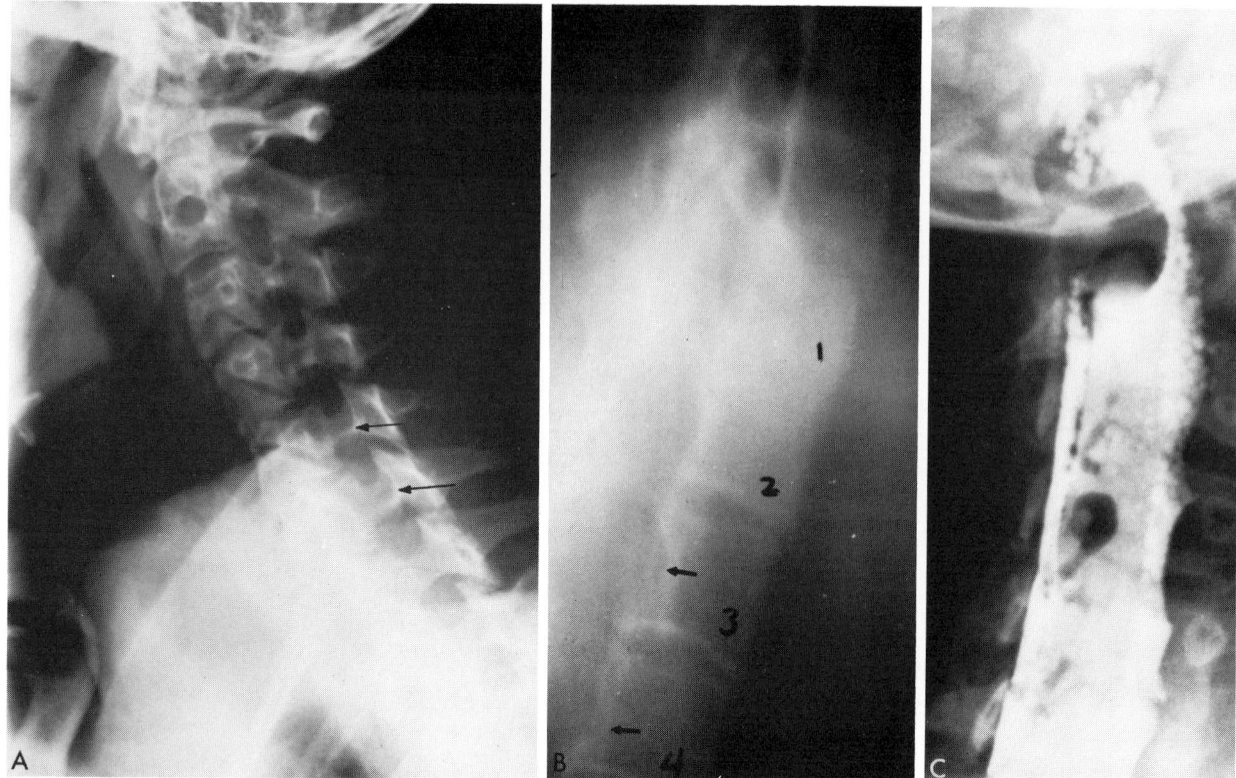

Figure 14–78. Neurofibromatosis. **A,** *Enlargement of multiple neural foramina (arrows) can be seen in this patient with neurofibromatosis.* **B,** *Posterior vertebral body scalloping is present at multiple vertebral levels (arrows).* **C,** *Several of the multiple neurofibromas are seen at myelography.*

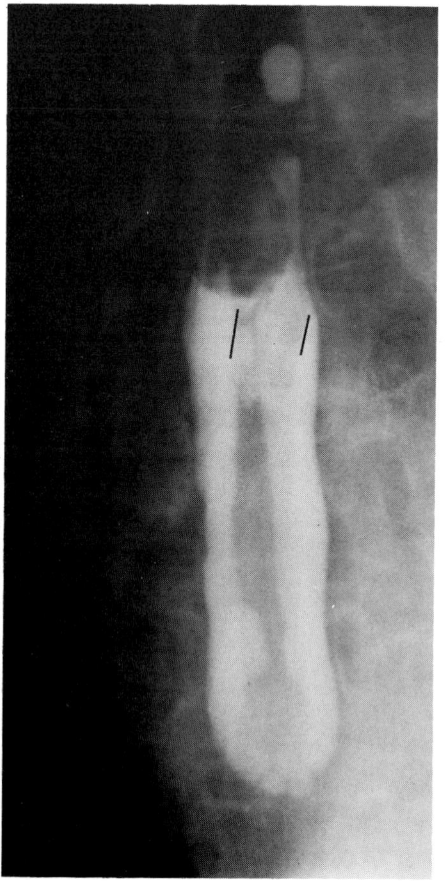

Figure 14–79. *Thoracic meningioma. Contrast medium caps a large thoracic meningioma, which displaces the spinal cord to the left. Note the narrowing of the subarachnoid space on the left side as the cord is pushed away from the tumor mass. (The black lines indicate the borders of the spinal cord.)*

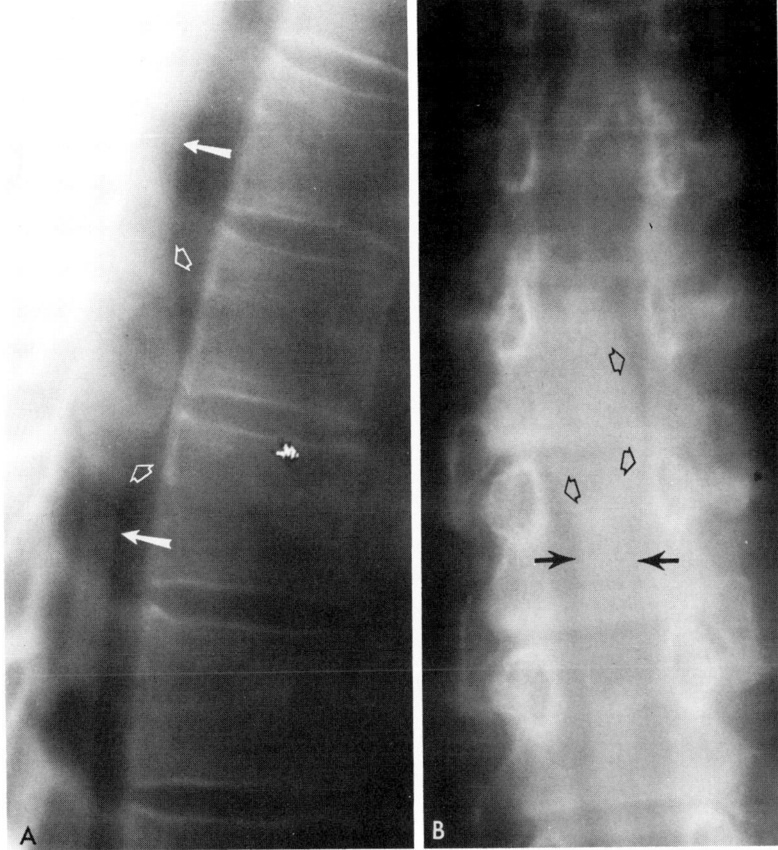

Figure 14–80. *Ependymoma. The fusiform enlargement of the thoracic spinal cord seen on this gas myelogram was due to an ependymoma. (Solid arrows, normal spinal cord borders; open arrows, tumor margins.)*

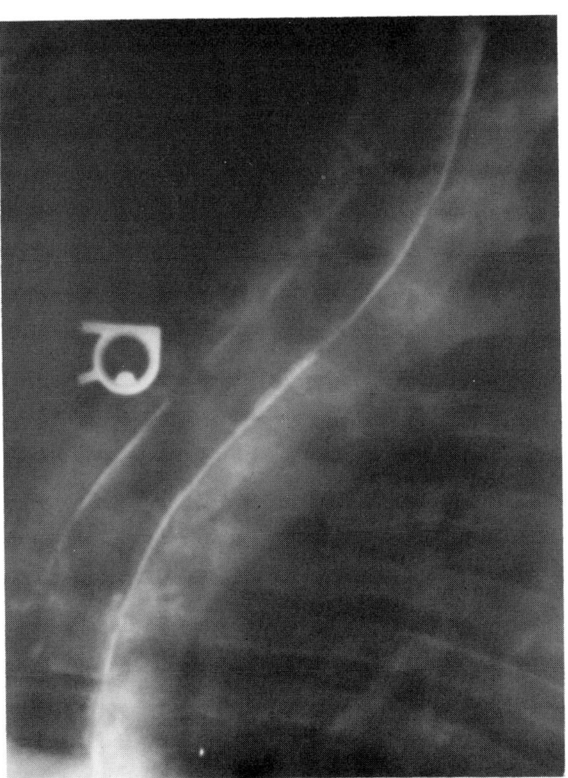

Figure 14–81. *Astrocytoma. An intramedullary astrocytoma involves virtually the entire spinal cord, enlarging it and filling most of the subarachnoid space.*

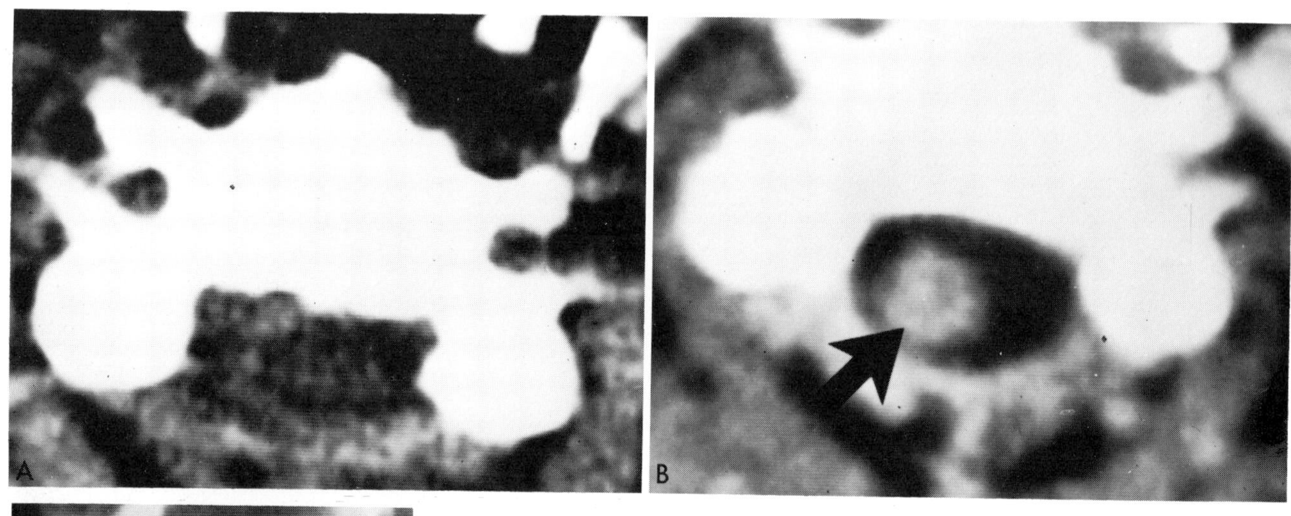

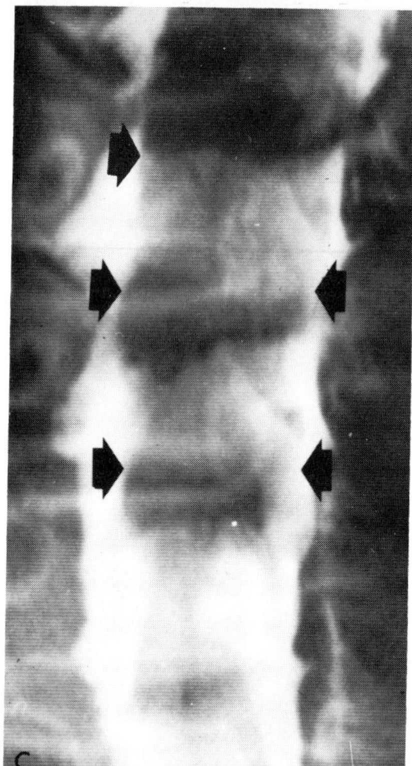

Figure 14–82. *Astrocytoma. A CT scan without* **(A)** *and with* **(B)** *intravenous contrast medium demonstrates an intramedullary astrocytoma (arrow).* **C,** *The myelogram demonstrates widening of the cervical spinal cord due to the astrocytoma (arrows). (From Handel S: J Comput Assist Tomogr 2:227, 1978. Courtesy of the Raven Press, New York.)*

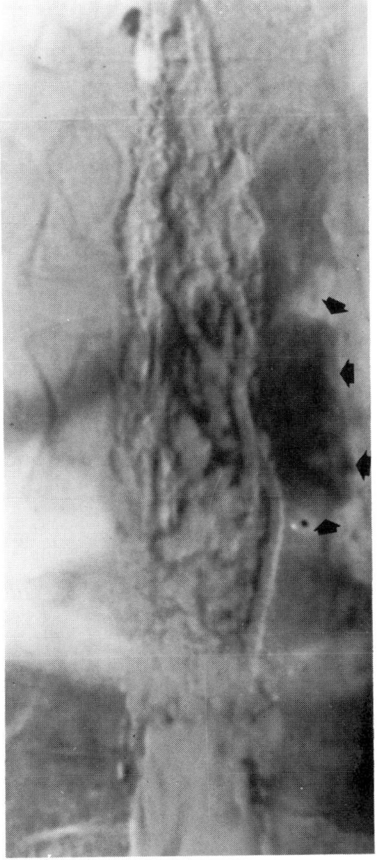

Figure 14–83. Hemangioblastoma. Subtraction film from a spinal arteriogram demonstrates a large tumor blush extending eccentrically away from the spinal cord (arrows). This appearance is seen most often with hemangioblastomas and rarely with other primary tumors of the spinal cord.

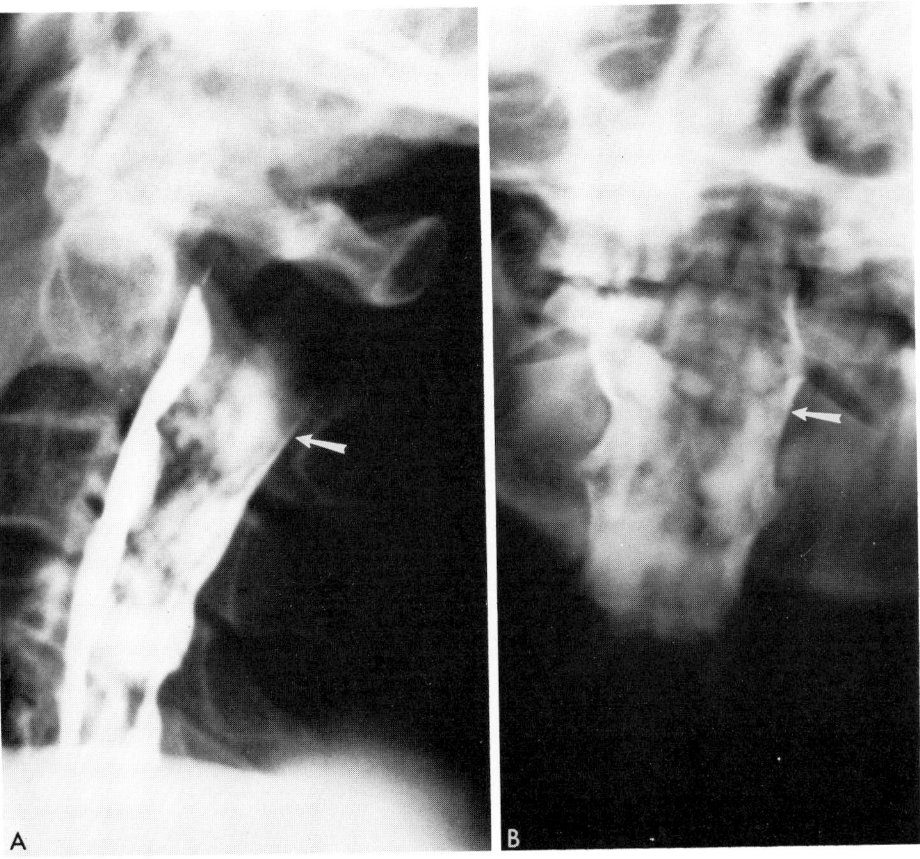

Figure 14–84. Intramedullary metastatic tumor. There is focal enlargement of the spinal cord as seen in both lateral and frontal projections. This is due to intramedullary metastasis from prostatic carcinoma. Note the symmetric narrowing of the contrast column as the cervical cord widens (arrow).

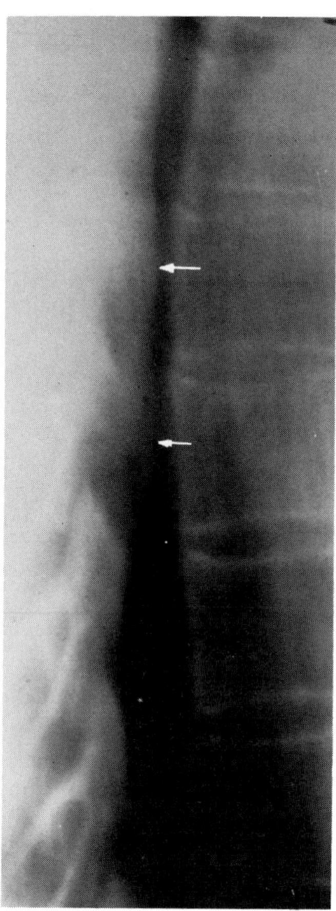

Figure 14–85. Intramedullary metastatic tumor. A gas myelogram reveals focal enlargement of the midthoracic spinal cord due to intramedullary involvement with metastatic breast carcinoma (arrows).

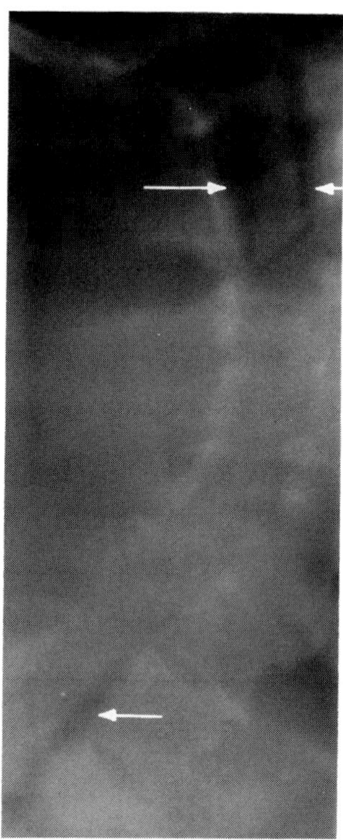

Figure 14–86. Intramedullary metastatic tumor. The lower cervical spinal cord virtually fills the spinal canal from C3 to C6 on this air myelogram. This was an intramedullary metastatic bronchogenic carcinoma. Air (arrows) is seen above and below the cord expansion.

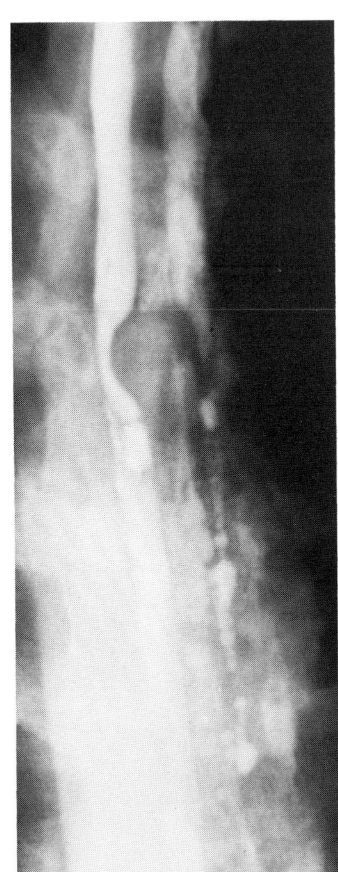

Figure 14–87. *Intramedullary neurinoma. An unusual intramedullary neurinoma focally enlarges the midthoracic spinal cord.*

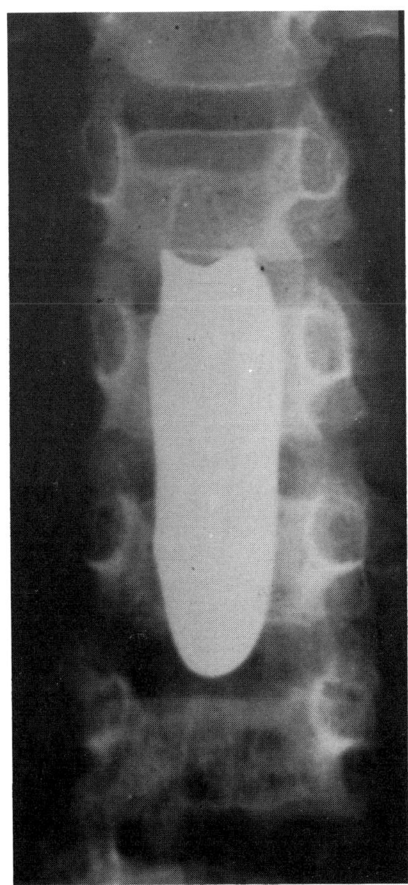

Figure 14–88. *Dermoid. A congenital dermoid enlarges the conus medullaris and obstructs the contrast column. Note the smooth singular contour of its outline compared with that of the ependymoma in Figure 14–75.*

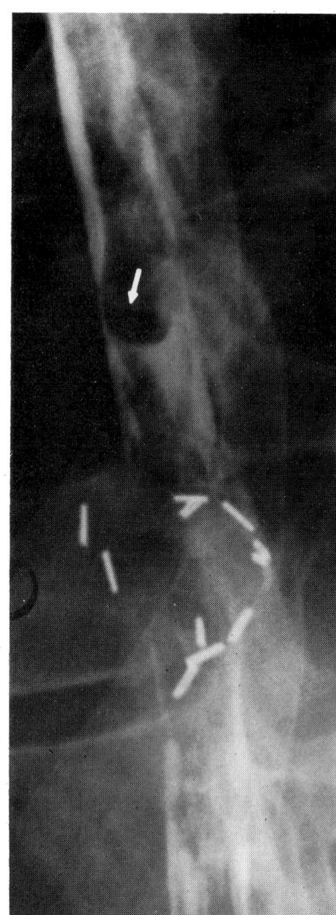

Figure 14–89. Neurofibroma. A postoperative myelogram demonstrates a second neurofibroma involving the spinal cord above the surgical site (arrow). This area was not evaluated preoperatively by myelography because a total block was demonstrated below the lesion.

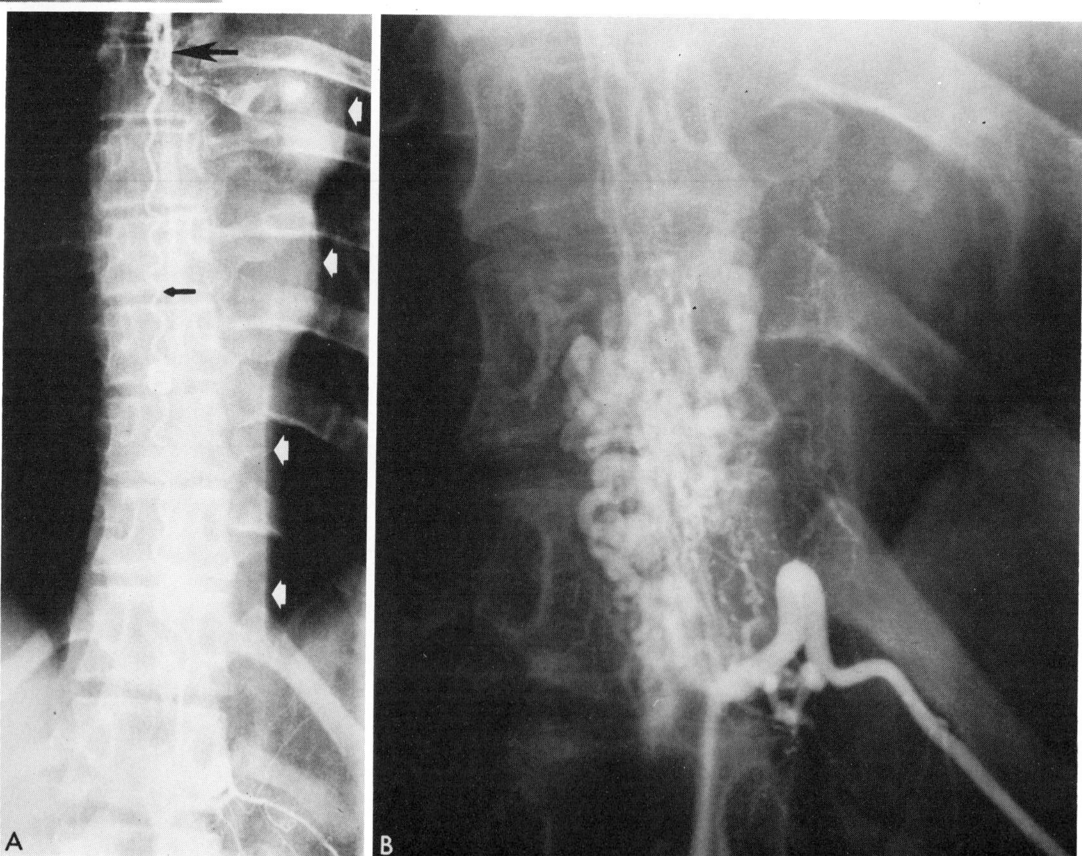

Figure 14–90. Arteriovenous malformation. **A,** There is a markedly enlarged spinal artery (small arrow) feeding an arteriovenous malformation (large arrow). In addition, a large soft tissue mass is seen in the paravertebral space (white arrows). **B,** Numerous tortuous and dilated arteries feed a massive spinal and paraspinal malformation. This patient had systemic angiomatosis (Ullmann's syndrome). (From Coel M, Alksne J: Vasc Surg 12:336, 1978.)

affected (90 per cent). Cutaneous angiomas may be found in the same segmental dermatome,[78] perhaps supplied by the same intercostal or lumbar artery that is feeding the spinal lesion. Arteriovenous malformations are often detected as part of a neurocutaneous syndrome[79] (Fig. 14–90). In these cases, high output failure may be the presenting manifestation.[80]

Most of the vascular abnormalities of the spinal cord are arteriovenous malformations, in which case there is no significant capillary bed between the involved arteries and veins. The blood is "stolen" from the normal arteries and passes rapidly through the malformation (Fig. 14–91). Venous angiomas (varices or varicose veins) of the spinal cord are associated with slower blood flow than that in an arteriovenous malformation. Both the arteriovenous malformation and the venous angioma are most frequently located on the surface of the spinal cord, especially the dorsal surface; 90 per cent of arteriovenous malformations occur in the thoracic and lumbar regions, with only a few involving the cervical cord (Fig. 14–92). Cavernous hemangiomas, on the other hand, may be deep within the cord, and hemorrhage (hematomyelia) in these lesions may require palliative surgical decompression.

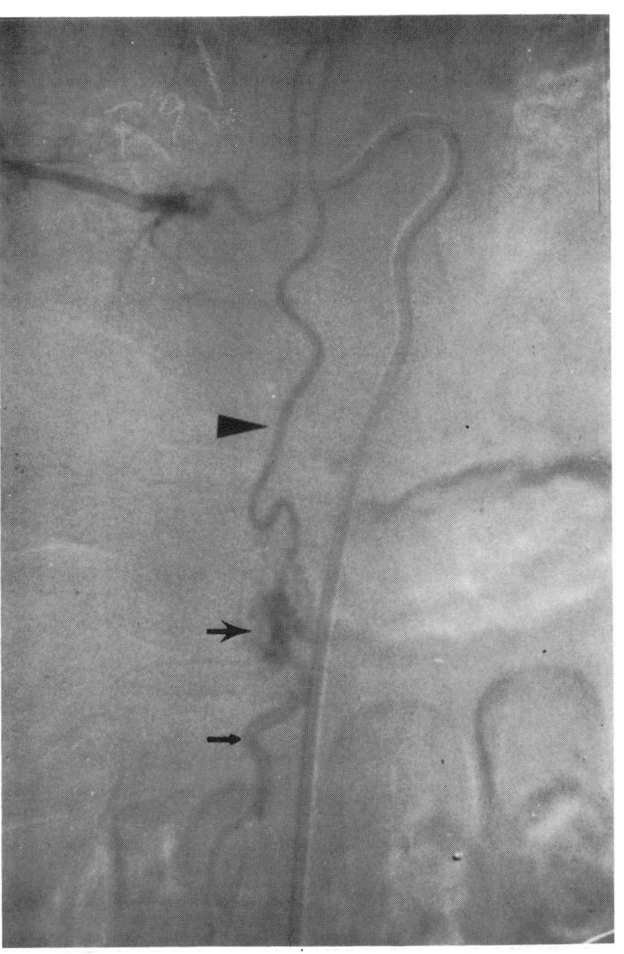

Figure 14–91. *Arteriovenous malformation. An enlarged artery of Adamkiewicz (arrowhead), with its characteristic cranial loop, feeds a malformation of the conus medullaris (arrow) and is drained by a dilated spinal vein (small arrow). This rapid shunting of blood is characteristic of arteriovenous malformations.*

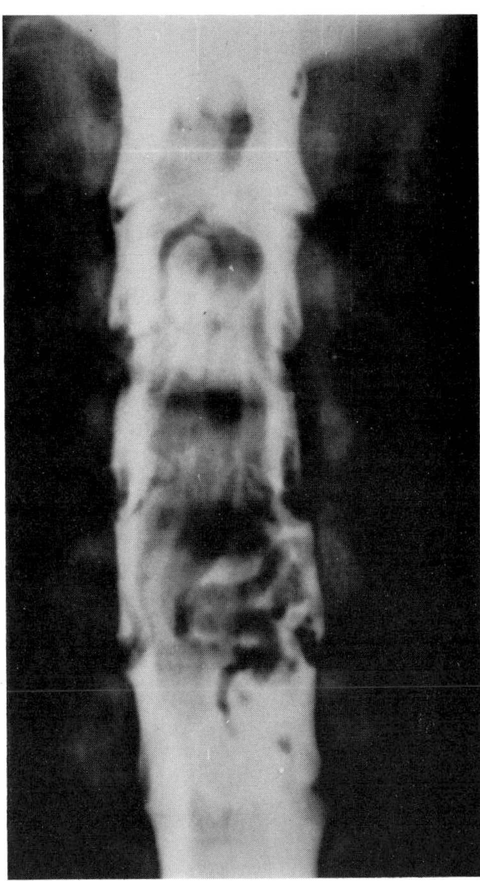

Figure 14–92. *Arteriovenous malformation. An iophendylate cervical myelogram demonstrates tortuous vessels, as arteries and veins supply an arteriovenous malformation. What appears to be massive spinal cord widening is in reality enlarged veins.*

There are no plain film findings that are diagnostic of a vascular malformation of the spinal cord. On rare occasions, a paraspinal mass may be found, representing extension of hemorrhage into the adjacent soft tissues (Fig. 14–90). The optimal method for demonstrating these lesions is selective spinal arteriography. The many arteries that feed the spinal cord must be injected to fully evaluate the length and possible multiplicity of these lesions, as well as to identify the blood supply of the malformation for the neurosurgeon. In recent years, embolization of these malformations has been accomplished with considerable success (Fig. 14–93), although occlusion of the feeding vessels will not permanently destroy the malformation.[81-83] In order to prevent recurrence of the lesion, emboli must be placed within the nidus of the malformation.

Malformations can be identified with positive contrast myelography, although the examination must be performed meticulously. The contrast column must cover the dorsal aspect of the spinal cord,

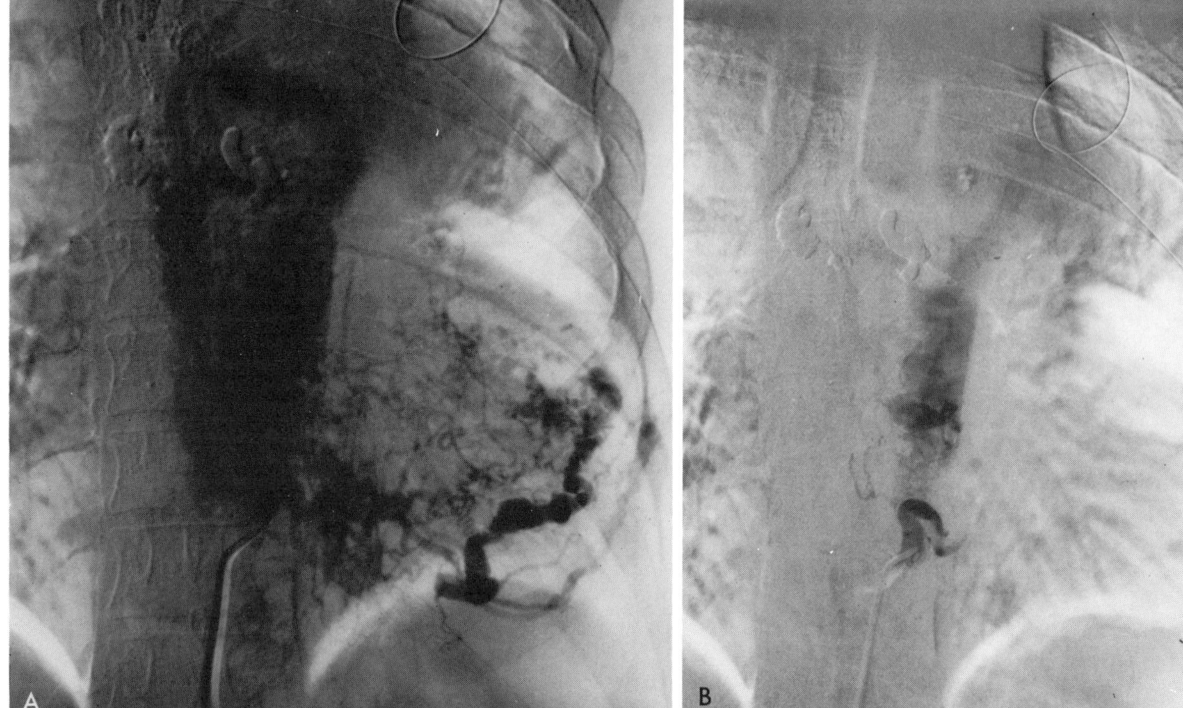

Figure 14–93. *Arteriovenous malformation.* **A,** *A massive arteriovenous malformation involves the spinal cord, paraspinal tissues, and the chest wall.* **B,** *In order to diminish the exaggerated cardiac output due to the rapid arteriovenous shunting, embolization of several malformations was performed. In this case cardiac output dropped from 20 liters per min at rest to 13 liters per min. (From Coel M, Alksne J: Vasc Surg 12:336, 1978.)*

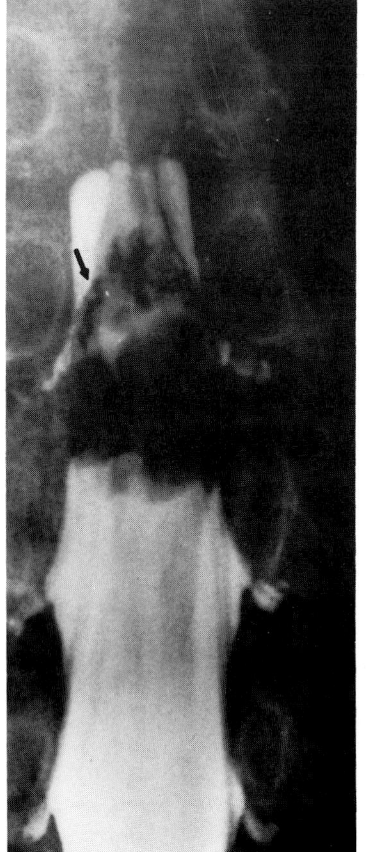

Figure 14–94. *Neurinoma. A lobulated neurinoma of the cauda equina obstructs venous drainage (arrow).*

which requires removal of the needle and placement of the patient in a supine position. The nidus of the malformation may still not be identified, as it produces virtually no mass effect on the spinal cord. The tortuous vessels feeding and draining the malformation will, however, be evident. Any mass effect that is detected is usually due to hematoma formation.

On occasion, a mass lesion compressing the spinal cord will obstruct the vascular drainage to such a degree as to cause dilatation and tortuosity of veins. This myelographic appearance must not be confused with that of a malformation, which has no mass effect (Figs. 14–19 and 14–94). In general, the enlarged, tortuous vessels of a malformation are greater in size than those found in association with mass lesions.

Syringomyelia

Syringomyelia is an intramedullary cavitation that has a lining composed of glial tissue. Syringomyelia may occur as an isolated lesion or in association with other congenital anomalies or intramedullary tumors. In the latter case, the cavitation is thought to result from compromise of spinal cord vascularity, with subsequent necrosis and cavity formation. The true syrinx remains isolated to a localized segment of the spinal cord or elongates, involving the entire cord. Clinical findings, such as muscle weakness and wasting, usually appear early in life, although some patients do not become affected until middle age.

A closely related condition is hydromyelia, which is thought to represent a dilatation of the central canal of the spinal cord, with communication with the fourth ventricle. Some pathologists believe that syringomyelia and hydromyelia are in reality the same condition, appearing with slightly different presentations. Syringomyelia and hydromyelia represent flaccid cysts that do not result from trauma, spontaneous hemorrhage, primary vascular occlusion, or tumor necrosis. Occasionally, the cyst may be tense and may not partially collapse with position change. Affected patients may present with neuropathic joint disease, particularly of the upper limbs.

Routine radiographic findings relate to the presence of an enlarged spinal cord leading to widening of the bony spinal canal (Fig. 14–95). Increased cervical lordosis may be secondary to muscle weak-

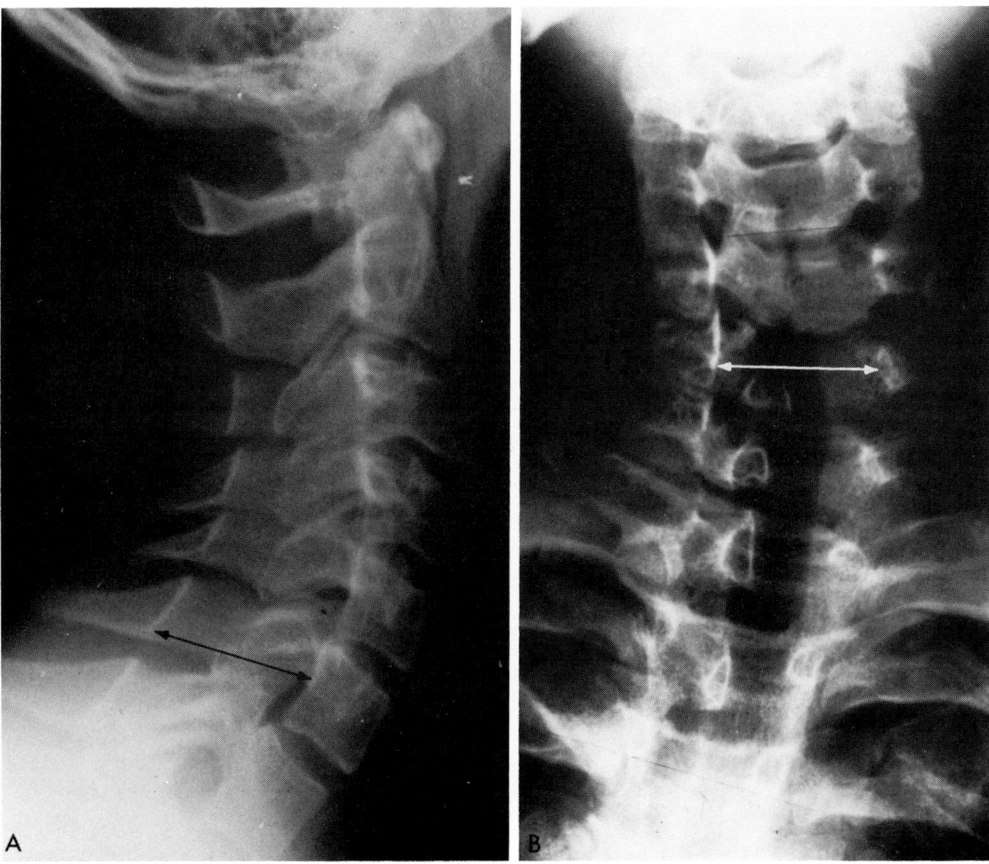

Figure 14–95. Syringomyelia. **A,** *The anteroposterior diameter of the cervical spinal canal has been widened (arrows). There is no evidence of bony erosion, thus indicating a long-standing process.* **B,** *There is widening of the interpedicular distances of the cervical vertebrae, with thinning of the pedicles (arrows). (See Fig. 14–98.)*

ness. Neuroarthropathic abnormalities, especially in the articulations of the upper extremity, may also be noted (see Chapter 70).

Myelography can be performed with either positive contrast media (iophendylate, metrizamide) or gas (air, oxygen). As the majority of these intramedullary cysts are flaccid, only the dependent portion of the lesion will be distended. Thus, myelography must be accomplished with the area of interest in both dependent and elevated attitudes, so that comparison of the spinal cord size in each of these positions is possible (Fig. 14–96). Typically, the lesions involve the cervical region, with enlargement of the spinal cord occurring in the Trendelenburg position and narrowing in the upright position. As the cranial portion of the cyst collapses, the spinal cord becomes smaller than normal, indicating a degree of atrophy (Figs. 14–96 and 14–97). If there is no change in the size with change in the patient's position, a distended cyst cannot be distinguished from a solid intramedullary tumor (Figs. 14–59, 14–81, and 14–98). In these cases, cyst puncture and introduction of contrast medium should be attempted (Fig. 14–99). The appearance of contrast medium in the fourth ventricle indicates direct communication (i.e., hydromyelia), rather than a localized cystic lesion (i.e., syringomyelia).

In patients with syringomyelia and hydromyelia, computed tomography may demonstrate a large area of diminished attenuation ("radiolucency") surrounded by a thin rim of normal-appearing neural tissue (Fig. 14–100).

Congenital Lesions

General Features. The term spinal dysraphism is utilized to describe abnormalities associated with incomplete development of the posterior neural arches. Included in these abnormalities are spina bifida occulta, diastematomyelia, low spinal cord (tethered cord), meningocele, myelomeningocele, subcutaneous and intrathecal lipoma (hamartoma), dermoid cyst, teratoma, neurenteric cyst, and spinal cutaneous fistula (pilonidal cyst).[84] Most patients with these disorders present early in life, although there is a small percentage of patients with

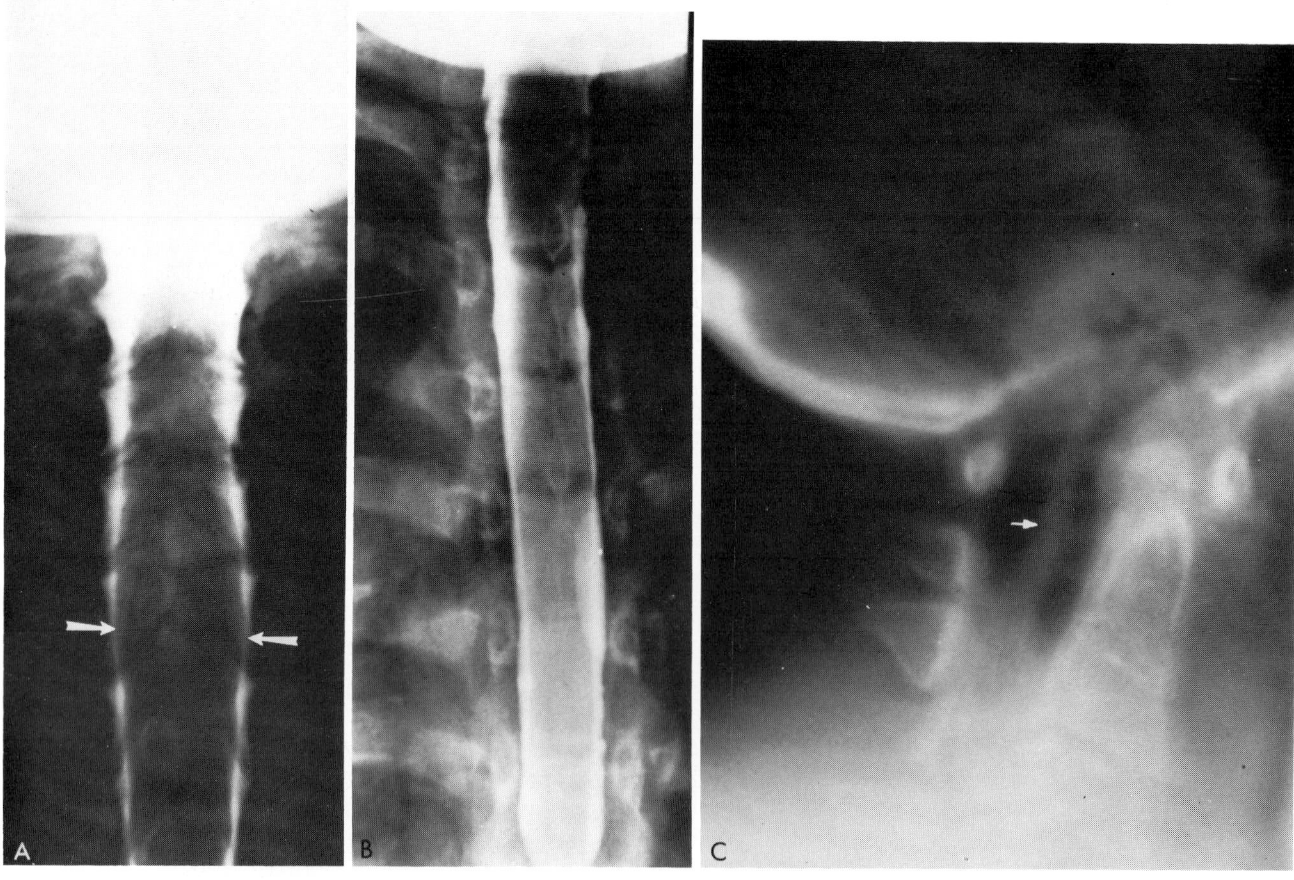

Figure 14–96. Syringomyelia. **A,** *A Pantopaque myelogram with the patient's head in a dependent position demonstrates widening of the cervical spinal cord (arrows).* **B,** *The dilatation of the spinal cord continues caudally through the thoracic region.* **C,** *On gas myelography with the head in an upright position, the collapse of the cervical portion of the syrinx can be seen as a markedly narrowed (atrophic) spinal cord (arrow).*

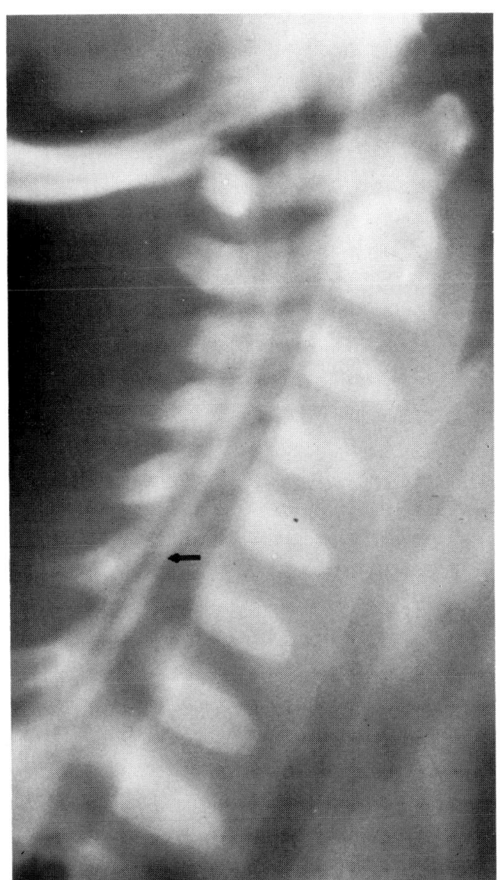

Figure 14–97. *Spinal cord atrophy. There is marked atrophy of the spinal cord (arrow) in a patient with syringomyelia who was examined by gas myelography in the upright position.*

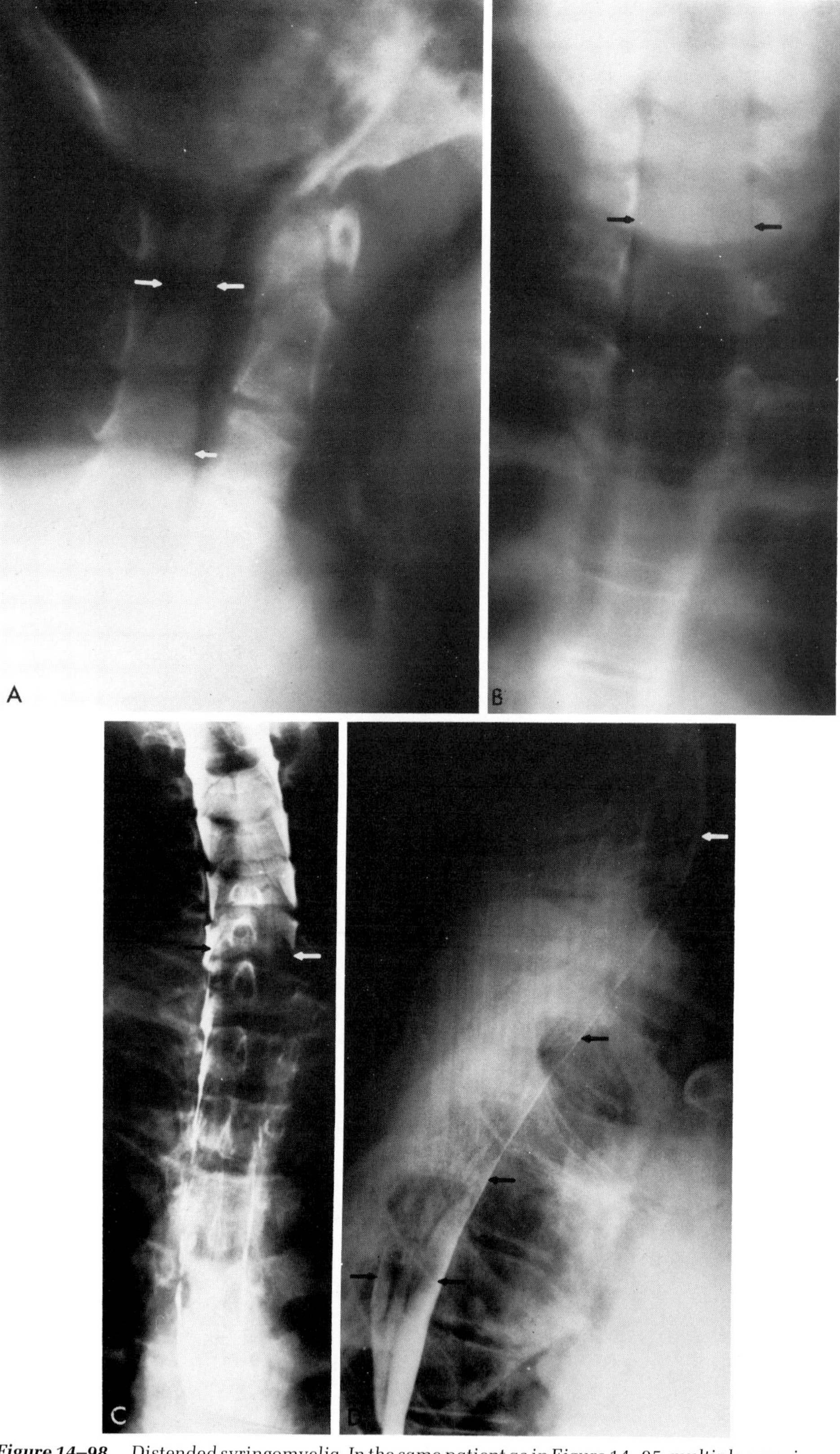

Figure 14–98. *Distended syringomyelia. In the same patient as in Figure 14–95, multiple examinations with position changes did not demonstrate any collapse of the distended syringomyelia. Radiographically, this was indistinguishable from a solid intramedullary mass.* **A,** *A gas myelogram in the upright position demonstrates widening of the medulla and cervical spinal cord (lateral projection) (arrows).* **B,** *The anteroposterior projection also demonstrates the widening of the spinal cord (arrows). This is diagnostic of an intramedullary mass without specific characteristics of a syrinx.* **C,** *Dependent iophendylate myelogram reveals widening of the spinal cord (arrows), an appearance that is unchanged from the upright gas myelogram.* **D,** *Lateral projection of the iophendylate myelogram again confirms the presence of an intramedullary mass lesion (arrows).*

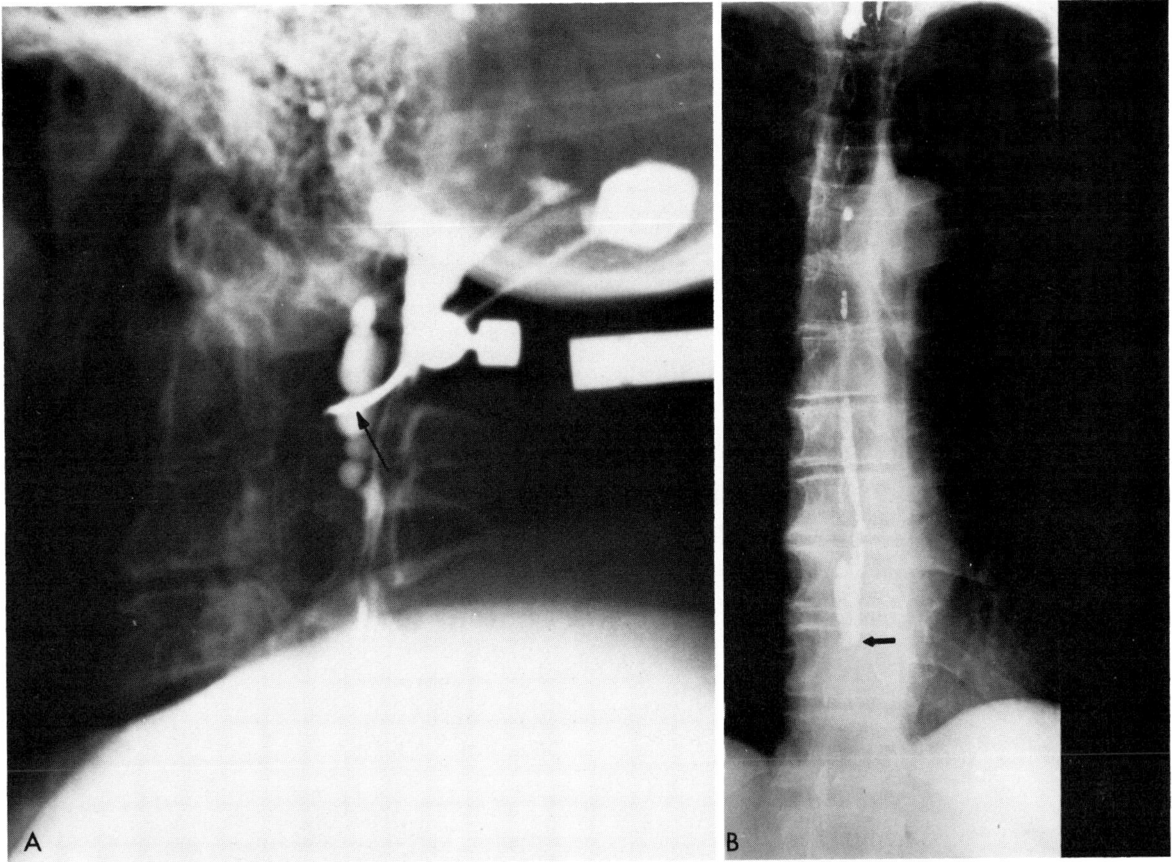

Figure 14–99. *Syringomyelia with cystogram. In a middle-aged patient with syringomyelia, a needle puncture is both diagnostic and therapeutic.* **A,** *The needle has been introduced into the cyst (arrow) and a few drops of iophendylate have been administered.* **B,** *The patient is placed in an upright position and the iophendylate has dropped to the bottom of the cyst, defining the cyst's full extent (arrow). At periodic intervals, fluid may be removed by cyst puncture to relieve some of the symptoms. (Residual iophendylate from myelography can be seen at the top and bottom of the radiograph.)*

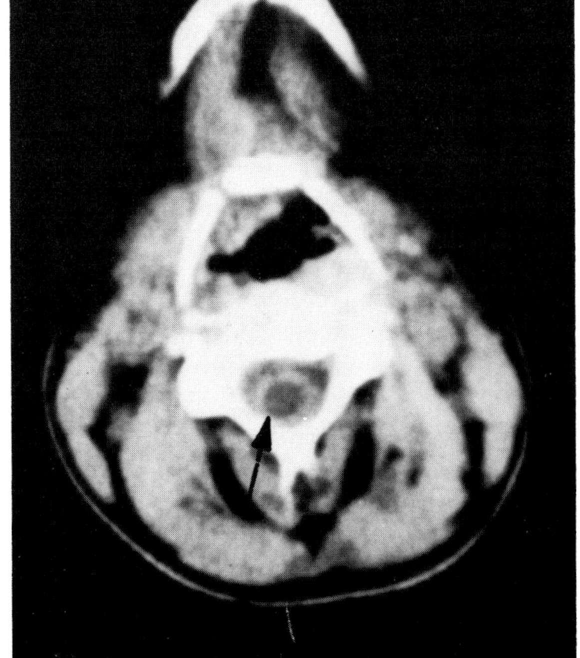

Figure 14–100. *Syringomyelia. CT examination of a patient with syringomyelia demonstrates the central radiolucent area of the intramedullary cyst (arrow) surrounded by normal spinal cord tissue. (Courtesy of Dr. Michael Wells.)*

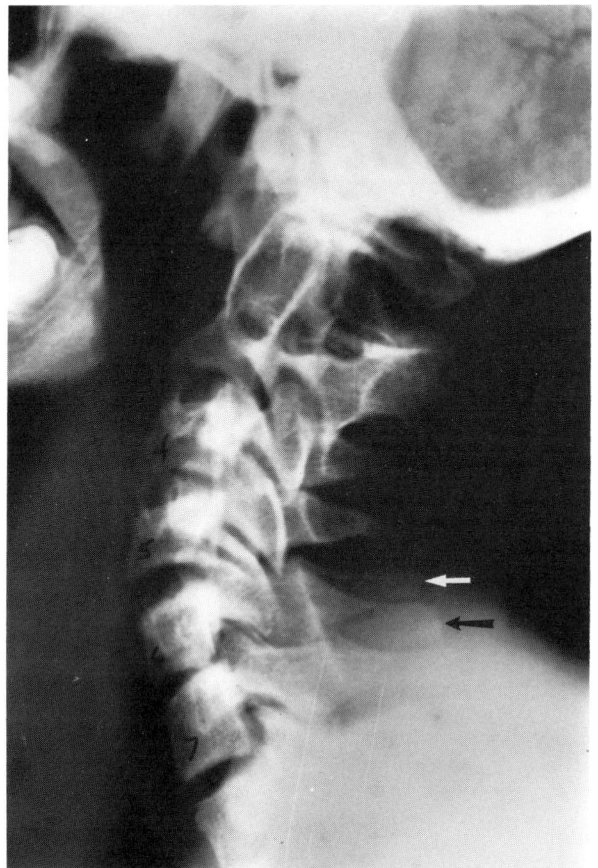

Figure 14–101. Syringomyelia. In a patient with syringomyelia, nonfusion of the posterior spinal arch can be seen at C6 and C7 (arrows). On this lateral projection, other bony anomalies involving craniovertebral junction are also noted.

spinal dysraphism who develop problems in adulthood and even as late as the seventh decade of life.[85] In these latter patients, it is not known why these lesions become symptomatic in the later years, although it has been postulated that it may be due to the continued slow growth of some of the mass lesions[86] or to the development of acquired spinal stenosis superimposed upon the congenital defect.[77]

Plain film radiographic examination may reveal a widened spinal canal, an abnormal spinal curvature in the affected region, defects of the posterior neural arch (spina bifida, spina bifida occulta) (Fig. 14–101), midline bony spurs (diastematomyelia), or vertebral body scalloping. Soft tissue masses such as myeloceles and meningomyeloceles are usually evident clinically, although presacral or intrasacral masses may first be detected radiographically. Myelography can be used to diagnose and evaluate the extent of many of the congenital lesions.

Diastematomyelia. Diastematomyelia is a congenital anomaly in which an osseous or fibrocartilaginous septum covered by dura mater splits and fixes the spinal cord in the sagittal plane. The septum is attached anteriorly to the vertebral bodies and posteriorly to the dura, passing through the spinal cord. This congenital defect may represent a remnant of the connection between the primitive neural and enteric tubes. The most common location of this abnormality is in the thoracolumbar canal. Neurologic examination may reveal only mild aberrations, including abnormal gait, bladder and bowel dysfunction, or cutaneous alterations, such as a skin dimple, nevus, or patch of hair on the lower back. Spinal roentgenograms in the frontal projection may show the ossified septum, a local widening of the vertebral canal, and defects of the vertebral arch (Fig. 14–102). Abnormalities of vertebral bodies and scoliosis are present in over 50 per cent of patients.[87] In some cases, tomography is necessary to demonstrate a faintly ossified septum or deformity of the laminae. Myelography and computed tomography[88] (Fig. 14–103) will reveal a split in the column of contrast medium as it deviates around the septum, "duplication of the spinal cord," and, in many cases, a low-lying conus medullaris with a thickened filum terminale. Surgical repair consists of removal of the septum and release of the tension on the spinal cord, procedures that may prevent the progression of the neurologic deficits and scoliosis.

Tethered Cord. The tethered cord syndrome is one entity that commonly becomes apparent in early life, but which may not be associated with significant defects until later life.[86] Neurologic deficits include bladder and bowel dysfunction, gait disturbance (usually due to muscle weakness), numbness or paresthesia of the legs and feet, and lower extremity radicular pain in those patients with associated lumbosacral lipomas.

Plain film examination may reveal posterior defects in the sacrum associated with a subcutaneous lipoma (Figs. 14–104 and 14–105), or, less frequently, enlargement of the spinal canal, scalloping of the vertebral bodies, and destruction of the pedicles. Air myelography, which should be utilized when a tethered cord is suspected, will demonstrate the low-lying conus medullaris and the thickened filum terminale (Fig. 14–106). A lipoma of the filum terminale and intrathecal bands may also be identified (Figs. 14–105, 14–107, and 14–108). Computed tomography may be an additional helpful modality in evaluating this condition.[89] There is some question as to the reparative value of surgical release of the tethering,[86] although severing the thickened filum terminale may prevent progression of the neurologic deficits.

Meningocele and Meningomyelocele. Meningoceles are outpockets or diverticula of the leptomeninges that extend through a developmental defect in the dura mater. The more common form of meningocele presents posteriorly under the skin as the subarachnoid space protrudes through a defect in the lamina. The adjacent vertebral canal is widened, with flattening of the pedicles and, rarely, vertebral body erosion. On occasion, anterior defects

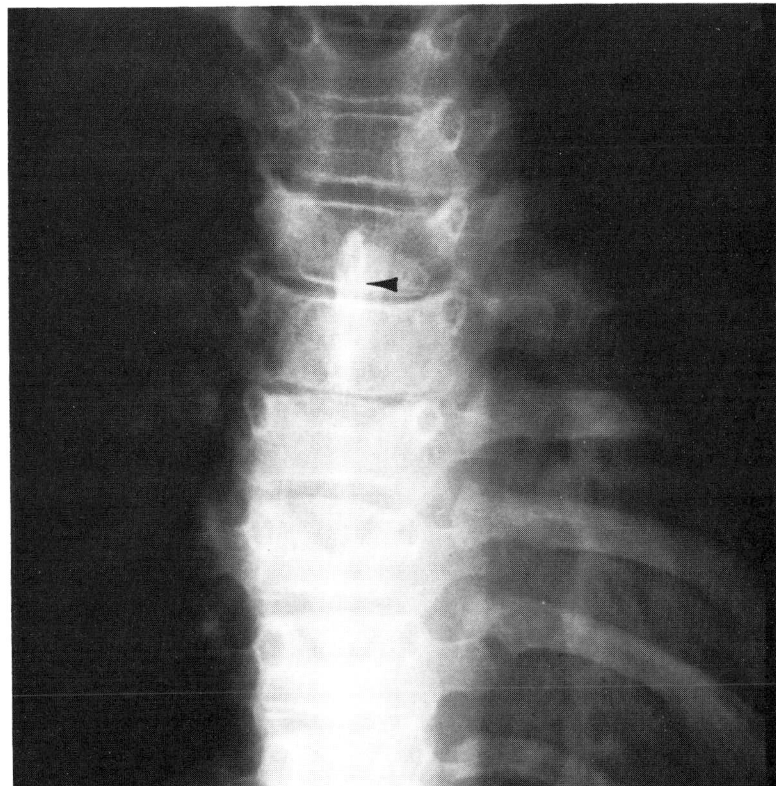

Figure 14–102. *Diastematomyelia. A midthoracic diastematomyelia is seen with plain film findings including an ossified septum (arrowhead) and local widening of the spinal canal.*

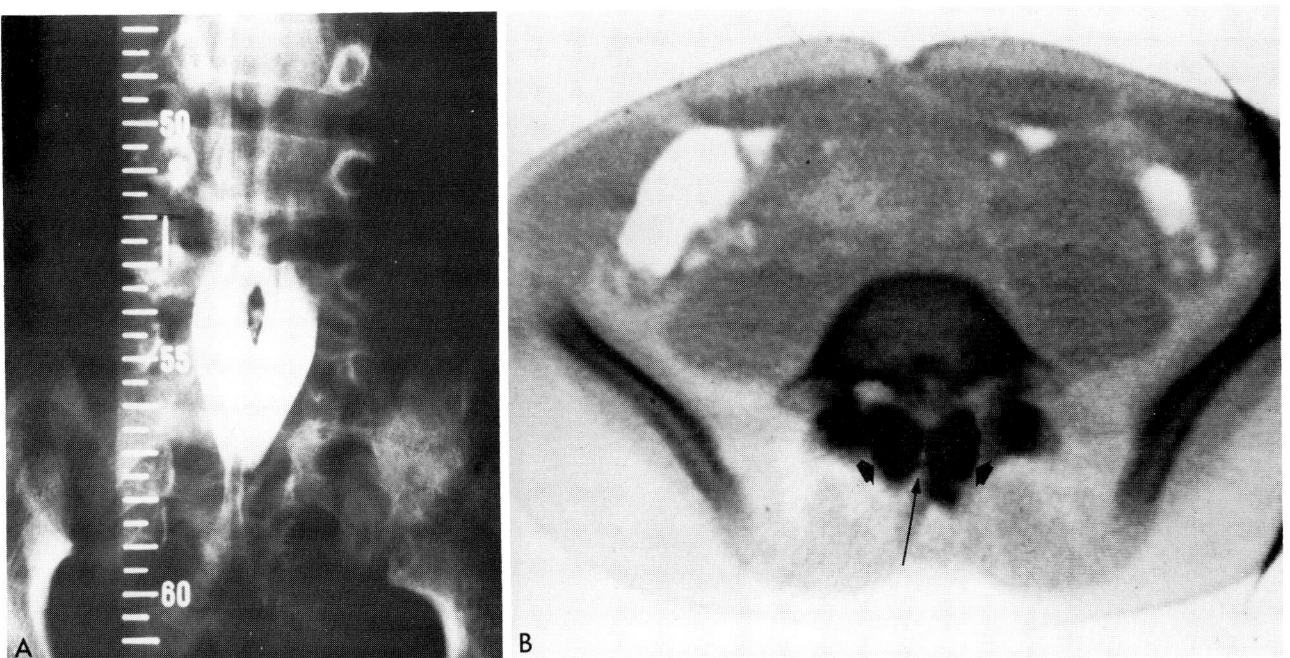

Figure 14–103. *Diastematomyelia. An unusual lower lumbar diastematomyelia is demonstrated on both myelography and computed tomography.* **A,** *At myelography, the septum can be seen splitting the contrast column. In addition, there is local widening of the entire lower lumbar spinal canal.* **B,** *With water-soluble contrast medium within the subarachnoid space (short arrows), computed tomography (with reversal of black and white) reveals a splitting of the subarachnoid space in its entire sagittal diameter by a nonossified septum (long arrow). (Courtesy of Dr. Derek Harwood-Nash, Hospital for Sick Children, Toronto, Ontario, Canada.)*

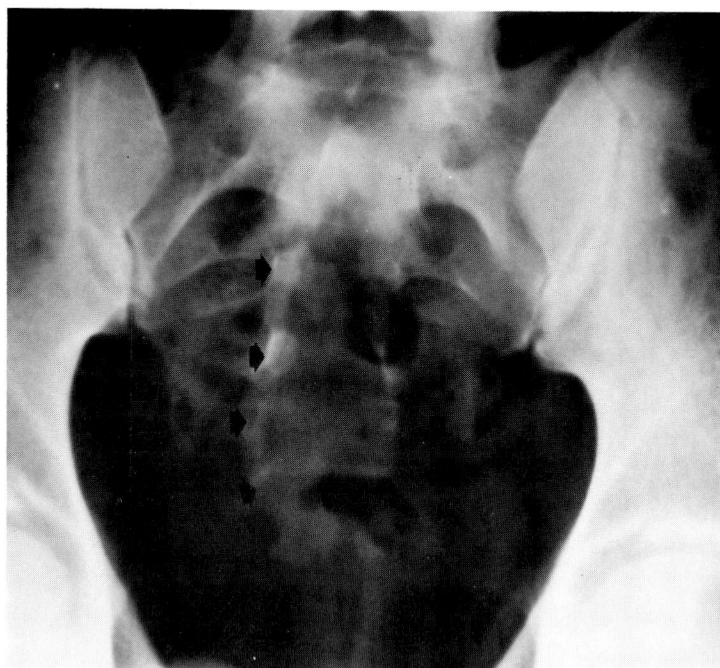

Figure 14–104. Tethered cord. There is nonfusion of the posterior bony elements of the sacrum (arrows) in a patient with a tethered cord and an intraspinal lipoma.

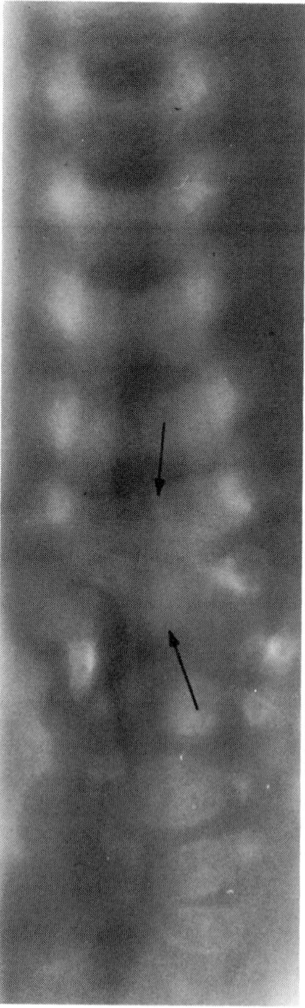

Figure 14–105. Tethered cord with intraspinal lipoma. The intraspinal lipoma at the lumbosacral junction is associated with local widening of the spinal canal and disordered spinal column development. The lipoma can be seen as a soft tissue defect surrounded by the gas (arrows).

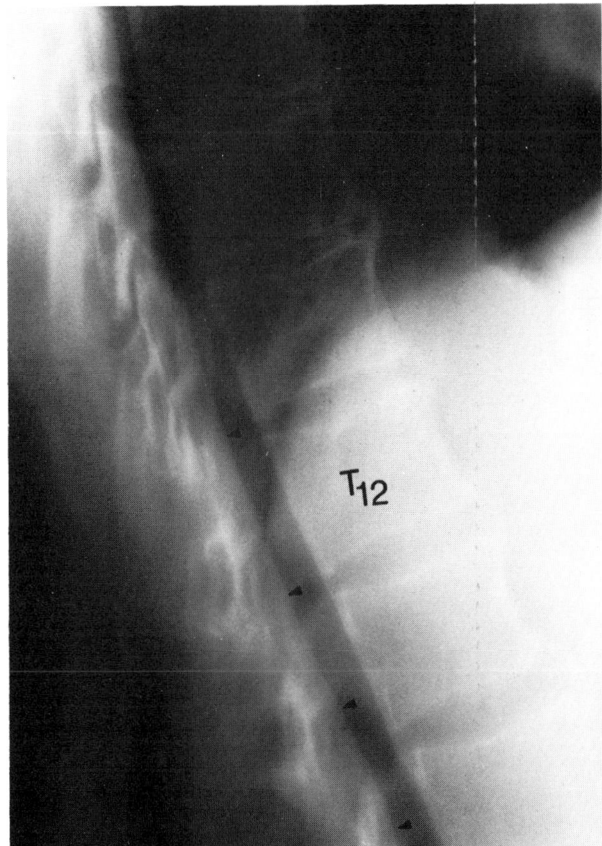

Figure 14–106. *Tethered cord. In a patient with tethered cord, the low-lying conus medullaris and thickened filum terminale are indistinguishable, as the soft tissue density of the cord (arrowheads) continues below the normal level.*

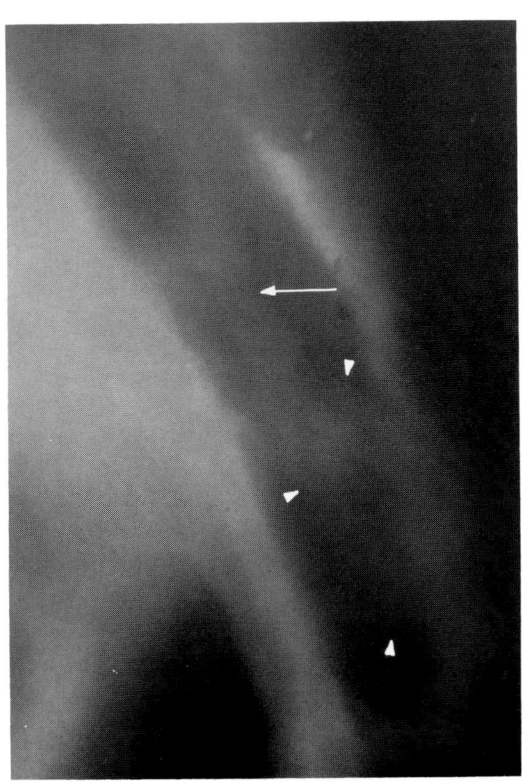

Figure 14–107. *Tethered cord with intraspinal lipoma. The thick fibrous band (arrow) tethering the spinal cord to an intrasacral and subcutaneous lipoma (arrowheads) is well demonstrated at gas myelography.*

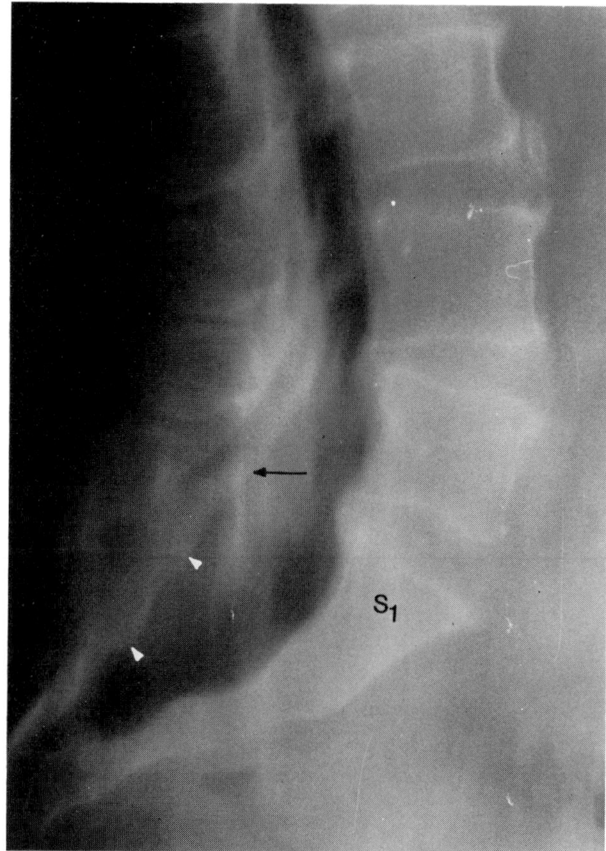

Figure 14–108. *Tethered cord with intraspinal and extraspinal lipoma. In the same patient as in Figure 14–104, the thickened band (arrow) connects the subcutaneous and intraspinal lipoma (arrowheads) via the sacral bony defects.*

of the sacrum allow intrapelvic protrusion of a subarachnoid sac. Virtually all meningoceles become apparent in childhood, especially those that involve neural tissue (spinal cord or nerve roots of the cauda equina). These latter structures are called meningomyeloceles. The spinal subarachnoid space communicates with all meningoceles, although the communicating channel may be small and difficult to demonstrate at myelography. It is for this reason that water-soluble contrast media are the agents of choice in demonstrating the communication. Lateral meningoceles associated with neurofibromatosis may present as large posterior mediastinal masses. Myelography usually demonstrates the communication and nature of the entity prior to surgery (Fig. 14–109).

Extradural Cyst. Extradural cysts are meningoceles whose communication has been obliterated. These occur in early life and are located almost exclusively in the thoracic region. The spinal canal is widened, with erosion or thinning of the medial borders of the pedicles. The posterior borders of the

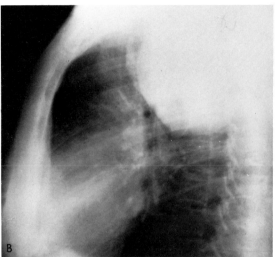

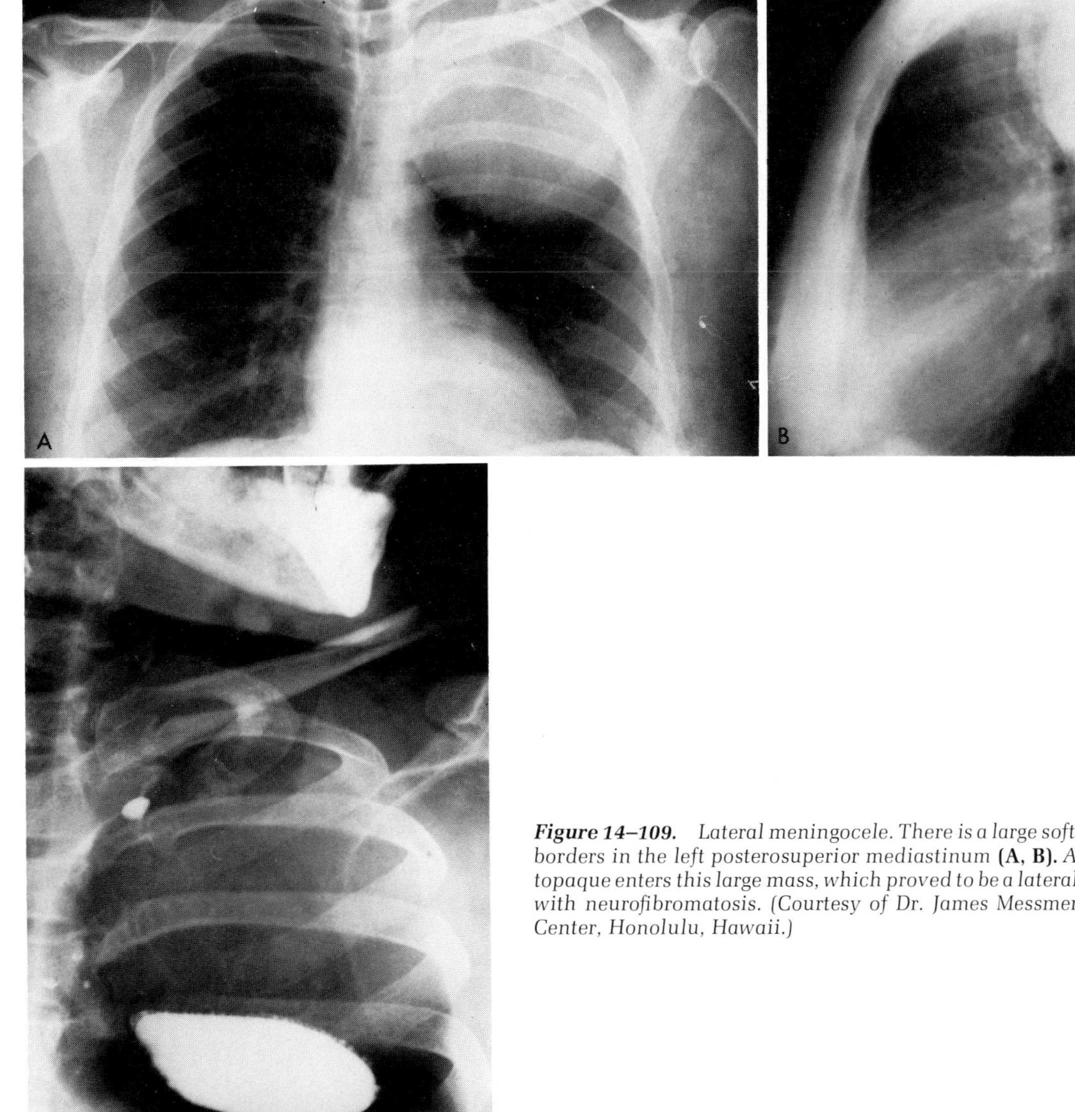

Figure 14–109. *Lateral meningocele. There is a large soft tissue mass with smooth borders in the left posterosuperior mediastinum* **(A, B).** *At myelography* **(C),** *Pantopaque enters this large mass, which proved to be a lateral meningocele associated with neurofibromatosis. (Courtesy of Dr. James Messmer, Tripler Army Medical Center, Honolulu, Hawaii.)*

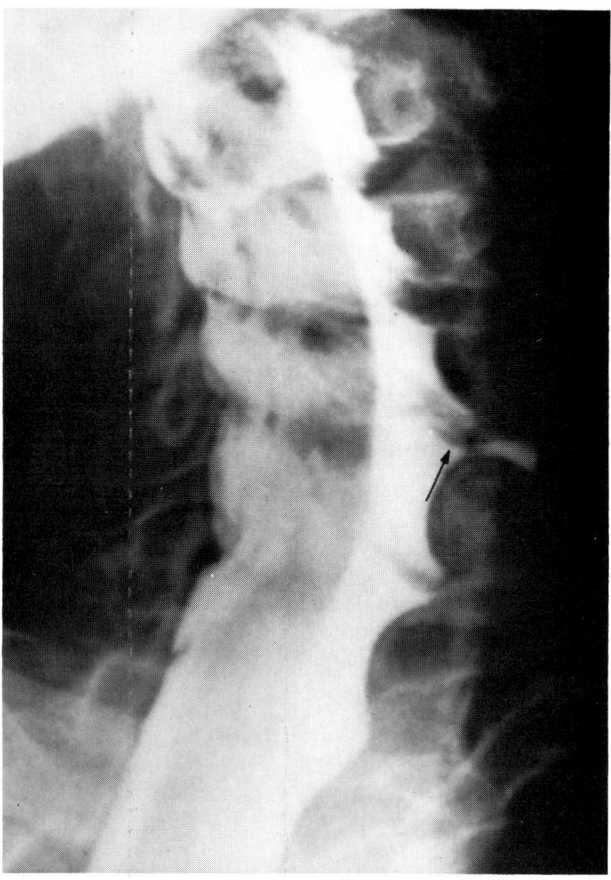

Figure 14–110. Nerve root sleeve "cyst." A single cervical nerve root cyst or diverticulum can be seen. The nerve roots enter the subarachnoid space outpouching (arrow), distinguishing this developmental variation from posttraumatic meningoceles.

vertebral bodies may be deviated anteriorly and the laminae may be thin. At myelography, no apparent communication between spinal canal and cyst is found, although, on occasion, the contrast medium will enter the sac, demonstrating that the lesion is a true intraspinal meningocele. Although these congenital lesions are virtually confined to the thoracic region,[90, 91] extradural cysts may develop after surgery,[92] particularly after the dura has been violated. The pulsations of the cerebrospinal fluid then create an intraspinal meningocele; the intactness of the arachnoid prevents a cerebrospinal fluid leak. If the arachnoid is severed as well, a pseudomeningocele will form, with dissection of cerebrospinal fluid into the surrounding tissues. Eventually this pocket will become relined with arachnoid tissue (Fig. 14–58).

Nerve Root Sleeve Cyst. Nerve root sleeve cysts or diverticula may exist in the cervical or lumbar region. These dilated subarachnoid spaces have no clinical significance and are differentiated from the posttraumatic root sleeve cyst or meningocele by the presence of nerve roots within the sac (Figs. 14–110 and 14–111).

Arnold-Chiari Malformation. Myelography can be used to evaluate the patient with an Arnold-Chiari malformation. This malformation represents a dysgenesis of the cerebellum. It is associated with downward displacement of the cerebellum, the cerebellar tonsils, and the medulla (Fig. 14–112). Meningoceles and meningomyeloceles with spina bifida accompany the more severe forms of Arnold-Chiari malformation.[93] Hydrocephalus is evident in a high percentage of these patients owing to outlet obstruction of the fourth ventricle from a contracted foramen magnum or outlet obstruction of the third ventricle by aqueductal stenosis. Hydromyelia may also be associated with these malformations.[94] Severe forms of this entity become evident early in life, producing cerebellar and brain stem signs. More mild forms may simulate disseminating sclerosis, cerebellar, brain stem, or cervical cord tumors, or syringomyelia.

Routine radiographic findings may include bony abnormalities of the occiput or cervical spine as well as osseous defects associated with the accompanying myeloceles. During myelography, the low-lying cerebellar tonsils will be demonstrated in the cervical canal. The tonsils have rounded, lobulated margins, and are located dorsal to the cervical spinal cord. Lobulated tumors of the foramen magnum (e.g., meningioma) or chronic tonsillar herniation from elevated intracranial pressure may simulate the appearance of the low-lying tonsils .of an Arnold-Chiari malformation.

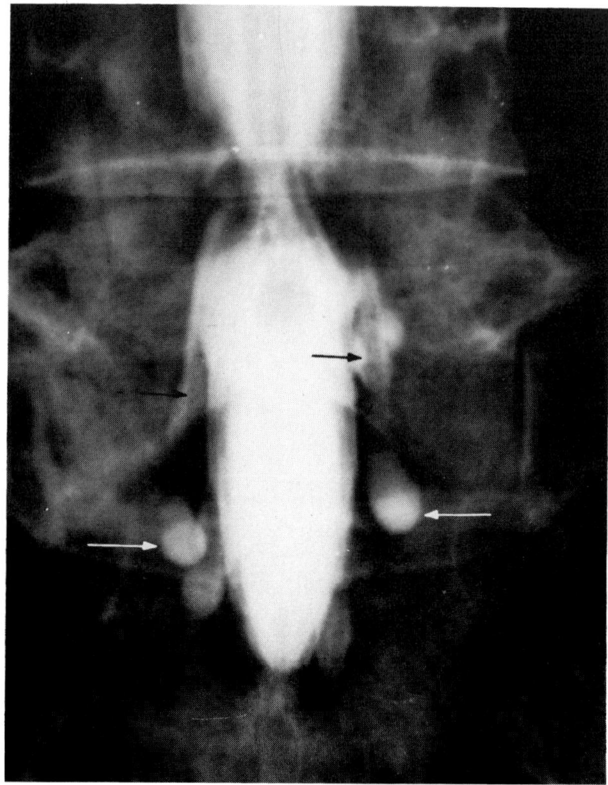

Figure 14–111. Nerve root sleeve "cysts" (white arrows) are frequently seen in the lumbosacral region. Nerve roots (black arrows) can be seen entering these diverticula. These are asymptomatic and are incidental findings in patients who are being examined for other pathologic conditions—e.g., herniated intervertebral discs (seen here at L4-L5).

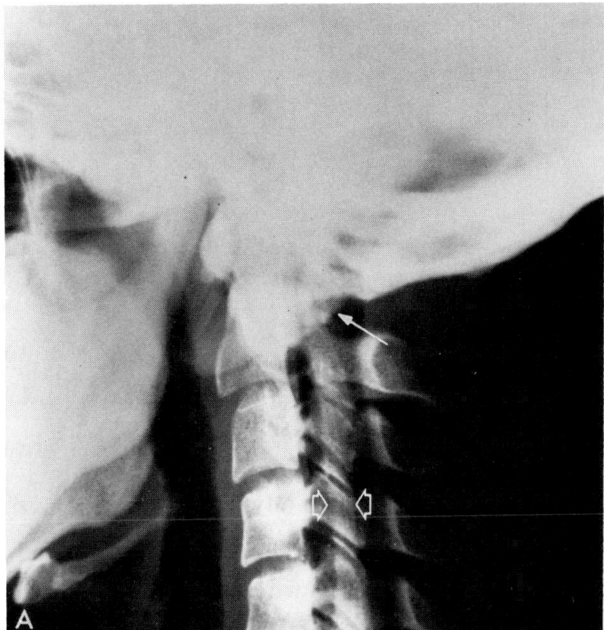

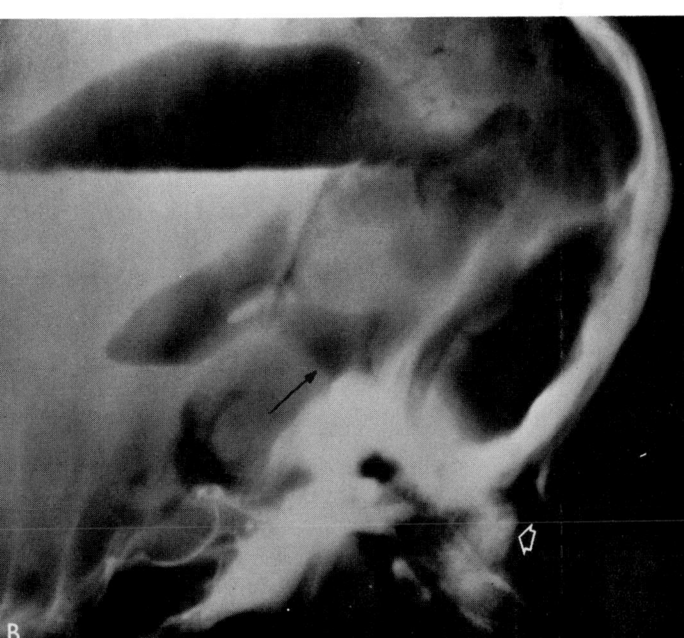

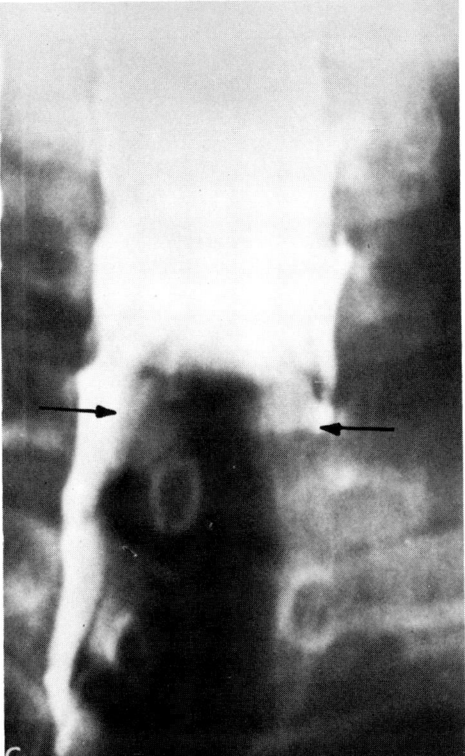

Figure 14–112. *Arnold-Chiari malformation.* **A,** *At gas myelography and pneumoencephalography, the low-lying cerebellar tonsils can be seen at the level of C2 (arrow). In addition, the cervical spinal cord is abnormally narrow (open arrows).* **B,** *The fourth ventricle (arrow) is in a low-lying position owing to dysgenesis of the cerebellum. The low-lying tonsils can again be seen (open arrow).* **C,** *At iophendylate myelography, with the head in a dependent position, the cervical spinal cord is widened (arrows). This finding, in association with the narrowed cord as seen in* **A,** *indicates a collapsing syringomyelia, or hydromyelia, associated with the Arnold-Chiari malformation. (Courtesy of Dr. David Feigin, University of California, San Diego.)*

Inflammatory Lesions

Arachnoiditis. Inflammatory lesions of the spine can be divided into two categories: infectious and noninfectious. A noninfectious inflammatory lesion, arachnoiditis, is common, representing a reaction to a stimulus that is known or cryptic. Arachnoiditis may result from infection, intrathecal drugs (including spinal anesthesia and myelographic contrast media)[6] and subarachnoid blood (spontaneous hemorrhage, trauma, or surgery) (Fig. 14–113). Occasionally, patients develop arachnoiditis in association with herniated intervertebral discs (Fig. 14–114). These changes may be due to an inflammatory response to the herniated nucleus pulposus. In many patients, however, arachnoiditis is idiopathic in nature (Fig. 14–115).

Acute arachnoiditis may lead to symptoms and signs within a few days of the insult to the leptomeninges.[6] Bladder and peripheral muscular paralysis as well as headache, nausea, vomiting, and neurosensory deficits may all occur. Chronic arachnoiditis usually follows asymptomatic acute inflammation. Leptomeningeal adhesions develop with thickening of the arachnoid membrane. In these cases, symptoms develop insidiously, with cord and root signs not limited to a single level.

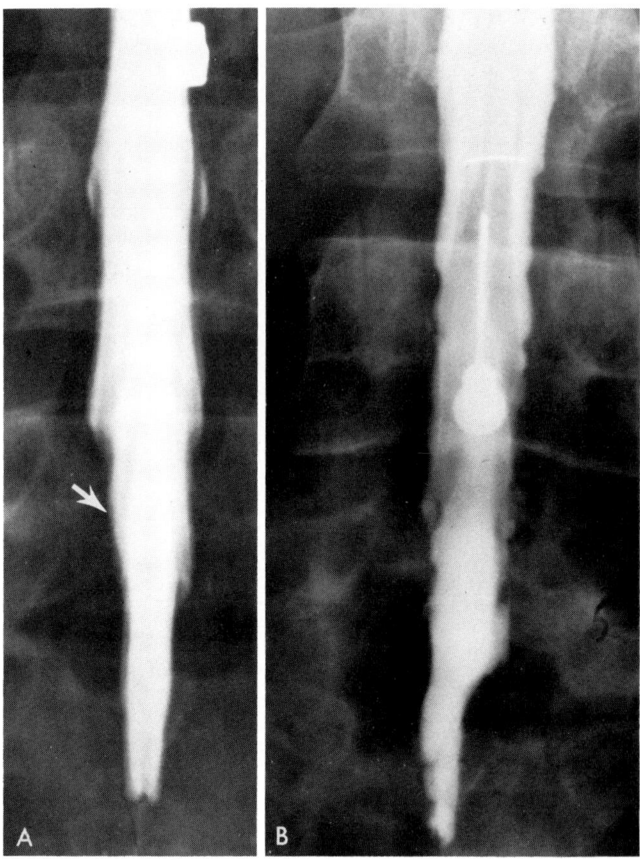

Figure 14–113. *Postsurgical arachnoiditis.* **A,** *Preoperative myelogram demonstrates impression upon the subarachnoid space and amputation of the L5-S1 nerve root sleeve (arrow). Large fragments of an L5 disc were removed at surgery.* **B,** *One year following surgery, the patient returned with recurrent symptoms. Myelography at that time demonstrated marked irregularity of the subarachnoid space, compatible with postoperative arachnoiditis.*

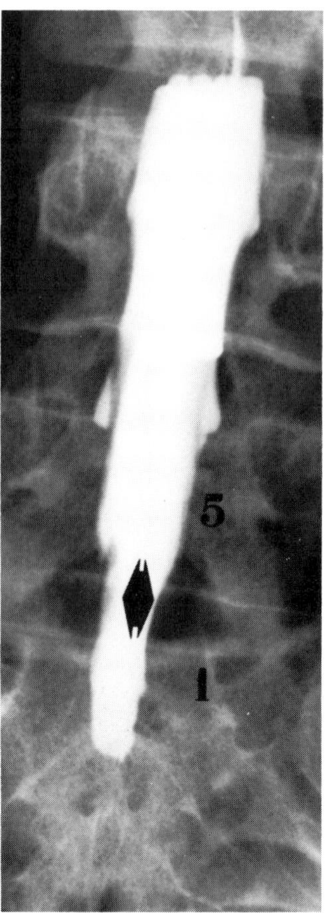

Figure 14–114. *Arachnoiditis secondary to herniated disc. Preoperative myelogram demonstrates symmetric narrowing of the subarachnoid space at L5 and S1 (arrow). At surgery, in addition to a small discal fragment on the right, there was marked thickening of the coverings surrounding the caudal sac. This arachnoiditis was presumed to be due to irritation and inflammation secondary to the herniated nuclear fragment.*

Positive contrast myelography plays a major role in the diagnosis of arachnoiditis. Myelographic findings vary from total obstruction to mild irregularities of the contrast-filled subarachnoid space. Irregular streaking is related to the adhesions that connect the dura and the arachnoid to the nerve roots (Figs. 14–114 and 14–115). Amputated nerve root sleeves may also be detected, simulating the appearance of a herniated intervertebral disc. Contrast media may collect in "subarachnoid cysts," which are merely pockets of arachnoid that are isolated by adhesions and scarring.

On rare occasions, myelographic abnormalities associated with other lesions may resemble those seen in arachnoiditis. Neurofibromatosis (Fig. 14–116) and metastatic deposits in the cauda equina (Fig. 14–117) are two such lesions.

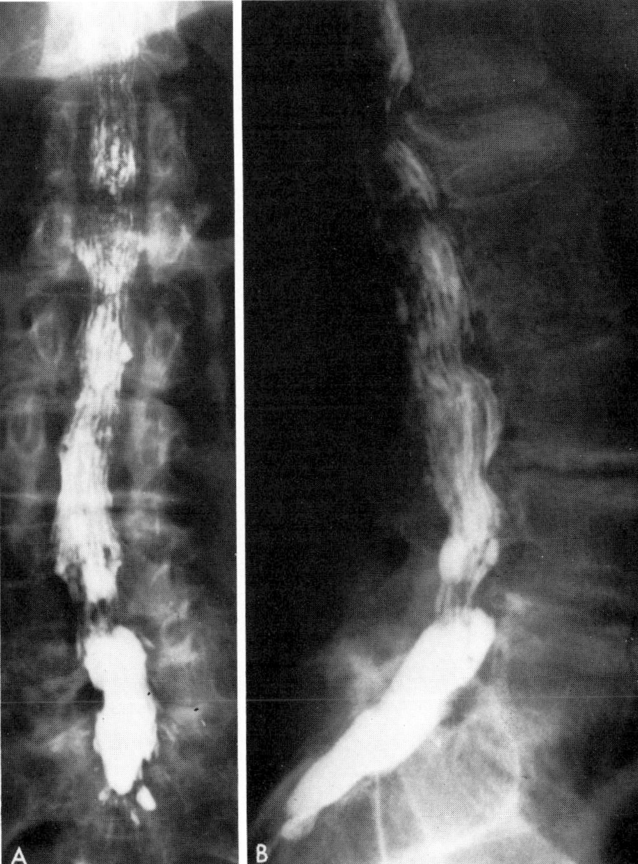

Figure 14–115. *Idiopathic arachnoiditis. Severe arachnoiditis of unknown etiology is demonstrated on iophendylate myelography as irregular streaking, thickening of the nerve roots, encystment of the contrast medium, and narrowing and irregularity of the subarachnoid space.*

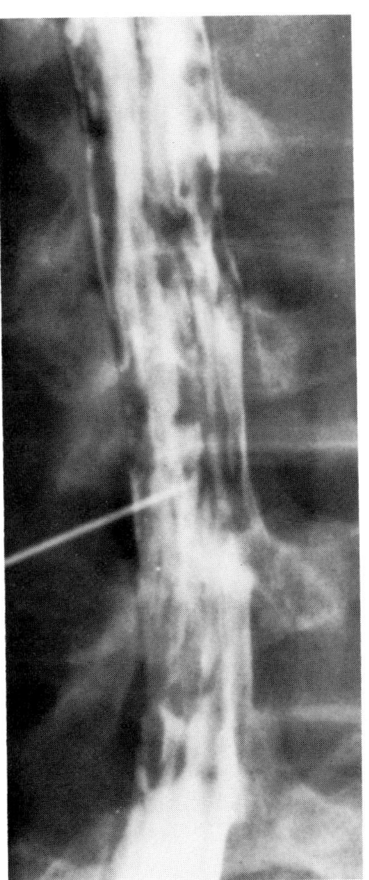

Figure 14–116. *Neurofibromatosis simulating arachnoiditis. A lesion with the appearance of arachnoiditis at myelography is in reality severe neurofibromatosis.*

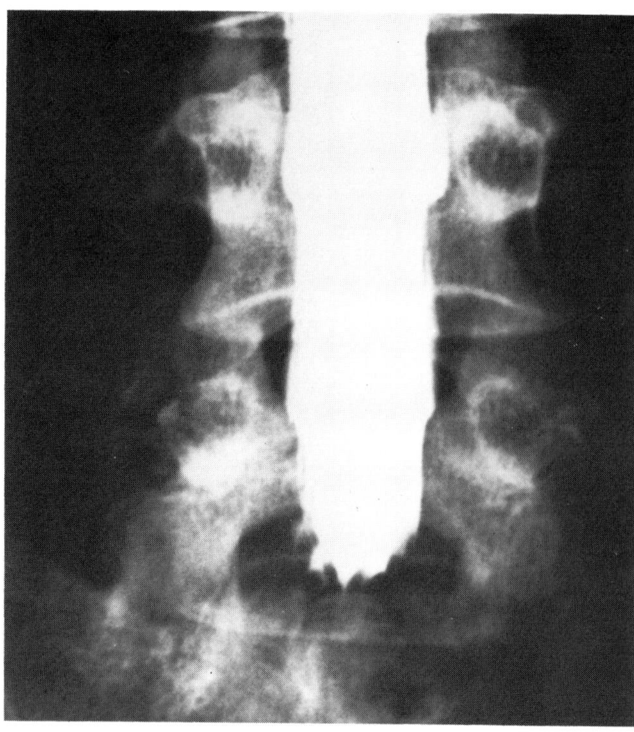

Figure 14–117. Metastasis simulating arachnoiditis. The irregularity at the bottom of the caudal sac in this case is due to metastatic deposits of lung carcinoma rather than arachnoiditis.

Infection. Spinal infections are most commonly located in the extradural space, arising by direct extension from a contaminated vertebral body or paravertebral focus. Rarely, hematogenous spread of infection to the epidural compartment is evident. This latter situation is noted in drug addicts, in patients with urinary tract infections, and in diabetic individuals. Postoperative infections may also occur.[95] On rare occasions, infections may involve the spinal cord itself, producing an intramedullary abscess or granuloma.

Patients may present with acute symptoms or signs of systemic or vertebral infection. Rapid progression of clinical manifestations is frequent in conjunction with staphylococcal and gram-negative bacterial infections. Initial films may reveal vertebral osteomyelitis and soft tissue swelling. Myelography, which may be performed as long as the needle puncture is distant from the infected site, and computed tomography are the diagnostic modalities of choice. The extradural defect resembles that of a tumor, extending across a vertebral body (Fig. 14–118). Complete blockage to the flow of contrast medium can be seen in many of these cases. An intramedullary abscess will create a typical mass.

Chronic nonspecific extradural granuloma probably represents a postinflammatory lesion with histologically evident reactive fibrosis and inflammatory infiltration. Occasionally organisms may be recovered from these lesions. Symptoms and signs usually develop slowly. Routine radiographs reveal narrowing of the intervertebral disc space or vertebral body erosions, with or without a paravertebral soft tissue mass. Myelography will demonstrate an extradural defect adjacent to an area of bony destruction.

Tuberculosis must be considered as one cause of an extradural granuloma.[96] Although spinal tuberculosis is not as frequent as it was in the past, it still occurs, and may lead to osseous destruction without acute, rapidly progressive neurologic deficits. In the patient with tuberculous gibbus deformity, myelography or computed tomography is performed to determine the degree of bony impingement upon the spinal cord.

SUMMARY

The radiographic examination for intraspinal pathology requires detailed attention to the clinical situation, as well as technical precision. A working knowledge of the various modalities — e.g., myelography, epidural venography, computed tomography, and so forth — allows the examiner to choose the

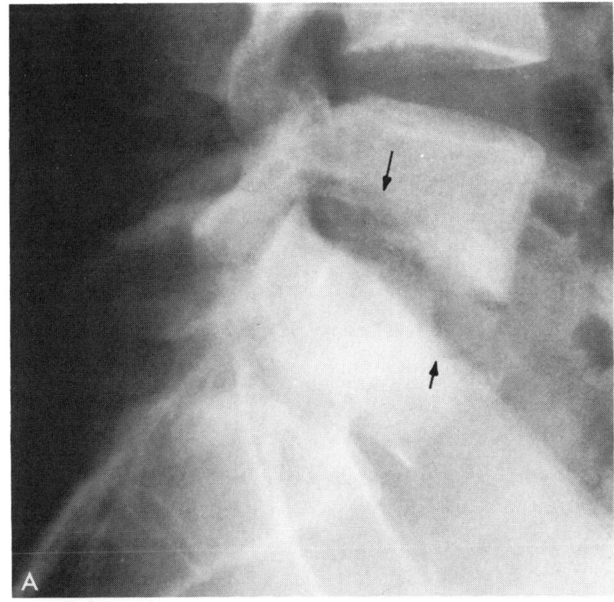

Figure 14–118. Epidural abscess. **A**, Bone destruction on both sides of the intervertebral disc space (arrows) is indicative of infection. An abscess due to infection by staphylococcus organisms was found in this patient. **B**, The subarachnoid space is posteriorly displaced (arrow) by the extradural mass extending over several vertebral segments. **C**, The anteroposterior projection demonstrates bilateral compression of the subarachnoid space by this epidural abscess.

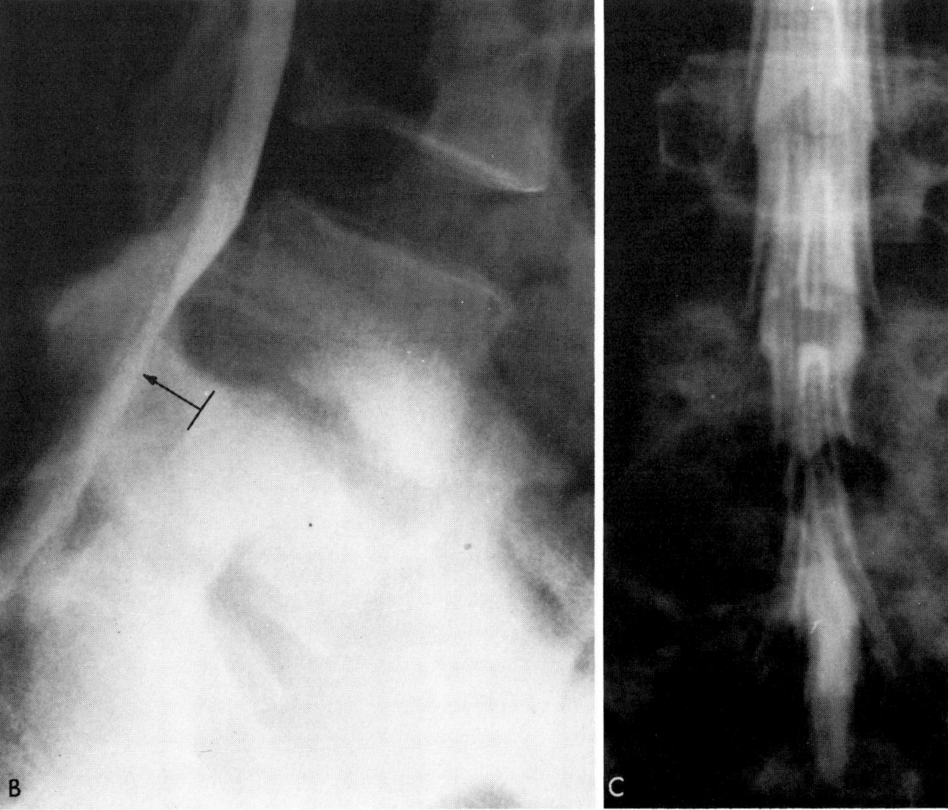

appropriate test for each clinical situation. Myelography remains the standard against which each of the other modalities is measured. Only if surgery is contemplated should myelography be performed. Computed tomography and epidural venography are alternative techniques that are of minimal risk, and which may be used in the clinical situation that does not seem to warrant immediate surgery.

REFERENCES

1. Jacobeus HC: On insufflation of air into the spinal canal for diagnostic purposes in cases of tumors in the spinal cord. Acta Med Scand *55*:555, 1921.
2. Dandy W: Roentgenography of the brain after the injection of air into the spinal canal. Ann Surg *70*:397, 1919.
3. Arnell S, Lidström F: Myelography with Skiodan (Abrodil). Acta Radiol *12*:287, 1931.
4. Strain WH, French JD, Jones GE: Iodinated organic compounds as contrast media for diagnoses. V. Escape of Pantopaque from intracranial subarachnoid space in dogs. Radiology *47*:47, 1946.
5. Ferry DW Jr, Gooding R, Standefer JC, Wiese GM: Effect of Pantopaque myelography on cerebrospinal fluid fractions. J Neurosurg *38*:167, 1973.
6. Mortara R, Brooks W: Chronic arachnoiditis after a Pantopaque study of the posterior fossa. South Med J *69*:520, 1976.
7. Tarlov IM: Pantopaque meningitis disclosed at operation. JAMA *129*:1014, 1945.
8. Hansen E, Fahrenkrug A, Praestholm J: Late meningeal effects of myelographic contrast media with special reference to metrizamide. Br J Radiol *51*:321, 1978.
9. Praestholm J, Klee JG, Klinken L: Histological changes in the central nervous system following intraventricular administration of oil soluble contrast media. Radiology *119*:391, 1976.
10. Holtermann H: Metrizamide. Acta Radiol (Suppl) *335*:1, 1973.
11. Skalpe IO, Amundsen P: Thoracic and cervical myelography with metrizamide. Radiology *116*:101, 1975.
12. Ahlgren P: Amipaque myelography: The side effects compared with Dimer-X. Neuroradiology *9*:197, 1975.
13. Haughton VM, Ho K-C, Larson SJ, Unger GF, Correa-Paz F: Experimental production of arachnoiditis with water soluble myelographic media. Radiology *123*:681, 1977.
14. Baker RA, Hillman BJ, McLennan JE, Strand R, Kaufman S: Sequelae of metrizamide myelography in 200 examinations. Am J Roentgenol *130*:499, 1978.
15. Sackett JF, Strother CM, Quaglieri CE, Javid, M, Levin A, Duff T: Metrizamide: CSF contrast medium. Radiology *123*:779, 1977.
16. Dullerud R, Morland TJ: Adhesive arachnoiditis after lumbar radiculography with Dimer-X and Depo-Medrol. Radiology *119*:153, 1976.
17. Eldevik OP, Haughton V, Ho KC, Williams AL, Unger G, Larson S: Ineffectiveness of prophylactic intrathecal methylprednisolone in myelography with aqueous media. Radiology *129*:99, 1978.
18. Tourtellotte W, Henderson W, Tucker RP, Gilland O, Walker J, Kokman E: A randomized double blind clinical trial comparing the 22 versus 26 gauge needle in the production of the post-lumbar puncture syndrome in normal individuals. Headache *12*:73, 1972.
19. Kelly DL, Alexander E Jr: Lateral cervical puncture for myelography. Technical Note. J Neurosurg *29*:106, 1968.
20. Deisenhammer E, Hammer B: Clinical and experimental studies on headache after myelography. Neuroradiology *9*:99, 1975.
21. Chynn KY: Painless myelography: Introduction of a new aspiration cannula and review of 541 consecutive studies. Radiology *109*:361, 1973.
22. Rice AC, Coyle GF: Oblique projections in cervical myelography. Radiology *113*:216, 1974.
23. Lindgren E: On the diagnosis of tumors of the spinal cord by the aid of gas myelography. Acta Chir Scand *82*:303, 1939.
24. Feria L, Rådberg C: Complete gas myelography via lumbar injection under pressure. Radiology *88*:917, 1967.
25. Heinz ER, Goldman R: The role of gas myelography in neuroradiologic diagnosis. Radiology *102*:629, 1972.
26. Simon J, Garrec A, Guégan Y: Hemorrhagic eye complications of gas myelography. J Radiol Electrol Med Nucl *54*:675, 1973.
27. Batson OV: The function of the vertebral veins and their role in the spread of metastases. Ann Surg *112*:138, 1940.
28. Vogelsang H: Intraosseous Spinal Venography. Baltimore, Williams & Wilkins, 1970.
29. Gargano F, Meyer J, Sheldon J: Transfemoral ascending lumbar catheterization of the epidural veins in lumbar disc disease. Radiology *111*:329, 1974.
30. O'Dell CW, Coel MN, Ignelzi RJ: Ascending lumbar venography in lumbar disc disease. J Bone Joint Surg *59A*:159, 1977.
31. Lasser EC: Personal communication.
32. Theron J, Djindjian R: Cervicovertebral phlebography using catheterization. Radiology *108*:325, 1973.
33. Théron J: Cervicovertebral phlebography: Pathological results. Radiology *118*:73, 1976.
34. Théron J, Moret J: Spinal Phlebography: Lumbar and Cervical Techniques. New York, Springer-Verlag, 1978.
35. LePage J: Transfemoral ascending lumbar catheterization of the epidural veins: Exposition and technique. Radiology *111*:337, 1974.
36. Guistra P, Wickenden J, Furman R, Wickenden R, Killoran P: Multiple contrast injections in epidural venography. Am J Roentgenol *131*:485, 1978.
37. Gargano FP: Extradural venography. *in* R Shapiro (Ed): Myelography. 3rd Ed. Chicago, Year Book Medical Publishers, 1975, p 566.
38. Gershater R, St Louis E: Lumbar epidural venography. Radiology *131*:409, 1979.
39. Grossman Z, Wistow B, Wallinga H, Heitzman ER: Recognition of vertebral abnormalities in computed tomography of the chest and abdomen. Radiology *121*:369, 1976.
40. Hammerschlag S, Wolpert S, Carter B: Computed tomography of the spinal canal. Radiology *121*:361, 1976.
41. Nickel A, Salem J: Clinical experience in North America with metrizamide: Evaluation of 1850 subarachnoid examinations. Acta Radiol (Suppl) *355*:409, 1977.
42. Tarlov IM: Spinal extradural hemangioblastoma roentgenographically visualized with Diodrast at operation and successfully removed. Radiology *49*:717, 1947.
43. DiChiro G, Wener L: Angiography of the spinal cord. J Neurosurg *39*:1, 1973.
44. Voigt K, Hoogland PH, Stoeter P, Djindjian R: Diagnostic value and limitations of selective spinal angiography in different lesions of the vertebral bones. Radiol Clin Biol *47*:73, 1978.
45. Gabrielsen TO, Seeger JF: Vertebral angiography in the diagnosis of intraspinal masses in upper cervical region. Neuroradiology *5*:7, 1973.
46. Djindjian R, Theron J, Merland J: Embolisation dans les malformations et tumeurs cervico-thoraciques et rachidiennes. J Neuroradiol *2*:39, 1975.
47. Benati A, DaPian R, Mazza C, Maschio A, Perini S, Bricolo A, Dalle Ore G: Preoperative embolization of a vertebral haemangioma compressing the spinal cord. Neuroradiology *7*:181, 1974.
48. Doppman J, DiChiro G, Ommaya A: Percutaneous embolization of spinal cord arteriovenous malformations. J Neurosurg *34*:48, 1971.
49. Wener L, DiChiro G, Gargour GW: Angiography of cervical cord injuries. Radiology *112*:597, 1974.
50. Bussat P, Rossier AB, Djindjian R, Vasey H, Berney J: Spinal cord angiography in dorsolumbar vertebral fractures with neurological involvement. Radiology *109*:617, 1973.
51. Albertson K, Doppman J, Ramsey R: Spinal seizures induced by contrast media. Radiology *107*:349, 1973.
52. DiChiro G: Unintentional spinal cord arteriography: A warning. Radiology *112*:231, 1974.
53. Lindblom K: Diagnostic puncture of intervertebral disks in sciatica. Acta Orthop Scand *17*:231, 1948.
54. Bromage PR, Bramwell RSB, Catchlove RF, Belanger G, Pearce CG: Peridurography with metrizamide: Animal and Human Studies. Radiology *128*:123, 1978.
55. Roberson GH, Hatten HP Jr, Hesselink JH: Epidurography: Selective catheter technique and review of 53 cases. Am J Roentgenol *132*:787, 1979.
56. Jabbari B, Pierce J, Boston S, Echols D: Brown-Séquard syndrome and cervical spondylosis. J Neurosurg *47*:556, 1977.
57. McIvor GWD, Kirkaldy-Willis WH: Pathological and myelographic changes in the major types of lumbar spinal stenosis. Clin Orthop *115*:72, 1976.
58. Kirkaldy-Willis WH, Pain KWE, Cauchoix J, McIvor G: Lumbar spinal stenosis. Clin Orthop *99*:30, 1974.
59. Salibi B: Neurogenic intermittent claudication and stenosis of the lumbar spinal canal. Surg Neurol *5*:269, 1976.
60. Roberson G, Llewellyn H, Tavaras J: The narrow lumbar spinal canal syndrome. Radiology *107*:89, 1973.
61. Eisenstein S: Measurements of the lumbar spinal canal in two racial groups. Clin Orthop *115*:42, 1976.

62. Epstein J, Epstein B, Lavine L, Carras R, Rosenthal A: Cervical myeloradiculopathy caused by arthritic hypertrophy of the posterior facets and laminae. J Neurosurg *49*:387, 1978.
63. Harris P: Cervical spine stenosis. Paraplegia *15*:125, 1977.
64. Devadiga KV, Gass HH: Chronic lumbar extradural haematoma simulating disc syndrome. J Neurol Neurosurg Psychiatry *36*:255, 1973.
65. Locke G, Giorgio A, Biggers S Jr, Johnson AP, Salem F: Acute spinal epidural hematoma secondary to aspirin-induced prolonged bleeding. Surg Neurol *5*:293, 1976.
66. Sokoloff J, Coel M, Ignelzi R: Spinal subdural hematoma. Radiology *120*:116, 1976.
67. Scher AT: Syringomyelia secondary to paraplegia due to fractures of the thoracic spine. S Afr Med J *50*:1406, 1976.
68. Komaki S: Localized spinal cord atrophy: Significance of its demonstration. Radiology *121*:111, 1976.
69. Shapiro R: Myelography. Chicago, Year Book Medical Publishers, 1975.
70. Epstein B, Epstein J: Extrapleural intrathoracic apical traumatic pseudomeningocele. Am J Roentgenol *120*:887, 1974.
71. Rocha-Campos B, Silva L, Ballalai N, Negrão M: Traumatic subarachnoid-pleural fistula. J Neurol Neurosurg Psychiatry *37*:269, 1974.
72. Kirks D, Berger P, Fitz C, Harwood-Nash D: Myelography in evaluation of paravertebral mass lesions in infants and children. Radiology *119*:603, 1976.
73. Banna M, Gryspeerdt G: Intraspinal tumors in children (excluding dysraphism). Clin Radiol *22*:17, 1971.
74. Hatam A, Hindmarsh T, Greitz T: Myelography in metastatic lesions. Acta Radiol (Diagn) *16*:321, 1975.
75. Lally J, Cossrow J, Dalinka M: Odontoid fractures in metastatic breast carcinoma. Am J Roentgenol *128*:817, 1977.
76. Twersky J, Kassner EG, Tenner M, Camera A: Vertebral and costal osteochondromas causing spinal cord compression. Am J Roentgenol *124*:124, 1975.
77. Edelson R, Deck M, Posner J: Intramedullary spinal cord metastases. Neurology *22*:1222, 1972.
78. Pia HW: Diagnosis and treatment of spinal angiomas. Acta Neurochir *28*:1, 1973.
79. Doppman J, Wirth F, DiChiro G, Ommaya A: Value of cutaneous angiomas in the arteriographic localization of spinal cord arteriovenous malformations. N Engl J Med *281*:1440, 1969.
80. Coel M, Alksne J: Embolization to diminish high output failure secondary to systemic angiomatosis (Ullmann's syndrome). Vasc Surg *12*:336, 1978.
81. Newton T, Adams J: Angiographic demonstration and non-surgical embolization of spinal cord angioma. Radiology *91*:873, 1968.
82. Doppman J: The nidus concept of spinal cord arteriovenous malformations. Br J Radiol *44*:758, 1971.
83. Kerber CW, Cromwell LD, Sheptak PE: Intra-arterial cyanoacrylate: An adjunct in the treatment of spinal/paraspinal arteriovenous malformations. Am J Roentgenol *130*:99, 1978.
84. James H, Oliff M, Mulcahy J: Spinal dysraphism: A comprehensive diagnostic approach. Neurosurgery *2*:15, 1978.
85. Sostrin R, Thompson J, Rouhe S, Hasso A: Occult spinal dysraphism in the geriatric patient. Radiology *125*:165, 1977.
86. Thomas J, Miller R: Lipomatous tumors of the spinal canal: A study of their clinical range. Mayo Clin Proc *48*:393, 1973.
87. Hilal S, Marton D, Pollack E: Diastematomyelia in children, Radiology *112*:609, 1974.
88. Weinstein M, Rothner AD, Duchesneau P, Dohn D: Computed tomography in diastematomyelia. Radiology *117*:609, 1975.
89. James H, Oliff M: Computed tomography in spinal dysraphism. J Comput Assist Tomogr *1*:391, 1977.
90. Taveras J, Wood E: Diseases of the spinal cord. *In* Diagnostic Neuroradiology. Vol II. 2nd Ed. Baltimore, Williams & Wilkins Co, 1976, p 1114.
91. Duncan A, Hoare R: Spinal arachnoid cysts in children. Radiology *126*:423, 1978.
92. Quencer R, Tenner M, Rothman L: The postoperative myelogram. Radiology *123*:667, 1977.
93. Shapiro R: Congenital lesions. *In* R Shapiro (Ed): Myelography, Chicago, Year Book Medical Publishers, 1975.
94. Harwood-Nash D, Fitz C: Myelography and syringohydromyelia in infancy and childhood. Radiology *113*:661, 1974.
95. Baker A, Ojemann R, Swartz M, Richardson E: Spinal epidural abscess. N Engl J Med *293*:463, 1975.
96. Marcq M, Sharma O: Tuberculosis of the spine: A reminder. Chest *63*:403, 1973.

ARTHROGRAPHY, TENOGRAPHY AND BURSOGRAPHY

by Donald Resnick, M.D.

15

Contrast opacification of joint cavities (arthrography), tendon sheaths (tenography), and bursae (bursography) is a useful procedure for evaluation of articulations and surrounding tissues. This chapter describes the indications, techniques, and normal and abnormal findings of this examination at specific locations in the body. Arthrographic abnormalities in patients with joint prostheses are summarized elsewhere in the book.

WRIST AND HAND

Arthrography of the Wrist

Arthrography of the wrist (Tables 15–1 and 15–2) is a safe procedure, which is useful in the diagnosis of traumatic and articular disorders.[1-5]

Technique (Fig. 15–1). Under fluoroscopic control, a 22 gauge, 1.5 inch long needle is introduced into the wrist from a dorsal approach. The

Table 15–1

WRIST ARTHROGRAPHY: KEY TO NUMBERS USED TO IDENTIFY STRUCTURES

1. Radiocarpal compartment
2. Inferior radioulnar compartment
3. Prestyloid recess
4. Extensor tendons and sheaths
5. Lymphatics
6. Midcarpal compartment
7. Common carpometacarpal compartment
8. Volar radial recesses
9. Pisiform-triquetral compartment

Table 15–2

INDICATIONS FOR WRIST ARTHROGRAPHY

Evaluation of:
- Presence and extent of synovial inflammation
- Injuries to the triangular fibrocartilage, interosseous ligaments, and joint capsule
- Soft tissue masses

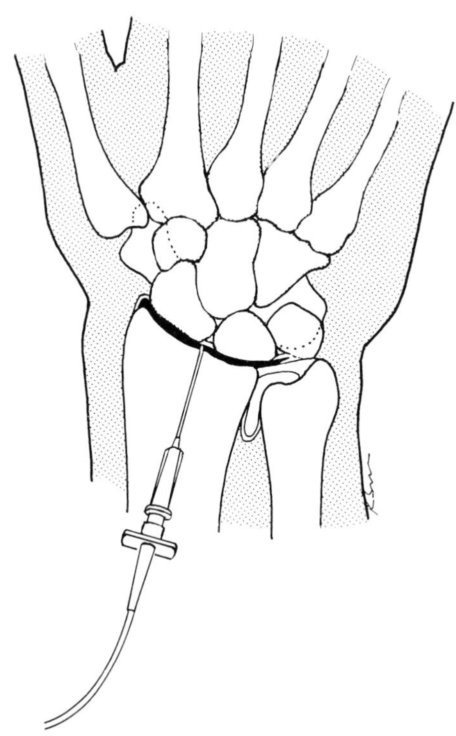

Figure 15–1. *Wrist arthrography: Technique. A needle is introduced into the radiocarpal compartment from a dorsal approach and 1.5 to 2.5 ml of contrast material is injected.*

needle is guided under the radial lip, entering the radiocarpal compartment between the scaphoid and the radius. Occasionally, this compartment must be entered at the junction of scaphoid, lunate, and radius, but at this site, care must be taken not to place the needle too distally, such that the scaphoid-lunate interosseous ligament is violated. A total of 1.5 to 2.5 ml of 60 per cent methylglucamine diatrizoate (Renografin) is administered. Anteroposterior, lateral, and oblique radiographs are obtained before and after mild exercise.

Normal Wrist Arthrogram (Figs. 15–2 and 15–3). Contrast opacification of the radiocarpal compartment reveals a concave sac with smooth synovial surfaces extending between the distal radius and proximal carpal row. The prestyloid recess appears as a finger-like projection that approaches the ulnar styloid process from the ulnar limit of the radiocarpal joint. One or more volar radial recesses are located beneath the distal radius.

As indicated in Chapter 3, communication between the radiocarpal compartment and other compartments in the wrist during arthrography may be observed in "normal" individuals or cadavers. The

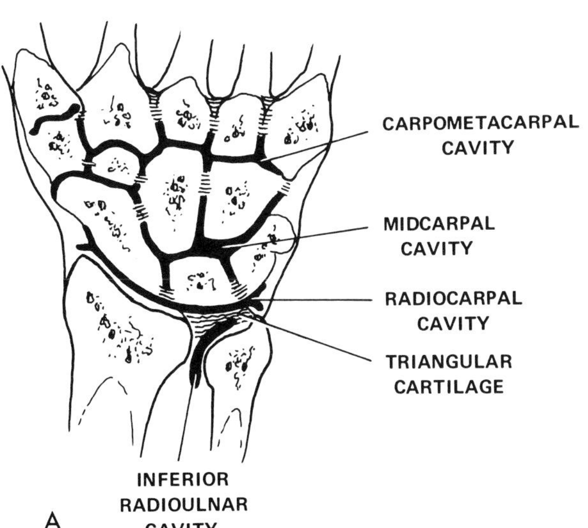

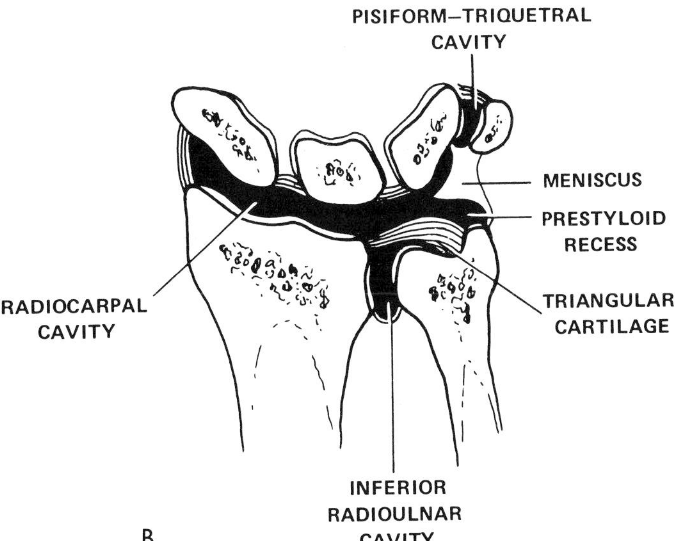

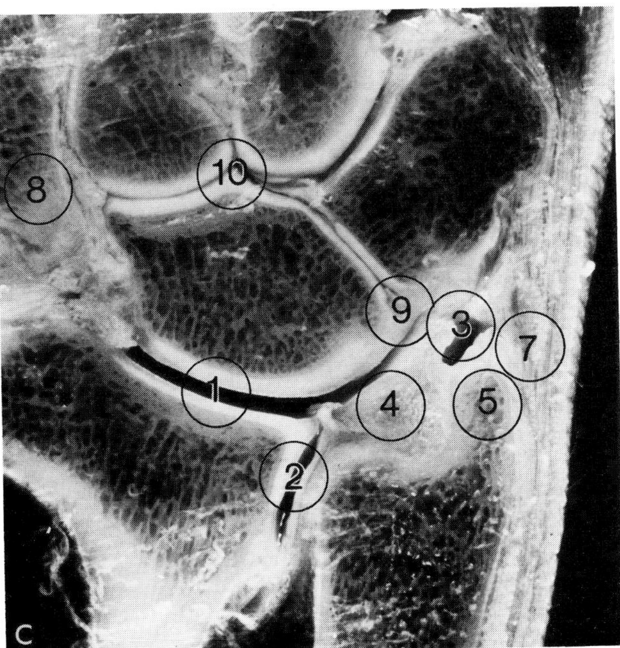

Figure 15–2. *Wrist arthrography: Normal anatomy.*

A *Drawing of a coronal section of the wrist. Observe the radiocarpal cavity, which is separated from the inferior radioulnar cavity by the triangular fibrocartilage, and which is separated from the midcarpal cavity by interosseous ligaments extending between bones of the proximal carpal row. A (common) carpometacarpal cavity is indicated between the bones of the distal carpal row and bases of the four ulnar metacarpals. This compartment extends distally between the metacarpal bases as intermetacarpal compartments. The first carpometacarpal compartment is also indicated between the trapezium and base of the first metacarpal.*

B *Detailed drawing of the radiocarpal compartment. Note its "C" shape with a Y-shaped ulnar limit produced by the meniscus. The proximal limb or diverticulum at the ulnar limit of the radiocarpal compartment is the prestyloid recess, which is intimate with the ulnar styloid. The distal limb extends along the triquetrum and may, in some instances, communicate with the pisiform-triquetral compartment.*

C *Coronal section of cadaveric wrist. Identified structures are the radiocarpal compartment (1), inferior radioulnar compartment (2), prestyloid recess (3), triangular fibrocartilage (4), ulnar styloid (5), ulnar collateral ligament (7), scaphoid (8), interosseous ligament between lunate and triquetrum (9), and midcarpal compartment (10).*

(**B, C** *From Resnick D: Radiology 113:331, 1974.*)

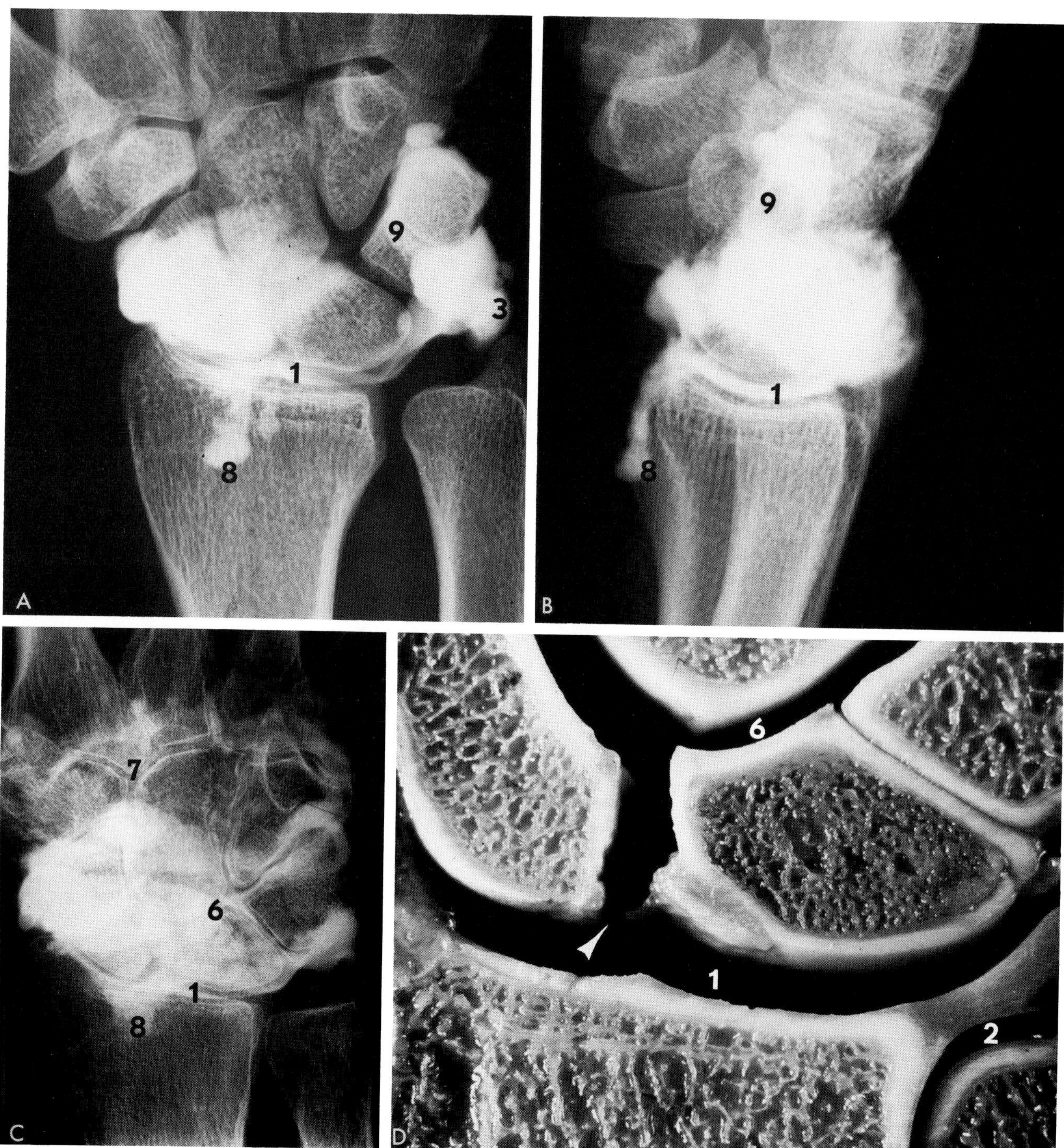

Figure 15–3. Wrist arthrography: Normal arthrogram.

A, B *Frontal and lateral views. Observe the contrast-filled radiocarpal compartment (1), which is communicating with the pisiform-triquetral compartment (9). Also note the prestyloid recess (3) and volar radial recesses (8).*

C, D *Radiocarpal–midcarpal compartment communication. A frontal radiograph following opacification of the radiocarpal compartment (1) reveals its communication with the midcarpal (6) and common carpometacarpal (7) compartments. This communication is possible when a defect exists in the interosseous ligament extending between bones of the proximal carpal row. On a photograph of a coronal section of a cadaveric wrist, observe disruption of the scapholunate ligament (arrowhead). The inferior radioulnar compartment (2) and volar radial recesses (8) are also indicated.*

Illustration continued on the opposite page

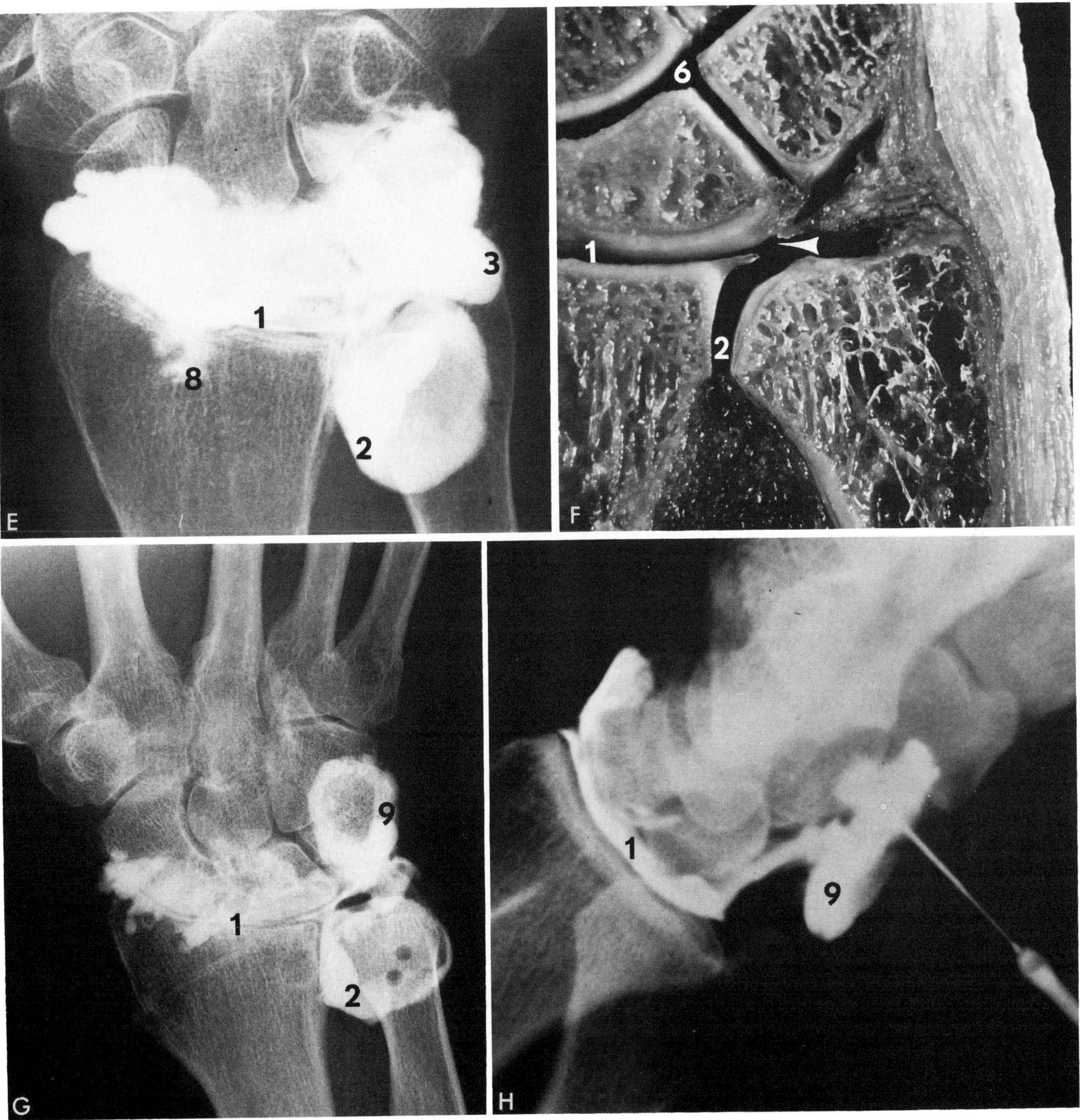

Figure 15–3. Continued

E, F *Radiocarpal–inferior radioulnar compartment communication. A frontal radiograph following opacification of the radiocarpal compartment (1) reveals its communication with the inferior radioulnar compartment (2). This communication is possible when a defect exists in the triangular fibrocartilage. Such a defect (arrowhead) is illustrated on a photograph of a coronal section of the wrist. Other indicated structures are the midcarpal compartment (6), volar radial recesses (8), and prestyloid recess (3).*

G, H *Radiocarpal compartment–pisiform-triquetral compartment communication. A frontal radiograph following introduction of contrast material into the radiocarpal compartment (1) demonstrates its communication with the pisiform-triquetral compartment (9) and inferior radioulnar compartment (2). On an oblique radiograph in another patient, a needle has been inserted into the pisiform-triquetral compartment (9). Overdistention of this cavity allows contrast to flow into the radiocarpal compartment (1).*

radiocarpal compartment may communicate with the midcarpal compartment in 13 to 47 per cent of the population and with the inferior radioulnar compartment in 7 to 35 per cent.[2, 3, 6] Arthrographic communication between the radiocarpal and pisiform-triquetral compartments is frequent, particularly with forceful injection of contrast material into either compartment.[5, 7]

Opacification of tendon sheaths and lymphatics is generally not observed in "normal" wrist arthrograms,[2] although Trentham and associates[6] indicated that tendon sheath visualization may be apparent in 6 per cent of such normal examinations.

Rheumatoid Arthritis (Figs. 15–4 to 15–6) (Table 15–3). Injection of contrast material into the radiocarpal compartment in patients with rheuma-

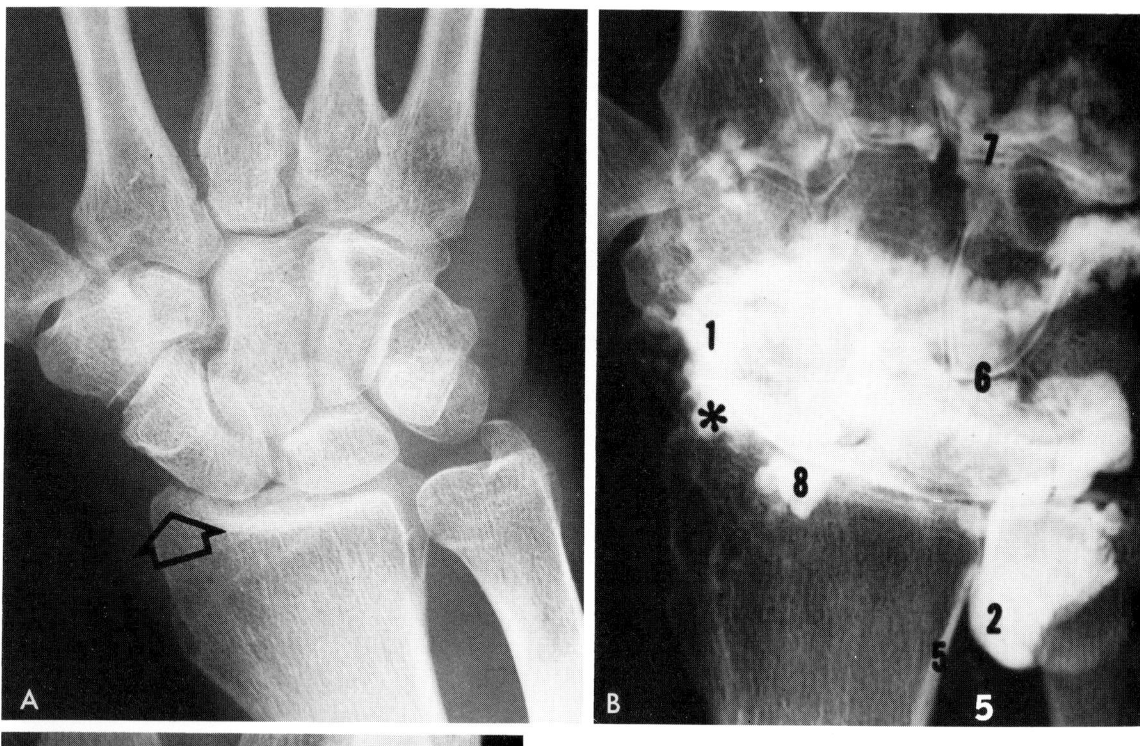

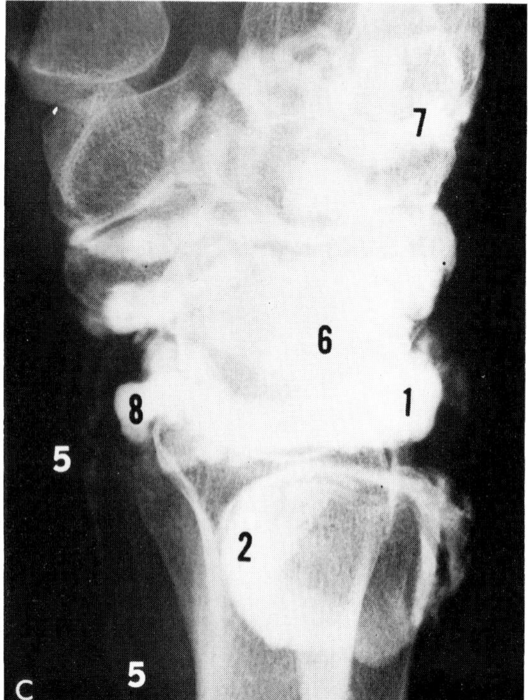

Figure 15–4. *Wrist arthrography: Rheumatoid arthritis.*

A *On the initial film, a small erosion of the radial styloid is evident (arrow).*

B, C *Posteroanterior* **(B)** *and oblique* **(C)** *views following arthrography demonstrate severe synovial irregularity or corrugation (asterisk), radiocarpal compartment (1) communication with the inferior radioulnar (2), midcarpal (6), and common carpometacarpal (7) compartments, lymphatic filling (5), and prominent volar radial recesses (8).*

(From Resnick D: Radiology 113:331, 1974.)

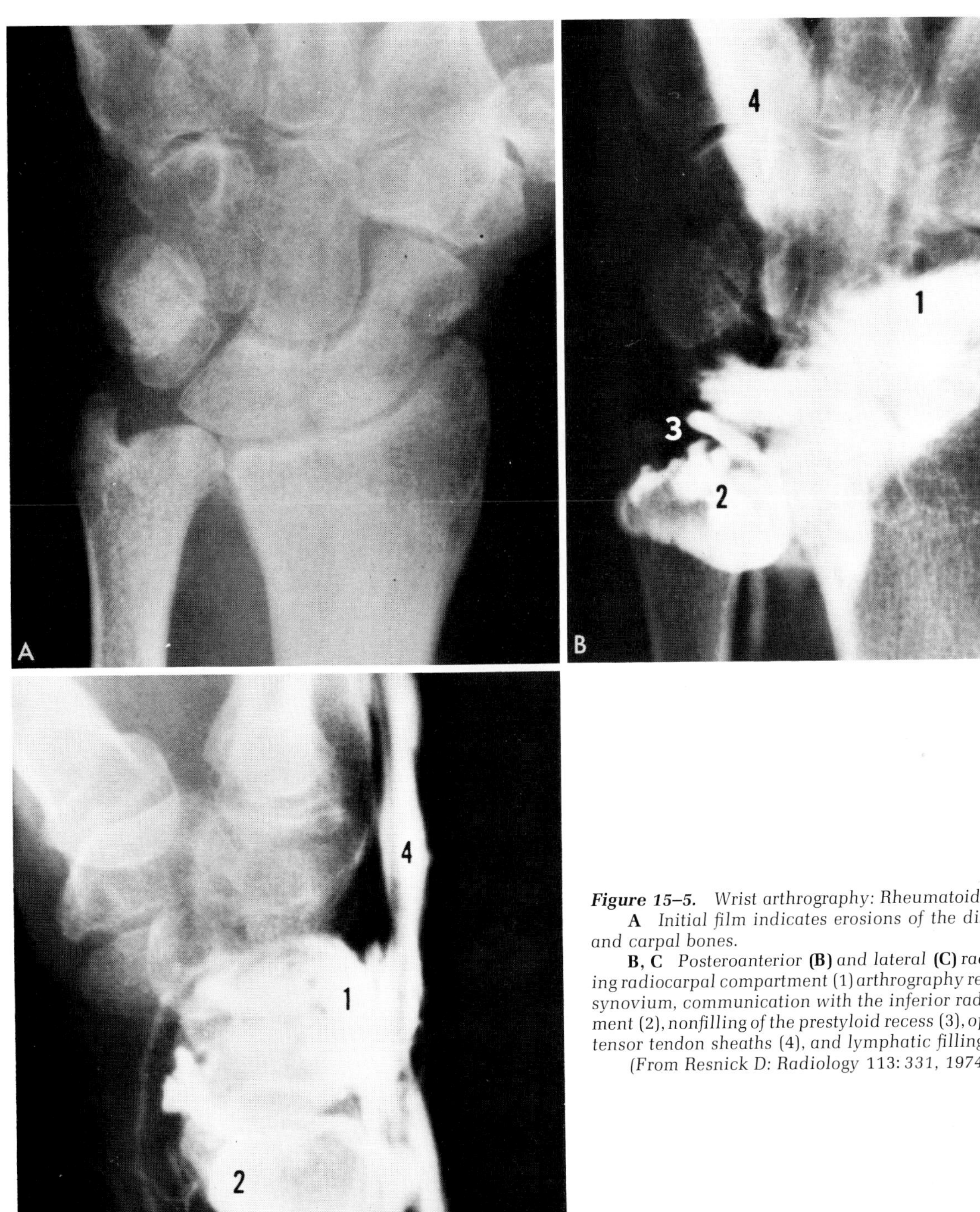

Figure 15–5. *Wrist arthrography: Rheumatoid arthritis.*

A *Initial film indicates erosions of the distal radius, ulna, and carpal bones.*

B, C *Posteroanterior* **(B)** *and lateral* **(C)** *radiographs following radiocarpal compartment (1) arthrography reveal a corrugated synovium, communication with the inferior radioulnar compartment (2), nonfilling of the prestyloid recess (3), opacification of extensor tendon sheaths (4), and lymphatic filling (5).*

(From Resnick D: Radiology 113: 331, 1974.)

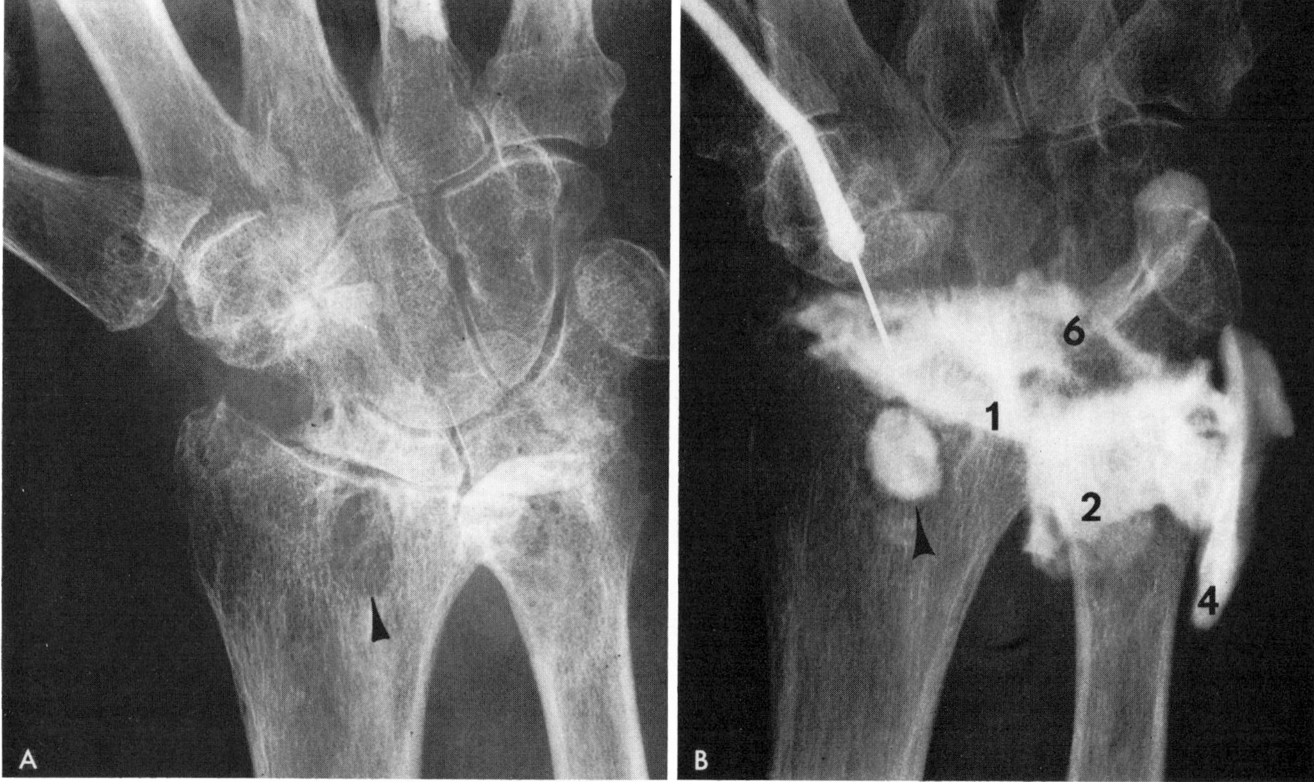

Figure 15–6. Wrist arthrography: Rheumatoid arthritis.

A The initial film demonstrates severe rheumatoid involvement of the wrist with erosions, subchondral cysts (arrowhead) and subluxation.

B Following radiocarpal compartment (1) arthrography, observe filling of the inferior radioulnar (2) and midcarpal (6) compartments and opacification of the extensor carpi ulnaris tendon sheath (4) and radial cyst (arrowhead). The synovium is slightly irregular.

Table 15–3
RHEUMATOID ARTHRITIS: ARTHROGRAPHIC FEATURES (40 WRISTS)

Finding	Frequency (Per Cent)	Frequency in Previous Study* (Per Cent)
Synovial Irregularity	90	90
Minimal	40	
Moderate to severe	50	
Prestyloid recess	80	
Compartment Communication	80	
Inferior radioulnar	55	70
Midcarpal	65	70
Carpometacarpal	53	
Pisiform-triquetral	50	
Tendon Communication	28	21
Extensor tendons	28	21
Flexor tendons	0	2
Lymphatic Communication	38	33

*Data from Harrison M et al: Am J Roentgenol *112*:480, 1971.

Table 15–4

FREQUENCY OF ARTHROGRAPHIC ABNORMALITIES IN ARTHRITIC DISORDERS OF THE WRIST

	Abnormality				
	SYNOVIAL IRREGULARITY				
Disorder	*Corrugated*	*Noncorrugated*	*LYMPHATIC FILLING*	*COMPARTMENT COMMUNICATION*	*TENDON COMMUNICATION*
Rheumatoid arthritis	+++		++	+++	+
Posttraumatic arthritis		+	−	++	+
Rheumatoid "variant" disorders	+++		++	+++	−
Neuropathic disease		++	−	++	+
Occupation-induced arthritis	++		+	++	−
Gout	++		+	++	+
Septic arthritis	++		++	++	+

+ = Mild abnormalities; ++ = moderate abnormalities; +++ = severe abnormalities; − = no abnormality.

toid arthritis reveals certain abnormalities.[2, 5, 6, 8] The most characteristic changes are corrugated irregularity of the contrast material (25 to 90 per cent) and opacification of lymphatic vessels (30 to 38 per cent). These two findings are not specific for rheumatoid arthritis but are reliable indicators of synovial inflammation. The corrugated pattern suggests villous hypertrophy of the synovial membrane and may initially be evident at specific sites in the radiocarpal compartment, such as the prestyloid or volar radial recesses.[8, 9] The basis of the lymphatic filling is not entirely known. The synovial membrane contains lymphatics, particularly along the volar aspect of the wrist. Synovial inflammation and hypertrophy in rheumatoid arthritis and related disorders may increase the permeability of the synovial membrane, allowing greater and more rapid absorption of contrast material by both vascular and lymphatic channels. This has been substantiated by radioisotopic studies revealing more rapid clearance of contrast material from rheumatoid articulations than from traumatic articulations.[10] Lymphatic hyperplasia is well recognized in rheumatoid arthritis,[11] and lymphatic filling has been observed in other rheumatoid joints during arthrography.[12, 13] Lymphatic filling may occasionally be seen in normal individuals with overdistention of the articular cavity during arthrography of the wrist or other joints.

Communication between the radiocarpal compartment and other compartments in the rheumatoid wrist is frequent (less than 80 per cent). This communication, which may occur between radiocarpal and midcarpal compartments (35 to 70 per cent), radiocarpal and inferior radioulnar compartments (55 to 70 per cent), radiocarpal and common carpometacarpal compartments (53 per cent), and radiocarpal and pisiform-triquetral compartments (50 per cent), lacks specificity as a finding of rheumatoid arthritis because of its common occurrence in normal individuals[2, 3, 6] and in patients with other types of articular disease.[5]

Tendon sheath visualization following radiocarpal compartment arthrography is observed in 20 to 28 per cent of rheumatoid wrists, presumably related to inflammatory synovial tissue or pannus within the articular cavity and tendon sheaths. This visualization is more frequently observed on the dorsum of the wrist related to filling of the sheaths about the extensor tendons. Tendon sheath visualization is not a reliable indicator of rheumatoid arthritis because of its occasional occurrence in other articular diseases[5] and normal individuals.[6]

In summary, wrist arthrography in patients with rheumatoid arthritis reveals certain abnormalities that suggest the presence of synovial inflammation. These abnormalities, particularly a corrugated synovial pattern and lymphatic filling, are not specific for rheumatoid arthritis, as they occur in other disorders with fundamental or predominant synovial hypertrophy. Therefore, wrist arthrography is not useful in diagnosing rheumatoid arthritis but may be helpful in indicating the presence and extent of synovial inflammation and its response to treatment (Table 15–4).

TRAUMA. Arthrographic abnormalities following wrist trauma most frequently are compartmental communications, tendon sheath visualization, and mild synovial irregularity,[4, 5, 14, 335] These abnormalities may follow a single traumatic episode or relate to repetitive trauma. In this latter situation, occupational trauma, such as occurs in pneumatic drillers or boxers, may produce similar arthrographic alterations[5] (Fig. 15–7).

The pattern of compartmental communication is dependent upon the site of trauma. With injuries to the triangular fibrocartilage or ulnar styloid, communication between the radiocarpal and inferior radioulnar compartments is observed (Fig. 15–8). In these instances, the capsule about the inferior radioulnar joint may also be disrupted with soft tissue extravasation of contrast material. With scaphoid fractures or injuries to the interosseous ligaments between the bones of the proximal carpal row, one sees communication between the radiocarpal and

Text continued on page 524

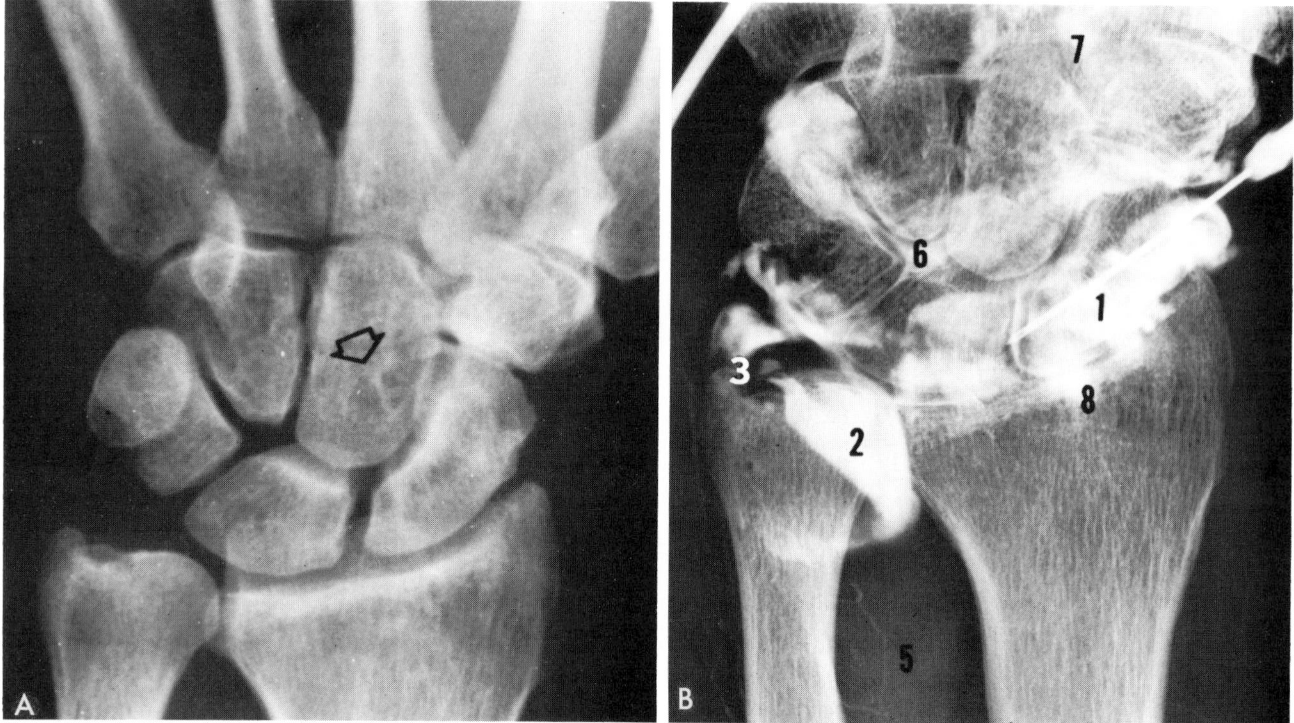

Figure 15–7. Wrist arthrography: Occupational trauma—driller's disease. This 61 year old man had worked as a pneumatic driller for 35 years and had intermittent wrist pain and swelling.

A The initial film reveals extensive cystic abnormality throughout the carpal bones (arrow).

B Following opacification of the radiocarpal compartment (1), contrast material outlines the inferior radioulnar (2), midcarpal (6), and common carpometacarpal (7) compartments, volar radial recesses (8), prestyloid recess (3), and lymphatics (5).

(From Resnick D: Radiology 113:331, 1974.)

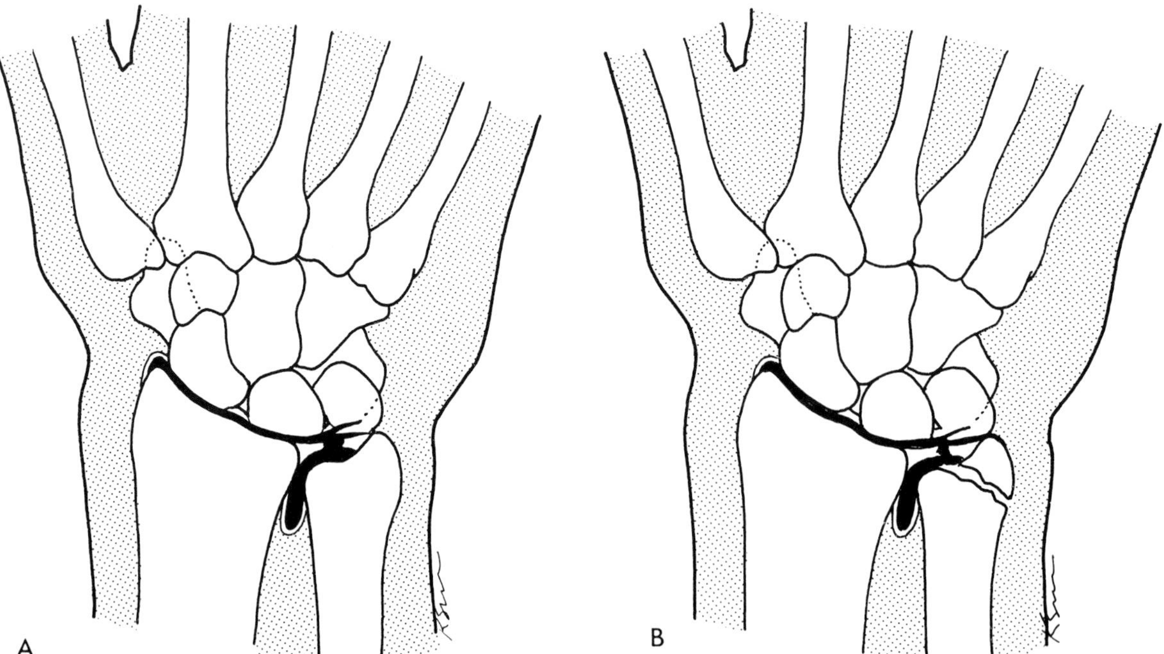

Figure 15–8. Wrist arthrography: Injuries of triangular fibrocartilage, ulnar styloid, and inferior radioulnar joints.

A, B Diagrams indicate the pattern of compartmental communication that may be seen following isolated injury to the triangular fibrocartilage **(A)** or ulnar styloid **(B)**. In both instances, contrast introduced into the radiocarpal compartment will opacify the inferior radioulnar compartment through defects in the triangular fibrocartilage.

Illustration continued on the opposite page

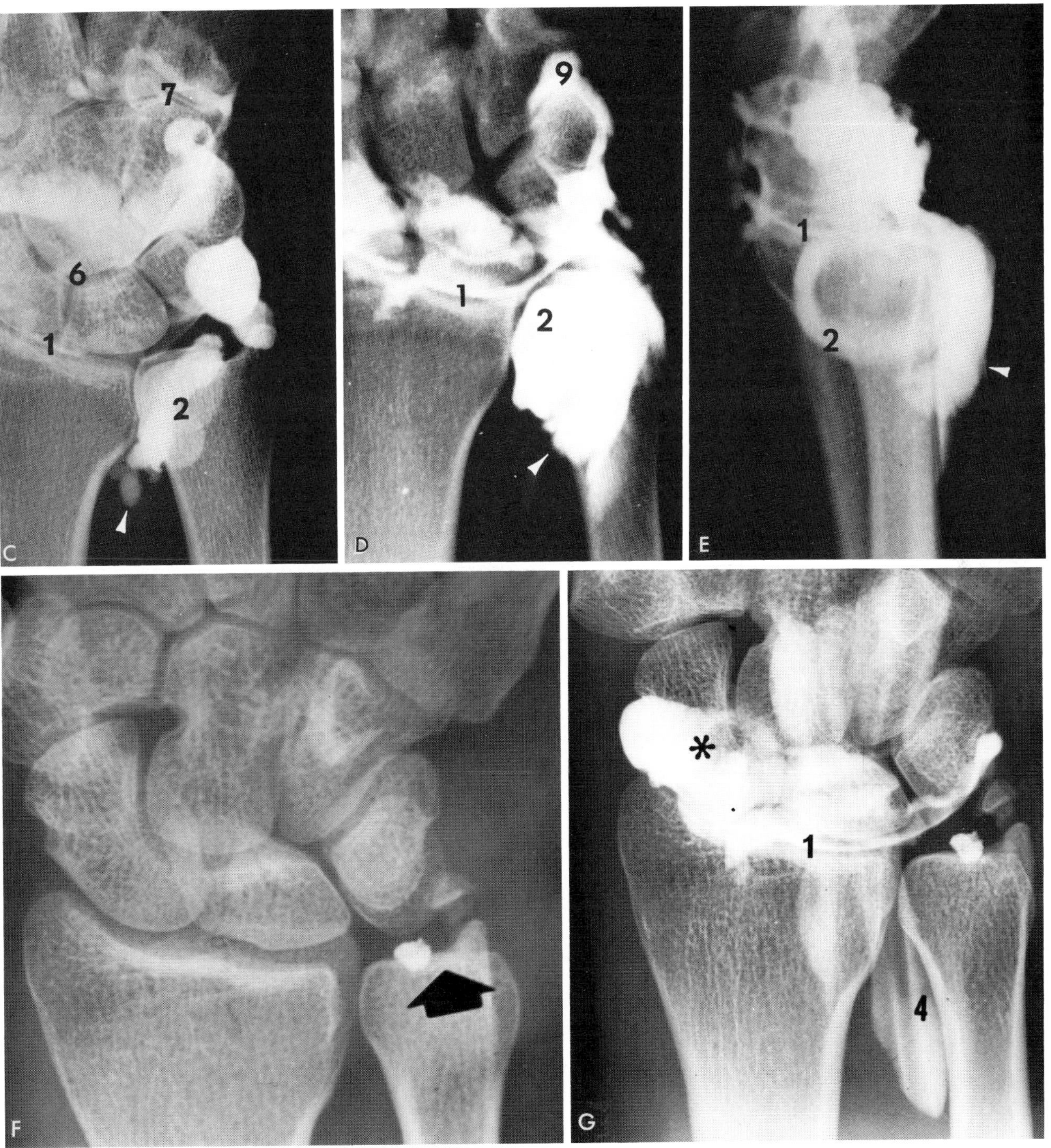

Figure 15–8. Continued

C *Triangular fibrocartilage injury. This young man developed pain over the distal ulna following an injury. A wrist arthrogram reveals communication between the radiocarpal compartment (1) and inferior radioulnar compartment (2). The midcarpal (6) and common carpometacarpal (7) compartments are also opacified. Small contrast-filled diverticula near the proximal aspect of the inferior radioulnar joint (arrowhead) may indicate a capsular tear.*

D, E *Triangular fibrocartilage and inferior radioulnar capsular injury. Another young patient with significant disability following an accident. Frontal* **(D)** *and lateral* **(E)** *radiographs following arthrography reveal communication of the radiocarpal compartment (1) with the inferior radioulnar (2) as well as the pisiform-triquetral compartment (9). Note soft tissue extravasation of contrast material from the inferior radioulnar compartment (arrowhead) indicating a capsular tear.*

F, G *Ulnar styloid injury. The initial film indicates a previous fracture of the ulnar styloid and a metallic fragment (arrow). The arthrogram outlines contrast within the radiocarpal compartment (1), which is smooth in outline, opacification of extensor tendon sheaths (4), and a cartilaginous loose body (asterisk) producing a persistent filling defect.*

(**F, G,** *From Resnick D: Radiology 13:331, 1974.*)

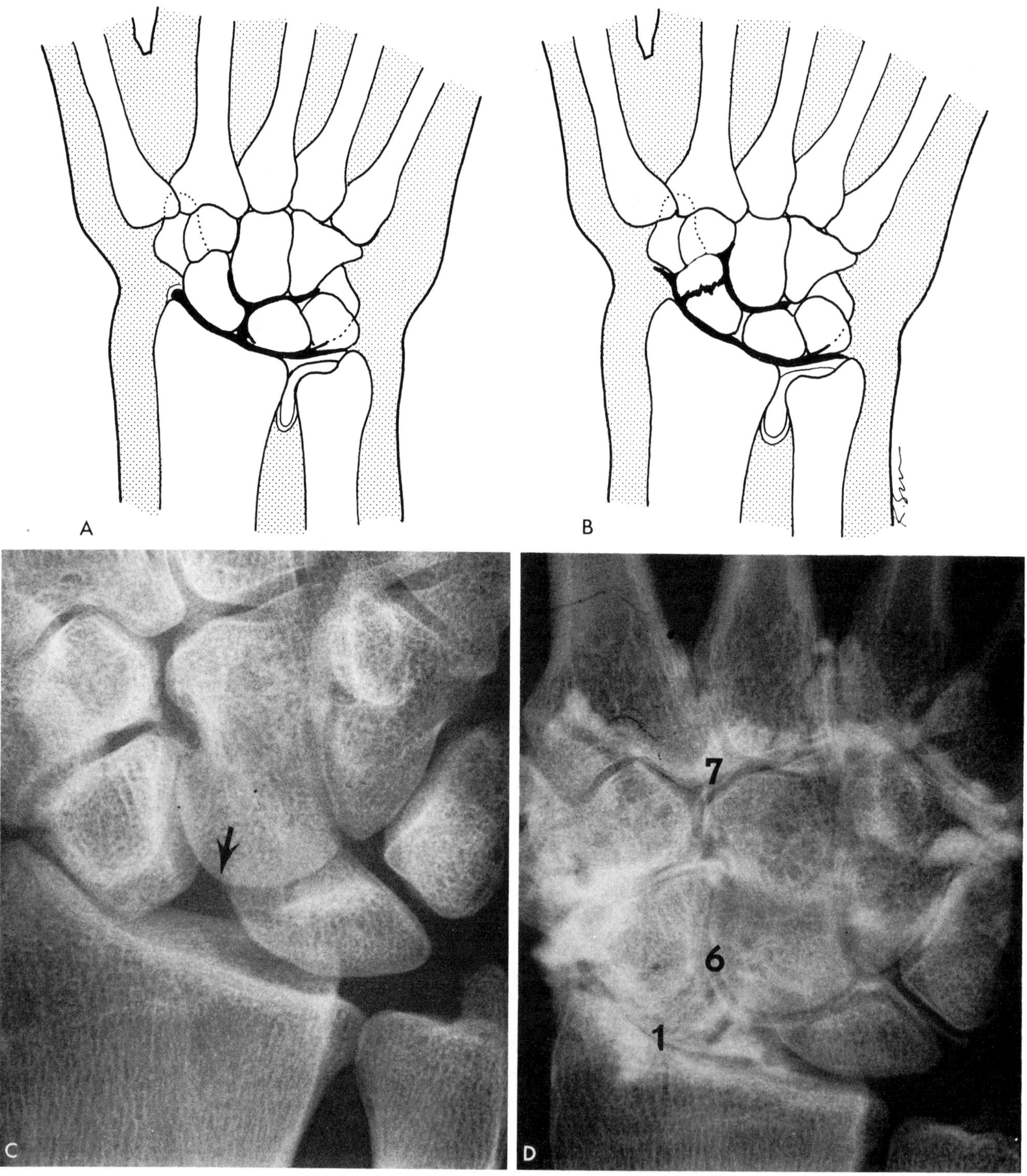

Figure 15–9. *Wrist arthrography: injuries of the scaphoid and interosseous ligaments of the proximal carpal row.*

A, B *Injury to the interosseous ligament between scaphoid and lunate* **(A)** *allows communication between the radiocarpal and midcarpal compartments. Similar communication may occur through a fracture of the scaphoid* **(B).**

C, D *Scaphoid-lunate dissociation with disruption of the scaphoid-lunate ligament. The initial film* **(C)** *reveals widening of the scaphoid-lunate space (arrow) and foreshortening of the scaphoid. Secondary degenerative joint disease of the radiocarpal compartment is seen. Following arthrography* **(D)** *contrast material has flowed from the radiocarpal compartment (1) into the midcarpal (6) and comon carpometacarpal (7) compartments. Contrast material overlies the scaphoid-lunate space.*

Illustration continued on the opposite page

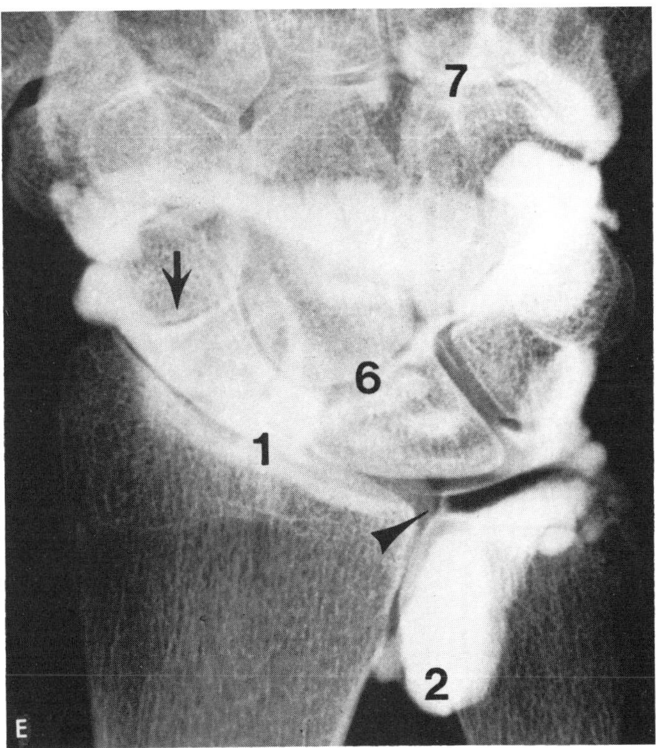

Figure 15–9. Continued
E *Fracture of the scaphoid. A wrist arthrogram outlines communication between the radiocarpal (1) and midcarpal (6) compartments through a scaphoid fracture (arrow). The common carpometacarpal (7) and inferior radioulnar (2) compartments are also opacified. Opacification of the latter compartment occurs via a defect (arrowhead) in the triangular fibrocartilage.*

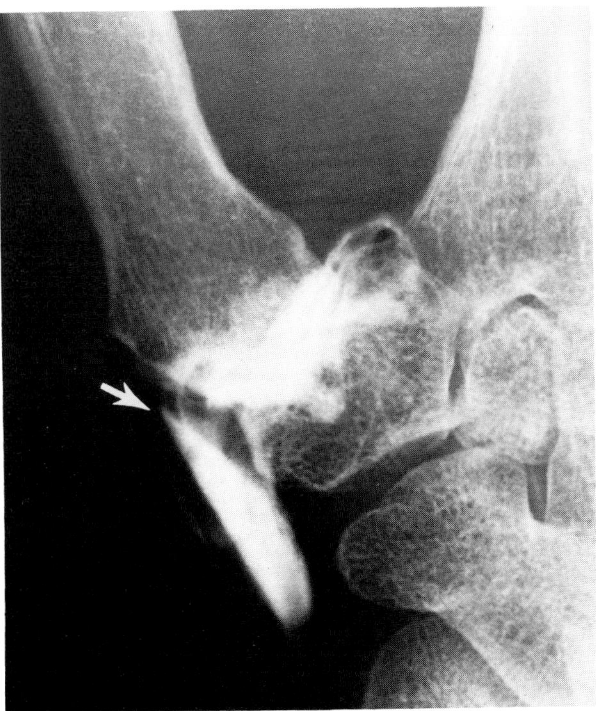

Figure 15–10. *Wrist arthrography: Injury of the capsule about the first carpometacarpal articulation. Following direct opacification of this compartment, extravasation of contrast material on the radial aspect of the wrist (arrow) indicated a capsular injury.*

midcarpal compartments (Fig. 15–9). Direct arthrographic opacification of other compartments of the wrist may delineate capsular injuries (Fig. 15–10).

Synovial irregularity is absent or localized on wrist arthrograms following trauma.[5] Tendon sheath communication may be observed but lymphatic filling is generally absent.

Wrist arthrography has a definite role in identifying the cause of the patient's symptoms and signs following trauma. This role is better established in young individuals, in whom compartmental communication may provide presumptive evidence of the site of soft tissue injury when initial radiographs are normal. In older patients, the frequency of such communication in "normal" persons limits the value of wrist arthrography.

Other Articular Disorders. Arthrographic alterations in patients with other articular disorders are consistent with the pathogenesis of these disease processes. Reported findings in gout are compartmental and tendon sheath communications, lymphatic visualization, and synovial irregularity.[6] In this disease, communication between the radiocarpal and inferior radioulnar compartments is unusual, whereas communication between the radiocarpal and midcarpal compartments is more common (Fig. 15–11). Perhaps the less aggressive synovial inflammation associated with gout compared with rheumatoid arthritis is able to penetrate the relatively weak interosseous carpal ligaments protecting the midcarpal compartment rather than the tough triangular fibrocartilage protecting the inferior radioulnar compartment.[6] Lymphatic visualization (27 per cent) and corrugated synovial irregularity (17 per cent), indicating synovial inflammation, simulate the findings of rheumatoid arthritis.

It is expected that wrist arthrography in patients with rheumatoid "variant" disorders, such as psoriasis, Reiter's syndrome, and ankylosing spondylitis, would reveal abnormalities similar to those of rheumatoid arthritis. This has been documented in patients with ankylosing spondylitis, in whom wrist arthrograms demonstrate corrugated synovial irregularity, lymphatic filling, and compartmental and tendon sheath communication[5] (Fig. 15–12). In neuroarthropathy, reported findings are noncorrugated synovial irregularity and compartmental and tendon sheath communication[5] (Fig. 15–13). In this disorder, localized synovial inflammation related to areas at which the synovial membrane is reflected over abnormal bone or intra-articular pieces of cartilage and bone, some embedded in the membrane itself, produces contrast irregularity. Compartmental and tendon sheath visualization is expected in neuroarthropathy related to capsular and soft tissue disruption.

Wrist arthrography in patients with septic arthritis allows documentation of intra-articular needle placement for aspiration of joint contents. Subsequent contrast opacification will reveal findings similar to those of rheumatoid arthritis.[5]

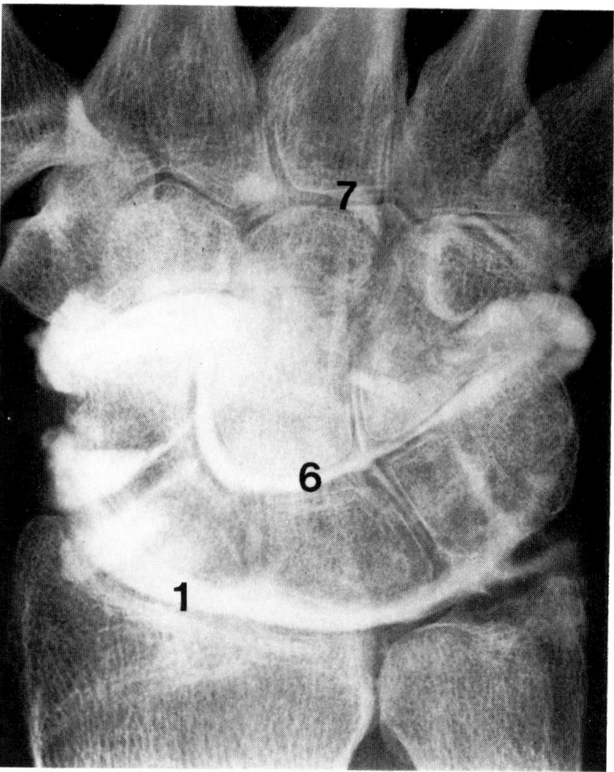

Figure 15–11. *Wrist arthrography: Gouty arthritis. A wrist arthrogram in a patient with gout demonstrates communication between the radiocarpal (1), midcarpal (6), and common carpometacarpal (7) compartments. The inferior radioulnar compartment does not opacify. The degree of synovial irregularity is mild.*

Evaluation of Soft Tissue Masses. Wrist arthrography can provide useful information for the surgeon who is evaluating a patient with an adjacent soft tissue mass.[5, 15, 16] These masses may represent synovial cysts, ganglions, or enlarged tendon sheaths.

In the evaluation of wrist ganglions, contrast material injected directly into the swelling may fail to opacify the wrist, whereas contrast material injected into the wrist may reveal its communication with the soft tissue mass[15] (Fig. 15–14). This phenomenon of a "one-way valve" between the ganglion and articular cavity is similar to that noted with synovial cysts about any articulation. It is therefore logical to first inject the joint itself. This will usually demonstrate the site of communication with filling of the soft tissue mass, although, in some cases, it is necessary to decompress the cyst initially. If, in fact, an arthrogram does not opacify the cystic mass, a second injection directly into the mass can be attempted.

Synovial cysts or herniations about the wrist are particularly frequent in rheumatoid arthritis, although they may accompany other articular disorders[16] (Fig. 15–15). As elsewhere, these cysts con-

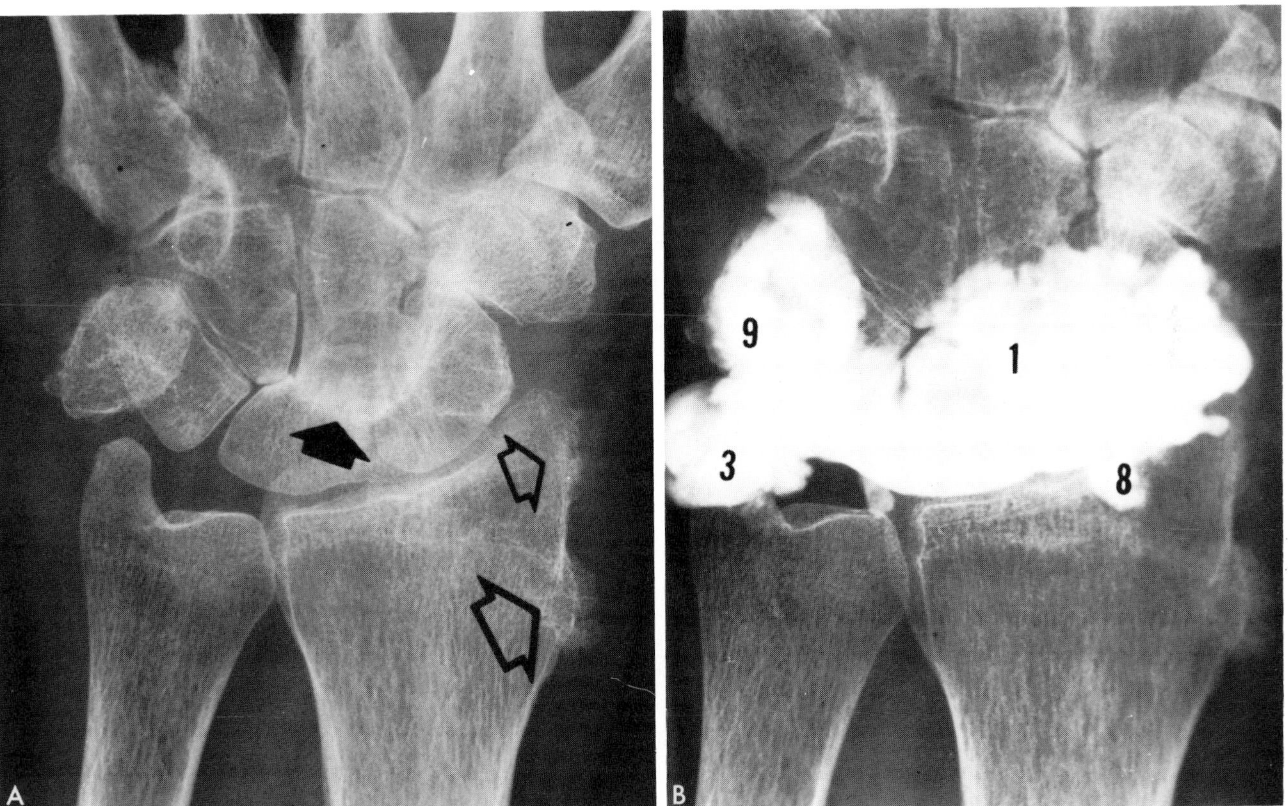

Figure 15–12. *Wrist arthrography: Ankylosing spondylitis. A middle-aged man with ankylosing spondylitis and peripheral joint disease. On clinical examination, marked synovitis of the wrist was evident.*

A *The initial film demonstrates mild osteoporosis, irregular new bone formation in the distal radius (open arrows) and midcarpal joint space narrowing (solid arrow).*

B *A frontal view following arthrography indicates mild to severe corrugated synovial irregularity within the radiocarpal compartment (1), pisiform-triquetral compartment (9), pre-styloid recess (3), and volar radial recesses (8).*

(From Resnick D: Radiology 113:331, 1974.)

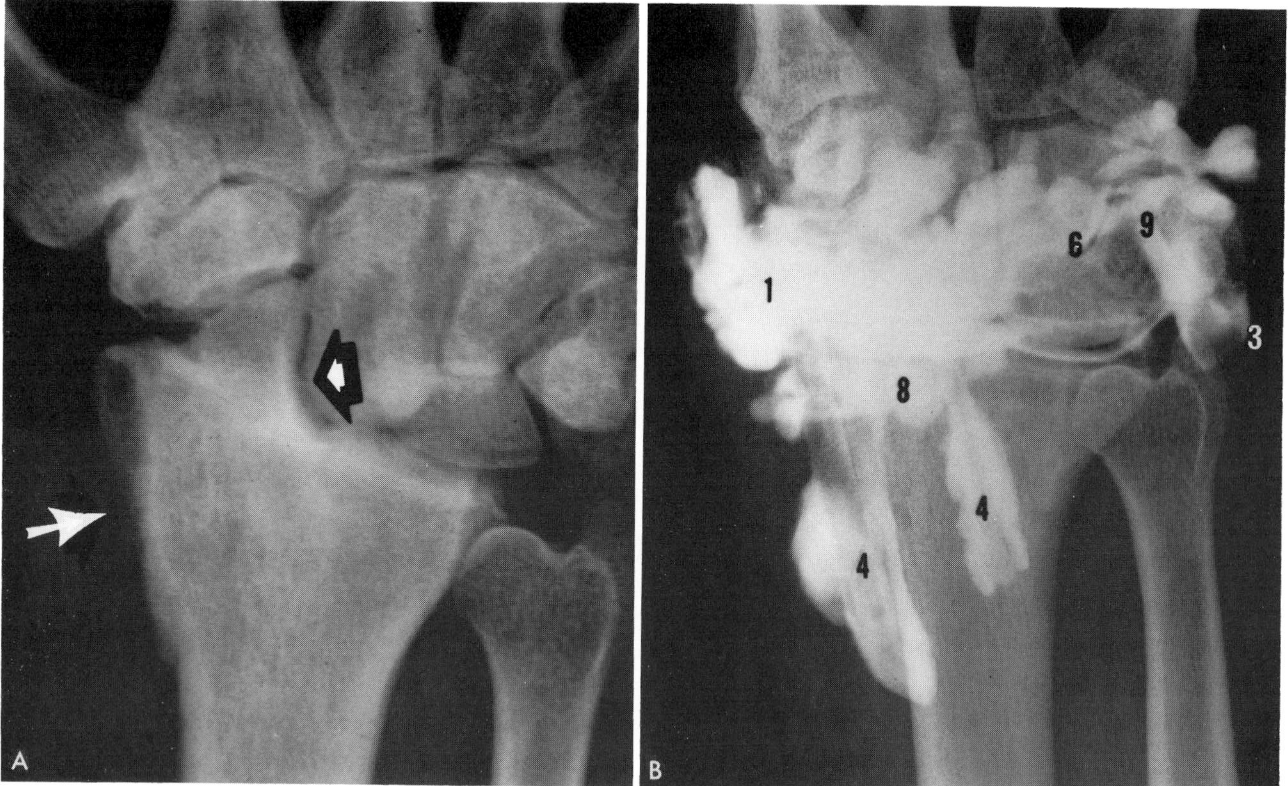

Figure 15–13. *Wrist arthrography: Neuroarthropathy. A 49 year old man with severe diabetes, peripheral neuropathy, and probable neuropathic disease of the wrist as well as the ipsilateral elbow and shoulder.*

A *The plain film indicates extensive sclerosis of the distal radius and scaphoid (arrows) and extreme joint space narrowing. Although the deformity of the distal radius suggested a previous fracture, the patient denied a history of trauma.*

B *The arthrogram reveals localized synovial irregularity and capsular disruption of the radiocarpal compartment (1), communication with the midcarpal (6) and pisiform-triquetral (9) compartments, prominent volar radial recesses (8), opacification of the extensor tendon sheaths (4), and a persistent filling defect in the prestyloid recess (3).*

(From Resnick D: Radiology 113:331, 1974.)

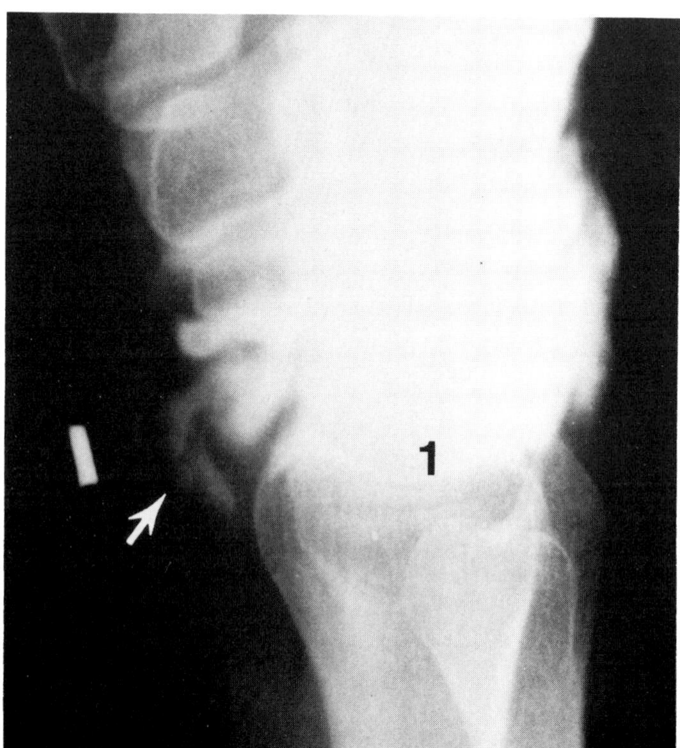

Figure 15–14. *Wrist arthrography: Ganglion. Following injection of contrast material into the radiocarpal compartment (1), a volar ganglion has opacified (arrow beneath metal marker) whose origin could be traced to the scaphoid-lunate space at surgery. Other wrist compartments have also filled with contrast material.*

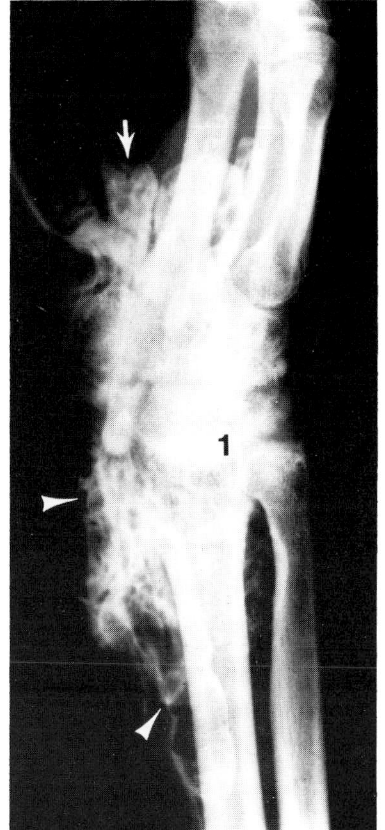

Figure 15–15. *Wrist arthrography: Synovial cyst. Following injection of the radiocarpal compartment (1) in this patient with rheumatoid arthritis, a large contrast-filled volar synovial cyst can be seen (arrowheads) which communicates with tendon sheaths (arrow).*

(Courtesy of Dr. Jack Bowerman, Johns Hopkins Hospital, Baltimore, Maryland.)

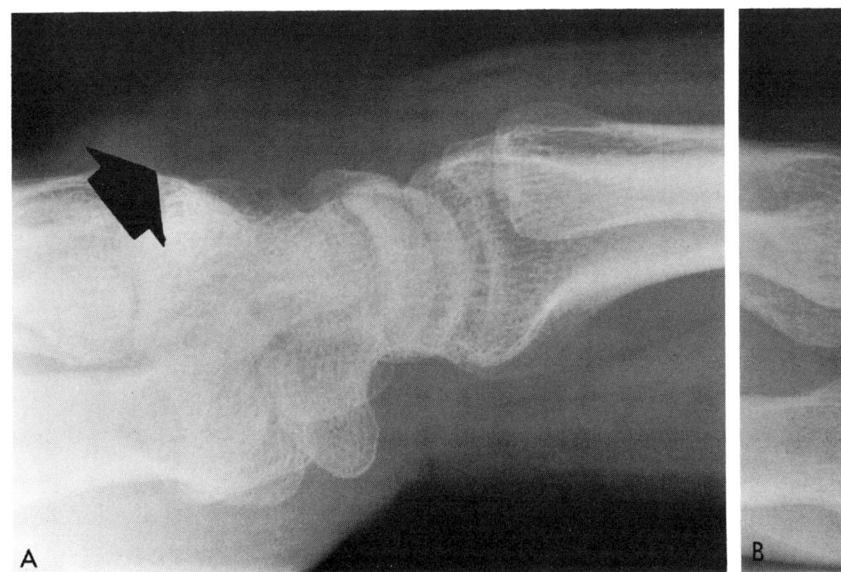

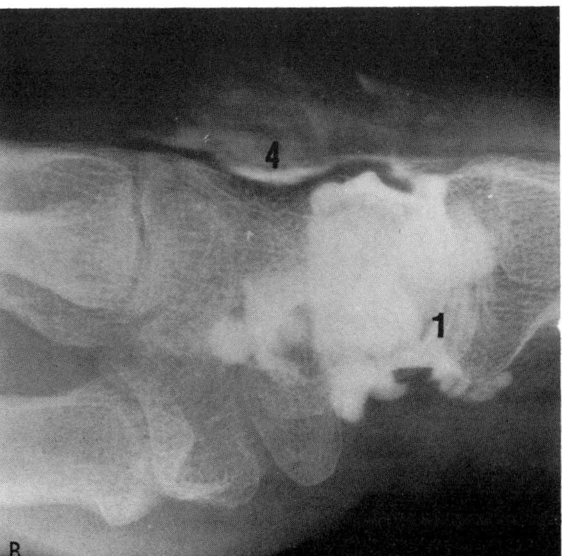

Figure 15–16. *Wrist arthrography: Enlarged tendon sheath. A 28 year old man presented with a painful mass on the dorsum of the wrist. Following radiography and arthrography, surgery was performed. At operation, 3 to 5 cm of hypertrophied gray synovium was noted in the extensor tendon sheaths. Microscopic evaluation demonstrated chronic synovial inflammation with cellular infiltration by lymphocytes and plasma cells as well as noncaseating granulomas.*

A *The initial film reveals considerable soft tissue swelling on the dorsum of the wrist (arrow).*

B *The arthrogram demonstrates communication of the radiocarpal compartment (1) with an irregular extensor tendon sheath (4).*

tain synovial fluid and may result from elevation of intra-articular pressure.

Cystic swelling about the wrist can indicate an enlarged tendon sheath (Fig. 15–16). In this situation, contrast opacification of the wrist may reveal communication with the sheath, allowing accurate diagnosis.[5]

Arthrography of the Metacarpophalangeal and Interphalangeal Joints of the Hand

Arthrography of the metacarpophalangeal and interphalangeal joints is not commonly performed. It may occasionally be useful in defining the extent of articular involvement in joint diseases, such as rheumatoid arthritis, or in delineating the presence and type of articular soft tissue injury.

TECHNIQUE (Fig. 15–17). Injection of the metacarpophalangeal joint of any of the four ulnar digits is best attempted under fluoroscopy with the digit flexed as much as 90 degrees.[17] The space between the metacarpal head and proximal phalanx can then be palpated and entered with a 22 or 26 gauge needle from a dorsolateral approach, adjacent to the extensor tendon. One to 1.5 ml of contrast material (methylglucamine diatrizoate [Renografin]) is injected. An alternative method consists of injecting the metacarpophalangeal joint with the finger in extension by inserting the needle from a radial (lateral) approach between the extensor apparatus and the articular surface. Injection of the first metacarpophalangeal joint is performed under fluoroscopic control from a dorsoradial approach with a 22 or 26 gauge needle, utilizing 1 to 1.5 ml of contrast material.[18-20]

Injection of the proximal interphalangeal or distal interphalangeal joints of the four ulnar digits and the interphalangeal joint of the thumb is accomplished under fluoroscopy from a dorsolateral approach adjacent to the extensor tendon utilizing a 26 gauge needle and 0.5 to 1 ml of contrast material.

NORMAL ARTHROGRAM (Fig. 15–18). Contrast opacification of the metacarpophalangeal joint reveals a linear collection between the metacarpal head and proximal phalanx with proximal recesses or extensions at the radial, ulnar, dorsal and volar aspects of the articulation. At the first metacarpophalangeal joint, large proximal dorsal and volar recesses are again evident (10 to 20 mm in length), whereas the distal recesses are smaller (1 to 5 mm in length). The collateral ligaments produce small indentations at the joint line. Arthrography of the interphalangeal joints produces a similar pattern with contrast material between the phalanges, larger proximal and smaller distal recesses, and waist-like defects at the sides related to the collateral ligaments.

ABNORMAL ARTHROGRAM. In rheumatoid arthritis and other synovial disorders, arthrographic findings include an irregular corrugated pattern of contrast material, enlarged articular cavities, perforations or retractions of the joint capsule, cartilage lesions, and lymphatic filling[21, 22] (Fig. 15–19).

Following injury, opacification of the articular cavity may reveal disruption of the capsule and adjacent ligaments with soft tissue extravasation of contrast material. Opacification is particularly helpful at the first metacarpophalangeal joint in the evaluation of injuries on the ulnar aspect of the articulation, the "gamekeeper's thumb"[18-20, 23-26] (Fig. 15–20). In this clinical situation, damage to the ulnar collateral and accessory collateral ligaments, volar plate, and capsule may be observed. Arthrographic

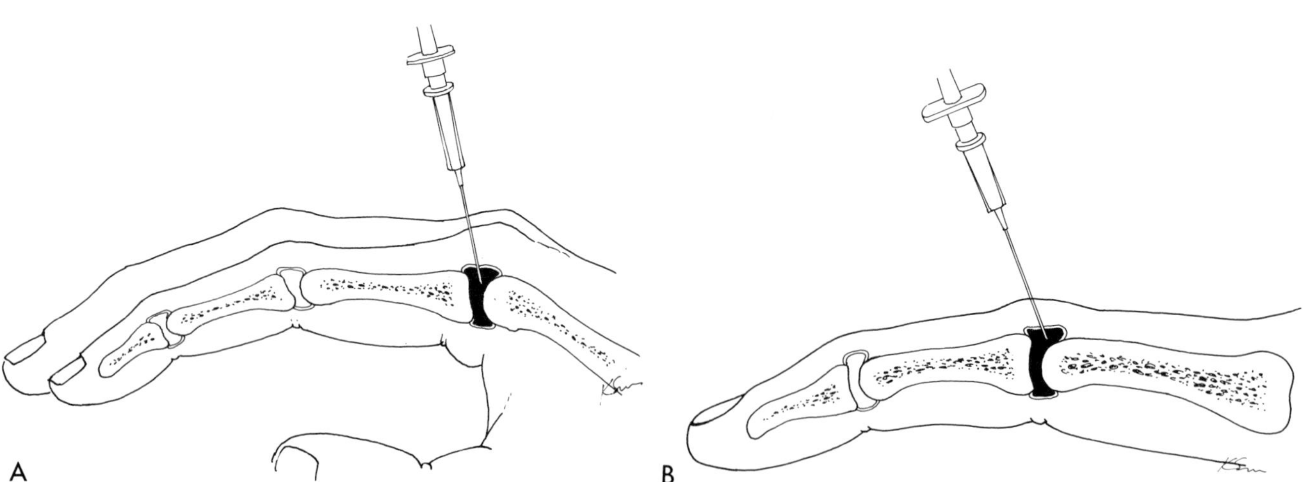

Figure 15–17. *Metacarpophalangeal and interphalangeal joint arthrography: Technique.*
A, B *Injection into either the metacarpophalangeal* **(A)** *or interphalangeal* **(B)** *joints of the hand is best accomplished from a dorsal approach under fluoroscopic control.*

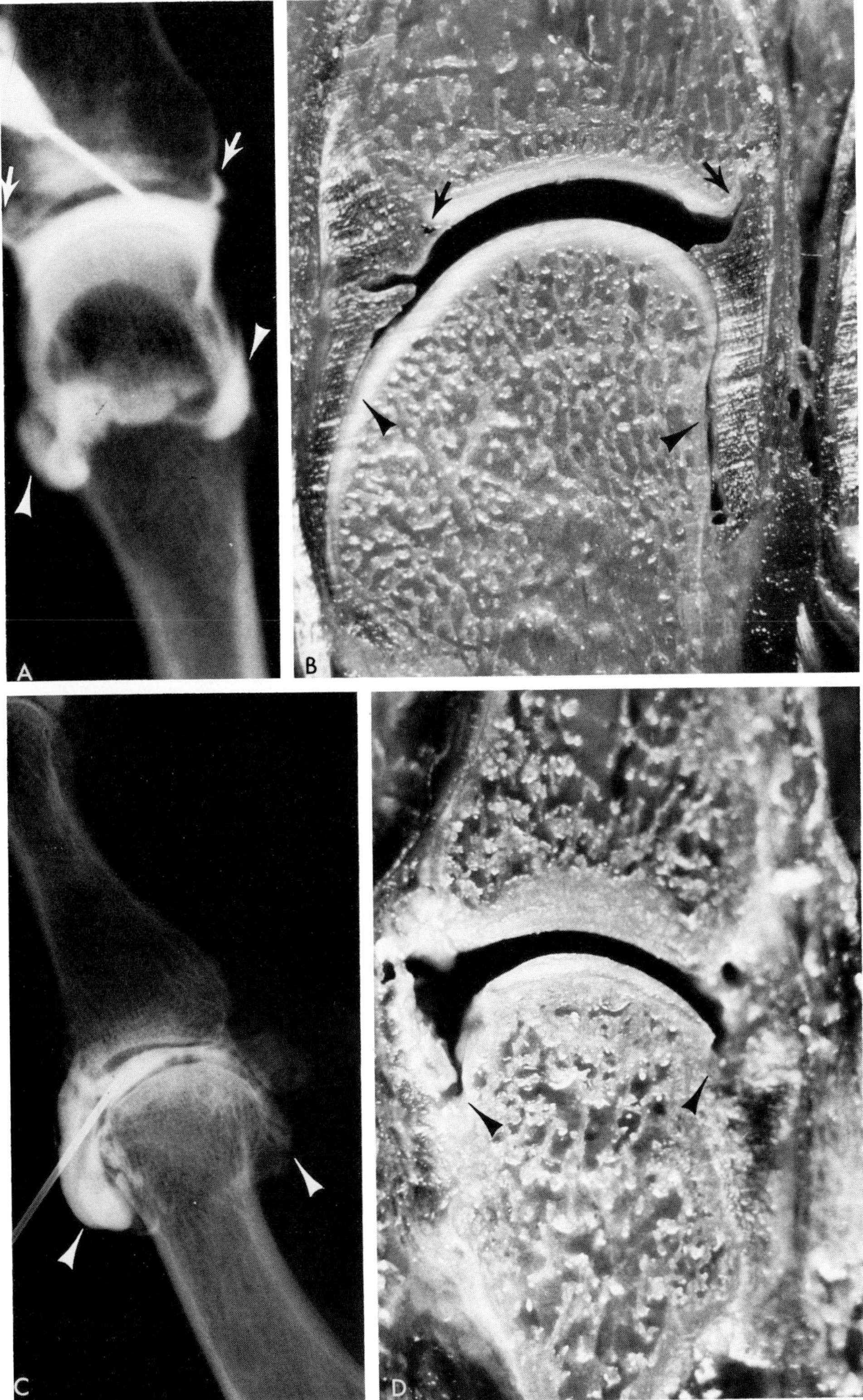

Figure 15–18. *Metacarpophalangeal and interphalangeal joint arthrography: Normal arthrogram.*

A, B *Second metacarpophalangeal joint. Contrast opacification of this articulation* **(A)** *reveals a smooth layer of radiopaque material between the metacarpal head and proximal phalanx and prominent proximal recesses (arrowheads) compared to distal recesses (arrows). A coronal section* **(B)** *through the joint demonstrates the large proximal extent of the articular cavity (arrowheads) compared to the distal extent (arrows).*

C, D *First metacarpophalangeal joint. Contrast opacification of this articulation* **(C)** *outlines a smooth synovial cavity with large proximal volar and dorsal recesses (arrowheads). On a coronal section* **(D)**, *the extent of the proximal recesses can be seen (arrowheads).*

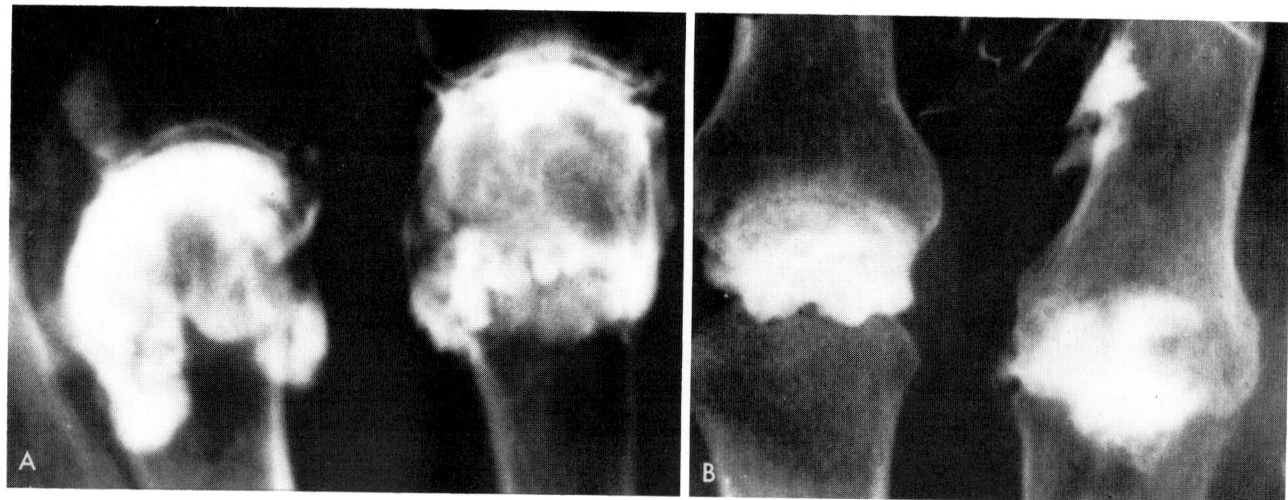

Figure 15–19. *Metacarpophalangeal joint arthrography: Rheumatoid arthritis.*

A, B *In two patients with rheumatoid arthritis, opacification of the metacarpophalangeal joints demonstrates irregularity and filling defects consistent with synovial inflammation* **(A)** *and decreased joint capacity consistent with synovial fibrosis* **(B).**

(Courtesy of Dr. M. Laval-Jeantet, Paris, France.)

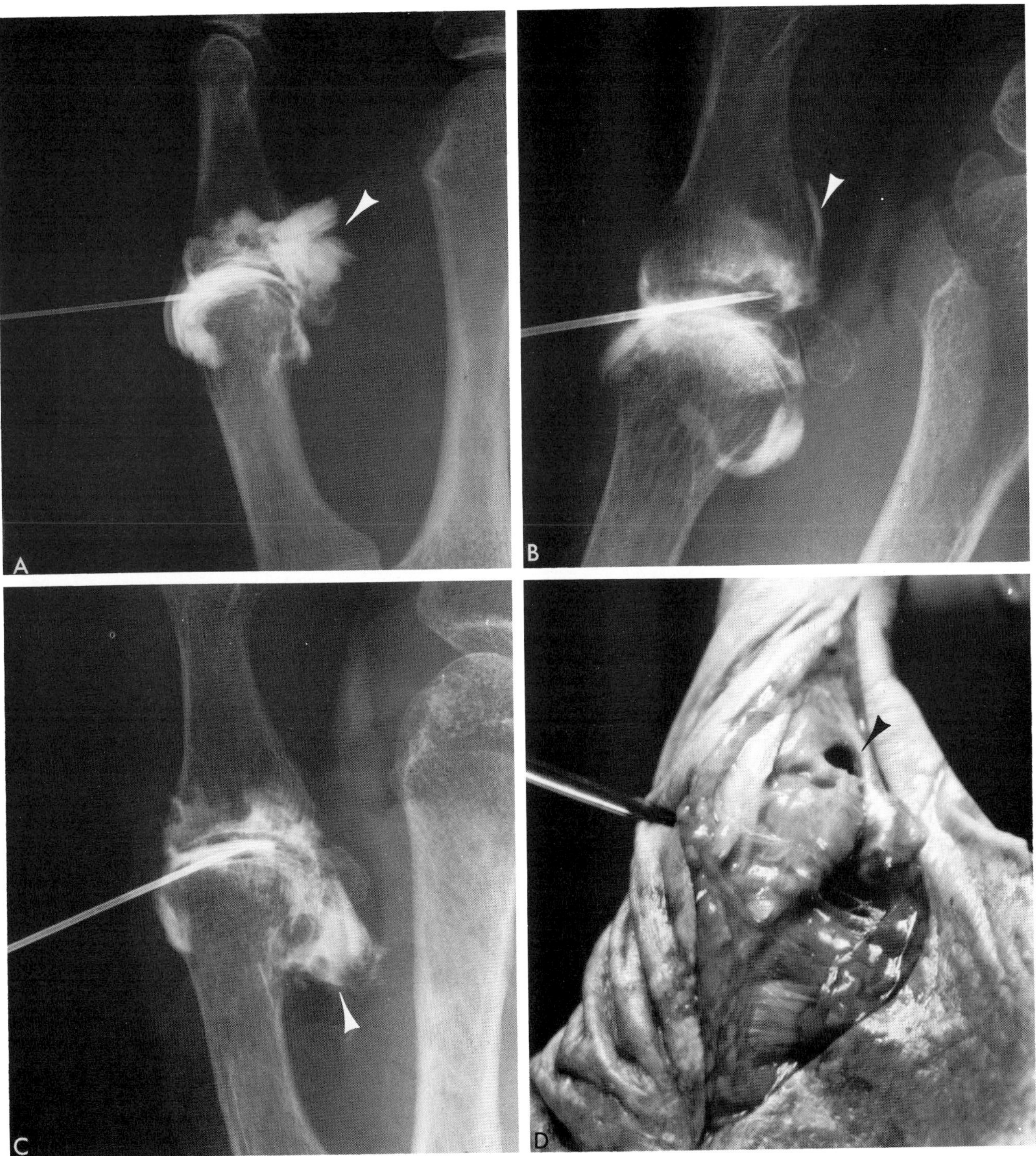

Figure 15–20. *Metacarpophalangeal joint arthrography: Gamekeeper's thumb.*

A–D *Following injury to the ulnar aspect of the first metacarpophalangeal joint, arthrography may reveal extravasation of contrast material.* **A–C,** *In these three cadavers, note the various patterns of contrast extravasation (arrowhead) along the ulnar side of the metacarpal head and proximal phalanx.* **D,** *A photograph of a dissection of cadaver* **C** *outlines the space between the avulsed ligament and its origin on the proximal phalanx (arrowhead).*

(From Resnick D, Danzig L: Am J Roentgenol 126:1046, 1976. Copyright 1976, American Roentgen Ray Society.)

findings include extravasation of variable size along the ulnar aspect of the joint[18-20] and a filling defect produced by interposition of the dorsal aponeurosis between the torn ligament and its phalangeal attachment.[19, 20, 25] These findings may be associated with plain film abnormalities, such as fractures of the proximal phalanx and stress film changes of increased joint laxity, although arthrographic alterations may be the only radiographic abnormalities.

Tenography and Bursography of the Hand and Wrist

Contrast opacification of tendon sheaths (tenography) and bursae (bursography) is a relatively simple radiographic procedure with limited clinical application. Tenography in rheumatoid arthritis allows accurate appraisal of the distribution and extent of synovial involvement of the tendon sheaths on the volar or dorsal aspect of the hand and wrist.[27-29] Outlining the synovial sheaths within the carpal tunnel may demonstrate local mechanical factors producing the carpal tunnel syndrome,[30] whereas visualization of sheaths or bursae on the volar aspect of the hand and wrist may provide insight into the pathogenesis and appearance of infections.[31]

Technique (Fig. 15–21). Evaluation of flexor tendon sheaths of the fingers is accomplished by injecting 0.5 to 3 ml of methylglucamine diatrizoate (Renografin).[30] A 22 gauge, 1.5 inch needle is introduced under fluoroscopy through the palmar skin overlying the distal one third of the proximal phalanx of the second through fifth digits. The needle is advanced in a proximal direction until increased resistance is encountered when the tip enters the tendon. The needle is withdrawn slightly, creating a sudden drop in resistance, and is advanced in a more shallow angle within the sheath. The injection of the sheath of the flexor pollicis longus is accomplished by flexing the terminal phalanx of the thumb, palpating the tendon, and inserting the needle directly into the sheath.

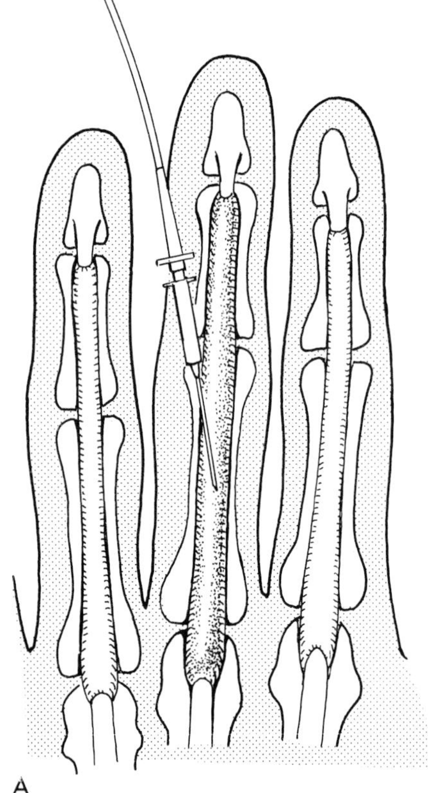

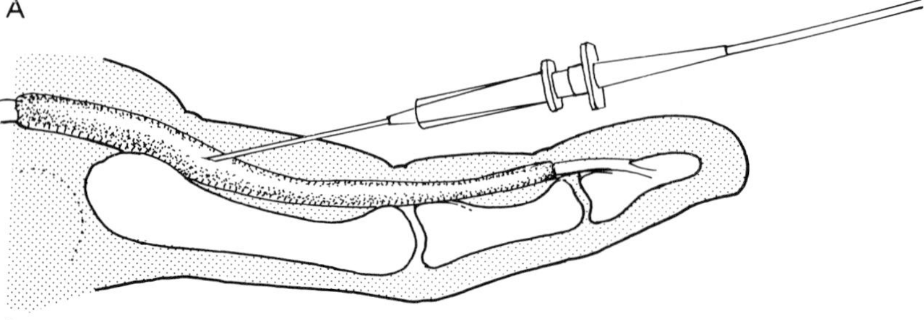

Figure 15–21. *Tenography of the hand and wrist: Technique of injecting the distal flexor tendon sheaths.*

A, B *These drawings indicate the technique of injecting the flexor tendon sheaths of the fingers. A palmar approach is utilized and a 22 gauge needle is placed within the sheath at the approximate level of the midportion of the proximal phalanx.*

Contrast opacification of the extensor tendon sheaths on the dorsum of the wrist can be accomplished by palpating the tendons and advancing the needle into the sheath through the dorsal carpal ligament.[30]

Direct puncture of the bursae on the volar aspect of the wrist has been described. Five milliliters of contrast material can be injected into the ulnar bursa, outlining its normal communication with the digital flexor tendon sheaths.[32, 33]

Normal Tenogram

Digital Flexor Tendon Sheaths (Fig. 15–22). The flexor tendons of the fingers, the sublimis digitorum and profundus digitorum, are enveloped by digital sheaths from a line of insertion of the flexor profundus to a line 1 cm proximal to the proximal border of the deep transverse ligament.[34] This arrangement, which is not constant, is most frequent in the index, middle, and ring fingers.[35] Any of these three sheaths may extend to the wrist.[36] The flexor sheath of the thumb extends from the terminal phalanx to a point 2 to 3 cm proximal to the proximal volar crease of the wrist, although on occasion a septum separates proximal and distal halves of the sheath.[35] The synovial sheath of the little finger also commences at its terminal phalanx. It may end near the deep transverse ligament or continue into the palm, expanding to envelop the adjacent tendons of the second, third, and fourth fingers.[34, 35, 37]

The relationship of the digital flexor tendon sheaths and the joints of the second, third, fourth, and fifth fingers is of clinical importance. There is a considerable amount of fibrous tissue between the metacarpophalangeal joint of each of these fingers and the sheath.[37] Slightly more distally, near the base of the proximal phalanx, the sheath and bone are more intimate; at the proximal interphalangeal joint, more fibrous tissue separates the sheath and synovial cavity, as at the metacarpophalangeal joint.[37] Sections reveal that the axial portion of the joint capsule at the proximal interphalangeal joint is indistinguishable from the fibrous tendon sheath.[38]

The digital sheath of the thumb lies distally near the proximal phalanx, but as it ascends toward the palm it separates from the metacarpal head. Thus, the sheath is separated from the first metacarpophalangeal joint by considerable fibrous tissue.[37]

Synovial Sacs of the Palm (Fig. 15–23). Communication between the individual digital tendon sheaths and synovial sacs or bursae in the palm is not constant;[36] most frequently, such continuation is noted involving the first digit. Not uncommonly the

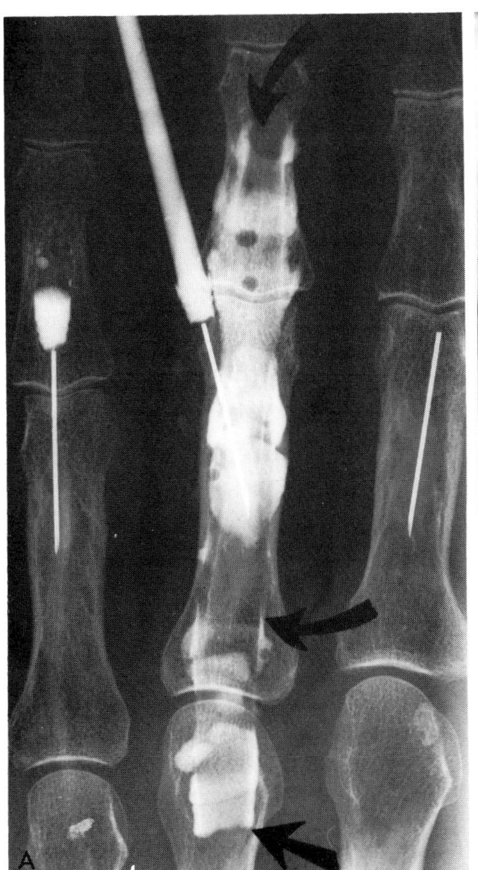

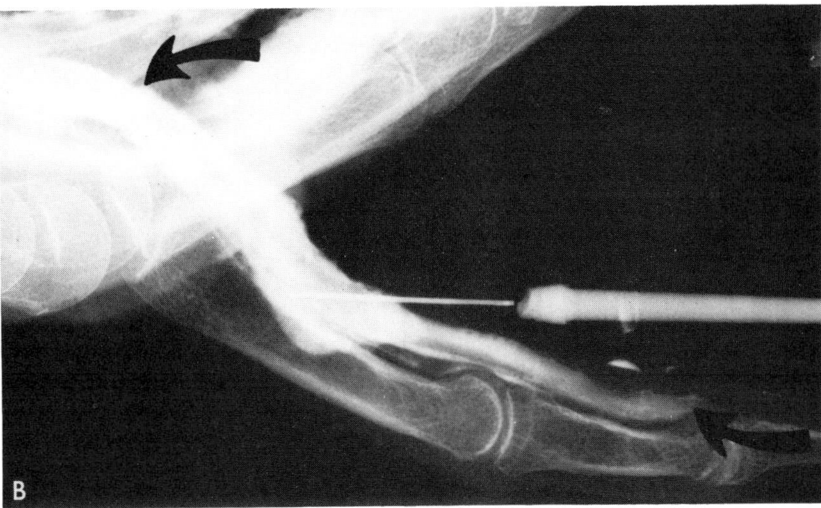

Figure 15–22. *Tenography of the hand and wrist: Normal tenogram of the digital flexor tendon sheaths.*

A, B *Contrast medium within the synovial sheath (arrows) extends from a site close to the distal interphalangeal joint to another site proximal to the metacarpophalangeal joint. No communication with the palmar synovial sacs is seen.*

(From Resnick D: Am J Roentgenol 124:44, 1975. Copyright 1975, American Roentgen Ray Society.)

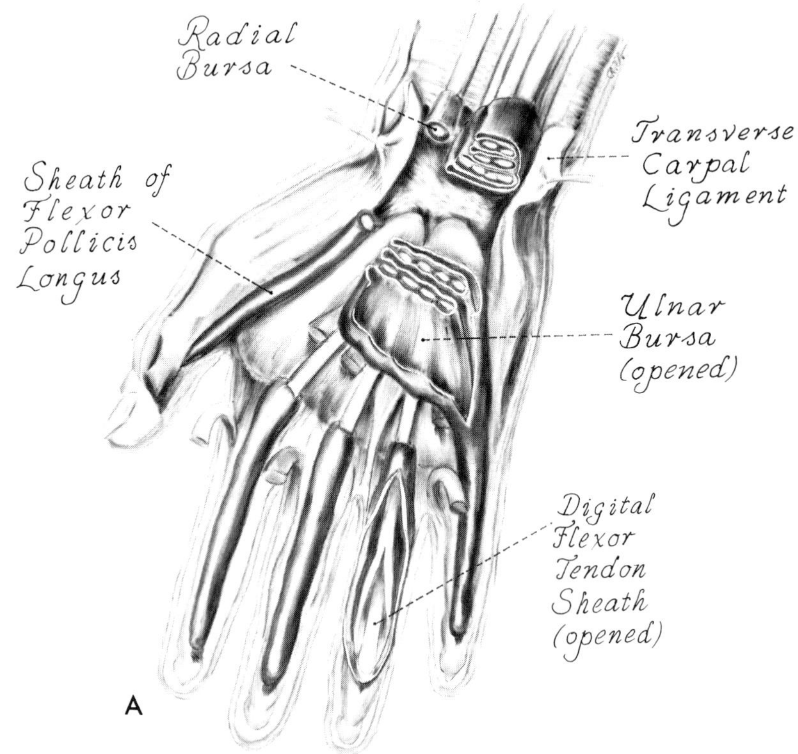

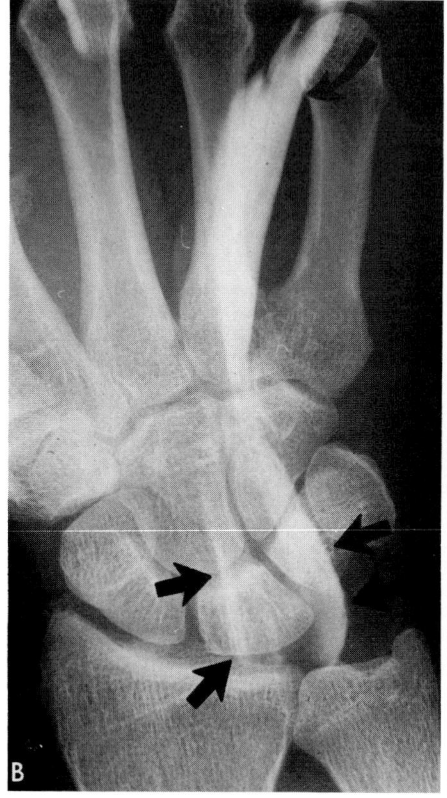

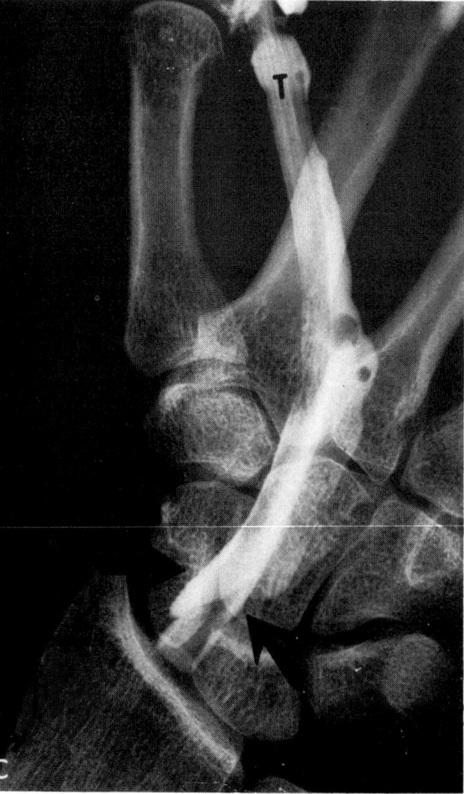

Figure 15–23. *Tenography of the hand and wrist: Normal appearance of synovial sacs of the palm.*

A *The digital flexor tendon sheaths of the second through fourth fingers terminate proximal to the metacarpophalangeal joint. That of the fifth finger communicates with the ulnar bursa. The sheath of the flexor pollicis longus is continuous with the radial bursa. Note the three invaginations of the ulnar bursa and, in this drawing, absence of communication between radial and ulnar bursae.*

B *Injection of the digital sheath of the fifth finger (curved arrow) reveals communication with the ulnar bursa (straight arrows).*

C *The synovial sheath of the flexor pollicis longus (T) is continuous with the radial bursa (arrows).*

Illustration continued on the opposite page

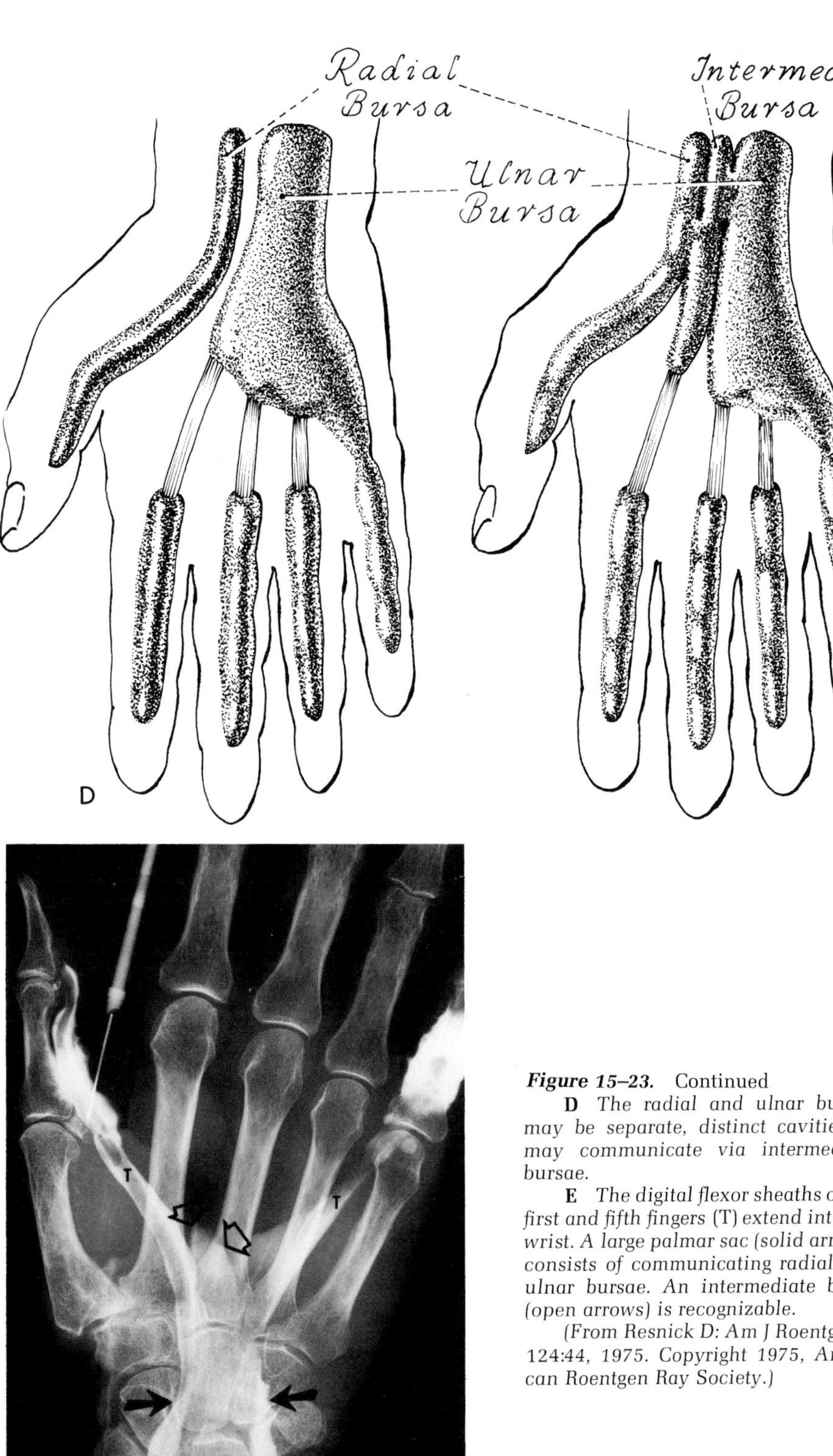

Figure 15–23. Continued

D *The radial and ulnar bursae may be separate, distinct cavities or may communicate via intermediate bursae.*

E *The digital flexor sheaths of the first and fifth fingers* (T) *extend into the wrist. A large palmar sac (solid arrows) consists of communicating radial and ulnar bursae. An intermediate bursa (open arrows) is recognizable.*

(From Resnick D: Am J Roentgenol 124:44, 1975. Copyright 1975, American Roentgen Ray Society.)

digital sheath of the fifth finger also continues into the palm.[35] Such communication is uncommon in the second, third, and fourth fingers.

The ulnar bursa on the medial aspect of the palm is composed of three communicating invaginations;[34, 35] a superficial extension lies in front of the flexor sublimis, a middle one between the tendons of the sublimis and the profundus, and a deep extension is found behind the flexor profundus. The bursa, beginning at the proximal end of the digital sheaths, spreads out proximally, overlying the third, fourth, and fifth metacarpals. A statistical analysis of the tendon sheath patterns in the hand using air insufflation techniques in 367 cases demonstrated that the ulnar bursa communicated with the sheaths of the little finger in 81 per cent, of the index finger in 5.1 per cent, of the middle finger in 4.0 per cent, and of the ring finger in 3.5 per cent of cases.[36]

The radial bursa is the expanded proximal continuation of the digital sheath of the flexor pollicis longus. It is found on the radial aspect of the palm overlying the second metacarpal. It continues prox-

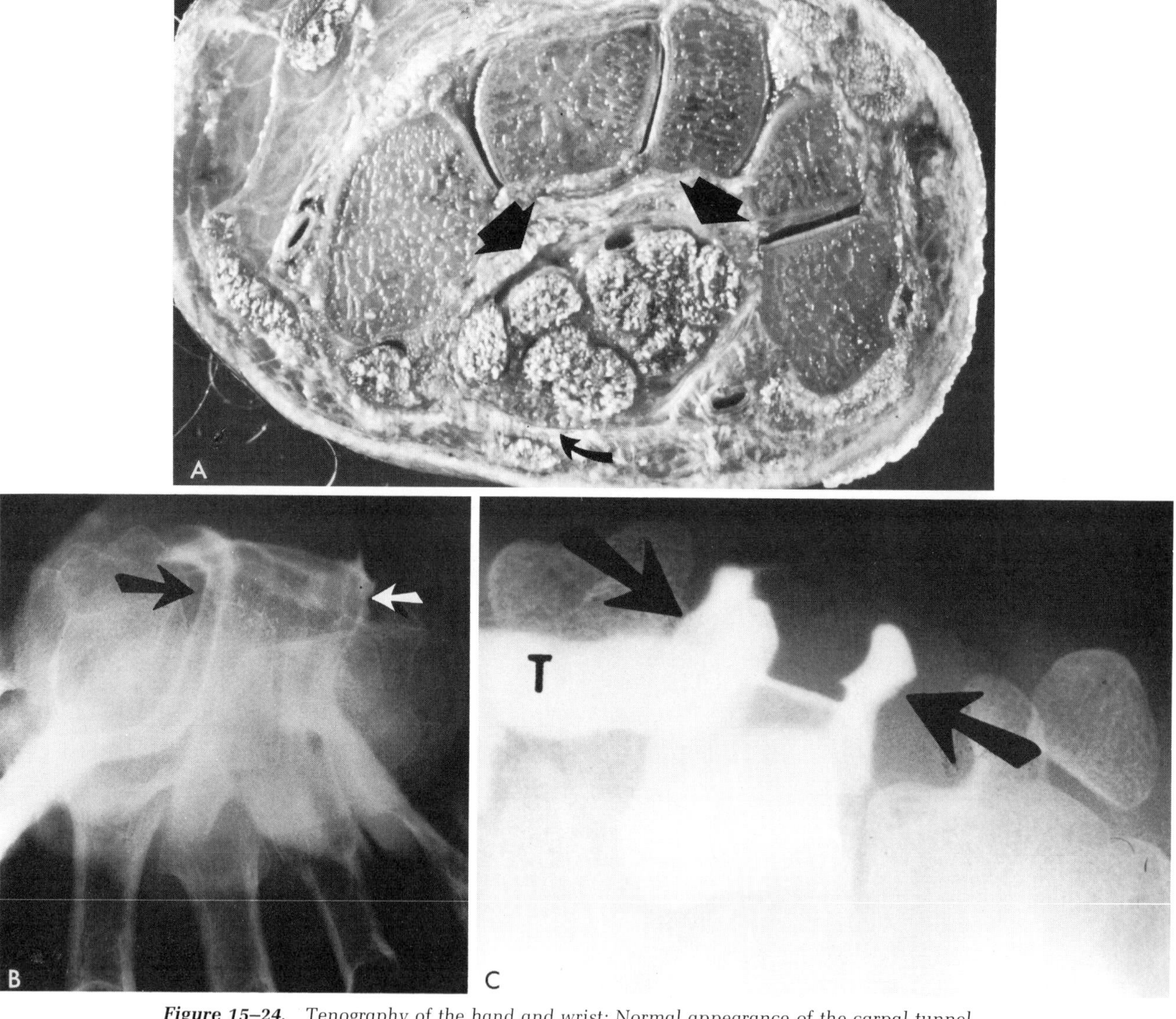

Figure 15–24. *Tenography of the hand and wrist: Normal appearance of the carpal tunnel.*

A *A transverse cross section through the carpal bones outlines the flexor tendons and sheaths within the carpal canal (large arrows). The transverse carpal ligament (curved arrow) is apparent.*

B *Contrast medium within the communicating radial and ulnar bursae delineates many flexor tendons within the carpal tunnel (arrows).*

C *An injection of the sheath of the flexor pollicis longus (T) outlines a noncommunicating radial bursa (arrows) within the carpal tunnel.*

(From Resnick D: Am J Roentgenol 124: 44, 1975. Copyright 1975, American Roentgen Ray Society.)

imally along the volar radial aspect of the wrist, terminating about 2 cm above the transverse carpal ligament.[34]

Intercommunications between the ulnar and radial bursae may be noted in 50 per cent of cases. Such connection is made via intermediate bursae. These accessory synovial sacs may be posterior in location, between the carpal canal and flexor profundus digitorum of the index finger, or, less commonly, anterior in location, between the superficial and deep tendons of the index finger. A separate carpal sheath that does not communicate with either radial or ulnar bursa may be found enveloping the index flexor tendons.[34] Additionally, a small synovial sac may enclose the tendon of the flexor carpi radialis as it passes under the crest of the trapezium.[34]

Carpal Tunnel (Fig. 15–24). Tendons, vessels, and nerves passing from the forearm to the hand must traverse a canal on the volar surface of the wrist formed between a deep excavation on the undersurface of the carpal bones and the transverse volar carpal ligament. The latter extends in the wrist from the radial side (inserting on the trapezium, scaphoid, and occasionally the radial styloid) to the ulnar side (inserting into the pisiform and hook of the hamate). On its radial aspect, a small opening in the volar carpal ligament as it bridges the trapezium produces a tunnel for the flexor carpi radialis tendon. Through the canal proper, which is triangular in transverse section, pass the digital flexor tendons and sheaths and the median nerve. Compression of the latter may result in the carpal tunnel syndrome; this may be associated with local or systemic diseases.[39, 40]

Extensor Tendon Sheaths (Fig. 15–25). Several synovial sheaths are located in the dorsum of the wrist beneath the dorsal carpal ligament; they extend for a short distance proximal and distal to that ligament. By insular attachments of the dorsal carpal ligament on the posterior and lateral surfaces of the radius and ulna, six distinct avenues are created for transport of ligamentous structures. The most medial compartment (sixth compartment) contains the extensor carpi ulnaris tendon and sheath (4 to 5 cm in length), lying at the dorsomedial aspect of the distal ulna. In the fifth compartment, a long sheath (6 to 7 cm in length) covers the extensor digiti quinti proprius, which lies in close proximity to and may communicate with the inferior radioulnar joint. The fourth compartment on the posteromedial aspect of the radius contains a large sheath (5 to 6 cm in length) enclosing the tendons of the extensor digitorum communis and the extensor indicis proprius. In the third compartment are the sheath (6 to 7 cm in length) and tendon of the extensor pollicis longus. The sheath may extend as far distally as the trapezium or first metacarpal bone. Lateral to this in the second compartment are sheaths (5 to 6 cm in length) covering the extensor carpi radialis longus and extensor carpi radialis brevis, which may communicate with the sheath of the extensor pollicis longus. Finally, a compartment along the lateral aspect of the radius (first compartment) contains a

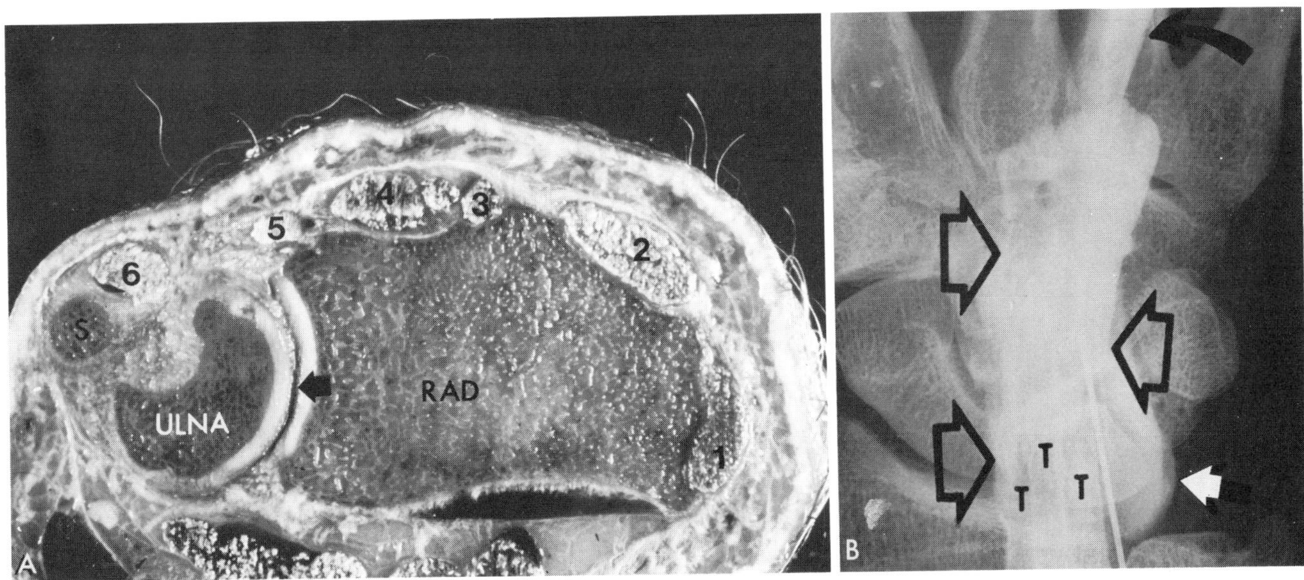

Figure 15–25. *Tenography of the hand and wrist: Normal appearance of extensor tendon sheaths.*

A *A transverse cross section through the distal radius (RAD), ulna, ulnar styloid (S), and inferior radioulnar joint (arrow) reveals the six compartments of the extensor tendons and sheaths.*

B *An injection has been made into the sheath (open arrows) enclosing the tendons (T) of the extensor digitorum communis and extensor indicis proprius. Previous injection in the flexor digiti minimi brevis sheath of the fifth finger (curved arrow) introduced contrast material, which continued into the ulnar bursa (straight arrow).*

(From Resnick D: Am J Roentgenol 124:44, 1975. Copyright 1975, American Roentgen Ray Society.)

common synovial sheath (5 to 6 cm in length) enclosing the abductor pollicis longus and extensor pollicis brevis.

Abnormal Tenogram. Rheumatoid arthritis and related disorders are associated with inflammation of the synovium-lined tendon sheaths and tendons. Effusions related to fluid production within the sheaths may produce distention, and villous hypertrophy of the synovial lining can lead to thickening and irregularity of the tendon sheath wall, a nodular corrugated pattern of the contrast material, and, on some occasions, interference with normal communicating pathways.[27-29] Displacement of the sheaths and lymphatic filling may occur.[22, 28] Sacculations and pseudodiverticula of the sheath may be outlined.[22, 29] Although tenography is not particularly beneficial in establishing a diagnosis of rheumatoid arthritis, as the presence of this disease is generally apparent on clinical examination, this procedure, by outlining the extent of synovial disease, may aid the surgeon who is contemplating operative intervention and the internist who is evaluating a therapeutic regimen.

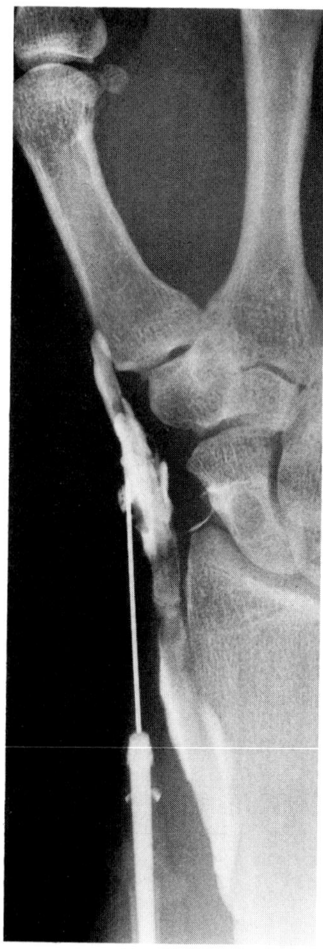

Figure 15–26. *Tenography of the hand and wrist: Tenosynovitis. Contrast material mixed with lidocaine has been injected into the most lateral extensor compartment in a patient with de Quervain's syndrome. Prompt relief of pain ensued.*

The tendon sheaths and bursae represent an important pathway for dissemination of infections in the hand.[31, 37] Their selective catheterization and visualization may be useful in detecting the extent of tissue contamination and providing an understanding of the infectious process. Furthermore, it is anticipated that in selected cases of carpal tunnel syndrome, tenography may reveal displacement of synovial sheaths by neighboring masses or edema. Finally, the injection of contrast material containing a small amount of lidocaine into an abnormal tendon sheath may lead to relief of clinical manifestations, confirming the origin of specific clinical findings (Fig. 15–26).

ELBOW

Elbow Arthrography

Arthrography of the elbow (Table 15–5) is not a commonly performed procedure.[336] It is a safe, relatively easy examination that may be utilized to outline the nature and extent of intra-articular disorders and the etiology of adjacent soft tissue masses.[41-46]

Technique (Fig. 15–27). The patient is seated adjacent to the radiographic table and the elbow is flexed to approximately 90 degrees, semipronated, and positioned beneath the fluoroscope. With an opaque metal marker, a mark is placed over the articular cavity between the radial head and capitellum of the humerus for appropriate localization. Six to 10 ml of contrast material alone (60 per cent methyglucamine diatrizoate [Renografin]), 0.5 to 1 ml of contrast material and 6 to 10 ml of air, or 8 to 12 ml of air alone are utilized for injection, depending upon the indication for the study. The injection of contrast material alone is particularly useful for outlining the presence and extent of synovial disorders, capsular integrity, and synovial cysts, whereas the double contrast study with contrast material and air or the single contrast study with air alone may be superior in demonstrating cartilaginous and osseous defects and "loose" intra-articular bodies.[41, 310] Following injection, anteroposterior, oblique, and lateral roentgenograms are obtained, supplemented with tomography when necessary.[311]

Normal Elbow Arthrogram (Fig. 15–28). On frontal radiographs, a thin layer of contrast

Table 15–5

INDICATIONS FOR ELBOW ARTHROGRAPHY

Evaluation of:
Presence and extent of synovial inflammation
Intra-articular cartilaginous and osseous bodies
Soft tissue masses

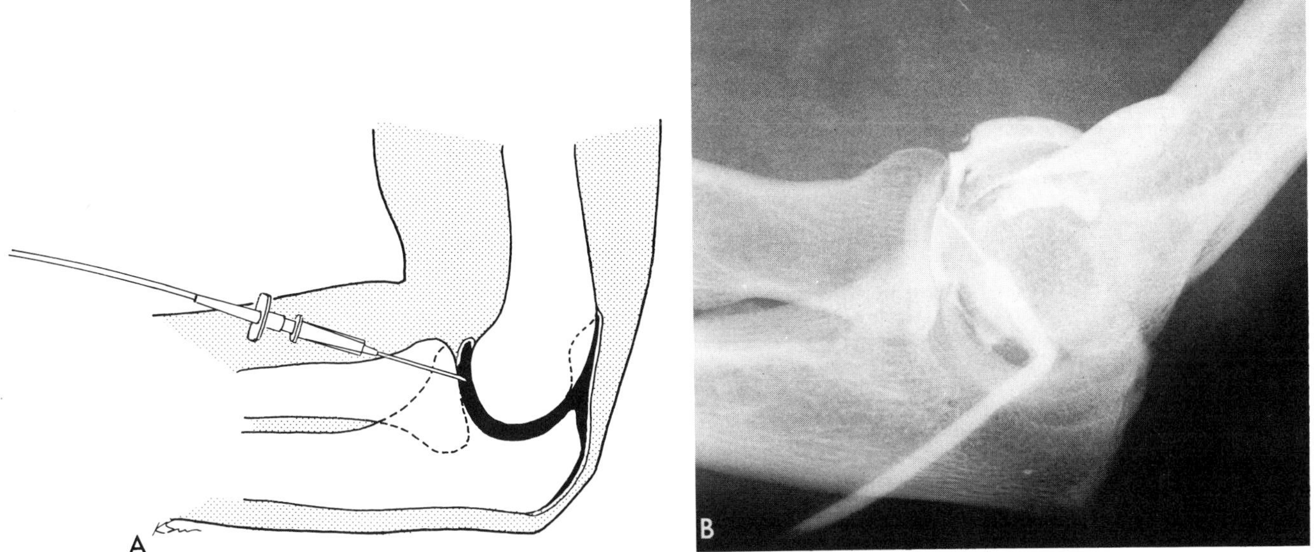

Figure 15–27. *Elbow arthrography: Technique. Under fluoroscopic control, a needle is directed between the radial head and capitellum into the elbow joint from a lateral (radial) approach.*

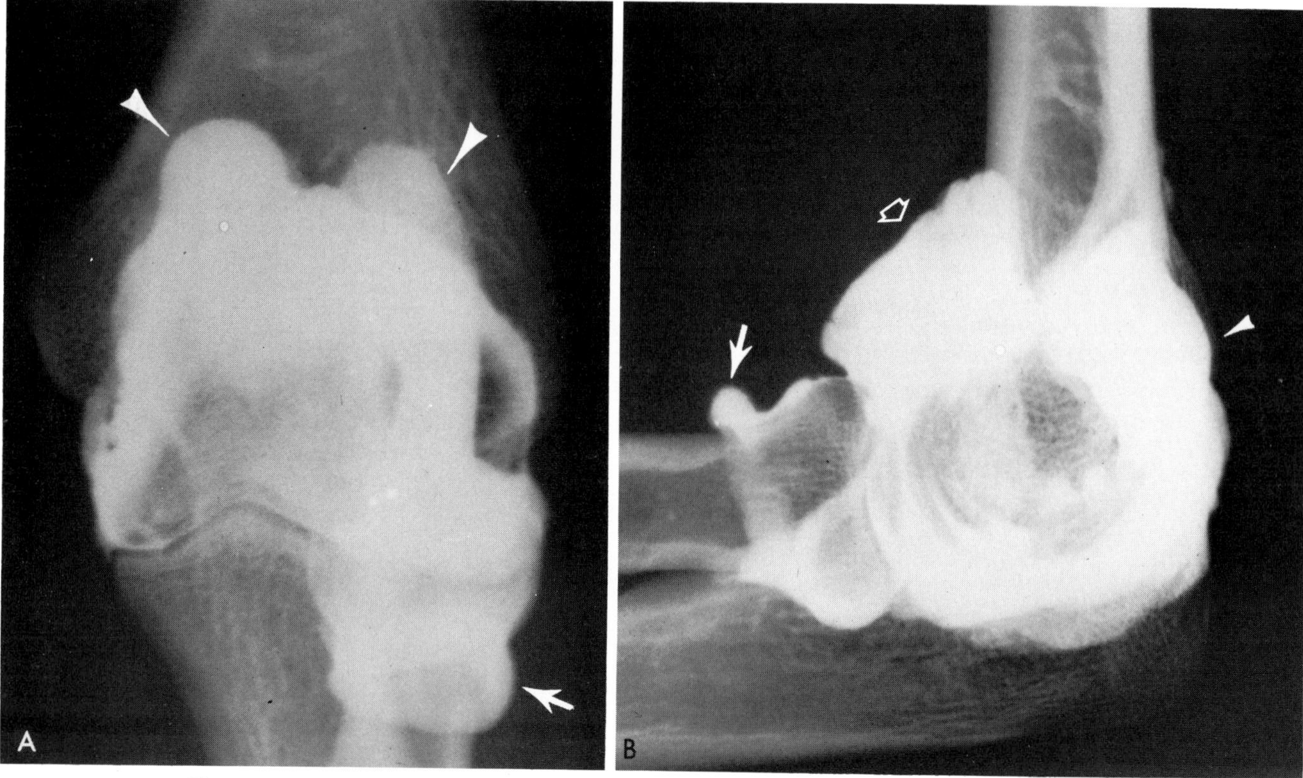

Figure 15–28. Elbow arthrography: Normal arthrogram.

A Anteroposterior radiograph. Observe the thin layer of contrast material between humerus and ulna, the proximal extension of material in front of the humerus resembling the ears of a rabbit (arrowheads), and the periradial or annular recess (arrow).

B Lateral radiograph. Note the peripheral or annular recess (arrow), the coronoid or anterior recess (open arrow), and the olecranon or posterior recess (arrowhead).

material or air is observed between the humerus, radius, and ulna. A periradial prolongation or recess is apparent about the proximal radius, which is indented where the annular ligament surrounds the bone. Proximal extension of contrast material along the anterior surface of the humerus may resemble the ears of a rabbit, the "Bugs Bunny" sign.[22] On a lateral radiograph, the periradial or annular recess is again apparent. In addition, coronoid (anterior) and olecranon (posterior) recesses are seen. The borders of all recesses and the remainder of the articular cavity appear smooth in configuration with two exceptions: The anterior border of the coronoid recess may be slightly wrinkled in flexion, and the medial border adjacent to the collateral ligament is irregular.[41] Smooth articular cartilage is observed on the humerus, radial head, and ulna; it is of uniform thickness except for a portion of the trochlear notch of the ulna, which lacks cartilage.

Rheumatoid Arthritis and other Synovial Disorders. Synovial inflammation with hypertrophy and villous transformation accounts for an irregular outline of contrast material, which may be apparent in rheumatoid arthritis[47] (Fig. 15–29) and disorders such as juvenile chronic polyarthritis,[22] ankylosing spondylitis, neuroarthropathy (Fig. 15–30), and septic arthritis. Lymphatic visualization is common and capsular distention, sacculation, and cystic swelling may be observed.[22, 30] Capsular rupture and synovial cyst formation are also seen.[48-50] Cysts, which may become large, occur anteriorly, medially, laterally, or even posteriorly over the olecranon, and are more frequent in patients with elbow flexion contractures. These cysts most frequently occur when the articulation itself is extensively involved in the rheumatoid process, but on occasion they may represent a relatively early sign of the disease. Altered dynamics at the proximal radioulnar joint and elbow may be contributing factors in the production of these cysts and the caput ulnae syndrome is frequently apparent in the ipsilateral wrist.[48, 51] Cysts in the antecubital fossa may produce swelling of the forearm and compress the interosseous nerve.[16]

Nodular filling defects within the contrast-filled elbow joint may represent hypertrophied synovium, as in rheumatoid arthritis, or synovial masses associated with pigmented villonodular synovitis and idiopathic synovial osteochondromatosis (Fig. 15–31).

Trauma. Opacification of the traumatized elbow joint, particularly after the introduction of air

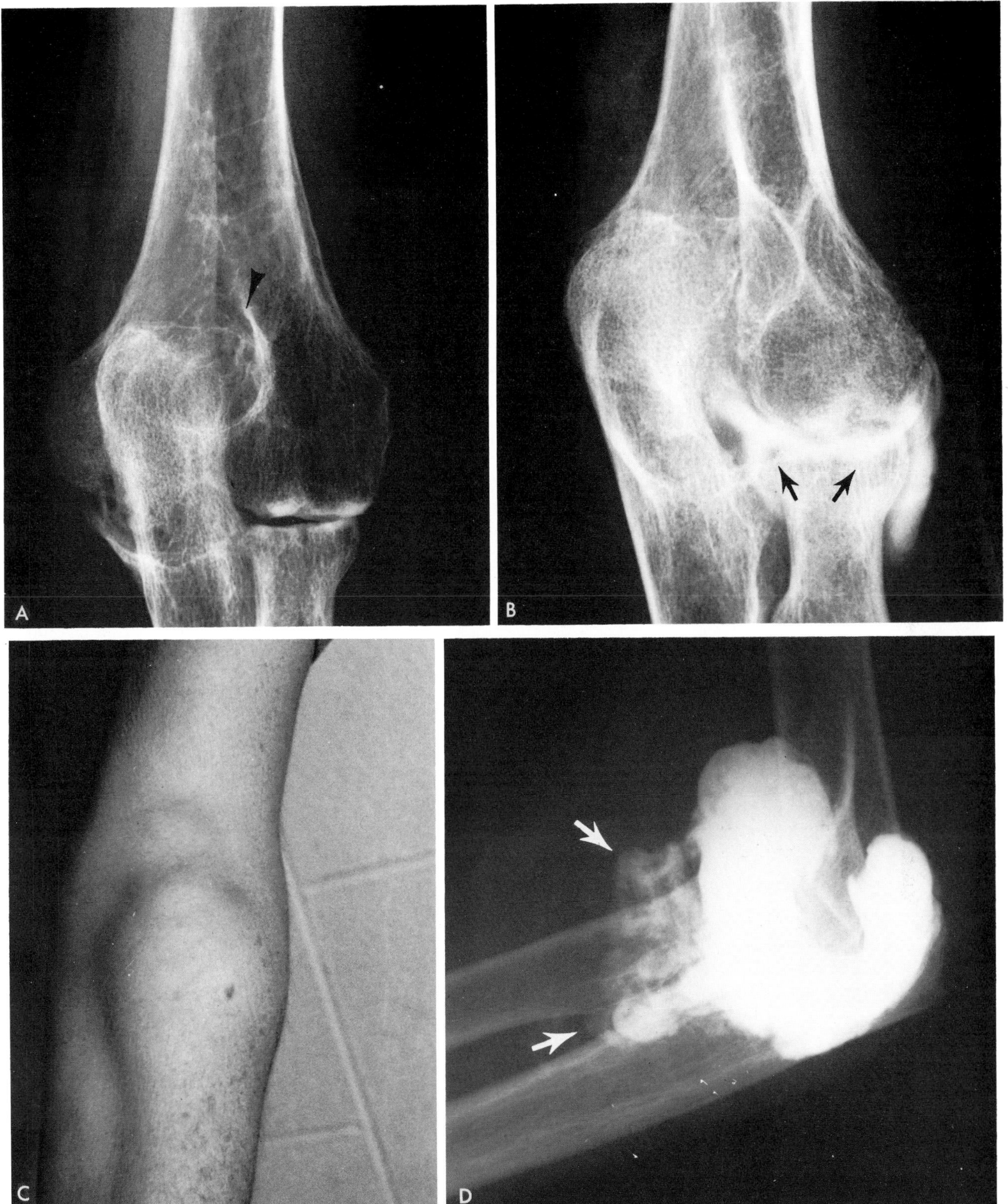

Figure 15–29. *Elbow arthrography: Rheumatoid arthritis.*

A, B *Plain film* **(A)** *and arthrogram* **(B)** *in a patient with long-standing rheumatoid arthritis. The initial radiograph reveals joint space narrowing, erosion, sclerosis, and a large cystic lesion of the distal humerus (arrowhead). The arthrogram indicates a reduced articular volume due to synovial fibrosis. Only a small amount of contrast material could be introduced, which flows between distal humerus and radial head (arrows).*

C, D *Clinical photograph* **(C)** *and arthrogram* **(D)** *from a 50 year old man with rheumatoid arthritis and a periarticular mass due to a synovial cyst. The photograph reveals the mass on the anterior surface of the elbow. The arthrogram outlines the distal cystic dilatation of the articular cavity with irregular synovium (arrows).*

Illustration continued on the following page

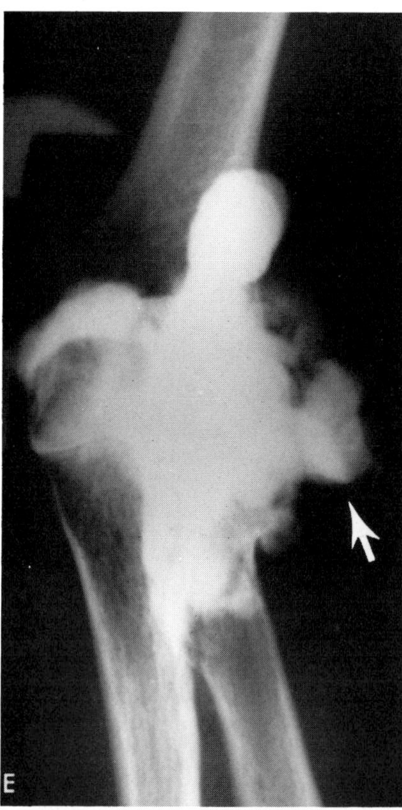

Figure 15–29. Continued

E *An arthrogram from a 56 year old woman with rheumatoid arthritis. Observe the cystic dilatation of the articular cavity (arrow).*

(**C–E,** From Ehrlich GE: *J Bone Joint Surg* 54A:165, 1972.)

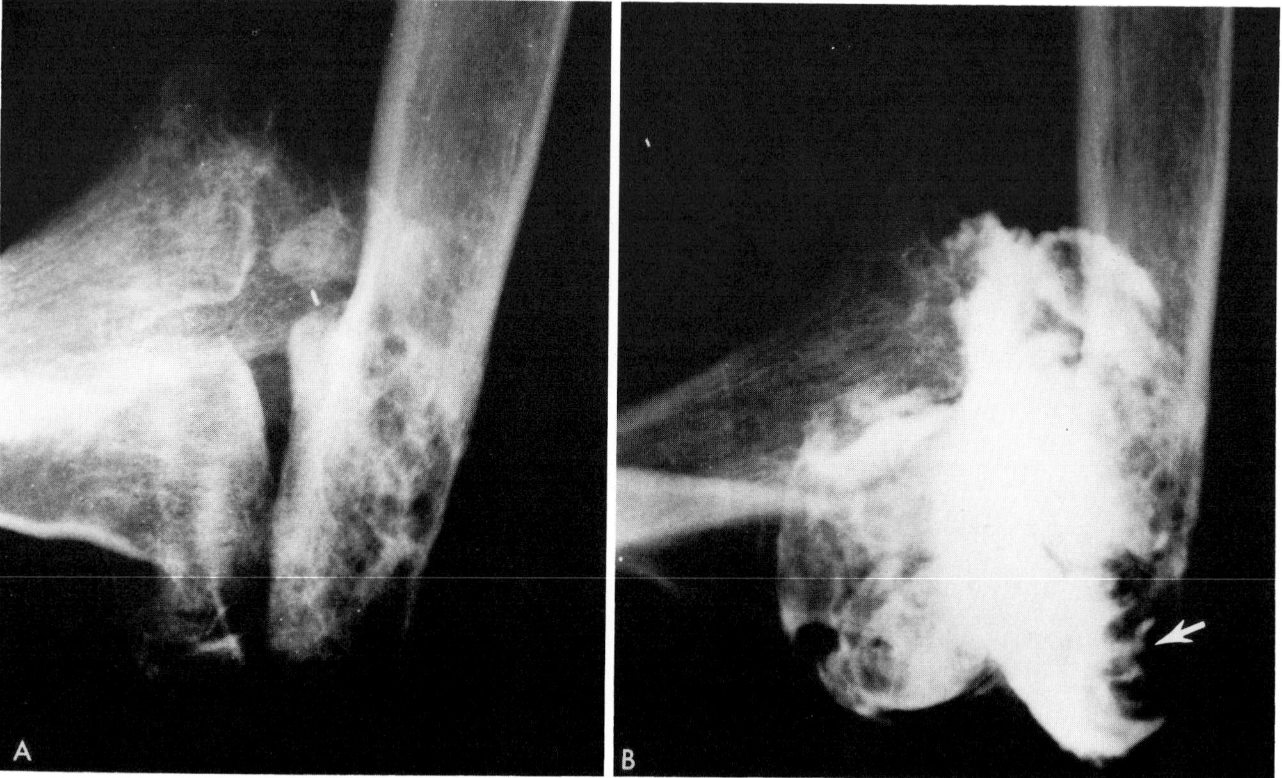

Figure 15–30. *Elbow arthrography: Neuroarthropathy.*

A *The plain film outlines severe flattening of the distal humerus, deformity of the ulna and radial head, sclerosis, fragmentation, and subluxation.*

B *Arthrography confirms articular deformity. The synovium is moderately corrugated or irregular in outline, particularly proximally (arrow). Some filling defects relate to intra-articular osseous bodies.*

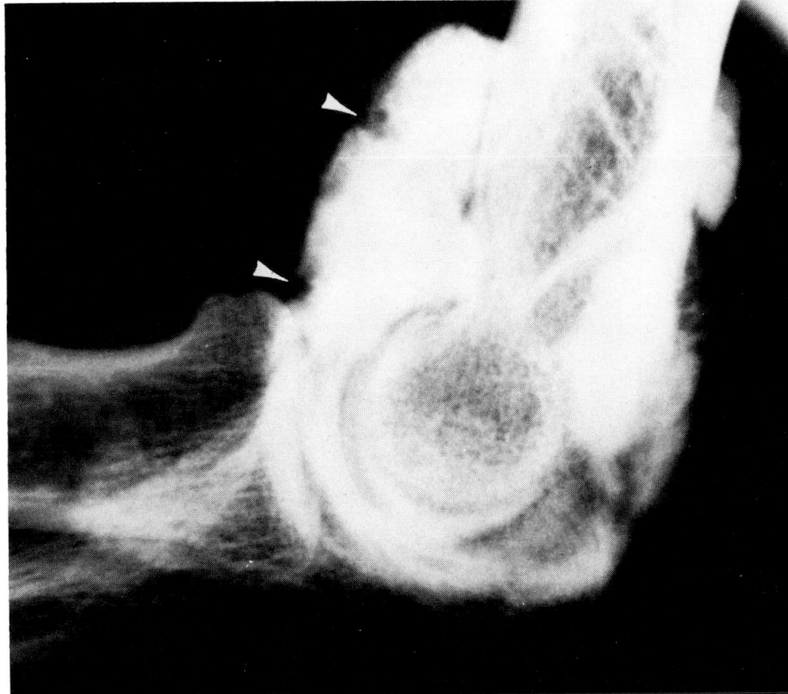

Figure 15–31. *Elbow arthrography: Idiopathic synovial osteochondromatosis. A lateral view following arthrography delineates irregular nodular filling defects (arrowheads), which represent cartilaginous foci resulting from synovial metaplasia.*

or air and contrast material, may reveal cartilaginous and osseous defects associated with osteochondritis dissecans (transchondral fractures) (Fig. 15–32). In these instances, contrast may dissect beneath the adjacent osseous fragment or reveal "loose" or embedded bodies elsewhere in the joint cavity.[41] Localized areas of synovial irregularity, capsular rupture, and soft tissue dissection of contrast material are additional findings following elbow trauma.[45] Intra-articular hematomas may be evident.[46] Following

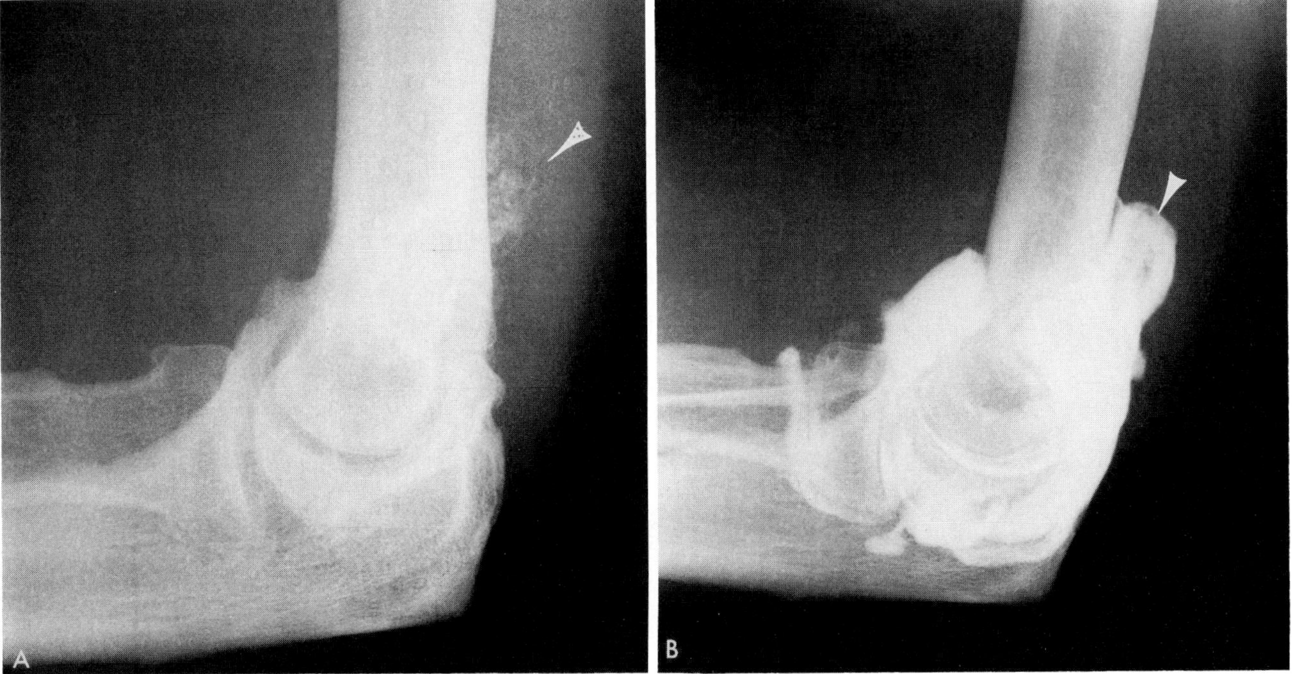

Figure 15–32. *Elbow arthrography: Intra-articular osseous bodies.*

A *The initial film reveals osseous densities behind the distal humerus (arrowhead).*

B *The intra-articular location of these bodies is documented during arthrography as defects (arrowhead), which can be seen in the contrast-filled joint cavity.*

gunshot injury of the elbow, metallic fragments may produce a "lead" arthrogram (see Fig. 15–83*E*).[52]

Olecranon Bursography

Injection of the olecranon bursa is readily accomplished and may delineate the nature of soft tissue masses in this area.[53]

Technique (Fig. 15–33). The olecranon bursa lies superficially like a cap about the olecranon process. Under fluoroscopy with the elbow flexed, a needle is placed into the bursa approximately 2 cm distal to the tip of the olecranon. Several milliliters of contrast material may be injected.

Normal and Abnormal Olecranon Bursogram (Figs. 15–34 to 15–36). A half-moon–shaped collection of contrast material is identified during the normal olecranon bursogram.[22, 53] In rheumatoid arthritis and related disorders, sacculation, distention, or protrusion along the dorsal aspect of the forearm can be identified. The olecranon bursa may communicate with the elbow joint under these abnormal conditions.

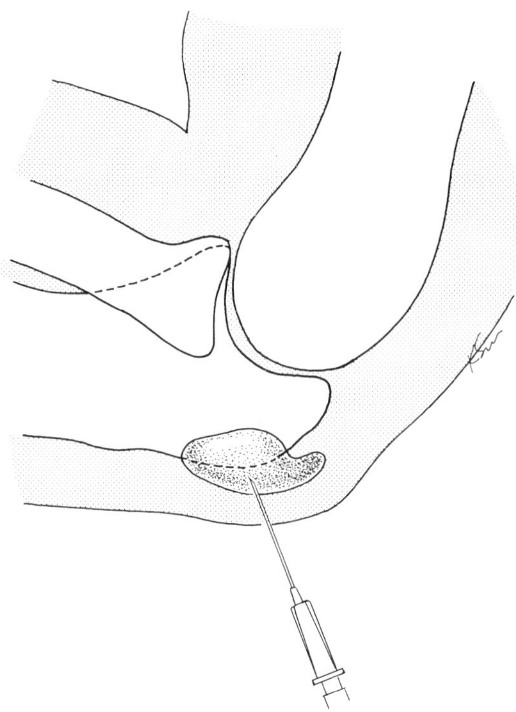

Figure 15–33. *Olecranon bursography: Technique. A needle is inserted into the bursa approximately 2 cm distal to the olecranon tip.*

SHOULDER

Arthrography of the Glenohumeral Joint

Contrast opacification of the glenohumeral joint (Table 15–6) as an aid to the diagnosis of rotator cuff tear, adhesive capsulitis, previous dislocation, articular disease, and bicipital tendon abnormalities has been a subject of a great number of articles.[54-64] The examination is readily performed and the arthrographic findings are reliable.[358]

Technique (Fig. 15–37). Two basic techniques have been advocated for shoulder arthrography: single contrast examination and double contrast examination.

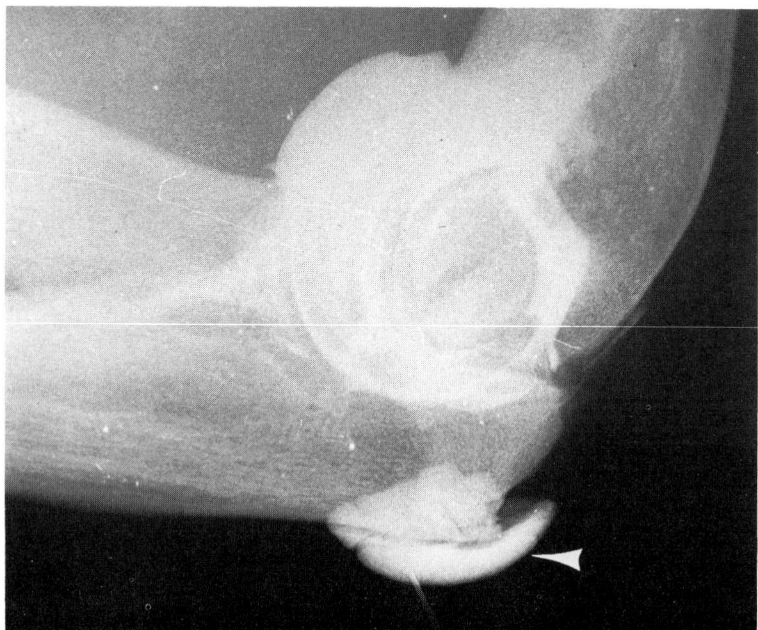

Figure 15–34. *Olecranon bursography: Normal examination. A lateral view reveals contrast material within a normal olecranon bursa (arrowhead). Note how the bursa is situated like a cap about the ulnar olecranon. An elbow arthrogram has also been performed. (Courtesy of Dr. W. J. Weston, Hutt Hospital, Lower Hutt, New Zealand.)*

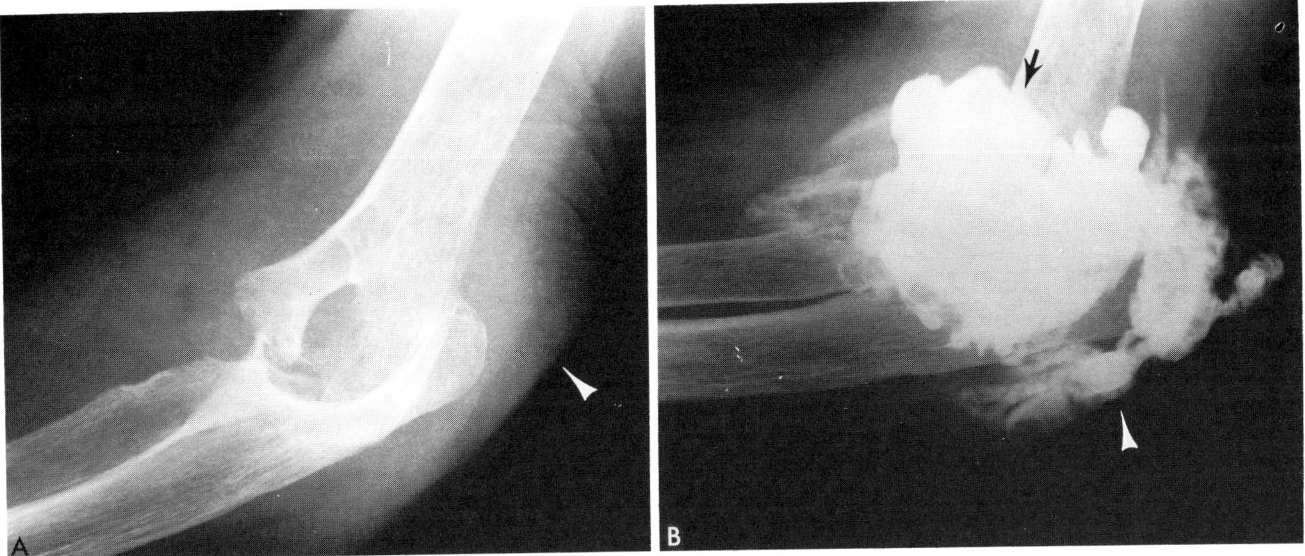

Figure 15–35. Olecranon bursography: Rheumatoid arthritis. This patient presented with a swollen olecranon bursa.

A An initial radiograph outlines the soft tissue swelling over the ulnar olecranon (arrowhead) and severe destruction of the elbow joint.

B Following injection of the bursa (arrowhead), contrast flowed into the elbow joint (arrow). Observe the enlarged articular and bursal cavities and the nodular, corrugated synovium.

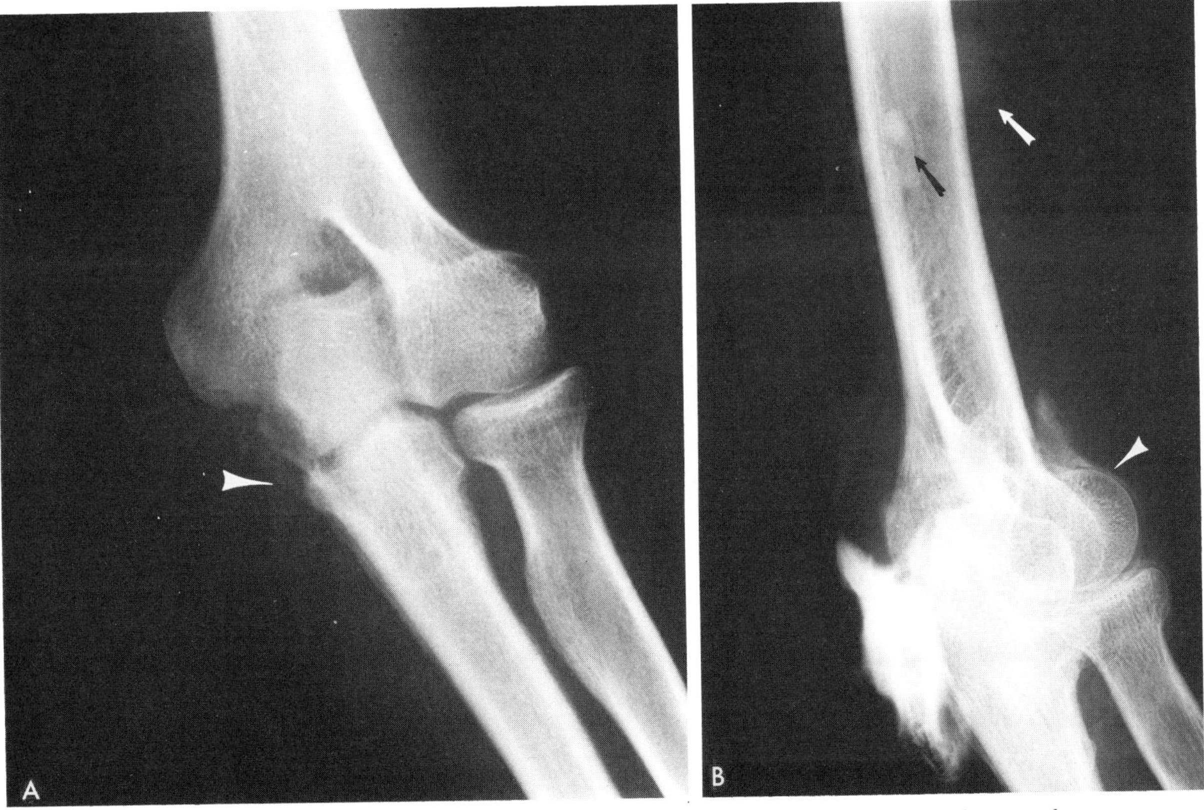

Figure 15–36. Olecranon bursography: septic arthritis. This patient developed a soft tissue abscess over the olecranon region and progressive pain and swelling of the elbow. Cultures revealed staphylococci.

A A plain film delineates osseous erosion and periostitis of the medial aspect of the humerus and ulna (arrowhead).

B Aspiration followed by contrast injection of the bursa reveals its irregular outline, proximal extension of the contrast material adjacent to the distal humerus (arrows), and communication with the articular cavity (arrowhead).

Table 15–6
INDICATIONS FOR GLENOHUMERAL JOINT ARTHROGRAPHY

Evaluation of:
Rotator cuff tears
Adhesive capsulitis
Bicipital tendon abnormalities
Previous dislocations
Presence and extent of synovial inflammation

Single Contrast Examination. After preliminary radiographs of the shoulder are obtained, the patient is positioned supine under the fluoroscope with the hand in external rotation, anchored with a sandbag. Some people advocate an oblique position, but the anteroposterior position is generally preferred.[65] A lead marker is placed over the subchondral border of the humerus (medial margin) at the junction of the middle and distal thirds of the glenoid cavity, although a grid may be used rather than a lead marker.[66] A 3 inch, 18 or 20 gauge spinal needle is inserted in a vertical direction toward the glenohumeral joint utilizing fluoroscopic guidance. The needle may contact the extreme medial margin of the humeral head, at which point it is elevated slightly and directed more medially, or it may pass directly into the articular cavity. Ten to 15 ml of 60 per cent methylglucamine diatrizoate (Renografin) is injected which, with accurate needle placement, should flow away from the needle tip. The needle is withdrawn and following mild exercise, anteroposterior roentgenograms are obtained in internal and external rotation, and axillary and tangential bicipital groove radiographs are also performed. This series of radiographs is repeated following moderate exercise.

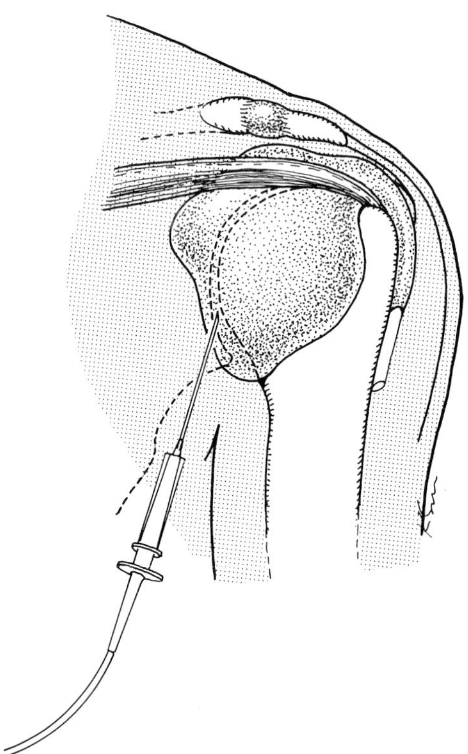

Figure 15–37. Glenohumeral joint arthrography: Technique. An anterior approach is utilized. A needle is inserted into the articulation at the level of the junction of the middle and lower thirds of the glenoid cavity. (Schematic drawing.)

Double Contrast Examination. More recently, double contrast shoulder arthrography has been advocated utilizing approximately 4 ml of Renografin and 10 ml of air.[67, 68] The needle placement is performed in a manner identical to that previously outlined. Following injection and withdrawal of the needle, the patient is placed upright with a 2.3 kg (5 lb) sandbag in his hand. Radiographs in internal and external rotation are obtained with or without a spot film device. The patient is then returned to the supine position and internal rotation, external rotation, axillary, and bicipital groove films are made. These roentgenograms can be repeated after mild exercise. The proponents of the double contrast technique observe that, with this technique, the width of the rotator cuff tear and the integrity of cuff tendons can be assessed, allowing the surgeon to more accurately plan the operative technique. Furthermore, the internal structures of the joint, including the glenoid labrum, are better identified.[337]

We have utilized both single and double contrast arthrography and agree that the double contrast study is superior, although it is more difficult to interpret, requiring a good deal of experience. In addition, we believe that 2 to 3 ml of lidocaine should be injected with the contrast material during shoulder arthrography as this procedure may be associated with mild immediate or delayed discomfort.

NORMAL GLENOHUMERAL JOINT ARTHROGRAM (Fig. 15–38). Contrast material is identified between the humeral head and the glenoid. In external rotation, the contrast substance ends abruptly laterally at the anatomic neck of the humerus. In this view, an axillary pouch may be opacified on the undersurface of the humeral head. In internal rotation, a prominent subscapular recess is observed overlying the glenoid and lateral scapular region. The axillary and subscapular recesses are not continuous, as a definite indentation is observed between them. The tendon of the long head of the biceps is visible as a radiolucent filling defect within the articular cavity and can be traced for a variable distance within the contrast-filled tendon sheath into the bicipital groove and along the metaphysis of the humerus.

In the axillary view, contrast material is identified between glenoid cavity and humeral head, anterior to the scapula (subscapular recess), and within the bicipital tendon sheath. The cartilaginous surfaces of glenoid and humerus, as well as the

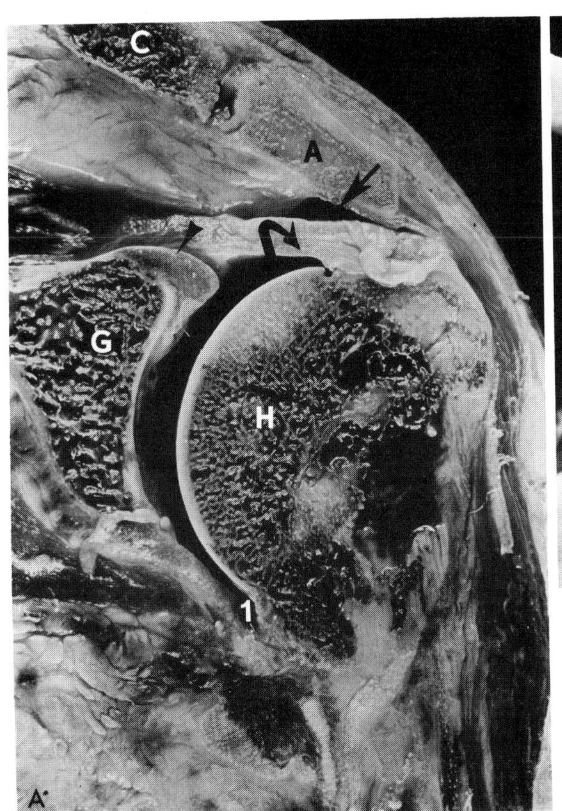

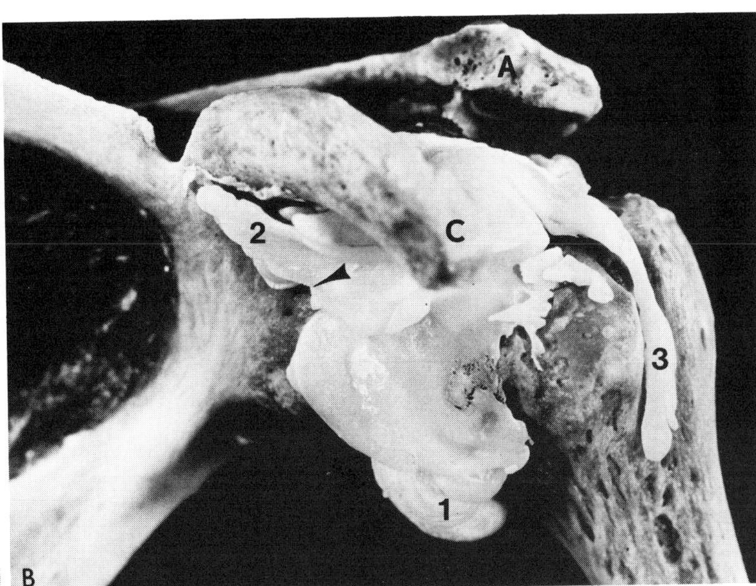

Figure 15–38. *Glenohumeral joint arthrography: Anatomy and normal arthrogram.*

A *Coronal section of the glenohumeral joint. Observe the glenoid (G), humeral head (H), distal clavicle (C), acromion (A), subacromial (subdeltoid) bursa (straight arrow), rotator cuff (curved arrow), and glenoid labrum (arrowhead). The joint cavity is seen extending inferiorly as the axillary pouch (1).*

(From Armbuster T et al: Am J Roentgenol 129:667, 1977. Copyright 1977, American Roentgen Ray Society.)

B *Anterior view of macerated specimen following glenohumeral joint arthrography utilizing methylmethacrylate. A model of the distended joint has been created. Note the axillary pouch (1), subscapular recess (2), indentation between these latter two structures (arrowhead), bicipital tendon sheath (long head of the biceps) (3), acromion (A), and coracoid process (C).*

Illustration continued on the following page

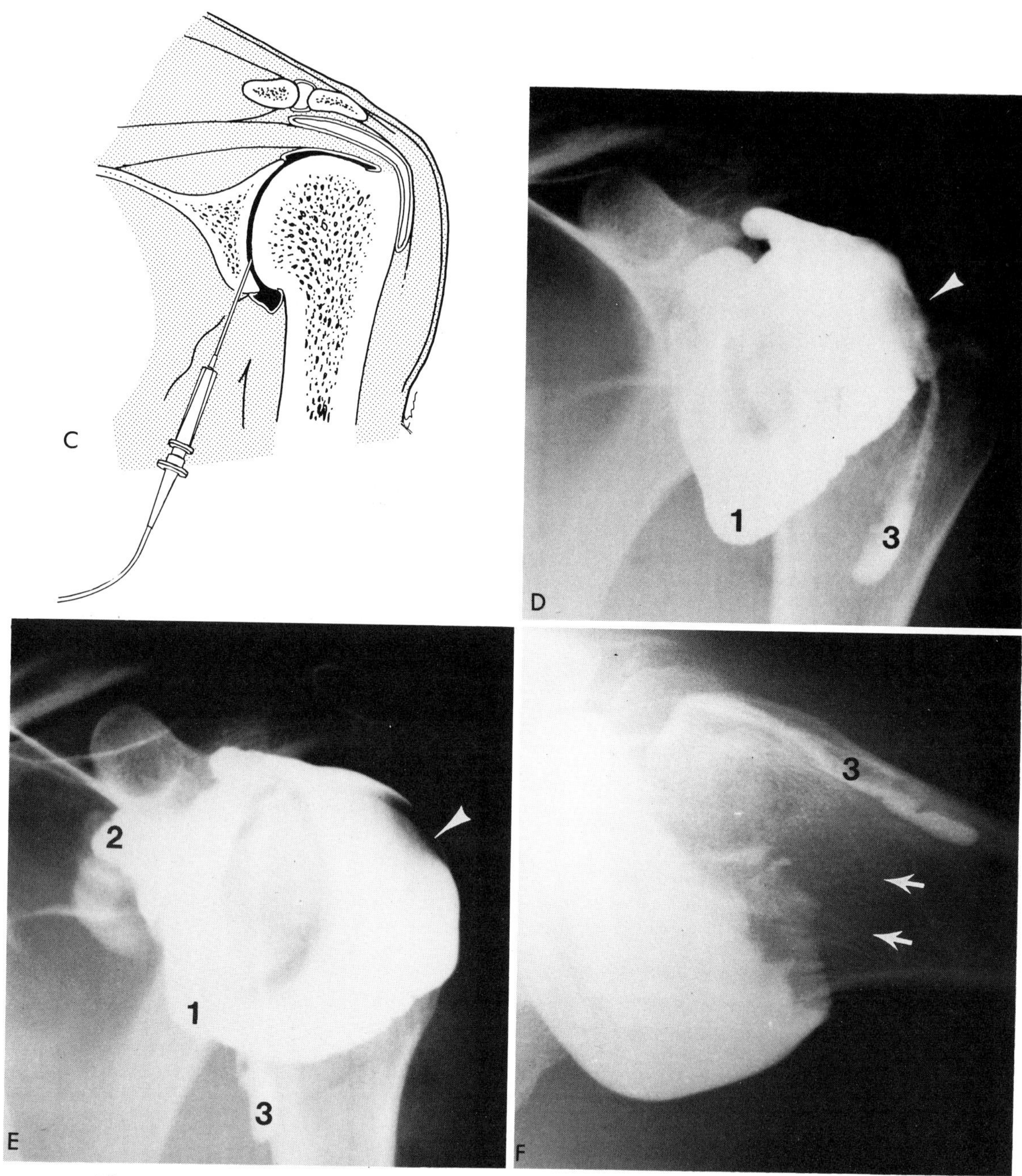

Figure 15–38. Continued

C *Diagram of normal arthrogram. Observe that the contrast material flows up to the greater tuberosity, below the rotator cuff.*

D *Normal arthrogram: External rotation. Visualized structures include the axillary pouch (1) and bicipital tendon sheath (3). Note that the subscapular recess is not well seen and the contrast material ends abruptly laterally at the anatomic neck of the humerus (arrowhead).*

E *Normal arthrogram: Internal rotation. Observe the prominent subscapular recess (2), axillary pouch (1), and bicipital tendon sheath (3). The articular cartilage of the humeral head is well seen (arrowhead). Minimal extravasation of contrast material has occurred in the axilla near the injection site.*

F *Normal arthrogram: axillary view. Observe the bicipital tendon (3) and the absence of contrast material over the surgical neck of the humerus (arrows).*

glenoid labrum, are seen. In this projection, contrast material should not overlie the surgical neck of the humerus. The tangential view of the bicipital groove demonstrates an oval filling defect within the contrast-filled sheath, representing the biceps tendon.

Complete and Incomplete Tears of the Rotator Cuff. Tears in the rotator cuff musculature may involve the entire thickness of the cuff (complete tear) or a portion of the cuff (incomplete or partial tear).

Complete Tear (Fig. 15–39). In this situation, abnormal communication exists between the glenohumeral joint cavity and the subacromial (subdeltoid) bursa. Contrast material can be identified within the bursa as a large collection superior and lateral to the greater tuberosity and adjacent to the undersurface of the acromion. The contrast material in the bursa is separated from the articular cavity by a lucency of varying size, representing the rotator cuff itself. If the musculature is thick, this lucency is quite large, whereas if the musculature is atrophic, the lucency is small or even absent. In the presence of a complete rotator cuff tear, contrast material is identified as a "saddle-bag" radiodense area across the surgical neck of the humerus on the axillary view. In

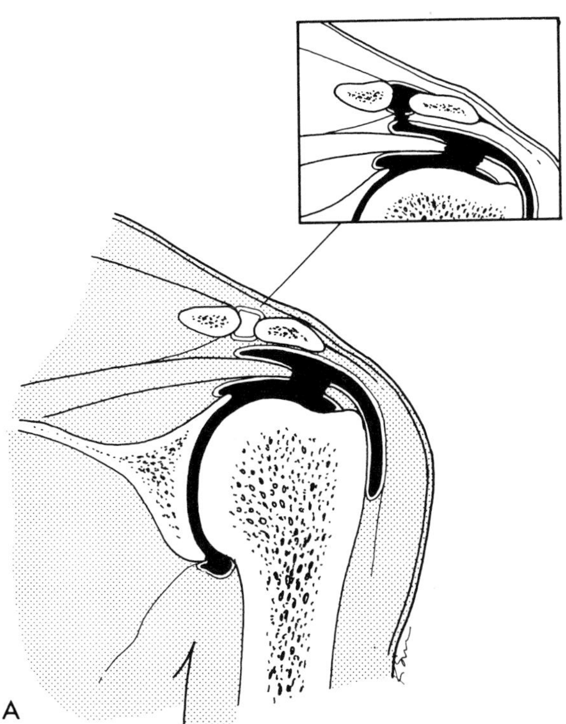

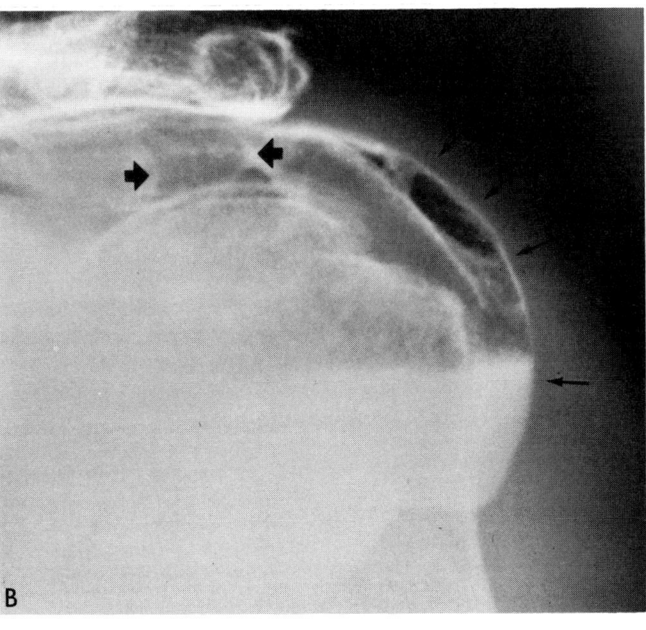

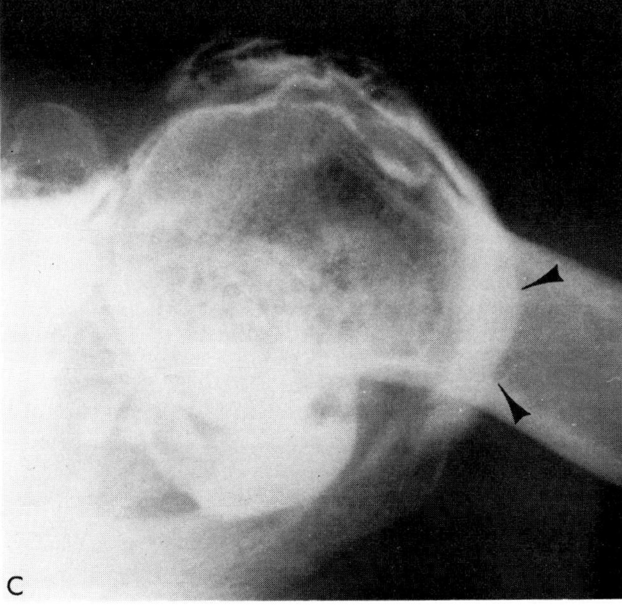

Figure 15–39. *Glenohumeral joint arthrography: Complete rotator cuff tear.*

A *The arthrographic findings of a complete tear of the rotator cuff. Contrast material extends from the glenohumeral joint through the rotator cuff into the subacromial (subdeltoid) bursa. The inset reveals contrast material extending from the glenohumeral joint through the rotator cuff into the subdeltoid bursa, and from there into the acromioclavicular joint.*

B, C *Double contrast arthrography. The external rotation view* **(B)** *demonstrates that contrast material has extended from the glenohumeral joint into the subacromial (subdeltoid) bursa (thin arrows). The width of the tear of the rotator cuff can be seen (between heavy arrows). In another patient with a rotator cuff tear, an axillary view* **(C)** *reveals a "saddle-bag" configuration, with contrast material overlying the surgical neck of the humerus (arrowheads).* **B,** *Courtesy of Dr. Jerrold Mink, Cedars-Sinai Medical Center, Los Angeles, California.)*

Illustration continued on the following page

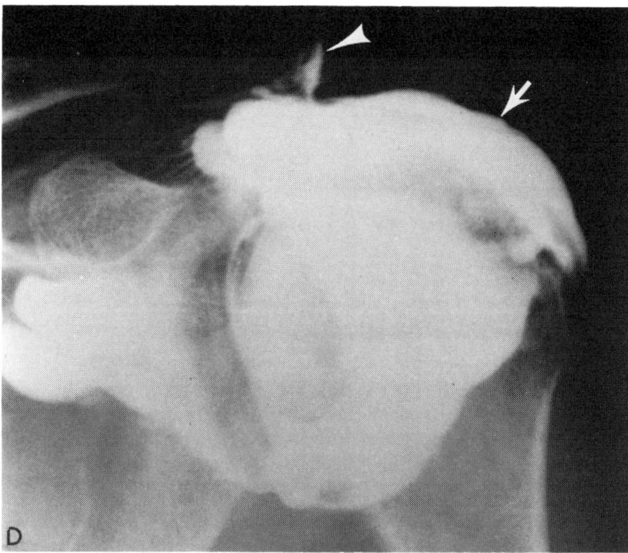

Figure 15–39. Continued
D *Single contrast arthrography. In this patient with a rotator cuff tear, contrast material in the subdeltoid bursa (arrow) has opacified the acromioclavicular joint (arrowhead).*

some patients with complete tears, the contrast material will pass from the subacromial bursa into the acromioclavicular joint.

Utilizing double-contrast shoulder arthrography, the degree of degeneration of the torn rotator cuff can be recognized.[68] Furthermore, the width of the tear itself is identified. The location of the disrupted tendons is apparent as the tendinous ends are coated by positive contrast material. In some patients, the torn rotator cuff tendons are either absent or consist of only a few small pieces, prohibiting adequate surgical repair or, at the very least, requiring an alternative method of surgery.[69-71]

Killoran and associates[54] have emphasized three potential sources of error in the diagnosis of a complete rotator cuff tear: Inadequate distribution of opaque material within the joint may prevent adequate visualization of the subacromial bursa; the contrast-filled sheath of the biceps tendon may project slightly lateral to the greater tuberosity on external rotation, simulating filling of the subacromial bursa; inadvertent bursal injection may simulate a complete tear unless one recognizes that the articular cavity is not opacified.

Incomplete Tear (Fig. 15–40). A partial tear may involve the deep surface of the rotator cuff, the superficial surface, or the interior substance of the tendon. Tears within the substance of the cuff will generally escape arthrographic detection but may not require operative repair.[72] Tears involving the superior surface of the cuff will also not be demonstrated on glenohumeral joint arthrography, although they may rarely be seen with direct subacromial bursography.[64] Tears on the inferior surface of the rotator cuff can be diagnosed on arthrography. In these cases, an ulcer-like circular or linear collection of contrast material may be identified above the opacified joint cavity, near the anatomic neck of the humerus.[54, 68] The intact superficial fibers prevent opacification of the subacromial bursa.[64] A false negative arthrogram in the presence of a partial tear of the rotator cuff can indicate that the tear is too small for recognition or that a fibrous nodule has occluded the defect.

Adhesive Capsulitis. Glenohumeral joint arthrography has been utilized in the diagnosis and treatment of adhesive capsulitis.[73, 74]

Diagnosis (Fig. 15–41). Adhesive capsulitis prevents normal distention of the glenohumeral joint. Its pathologic basis is unknown; the condition may relate to capsular thickening,[75] adhesions between the capsule and bicipital tendon,[76] and adhesions in the subacromial bursa and beneath the coracoid process.[77] Adhesive capsulitis generally follows shoulder trauma, either to the soft tissues or to the osseous structures.[78] Usually, the entire joint capsule is involved, abnormalities being initially detected in the fibrous layer of the capsule, with obliteration of dependent recesses. Adhesive capsulitis has been described in other joints as well.[79]

The main arthrographic abnormality in adhesive capsulitis of the glenohumeral articulation is a joint of low capacity evidenced by increased resistance to injection and a "tight" feel. Only a small amount of fluid (5 to 8 ml) may be injected successfully, and when the hand is released from the plunger, the fluid may quickly return to the syringe. The subscapular and axillary recesses are small or absent. Filling of the bicipital tendon sheath is variable; in some cases it appears normal, whereas in others it fills poorly or not at all, or contrast may leak from the sheath. Contrast also commonly leaks elsewhere in the joint, particularly from the subscapular recess. An additional finding is irregularity of the capsular insertion.

Treatment (Fig. 15–42). Joint distention during arthrography, the "brisement" procedure,[74] may aid in treatment of this condition.[312] This technique requires slow, intermittent injection of larger and larger volumes of contrast material (mixed with sa-

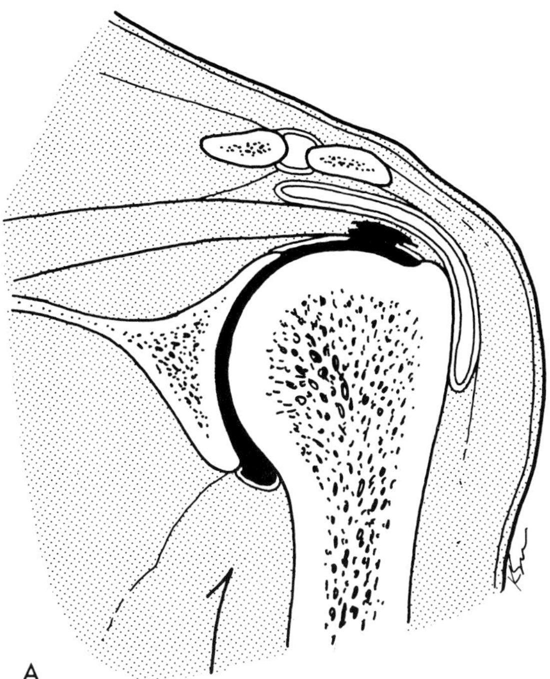

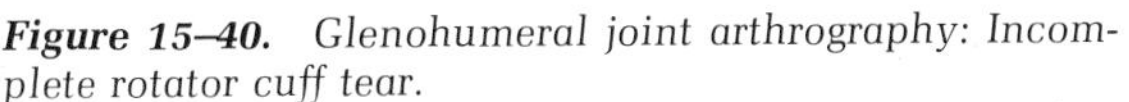

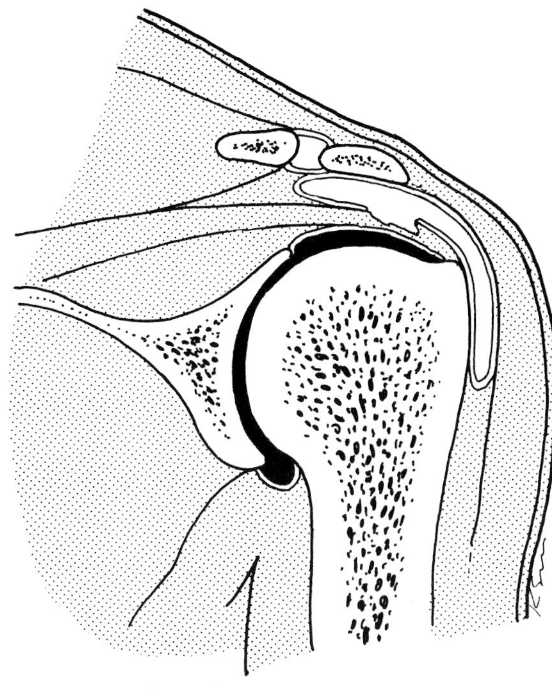

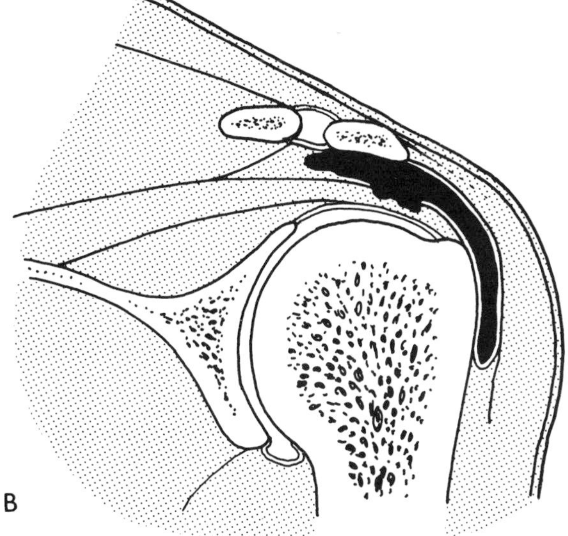

Figure 15–40. Glenohumeral joint arthrography: Incomplete rotator cuff tear.

A *Diagram illustrating that a tear on the undersurface of the rotator cuff can produce an ulcer-like collection of contrast material following opacification of the glenohumeral joint.*

B *In the presence of a partial tear on the superior surface of the rotator cuff, glenohumeral joint arthrography (top drawing) is unrewarding. Subacromial bursography (lower drawing) may demonstrate an ulcer-like collection of contrast material.*

C *A double-contrast arthrogram reveals a partial tear (arrowhead) on the undersurface of the rotator cuff. (Courtesy of Dr. Jerrold Mink, Cedars-Sinai Medical Center, Los Angeles, California.)*

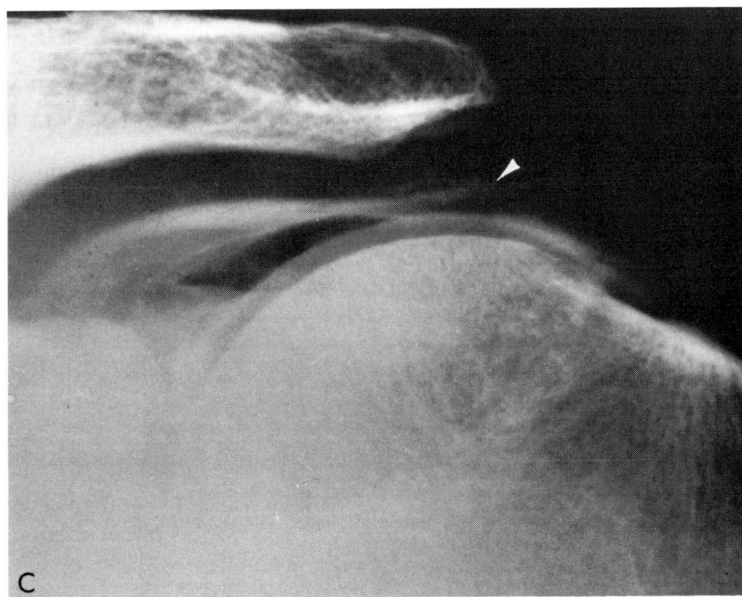

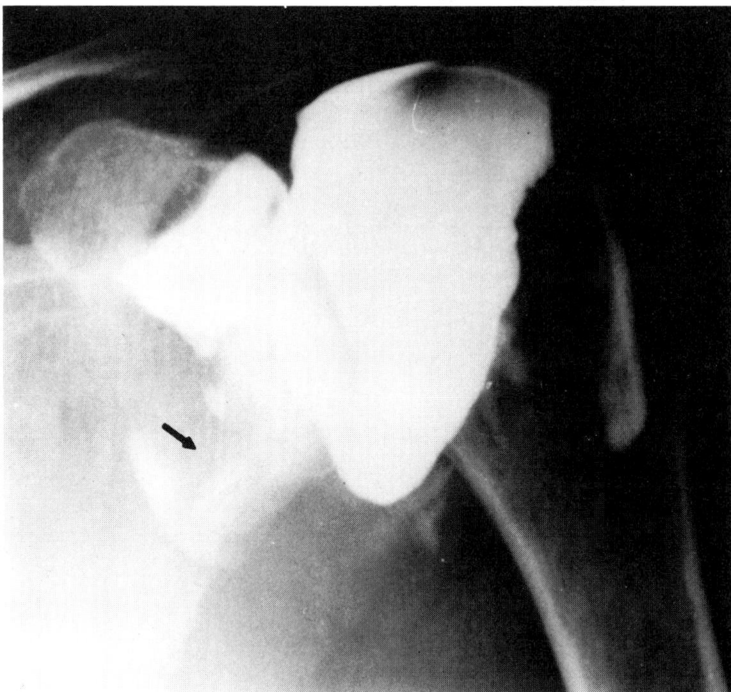

Figure 15–41. Glenohumeral joint arthrography: Diagnosis of adhesive capsulitis. Following the introduction of 6 ml of contrast material, the patient complained of pain and there was increased resistance as an additional 4 ml was injected. A radiograph reveals a "tight-looking" articulation with contrast extravasation medially (arrow).

line and lidocaine), allowing some of the fluid to return into the syringe after each injection. The patient is instructed to move his arm carefully during the procedure. In some patients, 100 ml of fluid may eventually be injected, although free extravasation, particularly at the subscapular recess or the bicipital tendon sheath, frequently occurs with extensive distention, and the procedure is halted. Our investigation with this technique in approximately 15 patients has revealed favorable results. With severe capsular restriction, the brisement procedure is less beneficial, and in all patients, symptoms may return, requiring repeated examinations.

Abnormalities of the Bicipital tendon (Fig. 15–43). Certain abnormalities of the bicipital tendon, such as complete rupture, are easy to recognize clinically and do not require arthrography for documentation, whereas others may produce nonspecific shoulder symptoms and signs, in which case arthrography can indeed be helpful.[313] These latter

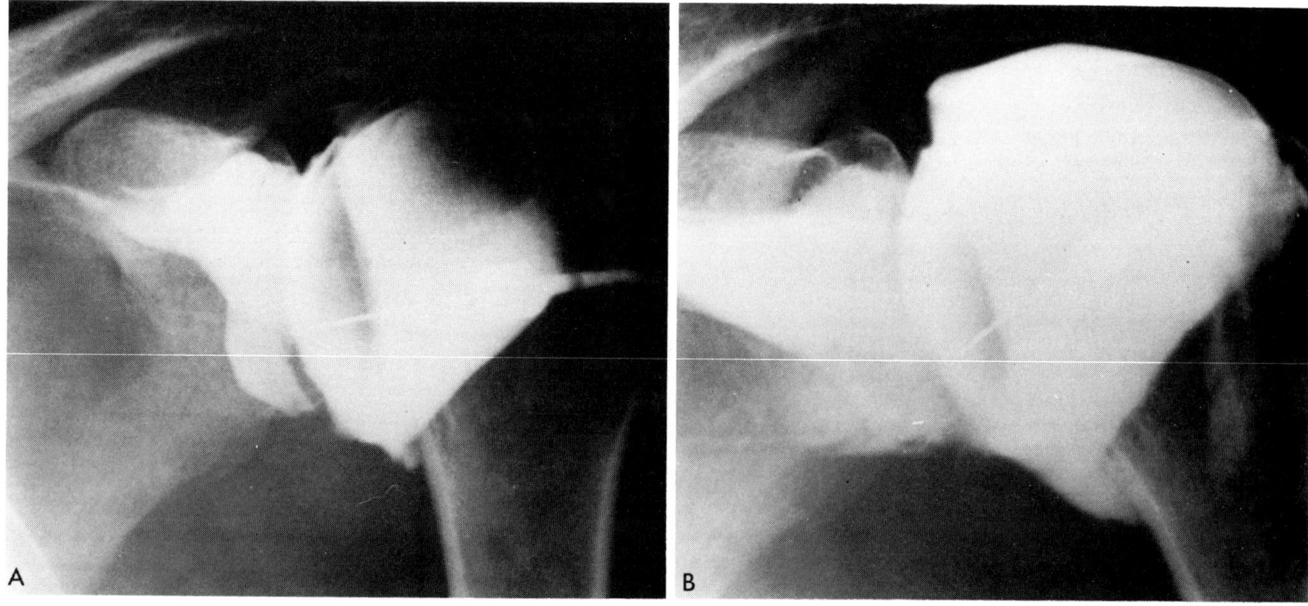

Figure 15–42. Glenohumeral joint arthrography: Treatment of adhesive capsulitis. Radiographs exposed during the "brisement" procedure indicate joint distention in a patient with adhesive capsulitis following injection of 15 ml **(A)** and 50 ml **(B)** of contrast material.

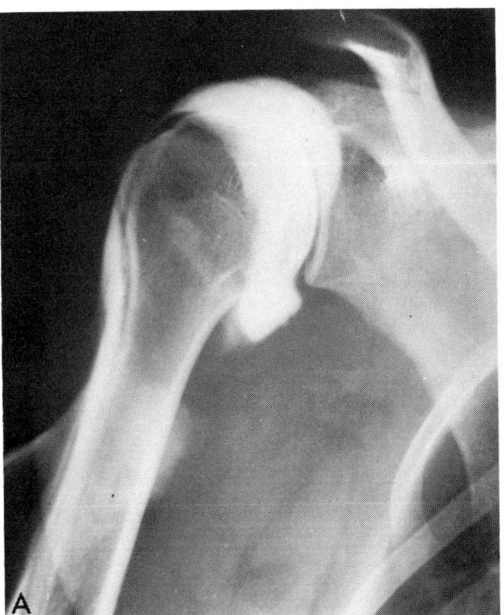

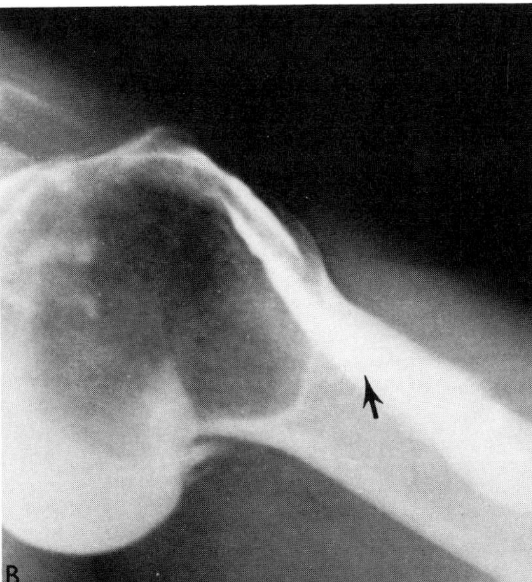

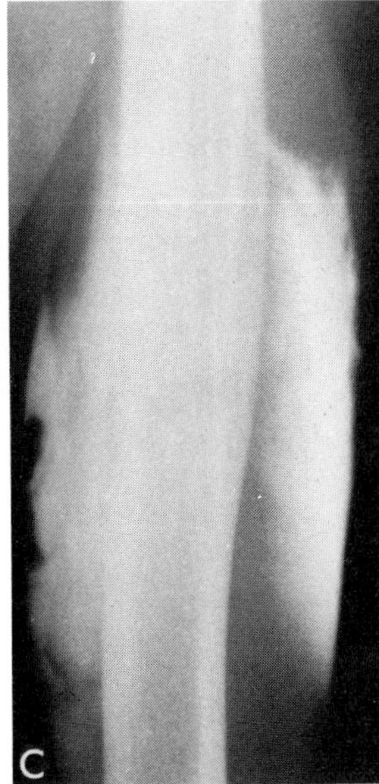

Figure 15–43. *Glenohumeral joint arthrography: Abnormalities of the bicipital tendon.*

A *Tear of the transverse bicipital ligament. Note contrast extension for a considerable distance along the course of the bicipital tendon with soft tissue extravasation. (Courtesy of Dr. Jerrold Mink, Cedars-Sinai Medical Center, Los Angeles, California.)*

B, C *Bicipital tendon rupture. Axillary* **(B)** *and frontal* **(C)** *views in a patient with known rupture of the bicipital tendon reveal contrast extension along the course of the bicipital tendon and extravasation into the soft tissues of the arm. The normal lucency of the bicipital tendon itself is not seen within the contrast-filled sheath (arrow).*

abnormalities include partial tears, dislocation, and tenosynovitis.

In the normal glenohumeral joint arthrogram, visualization of the tendon sheath and tendon of the long head of the biceps is not constant. Therefore, although the absence of visualization may indeed represent a tear of the biceps, it is not a reliable sign. Occasionally, following exercise, the tendon sheath will be seen when it was not apparent on preexercise films. Furthermore, leakage of contrast material from the biceps sleeve can be seen in normal individuals,[54] although some investigators regard it as a sign of disruption of the transverse bicipital ligament,[55, 59] rupture of the bicipital tendon itself,[56] or overdistention of the articular cavity.[80]

Considering the wide variation in the arthrographic appearance of the bicipital tendon and sheath in normal individuals, one must not rely too heavily on the arthrogram in establishing a significant abnormality. When a complete bicipital tendon rupture is apparent clinically, arthrography may confirm the diagnosis, demonstrating distortion of the synovial sheath and failing to identify the tendon within the opacified sheath. The arthrographic diagnosis of complete rupture is more accurate in cases of acute tears; with less acute ruptures, shrinkage of adjacent tissues may obscure the abnormal findings.[61] Incomplete tears of the bicipital tendon produce increased width of the tendon and distortion of the synovial sheath.[68] Medial dislocation of the tendon and sheath from their normal positions in the intertubercular groove can be suggested when the positions of these structures do not change on the internal and external rotation roentgenograms.[68] This finding can be verified on the bicipital groove radiograph.

Patients with Previous Dislocations (Fig. 15–44). Anterior dislocations of the glenohumeral joint are associated with soft tissue damage. As the dislocating humeral head moves anteriorly, it detaches or lifts the articular capsule from the glenoid and neck of the scapula, producing an abnormal recess of variable size between the subscapular and axillary recesses. On arthrography, the abnormal recess fills with contrast material, obscuring the indentation that is normally present between the subscapular and axillary recesses. This finding is more evident on radiographs taken in internal rotation.

Additional findings related to anterior dislocation are injuries of cartilage and bone. The Bankart deformity involves an avulsion or compression defect of the anteroinferior rim of the glenoid and may be purely cartilaginous in nature.[81] The arthrogram, particularly when performed with double contrast technique, may outline the cartilaginous abnormalities about the glenoid labrum.[314] The second defect associated with previous anterior dislocation is a Hill-Sachs compression deformity on the posterolateral aspect of the humeral head. This finding is generally evident on plain films but may require arthrography for demonstration if the defect is small or involves only cartilage.

Rheumatoid Arthritis and Other Synovial Disorders (Figs. 15–45 and 15–46). Synovial, cartilaginous, osseous and soft tissue changes of

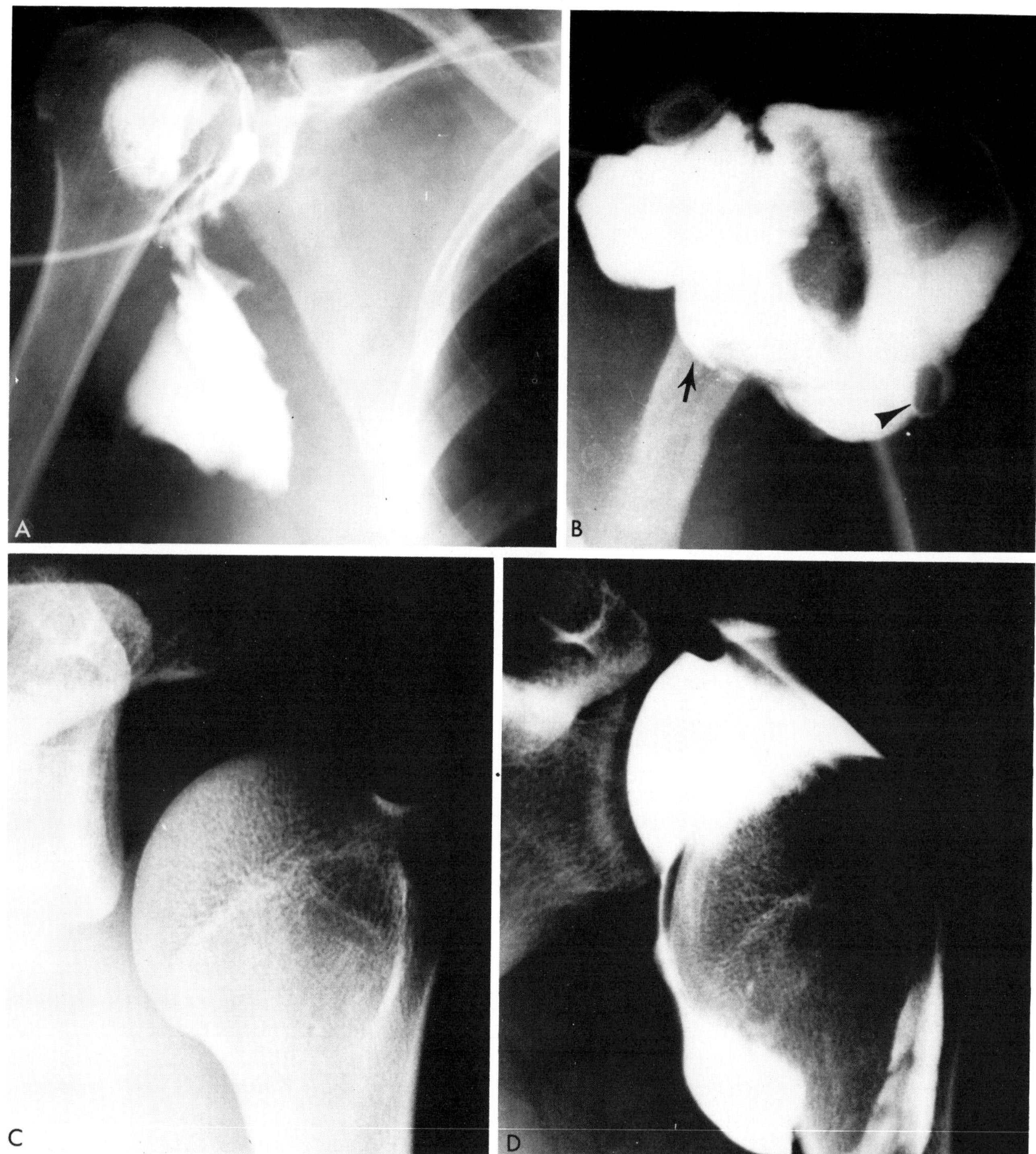

Figure 15–44. *Glenohumeral joint arthrography: Previous dislocation and subluxation.*

A *Following an acute anterior dislocation of the glenohumeral joint with an associated fracture of the greater tuberosity, arthrography outlines an anterior capsular tear with soft tissue extension of contrast material. (Courtesy of Dr. Jerrold Mink, Cedars-Sinai Medical Center, Los Angeles, California.)*

B *In a patient with previous anterior dislocations of the glenohumeral joint, arthrography demonstrates an abnormal recess (arrow) between the axillary pouch and subscapular recess and an intra-articular "loose" body (arrowhead).*

C, D *In a patient with voluntary inferior subluxation of the glenohumeral joint, the initial film* **(C)** *reveals the depressed position of the humeral head with respect to the glenoid. Arthrography* **(D)** *outlines the distorted joint cavity and stretched bicipital tendon.*

rheumatoid involvement of the glenohumeral joint can be identified on arthrography.[82-85] These findings include a corrugated, enlarged synovial cavity, nodular filling defects, cartilage loss, contrast filling of osseous erosions, lymphatic filling, enlarged axillary lymph nodes, capsulitis with a restricted joint cavity, and rotator cuff tear. The latter abnormality, reported by DeSmet and co-workers[82] in 5 of 13 patients with rheumatoid arthritis (38 per cent), is probably related to erosion of the inner aspect of the tendon by the inflamed synovium.[83] It should be expected that other disorders characterized by synovial inflammation could also lead to rupture of the rotator cuff, a speculation which is substantiated by observation of this complication in septic arthritis of the glenohumeral joint.[86] In the presence of a rotator cuff tear in patients with rheumatoid arthritis, arthrography of the glenohumeral joint may lead to opacification of an

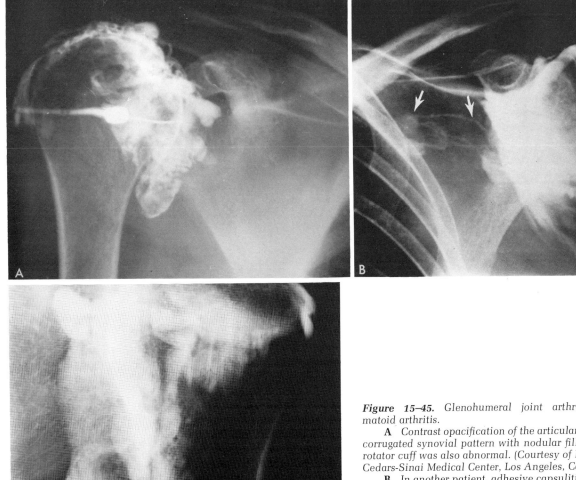

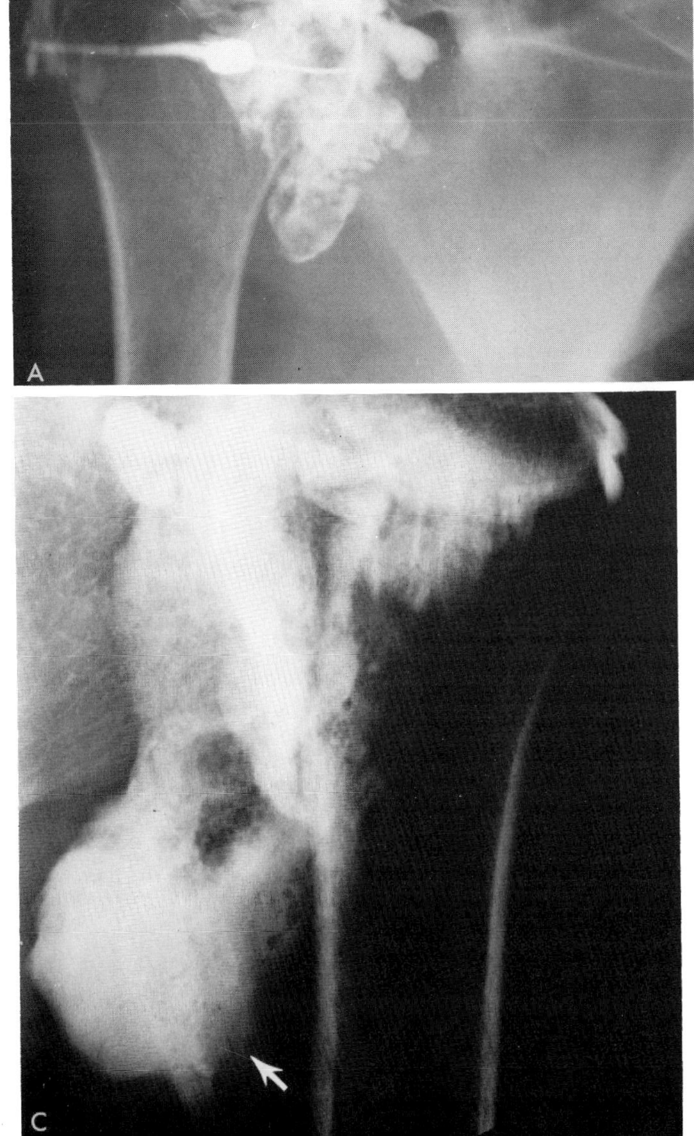

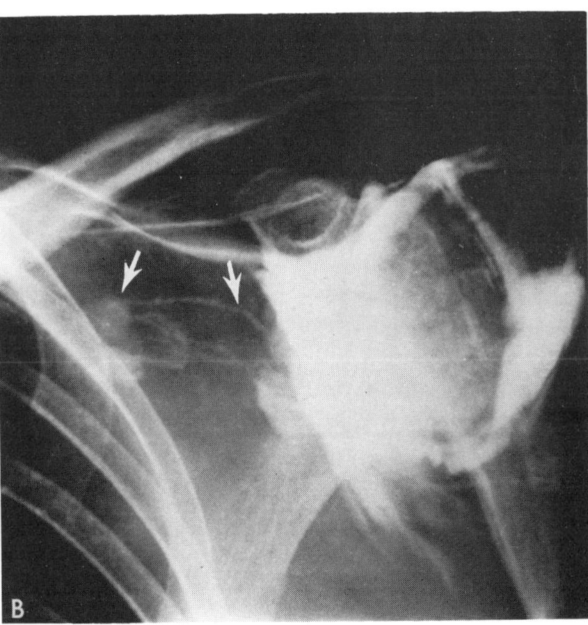

Figure 15–45. *Glenohumeral joint arthrography: Rheumatoid arthritis.*

A *Contrast opacification of the articular cavity reveals a corrugated synovial pattern with nodular filling defects. The rotator cuff was also abnormal. (Courtesy of Dr. Jerrold Mink, Cedars-Sinai Medical Center, Los Angeles, California.)*

B *In another patient, adhesive capsulitis is present with nonvisualization of the normal axillary pouch and subscapular recess. Observe filling of the lymphatic vessels (arrows).*

C *A large axillary synovial cyst (arrow) can be seen in a third patient with rheumatoid arthritis.*

enlarged subacromial bursa containing radiolucent masses.[87] These masses represent lobulated fatty tissue, which may be attached to the synovial lining.

In rheumatoid arthritis and other synovial disorders, synovial cysts about the glenohumeral joint may be documented by arthrography, as these cysts frequently communicate with the joint cavity. They may be filled with blood.[88]

Septic arthritis of the glenohumeral joint may lead to synovial irregularity and capsular and rotator

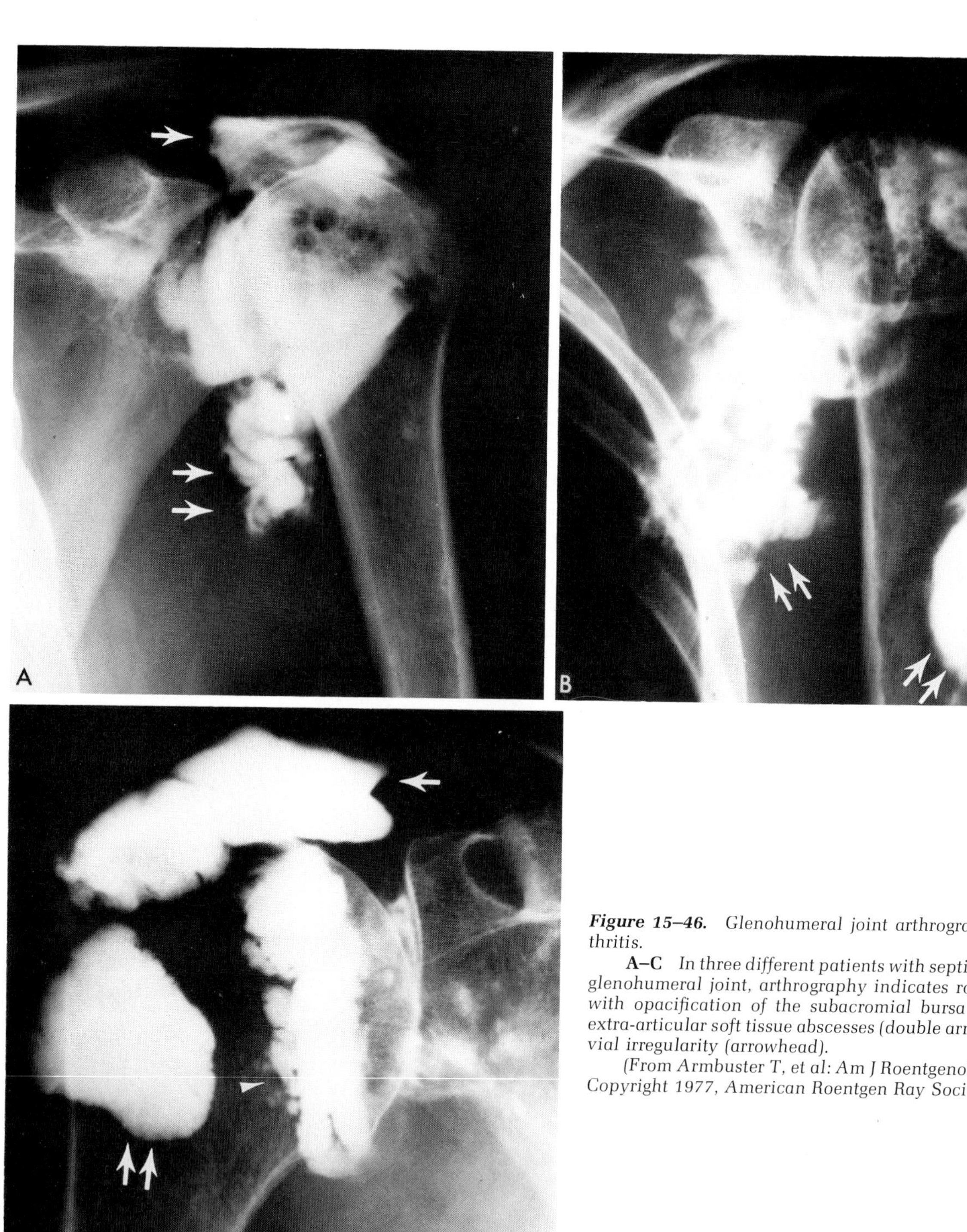

Figure 15–46. *Glenohumeral joint arthrography: Septic arthritis.*

A–C *In three different patients with septic arthritis of the glenohumeral joint, arthrography indicates rotator cuff tears with opacification of the subacromial bursa (single arrow), extra-articular soft tissue abscesses (double arrows), and synovial irregularity (arrowhead).*

(From Armbuster T, et al: Am J Roentgenol 129:667, 1977. Copyright 1977, American Roentgen Ray Society.)

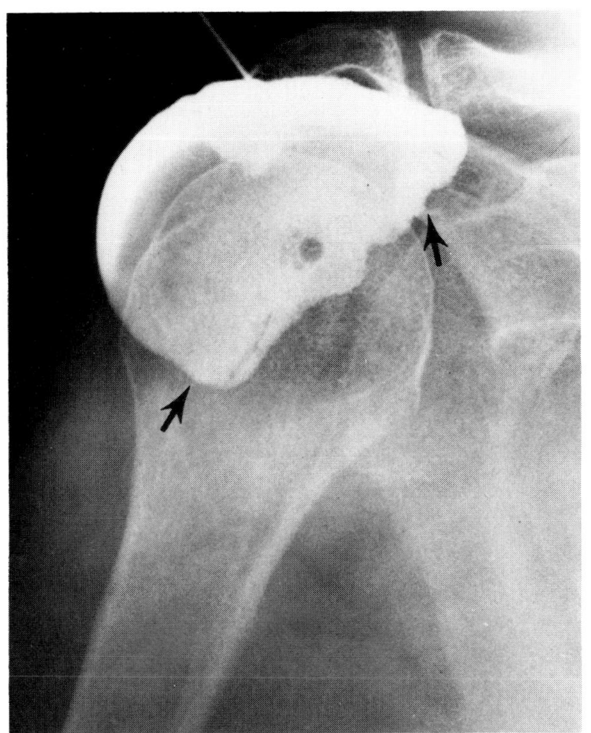

Figure 15–47. Subacromial bursography: Normal bursogram. A needle has been placed into the subacromial bursa. Contrast medium outlines the normal confines of this structure (arrows). (Courtesy of Dr. W. J. Weston, Hutt Hospital, Lower Hutt, New Zealand.)

cuff rupture, with the formation of soft tissue abscesses.[86] These abscesses appear as irregular contrast-filled cavities on glenohumeral joint arthrography.

Subacromial (Subdeltoid) Bursography

Although the subacromial bursa is occasionally injected inadvertently during attempted glenohumeral joint arthrography, it is only a potential space in normal individuals so that direct injection of this structure in the absence of subacromial bursal changes is difficult (Fig. 15–47). If the bursa is enlarged, it may indeed be opacified by placing a 22 gauge, 1.5 inch needle into it from a superolateral approach and introducing contrast medium. The typical synovial changes of rheumatoid arthritis can be identified in this fashion (Fig. 15–48). We have employed subacromial bursography with tomography in an attempt to identify partial tears of the superior surface of the rotator cuff. Because of the difficulties of accurate needle placement and the curvilinear shape of the bursa, this has not been successful in our hands. Subacromial bursography may identify a small bursa in association with adhesive capsulitis.[338]

Arthrography of the Acromioclavicular Joint

A previous report has outlined normal arthrographic findings of the acromioclavicular joint.[89] The technique involves puncturing the joint from the superior aspect under fluoroscopy, utilizing a 21 gauge needle (Fig. 15–49). One milliliter of contrast material will reveal an L-shaped articular cavity

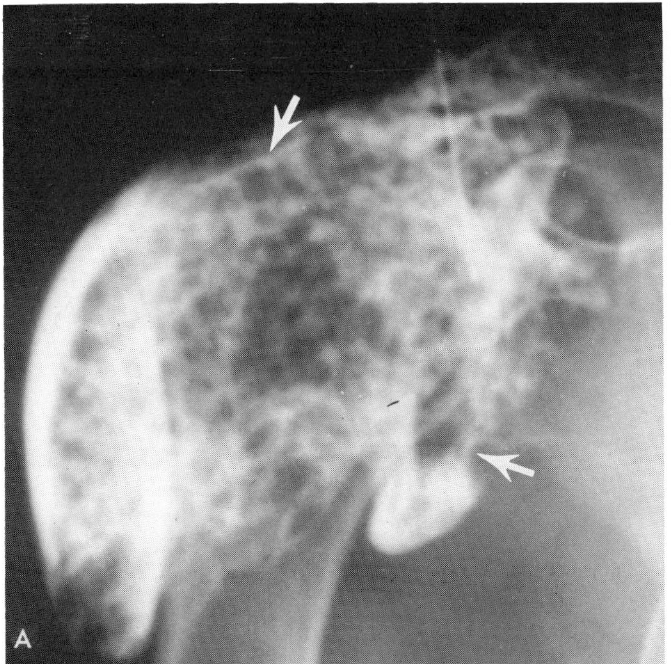

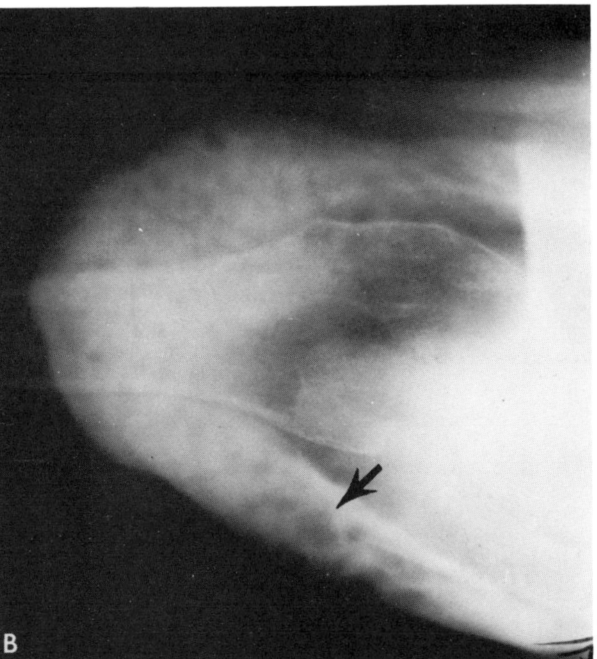

Figure 15–48. Subacromial bursography: Rheumatoid arthritis. Frontal **(A)** and axillary **(B)** views reveal an enlarged subacromial bursa with innumerable nodular filling defects (arrows). (Courtesy of Dr. W. J. Weston, Hutt Hospital, Lower Hutt, New Zealand.)

with a horizontal limb extending beneath the distal clavicle. Although acromioclavicular joint arthrography in rheumatoid arthritis could conceivably outline the degree of synovial irregularity, cartilaginous, discal, and osseous destruction, as well as the presence of a synovial cyst, there appears to be little clinical application for this procedure in this disease. However, a recent report has indicated that arthrography may provide useful information in dislocations of the acromioclavicular joint.[315] Leakage of contrast medium around the articulation and in the direction of the coracoid process may provide information regarding the severity of the injury to the ligaments.

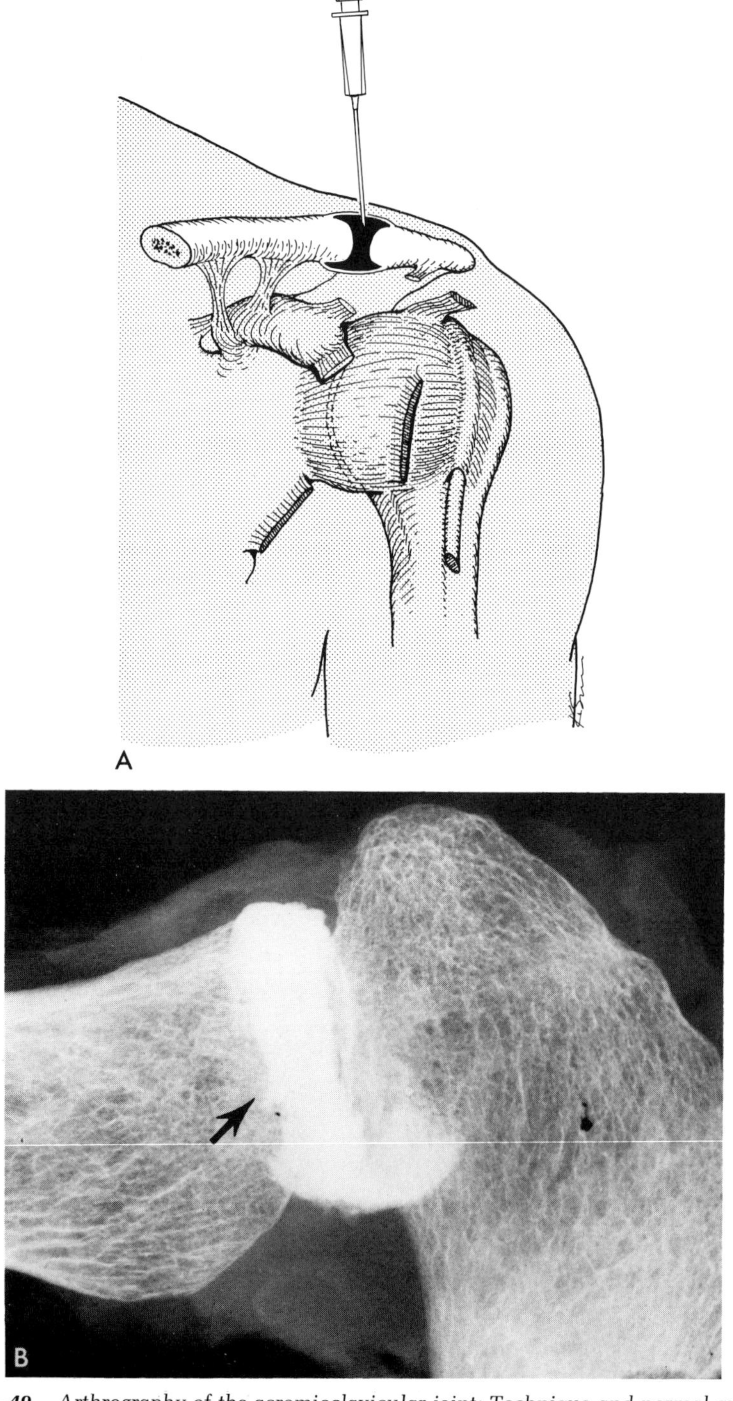

Figure 15–49. *Arthrography of the acromioclavicular joint: Technique and normal arthrogram.*

A *The joint is punctured from the superior aspect.*

B *In a cadaver, the normal contrast-filled articular cavity (arrow) is viewed in an inferosuperior radiographic projection. (Courtesy of Dr. W. J. Weston, Hutt Hospital, Lower Hutt, New Zealand.)*

HIP

Arthrography of the Hip

Although most descriptions of hip arthrography record its application in the investigation of patients with painful prostheses (which is discussed elsewhere in this book), this procedure may also be utilized in patients with congenital, traumatic, and articular disorders (Table 15–7).

Table 15–7

INDICATIONS FOR HIP ARTHROGRAPHY

Evaluation of:
- Congenital dislocation of the hip
- Septic arthritis and osteomyelitis with epiphyseal separation
- Epiphyseal dysplasia and osteonecrosis
- Certain synovial disorders
- Soft tissue masses

TECHNIQUE (Fig. 15–50). Many techniques exist for puncturing the hip joint. Some utilize a direct or angulated anterior approach,[90-93] whereas others describe lateral, superior,[94] or inferior[95, 316] approaches. The technique will vary somewhat in adults and in children. Fluoroscopy is mandatory.[96]

We use an anterior approach in performing hip arthrography. The patient is placed supine on the table with the legs stabilized in internal rotation by sandbags or a traction device. After preliminary films are obtained, the femoral artery is palpated in the groin and a metal marker is placed 2 cm lateral and 2 cm distal to this point. The position of the marker is checked under the fluoroscope; it should lie near the medial margin of the femoral neck. After skin preparation and adequate local anesthesia, an 18 gauge, 3 inch spinal needle is inserted in a superior direction with fluoroscopic guidance in order to contact the bone at the junction of the medial aspect of the femoral head and neck. This position is checked by turning the patient into a steep oblique projection. A joint aspirate may be sent to the laboratory; if no fluid is obtained, nonbacteriostatic saline solution is injected and then recovered, to be sent for analysis. Ten to 15 ml of contrast medium (60 per cent methylglucamine diatrizoate [Renografin]) is then injected, and the needle is withdrawn. Anteroposterior radiographs in internal and external rotation, a "frog-leg" view, and true lateral roentgenograms are obtained before and after mild exercise.

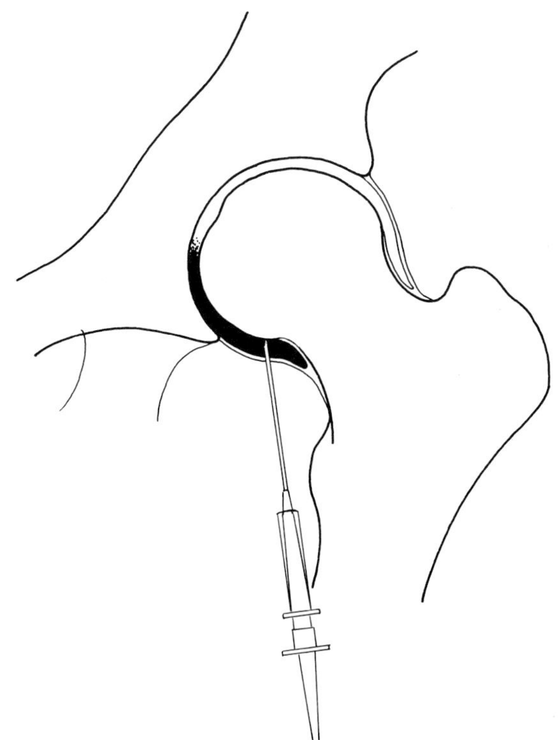

Figure 15–50. *Hip arthrography: Technique. The needle is inserted from an anterior approach and directed superiorly so as to contact the osseous surface at the junction of the femoral head and femoral neck.*

In infants and children, an anterolateral subepiphyseal plate site is ideal for contacting the bone.[96] This metaphyseal location is within the joint capsule yet distant from the femoral vessels, cartilaginous femoral head, and growth plate. Approximately 1.5 to 2 ml is injected in an infant and 5 to 8 ml in adolescents.

In performing hip arthrography in patients with joint prostheses, "subtraction" arthrography is frequently necessary so that contrast material can be differentiated from the radiopaque acrylic cement that is used to fix the prosthesis in place.[97]

NORMAL HIP ARTHROGRAM (Fig. 15–51). The normal hip arthrogram in adults consists of the following structures. The recess capitis is a thin, smooth collection of contrast material between the articular surfaces of acetabulum and femoral head.[98, 99] This recess is interrupted only at the site where the ligamentum teres enters the fovea centralis of the femoral head. The ligamentum transversum produces a radiolucent defect adjacent to the inferior rim of the acetabulum. An inferior articular recess exists as a pouch at the inferior base of the femoral head below the acetabular notch and ligamentum transversum. The superior articular recess extends cephalad around the acetabular labrum. The latter appears as a triangular radiolucent area adjacent to the superolateral lip of the acetabulum. The zona orbicularis is a circumferential lucent band around the femoral neck, which changes configuration during femoral rotation. The recess colli superior and recess colli inferior are poolings of contrast material beneath the zona orbicularis and the apex and base of the intertrochanteric line.

In children, similar arthrographic features are

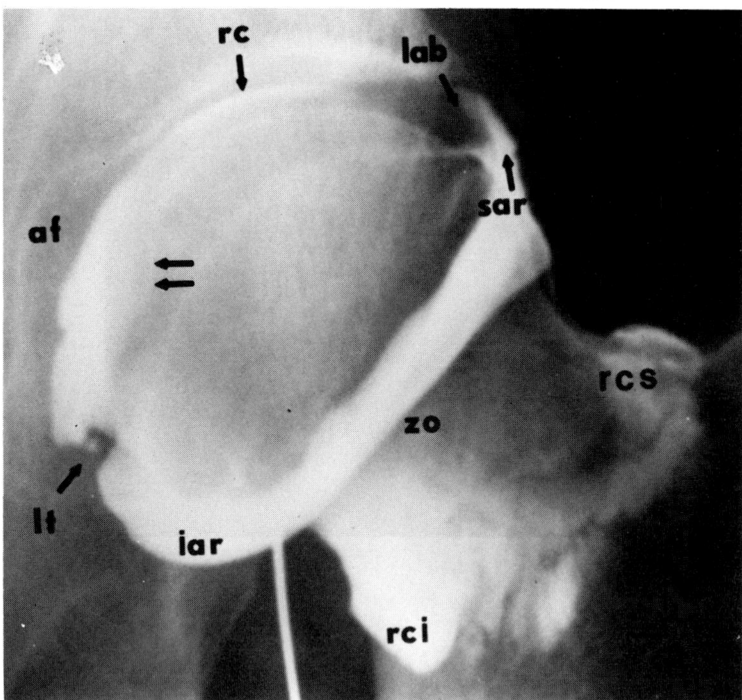

Figure 15–51. Hip arthrography: Normal arthrogram. The recess capitus (rc) is a thin, smooth collection of contrast medium between apposing articular surfaces and is interrupted only where the ligamentum teres (double arrows) enters the fovea centralis of the femoral head. The ligamentum transversum (lt) is seen as a radiolucent defect adjacent to the inferior rim of the acetabulum. The ligamentum teres bridges the acetabular notch and effectively deepens the acetabulum. The inferior articular recess (iar) forms a pouch at the inferior base of the femoral head below the acetabular notch and ligamentum transversum. The superior articular recess (sar) extends cephalad around the acetabular labrum (lab). The acetabular labrum is seen as a triangular radiolucent area adjacent to the superolateral lip of the acetabulum. The zona orbicularis (zo) is a circumferential lucent band around the femoral neck, which changes configuration with rotation of the femur. The recess colli superior (rcs) and recess colli inferior (rci) are poolings of contrast material at the apex and base of the intertrochanteric line and are the most caudad extensions of the synovial membrane. (From Guerra J Jr, et al: Radiology 128:11, 1978.)

apparent.[96] The cartilaginous tissue around the femoral head is abundant in amount, reflecting both articular cartilage and that portion of the femoral head that is not yet ossified.

Congenital Dislocation of the Hip (Fig. 15–52). In infants, hip arthrography may be useful in the evaluation of congenital hip dislocation, although it is generally not essential for diagnosing the condition.[92, 94, 95, 100, 101] Conventional arthrography is considered adequate by most investigators, although some advocate video-arthrography.[101]

In infants with congenital dislocation of the femoral head, the cartilaginous limbus will be apparent as a filling defect beneath the displaced head of the femur. In this situation, the head will deform or compress the limbus and the ligamentum teres is stretched, leading from the inferior margin of the acetabulum to the fovea of the dislocated femoral head. The capsule is also stretched around the head, and the opacified hip joint will have an hourglass configuration.[100]

The hip arthrogram may be used to evaluate the adequacy of reduction of a dislocated femoral head, particularly in the older infant or child.[95] In this situation, an inverted limbus may be interposed between the acetabulum and head, preventing complete reduction. Arthrography will outline the inverted limbus, and pooling of contrast material may be identified between the femoral head and medial acetabular wall. This information may aid the orthopedic surgeon in determining the need for surgery and in planning the operative procedure.

Septic Arthritis in Infants (Fig. 15–53). Hip arthrography is useful in the clinical setting of neonatal sepsis and an apparent dislocation of the femoral head.[105] In this situation, it is impossible to determine the exact position of the unossified femoral head on initial radiographs. Two possibilities exist: The hip is indeed dislocated, or there is a pathologic epiphyseal separation related to osteomyelitis with a normal relationship between cartilaginous head and acetabulum. A hip arthrogram will allow aspiration of joint contents and documentation of the position of the femoral head. The diagnosis of true dislocation or epiphyseal separation can then be made accurately.

Glassberg and Ozonoff[106] have also emphasized the use of arthrography in septic arthritis of the hip. This technique allows accurate placement of the needle for aspiration and assessment of the degree of cartilaginous destruction.

Epiphyseal Dysplasia, Legg-Calvé-Perthes Disease, and Related Conditions (Fig. 15–54). Hip arthrography has been employed to investigate the pathogenesis of multiple epiphyseal dysplasia, and spondyloepiphyseal dysplasia.[107] Although the study does not allow differentiation among the various dysplasias, it does reveal that the cartilaginous head is generally smooth despite the presence of irregular fragmented ossific densities within the femoral head, suggesting that these disorders relate to faulty, incomplete, or delayed epiphyseal ossification. The integrity of the articular cartilage can also be evaluated by using hip arthrography.

Hip arthrography may have more immediate clinical benefit in evaluating patients with Legg-Calvé-Perthes disease.[91, 109-111] In this condition, one

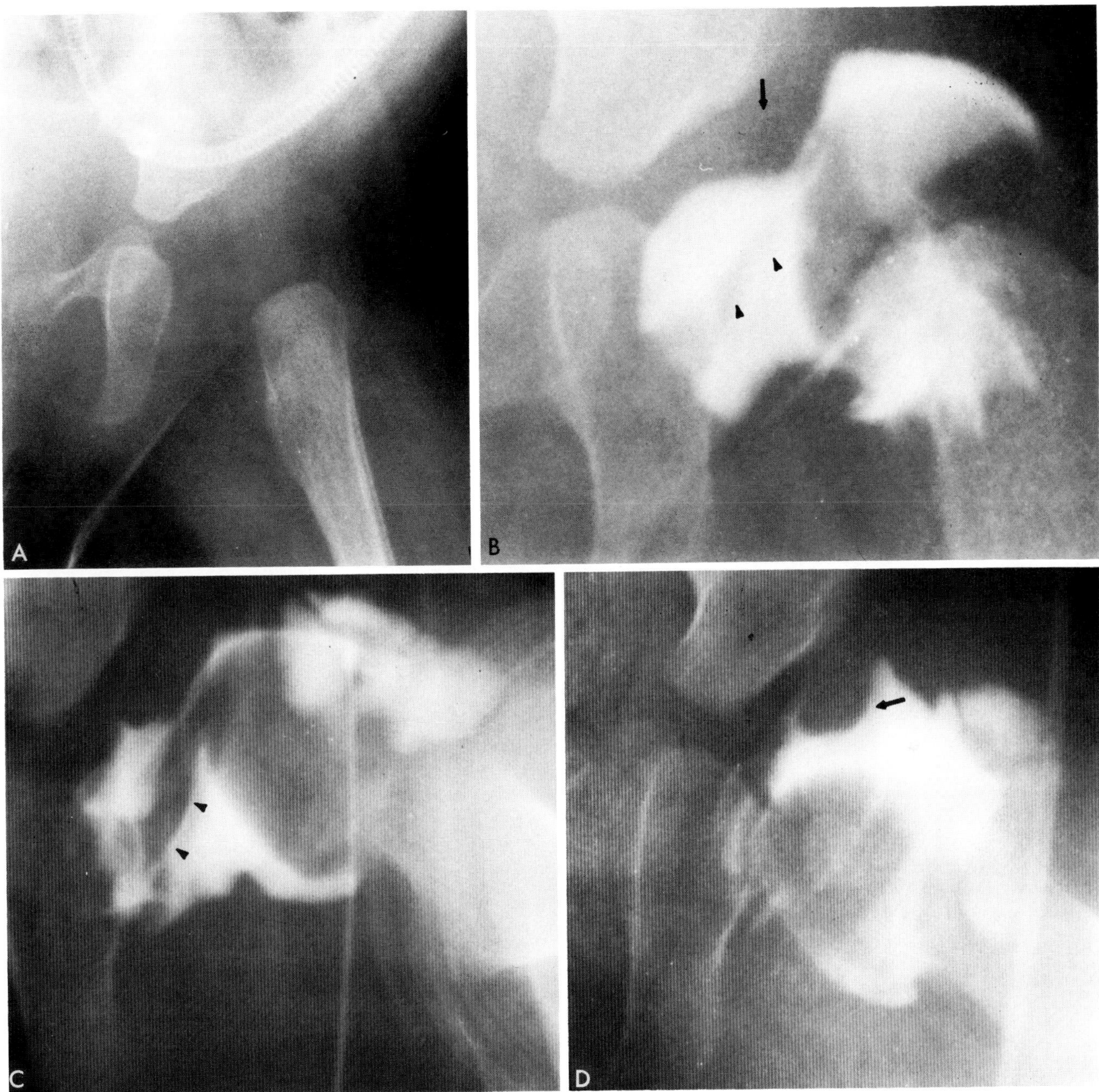

Figure 15–52. *Hip arthrography: Congenital dislocation of the hip.*

A, B *A 2 month old infant with hip dislocation. The initial film* **(A)** *reveals the lateral position of the femur with respect to the acetabulum. The arthrogram* **(B)** *obtained in neutral position outlines the radiolucent cartilaginous femoral head, a deformed limbus (arrow) between the displaced femoral head and acetabulum, and a stretched ligamentum teres (arrowheads). Because of the stretched capsule, the opacified hip joint has an hourglass configuration.*

C, D *A 1 year old infant with hip dislocation. On an initial arthrographic view* **(C)**, *observe the dislocated femoral head and stretched ligamentum teres (arrowheads). In another view obtained with 45 degrees of abduction, flexion, and traction, the limbus appears inverted (arrow).*

(From Kaye JJ, Winchester PH, Freiberger RH: Radiology 114:671, 1975.)

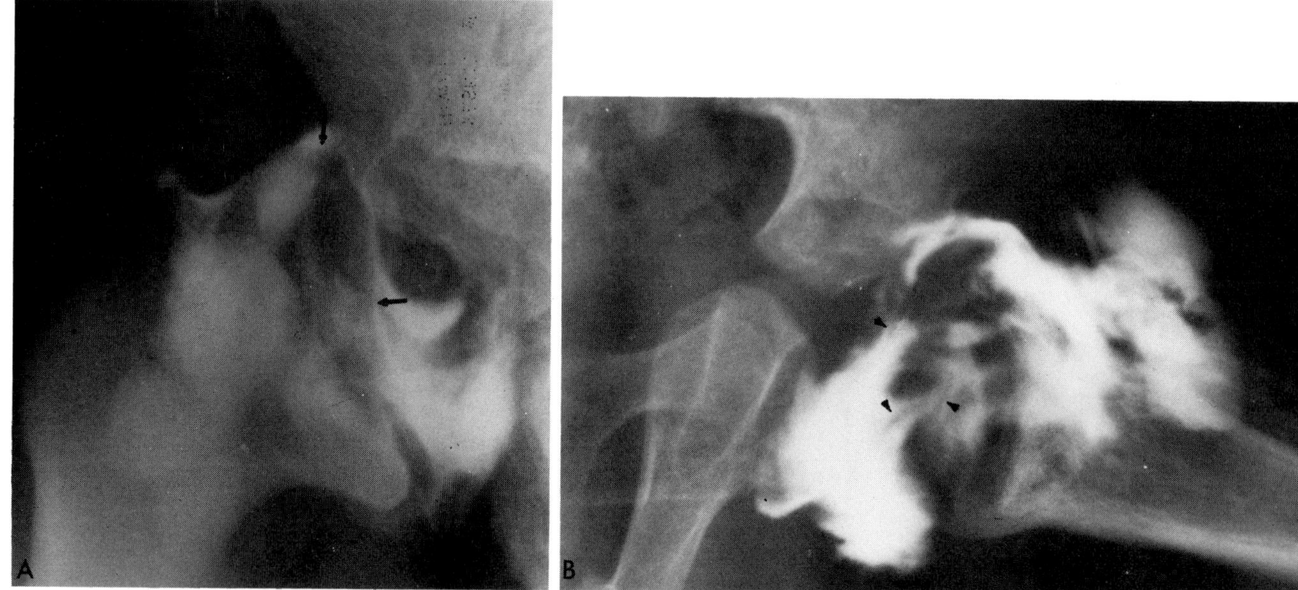

Figure 15–53. *Hip arthrography: Septic arthritis and osteomyelitis.*

A *Septic arthritis. In a male infant with septic dislocation of the femoral head, an arthrogram reveals severe cartilaginous deformity with a triangular cartilaginous head (arrows). Normal recesses are absent.*

B *Septic arthritis. In another male infant with septic dislocation of the femoral head, lateral subluxation and synovial adhesions with a swirled appearance of contrast material (arrowheads) are evident.*

(**A, B,** *From Glassberg GB, Ozonoff, MB: Radiology 128:151, 1978.*)

Illustration continued on the opposite page

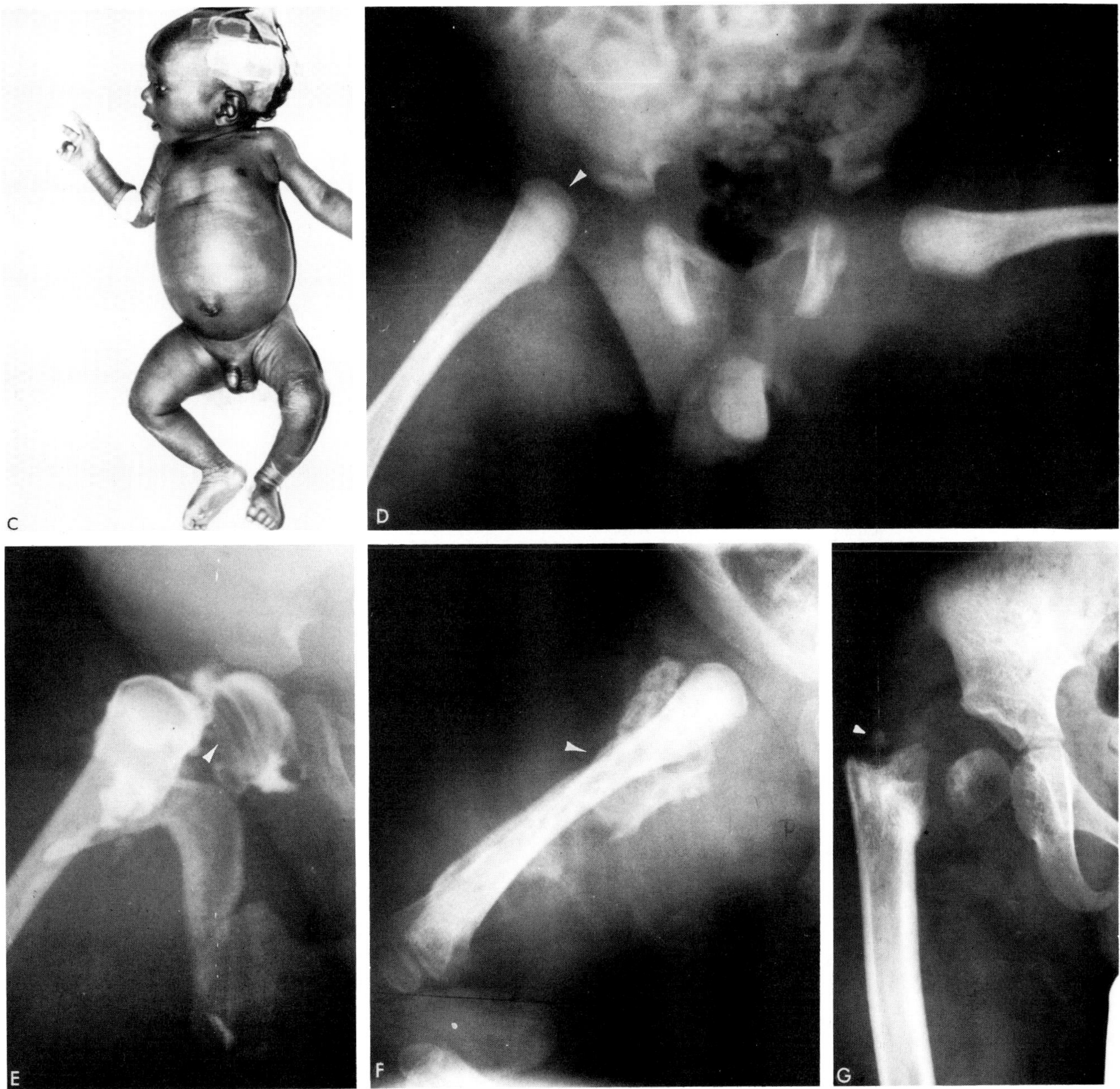

Figure 15–53. Continued
C–G *Osteomyelitis with epiphyseal separation. The clinical photograph* **(C)** *of this 10 day old black infant demonstrates a swollen right leg, held in abduction and flexion. An initial radiograph* **(D)** *reveals an apparent "dislocation" of the right hip because of the laterally displaced femoral metaphysis (arrowhead). An arthrogram* **(E)** *performed 4 days later outlines a radiolucent femoral head (arrowhead), which is in normal position with respect to the acetabulum, and a displaced femoral metaphysis indicating an epiphyseal separation. Several weeks later after treatment with a hip spica, metaphyseal bone destruction (arrowhead) indicates the presence of osteomyelitis.* **G,** *Radiograph made at 37 months of age delineates residual changes of the femoral metaphysis, varus deformity, a deformed, partially ossified femoral head within the acetabulum, acetabular flattening and a small ossification center of the greater trochanter (arrowhead).*

Illustration continued on the following page

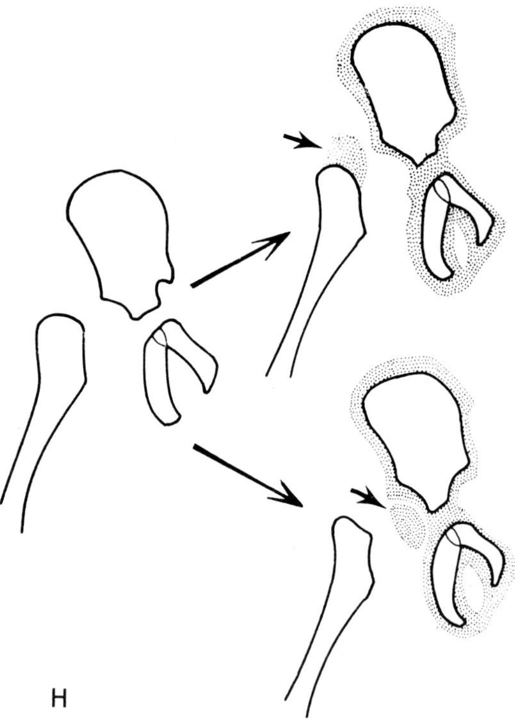

Figure 15–53. Continued

H *Septic arthritis versus osteomyelitis with epiphyseal separation. In either case, an initial radiograph (on left) will indicate a displaced metaphysis with respect to the acetabulum. With a true dislocation (top right) the cartilaginous epiphysis is displaced laterally (arrow). With an epiphyseal separation (bottom, right) the femoral head is normally placed in the acetabulum (arrow) (cartilaginous areas are stippled).*

(**C–H,** *From Kaye JJ, Winchester PH, Freiberger RH: Radiology 114:671, 1975.*)

arthrographic finding is an absolute enlargement of the femoral head related to hyperplasia of the epiphyseal cartilage. This finding suggests that the apparent noncontact of femoral head and medial acetabulum noted on initial plain film radiography in this condition is, in reality, related to cartilaginous hyperplasia,[110] so that subluxation is not present. This method of identifying the true position of the cartilaginous head may allow the surgeon to determine which position of the hip will be best during treatment of the condition. Bilateral hip arthrograms may be necessary in these individuals,

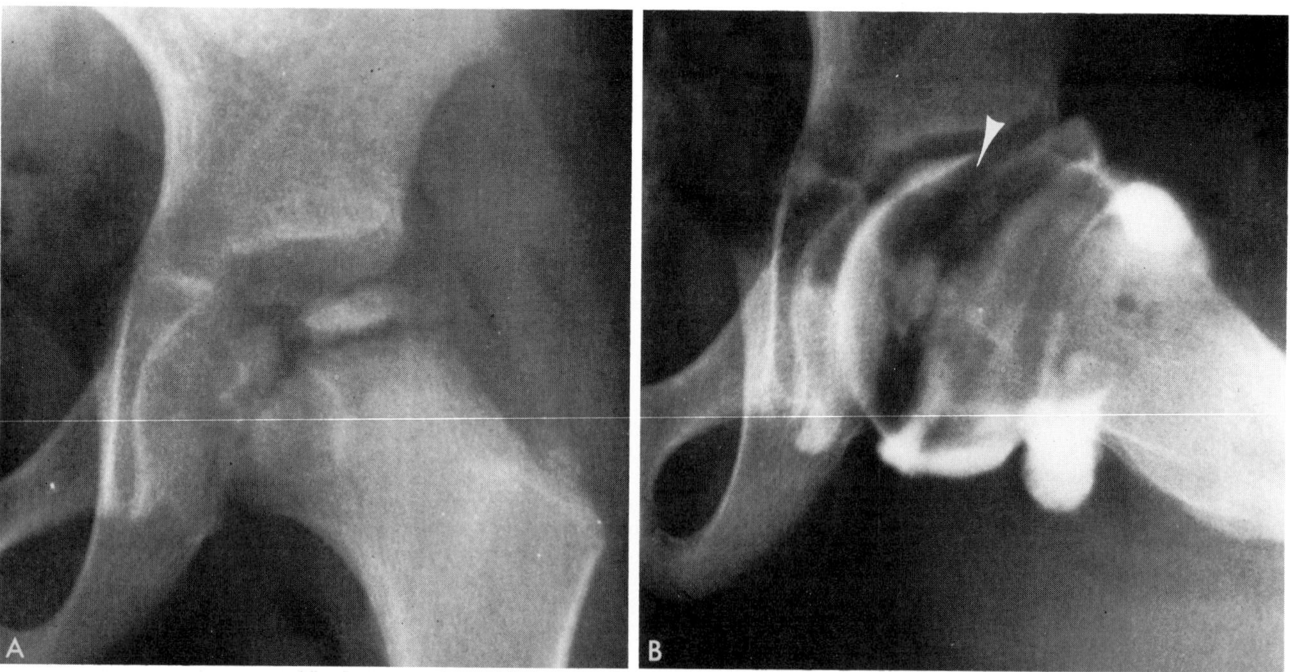

Figure 15–54. *Hip arthrography: Legg-Calvé-Perthes disease.*

A *On the initial film, epiphyseal fragmentation and metaphyseal irregularity are apparent.*

B *Arthrographic image in hip abduction indicates a relatively smooth radiolucent cartilaginous head (arrowhead), which is well covered by the acetabulum.*

enabling normal and abnormal sides to be compared.[359]

Arthrography in patients with transient synovitis of the hip has outlined similar thickening of articular cartilage.[110] Since many investigators suggest that synovitis may be etiologically related to Legg-Calvé-Perthes disease, the observation that synovitis can lead to cartilaginous hyperplasia is significant.

Arthrography of the hip in Legg-Calvé-Perthes disease has also been utilized to demonstrate the existence of an osteochondral fragment.[330] This uncommon complication relates to the presence of an unhealed necrotic fragment, which appears separate from the remainder of the femoral head. The arthrogram will delineate whether the necrotic fragment is loose; in this case, contrast material introduced into the hip will dissect under the osteochondral fragment.

ARTICULAR DISORDERS (Figs. 15–55 to 15–58). Contrast opacification of the hip may allow more accurate diagnosis of a variety of articular disorders. In idiopathic synovial osteochondromatosis or pigmented villonodular synovitis, the extent of synovial and capsular abnormality can be determined in this fashion.[112] This is important not only in outlining the severity of the disorder but also in establishing the correct diagnosis when plain films are not conclusive. In patients with septic arthritis, hip arthrography provides a vehicle for aspiration and culture and also a means of evaluating cartilaginous, osseous, and synovial abnormalities. Hip arthrography provides information regarding the origin and nature of intra-articular and para-articular radiodense areas.

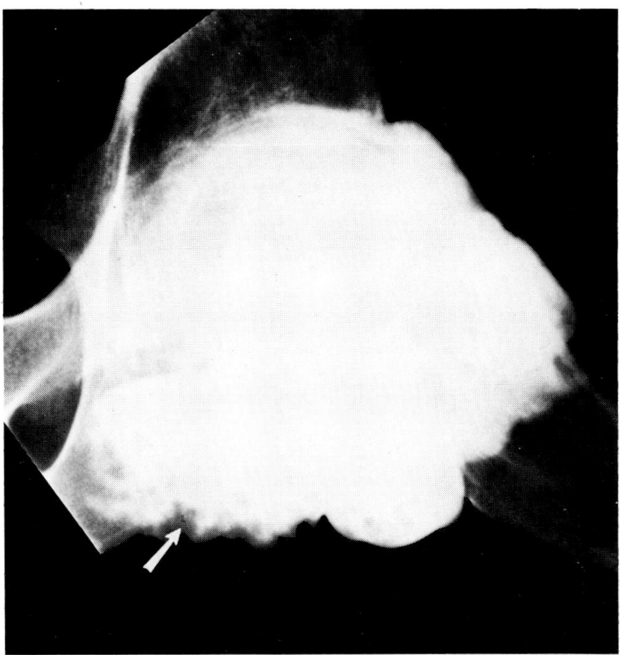

Figure 15–55. *Hip arthrography: Idiopathic synovial osteochondromatosis. Observe an enlarged, contrast-opacified hip joint with multiple filling defects (arrow) related to osteocartilaginous bodies.*

Hip arthrography in rheumatoid arthritis and other synovial disorders will reveal the degree of

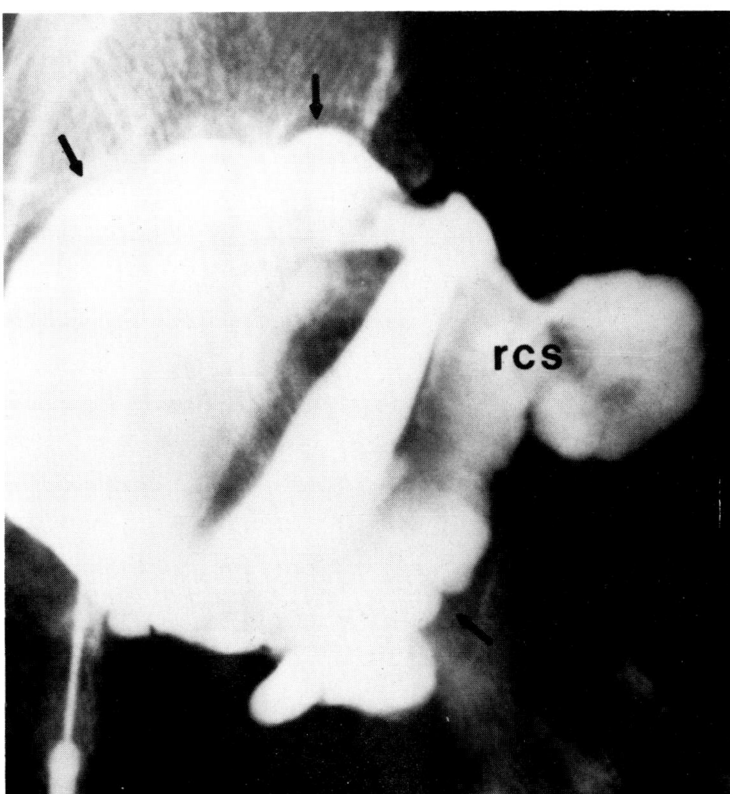

Figure 15–56. *Hip arthrography: Septic arthritis. Arthrography in a patient with septic arthritis demonstrates irregularity of contrast material and cartilage loss (arrows). The recess colli superior (rcs) is indicated. (From Guerra J, et al: Radiology 128: 11, 1978.)*

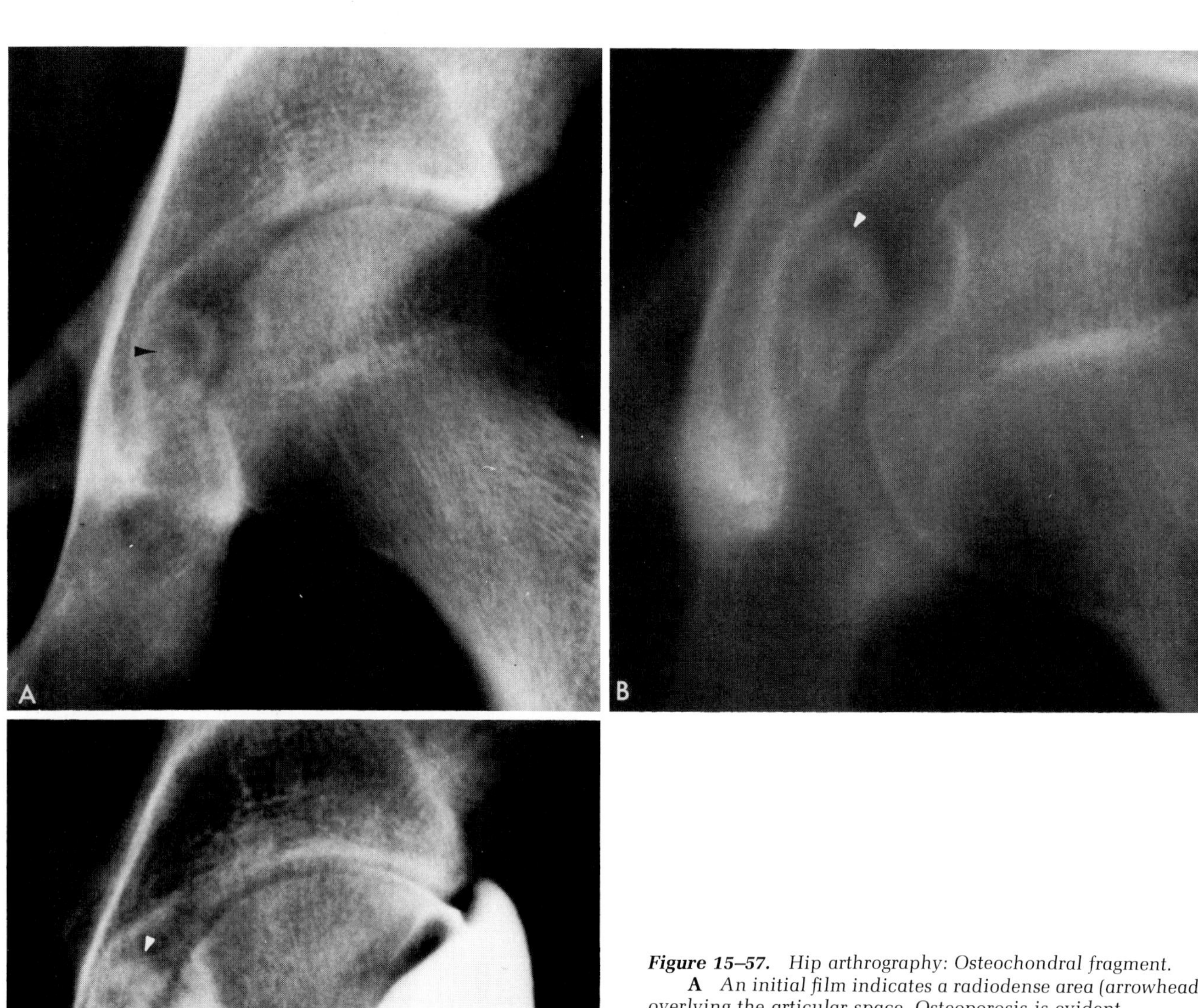

Figure 15–57. Hip arthrography: Osteochondral fragment.

A An initial film indicates a radiodense area (arrowhead) overlying the articular space. Osteoporosis is evident.

B On a tomogram, the radiodense lesion (arrowhead) is better delineated.

C Arthrography indicates that contrast material partially surrounds the osseous body (arrowhead). At surgery, an osteochondral fragment attached to the acetabulum was removed.

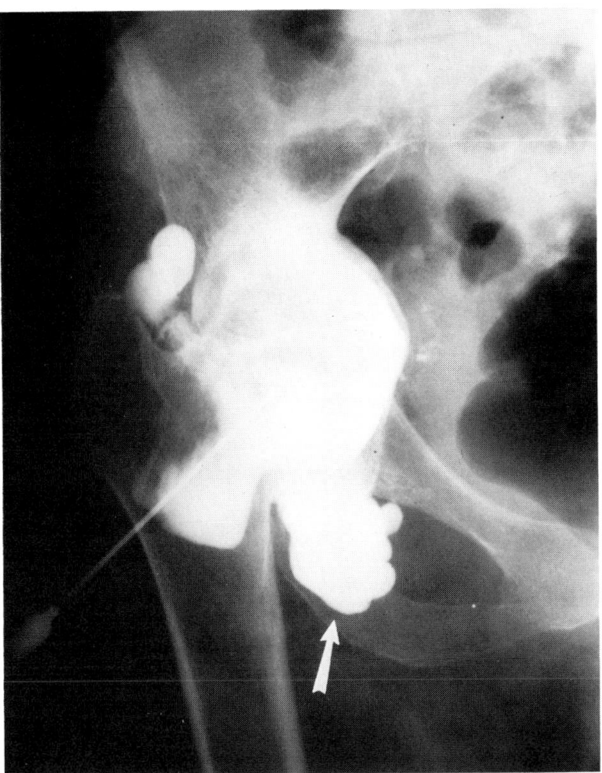

Figure 15–58. *Hip arthrography: Rheumatoid arthritis and synovial cyst formation. In this 65 year old woman with rheumatoid arthritis and an apparent "femoral hernia," arthrography indicates that the clinically evident soft tissue mass is related to a synovial cyst (arrow). Observe the sacculation of the articular cavity and a protrusio acetabuli defect.*

intra-articular alterations and the presence or absence of communicating synovial cysts. Opacification of the iliopsoas bursa may be identified and, although this is apparent in 15 per cent of normal hips,[113] communication of the hip and iliopsoas bursa in the presence of intra-articular diseases such as osteoarthritis, rheumatoid arthritis, pigmented villonodular synovitis, and idiopathic synovial osteochondromatosis may lead to bursal enlargement producing a mass in the ilioinguinal region that may simulate a hernia and produce obstruction of the femoral vein.[114, 115] A second potential communication that may allow decompression of a hip joint with elevated intra-articular pressure exists at the crossing of the iliofemoral and iliopubic ligaments, at which point fluid may dissect into the fat plane of the obturator externus muscle.[98]

KNEE

Arthrography of the Knee

The role of arthrography is most established for abnormalities of the knee as it is useful in evaluating this joint in a variety of clinical situations[116] (Table

Table 15–8

INDICATIONS FOR KNEE ARTHROGRAPHY

Evaluation of:
- Meniscal tears, cysts, and ossicles
- Discoid menisci
- Postmeniscectomy syndromes
- Ligamentous injuries
- Transchondral fractures
- Chondromalacia patellae
- Degenerative joint disease
- Intra-articular osseous and cartilaginous bodies
- Synovial disorders
- Blount's disease
- Soft tissue masses

15–8). The technique of examination has evolved through the years; single contrast examination utilizing air and oxygen[117] or radiopaque substances[118, 119] has been replaced, in large part, by double contrast examination utilizing air and radiopaque contrast material,[120] which is preferable for evaluation of subtle meniscal and articular cartilage abnormalities. However, some studies indicate that comparable results can be obtained with either technique.[317]

Technique (Fig. 15–59). In recent years, two double contrast examination techniques have been advocated. Both have advantages and disadvantages, although at present the fluoroscopic technique is much more widely utilized.

Horizontal Beam Technique. This technique relies upon horizontal beam radiography without the use of fluoroscopy.[120, 121] Its great advantage is improved meniscal and articular cartilage coating, which is produced as excess positive contrast material falls to the dependent portion of the knee, and air rises to envelop the contrast-covered cartilaginous structure. Its disadvantages are the need for special cassettes to hold the film and the inability to be certain that the radiographs are obtained in an ideal tangential projection. Furthermore, this technique is more time consuming than the fluoroscopic method and requires considerable expertise in patient positioning. Some patients are unable to assume all the necessary positions.

The patient is placed on the fluoroscopic table with the knee extended in the lateral position, and a straight line is drawn on the skin along the articular margin of the medial tibial plateau. The patient is then turned to the opposite lateral projection, and a second straight line is drawn along the articular margin of the lateral tibial plateau. These lines should meet at the front and back of the knee.

The knee is punctured from a medial or lateral approach with a 20 gauge needle and all intra-articular fluid is aspirated. If a previous patellectomy has been performed, an anterior approach is utilized, with the patient sitting on the edge of the table. Seven to 10 ml of 60 per cent methylglucamine

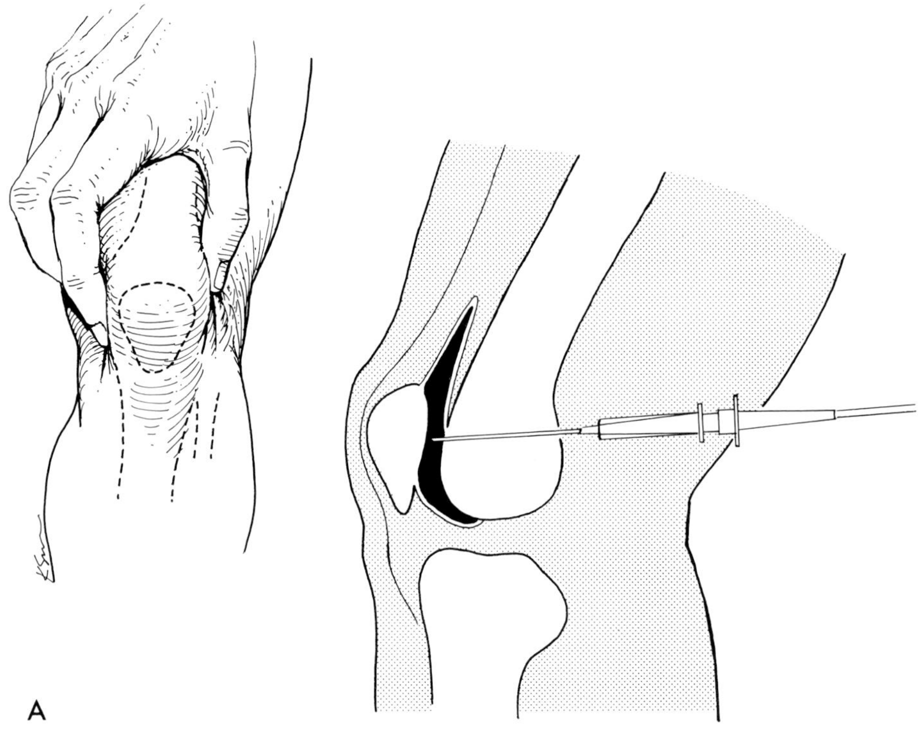

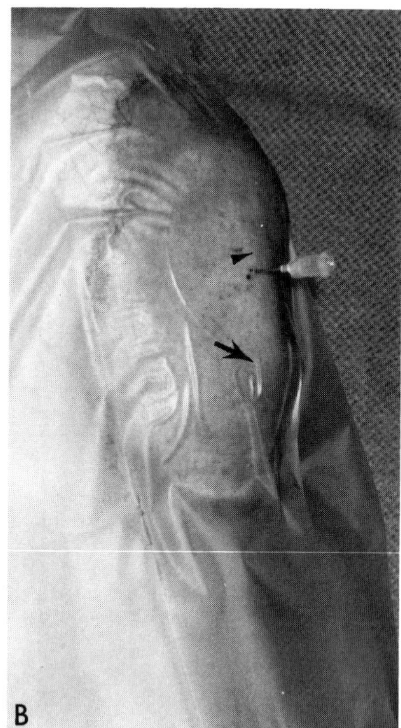

Figure 51–59. *Knee arthrography: Technique.*

A, B *Joint puncture. A medial or lateral approach may be utilized* **(A).** *The opposite side of the patella is manually depressed, increasing the space at the puncture site. If a patellectomy has previously been performed* **(B),** *an anterior approach may be used; the needle is advanced on either side of the infrapatellar tendon with the knee flexed and the patient sitting on the edge of the table. This photograph reveals the ideal entry point in the patellectomized patient. The tibial tuberosity (arrow) and infrapatellar tendon (arrowhead) are shown.*

Illustration continued on the opposite page

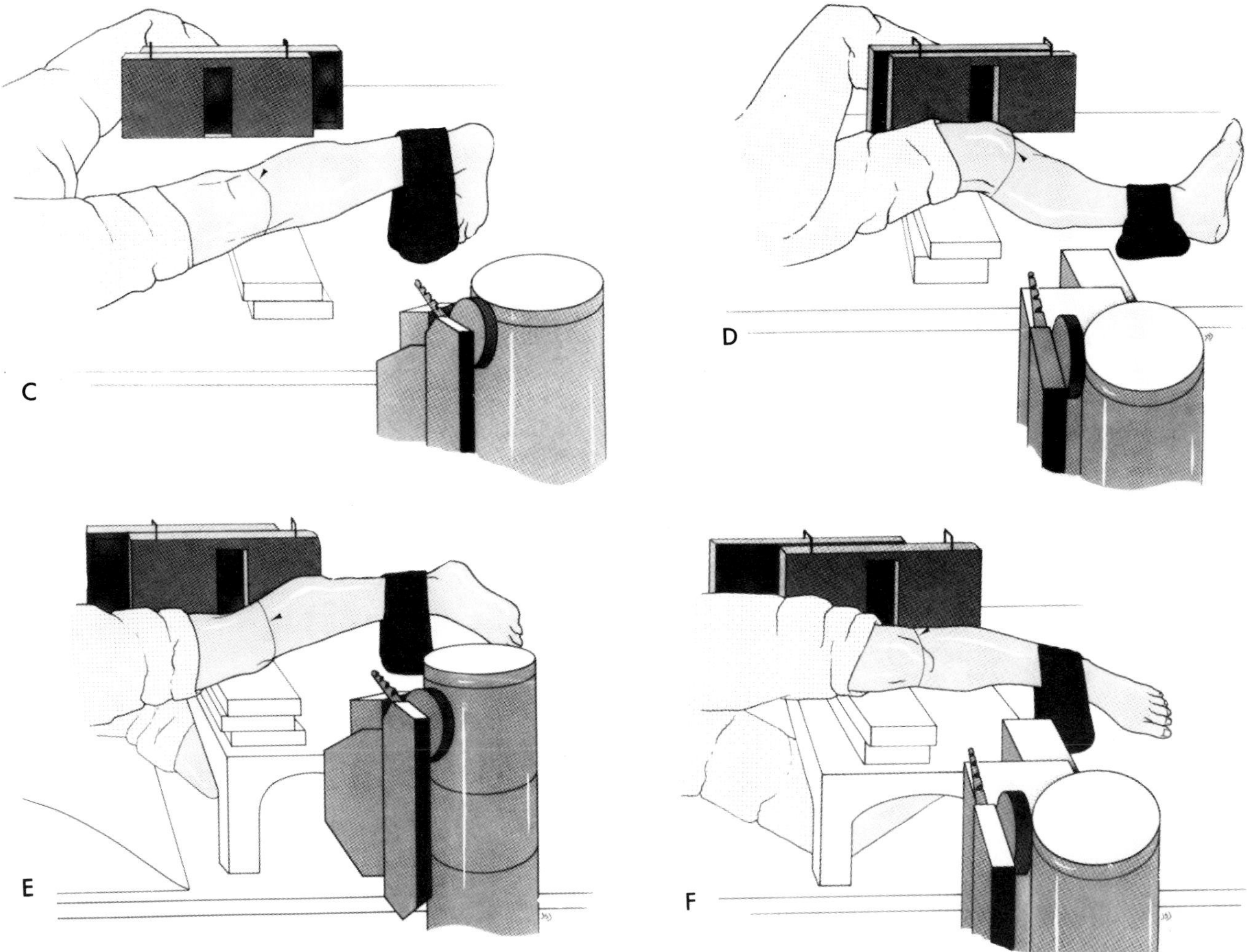

C

D

E

F

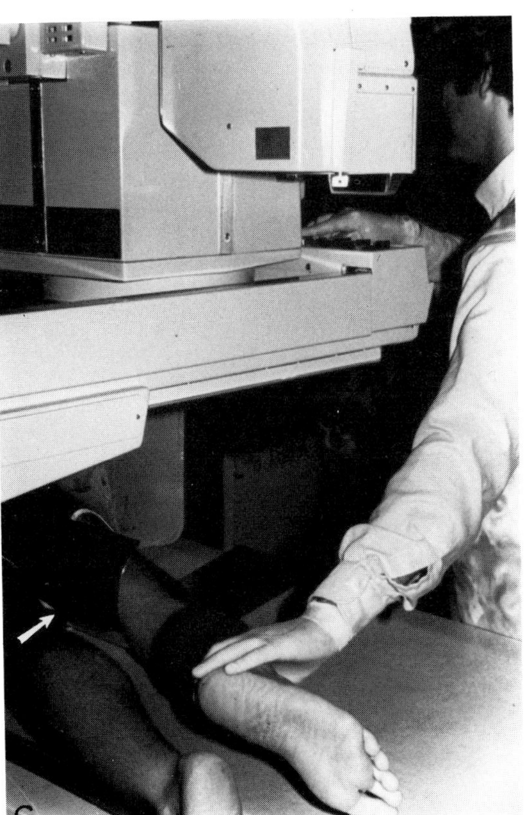

Figure 15–59. Continued

C–F *Horizontal beam technique with magnification. For examination of the posterior portion of the medial meniscus* **(C)**, *note the position of the leg. The x-ray beam is angled along the axis of the medial tibial plateau (arrowhead). Note the space between the patient's knee and film, allowing radiographic magnification. In the evaluation of the anterior portion of the medial meniscus* **(D)**, *a change in the patient's position is required. Again, the x-ray tube and beam are angled along the appropriate line (arrowhead). For evaluation of the posterior portion of the lateral meniscus* **(E)**, *the involved knee is placed above a small table and the patient rests on a support. The line of the lateral aspect of the tibial plateau is used (arrowhead). The midportion of the lateral meniscus* **(F)** *requires a different position. The upper line is again utilized for orientation of the x-ray beam (arrowhead).*

G *Fluoroscopic technique. In this photograph, the patient is positioned for evaluation of the anterior portion of the lateral meniscus. The metal brace (arrow) is utilized for appropriate stress. Other stress devices are also available.*

diatrizoate (Renografin) and 12 ml of air are injected. Following removal of the needle and mild exercise, filming is begun. Approximately 10 to 12 exposures are obtained of each meniscus, utilizing a horizontal x-ray tube, a cylindric pillow beneath the leg, a special cassette holder, and a sandbag over the ankle. During the filming of each meniscus, the patient lies first in the prone position and ends in the supine position. The incident beam is angled along the appropriate line drawn on the skin. For the medial meniscus, the beam is usually angulated toward the head, and for the lateral meniscus, the beam is usually angulated toward the feet. After each exposure, the leg is turned approximately 15 degrees, and the next exposure is obtained. For examining the lateral meniscus, a wooden table is necessary so that the opposite leg will not be in the field of the incident beam. Although this technique usually requires a target-film distance of 1.2 meter (48 in), magnification radiographs can be employed utilizing the same equipment and patient positioning, with increase in patient-film distance and decrease in focal spot–patient distance. After the spot films are obtained, overhead projections are also made to examine the patellar cartilage and cruciate ligaments and to determine whether a popliteal cyst is present.

Fluoroscopic Technique. This technique, which is more popular than the horizontal beam technique, relies upon vertical imaging with fluoroscopy.[122, 123] Its main advantage is direct monitoring of the menisci during the examination, allowing ideal tangential positioning. Furthermore, it is less time consuming than the horizontal beam technique. Because films are obtained in a vertical fashion, ideal mixing of contrast material and air is not obtained. In addition, two people are required to perform the examination properly; one individual operates the fluoroscope while the second provides appropriate stress on the knee.

Following puncture of the joint and aspiration of joint contents, 2 to 5 ml of contrast material (methylglucamine diatrizoate [Renografin]) and 30 ml of air are injected. Some investigators have utilized carbon dioxide in place of air,[122] although recent evidence suggests that this causes more postprocedural pain, owing to a decrease in joint pH.[369] The patient then undergoes moderate exercise and is placed beneath the fluoroscopic unit. Six to 12 exposures are made of each meniscus, utilizing slight changes in position and appropriate leg traction. A variety of traction devices have been described to provide appropriate varus and valgus stress during the examination.[124-129, 339, 340] Following fluoroscopy, overhead films are taken to evaluate articular cartilage and cruciate ligaments and to determine whether a popliteal cyst is present.

Additional Technical Considerations. Whether the horizontal beam or fluoroscopic method is utilized, certain conditions are important if high-quality results are to be obtained.

Equipment. Radiographic tubes with small focal spots are essential for quality roentgenograms. A 0.6 mm focal spot is satisfactory, although a 0.3 mm focal spot tube will produce superior images. With the fluoroscopic technique, proper coning of the x-ray beam is mandatory and the resulting images can be displayed on the film with a 4 on 1, 6 on 1, or 9 on 1 format. These should be numbered consecutively, usually proceeding from the posterior aspect of the meniscus to the anterior aspect.

Quality of Contrast Coating. It is imperative that most of the intra-articular fluid be aspirated. This may require a joint puncture with an 18 gauge needle when the aspirate is thick. When considerable intra-articular fluid is present, contrast coating of the menisci is less than ideal, and subtle tears will be missed. Removed fluid can also be studied.[370]

The examination must be performed in a rapid (albeit not rushed) manner, as the contrast coating will deteriorate as time elapses. The meniscus that is suspected of injury should be the one examined first.

The addition of intra-articular epinephrine (0.2 ml of 1:1000 solution) may enhance meniscal visualization by causing vasoconstriction of synovial vessels, decreasing both the amount of contrast absorbed from the joint cavity and the amount of intra-articular fluid formed.

Overhead Films and Tomography. Certain overhead films have been recommended following the procedure. These are obtained to evaluate the cruciate ligaments, articular cartilage, and synovial cavity. Lateral radiographs obtained in a cross-table supine projection and sitting position with one leg over the side of the table are useful. Anteroposterior views are also helpful and delayed films have been recommended.[130, 341] Special projections to evaluate the cruciate ligaments (which may require tomography) may be utilized. These will be discussed later in this chapter.

Normal Knee Arthrogram (Fig. 15–60)

Medial Meniscus (Fig. 15–61). The medial meniscus is identified as a sharply defined soft tissue triangular shadow. Its posterior horn is usually large, averaging 14 mm in width.[119] Its midportion is somewhat smaller, whereas the anterior horn is usually the smallest portion of the medial meniscus, averaging 6 mm in width.[119] Occasionally the anterior horn may be larger than the midportion of the medial meniscus.[131] The peripheral surface of the medial meniscus is firmly attached to the medial collateral ligament. Certain normal recesses about the medial meniscus produce focal pouch-like collections of air and contrast material.[132, 133] A superior recess is frequently present above the posterior horn

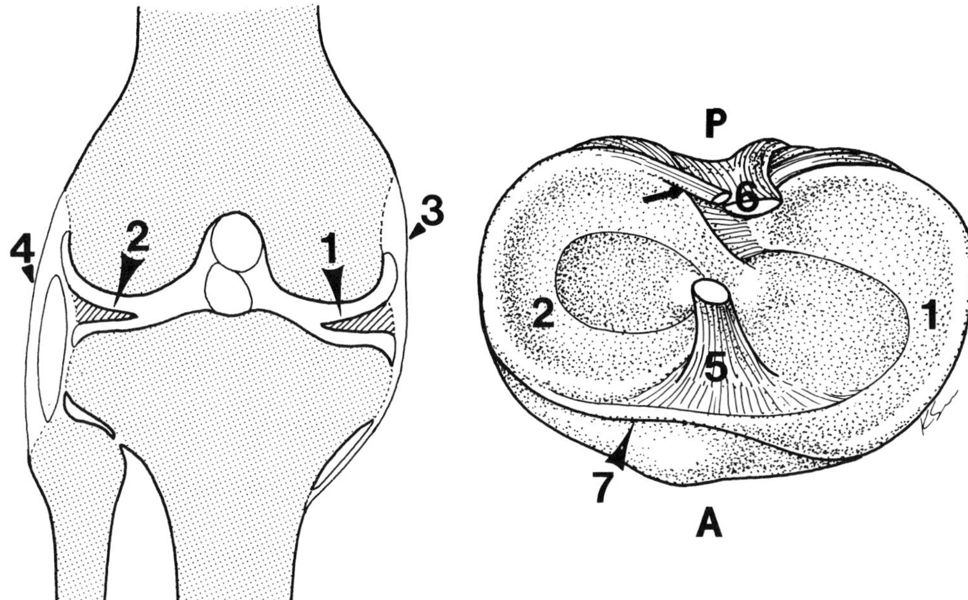

Figure 15–60. Knee arthrography: Pertinent anatomy. Coronal section (on left) and view of the upper portion of the tibia (on right). A, anterior; P, posterior. Visualized structures are the medial meniscus (1), lateral meniscus (2), medial collateral ligament (3), fibular collateral ligament (4), anterior cruciate ligament (5), posterior cruciate ligament (6), transverse ligament of the knee (7), and slip from the lateral meniscus to the posterior cruciate ligament (arrow). Observe the relatively large posterior horn of the medial meniscus and its firm attachment to the medial collateral ligament and the more circular configuration of the lateral meniscus with its relatively uniform size.

of the medial meniscus. A posterior inferior recess is less common, although the presence of such a recess beneath the anterior horn of the medial meniscus is more frequent. These inferior recesses beneath the medial meniscus are generally small, and some regard recesses that are greater than 2 mm in size as abnormal.[134] The anterior part of the medial meniscus is covered with the base of the infrapatellar fat pad, making evaluation of this region more difficult.

Lateral Meniscus (Fig. 15–62). The lateral meniscus is more circular in configuration than the medial meniscus. It too is projected as a sharply defined triangular radiodense area surrounded by air and contrast material. It changes little in size from its anterior to its posterior horn, averaging 10 mm in width.[135] Inferior recesses are frequent beneath both the anterior and posterior horns of the lateral meniscus. The anterior horn is attached to the lateral ligament, but the posterior horn of the lateral meniscus is separated from this ligament by the synovial sheath of the popliteus tendon. This sheath fills with air and contrast material and overlies the peripheral portion of the posterior horn of the lateral meniscus, producing variable arthrographic findings, which have received great attention.[133, 136-139, 331, 332, 342] Two delicate bands of connective tissue, termed struts or fascicles, connect the posterior horn of the lateral meniscus to the joint capsule around the popliteal tendon sheath. In any one view of this portion of the lateral meniscus, two struts may be observed with the intervening sheath, one strut may be apparent in conjunction with the sheath, or the sheath may be observed without visualization of either strut. Classically, however, arthrography of the most posterior aspect of the lateral meniscus will reveal an intact superior strut; a slightly more anterior view will reveal both struts, and a more anterior projection will reveal an inferior strut. The variability in appearance of the fascicles or struts of the lateral meniscus combined with the presence of an overlying air-filled tendon sheath makes difficult the evaluation of the posterior horn of the lateral meniscus. However, narrowing, compression or absence of the popliteus tendon sheath may indicate tears of the lateral meniscus, discoid menisci, adhesive capsulitis, prior surgery, or a rare congenital abnormality.[342]

MENISCAL ABNORMALITIES

Meniscal Tear. The arthrographic appearance of meniscal tears in both adults[116, 121, 122, 134, 140-142, 318] and children[143-145] has been well described. A classification of types of meniscal tears has been utilized,[121, 360] although specification of a particular type of tear during arthrography is often impossible and, even when possible, may have little clinical significance. The location of the tear in one aspect of the meniscus is of greater significance. A meniscal tear is more frequent on the medial side, involving particularly the posterior horn of the medial meniscus. The lateral meniscal tear most commonly involves the anterior horn.

***Vertical Concentric Tear* (Fig. 15–63).** A vertical radiodense line extending through the meniscus will be observed. The inner fragment may be displaced, producing a bucket-handle tear, and may lodge in the central portion of the articulation, where it may or may not be identified during arthrography.

***Vertical Radial Tear* (Fig. 15–64).** A vertical tear along the inner contour of the meniscus will produce a contrast-coated inner meniscal margin and a blunted meniscal shadow.

***Horizontal Tear* (Fig. 15–65).** Such tears, which

Text continued on page 578

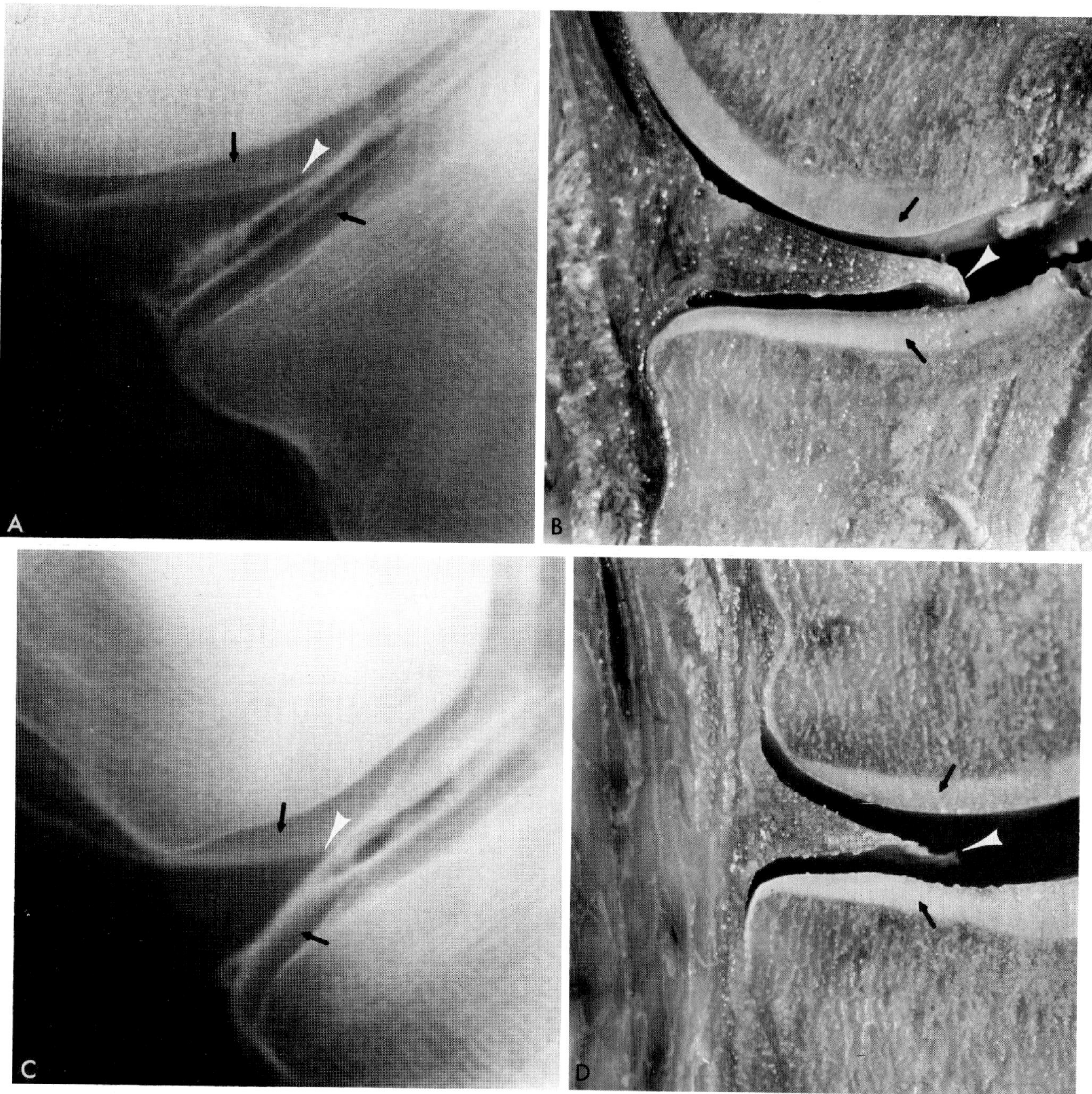

Figure 15–61. Knee arthrography: Anatomy and normal arthrography of the medial meniscus (arthrograms and pie-shaped longitudinal sections).

A, B Posterior horn of the medial meniscus. This segment is relatively large, extending for a considerable distance into the articular cavity (arrowhead). The adjacent articular recesses are small. The articular cartilage (arrows) is smooth.

C, D Midportion of the medial meniscus. This segment does not extend so far into the joint (arrowhead). The articular cartilage is again normal in appearance (arrows).

Illustration continued on the opposite page

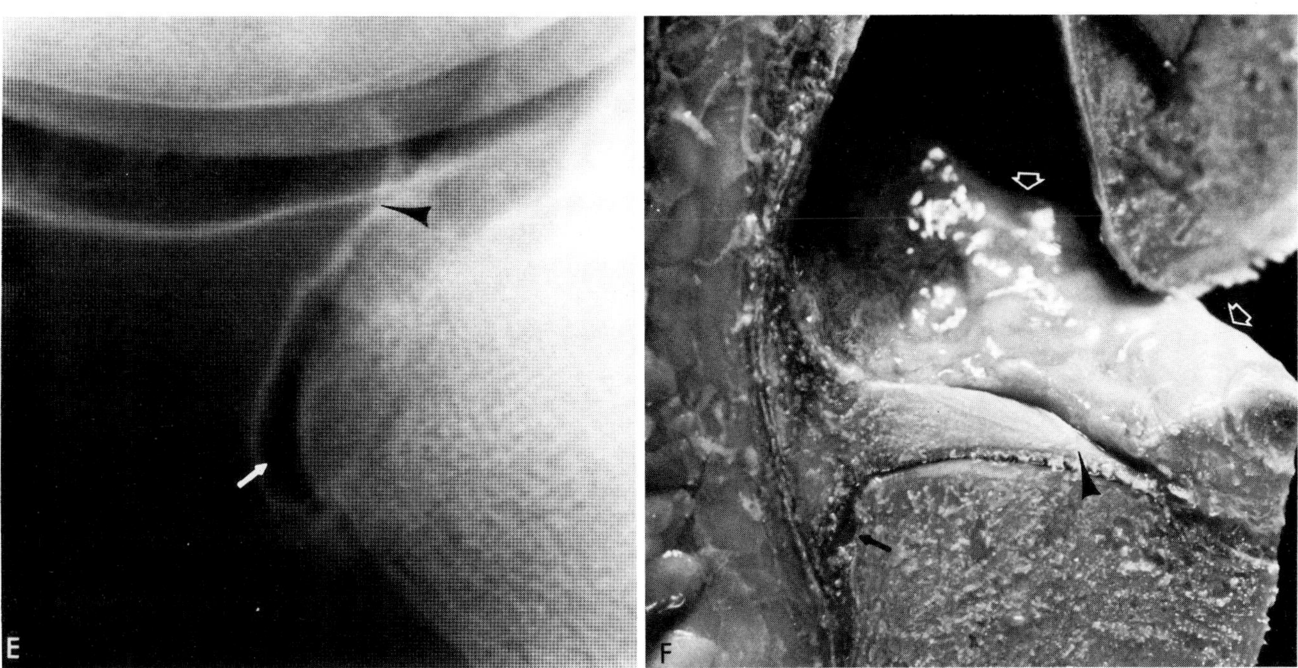

Figure 15–61. Continued

E, F *Anterior horn of the medial meniscus. The size of this segment is variable (arrowhead). Note the fat pad that overlies the meniscus (open arrows). An inferior recess is visualized (solid arrow).*

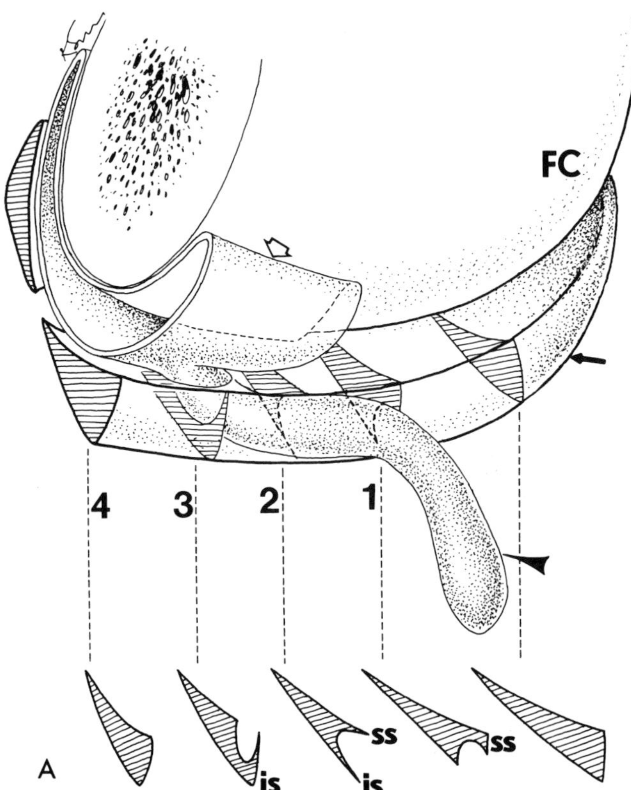

Figure 15–62. *Knee arthrography: Anatomy and normal arthrography of the lateral meniscus (arthrograms and pie-shaped longitudinal sections).*

A *Diagrammatic representation of the posterolateral aspect of the knee joint demonstrates relationships of the lateral meniscus (solid arrow) and popliteus tendon sheath (arrowhead). The very posterior aspect of the femoral condyle* (FC) *and synovial reflection (open arrow) are indicated. The popliteus muscle originates posteriorly and inferiorly on the tibia and extends obliquely, anteriorly, and superiorly to insert on the lateral aspect of the femur. The popliteus tendon enters the joint close to the posterior and lateral aspects of the meniscus and passes through an oblique tunnel. Anteroinferior and posterosuperior to the intra-articular portion of the popliteus tendon are recesses, which fill with contrast medium during arthrography. Two bands of connective tissue, termed struts or fascicles, connect the posterior horn of the lateral meniscus to the joint capsule around the popliteal tendon sheath. Classically, (1) the more posterior aspect of the lateral meniscus will reveal an intact superior strut* (ss); *(2) a slightly more anterior section will reveal both superior strut* (ss) *and inferior strut* (is); *(3) a more anterior section will reveal only an inferior strut* (is); *and (4) a still further anterior section (midportion of the lateral meniscus) depicts an intact meniscus with no visible popliteal tendon sheath.*

B, C *Posterior aspect of the lateral meniscus (section 2). In this arthrogram* **(B)** *and longitudinal section* **(C)**, *observe the popliteus tendon sheath (arrowheads), lateral meniscus (arrow), superior strut* (ss), *and inferior strut* (is). *The latter strut has been disrupted in the preparation of this section.*

D, E *Slightly more anterior aspect of the lateral meniscus (section 3). In this arthrogram* **(D)** *and longitudinal section* **(E)**, *note the popliteus tendon sheath (arrowhead), lateral meniscus (arrow) and inferior strut* (is). *A thin superior strut is visible on the arthrogram but is absent on the section.*

F, G *Anterior horn of the lateral meniscus. In this arthrogram* **(F)** *and longitudinal section* **(G)**, *the meniscus (solid arrow) is well shown. Observe the articular cartilage (arrowheads) and prominent recesses (open arrow).*

Illustration continued on the opposite page

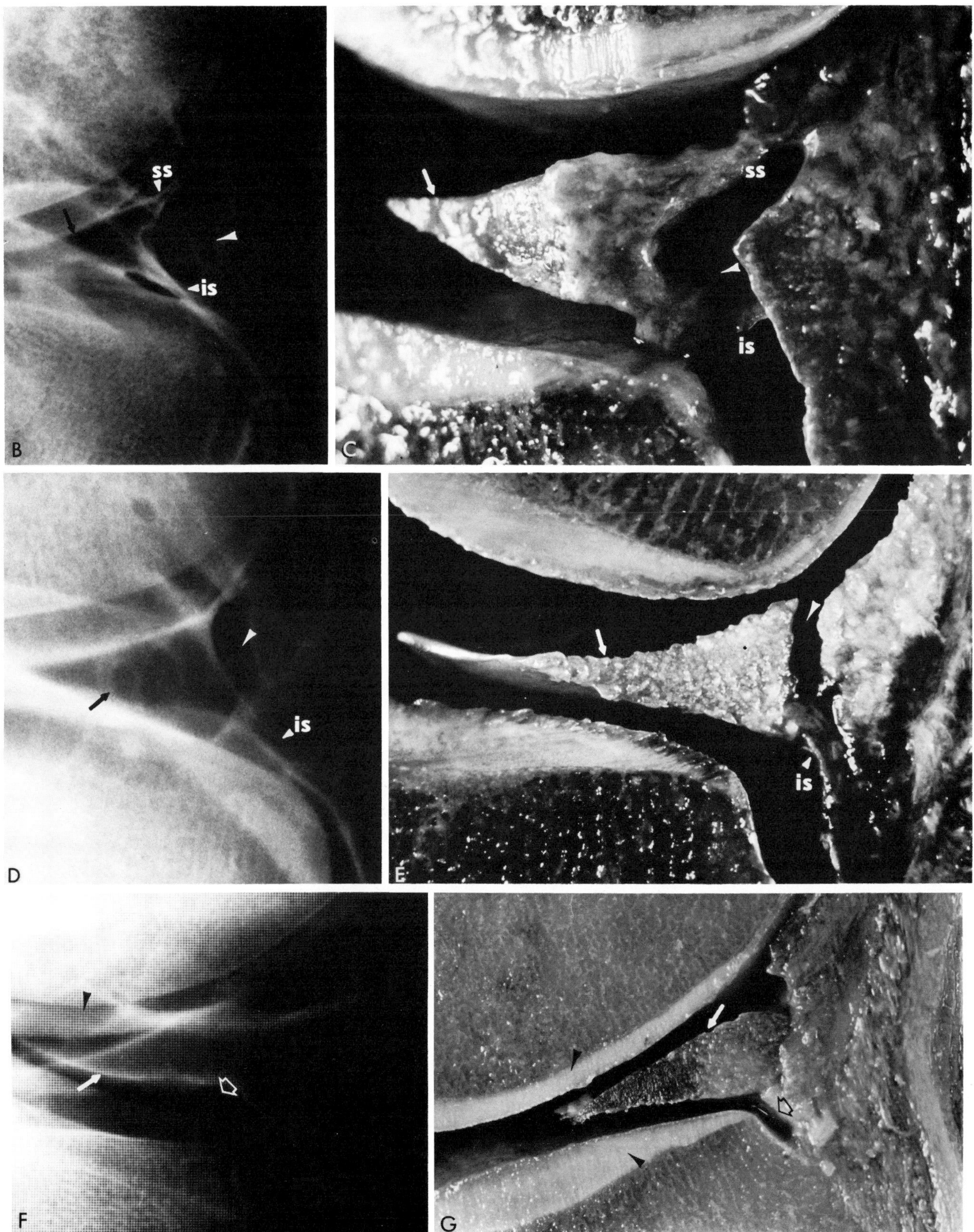

Figure 15–62. Continued

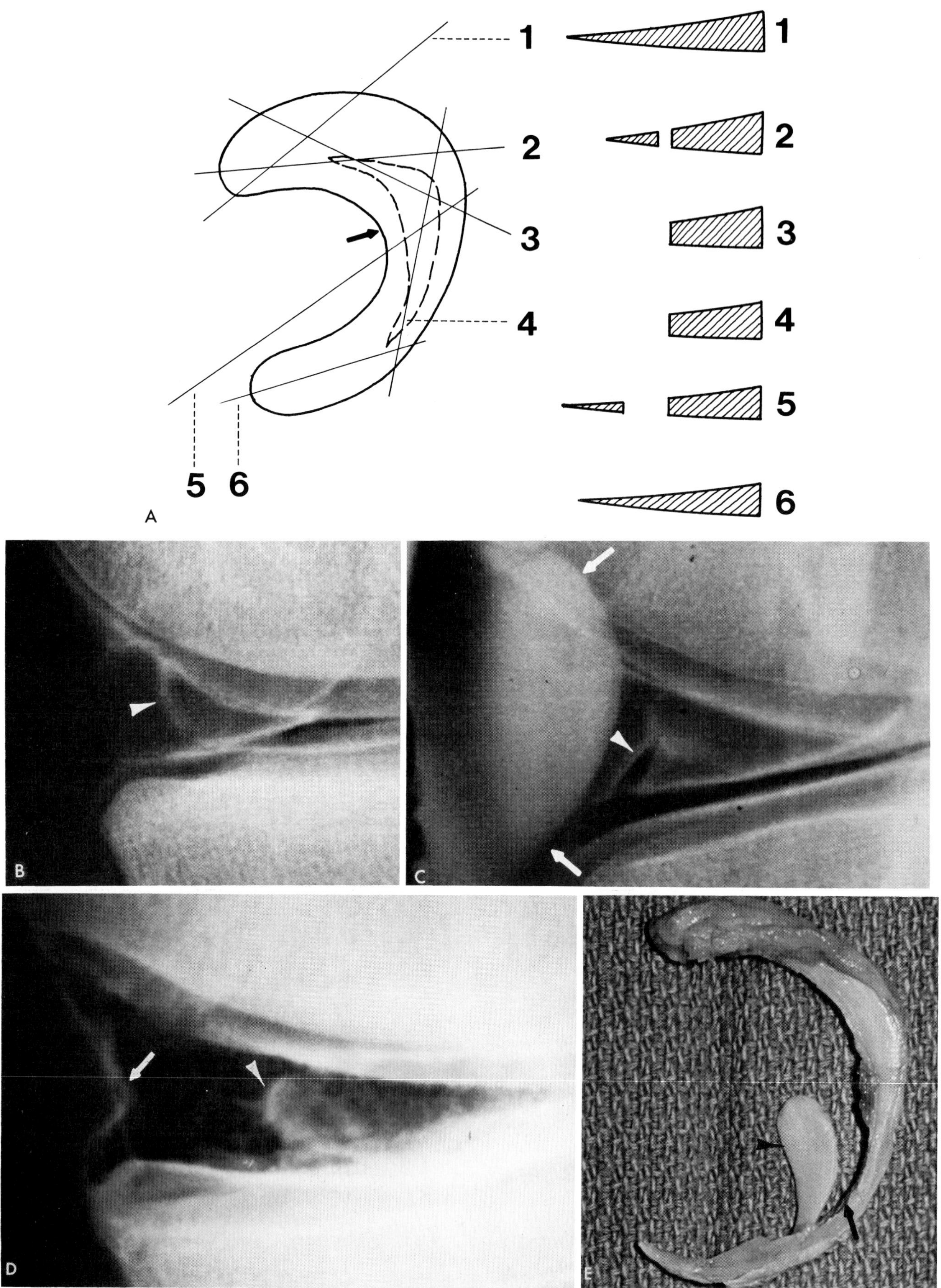

Figure 15–63. See legend on the opposite page

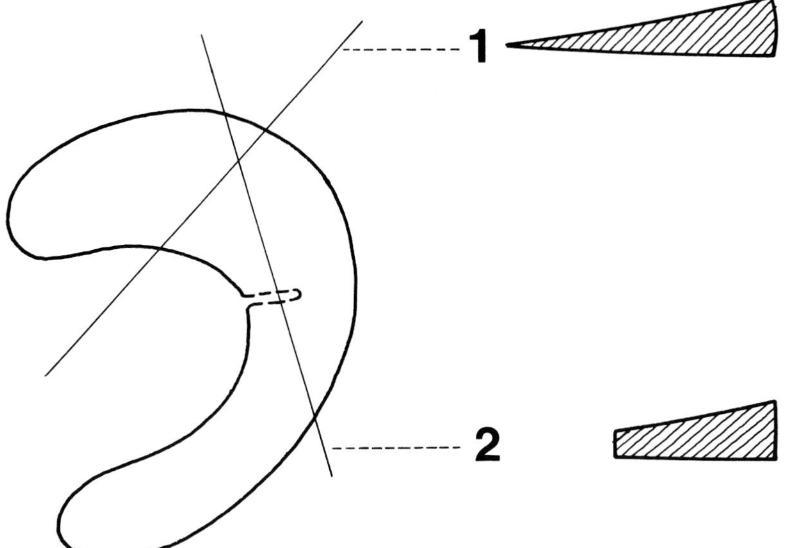

Figure 15–64. Knee arthrography: Vertical radial meniscal tear.

A *The medial meniscus is viewed from above. Its posterior horn is located superiorly. A vertical radial tear is evident on the inner contour of the meniscus. Some arthrographic views (1) will appear normal, whereas others passing through the tear (2) will reveal a blunted contrast-coated inner meniscal shadow.*

B *An arthrogram demonstrates such a radial tear (arrowhead) of the medial meniscus.*

C *In a different patient, the radial component (arrowhead) of the tear in the medial meniscus is evident. Elsewhere, the tear is more complex.*

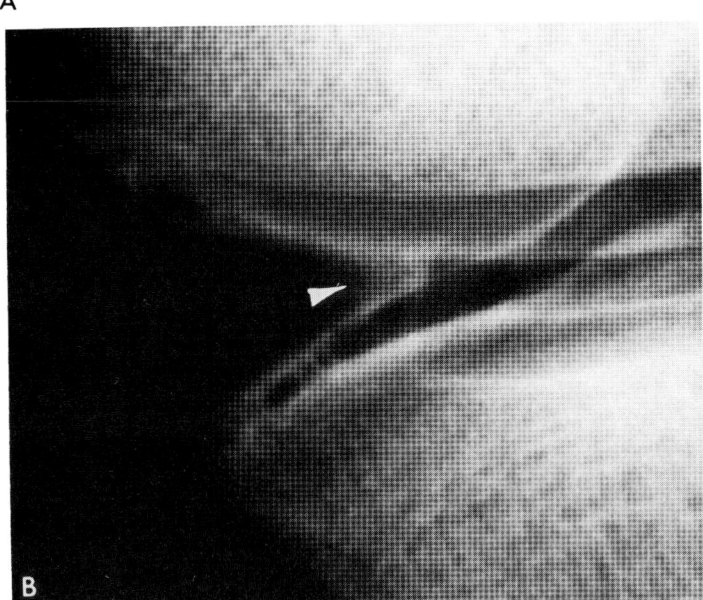

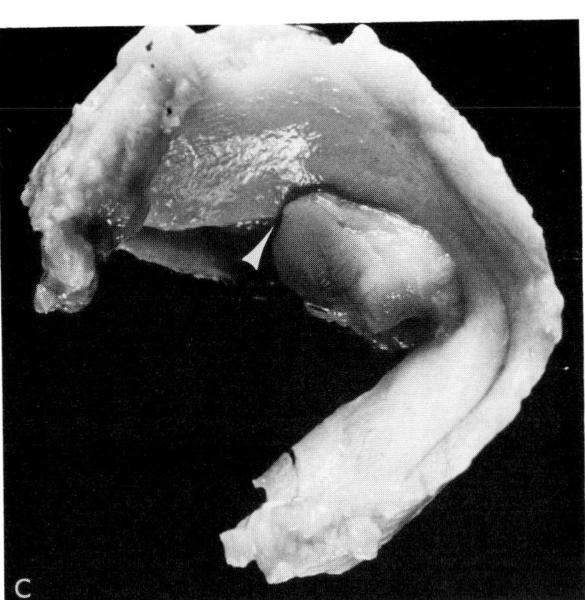

Figure 15–63. Knee arthrography: Vertical concentric meniscal tear.

A *Vertical concentric ("bucket-handle") tears. The medial meniscus is viewed from above with the posterior horn located superiorly. The vertical tear can be seen and the inner fragment is displaced centrally (arrow). The arthrographic appearance will depend upon the specific site of the tear. A view of the posterior aspect of the meniscus (1) will be normal. Slightly more anteriorly (2) a vertical tear will be apparent with minimal displacement of the fragment. At positions 3 and 4, an amputated meniscal shadow will be apparent. At position 5, significant displacement of the inner fragment is observed. The anterior horn of the meniscus (6) will appear normal.*

B, C *Vertical concentric tears — two examples of medial meniscal abnormalities. Observe the contrast or air-filled linear shadows (arrowhead) in the meniscus. A popliteal cyst is evident (arrows).*

D, E *Vertical concentric tears — "bucket-handle" type. An arthrogram* **(D)** *and photograph of a gross specimen* **(E)** *from two different patients. The arthrogram outlines amputation of the medial meniscus (arrow) with a displaced inner fragment (arrowhead) located in the central portion of the articulation. The gross photograph of a torn medial meniscus (posterior horn on top; anterior horn on bottom) demonstrates the amputated meniscus (arrow) and a displaced inner fragment (arrowhead).*

are more frequently observed in older individuals,[146] may also be present in younger patients without producing symptoms.[147] A radiopaque line of contrast material is apparent overlying the meniscal shadow, extending to the superior or inferior surface. The meniscus may lose its wedge-shaped configuration.

Combined Tears. Combinations of any of the above meniscal alterations can be observed.

Meniscal Cyst (Fig. 15–66). These cysts are multiloculated collections of mucinous material of unknown etiology which have predilection for the lateral aspect of the knee.[148-151] Most observers believe that these cysts develop following trauma, although others consider that degenerative or congenital factors may be important. The cysts are generally located at the peripheral meniscal margin and do not communicate with the joint cavity. In this location,

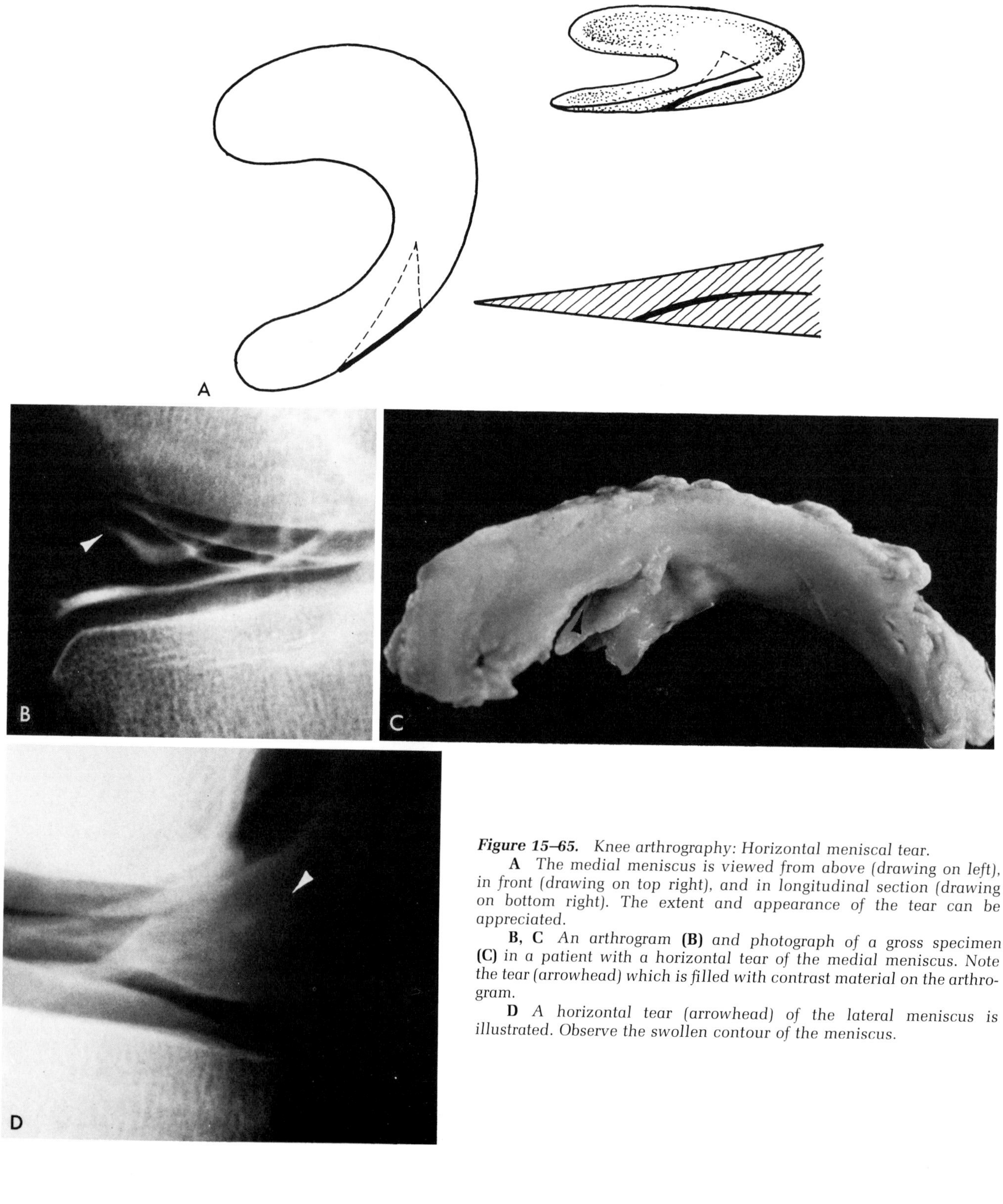

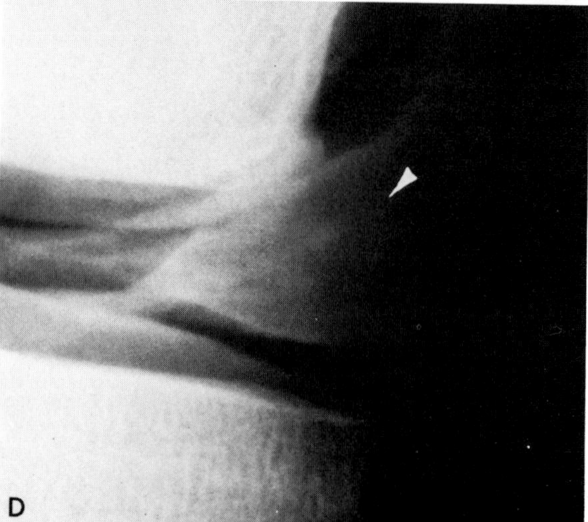

Figure 15–65. *Knee arthrography: Horizontal meniscal tear.*

A *The medial meniscus is viewed from above (drawing on left), in front (drawing on top right), and in longitudinal section (drawing on bottom right). The extent and appearance of the tear can be appreciated.*

B, C *An arthrogram* **(B)** *and photograph of a gross specimen* **(C)** *in a patient with a horizontal tear of the medial meniscus. Note the tear (arrowhead) which is filled with contrast material on the arthrogram.*

D *A horizontal tear (arrowhead) of the lateral meniscus is illustrated. Observe the swollen contour of the meniscus.*

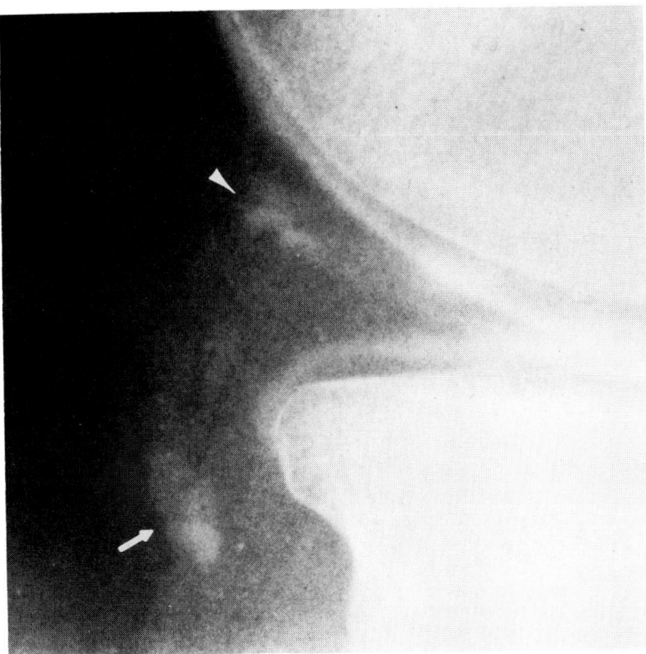

Figure 15–66. Knee arthrography: Meniscal cyst. A cyst of the medial meniscus is opacified (arrow) and associated with a horizontal tear of the meniscus (arrowhead).

they may produce few or no arthrographic changes. Cysts that are more centrally located may distort the menisci or, on rare occasions, may be opacified because of articular communication. Meniscal cysts frequently occur following meniscectomy. Rarely, they may erode bone.[321]

Gross and microscopic studies of excised menisci may reveal a surprisingly high (7 per cent) percentage of associated cysts.[319, 361] These menisci commonly reveal horizontal tears, and tracks may be identified leading from the tear to the cyst.[343] These facts coupled with the observation that fluid within the cyst histochemically resembles synovial fluid suggest that a pumping mechanism may exist that propels synovial fluid through the tears into the surrounding soft tissue, creating meniscal cysts. Thus, the cysts may not arise from primary myxoid degeneration. In fact, delayed roentgenograms following arthrography may reveal such communication.[320]

Discoid Meniscus (Fig. 15–67). A discoid meniscus has an altered shape. It is broad and disc-like in appearance rather than semilunar in configuration, although intermediate varieties of discoid menisci have been described.[152] These include the slab type (flat, circular meniscus), biconcave type (biconcave disc, thinner in its central portion), wedge type (large but normally tapered meniscus), anterior type (enlarged anterior horn), forme fruste (slightly enlarged meniscus), and grossly torn type (too deformed for accurate classification). A discoid lateral meniscus[153-158] is much more common than a discoid medial meniscus.[157-164]

The reported incidence of discoid lateral menisci varies from 0 to 2.7 per cent,[152, 165] although occasionally a higher incidence, determined by arthrography in children[143, 166] or by direct inspection during meniscectomy,[154, 157, 167] is cited. The usual age of patients at the time of clinical presentation is between 15 and 35 years, and men are more frequently affected. These patients commonly present with symptoms of a torn cartilage. Bilateral discoid menisci and a familial incidence of an abnormal meniscal shape[168] have also been noted.

An embryologic explanation for discoid menisci has not yet been determined. During development, undifferentiated mesenchymal tissue exists between the cartilaginous precursors of bone. This tissue subsequently cavitates, producing an articular cavity. In some articulations, a portion of the mesenchyme exists as fibrocartilaginous discs or menisci. In knee development, under normal circumstances, undifferentiated mesenchyme evolves into fetal cartilage, which by the tenth week is semilunar in shape, closely resembling the adult meniscus.[155, 162] This normal sequence of embryologic development does not, therefore, contain a stage in which either the medial or the lateral meniscus is discoid in shape; the appearance of such a meniscus in a child or adult cannot occur through persistence of a fetal stage.

Kaplan[155] has postulated that the discoid lateral meniscus is acquired after birth as a result of an abnormal attachment of its posterior horn to the tibial plateau. He suggested that a primary abnormality of the inferior strut or fascicle will eventually produce a discoid meniscus because of repetitive abnormal mediolateral and anteroposterior movement of the meniscus, with subsequent enlargement and thickening of meniscal tissue. Other investigators have noted that this strut is frequently poorly visualized or definitely abnormal in many patients with discoid lateral menisci, observations that lend support to Kaplan's theory.[152]

Initial plain films in patients with discoid menisci are generally unrewarding, although widening of the articular space in the ipsilateral compartment of the knee documented by weight-bearing radiography, a high fibular head, and an abnormally shaped lateral malleolus have been observed in patients with discoid lateral menisci. A discoid medial meniscus may be associated with irregularity of the medial margin of the proximal tibial epiphysis.[333] Arthrography reveals the abnormally large and elongated meniscus, frequently extending to the intercondylar notch. The margins of the body of the meniscus are relatively parallel rather than converging in configuration. An associated meniscal tear is frequently observed.[322]

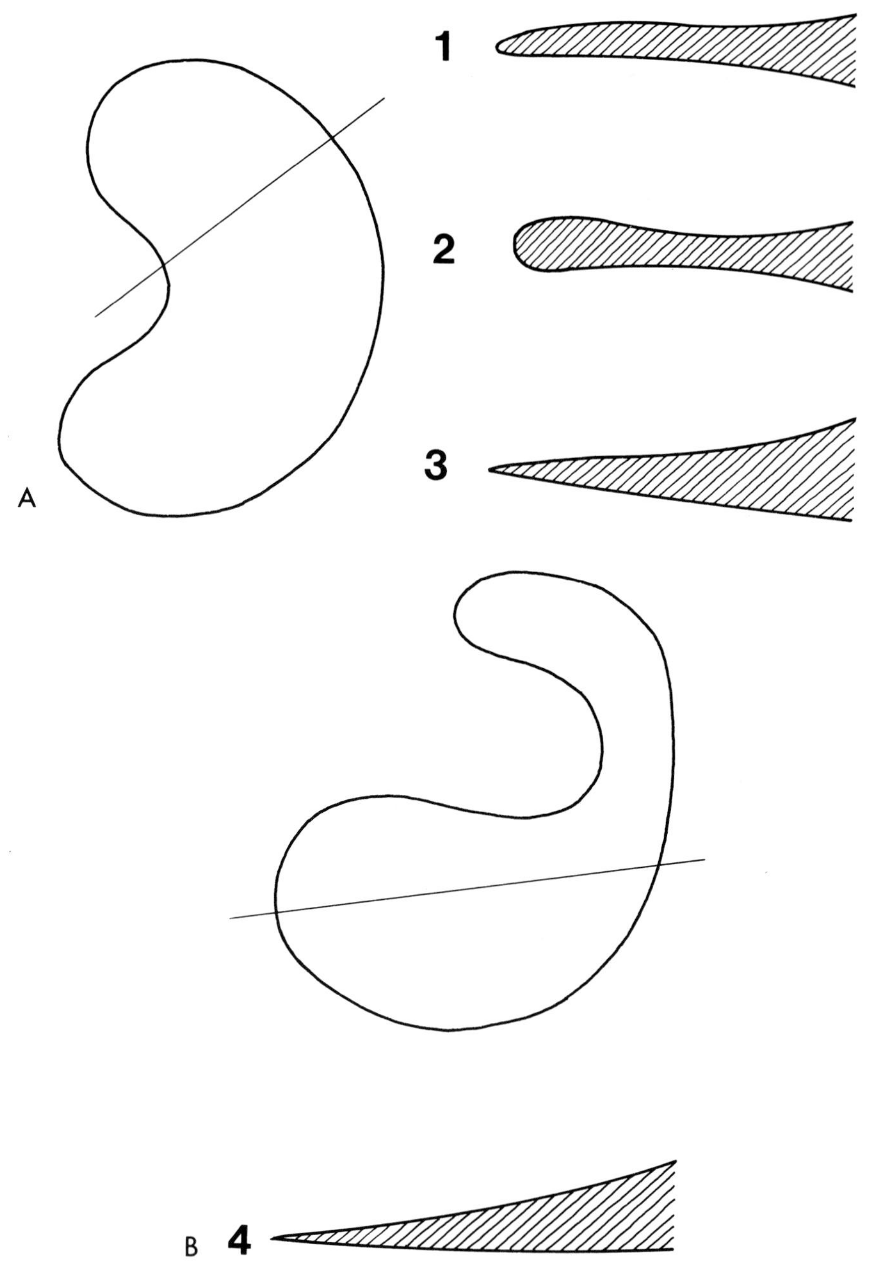

Figure 15–67. Knee arthrography: Discoid meniscus.

A, B *Types of discoid menisci include the slab type (1), biconcave type (2), wedge type (3), and anterior type (4).*

C *Discoid lateral meniscus (slab type) with tear. Observe that the meniscus extends far into the joint cavity (arrowheads). A vertical tear is evident (arrow).*

D *Discoid lateral meniscus (biconcave type). The central extension (arrowheads) and the thinner central portion (arrow) of the meniscus are observed.*

E, F *Discoid medial meniscus (slab type). The preoperative arthrogram* **(E)** *demonstrates the discoid meniscus extending far into the central portion of the joint (arrowhead), with a peripheral tear (arrow). The specimen photograph* **(F)** *confirms the discoid medial meniscus with a peripheral tear (arrowhead).*

Illustration continued on the opposite page

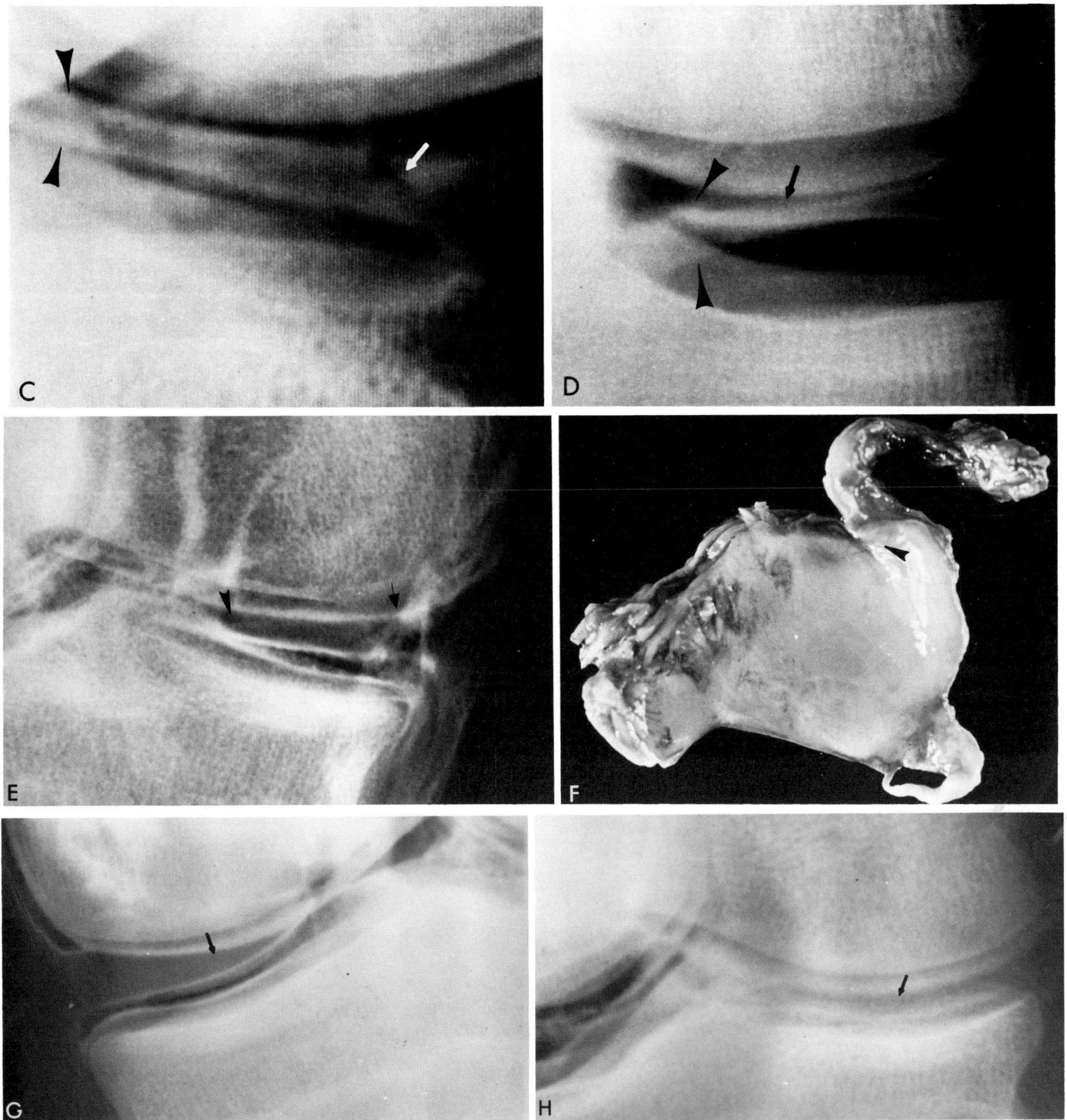

Figure 15–67. Continued

G *Discoid medial meniscus (wedge type). An apparently intact discoid meniscus (arrow) is noted.*

H *Discoid medial meniscus (slab type). During compression of the medial compartment of the knee, a discoid medial meniscus (arrow) is interposed between the tibia and the femur, preventing contact between the articular cartilages.*

*(**E–H,** From Resnick D, et al: 121:575, 1976.)*

Illustration continued on the following page

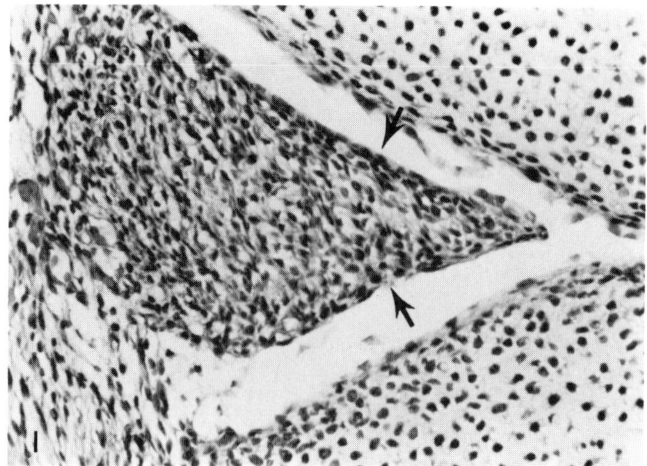

Figure 15–67. Continued

I *Embryologic development of the meniscus. Even in early fetal life, the undifferentiated mesenchymal tissue that is to become the knee meniscus is semilunar in shape (arrows) (100×). A discoid shape is not part of the normal sequence of embryologic development of the meniscus.*

Meniscal Ossicle (Fig. 15–68). Meniscal ossicles represent foci of ossification within the menisci. They are rarely observed in the human knee,[169-173] although they are a normal finding in the knees of certain rodents.[174] Ossicles represent hyaline cartilage enclosing lamellar and cancellous bone and marrow. Their origin in humans is controversial; some investigators believe they are vestigial structures,[171, 174] whereas others suggest they are acquired following trauma.[169] Patients with knee ossicles may be asymptomatic or have local pain and swelling.

Initial films reveal ossification of variable shape in the anterior or posterior portions of either the medial or the lateral meniscus.[344] Thus, the radiodense region is generally centrally located within the articular space. Arthrography confirms the location of the ossification within the meniscus.[173] The meniscus itself may be normal, contain associated tears,[169-171, 323] or be discoid in type.[175]

Meniscal ossicles must be differentiated from other causes of articular radiodensities, particularly intra-articular osteochondral fragments. These latter fragments are not central in location, may move in location from one examination to another, or may appear in the joint recesses. If a meniscal ossicle produces considerable symptoms, requiring meniscectomy, radiography of the removed meniscus will document the intrameniscal location of the ossification.

Meniscectomy (Fig. 15–69). Following the documentation of a meniscal abnormality, the orthopedic surgeon may elect to operate on the patient. A total or partial meniscectomy may be performed. If the former is chosen, the entire meniscus will be removed from

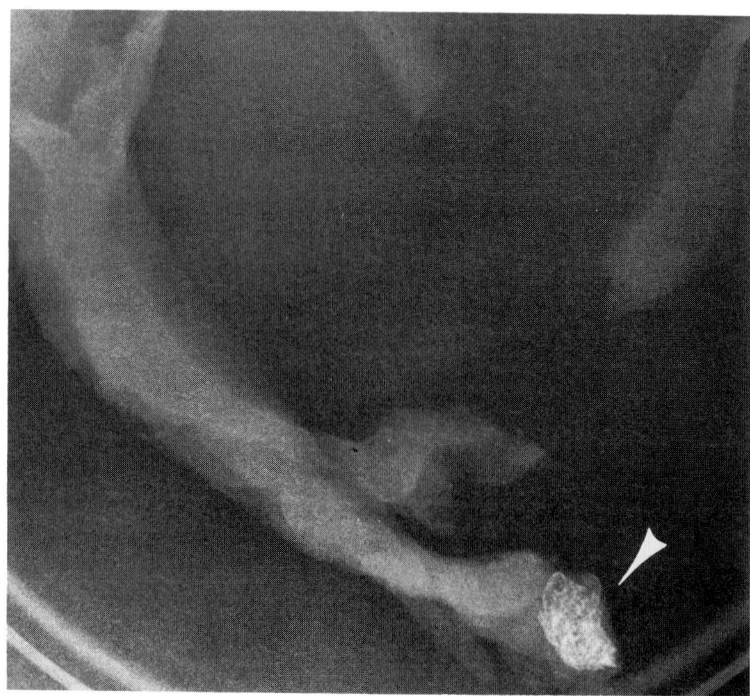

Figure 15–68. *Knee arthrography: Meniscal ossicle. A radiograph of a removed medial meniscus reveals a meniscal ossicle (arrowhead) which simulated an intra-articular osseous body on the initial plain films of the knee.*

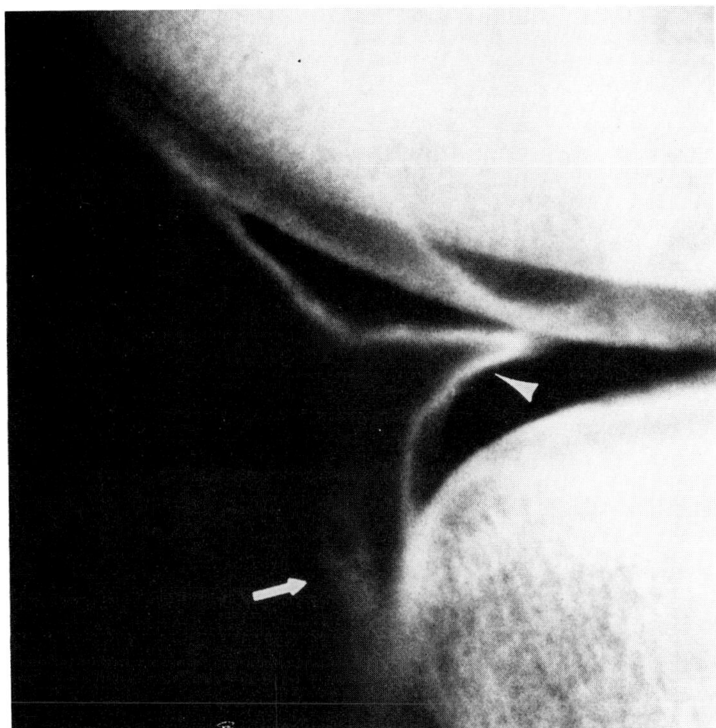

Figure 15–69. *Knee arthrography: Retained fragment following meniscectomy. This patient described recurrent symptoms following a partial medial meniscectomy. A retained posterior horn is apparent (arrowhead). A small collection of contrast material (arrow) may represent a partial separation of the meniscus from the medial collateral ligament.*

its capsular attachment. This may be accomplished through an anterior approach alone, although in some instances the posterior horn will be left behind, which, if recognized, will require a second incision for removal. There are two types of partial meniscectomies. The anterior two thirds of the abnormal meniscus may be removed, deliberately leaving the posterior horn in place. Alternatively, the torn portion of the meniscus may be removed, leaving the remainder of the meniscus intact. Following complete meniscectomy, fibrous regeneration of the meniscus occurs within 6 weeks to 3 months.[176] The regenerated meniscus is thinner and narrower than a normal meniscus, with a decreased surface area and diminished mobility. Tears through regenerated menisci, although reported,[177, 178] are rare.

Plain film radiographic findings following meniscectomy may include flattening of the ipsilateral femoral condyle, a spur projecting inferiorly from the margin of the femoral condyle at the meniscectomy site, and joint space narrowing.[334, 345] Arthrographic evaluation following complete or partial meniscectomy may reveal a retained fragment, a regenerated meniscus, a tear of the opposite meniscus, or additional abnormalities.[179-182]

Retained Fragment. The retained posterior horn following incomplete meniscectomy will resemble a normal posterior horn, although it may be irregular or contain an obvious tear. Following the removal of the inner fragment of a bucket-handle tear, the retained peripheral fragment will appear as a truncated shadow with rough, irregular surfaces.[180]

Regenerated Meniscus. With regeneration of the meniscus, a small triangular shadow resembling an equilateral (isosceles) triangle is observed, varying from 2 to 7 mm in width.[180] It possesses smooth, well-defined margins but is not associated with adjacent normal recesses at the meniscocapsular junction.

Tear of Opposite Meniscus. Arthrographic findings in this situation are no different from those associated with meniscal tears in patients who have not undergone meniscectomy. The torn meniscus may have been overlooked on preoperative arthrography or may have occurred following surgery.

Additional Abnormalities. A variety of additional causes exist for postmeniscectomy pain, including ligament injury, loose bodies, and cartilage ulceration. Some of these causes are unrelated to the previous meniscal surgery, whereas others, such as degenerative joint disease, may occur with increased frequency following meniscectomy.[183, 184, 346] Radiographic evidence of degenerative joint disease has been noted in 85 per cent of knees within 10 years following meniscectomy.[185] Other investigators reported such changes in 23 to 62 per cent of knees,[183, 186, 187] but the incidence will depend upon the length of postoperative clinical follow-up and the type of surgery,[188] as well as other factors.

Miscellaneous Meniscal Abnormalities (Fig. 15–70). The diagnosis of a hypermobile meniscus is open to question.[116] An abnormally mobile meniscus could conceivably occur when adjacent recesses are greater than 2 mm in size, with the exception of the

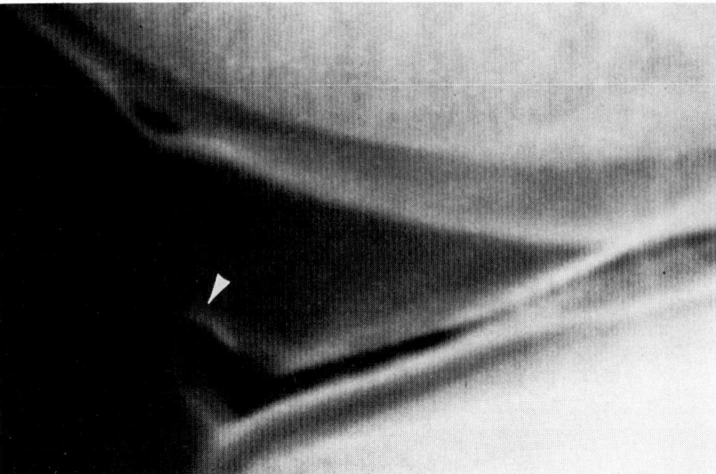

Figure 15–70. Knee arthrography: Mobile meniscus. A prominent inferior recess (arrowhead) beneath the posterior horn of the medial meniscus may lead to hypermobility, with clinical symptoms and signs.

inferior recess about the anterior horn of the lateral meniscus, which is frequently prominent in normal individuals.[134] Hypermobility may also be associated with previous peripheral meniscal tears or detachment.

Ligamentous Injury

Collateral Ligament Tears (Fig. 15–71). Injuries of the collateral ligaments may produce plain film radiographic findings, including widening of the joint space during varus or valgus stress and calcification, particularly near the femoral site of attachment of the medial collateral ligament (Pellegrini-Stieda syndrome). Recent tears of the collateral ligaments may be documented by arthrography. Contrast material introduced into the joint space will extravasate into the adjacent soft tissues. This finding is more readily apparent on the medial aspect of the knee, where a linear radiodense region may indicate a contrast-coated outer margin of the medial collateral ligament. Lateral collateral ligament injuries are more difficult to diagnose on arthrography because of the normal increased distance between the joint capsule and lateral collateral ligament.[134] An enlarged synovial fold between the tibial margin and meniscus may indicate a tear of the coronary ligament.[116]

Cruciate Ligament Injuries (Fig. 15–72). Several arthrographic techniques have been employed for the evaluation of cruciate ligament injuries, with varying degrees of success. Initial techniques utilizing double contrast arthrography were accurate in less than 50 per cent of cases,[121, 122] stimulating investigation with modified methods of examination. Some investigations report success utilizing a lateral view of the knee, flexed to 90 degrees over the edge of the table.[189] Others indicate approximately 75 to 90 percent accu-

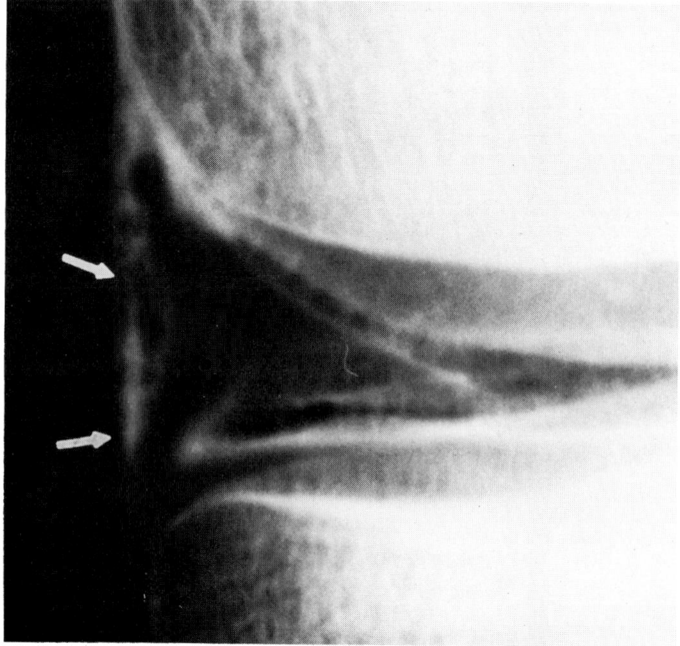

Figure 15–71. Knee arthrography: Collateral ligament injuries. A tear of the medial collateral ligament allows contrast material to pass from the articular cavity into the soft tissues, outlining the lateral aspect of the ligament (arrows).

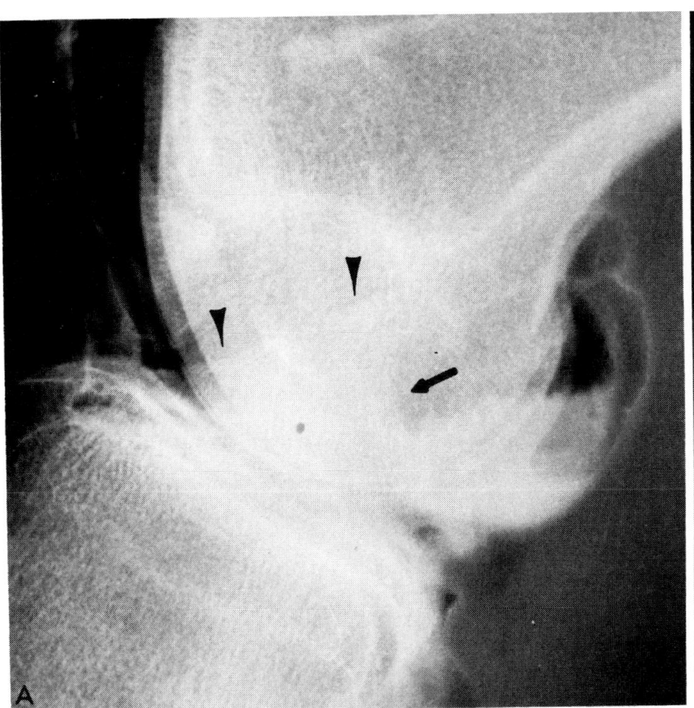

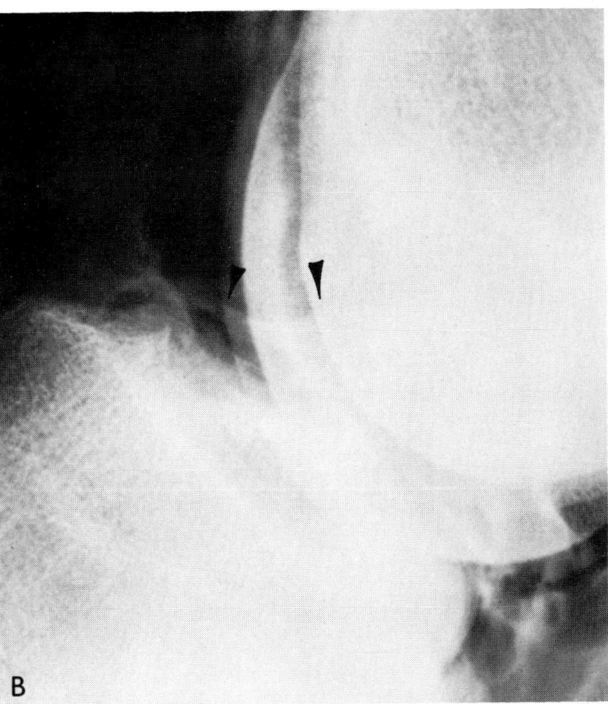

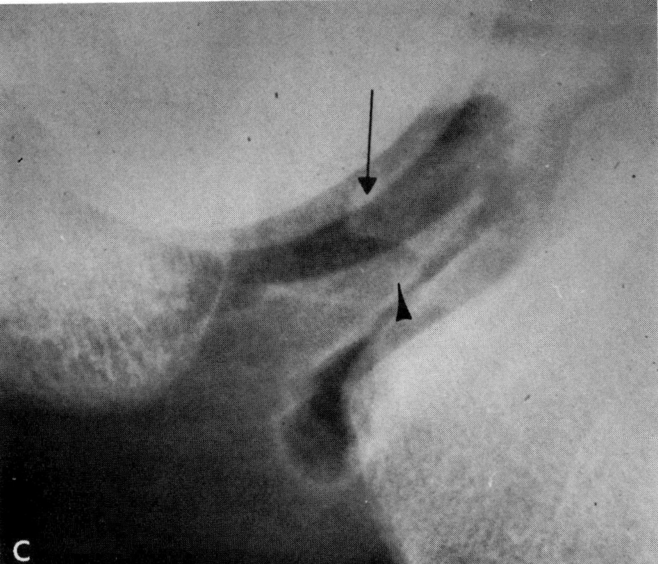

Figure 15–72. *Knee arthrography: Cruciate ligament injury.*

A *On this lateral view, the anterior cruciate (arrowheads) and posterior cruciate (arrow) ligaments are seen. Note their normal appearance and smooth contour.*

B *A torn anterior cruciate ligament is evident (arrowheads). Note the irregular coating and bowed appearance of the torn cruciate.*

C *In another patient, an intra-articular body (arrow) represents a contracted anterior portion of the detached anterior cruciate ligament. The meniscal shadow (arrowhead) can also be seen.*

*(**B, C,** From Dalinka MK, et al: CRC Crit Rev Radiol Sci 5:1, 1973.)*

Illustration continued on the following page

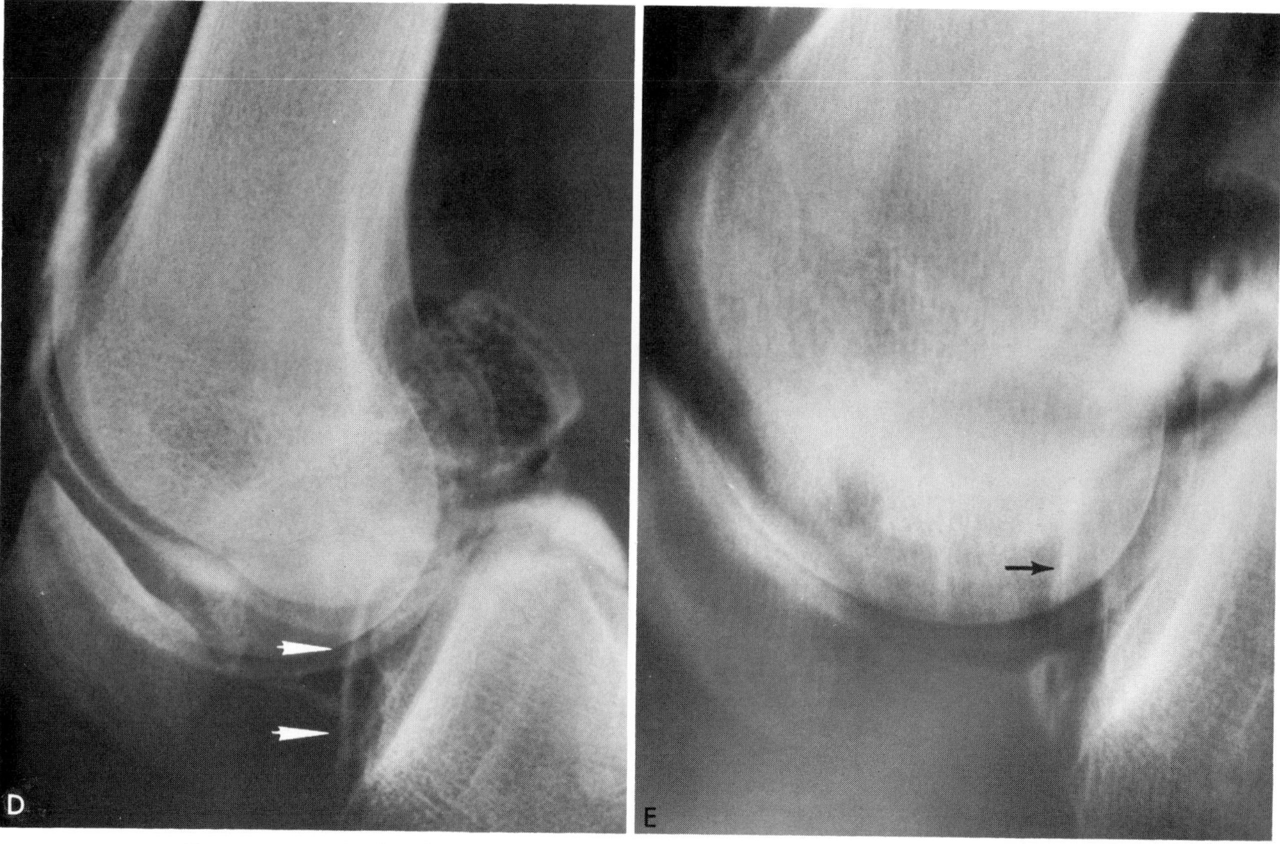

Figure 15–72. Continued

D, E *Infrapatellar synovial fold. On the initial lateral view* **(D)**, *coating of the infrapatellar synovial fold (arrows) simulates an intact anterior cruciate ligament. On the tomogram* **(E)**, *the infrapatellar fold is again evident (arrow). The density in the inferior aspect of the joint represents a coated, curled, and torn anterior cruciate ligament.*

*(***D, E,** *From Dalinka MK, Garofola J: Am J Roentgenol 127:589, 1976. Copyright 1976, American Roentgen Ray Society.)*

racy in diagnosing anterior cruciate tears using tomography.[190] This technique is improved if tomographic exposures are obtained immediately following injection, although this is time consuming, delaying the meniscal examination. More recently, specific radiographic positions have been employed to evaluate the cruciate ligaments at the conclusion of the meniscal study. The ligaments can be studied with patient supine[191] or sitting[192] by utilizing appropriate stress across the joint with traction devices. Under these circumstances, visualization of the posterior cruciate ligament without visualization of the anterior cruciate ligament is regarded as abnormal, the accuracy rate approaching 90 per cent. Recently, computed tomography has been advocated as an additional method for examination of the cruciate ligaments.[324]

The arthrographic abnormalities associated with anterior cruciate ligament tears include nonvisualization, a wavy irregular or bowed (concave or convex) ligamentous surface, and irregularity of the inferior attachment of the ligament.[190-192] The abnormal findings are frequently subtle, requiring of the examiner a good deal of experience and knowledge of adjacent anatomic structures such as the infrapatellar synovial fold, which may lead to confusion in interpretation.[193]

Lesions of Articular Cartilage. Contrast material within the joint cavity allows visualization of portions of articular cartilage. Because of the differences in shape of the articular surfaces of the femur and tibia, the tibial cartilage is more completely evaluated than the femoral cartilage. Knee arthrography with tomography may improve visualization of cartilaginous surfaces.[194] Abnormalities such as osteochondral fracture (osteochondritis dissecans) and chondromalacia may be identified. Cartilage thinning assciated with degenerative joint disease is discussed later in this chapter.

Osteochondral Fracture (Osteochondritis Dissecans) (Fig. 15–73 and 15–74). Transchondral fractures exist where tangential shearing forces are applied to the articular surface. In the knee, such fractures are most frequent on the lateral surface of the medial femoral condyle, although they may be noted elsewhere as well. The fracture fragment may consist of cartilage, cartilage and bone, or bone alone. It may remain in situ with relatively normal overlying

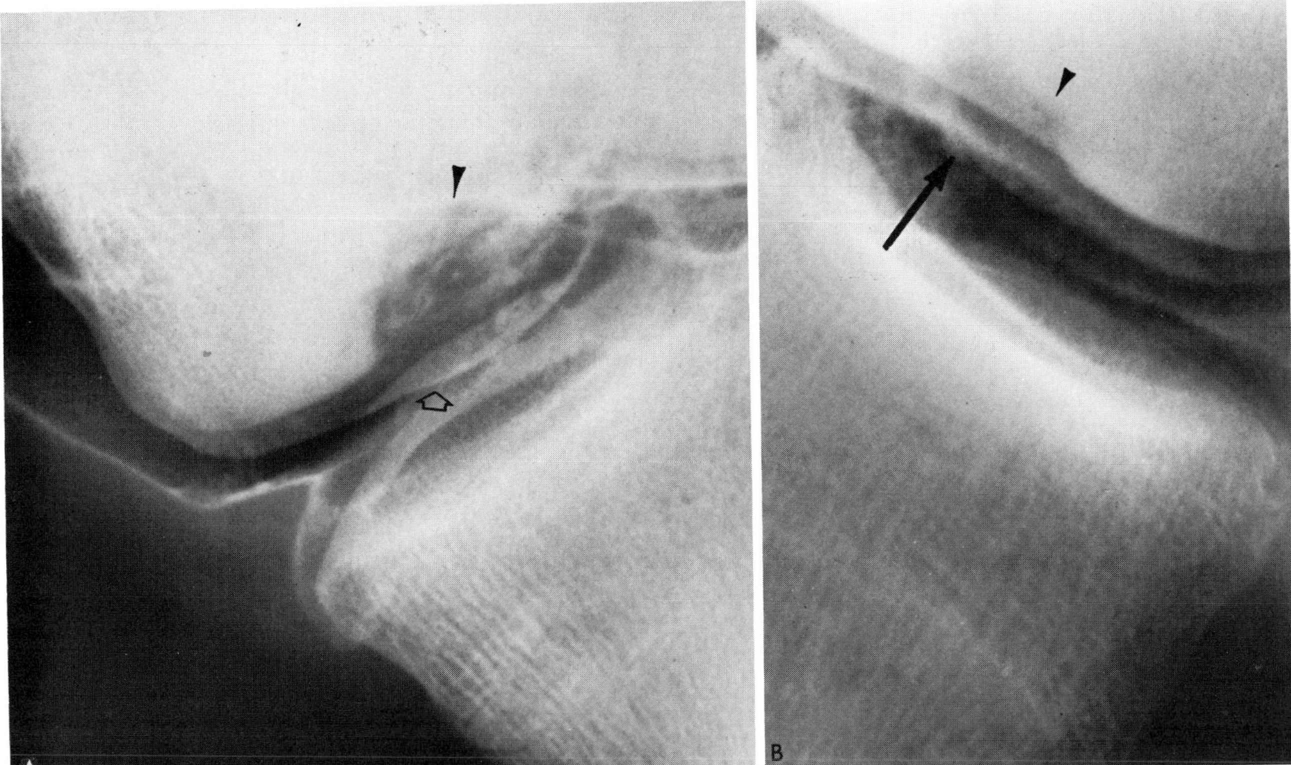

Figure 15–73. Knee arthrography: Osteochondral fractures.

A, B *Two examples of osteochondral fractures (arrowhead) evaluated with arthrography. One demonstrates swollen articular cartilage over the lesion (open arrow), and the other reveals irregular cartilaginous thinning (solid arrow).*

*(**A**, From Wershba M, et al: Clin Orthop 107:81, 1975; **B**, courtesy of Dr. M. K. Dalinka, University of Pennsylvania, Philadelphia, Pennsylvania.)*

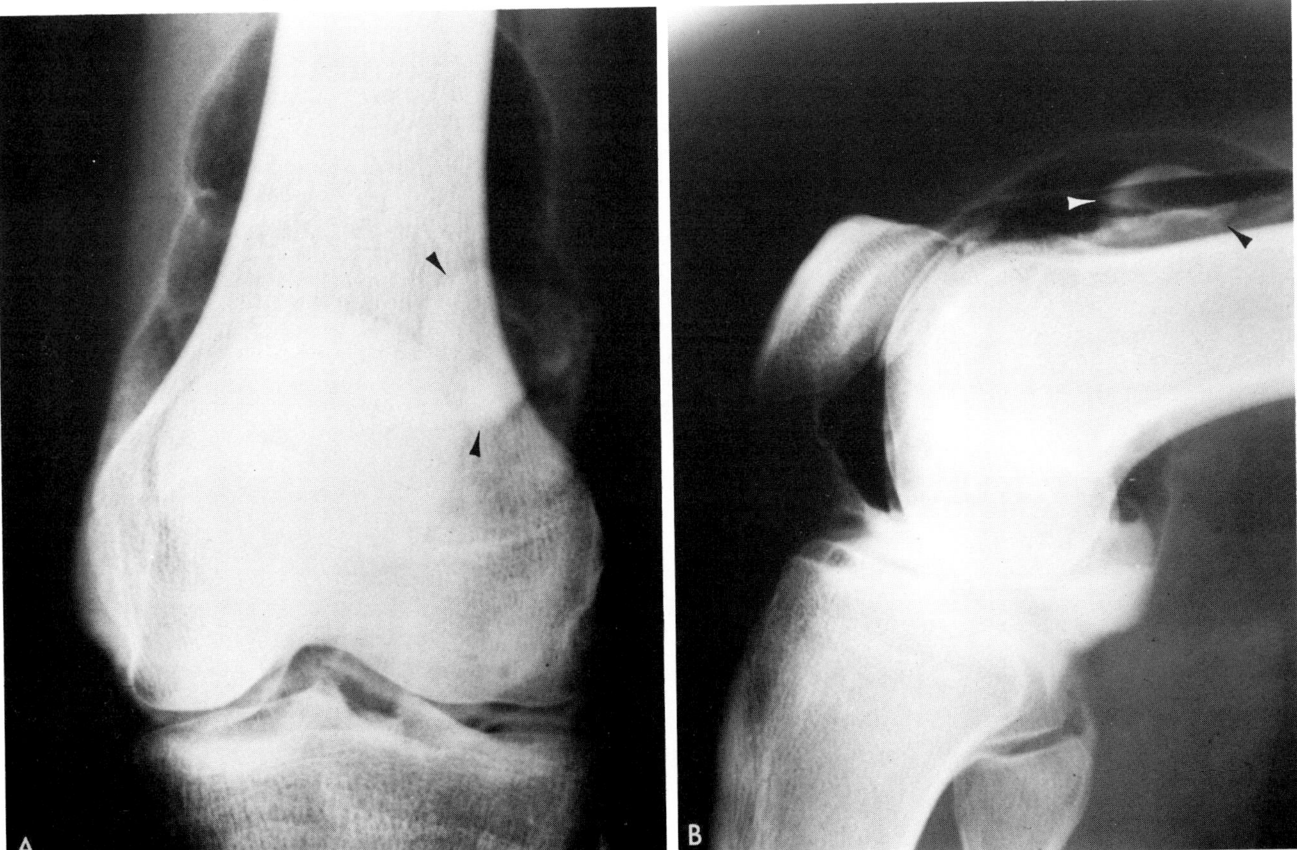

Figure 15–74. Knee arthrography: Chondral fragment. *After an injury, this patient continued to have pain and swelling of the knee. Plain films were unremarkable except for the presence of an effusion. Following arthrography, frontal **(A)** and lateral **(B)** films reveal a large contrast-coated cartilaginous fragment in the suprapatellar pouch (arrowheads).*

cartilage, become depressed with an indentation of the articular surface, or become detached, existing as a loose body in the articular cavity or as an attached body at a distant synovial site.

Arthrography will allow evaluation of the cartilaginous or osseous surface or both, at the fracture site.[195, 196] Contrast medium may outline a normal, swollen, or depressed cartilaginous surface, or it may dissect beneath the osteochondral fragment. The relative integrity of the cartilaginous surface can influence the need for and choice of surgical procedure.

Chondromalacia (Fig. 15–75). The role of arthrography in the diagnosis of chondromalacia of

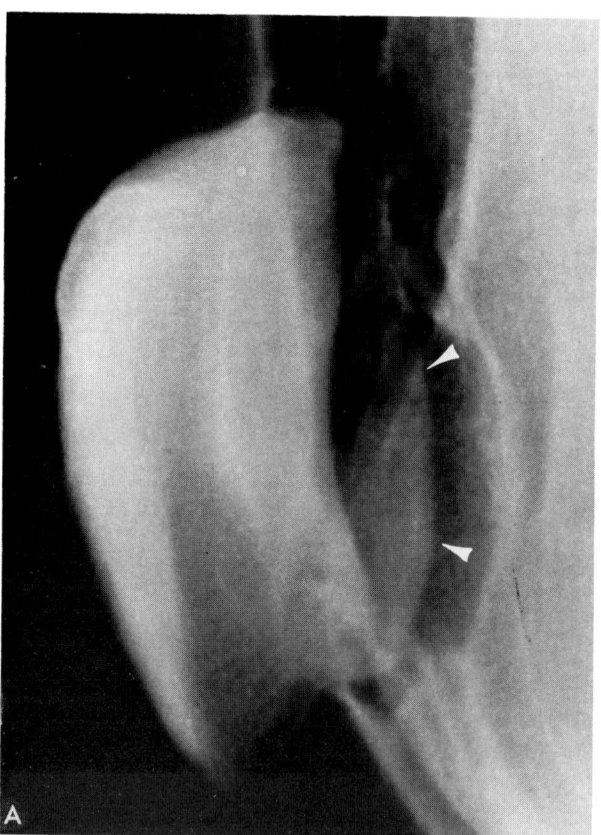

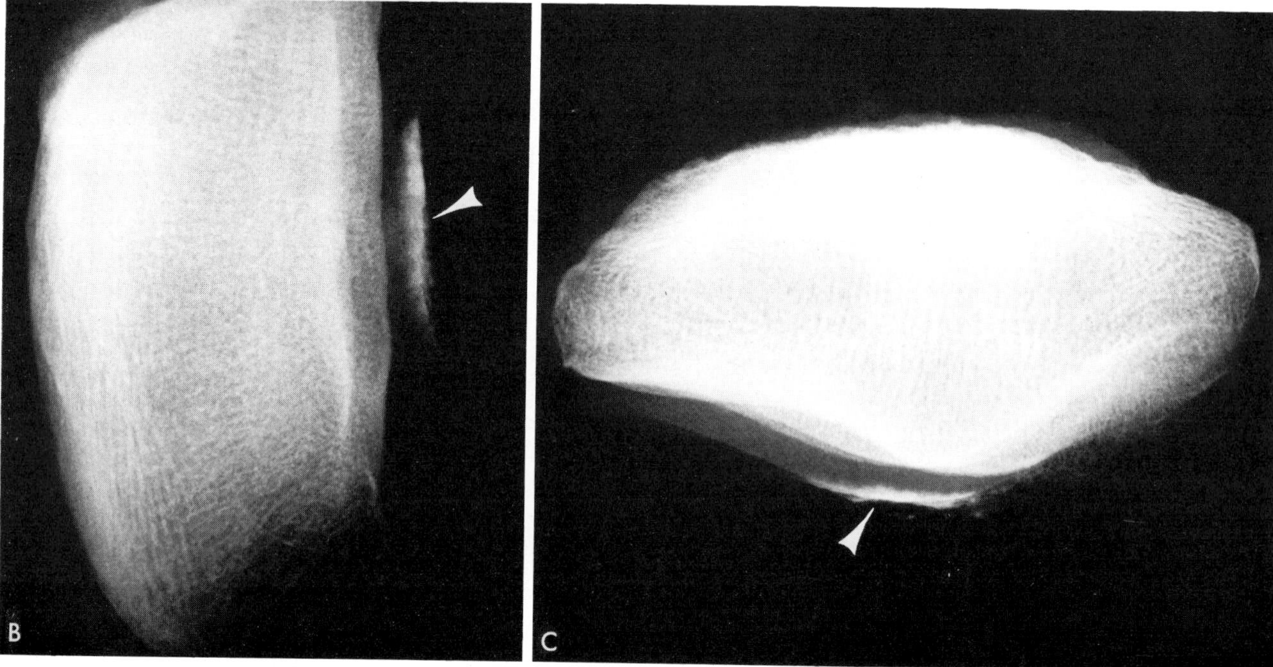

Figure 15–75. *Knee arthrography: Chondromalacia patellae.*

A *Normal appearance. A near-lateral projection following arthrography reveals the normal-appearing tangential surface of the lateral facet of the patella (arrowheads). Note its convex shape. The knee must be internally rotated to visualize the cartilage of the medial facet.*

B, C *On lateral* **(B)** *and axial* **(C)** *radiographs of an excised patella, contrast material has been applied to an area of cartilaginous erosion (arrowhead) to simulate the appearance of chondromalacia on knee arthrography.*

the patella has been the subject of debate. Most observers regard its role as minor or nonexistent,[134, 197] although others are more optimistic.[198, 199] The posterior surface of the patella is V-shaped, with medial and lateral facets separated by an osseous ridge. Routine lateral projections during arthrography demonstrate only a small amount of the patellar cartilaginous surface, that near the apex of the ridge. Axial projections increase the cartilaginous area that can be visualized, and oblique projections that are tangential to the medial and lateral facets may further improve this visualization.[325] If overhead and fluoroscopic filming is accomplished utilizing lateral, oblique, and axial positions supplemented with tomography, the diagnosis of chondromalacia may indeed be substantiated by arthrography in some patients.[362] Whether arthrographic diagnosis will ever be more accurate than clinical diagnosis of the disorder remains to be seen.

On arthrography, chondromalacia produces absorption or imbibition of contrast material by the patellar cartilage. Nodular elevation, fissuring, or diminution of the cartilaginous surface may be apparent.

Evaluation of Additional Bone or Soft Tissue Injuries

Quadriceps Tendon Rupture. The plain film radiographic findings associated with quadriceps tendon rupture have been summarized.[200] These include a suprapatellar soft tissue mass representing the retracted proximal portion of the disrupted tendon, absence of the normal quadriceps soft tissue shadow, effusion, and calcification or ossification within portions of an avulsed patella fragment. Arthrography in partial[201] or complete[202] quadriceps tendon rupture will substantiate the clinical and radiographic diagnosis. Contrast material introduced into the knee joint will reveal communication with the prepatellar or infrapatellar bursa.

Suprapatellar Bursa Rupture. Rupture of the suprapatellar bursa has been described.[203] Arthrographic findings include collection of contrast material near the apex of the bursa, with dissection into the thigh.

Tibial Plateau Fracture. Arthrography in patients with previous tibial plateau fractures has been employed to delineate the integrity of the cartilaginous surface.[204]

Miscellaneous Injury (Fig. 15–76). Following injury, adhesions may occasionally divide the articulation into two separate cavities. An inflammatory synovitis following trauma or other conditions can result in thickening of normal synovial folds or plicae, producing divisions of the articular space and clinical manifestations.[102-104, 108]

Articular Disorders (Table 15–9)

Degenerative Joint Disease (Fig. 15–77). Contrast examination of the knee in patients with degenerative joint disease delineates abnormalities of the articular cartilage and menisci and the presence of intra-

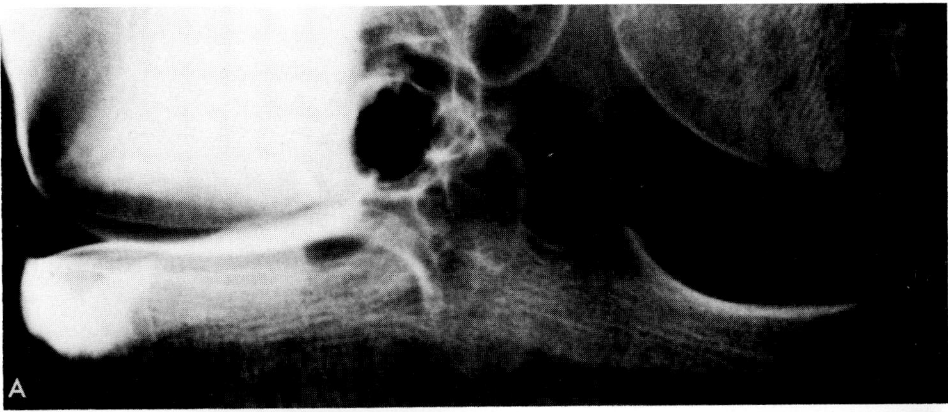

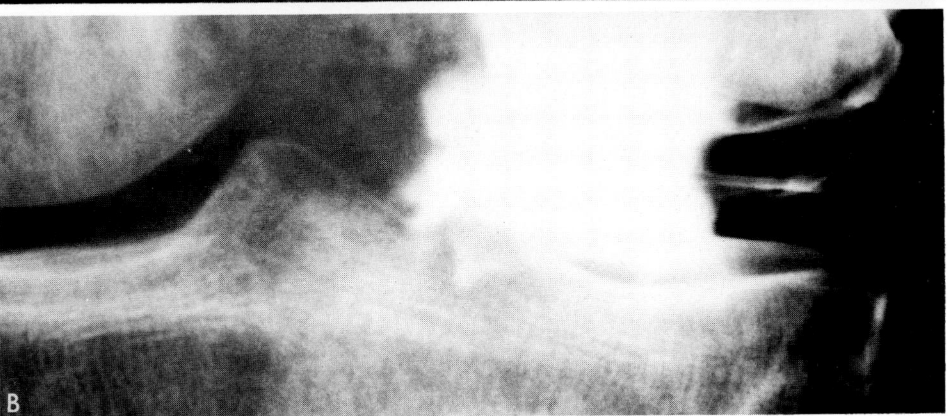

Figure 15–76. *Knee arthrography: Articular adhesions. This man had sustained a gunshot wound to the knee producing a femoral fracture and articular adhesions. Separate injections into the medial* **(A)** *and lateral* **(B)** *compartments were necessary to opacify the entire articular cavity.*

Table 15–9
MULTIPLE FILLING DEFECTS ON KNEE ARTHROGRAMS

Rheumatoid arthritis
Pigmented villonodular synovitis
Idiopathic synovial osteochondromatosis
Hemangioma/angioma
Lipoma aborescens

articular osseous bodies and popliteal cysts.[197] Arthrography in these individuals does have certain limitations: Proper positioning during arthrography in the elderly patient with degenerative disease can be extremely difficult and time consuming; tangential portions of the cartilaginous surface are the only areas that are adequately visualized; and evaluation of patellofemoral disease is difficult, as the patellar cartilage is not well delineated. Despite these shortcomings, arthrography may delineate generalized cartilaginous thinning or localized cartilaginous defects. A rough, irregular surface with imbibition of contrast material may be apparent.

When compared to routine and weight-bearing radiographic films, arthrography adds little additional information regarding alterations in the more involved femorotibial compartment.[197] In the less involved (contralateral) compartment, arthrography may reveal information regarding cartilaginous integrity not obtainable by these other examinations.

Meniscal alterations in patients with degenerative joint disease can include acute tears, similar in appearance to those occurring in patients without

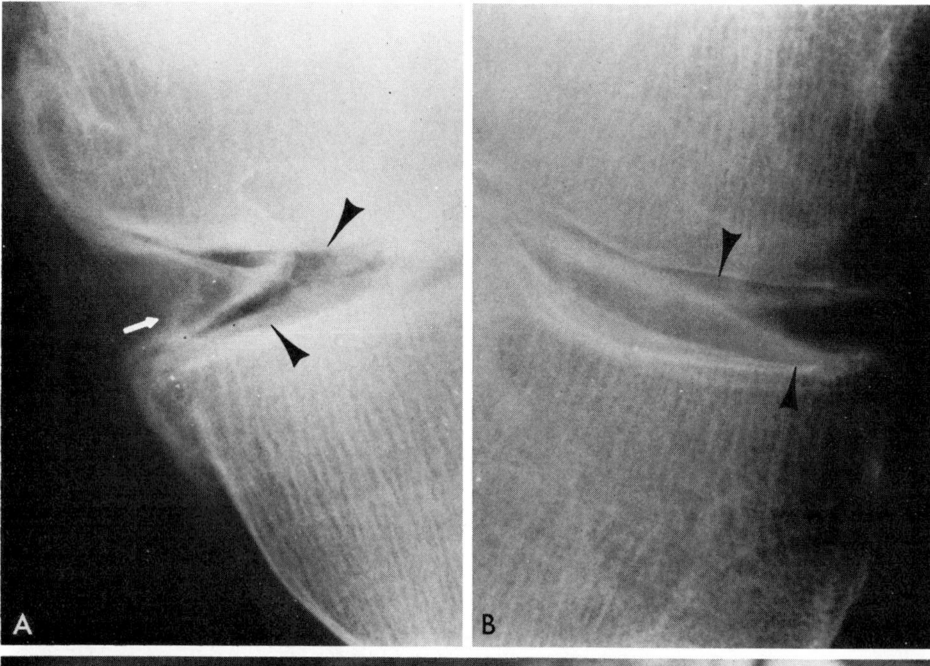

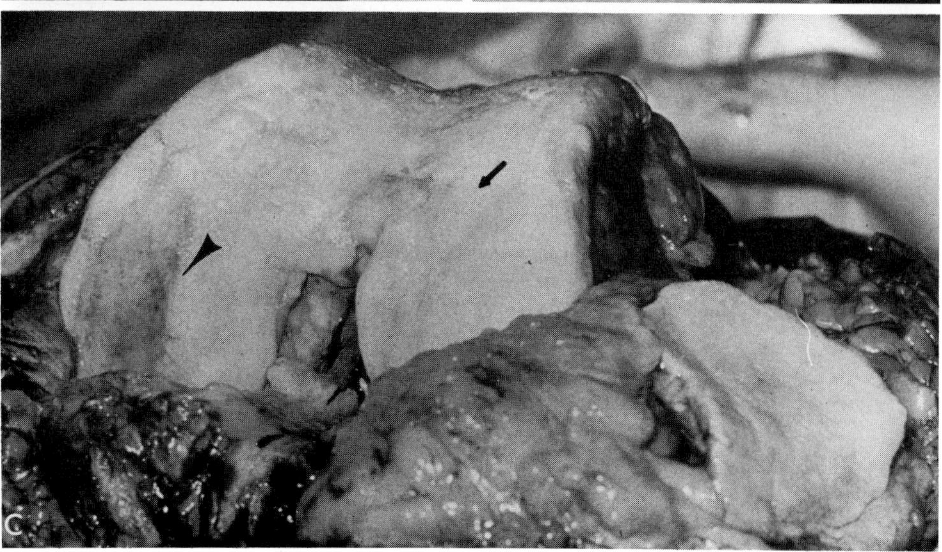

Figure 15–77. *Knee arthrography: Degenerative joint disease. A 56 year old man had left knee pain for 15 years. Initial films revealed more significant medial femorotibial compartment changes than lateral femorotibial compartment abnormalities. Arthrography was performed. In the medial compartment* **(A)** *findings included severe denudation of articular cartilage on both femur and tibia (arrowheads). The medial meniscus is swollen, with an incomplete vertical tear (arrow) and an irregular inner contour. In the lateral compartment* **(B)**, *moderate thinning of articular cartilage can be seen (arrowheads), although the meniscus appears normal. Radionuclide examination confirmed the presence of both medial and lateral compartment abnormalities. During a total knee replacement* **(C)**, *severe abnormalities of the medial compartment (arrowhead) and moderate abnormalities of the lateral compartment (arrow) were detected on the anterior surface of the femur.*

degenerative joint disease, or degenerative tears. These latter tears appear as swollen, irregular meniscal surfaces with fragmented inner contours, and imbibition of contrast material. Horizontal collections of contrast material within the involved meniscus represent degenerative crevices.

Loose or attached bodies in degenerative joint disease may be detected on arthrography. They result from surface disintegration or osteophyte fragmentation. These intra-articular osseous bodies may remain free in the joint cavity or attach at a distant synovial site.

Synovial cyst formation may complicate degenerative joint disease as well as other disorders. This complication is discussed later in this chapter.

Rheumatoid Arthritis (Fig. 15–78). Arthrographic findings have been documented in the knee in rheumatoid arthritis.[205-208] These include enlargement of the joint cavity or suprapatellar pouch, nodular irregularity or corrugation of the synovial membrane, filling defects within the joint cavity, lymphatic filling,[10, 12, 13, 207, 326] and synovial cyst formation. Following synovectomy, these findings may be less marked, although they frequently recur, often as early as 3 months after surgery.

Pigmented Villonodular Synovitis (Fig. 15–79 and 15–80). The knee arthrogram in diffuse pigmented villonodular synovitis reveals an enlarged synovial cavity, irregular synovial outline with "laking" or

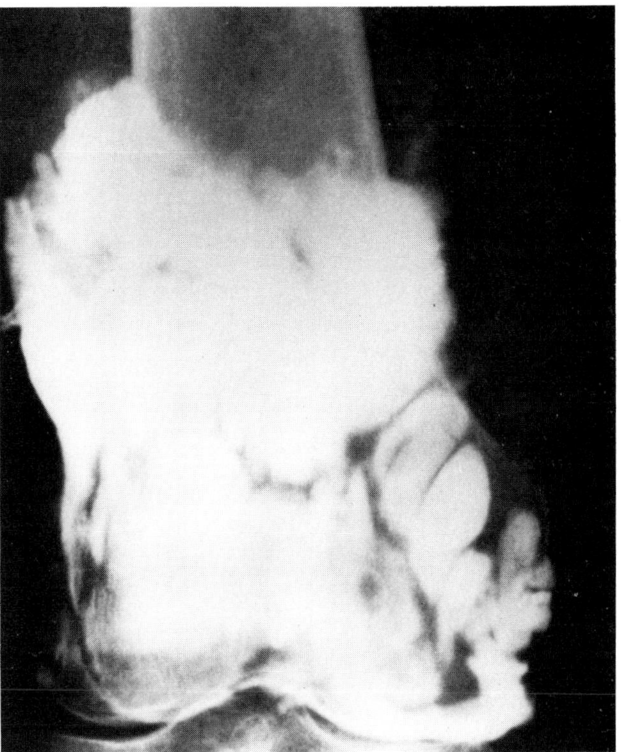

Figure 15–78. *Knee arthrography: Rheumatoid arthritis. Nodular and linear irregularity and pooling of contrast material reflect synovial hypertrophy.*

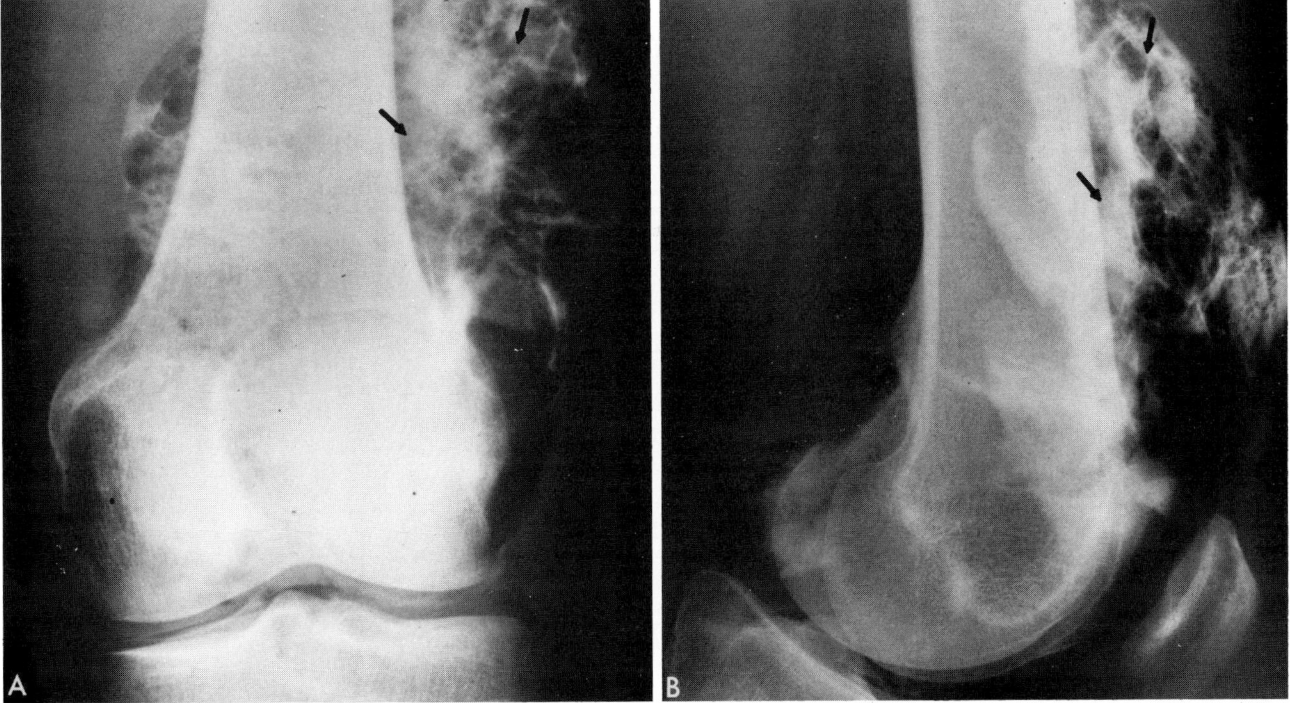

Figure 15–79. *Knee arthrography: diffuse pigmented villonodular synovitis. Observe the irregular distribution and appearance of contrast material (arrows) in the suprapatellar pouch. (From Dalinka MK, et al: CRC Crit Rev Radiol Sci 5:1, 1973.)*

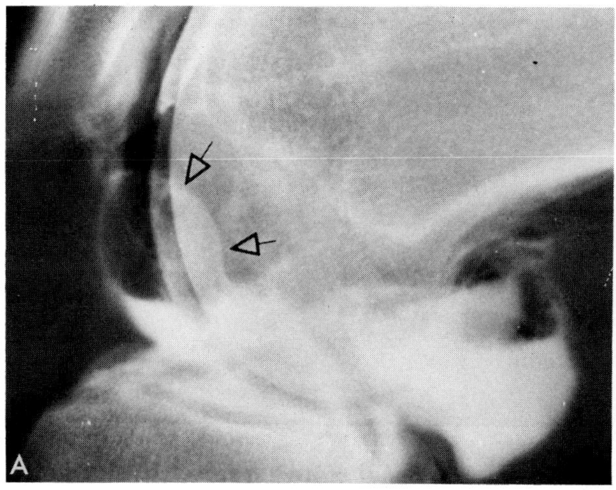
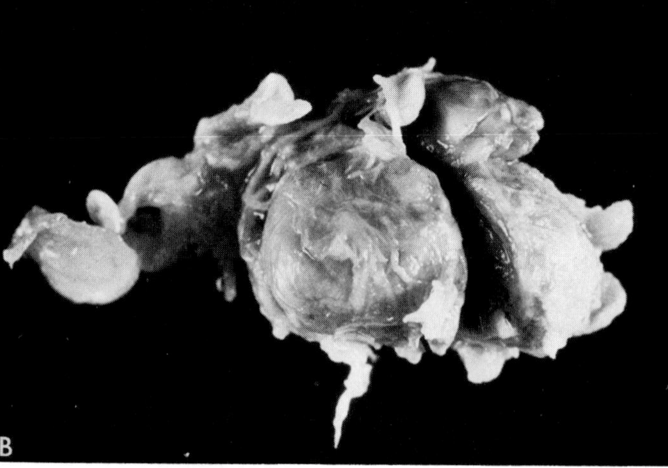
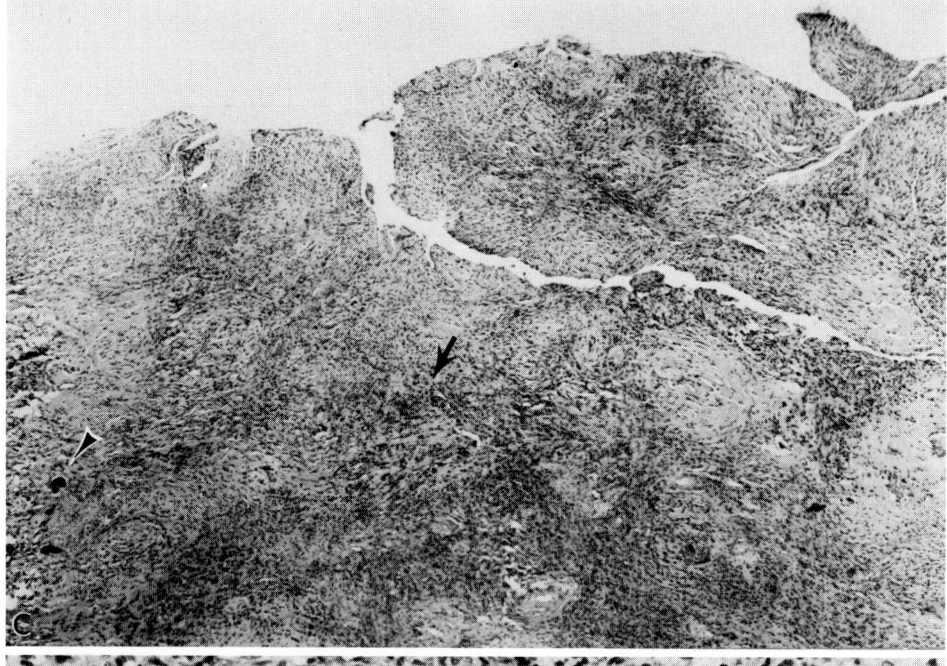
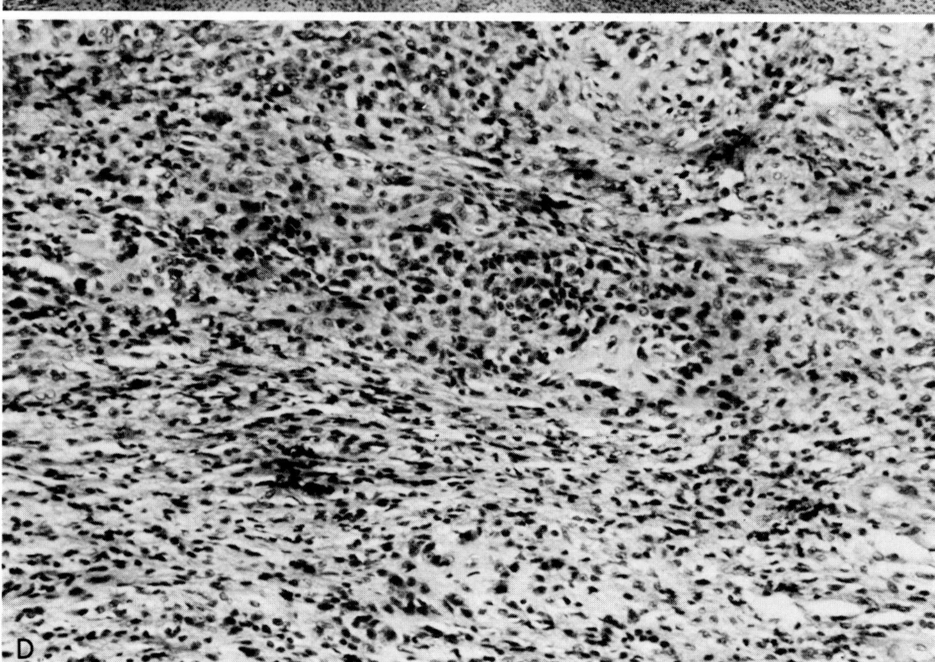

Figure 15–80. Knee arthrography: Localized nodular synovitis.

A, B *This 25 year old man complained of a popping sensation in his knee with intermittent locking. Arthrography* **(A)** *reveals a prominence in the region of the infrapatellar fat pad (arrows). A photograph* **(B)** *of the removed and sectioned specimen reveals a fibrous, well-circumscribed mass.*

C *A photomicrograph (135×) outlines fibrous proliferation with a villonodular pattern, pigmented cells (arrow), and occasional giant cells (arrowhead).*

D *At a higher magnification (540×), round and spindle-shaped cells are seen to be present, with scattered areas of pigmentation.*

Illustration continued on the opposite page

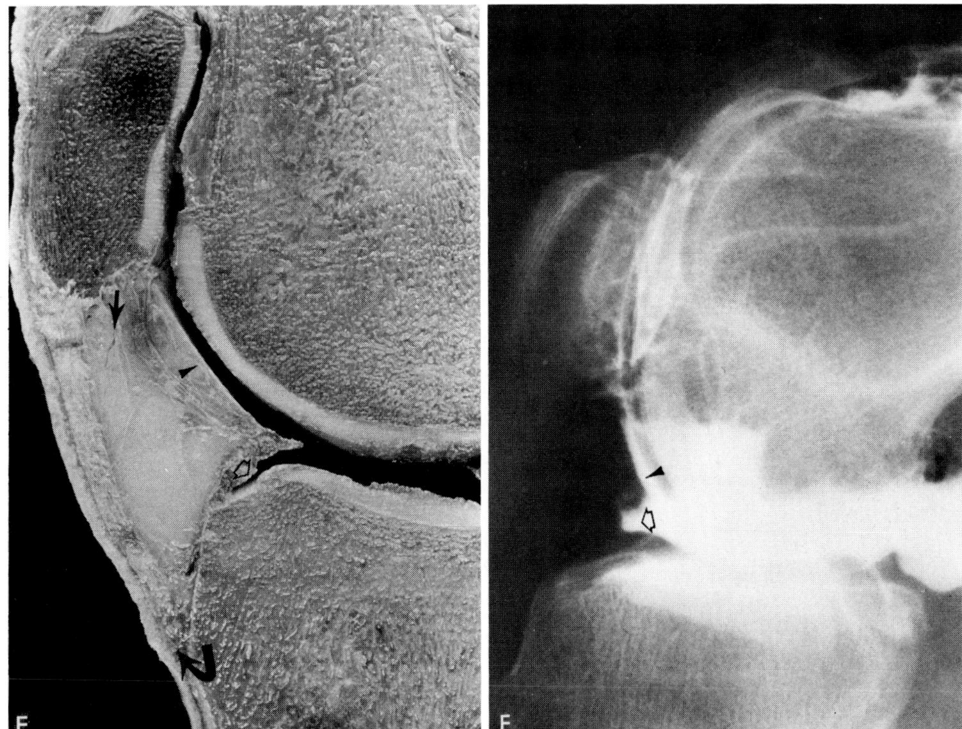

Figure 15–80. Continued

E, F *Anatomy and normal arthrography of the infrapatellar fat pad. A photograph* **(E)** *of a sagittal section of the knee demonstrates the infrapatellar fat pad (straight arrow) beneath the infrapatellar tendon (curved arrow). Synovium is reflected over the fat pad (arrowhead) and the small recess located beneath the fat pad (open arrow). A normal arthrogram* **(F)** *reveals a smooth synovial covering over the fat pad (arrowhead) and a small inferior synovial recess (open arrow) (compare with* **A**).

(From Goergen TG, et al: Am J Roentgenol 126:647, 1976. Copyright 1976, American Roentgen Ray Society.)

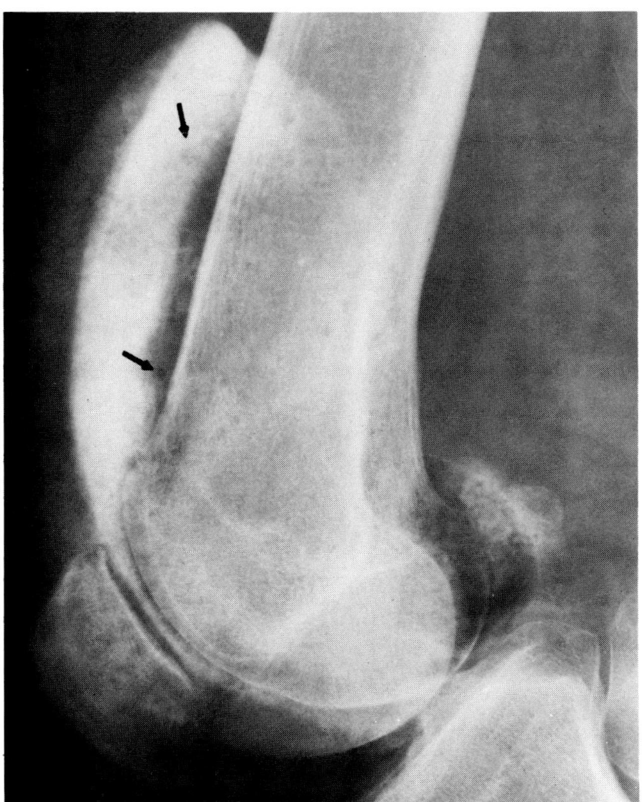

Figure 15–81. Knee arthrography: *Idiopathic synovial osteochondromatosis. Observe multiple sharply defined filling defects (arrows) throughout the articular cavity. (From Dalinka MK, et al: CRC Crit Rev Radiol Sci 5:1, 1973.)*

pooling of contrast material, and nodular filling defects.[209-211]

Arthrographic alterations associated with localized nodular synovitis of the knee may include a mass-like lesion coated with contrast material.[212] Identification of such a mass is important, as patients with this lesion may have symptoms and signs that suggest a mechanical problem.[213] Differential diagnosis of such a mass should include an enlarged infrapatellar fat pad, sometimes termed Hoffa's disease,[214] an intra-articular ganglion arising from the alar fold of synovium,[215] an uncalcified intra-articular body, and other rare synovial tumors, such as fibromas, hemangiomas, and giant cell tumors.[363]

Idiopathic Synovial Osteochondromatosis (Fig. 15–81). Knee arthrography in idiopathic synovial osteochondromatosis reveals an enlarged synovial cavity and multiple small, sharply defined filling defects.[216, 217] Occasionally larger defects are apparent. The nodular lesions of idiopathic synovial osteochondromatosis are better defined than those of pigmented villonodular synovitis.

Lipoma Arborescens. This is a rare intra-articular lesion of unknown etiology, most commonly located in the knee, consisting of focal deposits of fat beneath the swollen synovial lining.[218] Arthrography reveals numerous moderately well defined defects of variable size.[219, 365] Rarely, true lipomas may produce filling defects in the opacified knee.[327]

Synovial Hemangioma. Hemangiomas of the synovial membrane occur most frequently in the knee, although they are also apparent in other articulations, as well as in synovial tendon sheaths.[220-222] Initial radiographs may reveal soft tissue masses, calcified phleboliths, and a hemophilia-like arthropathy with osteoporosis and epiphyseal enlargment.[223] Arthrography may reveal single or multiple radiolucent defects, and arteriography will outline hypervascular tumors.[224] A synovial angioma may have a similar arthrographic appearance.[225]

Hemophilia. Reported arthrographic findings of the knee in hemophilia are synovial irregularity, focal areas of cartilage thinning, and osseous irregularities covered by relatively normal cartilage.[116, 226]

BLOUNT'S DISEASE (Fig. 15–82). Dalinka and co-workers[227] suggested that arthrography in patients with Blount's disease (tibia vara) reveals information that is necessary to evaluate and manage these patients. The plain film findings in this condition are well known and include varus deformity of the proximal tibia, cortical thickening of the medial tibial shaft, and the presence of a bony excrescence on the posteromedial aspect of the proximal tibial metaphysis. The medial aspect of the proximal tibia appears depressed. Arthrography allows analysis of the integrity of the unossified cartilage above the medial tibial plateau, information that can assist the surgeon.[228] If this cartilage is normal, a valgus osteotomy correcting the angular deformity is sufficient treatment; if significant cartilaginous depression is evident, additional surgery may be required to control ligament laxity, including elevation of the tibial plateau.

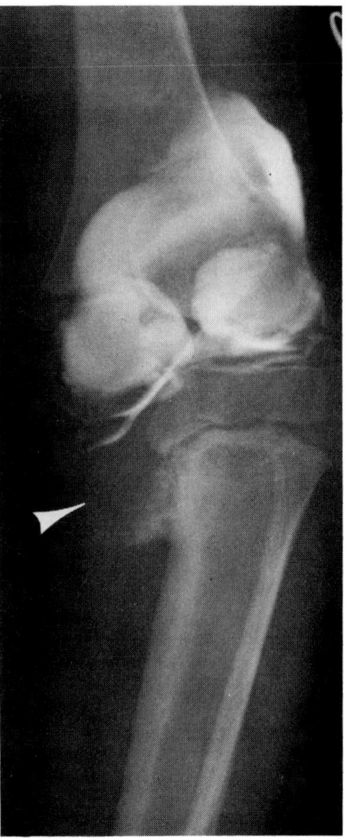

Figure 15–82. *Knee arthrography: Blount's disease. In this 5 year old child, knee arthrography reveals depression of epiphyseal cartilage and metaphyseal bone (arrowhead), with stress fractures of the metaphysis. A tibial osteotomy was performed, which was unsuccessful. (From Dalinka MK, et al: Radiology 113: 161, 1974.)*

PATIENTS WITH SYNOVIAL CYSTS (Fig. 15–83). Synovial cysts about the knee are most frequent in the popliteal region, where communication between the joint and normal posterior bursae can be identified.[229-232] The most commonly involved bursa is the gastrocnemio-semimembranosus bursa, located posterior to the medial femoral condyle between the tendons of the gastrocnemius and semimembranosus muscles, with an additional portion anterior to the medial head of the gastrocnemius. The anterior limit of this bursa abuts the posterior surface of the joint capsule and is relatively thin.[229] Communication between the bursa and the knee joint occurs in 35 to 55 per cent of cadavers[229, 231] and increases in frequency with advancing age. This communication occurs via a transverse slit, usually between 15 to 20 mm in size.[229] The opening may be covered with a fibrous membrane in approximately 70 per cent of cases.[229]

Swelling of this posterior bursa is termed a Baker's cyst.[233] The etiology of such cysts is not entirely clear, and various theories have been proposed: (1) Herniation of the synovial membrane of the knee through a weak area in the posterior joint capsule; (2)

rupture of the posterior joint capsule with extravasation of fluid into the soft tissues and secondary encapsulation; (3) rupture of the posterior joint capsule, producing communication with a normally occurring posterior bursa. Of these theories, the third theory seems most probable,[220-231, 234, 235] as direct observation has never documented a synovial herniation from the knee into a normal bursa nor a popliteal cyst completely separated from the articular cavity.

The presence of a slit between articular cavity and posterior bursa may be responsible for a ball-valve mechanism that has been noted in conjunction with synovial cysts[236, 237, 350]; fluid introduced into a cyst may not enter the joint cavity. Because of this one-way directional flow, arthrography rather than bursography is more accurate in defining the extent of a cyst and its connection with a neighboring joint.

In addition to the gastrocnemio-semimembrano-

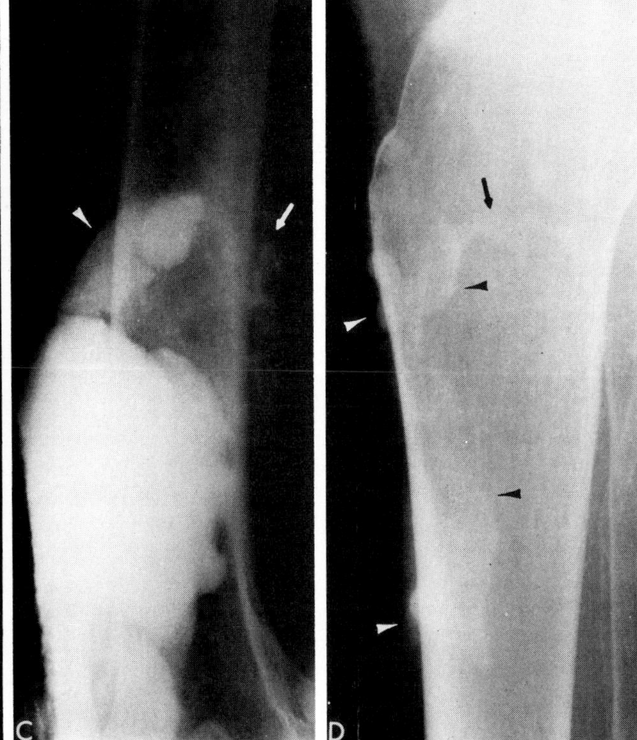

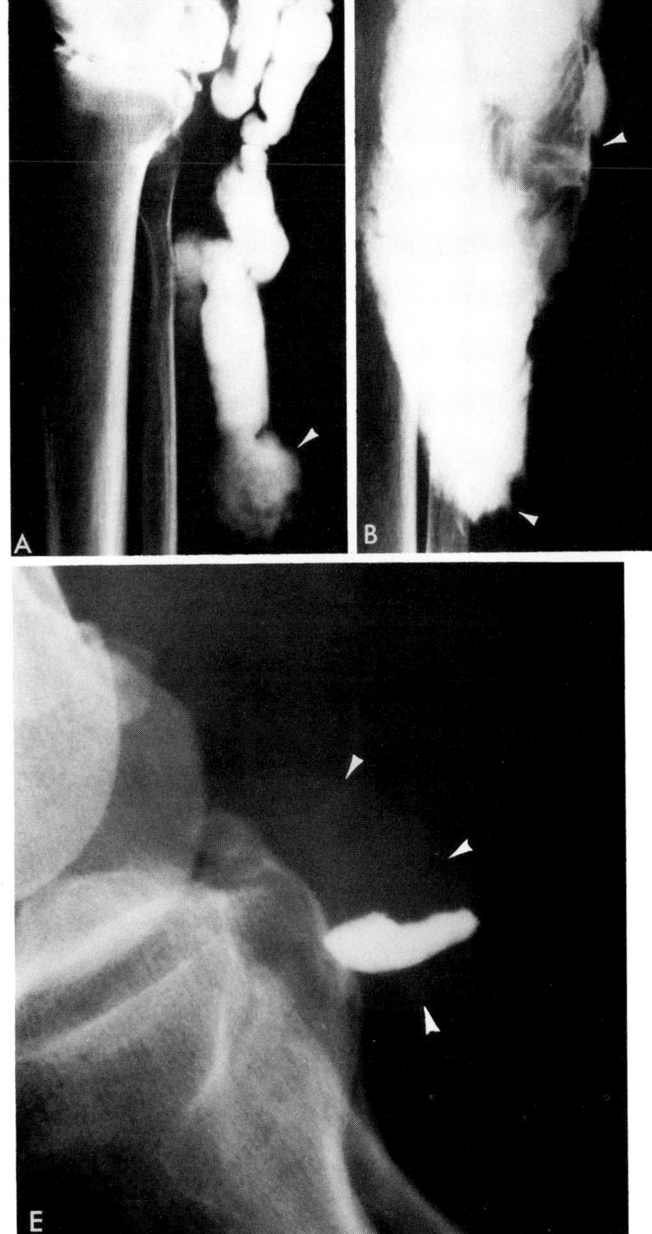

Figure 15–83. Knee arthrography: Synovial cyst formation.

A *Rheumatoid arthritis. A typical large popliteal cyst extending into the calf is filled with contrast material. It is slightly irregular in contour, particularly inferiorly (arrowhead), which may reflect synovial inflammation. No free extravasation into the soft tissues is seen.*

B *Rheumatoid arthritis. Another popliteal cyst extending behind the tibia. It has an irregular, feathery appearance (arrowheads) consistent with tissue extravasation.*

C *Rheumatoid arthritis. Extension of suprapatellar pouch. On this lateral view of the pouch following arthrography, note the cystic extension superiorly (arrowhead) with adjacent lymphatic filling (arrow).*

D *Rheumatoid arthritis. A synovial cyst has extended from the joint (arrow) along the anterior surface of the tibia (arrowheads).*

E *Bullet-induced "lead" bursogram. Dissolution of metallic particles has produced a spontaneous swelling of the bursa (arrowheads) following a gunshot wound.*

sus bursa, a second posterior bursa is located beneath the popliteal tendon,[232] which communicates less frequently with the joint. A third posterior bursa exists between the medial head of the gastrocnemius and the distal end of the biceps. A weak point occurs laterally beneath the popliteal tendon, which may represent an extended popliteal tendon sheath.[16, 232] Furthermore, communication may exist between the knee and proximal tibiofibular joint cavity in 10 per cent of adults. Occasionally, anterior, medial, and lateral synovial cysts may also be observed.[238, 347]

Any of these synovial cysts may enlarge, producing a mass with or without pain. Rupture of a cyst is associated with soft tissue extravasation of fluid contents. Ruptures occurring posteriorly can simulate thrombophlebitis,[348] and, in fact, the two conditions can coexist.[239-241, 328] Giant synovial cysts can extend into the calf, ankle, heel, and thigh.[242-245]

Arthrography of the knee is an accurate method of diagnosing synovial cysts,[246-251] although some investigators also recommend ultrasonic[252-257] or isotopic[258] examination in this clinical situation. Computed tomography appears of little value in diagnosing these cysts.[259] Routine overhead films after injection of contrast material will usually reveal the synovial cyst, although specialized techniques may be helpful, including radiography after Ace bandage wrapping of the suprapatellar pouch, exercise, and standing. Knee flexion will accentuate filling of the posterior bursae,[251] probably related to widening of the communicating slit between bursa and joint cavity and compression of the suprapatellar pouch between the quadriceps tendon and anterior surface of the femur. Cineradiography will document the "to-and-fro" movement of fluid between these two structures, although demonstration of a small posterior synovial cyst, particularly during knee flexion, may not indicate a pathologic situation and must be differentiated from the normal bulging of the posterior capsule of the knee joint that occurs in this position.[230]

The arthrographic appearance of an abnormal synovial cyst will vary. In most instances, a well-defined, lobulated structure filled with air and radiopaque contrast material will be revealed. It may have an irregular surface related to hypertrophy of its synovial lining and be associated with adjacent lymphatic filling. Alternatively, the entire cyst or a portion of it may rupture,[260, 261] with extravasation of contrast material into soft tissues posteriorly, or less commonly, superiorly or anteriorly.[238, 247, 250]

Any inflammatory, degenerative, traumatic, or neoplastic condition that produces a knee effusion can lead to synovial cyst formation. These conditions include rheumatoid arthritis, degenerative joint disease, gout, pigmented villonodular synovitis, and idiopathic synovial osteochondromatosis, as well as other localized or systemic articular conditions. In the absence of any obvious cause, one must search diligently for meniscal abnormality. Synovial cysts may be noted in children with juvenile chronic polyarthritis[262] or on a familial basis.[263] Surgical removal of synovial cysts without treatment of the underlying articular disease process is rarely successful, as the cyst will recur.[349, 364]

Accuracy of Knee Arthrography. The accuracy of this examination in detecting abnormalities of the knee, particularly meniscal alterations, depends primarily on the quality of the study and the expertise of the observer. In the hands of a skilled radiologist, the accuracy rate of diagnosing medial meniscal tears in patients who have these tears documented at surgery may reach 99 per cent; similarly, the accuracy in diagnosing lateral meniscal tears can approximate 93 per cent.[134] False negative arthrograms in patients with meniscal tears or false positive arthrograms in patients without tears are rare if the examination is performed carefully by experienced radiologists.[329] Since arthrography can be a safe and reliable procedure in diagnosing meniscal abnormalities, it should be preferred over arthroscopy in this clinical situation, or, at the very least, should be combined with arthroscopy.[351-353] Arthroscopy appears to be more accurate for meniscal lesions involving the central edge and anterior horn; arthrography is more sensitive to midbody and peripheral meniscal tears. The arthrographic diagnosis of other conditions, such as cruciate lesions and chondromalacia, is less accurate.

ANKLE AND FOOT

Ankle Arthrography (Table 15–10)

Injuries of the ankle are a common problem and may lead to considerable disability. Orthopedic surgeons do not agree on the proper mode of therapy for treatment of ankle ligament "sprains"; some recommend surgical intervention, whereas others advocate conservative treatment. It is because of this disagreement that the number of requests for ankle arthrography varies from one institution to another, the procedure being utilized particularly by physicians who believe in operative treatment of ankle sprains. Contrast opacification of the ankle allows identifica-

Table 15–10

INDICATIONS FOR ANKLE ARTHROGRAPHY

Evaluation of:
Ligamentous injuries
Transchondral fractures
Intra-articular osseous and cartilaginous bodies
Adhesive capsulitis

tion and delineation of ligamentous injuries and can be combined effectively with routine and stress radiography of the ankle.

TECHNIQUE (Fig. 15–84). Arthrographic technique[264-266] has been well described. Ideally, the examination should be performed within a few days of the acute injury as blood and tissue adhesions about the ligamentous tear may result in false negative examinations if the procedure is delayed.[264, 265]

The procedure is accomplished in the recumbent position under fluoroscopic control. Both supine and lateral fluoroscopy may be necessary. A metal marker is placed over the anteromedial portion of the ankle, approximately 1 cm below the joint line. A 20 gauge, 1.5 inch needle is introduced into the ankle under fluoroscopic guidance after cleaning the skin and applying local anesthesia. Six to 10 ml of 60 per cent methylglucamine diatrizoate (Renografin) is injected, which may be mixed with approximately 1 ml of lidocaine. The needle is withdrawn and radiographs are exposed in anteroposterior, oblique, and lateral projections following mild exercise of the ankle. Stress radiographs may also be obtained.

NORMAL ANKLE ARTHROGRAM (Fig. 15–85). Under normal circumstances, ankle arthrography results in opacification of the articular cavity without evidence of extra-articular leak except for filling of the tendon sheath of the flexor hallucis longus or the flexor digitorum longus, or both in approximately 20 per cent of patients.[264-268] The posterior subtalar joint will be opacified in approximately 10 per cent of patients. All other patterns of contrast extravasation are regarded as abnormal.

The normal ankle arthrogram reveals three recesses. In the region of the syndesmosis between distal tibia and fibula, a small vertical recess, best delineated on oblique radiographs, extends 1 to 2.5 cm in height and is approximately 4 mm in width.[267] Additional anterior and posterior recesses are best observed on lateral radiographs. All three recesses should be smooth and well delineated.

LIGAMENTOUS INJURIES (Fig. 15–86 and 15–87). Arthrographic abnormalities associated with ligamentous injuries have been well described[264-274] and require an understanding of pertinent anatomy of the ankle.[275]

Anterior Talofibular Ligament Injury. This ligament extends from the anterior surface of the distal fibula to the talar neck. It is most susceptible to injury. With tears, contrast material will be seen both inferior and lateral to the distal fibula on frontal radiographs and anterior to the distal fibula on lateral radiographs. Occasionally, on anteroposterior views, the contrast material will overlie the syndesmosis.

Calcaneofibular Ligament Injury. This strong ligament originates from the posterior aspect of the distal fibula and inserts on the superior aspect of the calcaneus. When this ligament is torn, contrast material fills the peroneal tendon sheaths as the inner aspect of the sheaths is also torn. Tears of the

Text continued on page 603

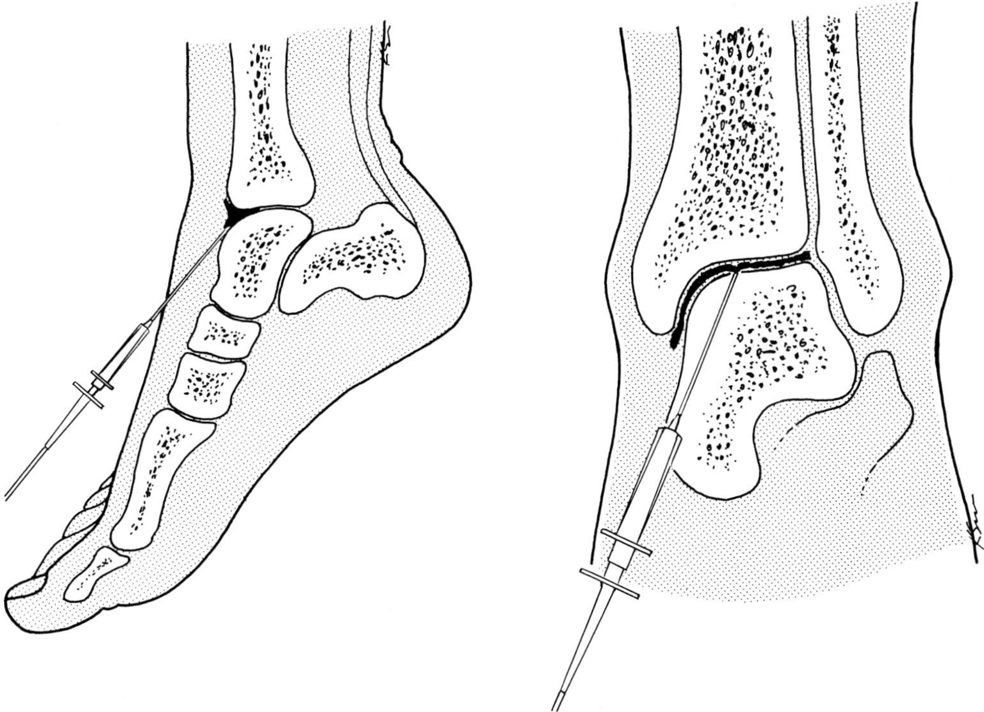

Figure 15–84. *Ankle arthrography: Technique. A needle is inserted from an anterior approach into the tibiotalar joint.*

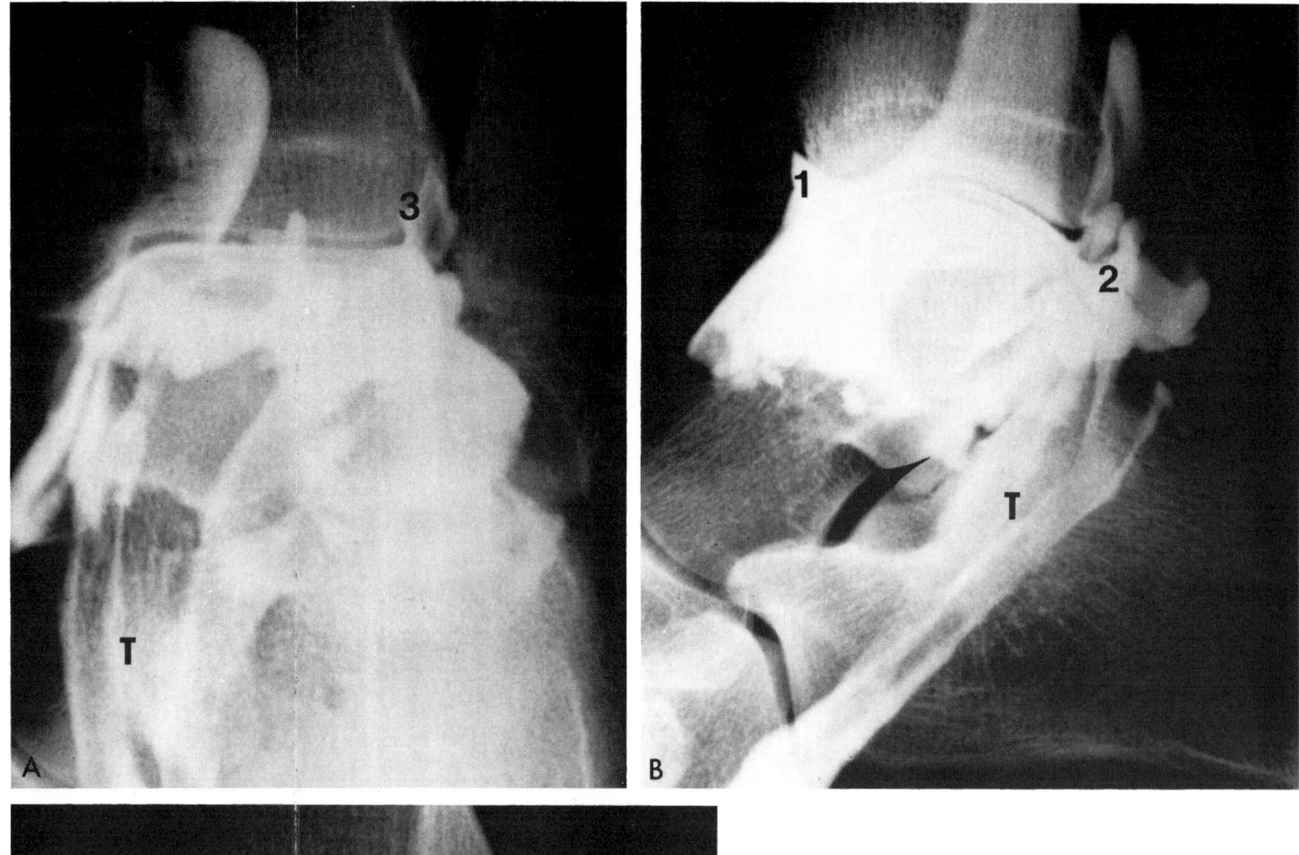

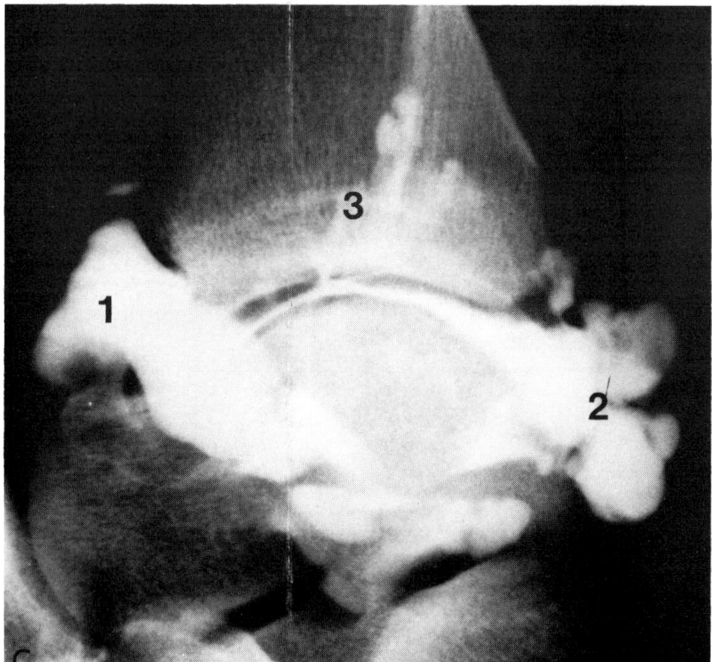

Figure 15–85. *Ankle arthrography: Normal arthrogram.*

A, B *Anteroposterior* **(A)** *and lateral* **(B)** *views. The tibiotalar joint has been opacified. Note the normal recesses: anterior recess (1), posterior recess (2), and syndesmotic recess (3). Filling of the medial tendon sheaths (T) and posterior subtalar joint (arrowhead) is a normal finding.*

C *Lateral view on another patient showing prominent (but normal) anterior (1), posterior (2), and syndesmotic (3) recesses.*

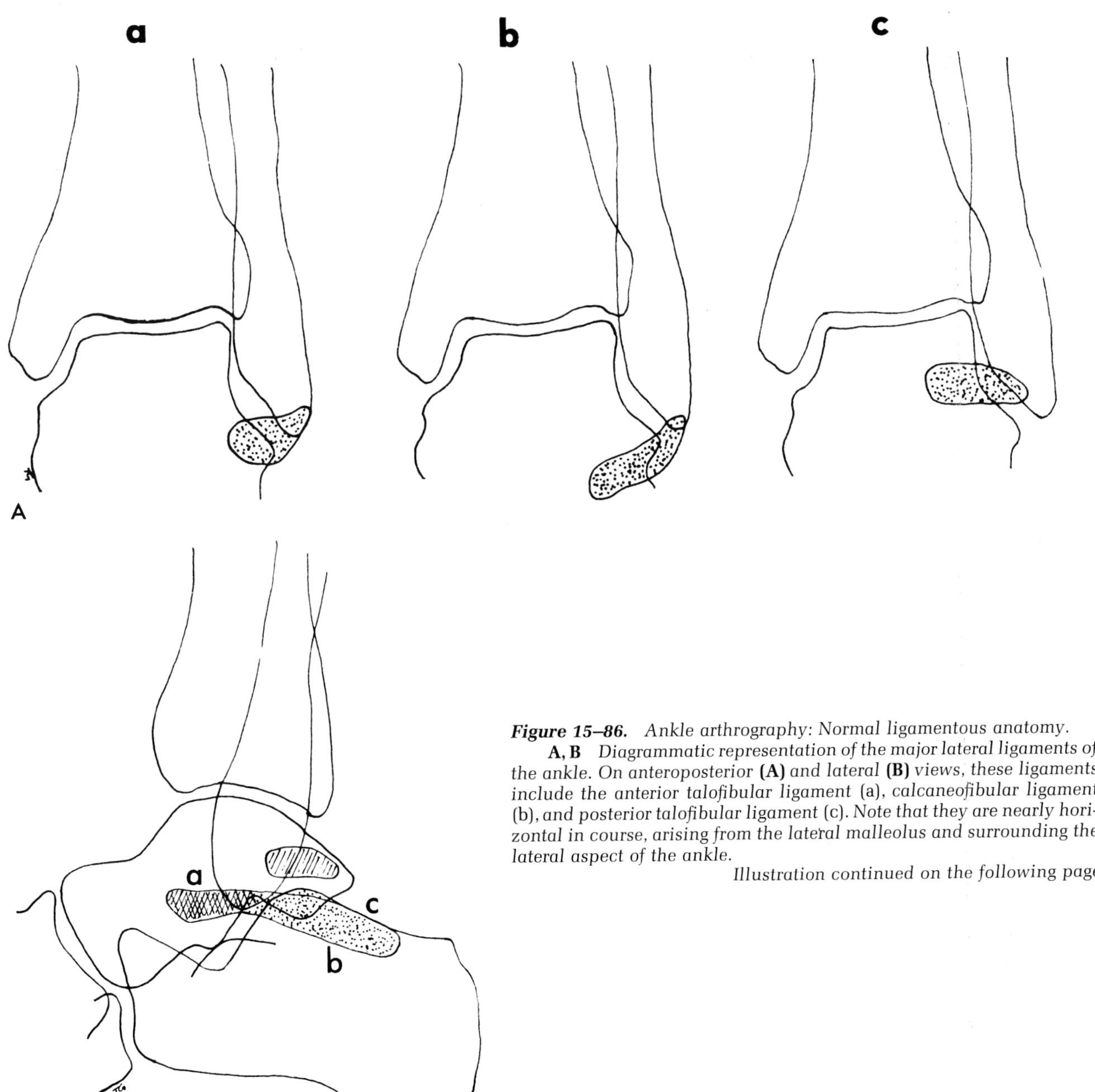

Figure 15–86. *Ankle arthrography: Normal ligamentous anatomy.*

A, B *Diagrammatic representation of the major lateral ligaments of the ankle. On anteroposterior* **(A)** *and lateral* **(B)** *views, these ligaments include the anterior talofibular ligament (a), calcaneofibular ligament (b), and posterior talofibular ligament (c). Note that they are nearly horizontal in course, arising from the lateral malleolus and surrounding the lateral aspect of the ankle.*

Illustration continued on the following page

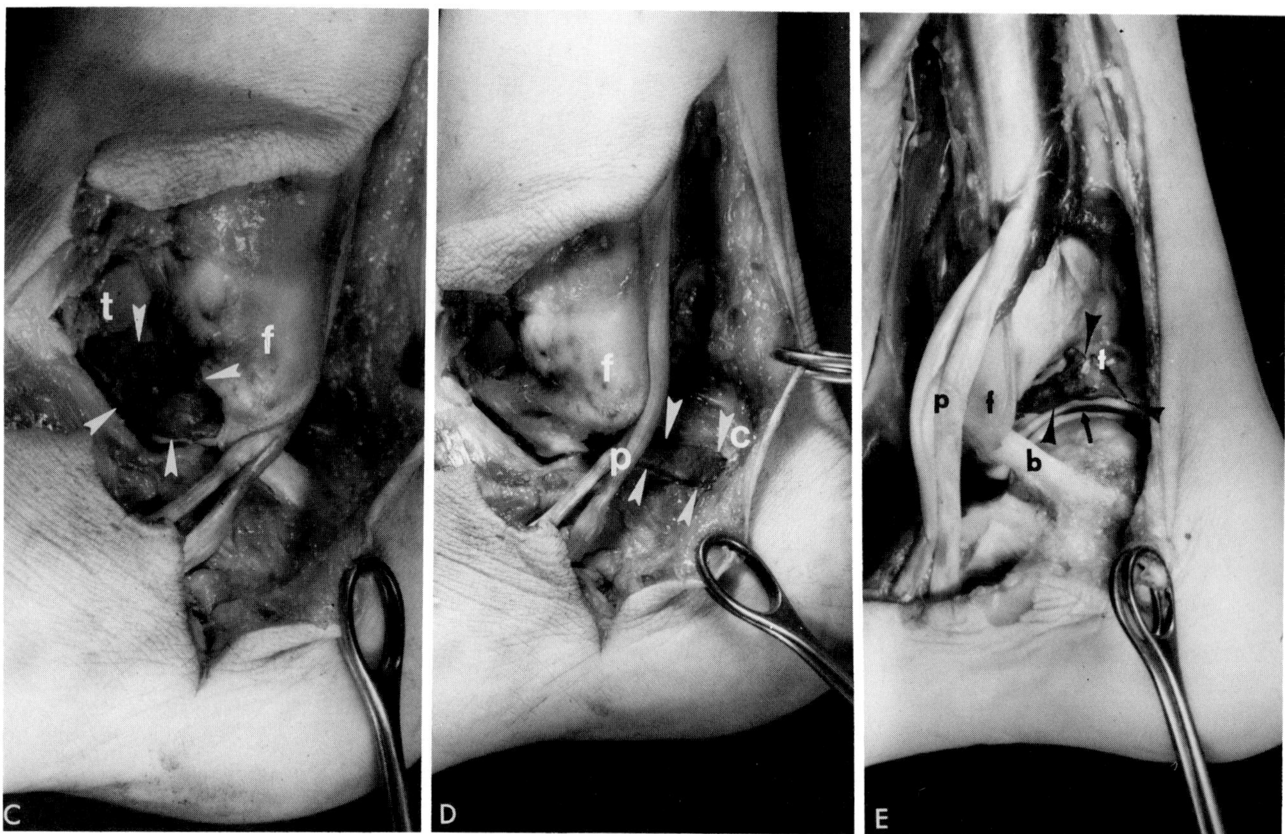

Figure 15–86. Continued

C–E *Dissection identifying the major lateral ligaments of the ankle (ligaments are painted with tantalum). The anterior talofibular ligament* **(C)** *(arrowheads) extends from the distal end of the fibula* (f) *to the talus* (t). *The calcaneofibular ligament* **(D)** *(arrowheads) originates from the posterior aspect of the distal fibula* (f) *and inserts on the superior aspect of the calcaneus* (c). *It is intimate with the tendons of the peroneal muscles* (p). *The posterior talofibular ligament* **(E)** *(arrowheads) extends from the fibula* (f) *to the talus* (t). *Note its relationship to the calcaneofibular ligament* (b), *peroneal tendons* (p), *and posterior subtalar joint (arrow).*

Illustration continued on the opposite page

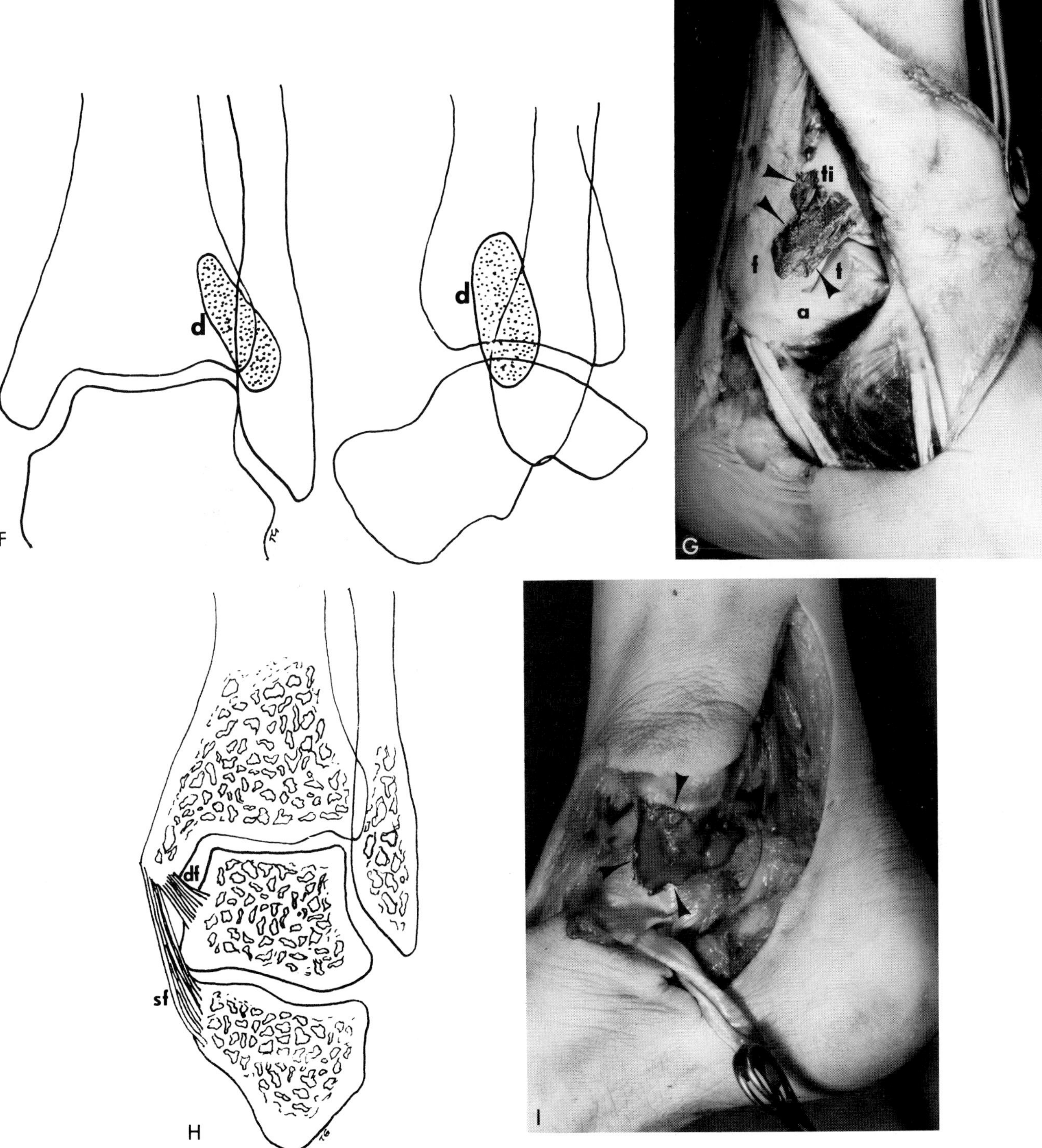

Figure 15–86. Continued

F *Diagrammatic representation of the distal anterior tibiofibular ligament* (d) *on anteroposterior and lateral views. This ligament extends from the anterior and lateral aspects of the distal tibia to the anterior portion of the distal fibula.*

G *Dissection of ankle to reveal the distal anterior tibiofibular ligament (arrowheads). In this anterior oblique view, the ligament can be traced from its origin on the tibia* (ti) *to its insertion on the fibula* (f). *It is located above the dome of the talus* (t) *and the anterior talofibular ligament* (a).

H *Diagrammatic representation of a coronal section through the deltoid ligament. Superficial* (sf) *and deep* (df) *fibers are evident.*

I *Dissection of ankle to reveal the deltoid ligament. On this lateral view, the tantalum-coated deep fibers of the ligament (arrowheads) are seen. The posterior tibial tendon and long flexor tendons are held by the clamp.*

(**A, B, F, H,** *Courtesy of Dr. T. Goergen, Palomar Memorial Hospital, Escondido, California;* **C–E, G, I,** *from Kaye JJ, Bohne WH: Radiology* 125: 659, 1977.)

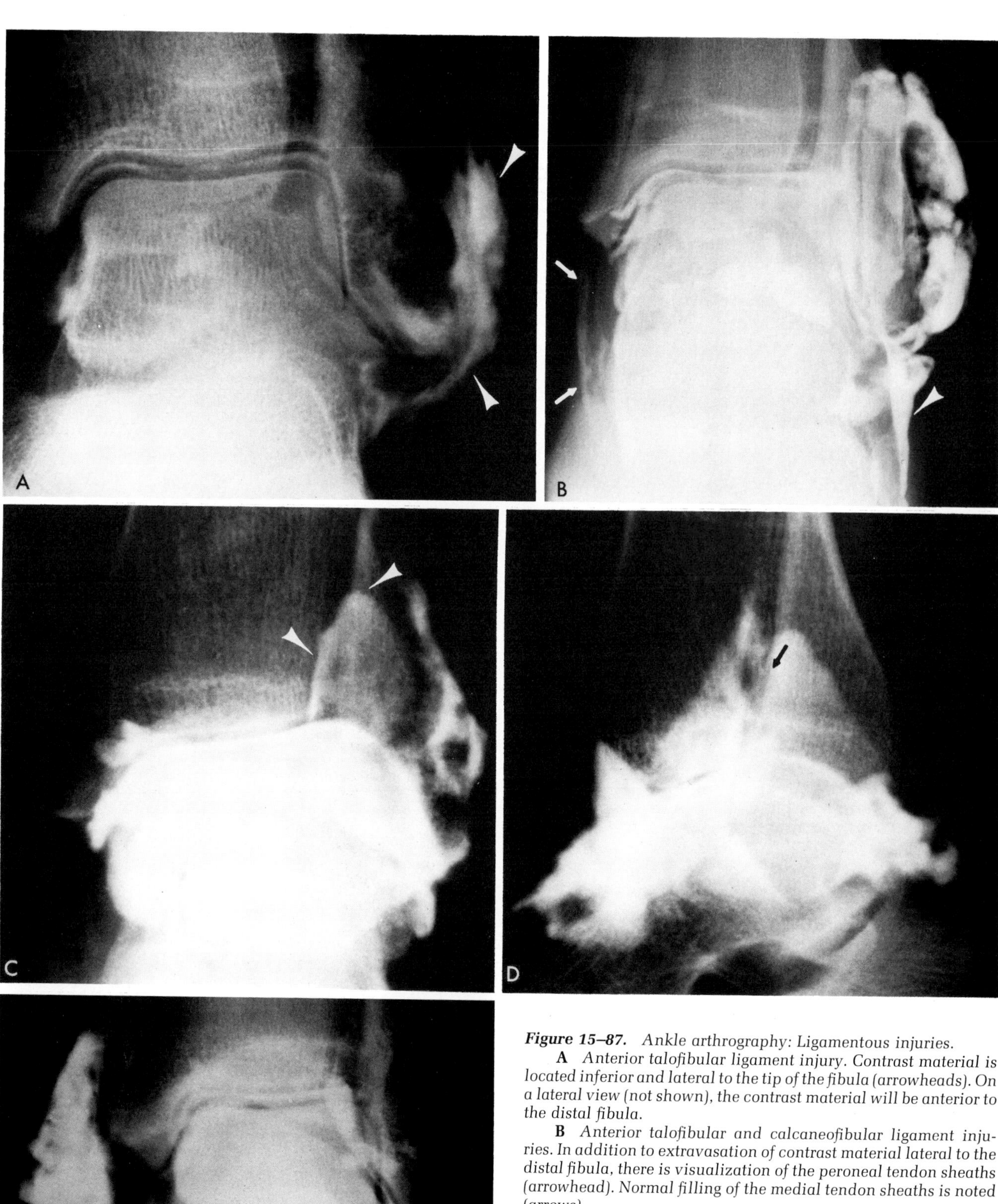

Figure 15–87. *Ankle arthrography: Ligamentous injuries.*

A *Anterior talofibular ligament injury. Contrast material is located inferior and lateral to the tip of the fibula (arrowheads). On a lateral view (not shown), the contrast material will be anterior to the distal fibula.*

B *Anterior talofibular and calcaneofibular ligament injuries. In addition to extravasation of contrast material lateral to the distal fibula, there is visualization of the peroneal tendon sheaths (arrowhead). Normal filling of the medial tendon sheaths is noted (arrows).*

C, D *Distal anterior tibiofibular ligament injury. Oblique* **(C)** *and lateral* **(D)** *views reveal extravasation between the distal tibia and fibula (arrowheads). The normal clear zone anterior to the distal fibula has been obliterated (arrow).*

E *Deltoid ligament injury. There is contrast material, which is extravasated beneath and medial to the medial malleolus (arrowhead).*

calcaneofibular ligament are associated with tears of the anterior talofibular ligament,[354] so that the arthrographic findings of both ligament injuries are apparent. A third ligament, the posterior talofibular ligament, may also be injured in these instances.

Distal Anterior Tibiofibular Ligament Injury. This structure extends from the anterior and lateral aspects of the distal tibia to the adjacent anterior portion of the distal fibula. After injury to this ligament, extravasation of contrast material occurs between distal tibia and fibula, beyond the syndesmotic recess.

Deltoid Ligament Injury. This ligament originates from the medial malleolus and extends to the talus and calcaneus. With tears of the deltoid ligament, contrast material extravasates beyond the medial confines of the joint.

The amount of contrast extravasation following any of these ligament tears is dependent upon many factors, including the volume of contrast material injected, the degree of surrounding soft tissue injury, the presence of scar tissue from previous injuries, and the length of time from injury to arthrography.[264] Arthrography performed after considerable delay may not reveal the presence of ligamentous injury; arthrography performed after appropriate conservative or operative therapy may not demonstrate previously evident abnormalities.[265]

Ankle arthrography is a reliable method of delineating these ligamentous injuries. Its reported accuracy is 75 to 90 per cent.[268, 269] Some observers report less success, particularly in diagnosing double injuries of the lateral ligaments.[266] In these cases, massive extravasation related to one injury may obscure extravasation related to a second injury.

Any of these ankle injuries may be associated with abnormalities on plain films, including soft tissue swelling and avulsion fractures at the osseous sites of attachment of the specific ligament. Furthermore, stress roentgenography may indicate ligament weakening by revealing abnormal widening of the joint.[366]

Other Traumatic Disorders

Transchondral Fracture (Fig. 15–88). Osteochondral fractures (osteochondritis dissecans) of the talar dome are not infrequent.[276-277] Arthrography in this situation will outline the integrity of the overlying cartilage and the presence of intra-articular cartilaginous bodies. The arthrographic technique should be modified so that air alone or air with 1 to 2 ml of radiopaque contrast material is utilized.

Soft Tissue and Bony Intra-articular Debris (Fig. 15–89). As noted above, arthrography may outline pieces of cartilage or cartilage and bone within the joint cavity following ankle trauma. In addition, a mass consisting of hyalinized connective tissue may lodge between fibula and talus following an inversion sprain,[278] leading to persistent or intermittent pain over the lateral aspect of the ankle. Arthrography can delineate the abnormal tissue in this condition.

Adhesive Capsulitis (Fig. 15–90). Posttraumatic adhesive capsulitis in the ankle has been described.[79, 355] This condition, which has classically been recognized as a complication of trauma about the shoulder, is not confined to the shoulder joint but may occur elsewhere. In the ankle, patients develop restricted motion following trauma to bone or soft tissue. Arthrography delineates a decrease in the articular capacity, with resistance to injection of contrast material, obliteration of normal anterior and

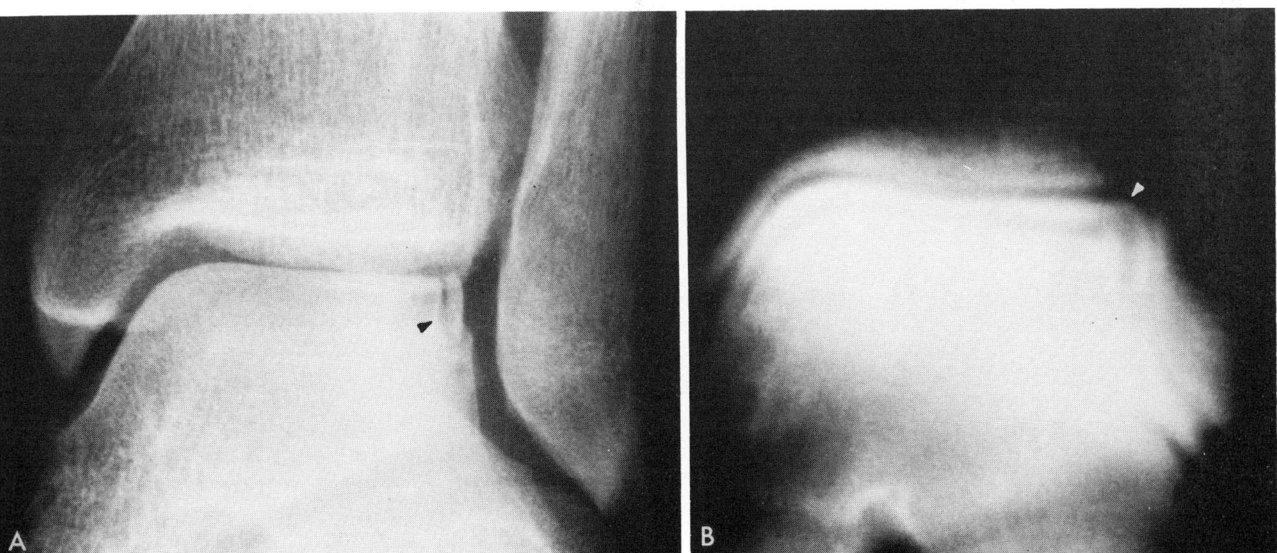

Figure 15–88. *Ankle arthrography: Transchondral fractures.*

A *A small bony density is seated within an osseous defect (arrowhead) on the lateral aspect of the talus.*

B *On arthrotomography, there is smooth articular cartilage over the lesion without evidence of separation of the fragment (arrowhead).*

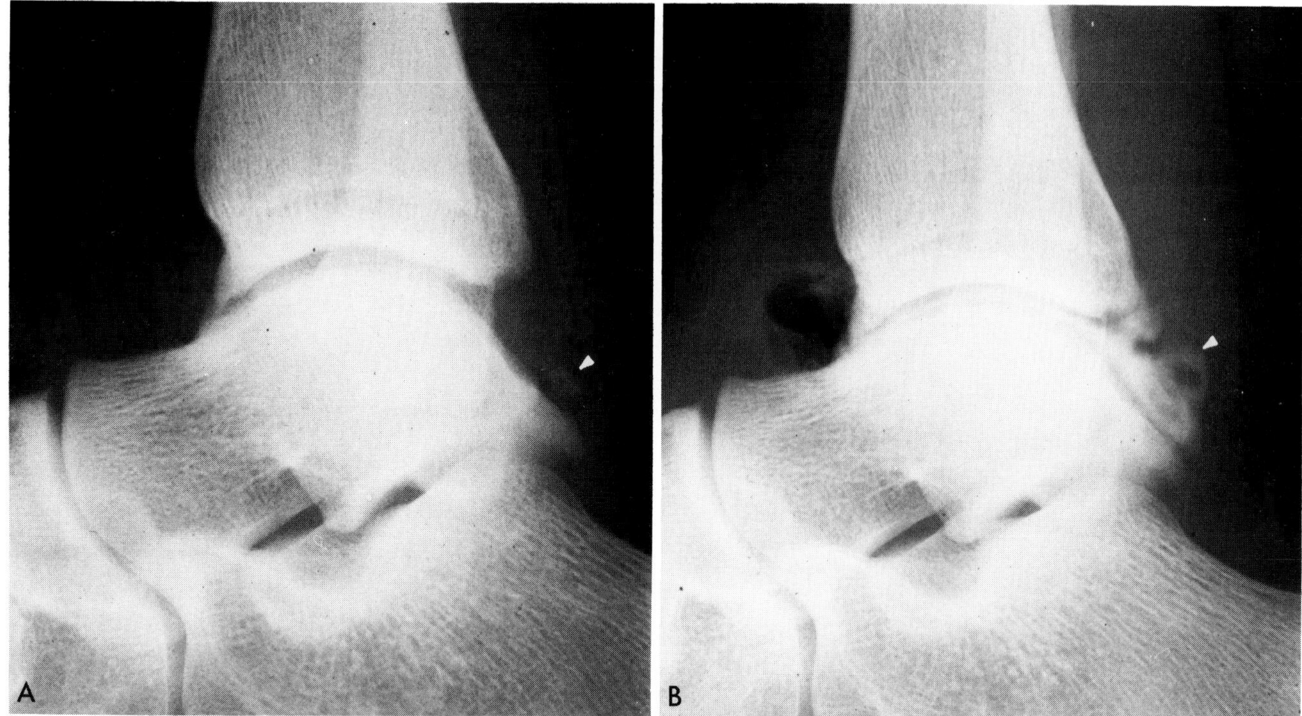

Figure 15–89. Ankle arthrography: Intra-articular osseous body.

A *An initial radiograph demonstrates an osseous dense area (arrowhead) adjacent to the talus.*

B *Arthrography confirms its intra-articular location, the dense region producing a filling defect (arrowhead) in the contrast-filled joint cavity.*

(Courtesy of Dr. M. K. Dalinka, University of Pennsylvania, Philadelphia, Pennsylvania.)

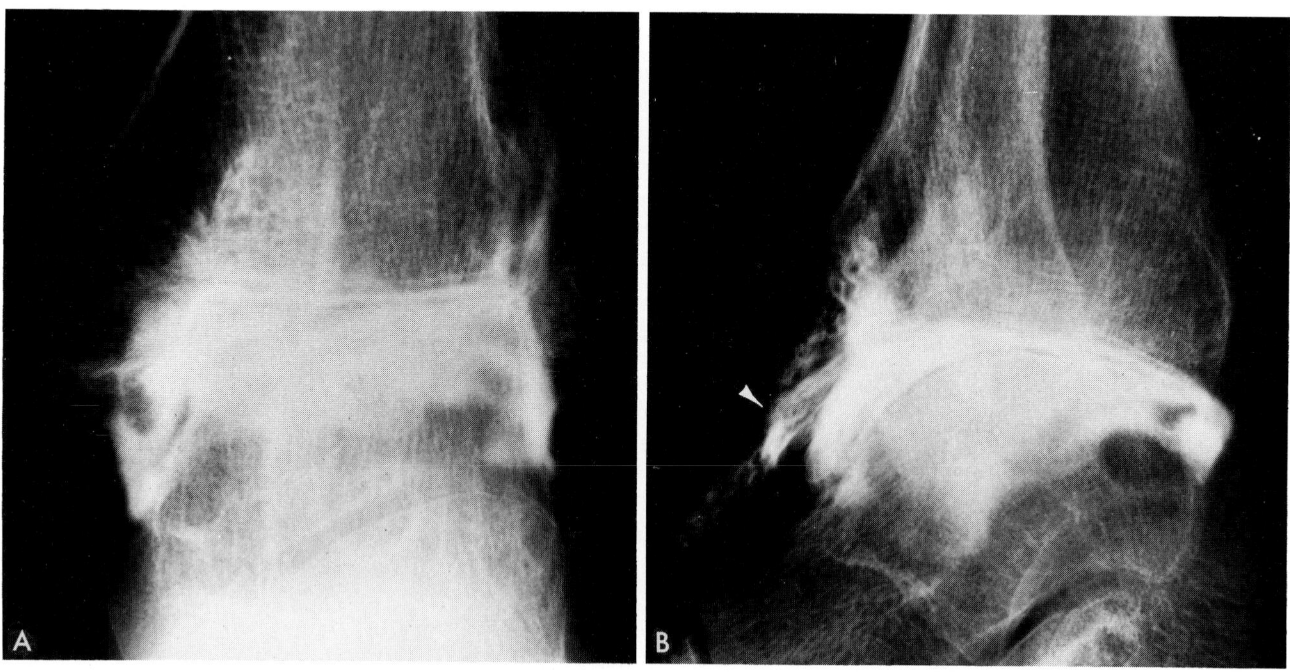

Figure 15–90. *Ankle arthrography: Adhesive capsulitis. The oblique view* **(A)** *reveals decreased joint volume and irregularities of capsular attachment. On the lateral view* **(B)**, *there is no filling of normal anterior and posterior recesses, and there is extravasation of contrast material along the needle track (arrowhead).*

posterior recesses or tibiofibular syndesmosis, and extravasation of contrast material along the needle tract.

RHEUMATOID ARTHRITIS. As in other joints, rheumatoid arthritis of the ankle may be delineated with arthrography.[22] A nodular corrugated synovial pattern, diminished cartilaginous surface, and lymphatic filling may be apparent. On rare occasions, synovial cysts may be delineated.

Peroneal Tenography

Contrast opacification of the peroneal tendons (peroneal tenography) may provide useful information in patients with articular or traumatic disorders.[279, 280, 356, 357]

TECHNIQUE. Following administration of local anesthesia, a 22 gauge, 1.5 inch needle is inserted into the common peroneal sheath above the lateral malleolus. The tendon can easily be palpated in this region, and the needle is advanced in an inferior direction until firm resistance is met. Under fluoroscopic control, 10 to 20 ml of methylglucamine diatrizoate (Renografin) is administered and traced as the material flows in an inferior and superior direction along the sheath. Radiographs are taken in anteroposterior, lateral, and oblique projections. An anteroposterior "tunnel" view is also obtained with forefoot inversion and the radiographic beam angled 45 degrees toward the head.[279] Contrast material can then be aspirated and lidocaine is injected.

NORMAL PERONEAL TENOGRAM (Fig. 15–91). The peroneus longus and peroneus brevis muscles occupy the lateral aspects of the leg and foot. The peroneus longus extends from the lateral condyle of the tibia, the head and upper two thirds of the lateral aspect of the fibula, and the intermuscular septae and fascia around the lateral malleolus obliquely across the sole of the foot to attach to the medial cuneiform and base of the first metatarsal. The peroneus brevis shares a common sheath with the peroneus longus as the two tendons pass around the lateral malleolus. It originates from the lower two thirds of the lateral surface of the fibula and adjacent intermuscular septae and inserts into the base of the fifth metatarsal.

The normal peroneal tenogram outlines the common sheath of the peroneus longus and peroneus brevis muscles and the point of bifurcation of this sheath into separate sheaths enclosing either tendon. These sheaths can be traced for variable distances in the foot, appearing smooth in outline, containing a radiolucent tendon, without displacement.

PERONEAL TENOGRAPHY FOLLOWING LOCAL TRAUMA (Fig. 15–92). Painful disability following calcaneal fractures may result from one of four major factors[281]: posttraumatic arthritis of the subtalar or talocalcaneonavicular joints; stenosing tenosynovitis of the peroneal tendons[282, 283]; excessive bone formation on the plantar aspect of the heel; and injury to the septae of the heel pad. In most instances, the clinical diagnosis is not difficult. For example, peroneal dysfunction may be suspected by deformity and widening of the lateral aspect of the calcaneus beneath the fibula. In some patients, however, the source of pain may be more obscure. In these patients, peroneal tenography is useful.

The tenogram may show several abnormal findings: (1) extrinsic compression and irregularity of the sheath; (2) lateral or anterior displacement of the tendons and sheath; (3) complete obstruction of contrast flow; and (4) tendon rupture.

Peroneal tenography and subtalar arthrography can be accompanied by lidocaine injection to localize the source of obscure pain in patients with previous calcaneal fractures.[280] This distinction may aid the surgeon; stenosing peroneal tenosynovitis may require only excision of a protruding calcaneal spicule, whereas subtalar arthritis may necessitate an extensive arthrodesis.

Acute peroneal tendon dislocation is an infrequent injury that usually results from skiing accidents.[284, 285] Following extreme dorsiflexion of the foot, strong contraction of the peroneal tendons may occur. This contraction tears the fibular periosteum and superior peroneal retinaculum and may dislodge a small fragment of fibular cortex. Initial radiographs will reveal soft tissue swelling and an osseous fragment in this clinical setting. Peroneal tenography might be useful in delineating the position of the displaced peroneal tendons.

A report has appeared of a recurrent ganglion about the lateral aspect of an ankle that was injected with contrast material.[286] Opacification of the peroneus longus tendon sheath was observed, which led to appropriate surgery.

Additional Tenography and Retrocalcaneal Bursography (Fig. 15–93)

Contrast opacification of additional tendon sheaths about the ankle and the retrocalcaneal bursa has been undertaken.[287-289] Opacification of the tendon sheaths is not difficult, particularly in patients with rheumatoid arthritis, and consists of introducing a 22 gauge, 1.5 inch needle directly into the distended structure and injecting several milliliters of contrast material. The retrocalcaneal bursa can be punctured with a 22 gauge, 1.5 inch needle introduced adjacent to the Achilles tendon. The needle is advanced until it contacts the upper posterior surface of the calcaneus. Up to 1 ml of contrast

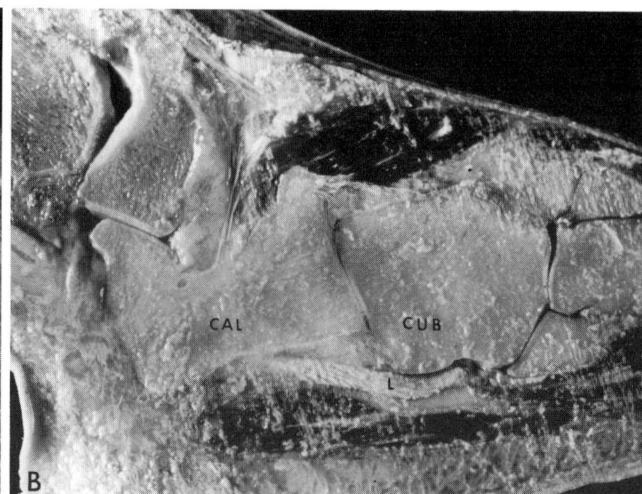

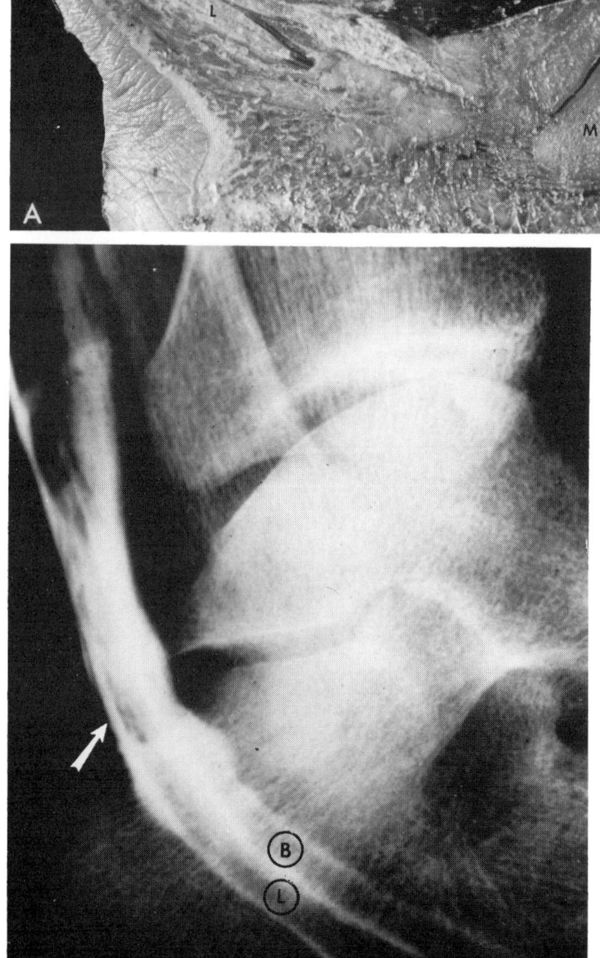

Figure 15–91. *Peroneal tenography: Anatomy and normal tenogram.*

A *A lateral sagittal section of the foot and ankle demonstrates the peroneus brevis (B) and peroneus longus (L) tendons passing around the lateral malleolus (arrowhead). The peroneus brevis can be followed close to the base of the fifth metatarsal (M).*

B *A slightly more medial sagittal section through the calcaneus (CAL) and cuboid (CUB) outlines the peroneus longus (L) tendon as it crosses underneath the foot.*

C *The normal peroneal tenogram reveals a smooth synovial sheath (arrow) separating into sheaths enclosing the peroneus brevis (B) and peroneus longus (L) tendons. No impingement or deviation of the contrast-filled sheaths can be seen.*

(From Resnick D, Goergen TG: Radiology 115:211, 1975.)

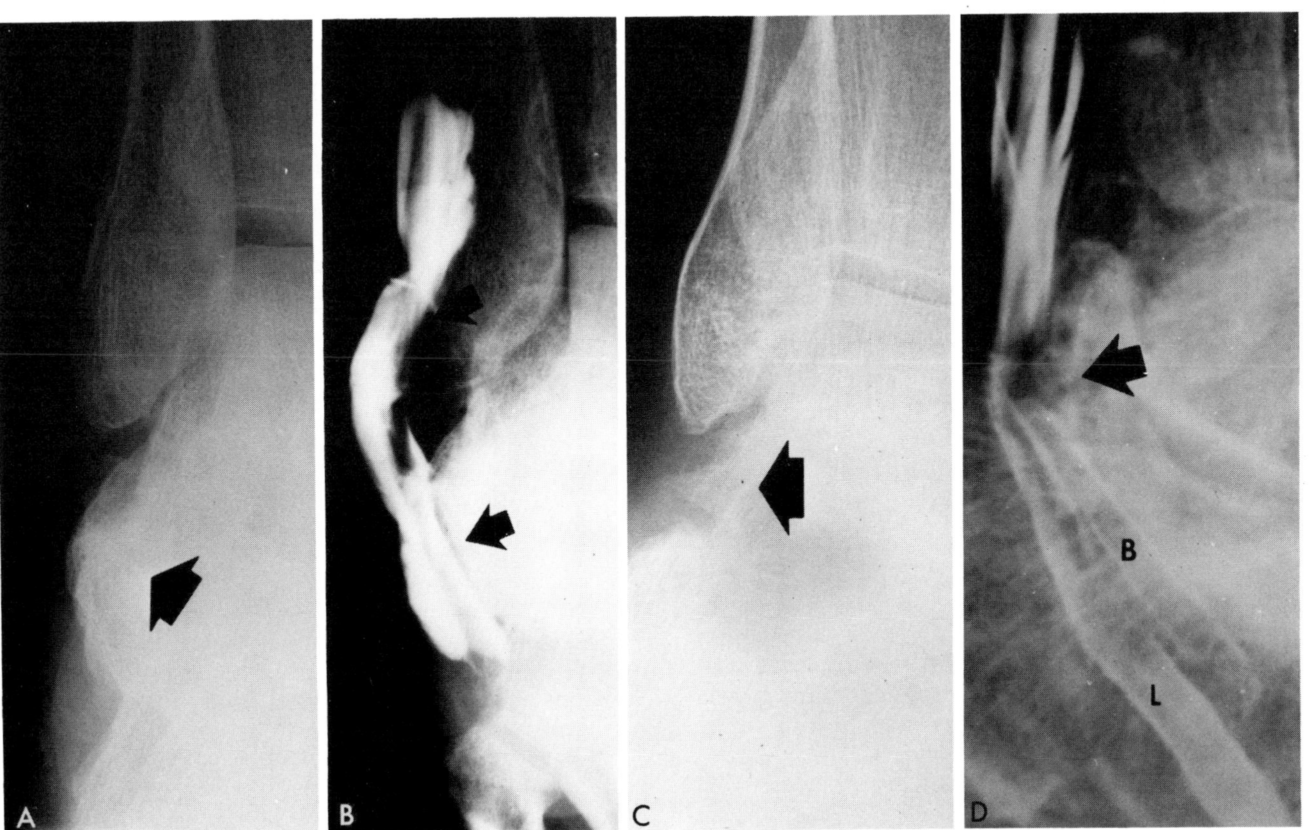

Figure 15–92. *Peroneal tenography: Abnormalities following trauma.*

A, B *Patient with previous calcaneal fracture. Initial radiograph* **(A)** *reveals deformity of the lateral surface of the calcaneus (arrow). The peroneal tenogram* **(B)** *indicates lateral displacement (upper arrow) and compression (lower arrow) of the peroneal tendons and sheath.*

C, D *A second patient with previous calcaneal fracture. The plain film* **(C)** *reveals a lateral calcaneal spicule (arrow) beneath the fibula. The peroneal tenogram* **(D)** *outlines impingement and compression of the sheath as it passes around the lateral malleolus (arrow) associated with incomplete filling of the peroneus brevis (B) and peroneus longus (L) sheaths.*

*(***B, D,** *From Resnick D, Goergen TG: Radiology 115:211, 1975.)*

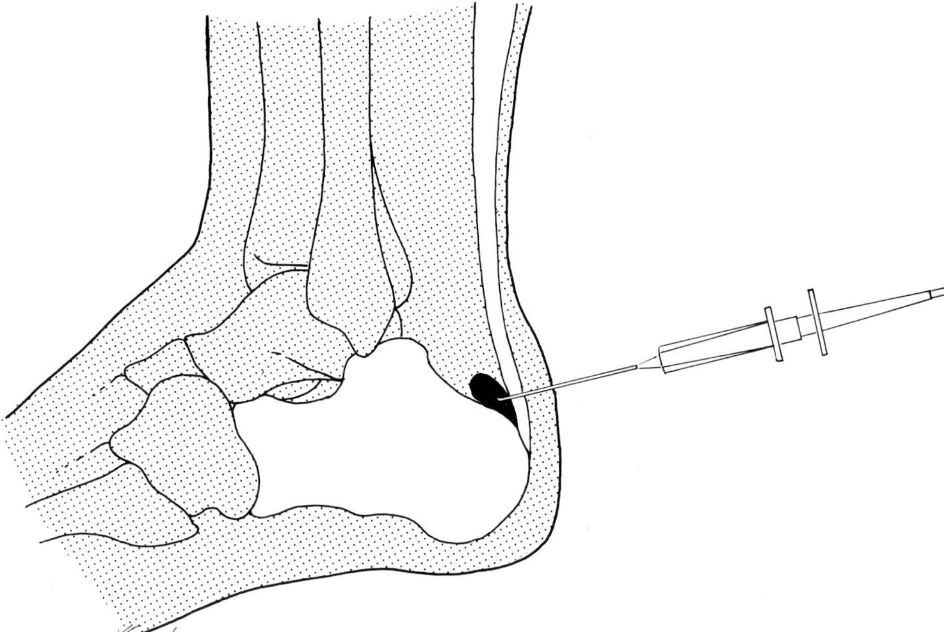

Figure 15–93. Retrocalcaneal bursography: Technique. The bursa is punctured from a posterior approach. The needle is inserted adjacent to the Achilles tendon and advanced until it contacts the upper posterior surface of the calcaneus.

material is then injected. In rheumatoid arthritis, irregularity and nodularity of the synovial lining of the sheath and bursa are observed.

Arthrography of Talocalcaneal Articulations

Arthrographic evaluation of either or both talocalcaneal articulations has been employed to investigate congenital, traumatic, and articular disorders. Injection of the talocalcaneonavicular joint is relatively easy; injection of the posterior subtalar joint is more difficult.[290]

Technique. Injection of the talocalcaneonavicular joint is accomplished under fluoroscopy utilizing a 22 gauge, 1.5 inch needle and 60 per cent methylglucamine diatrizoate (Renografin). The needle is introduced from a dorsal approach and aimed directly downward into the talonavicular space, approximately 1 cm medial to the dorsalis pedis artery. Upon entrance into the joint, 3 to 4 ml of contrast material is injected. Films are taken in anteroposterior, lateral, oblique, and axial projections.

Injection into the posterior subtalar joint can be made from a medial, posterior, or lateral approach. Utilizing the medial approach, one introduces a 22 gauge, 3.5 inch needle behind the medial malleolus, 1 cm posterior and inferior to the posterior tibial artery. The needle is advanced under fluoroscopic control in an anterosuperior direction into the space between the posterior aspects of the talus and calcaneus. With care taken not to introduce the needle through the interosseous ligament into the talocalcaneonavicular space, inject 1.5 to 2.5 ml of Renografin. Anteroposterior, oblique, lateral, and axial radiographs are obtained.

Normal Arthrography of Talocalcaneonavicular and Posterior Subtalar Joints (Fig. 15–94). The normal arthrogram of the talocalcaneonavicular joint demonstrates a smooth synovial cavity extending in a gradual curve, which is concave posteriorly, about the anterior aspect of the talus. The cavity extends dorsally to the talar neck and ventrally along the plantar aspect of the talus. It covers the sustentaculum tali. There is no communication with the calcaneocuboid, posterior subtalar, or cuneonavicular joints.

The contrast-filled posterior subtalar joint appears as a linear dense area between the posterior halves of talus and calcaneus along the lateral aspect of the foot. A recess appears as a sausage-shaped collection of contrast material at the posterior margin of the joint.[291] In 10 to 20 per cent of arthrograms, there is communication between the posterior subtalar joint and the ankle. Rarely is communication observed between the posterior subtalar joint and talocalcaneonavicular cavity.

Trauma (Fig. 15–95). Trauma may lead to abnormalities of the talocalcaneal articulations. Following calcaneal fractures, posttraumatic arthritis of the neighboring joints may cause significant disability. Selective injection of contrast material with lidocaine into each of the neighboring joints will lead to accurate appraisal as to the source of the symptoms.[280] Injections are made into one joint — the ankle, subtalar, or talocalcaneonavicular joint — and the patient is then asked to walk for approximately 30 minutes in order to determine if the lidocaine has relieved the pain. If the first injection

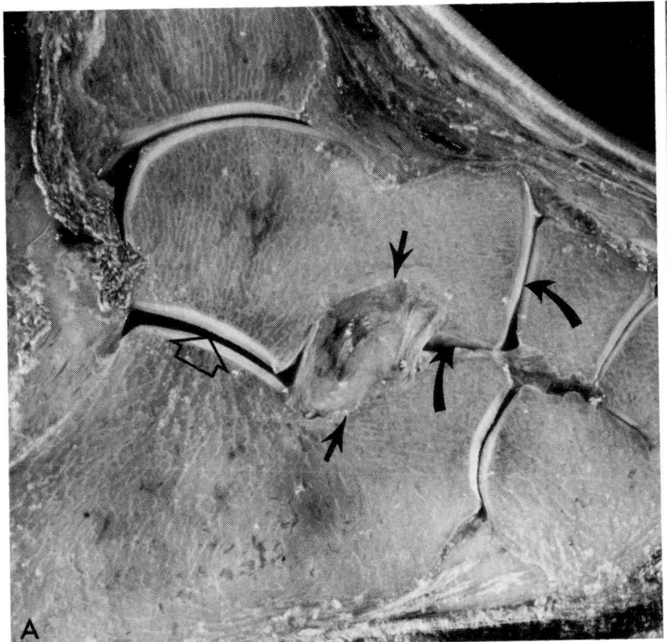

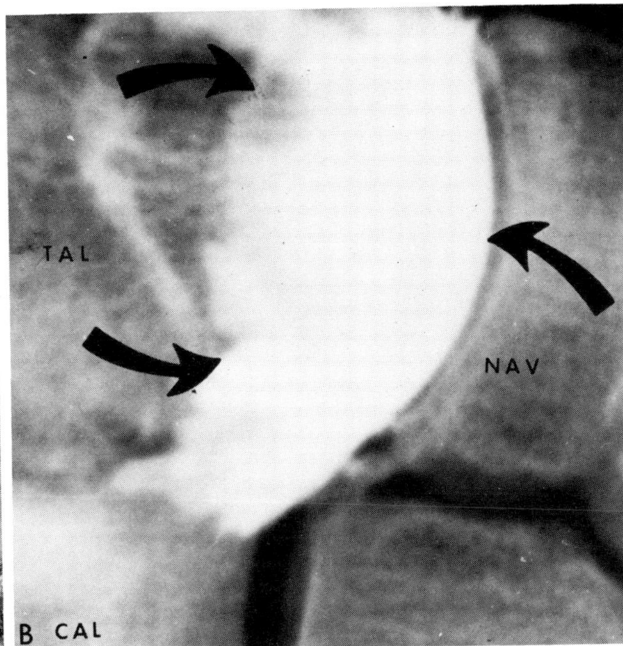

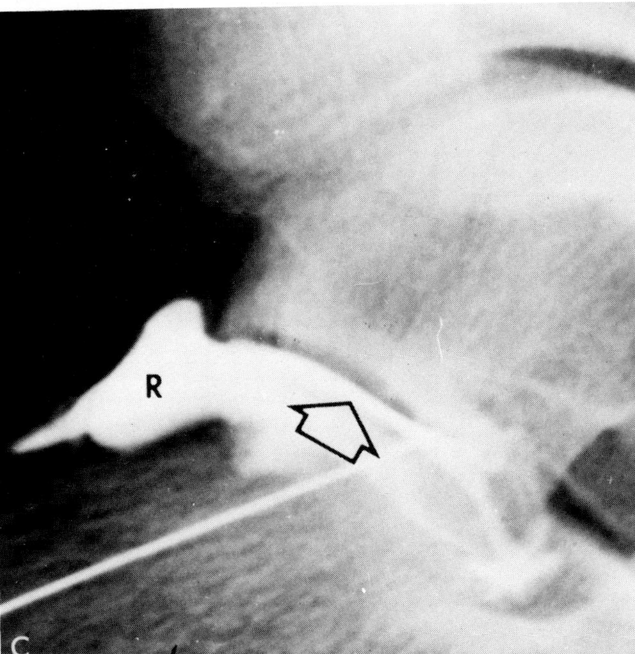

Figure 15–94. *Arthrography of the talocalcaneonavicular and posterior subtalar joints: Anatomy and normal arthrograms.*

A *Sagittal section of the ankle and foot. Observe the talocalcaneonavicular joint (curved arrows) between talus, navicular, and calcaneus, and the posterior subtalar joint (open arrow) between posterior facets of the calcaneus and talus. Interosseous ligaments (straight arrows) separate the two cavities.*

B *An oblique projection during arthrography of the talocalcaneonavicular joint. Note the partially filled articular cavity (arrows) between the talus (TAL), navicular (NAV), and calcaneus (CAL).*

C *A lateral projection during arthrography of the posterior subtalar joint reveals filling of the articular cavity (arrow) with visualization of a normal posterior recess (R). The talocalcaneonavicular joint does not opacify.*

(From Resnick D: Radiology 111:581, 1974.)

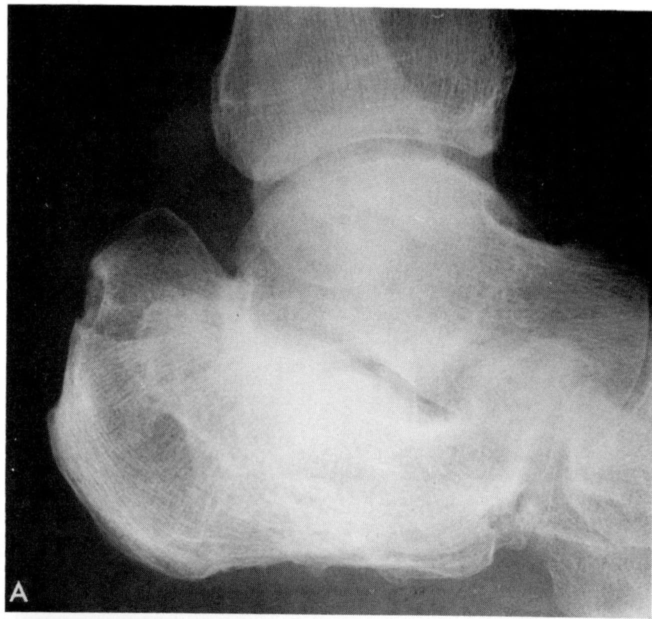

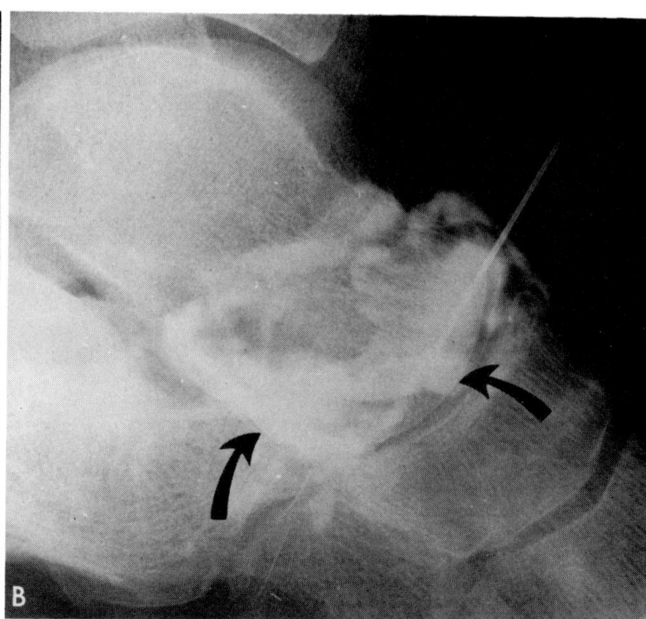

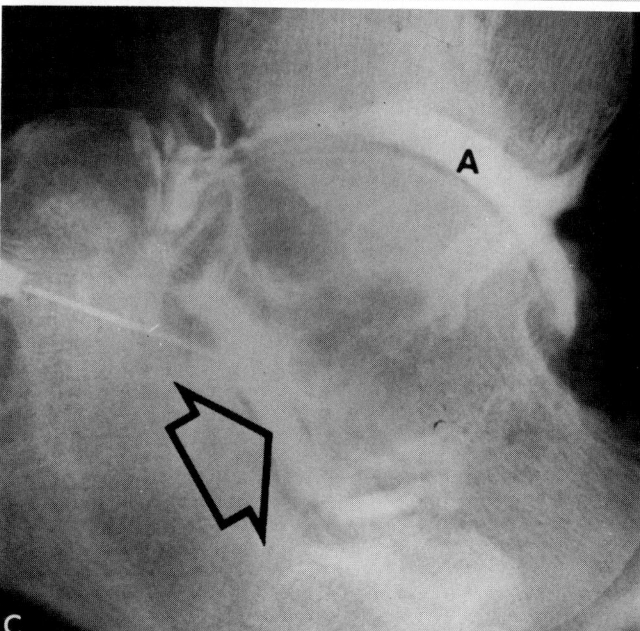

Figure 15–95. *Arthrography of the talocalcaneonavicular and posterior subtalar joints: Abnormalities following trauma.*

A–C *A patient with a previous calcaneal fracture and persistent heel pain. The initial film* **(A)** *indicates narrowing, sclerosis and deformity of the posterior subtalar joint, and flattening of the superior surface of the calcaneus. Injection of the talocalcaneonavicular joint* **(B)** *with a mixture of lidocaine and contrast material reveals irregularity of the articular cavity (arrows) and gave some temporary relief of pain. Similarly, injection of the posterior subtalar joint* **(C)** *(arrow) provided additional relief of pain, demonstrating posterior extravasation of contrast material as well. The ankle joint (A) has opacified. These findings indicated that the patient's symptoms were originating from both the talocalcaneonavicular and posterior subtalar joints. A triple arthrodesis might be the most appropriate therapy.*

Illustration continued on the opposite page

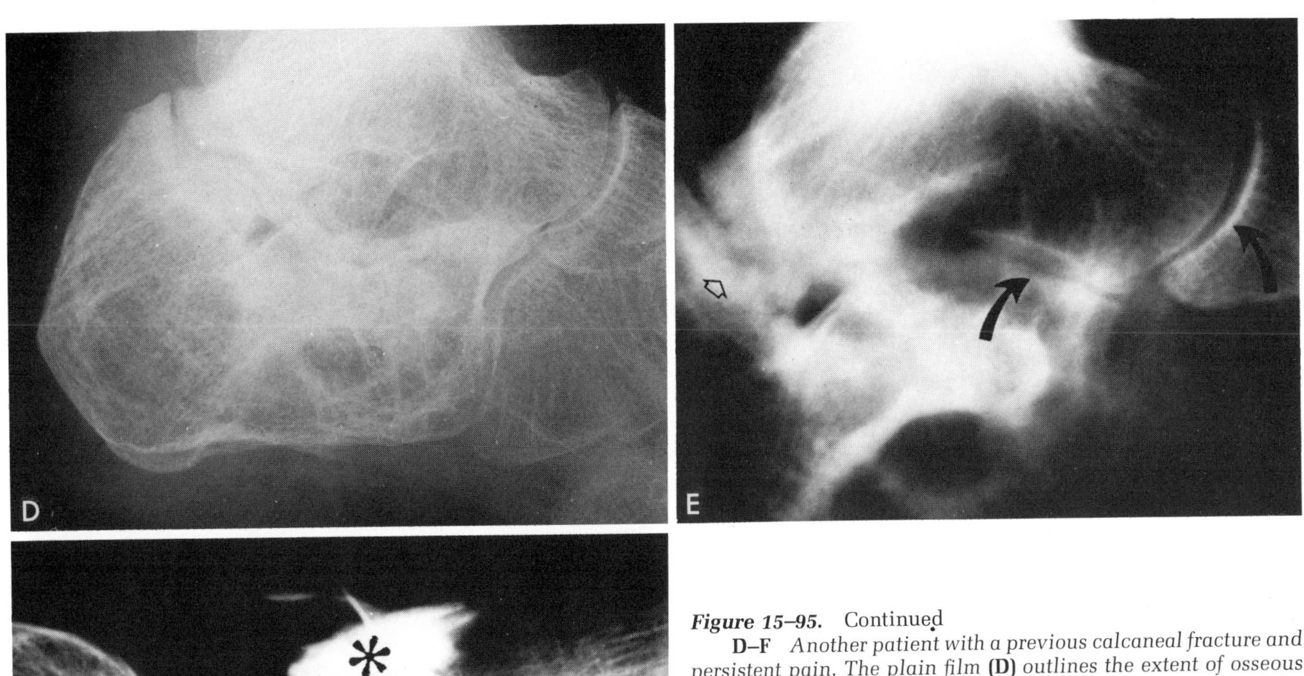

Figure 15–95. Continued

D–F *Another patient with a previous calcaneal fracture and persistent pain. The plain film* **(D)** *outlines the extent of osseous deformity and obliteration of the posterior subtalar joint, and the talocalcaneal portion of the talocalcaneonavicular joint. Tomography* **(E)** *further substantiates the severe joint space narrowing of the posterior subtalar joint (open arrow). The talonavicular and talocalcaneal portions of the talocalcaneonavicular joint appear narrowed but not fused (curved arrows). An arthrogram of the talocalcaneonavicular articulation* **(F)** *reveals opacification of the talonavicular portion of the joint space (arrows) and dorsal extravasation (asterisk). Failure to opacify the talocalcaneal portion of the talocalcaneonavicular joint is indicative of fibrous ankylosis.*

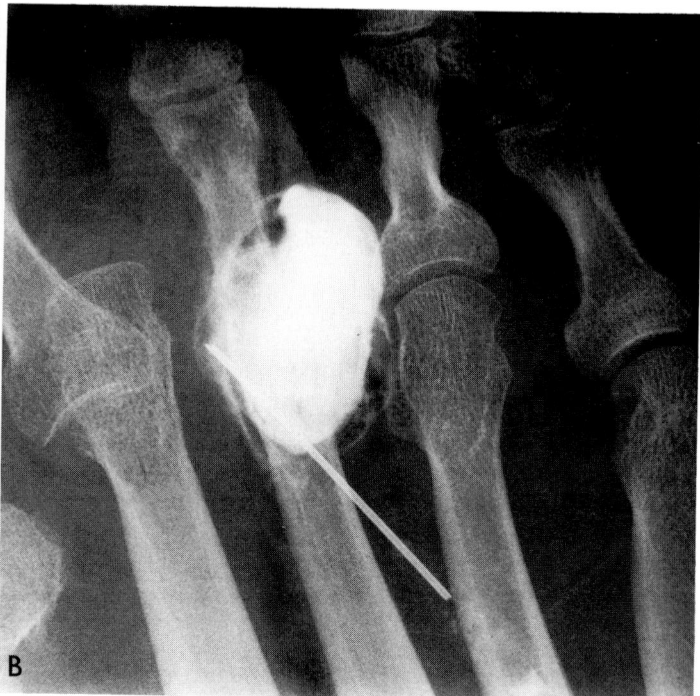

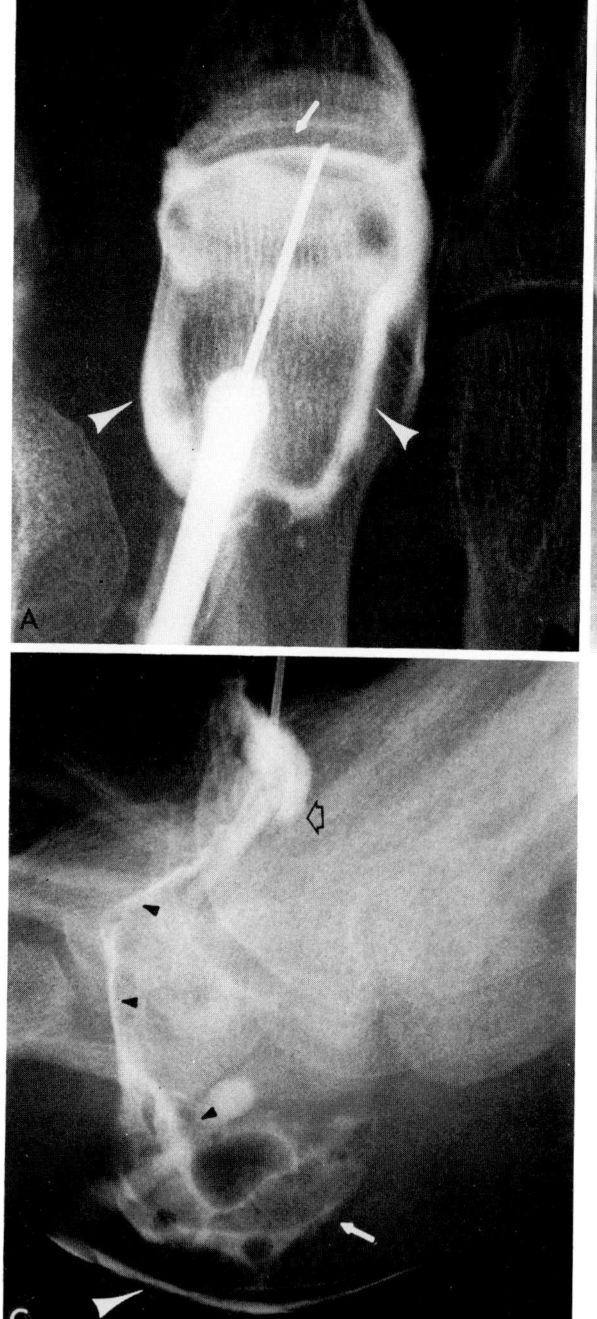

Figure 15–96. Arthrography of the forefoot: Normal and abnormal arthrograms.

A A normal arthrogram of the metatarsophalangeal joint reveals large proximal recesses (arrowheads) and smooth articular cartilage (arrow).

B Metatarsophalangeal joint arthrography in rheumatoid arthritis. Observe cystic dilatation of the articular cavity which, on lateral films, was located primarily on the plantar aspect of the joint. Typical rheumatoid erosions and subluxations are evident.

C Metatarsophalangeal joint arthrography in rheumatoid arthritis. A lateral view indicates the presence of a fistula with contrast opacification of the articular cavity (open arrow), fistulous tract (small arrowheads), plantar cyst (solid arrow), and skin surface (large arrowhead).

is unsuccessful, another articulation is injected, and the procedure is repeated until the painful articulation is localized. In some instances, incomplete contrast opacification of a specific articulation indicates posttraumatic fibrous ankylosis of the joint. On the basis of findings related to contrast and lidocaine arthrography, the surgeon can plan the most effective therapy for the patient.

Talocalcaneal joint arthrography may also be useful in studying patients with posttraumatic sinus tarsi syndrome.[292, 293] These patients develop pain in the midtarsal area over the lateral aspect of the sinus tarsi. It has been suggested that, in this condition, normal synovial folds of the posterior subtalar joint about the interosseous ligament are obliterated. These findings can be revealed by posterior subtalar arthrography, in which the normal recesses about the ligament are not opacified.[293] These changes are related to synovial hyperplasia and do not develop immediately after trauma. The arthrogram should be delayed for some time until the joint effusion diminishes and synovial hypertrophy has occurred. An associated rupture of the calcaneofibular ligament is common.

Developmental Disorders

Tarsal Coalition. Talocalcaneonavicular arthrography has been employed in patients with tarsal coalition.[294] Coalitions between the talus and sustentaculum tali of the calcaneus are frequently difficult to detect on initial radiographs. A tangential view of the area has been recommended, the Harris-Beath view.[295] On occasion, multiple tangential views with varying degrees of angulation of the incident beam and tomography are necessary. Osseous, fibrous, or cartilaginous sustentacular-talar coalition can be diagnosed with arthrography of the talocalcaneonavicular joint. Following introduction of contrast material, routine anteroposterior, lateral, and oblique views are supplemented by axial views taken with varying degrees of beam angulation (35 degrees, 45 degrees, 55 degrees). The normal sustentacular-talar articulation (middle facets of talocalcaneonavicular joint) will be filled with contrast material. In the presence of a coalition, this space will not be opacified.

Club Feet. Simultaneous arthrography of the ankle and talocalcaneonavicular joint has been advocated in studying children with club feet.[296-299] The degree of talar deformity is not readily determined on plain films because of the small size of the ossification centers in the infant's foot. By opacification of these two articular cavities, measurements of the length and width of the talus, the orientation of the talocalcaneonavicular joint, the trochlear curvature, and the talocrural recesses can be applied.[299] These measurements may allow selection of a more appropriate treatment in refractory or recurrent club feet.[367, 368]

Arthrography of the Midfoot and Forefoot

Opacification of the articulations of the midfoot and forefoot (Fig. 15–96) has been described in normal individuals[17, 22, 300, 301] and in patients with rheumatoid arthritis.[22, 287] In general, arthrography is easily accomplished by introducing a 22 gauge or 25 gauge needle directly into the articulation under fluoroscopic control. In rheumatoid arthritis, a typical corrugated synovial pattern may be seen, and saccular enlargement of the joint cavity, particularly on the plantar aspects of the metatarsophalangeal joints, can be observed. On rare occasions, a fistula between an involved metatarsophalangeal joint and the skin is delineated.

MISCELLANEOUS AREAS

Apophyseal Joints

Arthrography of the apophyseal joints of the lumbar spine may be accomplished by placing the patient in an oblique position under fluoroscopy and directing a needle downward into the articular cavity.[302] Opacification of these joints has revealed that defects associated with spondylolysis may communicate with the articular cavity. This communication may explain the high incidence of nonunion of these fractures.[303] Injection of lidocaine into these articulations may produce temporary relief of back pain.[304]

Interspinous Ligaments

Roentgenographic examination of the lumbar interspinous ligaments utilizing contrast material has been described.[305] The material is injected bilaterally. In normal situations, the ligament appears as a flat, spindle-shaped filling defect surrounded by contrast material; in abnormal cases, the contrast material penetrates the ligament itself.

Craniocervical Joints

Arthrography of the normal articulations between the occiput, atlas, and axis has been performed.[306] No clinical application has yet been documented for this procedure but utilization of this technique in patients with rheumatoid arthritis may be helpful in their management.

COMPLICATIONS OF ARTHROGRAPHY

Arthrography is considered a safe procedure. Initial reports describing pneumoarthrography included occasional examples of complications, such as pain, swelling, and subcutaneous emphysema.[307, 308] The most serious complication was reported by Kleinberg in 1927.[309] In this report, a 19 year old youth was subjected to pneumoarthrography of the knee because of a possible intra-articular fragment. After being inserted in a less than careful fashion, the needle was connected to an oxygen tank and oxygen was administered. The patient immediately complained of chest pain and a feeling of "dying." He subsequently became pulseless with widely dilated pupils, absent respirations, and an inaudible heart beat. At this point, the patient was "apparently dead." Artificial respiration and intracardiac injection of epinephrine revived the patient and he was discharged from the hospital 10 days after the procedure. Since a knee radiograph obtained shortly after the procedure failed to reveal intra-articular or periarticular gas, it was suggested that a stream of oxygen was forced directly into the bloodstream, occluding vessels in the lungs and producing cardiac failure.

As currently performed, arthrography is rarely associated with significant complications. Mild pain and discomfort may be encountered during the procedure. Transient synovitis with pain and swelling is occasionally apparent, particularly in patients with preexisting synovial inflammation. This complication is generally transient, disappearing within a day or two. Joint sepsis is rarely observed if proper sterile technique is employed. A vasovagal response may result in temporary lightheadedness and hypotension, but these symptoms quickly disappear. Hypersensitivity reaction to iodinated contrast agent is rarely observed.

SUMMARY

This chapter has stressed the many indications for contrast opacification of joint cavities, tendon sheaths, and bursae. These procedures generally are simple to perform, and the information they provide may be essential for proper diagnosis and treatment.

REFERENCES

1. Ranawat CS, Freiberger RH, Jordan LR, Straub LR: Arthrography in the rheumatoid wrist joint. A preliminary report. J Bone Joint Surg *51A*:1269, 1969.
2. Harrison MO, Freiberger RH, Ranawat CS: Arthrography of the rheumatoid wrist joint. Am J Roentgenol *112*:480, 1971.
3. Kessler I, Silberman Z: Experimental study of the radiocarpal joint by arthrography. Surg Gynecol Obstet *112*:33, 1961.
4. Ranawat CS, Harrison MO, Jordan LR: Arthrography of the wrist joint. Clin Orthop Rel Res *83*:6, 1972.
5. Resnick D: Arthrography in the evaluation of arthritic disorders of the wrist. Radiology *113*:331, 1974.
6. Trentham CE, Hamm RL, Masi AT: Wrist arthrography: Review and comparison of normal, rheumatoid arthritis and gout patients. Semin Arthritis Rheum *5*:105, 1975.
7. Resnick D: Early abnormalities of the pisiform and triquetrum in rheumatoid arthritis. Ann Rheum Dis *35*:46, 1976.
8. Resnick D: Rheumatoid arthritis of the wrist. The compartmental approach. Med Radiogr Photogr *52*:50, 1976.
9. Resnick D: Rheumatoid arthritis of the wrist: Why the ulnar styloid? Radiology *112*:29, 1974.
10. Stenström R, Wegelius O: Clearance of ^{125}I-labelled urographin from knee joints in rheumatoid arthritis. Acta Rheum Scand *16*:151, 1970.
11. Wiljasalo M, Julkunen H, Salven I: Lymphography in rheumatic diseases. Ann Med Intern Fenn *55*:125, 1966.
12. Lewin JR, Mulhern LM: Lymphatic visualization during contrast arthrography of the knee. Radiology *103*:577, 1972.
13. Weston WJ: Lymphatic filling during positive contrast arthrography in rheumatoid arthritis. Australas Radiol *13*:368, 1969.
14. Rieunau G, Gay R, Martinez C, Mansat M: Lesions de l'articulation radio-cubitale inférieure dans les traumatismes de l'avant-bras et du poignet. Intérêt de l'arthrographie. Rev Chir Orthop *57* (Suppl 1):253, 1971.
15. Andrén L, Eiken O: Arthrographic studies of wrist ganglions. J Bone Joint Surg *53A*:299, 1971.
16. Gerber NJ, Dixon AS: Synovial cysts and juxta-articular bone cysts (geodes). Semin Arthritis Rheum *3*:323, 1974.
17. Weston WJ: The normal arthrograms of the metacarpophalangeal, metatarsophalangeal and interphalangeal joints. Australas Radiol *13*:211, 1969.
18. Resnick D, Danzig LA: Arthrographic evaluation of injuries of the first metacarpophalangeal joint: Gamekeeper's thumb. Am J Roentgenol *126*:1046, 1976.
19. Bowers WH, Hurst LC: Gamekeeper's thumb. Evaluation by arthrography and stress roentgenography. J Bone Joint Surg *59A*:519, 1977.
20. Linscheid RL: Arthrography of the metacarpophalangeal joint. Clin Orthop Rel Res *103*:91, 1974.
21. Glogowski A, Laval-Jeantet M, Stora P: Arthrographie des doigts et du carpe dans les rhumatismes inflammatoires. J Radiol Electrol Med Nucl *57*:873, 1976.
22. Weston WJ, Palmer DG: Soft Tissues of the Extremities. A Radiologic Study of Rheumatic Disease. New York, Springer-Verlag, 1977.
23. Moberg E, Stener B: Injuries to the ligaments of the thumb and fingers. Diagnosis, treatment and prognosis. Acta Chir Scand *106*:166, 1954.
24. Neviaser RJ, Wilson JN, Lievano A: Rupture of the ulnar collateral ligament of the thumb (gamekeeper's thumb). Correction by dynamic repair. J Bone Joint Surg *53A*:1357, 1971.
25. Stener B: Displacement of the ruptured ulnar collateral ligament of the metacarpophalangeal joint of the thumb. A clinical and anatomical study. J Bone Joint Surg *44B*:869, 1962.
26. Schultz RJ, Fox JM: Gamekeeper's thumb. Result of skiing injuries. NY State J Med *73*:2329, 1973.
27. Brewerton DA: Tenography in the rheumatoid hand. Hand *2*:46, 1970.
28. Brewerton DA: Radiographic studies in the rheumatoid hand. Br J Radiol *42*:487, 1969.
29. Palmer DG: Dynamics of joint disruption. N Z Med J *78*:166, 1973.
30. Resnick D: Roentgenographic anatomy of the tendon sheaths of the hand and wrist: Tenography. Am J Roentgenol *124*:44, 1975.
31. Resnick D: Osteomyelitis and septic arthritis complicating hand injuries and infections: Pathogenesis of roentgenographic abnormalities. J Can Assoc Radiol *27*:21, 1976.
32. Weston WJ: The ulnar bursa. Australas Radiol *17*:216, 1973.
33. Weston WJ: The digital sheaths of the hand. Australas Radiol *13*:360, 1969.

34. Kaplan E: Functional and Surgical Anatomy of the Hand. 2nd Ed. Philadelphia, JB Lippincott Co, 1965.
35. Lampe E: Surgical anatomy of the hand with special reference to infections and trauma. Clin Symp *21*:66, 1969.
36. Scheldrup E: Tendon sheath patterns in hand. Surg Gynecol Obstet *93*:161, 1951.
37. Kanavel A: Infections of the Hand: A Guide to the Surgical Treatment of Acute and Chronic Suppurative Processes in the Fingers, Hand and Forearm. 7th ed. Philadelphia, Lea & Febiger, 1939.
38. Gad P: Anatomy of the volar part of the capsules of the finger joints. J Bone Joint Surg *49B*:362, 1967.
39. Leach R, Odom J Jr: Systemic causes of carpal tunnel syndrome. Postgrad Med *44*:127, 1968.
40. Phalen G: Carpal tunnel syndrome: Seventeen years' experience in diagnosis and treatment of six hundred fifty-four hands. J Bone Joint Surg *48A*:211, 1966.
41. Eto RT, Anderson PW, Harley JD: Elbow arthrography with the application of tomography. Radiology *115*:283, 1975.
42. Arvidsson H, Johansson O: Arthrography of the elbow joint. Acta Radiol *43*:445, 1955.
43. Chirls M: Arthrography in the diagnosis of joint disease. J Med Soc NJ *63*:61, 1966.
44. Del Buono MS, Solarino GB: Arthrography of the elbow with double contrast media. Ital Clin Orthop *14*:223, 1962.
45. Mouterde P, Massare C, Deburge A: Luxation traumatique du coude de l'adulte étude arthrographique. Aspect clinique d'une série de 100 cas. Ann Chir *29*:743, 1975.
46. Haage H: Röntgendiagnostik der Gelenkschwellung des Ellenbogens. Fortschr Geb Roentgenstr Nuklearmed *118*:45, 1973.
47. Weston WJ: The synovial changes at the elbow in rheumatoid arthritis. Australas Radiol *15*:170, 1971.
48. Goode JD: Synovial rupture of the elbow joint. Ann Rheum Dis *27*:604, 1968.
49. Ehrlich GE, Guttmann GG: Valvular mechanisms in antecubital cysts of rheumatoid arthritis. Arth Rheum *16*:259, 1973.
50. Erhlich GE: Antecubital cysts in rheumatoid arthritis — a corollary to popliteal (Baker's) cysts. J Bone Joint Surg *54A*:165, 1972.
51. Bäckdahl M: The caput ulnae syndrome in rheumatoid arthritis. A study of the morphology, abnormal anatomy and clinical picture. Acta Rheumatol Scand Suppl *5*:5, 1963.
52. Weston WJ: The lead arthrogram — plumbography. Skel Radiol *2*:169, 1978.
53. Weston WJ: The olecranon bursa. Australas Radiol *14*:323, 1970.
54. Killoran PJ, Marcove RC, Freiberger RH: Shoulder arthrography. Am J Roentgenol *103*:658, 1968.
55. Kernwein GA, Roseberg B, Sneed WR Jr: Arthrographic studies of shoulder joint. J Bone Joint Surg *39A*:1267, 1957.
56. Lindblom K: Arthrography and roentgenography in ruptures of the tendons of the shoulder joint. Acta Radiol *20*:548, 1939.
57. Nelson DH: Arthrography of the shoulder. Br J Radiol *25*:134, 1952.
58. Neviaser JS: Arthrography of shoulder joint: Study of findings in adhesive capsulitis of shoulder. J Bone Joint Surg *44A*:1321, 1962.
59. Samilson R, Raphael RL, Post L, Noonan C, Siris E, Raney F: Arthrography of shoulder joint. Clin Orthop Rel Res *20*:21, 1961.
60. Reeves B: Arthrography of shoulder. J Bone Joint Surg *48B*:424, 1966.
61. Den Herder BA: Clinical significance of arthrography of humeroscapular joint. Radiol Clin Biol *46*:185, 1977.
62. Nelson CL: The use of arthrography in athletic injuries of the shoulder. Orthop Clin North Am *4*:775, 1973.
63. Nelson CL, Burton RI: Upper extremity arthrography. Clin Orthop Rel Res *107*:62, 1975.
64. Preston BJ, Jackson JP: Investigation of shoulder disability by arthrography. Clin Radiol *28*:259, 1977.
65. Schneider R, Ghelman B, Kaye JJ: A simplified injection technique for shoulder arthrography. Radiology *114*:738, 1975.
66. Dalinka MK: A simple aid to the performance of shoulder arthrography. Am J Roentgenol *129*:942, 1977.
67. Ghelman B, Goldman AB: The double contrast shoulder arthrogram: Evaluation of rotator cuff tears. Radiology *124*:251, 1977.
68. Goldman AB, Ghelman B: The double-contrast shoulder arthrogram. A review of 158 studies. Radiology *127*:655, 1978.
69. Debeyre J, Patte D, Elmelik E: Repair of ruptures of the rotator cuff of the shoulder with a note on advancement of the supraspinatus muscle. J Bone Joint Surg *47B*:36, 1965.
70. Wolfgang GL: Surgical repair of tears of the rotator cuff of the shoulder. Factors influencing the result. J Bone Joint Surg *56A*:14, 1974.
71. McLaughlin HL: Rupture of the rotator cuff. J Bone Joint Surg *44A*:979, 1962.
72. Neviaser JS: Ruptures of rotator cuff. Clin Orthop Rel Res *3*:92, 1954.
73. Weber J, Kecskés S: Arthrografie bei Periarthritis humeroscapularis. Fortschr Geb Roentgenstr Nuklearmed *124*:573, 1976.
74. Andrén L, Lundberg BJ: Treatment of rigid shoulders by joint distention during arthrography. Acta Orthop Scand *36*:45, 1965.
75. Neviaser JS: Adhesive capsulitis of the shoulder. A study of the pathological findings in periarthritis of the shoulder. J Bone Joint Surg *27*:211, 1945.
76. Lippmann RK: Frozen shoulder; periarthritis; bicipital tenosynovitis. Arch Surg *47*:283, 1943.
77. Lidström A: Den "frusna" skuldran. Nord Med *69*:125, 1963.
78. Lundberg BJ: The frozen shoulder. Clinical and radiographical observations. The effect of manipulation under general anesthesia. Structure and glycosaminoglycan content of the joint capsule. Local bone metabolism. Acta Orth Scand (Suppl) *119*:5, 1969.
79. Goldman AB, Katz MC, Freiberger RH: Post-traumatic adhesive capsulitis of the ankle: Arthrographic diagnosis. Am J Roentgenenol *127*:585, 1976.
80. Ennevaara K: Painful shoulder joint in rheumatoid arthritis: A clinical and radiologic study of 200 cases, with special reference to arthrography of the glenohumeral joint. Acta Rheum Scand Suppl *11*:1, 1967.
81. Bankart ASB: The pathology and treatment of recurrent dislocation of the shoulder joint. Br J Surg *26*:23, 1938.
82. DeSmet AA, Ting YM, Weiss JJ: Shoulder arthrography in rheumatoid arthritis. Radiology *116*:601, 1975.
83. Weiss JJ, Thompson GR, Doust V, Burgener F: Rotator cuff tears in rheumatoid arthritis. Arch Intern Med *135*:521, 1975.
84. Burgener FA, Weiss JJ, Doust V: Die Schulterarthrographie bei primär chronischer Polyarthritis. Fortschr Geb Roentgenstr Nuklearmed *116*:490, 1972.
85. Weston WJ: Enlarged axillary glands in rheumatoid arthritis. Australas Radiol *15*:55, 1971.
86. Armbuster TG, Slivka J, Resnick D, Goergen TG, Weisman M, Master R: Extraarticular manifestations of septic arthritis of the glenohumeral joint. Am J Roentgenol *129*:667, 1977.
87. Weston WJ: The intrasynovial fatty masses in chronic rheumatoid arthritis. Br J Radiol *46*:213, 1973.
88. DeSeze S, Hubault A, Rampon S: Senile haemorrhagic shoulder. Ann Rheum Dis *27*:292, 1968.
89. Weston WJ: Arthrography of the acromio-clavicular joint. Australas Radiol *18*:213, 1974.
90. Heubelin GW, Greene GS, Conforti VP: Hip joint arthrography. Am J Roentgenol *68*:736, 1952.
91. Katz JF: Arthrography in Legg-Calvé-Perthes disease. J Bone Joint Surg *50A*:467, 1968.
92. Severin E: Arthrography in congenital dislocation of the hip. J Bone Joint Surg *21*:304, 1939.
93. Kenin A, Levine J: A technique for arthrography of the hip. Am J Roentgenol *68*:107, 1952.
94. Mitchell GP: Arthrography in congenital displacement of the hip. J Bone Joint Surg *45B*:88, 1963.
95. Astley R: Arthrography in congenital dislocation of the hip. Clin Radiol *18*:253, 1967.
96. Ozonoff MB: Controlled arthrography of the hip: A technic of fluoroscopic monitoring and recording. Clin Orthop Rel Res *93*:260, 1973.
97. Salvati EA, Ghelman B, McLaren T, Wilson PD Jr: Subtraction technique in arthrography for loosening of total hip replacement fixed with radiopaque cement. Clin Orthop Rel Res *101*:105, 1974.
98. Guerra J Jr, Armbuster TG, Resnick D, Goergen TG, Feingold ML, Niwayama G, Danzig LA: The adult hip: An anatomic study. Part II. The soft tissue landmarks. Radiology *128*:11, 1978.
99. Razzano CD, Nelson CL, Wilde AH: Arthrography of the adult hip. Clin Orthop Rel Res *99*:86, 1974.
100. Freiberger RH: Congenital dislocation of the hip. *In* Hip diseases of infancy and childhood. Curr Prob Radiol *3*:4, 1973.
101. Grech P: Video-arthrography in hip dysplasia. Clin Radiol *23*:202, 1972.
102. Patel D: Arthroscopy of the plicae–synovial folds and their significance. Am J Sports Med *6*:217, 1978.
103. Pipkin G: Knee injuries: The role of the suprapatellar plica and suprapatellar bursa in simulating internal derangements. Clin Orthop Rel Res *74*:161, 1971.
104. Harty M, Joyce JJ III: Synovial folds in the knee joint. Orthop Rev *7*:91, 1977.
105. Kaye JJ, Winchester PH, Freiberger RH: Neonatal septic "dislocation" of the hip: True dislocation or pathological epiphyseal separation? Radiology *114*:671, 1975.
106. Glassberg GB, Ozonoff MB: Arthrographic findings in septic arthritis of the hip in infants. Radiology *128*:151, 1978.
107. Lachman RS, Rimoin DL, Hollister DW: Arthrography of the hip. A clue to the pathogenesis of the epiphyseal dysplasias. Radiology *108*:317, 1973.
108. Hardaker WT Jr, Whipple TL, Bassett FM III: Diagnosis and treatment of the plica syndrome of the knee. J Bone Joint Surg: *62A*:221, 1980.

109. Axer A, Schiller MG: The pathogenesis of the early deformity of the capital femoral epiphysis in Legg-Calvé-Perthes syndrome (LCPS). An arthrographic study. Clin Orthop *84*:106, 1972.
110. Gershuni DH, Axer A, Hendel D: Arthrographic findings in Legg-Calvé-Perthes disease and transient synovitis of the hip. J Bone Joint Surg *60A*:457, 1978.
111. Jonsäter S: Coxa plana, a histo-pathologic and arthrographic study. Acta Orthop Scand Suppl *12*:5, 1953.
112. Murphy WA, Siegel MJ, Gilula LA: Arthrography in the diagnosis of unexplained chronic hip pain with regional osteopenia. Am J Roentgenol *129*:283, 1977.
113. Armstrong P, Saxton H: Ilio-psoas bursa. Br J Radiol *45*:493, 1972.
114. Warren R, Kaye JJ, Salvati EA: Arthrographic demonstration of an enlarged iliopsoas bursa complicating osteoarthritis of the hip — a case report. J Bone Joint Surg *57A*:413, 1975.
115. O'Connor DS: Early recognition of iliopectineal bursitis. Surg Gynecol Obstet *57*:674, 1933.
116. Dalinka MK, Cohen GS, Wershba M: Knee arthrography. CRC Crit Rev Radiol Sci *4*:1, 1973.
117. Keats TE, Staatz DS, Bailey RW: Pneumoarthrography of the knee. Surg Gynecol Obstet *94*:361, 1952.
118. Lindblom K: The arthrographic appearance of the ligaments of the knee joint. Acta Radiol *19*:582, 1938.
119. Lindblom K: Arthrography of the knee, a roentgenographic and anatomical study. Acta Radiol Suppl *74*:7, 1948.
120. Andrén L, Wehlin L: Double contrast arthrography of the knee with horizontal roentgen ray beam. Acta Orthop Scand *29*:307, 1960.
121. Freiberger RH, Killoran PJ, Cardona G: Arthrography of the knee by double contrast method. Am J Roentgenol *97*:736, 1966.
122. Butt WP, McIntyre JL: Double contrast arthrography of the knee. Radiology *92*:487, 1969.
123. Angell FL: Fluoroscopic technique of double contrast arthrography of the knee. Radiol Clin North Am *9*:85, 1971.
124. Angell FL: A restraint device for arthrography of the knee. Radiology *98*:186, 1971.
125. Gelmon MI, Riding LJ: Arthrography of the knee. Appl Radiol *4*:19, 1975.
126. Gilula LA: A simplified stress device for knee arthrography. Radiology *122*:828, 1977.
127. Levinsohn EM: A new simple restraining device for fluoroscopically monitored knee arthrography. Radiology *122*:827, 1977.
128. Nicks AJ, Mihalko M: A simple device to open the knee joint space during double contrast arthrography. Radiology *122*:827, 1977.
129. Lee KR, Sanders WF: A practical stress device for knee arthrography. Radiology *127*:542, 1978.
130. O'Malley BP: Value of delayed films in knee arthrography. J Can Assoc Radiol *25*:144, 1974.
131. Ricklin P, Rüttimann A, Del Buono MS: Meniscus Lesions — Practical Problems of Clinical Diagnosis, Arthrography and Therapy. New York, Grune & Stratton, 1971.
132. Montgomery CE: Synovial recesses in knee arthrography. Am J Roentgenol *121*:86, 1974.
133. Russell E, Hamm R, LePage JR, Schoenbaum SW, Satin R: Some normal variations of knee arthrograms and their anatomical significance. J Bone Joint Surg *60A*:66, 1978.
134. Nicholas JA, Freiberger RH, Killoran PJ: Double contrast arthrography of the knee. Its value in the management of 225 knee derangements. J Bone Joint Surg *52A*:203, 1970.
135. Heiser S, LaBriola JH, Meyers MH: Arthrography of the knee. Radiology *79*:822, 1962.
136. McIntyre JL: Arthrography of the lateral meniscus. Radiology *105*:531, 1972.
137. Jelaso DV: The fascicles of the lateral meniscus: An anatomic-arthrographic correlation. Radiology *114*:335, 1975.
138. Wickstrom KT, Spitzer RM, Olsson HE: Roentgen anatomy of the posterior horn of the lateral meniscus. Radiology *116*:617, 1975.
139. Fetto JF, Marshall JL, Ghelman B: An anomalous attachment of the popliteus tendon to the lateral meniscus. Case report. J Bone Joint Surg *59A*:548, 1977.
140. Ringertz HG: Arthrography of the knee. I. Localization of lesions. Acta Radiol Diagn *14*:138, 1973.
141. Ringertz HG: Arthrography of the knee. II. Isolated and combined lesions. Acta Radiol Diagn *17*:235, 1976.
142. Hall FM: Buckled meniscus. Radiology *126*:89, 1978.
143. Bramson RT, Staple TW: Double contrast knee arthrography in children. Am J Roentgenol *123*:838, 1975.
144. Stenström R: Diagnostic arthrography of traumatic lesions of the knee joint in children. Ann Radiol *18*:391, 1975.
145. Saddawi ND, Hoffman BK: Tear of the attachment of a normal medial meniscus of the knee in a four year old child. J Bone Joint Surg *52A*:809, 1970.
146. Noble J, Hamblen, DL: The pathology of the degenerate meniscus lesion. J Bone Joint Surg *57B*:180, 1975.
147. Noble J: Lesions of the menisci. Autopsy incidence in adults less than fifty-five years old. J Bone Joint Surg *59A*:480, 1977.
148. Hernandez FJ: Cysts of the semilunar cartilage of the knee. A light and electron microscopic study. Acta Orthop Scand *47*:436, 1976.
149. Burgan DW: Arthrographic findings in meniscal cysts. Radiology *101*:579, 1971.
150. Wroblewski M: Trauma and the cystic meniscus: Review of 500 cases. Injury *4*:319, 1971.
151. Raine GET, Gonet LCL: Cysts of the menisci of the knee. Postgrad Med J *48*:49, 1972.
152. Hall FM: Arthrography of the discoid lateral meniscus. Am J Roentgenol *128*:993, 1977.
153. Haveson SB, Rein BI: Lateral discoid meniscus of the knee: Arthrographic diagnosis. Am J Roentgenol *109*:581, 1970.
154. Smillie IS: The congenital discoid meniscus. J Bone Joint Surg *30B*:671, 1948.
155. Kaplan EB: Discoid lateral meniscus of the knee joint. Nature, mechanism and operative treatment. J Bone Joint Surg *39A*:77, 1957.
156. Fisher AGT: The disk-shaped external semilunar cartilage. Br Med J *1*:688, 1936.
157. Cave EF, Staples OS: Congenital discoid meniscus. A cause of internal derangement of the knee. Am J Surg *54*:371, 1941.
158. Jeannopoulos CL: Observations on discoid menisci. J Bone Joint Surg *32A*:649, 1950.
159. Murdoch G: Congenital discoid medial semilunar cartilage. J Bone Joint Surg *38B*:564, 1956.
160. Riachi E, Phares A: An unusual deformity of the medial semilunar cartilage. J Bone Joint Surg *45B*:146, 1963.
161. Richmond DA: Two cases of discoid medial cartilage. J Bone Joint Surg *40B*:268, 1958.
162. Ross JA, Tough ICK, English TA: Congenital discoid cartilage. Report of a case of discoid medial cartilage with an embryological note. J Bone Joint Surg *40B*:262, 1958.
163. Weiner B, Rosenberg N: Discoid medial meniscus: Association with bone changes in the tibia. A case report. J Bone Joint Surg *56A*:171, 1974.
164. Resnick D, Goergen TG, Kaye JJ, Ghelman B, Woody PR: Discoid medial meniscus. Radiology *121*:575, 1976.
165. Philippon J: Étude des malformations congénitales méniscales par arthropneumographie. J Radiol Electrol Med Nucl *40*:1, 1959.
166. Moes CAF, Munn JD: The value of knee arthrography in children. J Can Assoc Radiol *16*:226, 1965.
167. Nathan PA, Cole SC: Discoid meniscus — a clinical and pathological study. Clin Orthop Rel Res *64*:107, 1969.
168. Dashefsky JH: Discoid lateral meniscus in three members of a family. J Bone Joint Surg *53A*:1208, 1971.
169. Symeonides PP, Ioannides G: Ossicles in the knee menisci. Report of three cases. J Bone Joint Surg *54A*:1288, 1972.
170. Weaver JB: Calcification and ossification of the menisci. J Bone Joint Surg *24*:873, 1942.
171. Rosen IE: Unusual intrameniscal lunulae. Three case reports. J Bone Joint Surg *40A*:925, 1958.
172. Glass RS, Barnes WM, Kells DU, Thomas S, Campbell C: Ossicles of knee menisci. Report of seven cases. Clin Orthop Rel Res *111*:163, 1975.
173. Bernstein RM, Olsson HE, Spitzer RM, Robinson KE, Korn MW: Ossicle of the meniscus. Am J Roentgenol *127*:785, 1976.
174. Pederson HE: The ossicles of the semilunar cartilages of rodents. Anat Rec *105*:1, 1949.
175. Suzuki K, Izawa T, Eguro H: Ossification of semilunar cartilage. Report of a case. J Jap Orthop Assoc *44*:467, 1970.
176. Doyle JR, Eisenberg JH, Orth MW: Regeneration of knee menisci: A preliminary report. J Trauma *6*:50, 1966.
177. Smillie IS: Observations on the regeneration of the semilunar cartilages in man. Br J Surg *31*:398, 1944.
178. Goldenberg RR: Refracture of a regenerated internal semilunar cartilage. J Bone Joint Surg *17*:1054, 1935.
179. Massare C, Bard M, Tristant H: Intérêt de l'arthrographie du genou dans les gonalgies après meniscectomie. Revue de 200 dossiers personnels. J Radiol Electrol Med Nucl *55*:401, 1974.
180. Debnam JW, Staple TW: Arthrography of the knee after meniscectomy. Radiology *113*:67, 1974.
181. Laasonen EM, Wilppula E: Why a meniscectomy fails. Acta Orthop Scand *47*:672, 1976.
182. Dandy DJ, Jackson RW: The diagnosis of problems after meniscectomy. J Bone Joint Surg *57B*:349, 1975.
183. Jackson JP: Degenerative changes in the knee after meniscectomy. Br Med J *2*:525, 1968.
184. Appel H: Late results after meniscectomy in the knee joint. A clinical

and roentgenologic follow-up investigation. Acta Orthop Scand (Suppl *133*):6, 1970.
185. Tapper EM, Hoover NW: Late results after meniscectomy. J Bone Joint Surg *51A*:517, 1969.
186. Gear MWL: The late results of meniscectomy. Br J Surg *54*:270, 1967.
187. Huckell JR: Is meniscectomy a benign procedure? A long term follow-up study. Can J Surg *8*:254, 1965.
188. McGinty JB, Geuss LF, Marvin RA: Partial or total meniscectomy. A comparative analysis. J Bone Joint Surg *59A*:763, 1977.
189. Mittler S, Freiberger RH, Harrison-Stubbs M: A method of improving cruciate ligament visualization in double contrast arthrography. Radiology *102*:441, 1972.
190. Dalinka MK, Gohel VK, Rancier L: Tomography in the evaluation of the anterior cruciate ligament. Radiology *108*:31, 1973.
191. Pavlov H, Torg JS: Double contrast arthrographic evaluation of the anterior cruciate ligament. Radiology *126*:661, 1978.
192. Pavlov H, Freiberger RH: An easy method to demonstrate the cruciate ligaments by double contrast arthrography. Radiology *126*:817, 1978.
193. Dalinka MK, Garofola J: The infrapatellar synovial fold: A cause for confusion in the evaluation of the anterior cruciate ligament. Am J Roentgenol *127*:589, 1976.
194. Anderson PW, Maslin P: Tomography applied to knee arthrography. Radiology *110*:271, 1974.
195. Wershba M, Dalinka MK, Coren GS, Cotler J: Double contrast knee arthrography in the evaluation of osteochondritis dissecans. Clin Orthop Rel Res *107*:81, 1975.
196. Horns JW: Single contrast knee arthrography in abnormalities of the articular cartilage. Radiology *105*:537, 1972.
197. Thomas RH, Resnick D, Alazraki NP, Daniel D, Greenfield R: Compartmental evaluation of osteoarthritis of the knee. A comparative study of available diagnostic modalities. Radiology *116*:585, 1975.
198. Horns JW: The diagnosis of chondromalacia by double contrast arthrography of the knee. J Bone Joint Surg *59A*:119, 1977.
199. Thijn CJP: Double contrast arthrography in meniscal lesions and patellar chondropathy. Radiol Clin Biol *45*:345, 1976.
200. Newberg A, Wales L: Radiographic diagnosis of quadriceps tendon rupture. Radiology *125*:367, 1977.
201. Smason JB: Post-traumatic fistula connecting prepatellar bursa with knee joint. Report of a case. J Bone Joint Surg *54A*:1553, 1972.
202. Jelaso DV, Morris GA: Rupture of the quadriceps tendon: Diagnosis by arthrography. Radiology *116*:621, 1975.
203. Duncan AM: Arthrography in rupture of the suprapatellar bursa with pseudocyst formation. Am J Roentenol *121*:89, 1974.
204. Anderson PW, Harley JD, Maslin PU: Arthrographic evaluation of problems with united tibial plateau fractures. Radiology *119*:75, 1976.
205. Taylor AR: Arthrography of the knee in rheumatoid arthritis. Br J Radiol *42*:493, 1969.
206. Taylor AR, Ansell BM: Arthrography of the knee before and after synovectomy for rheumatoid arthritis. J Bone Joint Surg *54B*:110, 1972.
207. Hall AP, Scott JT: Synovial cysts and rupture of the knee joint in rheumatoid arthritis; an arthrographic study. Ann Rheum Dis *25*:32, 1966.
208. Pinder IM: Treatment of the popliteal cyst in the rheumatoid knee. J Bone Joint Surg *55B*:119, 1973.
209. Wolfe RD, Giuliano VJ: Double-contrast arthrography in the diagnosis of pigmented villonodular synovitis of the knee. Am J Roentgenol *110*:793, 1970.
210. Greenfield MM, Wallace KM: Pigmented villonodular synovitis. Radiology *54*:350, 1950.
211. Sanderud A: Pigmented villonodular synovitis. Acta Orthop Scand *24*:155, 1955.
212. Goergen TG, Resnick D, Niwayama G: Localized nodular synovitis of the knee: A report of two cases with abnormal arthrograms. Am J Roentgenol *126*:647, 1976.
213. Granowitz SP, Mankin HJ: Localized pigmented villonodular synovitis of knee. J Bone Joint Surg *49A*:122, 1967.
214. Hoffa A: Uber Röntgenbilder nach Sauerstoffeinblasung in das Kniegelenk. Berl Klin Wschr *43*:940, 1906.
215. Muckle DS, Monahan P: Intra-articular ganglion of the knee. Report of two cases. J Bone Joint Surg *54B*:520, 1972.
216. Crittenden JJ, Jones DM, Santarelli AG: Knee arthrogram in synovial chondromatosis. Radiology *94*:133, 1970.
217. Prager RJ, Mall JC: Arthrographic diagnosis of synovial chondromatosis. Am J Roentgenol *127*:344, 1976.
218. Weitzman G: Lipoma arborescens of the knee. Report of a case. J Bone Joint Surg *47A*:1030, 1965.
219. Burgan DW: Lipoma arborescens of the knee: Another cause of filling defects on a knee arthrogram. Radiology *101*:583, 1971.
220. Brodsky AE: Synovial hemangioma of the knee joint. Bull Hosp Joint Dis *17*:58, 1956.
221. Coventry MB, Harrison EG Jr, Martin JF: Benign synovial tumors of the knee: A diagnostic problem. J Bone Joint Surg *48A*:1350, 1966.
222. Moon NF: Synovial hemangioma of the knee joint. A review of previously reported cases and inclusion of two new cases. Clin Orthop Rel Res *90*:183, 1973.
223. Resnick D, Oliphant M: Hemophilia-like arthropathy of the knee associated with cutaneous and synovial hemangiomas. Report of 3 cases and review of the literature. Radiology *114*:323, 1975.
224. Forrest J, Staple TW: Synovial hemangioma of the knee. Demonstration by arthrography and arteriography. Am J Roentgenol *112*:512, 1971.
225. Thomas ML, Andress MR: Angioma of the knee demonstrated by angiography and arthrography—report of a case. Acta Radiol (Diagn) *12*:217, 1972.
226. Salerno NR, Menges JF, Borns PF: Arthrograms in hemophilia. Radiology *102*:135, 1972.
227. Dalinka MK, Coren G, Hensinger R, Irani RN: Arthography in Blount's disease. Radiology *113*:161, 1974.
228. Siffert RS, Katz JF: The intra-articular deformity in osteochondrosis deformans tibiae. J Bone Joint Surg *52A*:800, 1970.
229. Lindgren PG, Willen R: Gastrocnemio-semimembranosus bursa and its relation to the knee joint. I. Anatomy and histology. Acta Radiol (Diagn) *18*:497, 1977.
230. Doppman JL: Baker's cyst and the normal gastrocnemio-semimembranosus bursa. Am J Roentgenol *94*:646, 1965.
231. Wilson PD, Eyre-Brook AL, Francis JD: Clinical and anatomical study of semimembranosus bursa in relation to popliteal cyst. J Bone Joint Surg *20*:963, 1938.
232. Burleson RJ, Bickel WH, Dahlin DC: Popliteal cyst: Clinico-pathologic survey. J Bone Joint Surg *38A*:1265, 1956.
233. Baker WM: Formation of synovial cysts in leg in connection with disease of knee joint. St Bartholomew's Hosp Rep *13*:245, 1877.
234. Gristina AG, Wilson PD: Popliteal cysts in adults and children: Review of 90 cases. Arch Surg *88*:357, 1964.
235. Hoffman BK: Cystic lesions of popliteal space. Surg Gynec Obstet *116*:551, 1963.
236. Jayson MIV, Dixon AS: Intra-articular pressure in rheumatoid arthritis of the knee. III. Pressure changes during joint use. Ann Rheum Dis *29*:401, 1970.
237. Taylor AR, Rana NA: A valve. An explanation of the formation of popliteal cysts. Ann Rheum Dis *32*:419, 1973.
238. Palmer DG: Anteromedial synovial cysts at the knee joint in rheumatoid disease. Australas Radiol *16*:79, 1972.
239. Schmidt MC, Workman JB, Barth WF: Dissection or rupture of a popliteal cyst. A syndrome mimicking thrombophlebitis in rheumatic diseases. Arch Intern Med *134*:694, 1974.
240. Swett HA, Jaffe RB, McIff EB: Popliteal cysts: Presentation as thrombophlebitis. Radiology *115*:613, 1975.
241. Solomon L, Berman L: Synovial rupture of knee joint. J Bone Joint Surg *54B*:460, 1972.
242. Iacano V, Gauvin G, Zimbler S: Giant synovial cyst of the calf and thigh in a patient with granulomatous synovitis. Clin Orthop Rel Res *115*:220, 1976.
243. Pallardy G, Fabre P, Ledoux-Lebard G, Delbarre F: L'arthrographie du genou dans l'etude des bursites et des kystes synoviaux. J Radiol Electrol Med Nucl *50*:481, 1969.
244. Shapiro RF, Resnick D, Castles JJ, D'Ambrosia R, Lipscomb PR, Niwayama G: Fistulization of rheumatoid joints. Spectrum of identifiable syndromes. Ann Rheum Dis *34*:489, 1975.
245. Perri JA, Rodnan GP, Mankin HJ: Giant synovial cysts of the calf in patients with rheumatoid arthritis. J Bone Joint Surg *50A*:709, 1968.
246. Lapayowker MS, Cliff MM, Tourtellotte CD: Arthrography in the diagnosis of calf pain. Radiology *95*:319, 1970.
247. Pastershank SP, Mitchell DM: Knee joint bursal abnormalities in rheumatoid arthritis. J Can Assoc Radiol *28*:199, 1977.
248. Wolfe RD, Colloff B: Popliteal cysts. An arthrographic study and review of the literature. J Bone Joint Surg *54A*:1057, 1972.
249. Bryan RS, DiMichele JD, Ford GL Jr: Popliteal cysts. Arthrography as an aid to diagnosis and treatment. Clin Orthop Rel Res *50*:203, 1967.
250. Grepl J: Beitrag zur positiven Arthrographie bei pathologischen Veränderungen der Bursae popliteae. Fortschr Geb Roentgenstr Nuclearmed *119*:84, 1973.
251. Clark JM: Arthrography diagnosis of synovial cysts of the knee. Radiology *115*:480, 1975.
252. Cooperberg PL, Tsang I, Truelove L, Knickerbocker J: Grey scale ultrasound in the evaluation of rheumatoid arthritis of the knee. Radiology *126*:759, 1978.
253. Ambanelli U, Manganelli P, Nervetti A, Ugolotti U: Demonstration of articular effusions and popliteal cysts with ultrasound. J Rheumatol *3*:134, 1976.
254. Carpenter JR, Hattery RR, Hunder GG, Bryan RS, McLeod RA: Ultrasound evaluation of the popliteal space. Comparison with arthrography and physical examination. Mayo Clin Proc *51*:498, 1976.

255. Rudikoff JC, Lynch JJ, Philipps E, Clapp PR: Ultrasound diagnosis of Baker cyst, JAMA *235*:1054, 1976.
256. Moore CP, Sarti DA, Lovie JS: Ultrasonographic demonstration of popliteal cysts in rheumatoid arthritis. A noninvasive technique. Arthritis Rheum *18*:577, 1975.
257. Meire HB, Lindsay DJ, Swinson DR, Hamilton EBD: Comparison of ultrasound and positive contrast arthrography in the diagnosis of popliteal and calf swellings. Ann Rheum Dis *33*:221, 1974.
258. Levin MH, Nordyke RA, Ball JJ: Demonstration of dissecting popliteal cysts by joint scans after intra-articular isotope injections. Arthritis Rheum *14*:591, 1971.
259. Cooper RA: Computerized tomography (body scan) of Baker's cyst. J Rheumatol *5*:184, 1978.
260. Dixon AS, Grast C: Acute synovial rupture in rheumatoid arthritis: Clinical and experimental observations. Lancet *1*:742, 1964.
261. Tait GBW, Bach F, Dixon AS: Acute synovial rupture: Further observations. Ann Rheum Dis *24*:273, 1965.
262. Barbaric ZL, Young LW: Synovial cyst in juvenile rheumatoid arthritis. Am J Roentgenol *116*:655, 1972.
263. Toyama WM: Familial popliteal cysts in children. Am J Dis Child *124*:586, 1972.
264. Olson RW: Arthrography of the ankle: Its use in the evaluation of ankle sprains. Radiology *92*:1439, 1969.
265. Broström L, Liljedahl SO, Lindvall N: Sprained ankles. II. Arthrographic diagnosis of recent ligament ruptures. Acta Chir Scand *129*:485, 1965.
266. Spiegel PK, Staples OS: Arthrography of the ankle joint: Problems in diagnosis of acute lateral ligament injuries. Radiology *114*:587, 1975.
267. Arner O, Ekengren K, Hulting B, Lindholm A: Arthrography of the talocrural joint: Anatomic, roentgenographic and clinical aspects. Acta Chir Scand *113*:253, 1957.
268. Fordyce AJW, Horn CV: Arthrography in recent injuries of the ligament of the ankle. J Bone Joint Surg *54B*:116, 1972.
269. Ala-Ketola L, Puranen J, Koivisto E, Puuperä M: Arthrography in the diagnosis of ligament injuries and classification of ankle injuries. Radiology *125*:63, 1977.
270. Mehrez M, El Geneidy S: Arthrography of the ankle. J Bone Joint Surg *52B*:308, 1970.
271. Fussell ME, Godley DR: Ankle arthrography in acute sprains. Clin Orthop Rel Res *93*:278, 1973.
272. Sanders HWA: Ankle arthrography and ankle distortion. Radiol Clin Biol *46*:1, 1977.
273. Gordon RB: Arthrography of the ankle joint. Experience in 107 studies. J Bone Joint Surg *52A*:1623, 1970.
274. Percy EC, Hill RO, Callaghan JE: The "sprained" ankle. J Trauma *9*:972, 1969.
275. Kaye JJ, Bohne WHO: A radiographic study of the ligamentous anatomy of the ankle. Radiology *125*:659, 1977.
276. Smith GR, Winquist RA, Allan NK, Northrop CH: Subtle transchondral fractures of the talar dome: A radiological perspective. Radiology *124*:667, 1977.
277. Berndt AL, Harty M: Transchondral fractures (osteochondritis dissecans) of the talus. J Bone Joint Surg *41A*:988, 1959.
278. Wolin I, Glassman F, Sideman S, Levinthal DH: Internal derangement of the talofibular component of the ankle. Surg Gynecol Obstet *91*:193, 1950.
279. Deyerle WM: Long term follow-up of fractures of the os calcis. Diagnostic peroneal synoviagram. Orthop Clin North Am *4*:213, 1973.
280. Resnick D, Goergen TG: Peroneal tenography in previous calcaneal fractures. Radiology *115*:211, 1975.
281. Garcia A, Parkes J: Fractures of the foot. *In* N Giannestras (Ed): Foot Disorders. Medical and Surgical Management. Philadelphia, Lea & Febiger, 1973.
282. Burman M: Stenosing tendovaginitis of the foot and ankle; studies with special reference to the stenosing tendovaginitis of the peroneal tendons at the peroneal tubercle. Arch Surg *67*:686, 1953.
283. Webster FS: Peroneal tenosynovitis with pseudotumor. J Bone Joint Surg *50A*:153, 1968.
284. Earle AS, Moritz JR, Tapper EM: Dislocation of the peroneal tendons at the ankle: An analysis of 25 ski injuries. Northwest Med *71*:108, 1972.
285. Church CC: Radiographic diagnosis of acute peroneal tendon dislocation. Am J Roentgenol *129*:1065, 1977.
286. Daffner RH, Whitfield PW: Recurrent ganglion cyst: The value of preoperative ganglionography. Am J Roentgenol *129*:345, 1977.
287. Palmer DG: Tendon sheaths and bursae involved by rheumatoid disease at the foot and ankle. Australas Radiol *14*:419, 1970.
288. Resnick D, Feingold ML, Curd J, Niwayama G, Goergen TG: Calcaneal abnormalities in articular disorders. Rheumatoid arthritis, ankylosing spondylitis, psoriatic arthritis and Reiter syndrome. Radiology *125*:355, 1977.
289. Weston WJ: The bursa deep to teno Achillis. Australas Radiol *14*:327, 1970.
290. Resnick D: Radiology of the talocalcaneal articulations. Anatomic considerations and arthrography. Radiology *111*:581, 1974.
291. Weston WJ: Traumatic effusions of the ankle and posterior subtaloid joints. Br J Radiol *31*:445, 1958.
292. Meyer JM: L'arthrographie de l'articulation sous-astragalienne postérieure et de l'articulation de Chopart. Thèse Méd Genève, No 3318, 1973.
293. Meyer JM, Lagier R: Post-traumatic sinus tarsi syndrome. An anatomical and radiological study. Acta Orthop Scand *48*:121, 1977.
294. Kaye JJ, Ghelman B, Schneider R: Talocalcaneonavicular joint arthrography for sustentacular-talar tarsal coalitions. Radiology *115*:730, 1975.
295. Harris RI, Beath T: Etiology of peroneal spastic flat foot. J Bone Joint Surg *30B*:624, 1948.
296. Sahlstedt B: Simultaneous arthrography of the talocrural and talonavicular joints in children. I. Technique. Acta Radiol (Diagn) *17*:545, 1976.
297. Hjelmstedt A, Sahlstedt B: Simultaneous arthrography of the talocrural and talonavicular joints in children. II. Comparison between anatomic and arthrographic measurements. Acta Radiol (Diagn) *17*:557, 1976.
298. Hjelmstedt A, Sahlstedt B: Simultaneous arthrography of the talocrural and talonavicular joints in children. II. Measurements on normal feet. Acta Radiol (Diagn) *18*:513, 1977.
299. Hjelmstedt A, Sahlstedt B: Simultaneous arthrography of the talocrural and talonavicular joints in children. IV. Measurements on congenital club feet. Acta Radiol (Diagn) *19*:223, 1978.
300. Weston WJ: Positive contrast arthrography of the normal midtarsal joints. Australas Radiol *13*:365, 1969.
301. Resnick D: Roentgen features of the rheumatoid mid and hindfoot. J Can Assoc Radiol *27*:99, 1976.
302. Glover JR: Arthrography of the joints of the lumbar vertebral arches. Orthop Clin North Am *8*:37, 1977.
303. Ghelman B, Doherty JH: Demonstration of spondylolysis by arthrography of the apophyseal joint. Am J Roentgenol *130*:986, 1978.
304. Mooney V, Robertson J: The facet syndrome. Clin Orthop Rel Res *115*:149, 1976.
305. Köhler R: Contrast examination of the lumbar interspinous ligaments. Preliminary report. Acta Radiol *52*:21, 1959.
306. Dirheimer Y, Ramsheyi A, Reolon M: Positive arthrography of the craniocervical joint. Neuroradiology *12*:257, 1977.
307. McGaw WH, Weckesser EC: Pneumarthrograms of the knee. A diagnostic aid in internal derangements. J Bone Joint Surg *27*:432, 1945.
308. Meschan I, McGaw WH: Newer methods of pneumoarthrography of the knee with an evaluation of the procedure in 315 operated cases. Radiology *49*:675, 1947.
309. Kleinberg S: Pulmonary embolism following oxygen injection of a knee. JAMA *89*:172, 1927.
310. Pavlov H, Ghelman B, Warren RF: Double-contrast arthrography of the elbow. Radiology *130*:87, 1979.
311. Roback DL: Elbow arthrography: Brief technical considerations. Clin Radiol *30*:311, 1979.
312. Gilula LA, Schoenecker PL, Murphy WA: Shoulder arthrography as a treatment modality. Am J Roentgenol *131*:1047, 1978.
313. Slätis P, Aalto K: Medial dislocation of the tendon of the long head of the biceps brachii. Acta Orthop Scand *50*:73, 1979.
314. El-Khoury GY, Albright JP, Abu Yousef MM, Montgomery WJ, Tuck SL: Arthrotomography of the glenoid labrum. Radiology *131*:333, 1979.
315. Zachrisson BE, Ejeskär A: Arthrography in dislocation of the acromioclavicular joint. Acta Radiol (Diagn) *20*:81, 1979.
316. Schwartz AM, Goldberg MJ: The medial adductor approach to arthrography of the hip in children. Radiology *132*:483, 1979.
317. Tegtmeyer CJ, McCue FC III, Higgins SM, Ball DW: Arthrography of the knee: A comparative study of the accuracy of single and double contrast techniques. Radiology *132*:37, 1979.
318. Hall FM: Further pitfalls in knee arthrography. J Can Assoc Radiol *29*:179, 1978.
319. Barrie HJ: The pathogenesis and significance of meniscal cysts. J Bone Joint Surg *61B*:184, 1979.
320. Buckwalter JA, Dryer RF, Mickelson MR: Arthrography in juxta-articular cysts of the knee. Two cases diagnosed by delayed roentgenograms. J Bone Joint Surg *61A*:465, 1979.
321. Enis JE, Ghandur-Mnaymneh L: Cyst of the lateral meniscus causing erosion of the tibial plateau. A case report. J Bone Joint Surg *61A*:441, 1979.
322. Berson BL, Hermann G: Torn discoid menisci of the knee in adults. Four case reports. J Bone Joint Surg *61A*:303, 1979.
323. Kossoff J, Naimark A, Corbett M: Case report 85. Skel Radiol *4*:45, 1979.
324. Pavlov H, Hirschy JC, Torg JS: Computed tomography of the cruciate ligaments. Radiology *132*:389, 1979.

325. Rau WS, Kauffmann G: Röntgendiagnostik des Knorpelschadens am Kniegelenk. Radiologe *18*:451, 1978.
326. Kormano M, Mäkelä P: Lymphatics filled at knee arthrography. Acta Radiol (Diagn) *19*:853, 1978.
327. Pudlowski RM, Gilula LA, Kyriakos M: Intra-articular lipoma with osseous metaplasia: Radiographic-pathologic correlation. Am J Roentgenol *132*:471, 1979.
328. Gordon GV, Edell S, Brogadir SP, Schumacher HR, Schimmer BM, Dalinka M: Baker's cysts and true thrombophlebitis. Report of two cases and review of the literature. Arch Intern Med *139*:40, 1979.
329. Gillies H, Seligson D: Precision in the diagnosis of meniscal lesions: A comparison of clinical evaluation, arthrography, and arthroscopy. J Bone Joint Surg *61A*:343, 1979.
330. Hallel T, Salvati EA: Osteochondritis dissecans following Legg-Calvé-Perthes disease. Report of three cases. J Bone Joint Surg *58A*:708, 1976.
331. Dalinka MK, Lally JF, Gohel VK: Arthrography of the lateral meniscus. Am J Roentgenol *121*:79, 1974.
332. Harley JD: An anatomic-arthrographic study of the relationships of the lateral meniscus and the popliteus tendon. Am J Roentgenol *128*:181, 1977.
333. Weiner B, Rosenberg N: Discoid medial meniscus: Association with bone changes in the tibia. A case report. J Bone Joint Surg *56A*:171, 1974.
334. Fairbank TJ: Knee joint changes after meniscectomy. J Bone Joint Surg *30B*:664, 1948.
335. Ganel A, Engel J, Ditzian R, Farin I, Militeanu J: Arthrography as a method of diagnosing sof-tissue injuries of the wrist. J Trauma *19*:376, 1979.
336. Hall FM: Elbow arthrography. Radiology *132*:775, 1979.
337. Mink JH, Richardson A, Grant TT: Evaluation of glenoid labrum by double-contrast shoulder arthrography. Am J Roentgenol *133*:883, 1979.
338. Mikasa M: Subacromial bursography. J Jap Orthop Assoc *53*:225, 1979.
339. Rosenthal DI, Murray WT, Jauernek RR, Butch R: Stressing the knee joint for arthrography. Radiology *134*:250, 1980.
340. Bowen AD III: Have you tried this knee arthrography stress device? Am J Roentgenol *134*:197, 1980.
341. Foote GA: Delayed films in double contrast knee arthrography. Australas Radiol *22*:273, 1978.
342. Pavlov H, Goldman AB: The popliteus bursa: An indicator of subtle pathology. Am J Roentgenol *134*:313, 1980.
343. Schuldt DR, Wolfe RD: Clinical and arthrographic findings in meniscal cysts. Radiology *134*:49, 1980.
344. Conforty B, Lotem M: Ossicles in human menisci: Report of two cases. Clin Orthop Rel Res *144*:272, 1979.
345. Vahvanen V, Aalto K: Meniscectomy in children. Acta Orthop Scand *50*:791, 1979.
346. Noble J, Erat K: In defense of the meniscus. A prospective study of 200 meniscectomy patients. J Bone Joint Surg *62B*:7, 1980.
347. Seidl G, Scherak O, Hofner W: Antefemoral dissecting cysts in rheumatoid arthritis. Radiology *133*:343, 1979.
348. Eyanson S, Macfarlane JD, Brandt KD: Popliteal cyst mimicking thrombophlebitis as the first indication of knee disease. Clin Orthop Rel Res *144*:215, 1979.
349. Rauschning W, Lindgren PG: Popliteal cysts (Baker's cysts) in adults. I. Clinical and roentgenological results of operative excision. Acta Orthop Scand *50*:583, 1979.
350. Lindgren PG, Rauschning W: Clinical and arthrographic studies on the valve mechanism in communicating popliteal cysts. Arch Orthop Traumat Surg *95*:245, 1979.
351. Ireland J, Trickey EL, Stoker DJ: Arthroscopy and arthrography of the knee. A critical review. J Bone Joint Surg *62B*:3, 1980.
352. Levinsohn EM, Baker BE: Prearthrotomy diagnostic evaluation of the knee: Review of 100 cases diagnosed by arthrography and arthroscopy. Am J Roentgenol *134*:107, 1980.
353. Korn MW, Spitzer RM, Robinson KE: Correlations of arthrography with arthroscopy. Orthop Clin N Am *10*:535, 1979.
354. Lindholmer E, Foged N, Jensen JT: Arthrography of the ankle. Value in diagnosis of rupture of the lateral ligaments. Acta Radiol (Diagn) *19*:585, 1978.
355. Moppes FI, Hoogenband CR, Greep JM: Adhesive capsulitis of the ankle (frozen ankle). Arch Orthop Traumat Surg *94*:313, 1979.
356. Abraham E, Stirnaman JE: Neglected rupture of the peroneal tendons causing recurrent sprains of the ankle. Case report. J Bone Joint Surg *61A*:1247, 1979.
357. Evans GA, Frenyo SK: The stress-tenogram in the diagnosis of ruptures of the lateral ligament of the ankle. J Bone Joint Surg *61B*:347, 1979.
358. Neviaser TJ: Arthrography of the shoulder. Orthop Clin North Am *11*:205, 1980.
359. Gershuni DH, Axer A, Hendel D: Arthrography as an aid to diagnosis, prognosis, and therapy in Legg-Calvé-Perthes' disease. Acta Orthop Scand *51*:505, 1980.
360. Ferrer-Roca O, Vilalta C: Lesions of the meniscus. Part I: Macroscopic and histologic findings. Clin Orthop Rel Res *146*:289, 1980.
361. Ferrer-Roca O, Vilalta C: Lesions of the meniscus. Part II: Horizontal cleavages and lateral cysts. Clin Orthop Rel Res *146*:301, 1980.
362. Reichelt A, Hehne HJ, Rau WS, Schlageter M: Die doppel Kontrast-arthrographie bei der Chondropathia patellae — klinische und experimentelle Studie zur Pathogenese und Diagnostik. Z Orthop *117*:746, 1979.
363. Beyer D, Fiedler V, Schütt H, Boehnke E: Hypertrophie des hoffaschen fettkörpers-eine arthrographische diagnose? Röntgen-Bl *32*:429, 1979.
364. Rauschning W, Lindgren PG: The clinical significance of the valve mechanism in communicating popliteal cysts. Arch Orthop Traumat Surg *95*:251, 1979.
365. Hermann G, Hochberg F: Lipoma arborescens: Arthrographic findings. Orthopedics *3*:19, 1980.
366. Van Moppes FI, VanEngelshoven JMH, Van de Hoogenband CR: Comparison between talar tilt, anterior drawer sign and ankle arthrography in ankle ligament lesions. J Belge Radiol *62*:441, 1979.
367. Hjelmstedt EA, Sahlstedt B: Arthrography as a guide in the treatment of congenital clubfoot. Acta Orthop Scand *51*:321, 1980.
368. Hjelmstedt A, Sahlstedt B: Talo-calcaneal osteotomy and soft tissue procedures in the treatment of clubfoot. Parts I, II. Acta Orthop Scand *51*:335, 349, 1980.
369. Mink JH, Dickerson R: Air or CO_2 for knee arthrography? Amer J Roentgenol *134*:991, 1980.
370. Sedgwick WG, Gilula LA, Lesker PA, Whiteside LA: Wear particles: Their value in knee arthrography. Radiology *136*:11, 1980.

16

ANGIOGRAPHY OF ARTICULAR AND PARA-ARTICULAR DISEASE

by
Joseph J. Bookstein, M.D.

Angiography ordinarily is unnecessary in the investigation of joint disease. In selected cases, however, angiography may be indicated for a variety of diagnostic or therapeutic purposes. Articular or para-articular disorders may be simulated by vascular disease. Examples include arterial aneurysm or venous thrombosis mimicking arthritis. Tumors of bone, such as giant cell tumor or osteosarcoma, may be hypervascular, and the nature and extent of the osseous abnormality can be investigated angiographically, particularly when a significant soft tissue component is suspected. Diagnosis and extent of para-articular soft tissue tumors, particularly angiomatous malformations, can be evaluated angiographically with reasonable accuracy. Joint trauma is not infrequently associated with vascular injury. When vascular injury is suspected clinically, angiography is indicated for definitive diagnosis and in estimating the need for, and extent of, surgery. Angiography may provide interesting information in various laboratory or clinical investigations, such as in defining the vascular supply of the hip in osteonecrosis. Finally, and very importantly, transcatheter therapy is becoming applicable in a variety of orthopedic conditions, such as in controlling hemorrhage from bone trauma, facilitating hemostasis during operation on hypervascular bone tumors, providing palliative relief from pain of bone tumors, or definitively treating vascular malformations of the soft tissues.

This chapter will consider in some detail the role of arteriography in the assessment of joint disease, including the following conditions:

A. Acute trauma

1. Diagnosis
2. Transcatheter therapy

B. Aneurysm and other primary arterial lesions

1. Atherosclerotic
2. Associated with osteochondroma
3. Popliteal artery cyst
4. Popliteal entrapment by gastrocnemius muscle
5. Hypothenar hammer syndrome

C. Neoplasms and other masses

1. Para-articular bone tumors, primary or secondary
2. Evaluating extent of soft tissue masses
3. Transcatheter therapy

D. Autoimmune diseases

1. Rheumatoid arthritis
2. Giant cell arteritis (polymyalgia rheumatica)
3. Scleroderma
4. Lupus erythematosus
5. Necrotizing arteritis (polyarteritis)

E. Venous disease

1. Thrombophlebitis
2. Popliteal bursal cyst simulating venous obstruction

F. Miscellaneous

1. Acro-osteolysis
2. Frostbite
3. Osteonecrosis of the hip

TRAUMA

Articular trauma may occur secondary to blunt or penetrating injury; in either case, vascular injury may be an associated finding (Figs. 16–1 to 16–4). Clinical examination usually demonstrates marked swelling, but differentiation of hemarthrosis, diffuse tissue hematoma, or pseudoaneurysm associated with arterial trauma is often impossible. Although the pulse is often absent distally and the limb may be cool in the presence of arterial injury, these findings are neither totally sensitive nor specific. Pulse loss, for example, may reflect compartment syndromes, rather than intrinsic arterial injury. From a practical viewpoint, arteriography should be performed whenever there is the slightest indication of arterial injury in association with skeletal trauma.[7, 28]

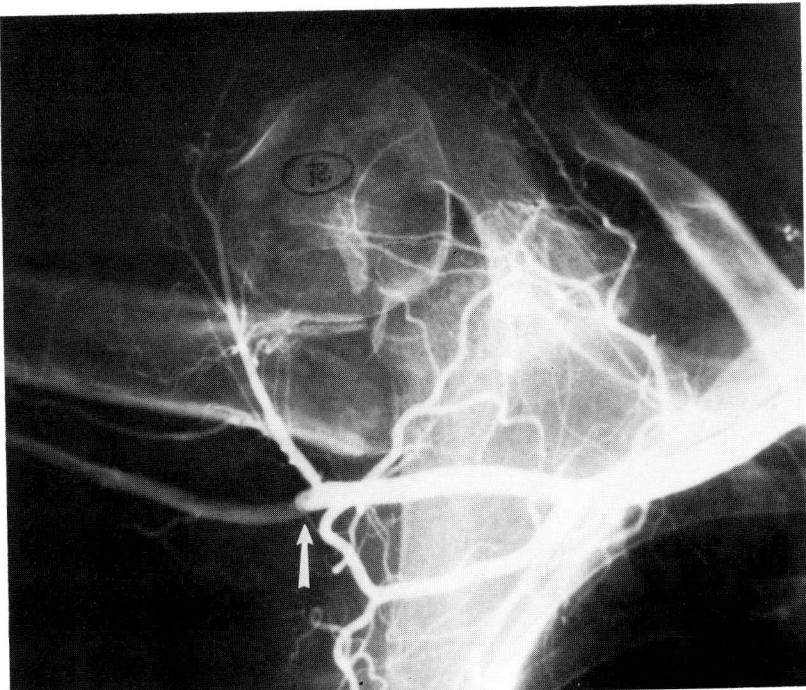

Figure 16–1. *Arterial injury associated with blunt trauma to the shoulder. After the patient suffered this displaced humeral neck fracture, the entire upper extremity became pulseless, pale, and cool. The angiogram demonstrates an intimal tear and partial obstruction of the high brachial artery (arrow).*

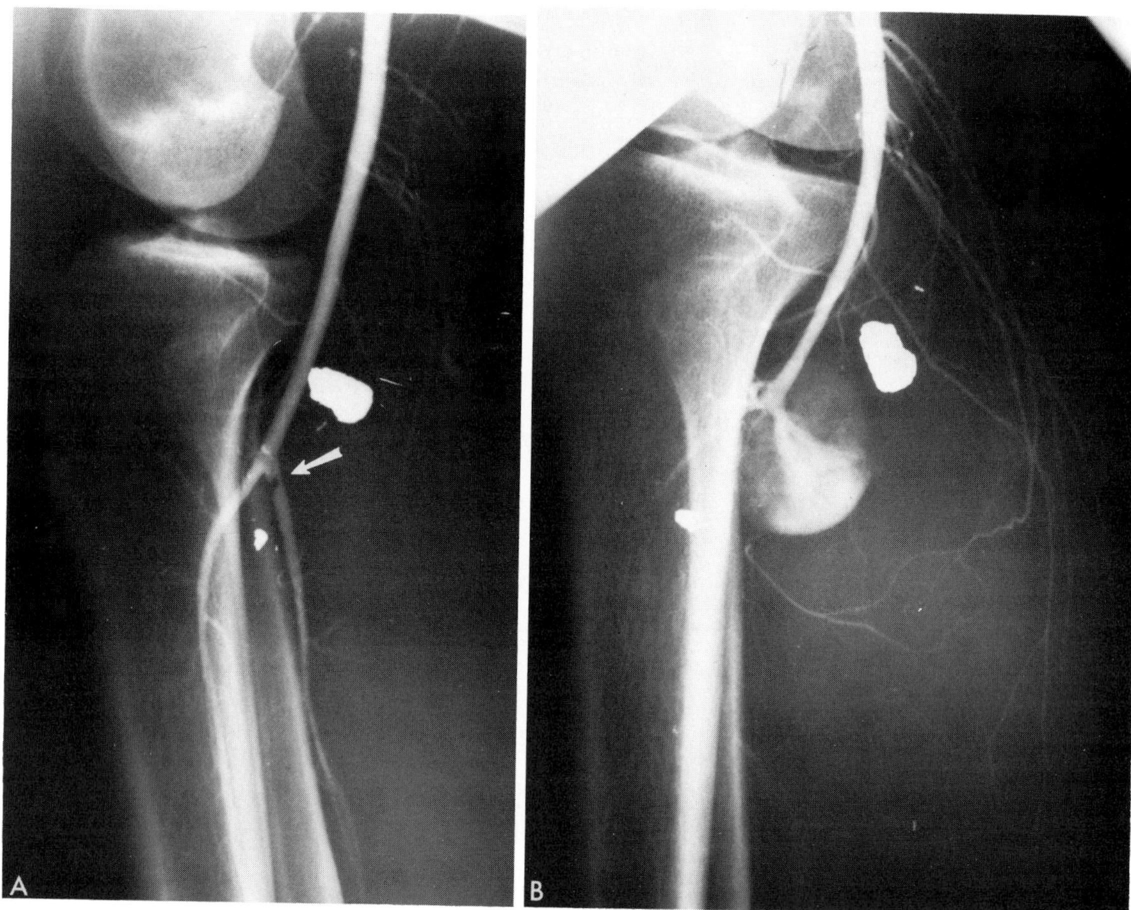

Figure 16–2. Traumatic mycotic aneurysm secondary to penetrating trauma. This 29 year old drug abuser, after being shot near the knee, had marked joint swelling and tenderness and a cool foot. After the initial arteriogram **(A)**, he developed a clostridial infection that was treated with hyperbaric oxygen. Following institution of heparin therapy a month after injury, he developed a sudden painful, pulsatile swelling in the right popliteal fossa, clinically thought to represent an abscess or aneurysm.

A Initial arteriogram demonstrates an intimal tear at the origin of the tibioperoneal trunk (arrow), and downstream compression of this artery by hematoma. Also, several bullet fragments are evident.

B Arteriogram taken 1 month later, after sudden development of popliteal swelling, shows a mycotic aneurysm.

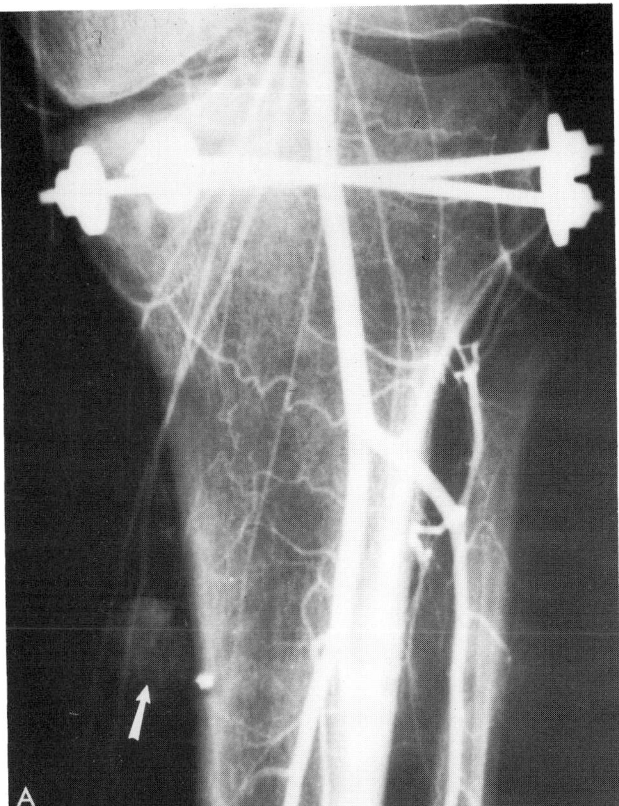

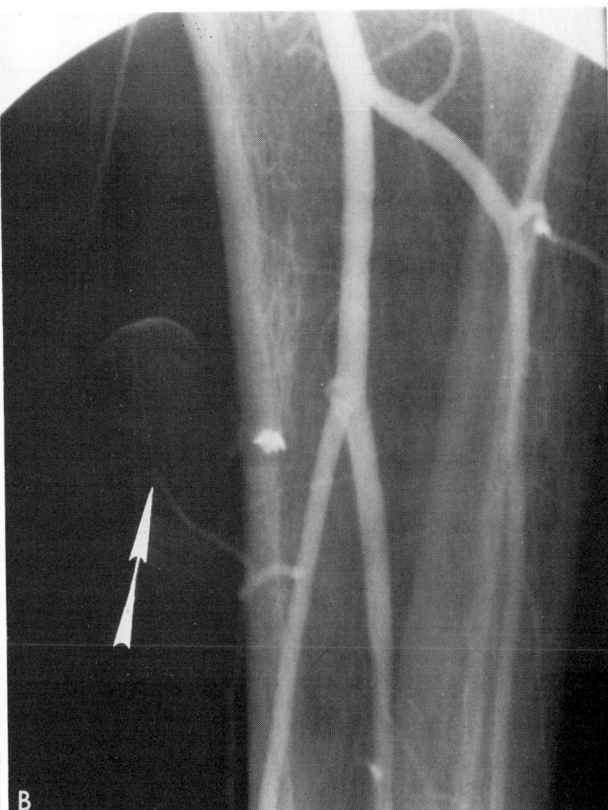

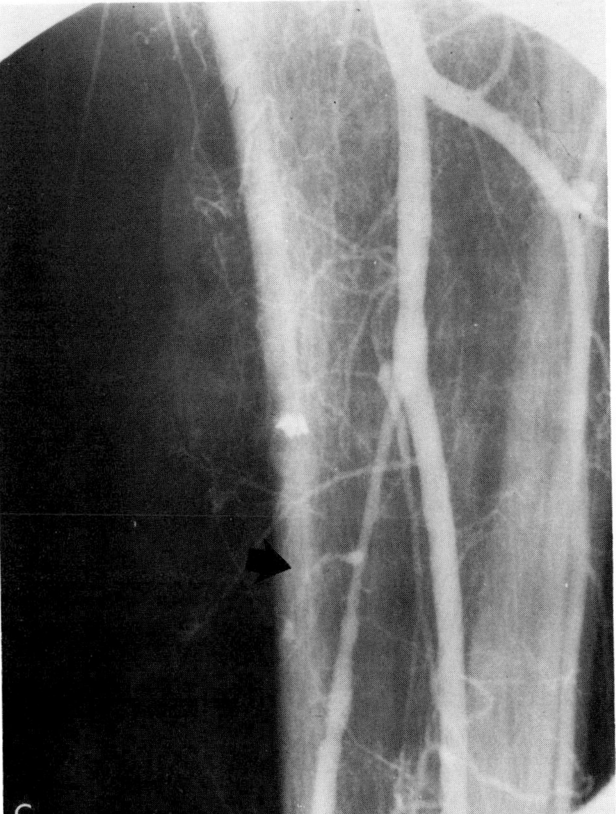

Figure 16–3. *Iatrogenic aneurysm incident to an orthopedic procedure. A tibial plateau fracture had previously been pinned more distally. After the pins were removed and replaced more proximally, intermittent bleeding developed at the site of the original pins. After transcatheter embolization, bleeding remained permanently controlled.*

A *Nonmagnified arteriogram demonstrating faint accumulation of contrast medium within an aneurysm (arrow). The source of bleeding was not shown.*

B *After selective injection into the popliteal artery, magnification arteriography demonstrates the actual bleeding artery as it briefly spurted into the high-pressure aneurysm (arrow).*

C *After selective catheterization and embolization of the feeding artery, bleeding stopped permanently (arrow).*

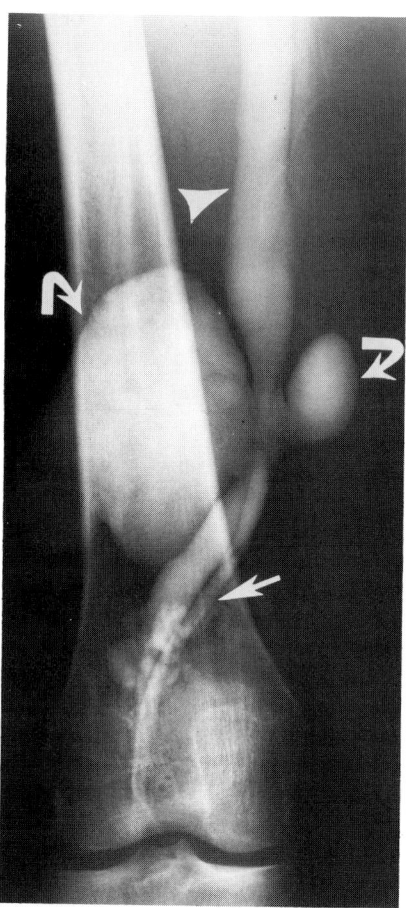

Figure 16–4. Pulsatile venous aneurysm and arteriovenous fistula after penetrating injury from an ice pick several years earlier. The arteriogram demonstrates two venous aneurysms at the site of fistula (curved arrows), early venous opacification of a somewhat dilated superficial femoral vein (arrowhead), and delayed flow in the small postfistulous popliteal artery (straight arrow).

TRANSCATHETER HEMOSTASIS

Hemorrhage may occur in and around joints, most frequently after trauma. Usually the hemorrhage is self-limited or is controlled surgically. Occasionally, however, control of the hemorrhage via transcatheter embolization may be an attractive alternative. For example, pelvic fractures, particularly those involving the pubic rami, may produce life-threatening hemorrhage. Selective catheterization and embolization of the appropriate internal iliac branches can be a simple life-saving measure.[36, 37, 56] Postoperative hemorrhage after orthopedic procedures, with or without associated infection, has been treated in the same manner.[39] Although not yet reported, transcatheter therapy of hemophilic hemarthrosis may be feasible. Figure 16–3 illustrates and aneurysm that bled after removal of a traction pin. After selective transcatheter embolization, the hemorrhage was permanently controlled.

ANEURYSM AND OTHER PRIMARY ARTERIAL DISEASES

Aneurysms

Aneurysms not infrequently involve the popliteal artery (Fig. 16–5), and produce a mass in the popliteal space that superficially simulates joint disease. Clinical examination almost always reveals intrinsic pulsation, however, and the aneurysm will not expand the suprapatellar bursa, as would a knee joint effusion. Because popliteal aneurysms may rupture, operative correction is generally warranted. Arteriography is indicated in planning surgery.

Several recent articles report the development of arterial aneurysms in association with osteochondromas about the knee joint.[14, 17] The usual proximity of the popliteal artery to the rough aspect of the osteochondroma, and the mechanical trauma secondary to motion of the knee joint combine to produce chronic arterial injury and eventual aneurysm. In the case illustrated in Figure 16–6, rapid expansion of the aneurysm simulated malignant transformation of the osteochondroma.

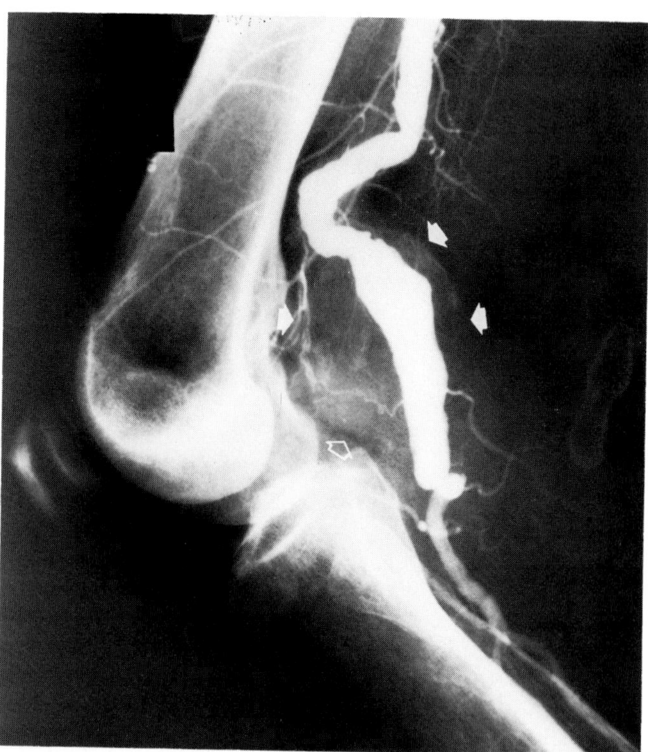

Figure 16–5. Ordinary atherosclerotic aneurysm in a patient with a cool left foot and barely pulsatile mass in left popliteal fossa. Note that much of the aneurysm is filled with nonopacified clot. The margin is demarcated by minimal intimal calcification (open and solid arrows). (Courtesy of Lewis Wexler, M.D.)

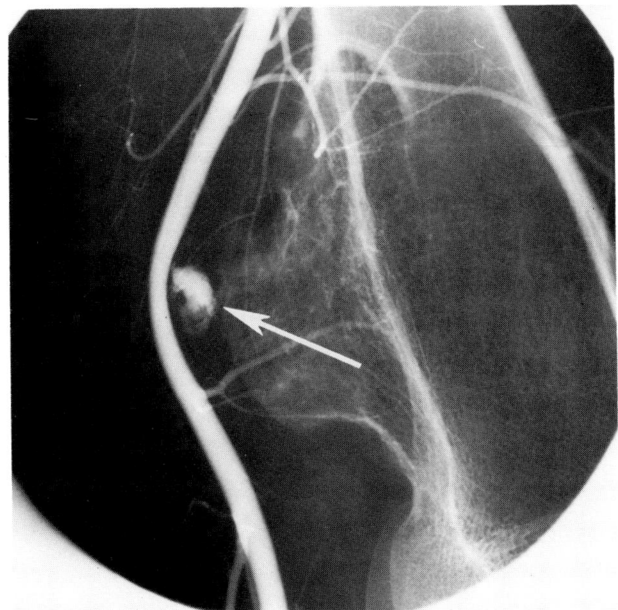

Figure 16–6. *Aneurysm secondary to femoral exostosis. This patient with multiple exostoses developed pain, tenderness, and enlargement over an exostosis near the knee, and malignant degeneration was suspected.*

Magnification arteriogram in lateral view shows no pathologic vessels in the region of exostosis to suggest malignancy. Instead, a pseudoaneurysm is beginning to opacify (arrow) at the site of chronic arterial injury from the exostosis.

Cystic Mucinous Degeneration

Cystic mucinous degeneration may involve the popliteal artery. The usual manifestations are ischemic, often of abrupt onset in young men, secondary to arterial obstruction by the cyst; rarely the mass is palpable, simulating a primary articular lesion. Hemorrhage into the cyst may occur, producing intramural hematoma. The etiology is unknown; a congenital origin is postulated by some because the condition may affect relatively young patients.[10, 40]

Popliteal Entrapment Syndrome

The popliteal entrapment syndrome is produced by compression of the popliteal artery by the medial head of the gastrocnemius muscle (Fig. 16–7). It is generally manifested as intermittent claudication in a young, otherwise normal patient. The compression may be due to either (a) abnormal position of the popliteal artery medial to the medial head of the gastrocnemius muscle, or (b) compression of a normally situated popliteal artery by an anomalous laterally inserting slip from the medial head of the gastrocnemius.[21, 22]

Hypothenar Hammer Syndrome

The hypothenar hammer syndrome is characterized by thrombosis, spasm, or aneurysm of the ulnar artery secondary to repetitive minor, usually occupational, trauma.[6] Because of the variability of the arterial supply to the fingers and the associated collateral circulation, any one finger or combination of fingers may show signs of ischemia. Arteriography demonstrates narrowing, occlusion, or aneurysm of the ulnar artery, usually adjacent to the hook of the hamate.[1] Most symptomatic patients will have multiple occlusions involving digital arteries, metacarpal arteries, and palmar arches. The distal occlusions are apparently secondary to emboli that have arisen within the ulnar artery (Fig. 16–8).

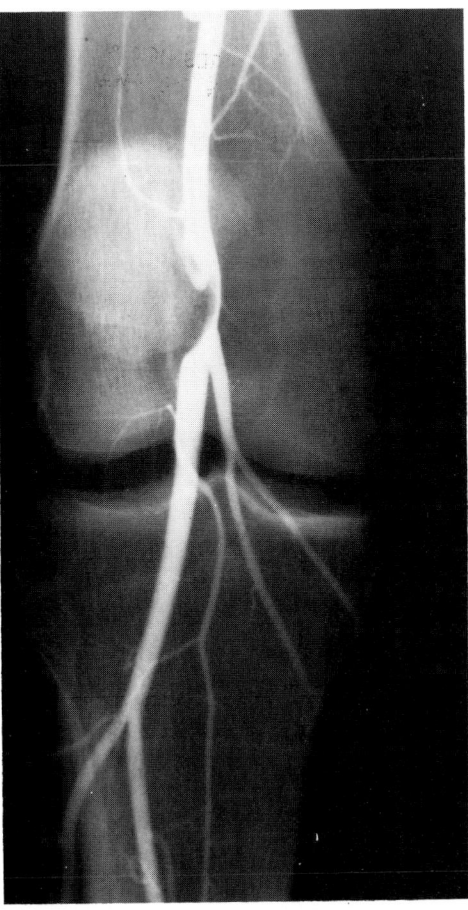

Figure 16–7. *Compression of the popliteal artery by the medial head of the gastrocnemius muscle. Twenty year old man who developed claudication while at work. The artery appears to be smoothly compressed from its lateral aspect. The normal course of the artery suggests that compression is due to an aberrant slip of the medial head of the gastrocnemius, not to an anomalous course of the popliteal artery medial to a normal gastrocnemius. There were some associated intimal changes noted at operation. (Though this was not mentioned, the possibility of some mural thickening due to cyst or hemorrhage is also suspected.) Operative release of the head of the gastrocnemius and endarterectomy resulted in relief of symptoms. (Courtesy of Dr. Andrew B. Crummy.)*

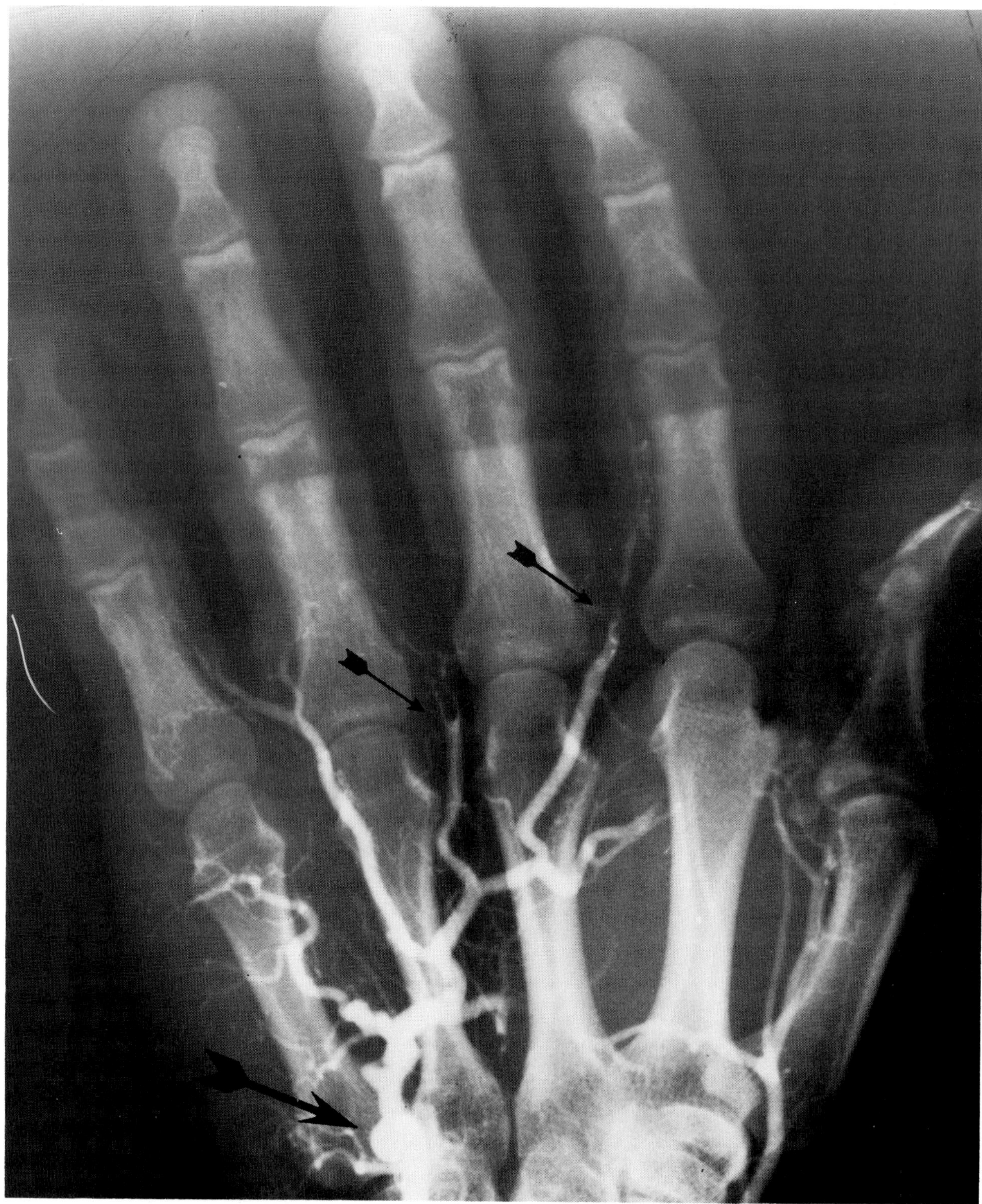

Figure 16–8. *Hypothenar hammer syndrome. This 30 year old tool and dye worker had symptoms of Raynaud's phenomenon. His occupation involved repeated minor trauma to the ulnar aspect of his hand.*

The arteriogram demonstrates minor irregularity and dilatation of the distal ulnar artery (large arrow). Multiple small emboli have originated in the ulnar artery and lodged in the proper digital arteries (small arrows).

TUMORS AND OTHER MASSES

Arteriography has been advocated in evaluating the type, extent, and behavioral characteristics of bone tumors.[18, 23, 26, 32, 51, 52] In my opinion, this advocacy should be somewhat tempered. Biopsy is much more reliable in evaluating behavioral characteristics, and plain films are generally adequate in determining extent. Giant cell tumor usually involves para-articular bone, most frequently the femoral condyles. The tumor is usually hypervascular and has been studied angiographically with some frequency.[13, 32] An example is shown in Figure 16–9. Angiography may be relatively helpful in cases in which there is an important soft tissue component.[32] Transcatheter embolization has been advocated in the palliative management of pain or hemorrhage of bone tumors[14, 48] (Fig. 16–9). Conceivably, angiography may become more applicable in the future, if effective chemotherapeutic agents are developed that require selective intra-arterial administration, or if transcatheter embolization proves to be effective in palliation.

Arteriography has assumed a larger role in evaluating the nature and extent of soft tissue masses.[12, 18, 20, 26, 27, 52] In my experience, the procedure is reliable only in the evaluation of arteriovenous malformations or hemangiomas, and even here

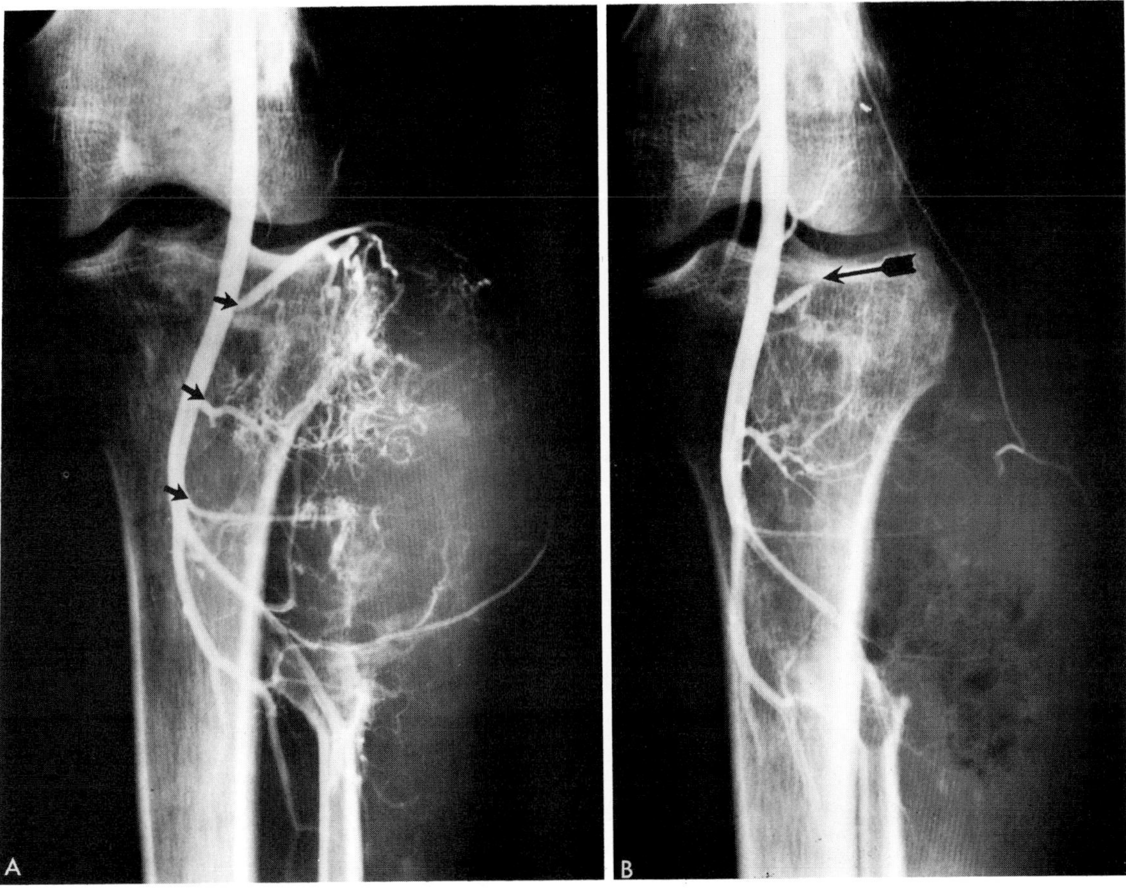

Figure 16–9. *Diagnostic and therapeutic arteriography of a giant cell tumor.*

Thirty-five year old man with giant cell tumor of the fibula. The patient had already had two other giant cell tumors removed from other sites, and had another tumor in the opposite leg. Bleeding had been severe and difficult to control after prearteriographic biopsy. Arteriography was performed as part of a plan to resect the multiple, histologically benign giant cell lesions while trying to avoid amputation and maintain locomotive ability.

A *Arteriogram demonstrates abundant tumor vessels of the fibular lesion (arrows). There also appears to be tumor vascularity within the tibia (subsequently confirmed by additional biopsy).*

B *Arteriogram after embolization demonstrates effective devascularization of the tumor. Gas in the soft tissues is secondary to an intervening biopsy. Arrow indicates the site of occlusion of the lateral inferior geniculate artery.*

(From Feldman F et al: Am J Roentgenol 123:130, 1975. Copyright 1975, American Roentgen Ray Society.)

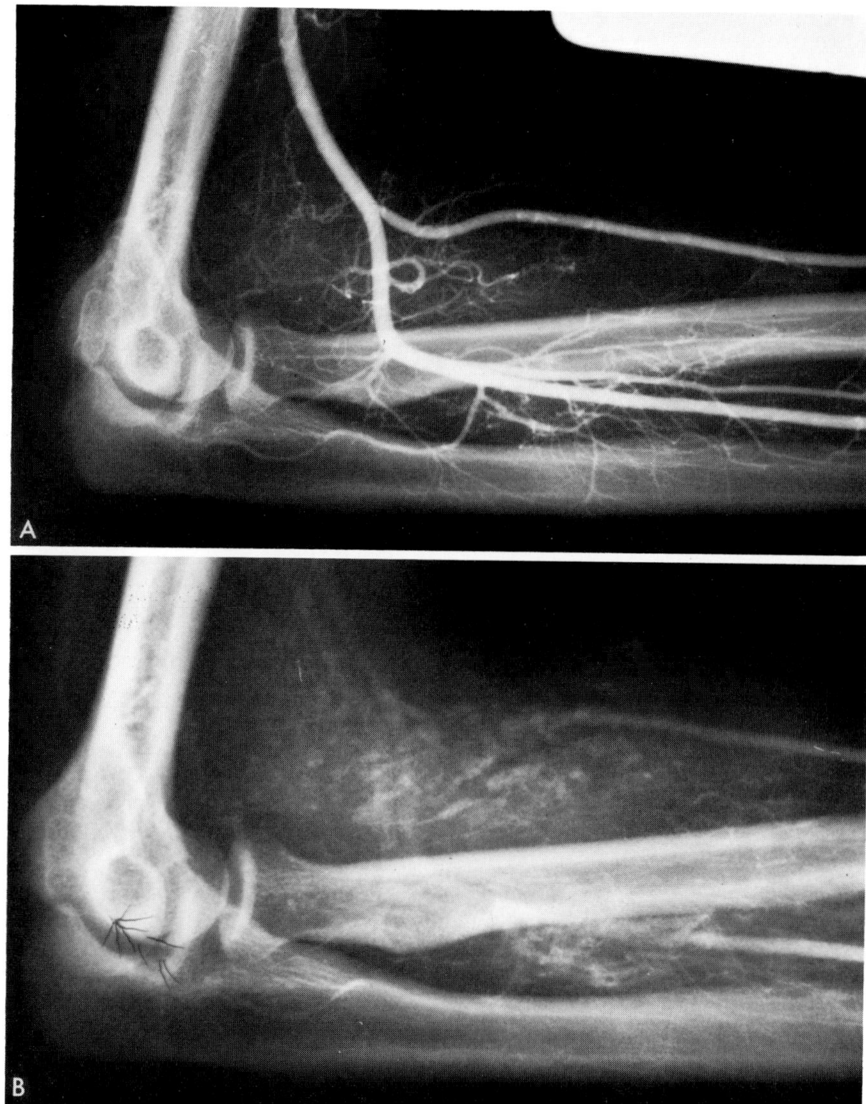

Figure 16–10. *Angiography of a para-articular soft tissue hemangioma. Thirty year old man with limited ability to extend the elbow. Minor soft tissue fullness was present on clinical examination. Prior operations had revealed infiltrating hemangioma.*

A *Arterial phase shows no definite abnormality.*

B *Parenchymal phase 15 minutes after intra-arterial injection of tolazoline (Priscoline) shows faint accumulations of contrast medium in the hemangioma. The striated pattern of accumulation indicates diffuse infiltration of muscle by the lesion, confirmed at exploratory operation.*

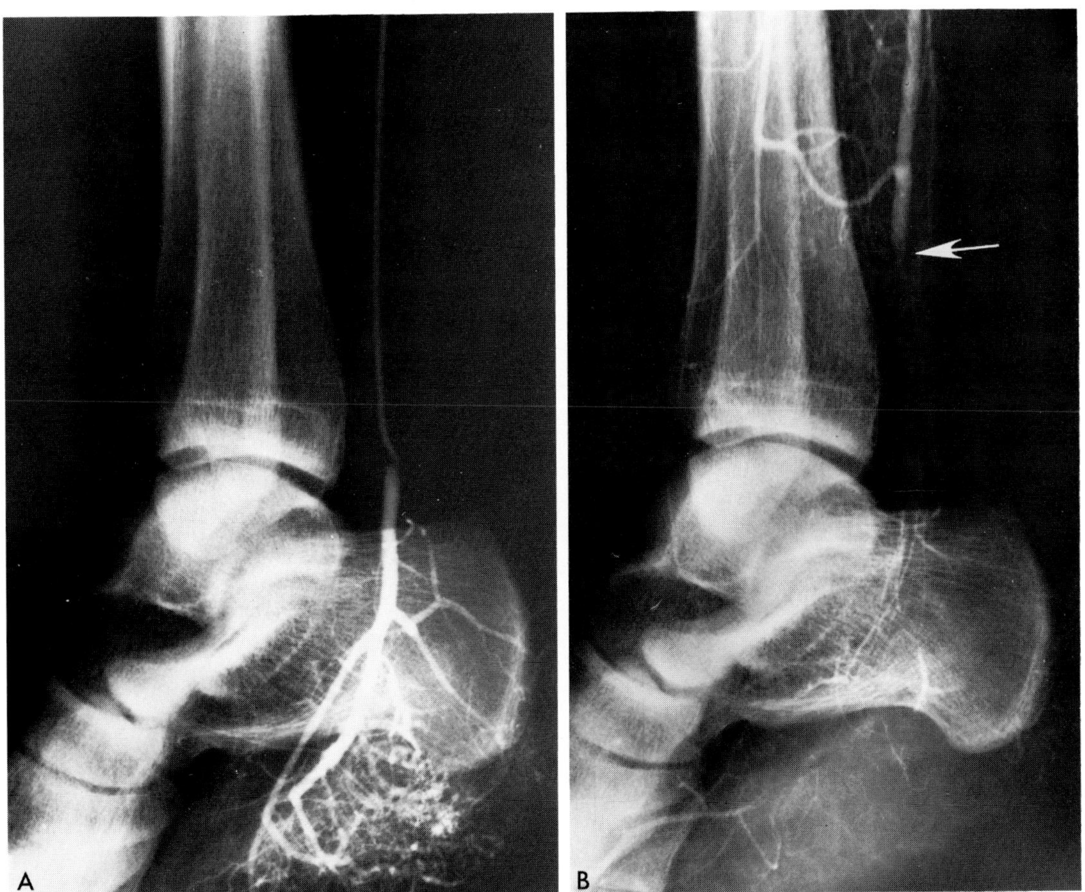

Figure 16–11. *Transcatheter therapy of a subcalcaneal hemangioma. This 16 year old boy had severe pain on walking owing to this hemangioma. Three prior operations had not provided permanent relief, and amputation was being considered.*

A *Posterior tibial arteriogram prior to embolization shows most of the hypervascular lesion.*

B *After embolization with both small and large particles of Ivalon (Unipoint, Inc., High Point, North Carolina), the hemangioma is poorly perfused. The posterior tibial artery became occluded (arrow) after the smaller emboli had been delivered into the lesion.*

Clinical status improved greatly, and the patient was relatively asymptomatic for 1 year, when pain again returned. Repeat arteriography demonstrated persistent occlusion of the embolized arteries, but additional collateral vessels to the lesion had developed, which were reembolized. Three separate embolic therapeutic sessions have now been held, with clinical improvement after each one. Each time, smaller Ivalon fragments were being used, in an effort to obliterate the lesion from within.

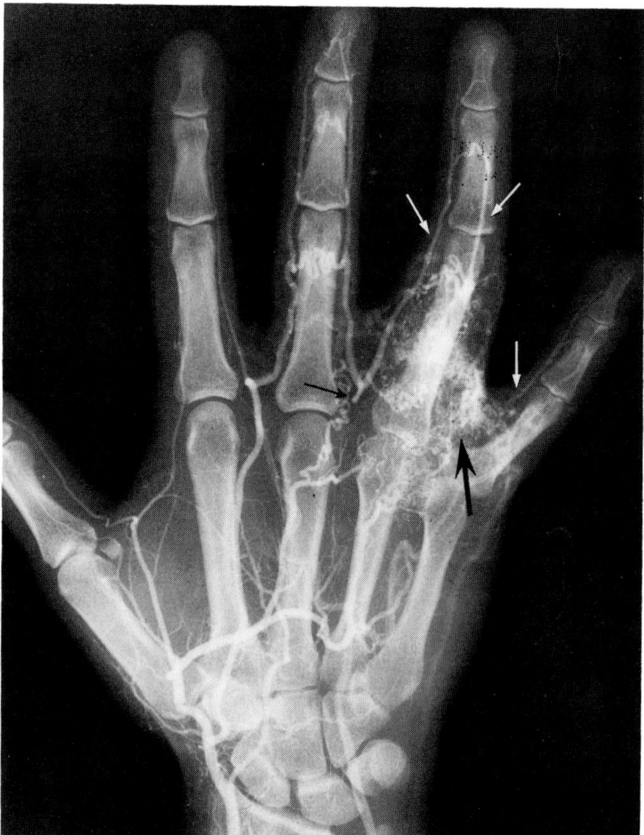

Figure 16–12. Angiography of typical arteriovenous malformation, which persisted after ligation of several feeding arteries. Arteriography was again performed in preparation for another attempt at removal of this para-articular mass, which limited mobility at the fourth metacarpophalangeal joint, and which bled intermittently. Despite prior surgical occlusion of all of the regional proper digital arteries (small arrows), these arteries as well as the lesion (large arrow) continue to opacify via collateral routes.

reliability is incomplete. Examples of vascular malformations are shown in Figures 16–10 to 16–12. In some of these vascular masses, extent cannot be well evaluated angiographically because all or portions of the lesion may not opacify, even after pharmacoangiography.[12, 18] Although histologic-arteriographic correlates of malignancy or benignancy have been described, their accuracy, in my opinion, is insufficient for clinical application.

Transcatheter therapy is being increasingly applied in the management of peripheral vascular malformations.[27, 29, 30, 44] Temporary control of pain, swelling, or hemorrhage can usually be achieved by obstructing major vessels leading to the malformation, but symptoms usually recur after a variable period of time owing to development of collateral circulation (Fig. 16–11). Efforts are currently being directed toward embolic obliteration of the small vessels within the lesion rather than the large feeding vessels outside the lesion, in order to prevent recurrences.

AUTOIMMUNE DISEASES

A considerable number of arterial diseases have been described that are loosely characterized by inflammation, proliferation, or destruction of components of the arterial wall. Polyarteritis nodosa, Takayasu's arteritis, and giant cell arteritis are examples of such diseases. It is generally believed that these diseases have an autoimmune basis[54] and are a response to intravascular deposition of immune complexes or to attachment of autoimmune antibodies to arterial and other tissues. These diseases have been classified by a variety of schema[19, 54, 55]: by histologic appearance (polyarteritis nodosa, giant cell arteritis, necrotizing arteritis, leukocytoclastic angiitis); by areas of involvement (temporal arteritis, polymyalgia rheumatica); by etiology (allergic arteritis); by acuteness of disease (Churg and Strauss arteritis); by size of vessel involved (aortitis, polyarteritis nodosa of medium-sized vessels); by constellation of involved organs or tissues (small vessels of lung and kidney — Wegener's disease; capillaries of lung and kidney — Goodpasture's syndrome; medium-sized arteries, synovial membranes, muscle tenderness — polymyalgia arteritica[31, 44]). Because of the lack of general agreement regarding classification as well as the tremendous overlap between diseases, and for want of a system based on fundamental objective criteria, I prefer to have the arteritides characterized by specifying all the above indicated features: acuteness; vessels, organs, and tissues involved; histologic evidence of necrosis, giant cells, aneurysms, or intimal proliferation; angiographic evidence of aneurysms or intimal proliferation.

Rheumatoid Arthritis

In this chapter, autoimmune diseases involving cross reactions between arterial and joint tissues are of prime concern. Rheumatoid arthritis is predominantly expressed as a disease of synovial membranes, but in a significant percentage of cases, vascular disease is also present, which occasionally becomes of clinical significance. Muscle biopsies have revealed arteritis in 8.8 per cent of cases of rheumatoid arthritis,[42] and active vasculitis has been noted in 25 per cent of an autopsied series.[8] Histologic features of rheumatic vasculitis include mild perivascular or adventitial inflammation, intimal thickening with little or no cellular reaction,[24, 25] arterial thromboses, and necrotizing arteriolar panarteritis.[49] Corticosteroid therapy has been implicated as a possible etiologic factor in those cases with necrotizing arteritis. Aortitis or aortic valvulitis is also an associated finding,[5] and spontaneous aortic rupture has been reported after steroid therapy for rheumatoid arthritis.[41] Arteriographic studies have been infrequent. Laws and co-workers[25] demonstrated arterial stenoses of the digital arteries in 26 of 38 patients with rheumatoid arthritis, with frequent collateral circulation. Nonspecific hyperemia was present in 22 of 37 patients, particularly near bony erosions or regions of synovial proliferation in joints or tendon sheaths.

Giant Cell Arteritis

Giant cell arteritis (also called temporal, cranial, or granulomatous arteritis) is a form of vasculitis characterized histologically by necrosis of the arterial wall and granulomatous vascular reaction with giant cells. Medium-sized arteries, such as the temporal, subclavian, or popliteal arteries, are most frequently involved, but virtually any artery, including the aorta, may be affected. Many extravascular manifestations are associated, including fatigue, fever, anorexia, weight loss, synovitis, and visual disturbances.[17]

Polymyalgia Rheumatica

Polymyalgia rheumatica (also called polymyalgia arteritica) is characterized by recurrent rheumatic discomfort involving muscles and joints, particularly of the shoulder and hip girdles, systemic manifestations of fever and malaise, elevated sedimentation rate, and, usually, associated arteritis of medium-sized vessels.[29,40] Two thirds of patients will have palpable synovial thickening or effusion at some point during their illness. Hands and sternoclavicular, acromioclavicular, sacroiliac, and pubic joints are predisposed to involvement. Joint biopsy will demonstrate nonspecific synovitis and capsulitis. Arterial biopsy will show arteritis in about 50 per cent of cases; usually giant cells are prominent, and the appearance and distribution of disease are generally indistinguishable from those of giant cell arteritis. The marked overlap between polymyalgia rheumatica and giant cell arteritis suggests that they are both manifestations of the same disease process.[2]

Scleroderma

Scleroderma (Figs. 16–13 and 16–14) is primarily expressed as a disease of small arteries, but joint involvement, often resembling rheumatoid arthritis, is not infrequent.[34,35] In a series of 24 patients with scleroderma who had arthritic symptoms, one or more skeletal abnormalities were present in the hands or wrists of each; in seven patients features resembled rheumatoid arthritis.[34] Histologic examination of digital arteries from patients with sclero-

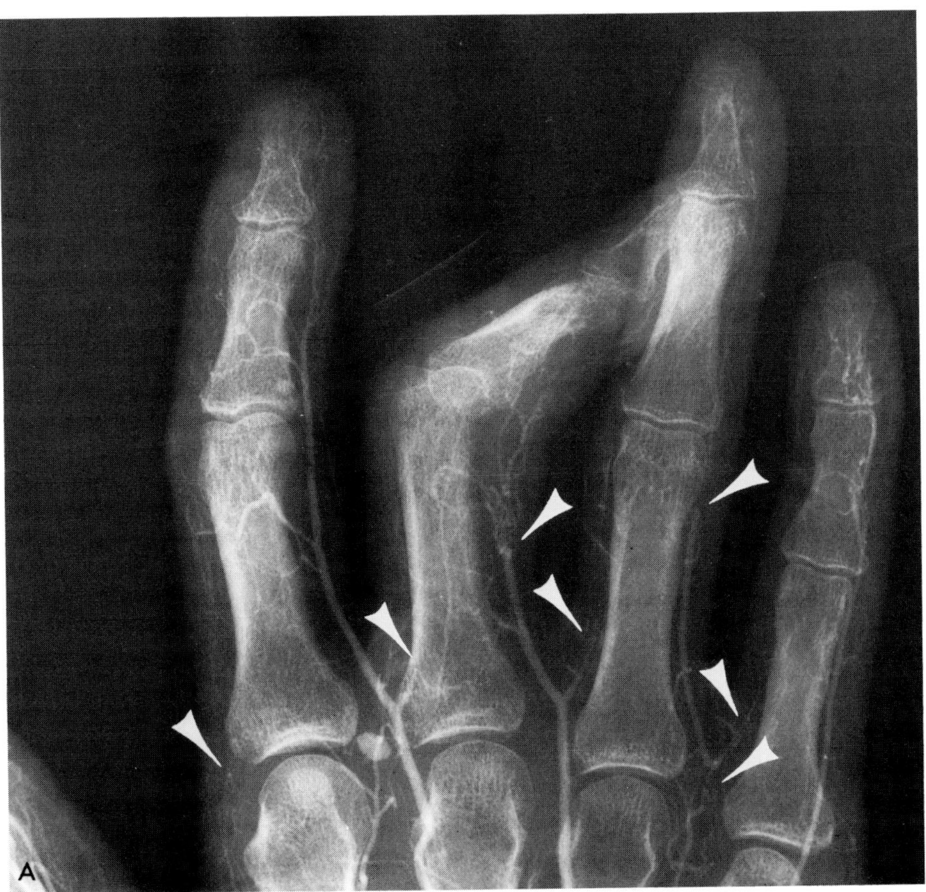

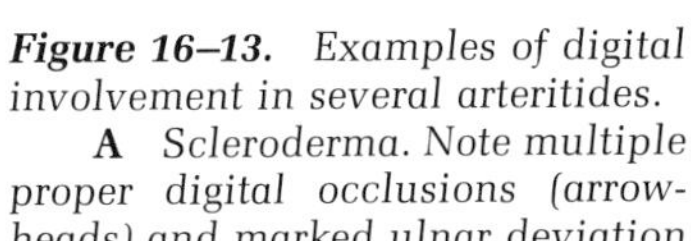

Figure 16–13. *Examples of digital involvement in several arteritides.*

A *Scleroderma. Note multiple proper digital occlusions (arrowheads) and marked ulnar deviation of the middle phalanx of the third finger due to scleroderma. Minor irregularities of the proper digital artery of the index finger are also present.*

Illustration continued on the following page

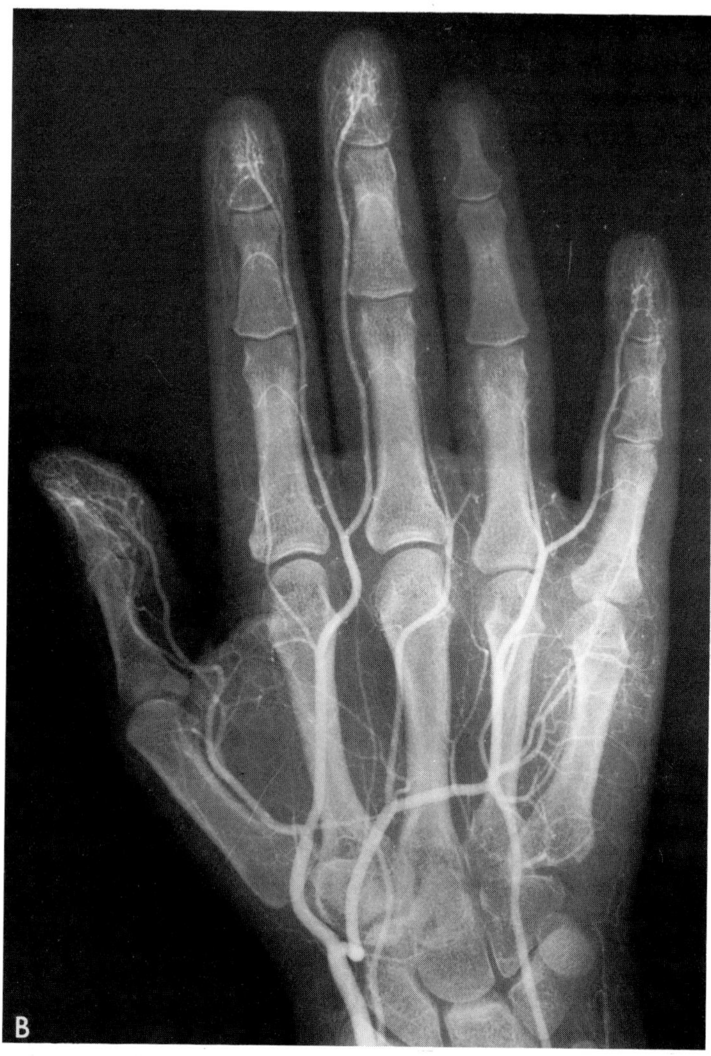

Figure 16–13. Continued

B *Lupus erythematosus. Ordinarily such large arteries are not involved in lupus, but in this patient the proper digital arteries of the second through fifth digits show occlusions indistinguishable from scleroderma.*

Illustration continued on the opposite page

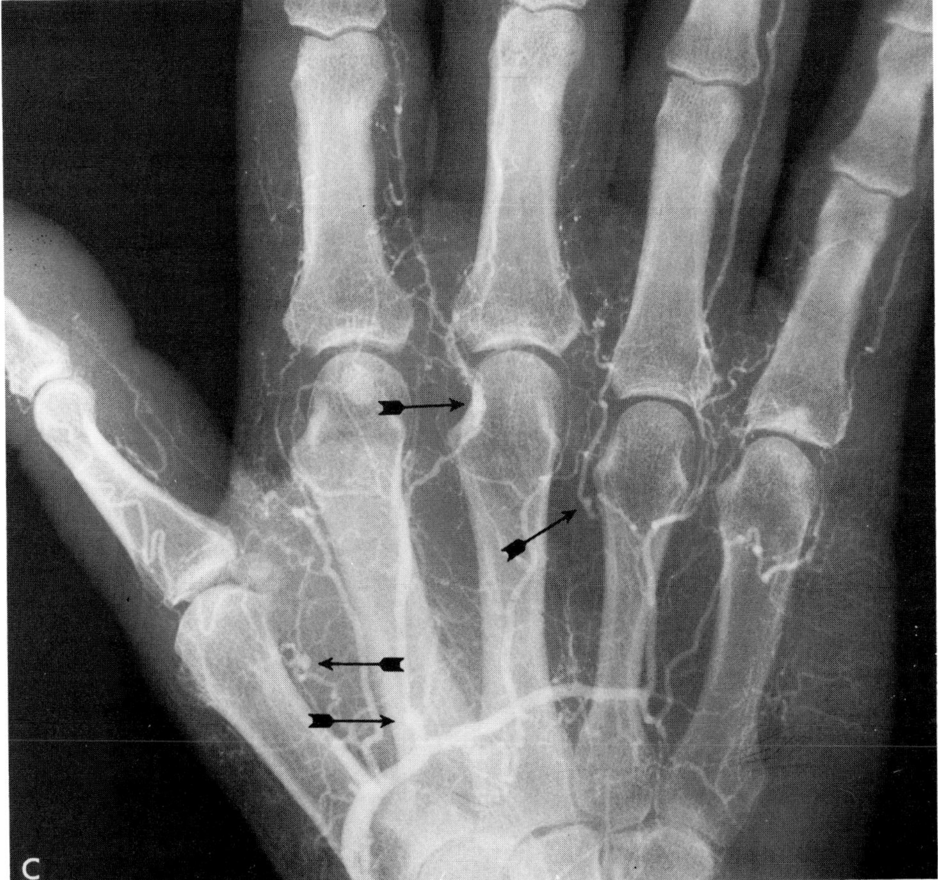

Figure 16–13. Continued

C *Polyarteritis nodosa. Multiple proper digital arteries and the ulnar artery are occluded, a distribution similar to that of scleroderma. However, the presence of a number of small aneurysms (arrows) suggests the possibility of a necrotizing arteritis.*

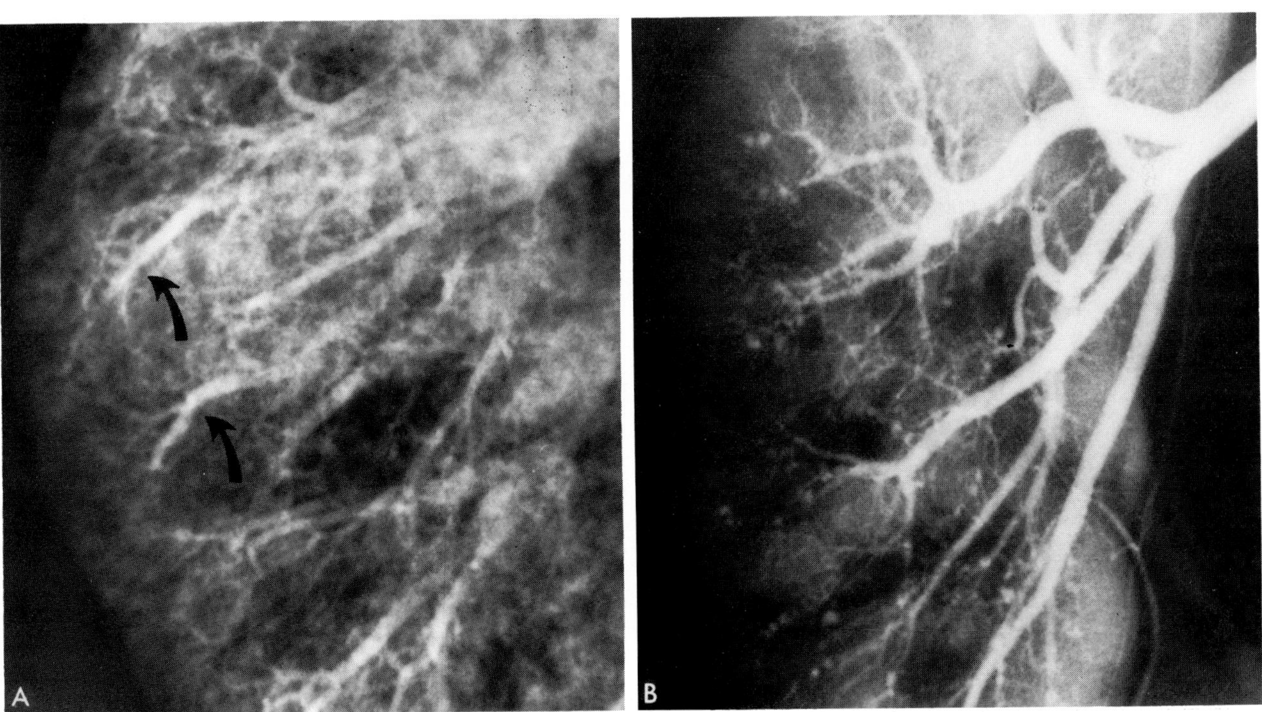

Figure 16–14. *Renal involvement in various arteritides.*

A *Scleroderma (3×). Arteries visualized (arrows) are the distal interlobar arteries. Interlobular arteries of the cortex are not seen, because they are either occluded or markedly narrowed. The coarse mottling of the nephrogram reflects multiple tiny scars due to microinfarcts.*

B *Polyarteritis (nonmagnified angiography). The disease tends to involve arteries of larger caliber than does scleroderma. Note multiple occlusions of distal interlobar arteries, with multiple associated aneurysms reflecting the presence of a necrotizing process.*

derma has consistently revealed uniquely extensive arterial disease.[25] Intimal arteriolar thickening is the most frequent manifestation, but panarteritis may also occur. Small arteries throughout the body may be involved. The kidneys are particularly predisposed, and small renal vessels, usually at the interlobular level, are involved in 90 per cent of those dying with the disease.[4]

Angiography reflects the severe arterial disease noted histologically. In a review of 31 digital arteriograms of patients with scleroderma,[9] severe stenoses or occlusions, usually multiple, were present in 29. Most commonly the proper digital arteries were involved in their middle or distal portions. The vascular beds of the terminal digits were often obliterated. In patients with clinical evidence of renal disease, renal arteriography usually demonstrates extensive obstructive and occlusive disease of interlobular arteries, and innumerable renal cortical microinfarcts and scars (Fig. 16–14).

Systemic Lupus Erythematosus

Systemic lupus erythematosus (SLE) (Fig. 16–13) is the most frequent of the collagen vascular disorders. Its features reveal significant overlap with those of rheumatoid arthritis. Approximately one third of patients with rheumatoid arthritis will show positive LE cell preparations, and an equal number of patients with SLE will have a positive test for rheumatoid factor.[15, 53] Most patients will have arthritic symptoms at some point in the course of disease, and roentgenographic signs of soft tissue or bony abnormalities are also frequent.[3, 48] For example, hand radiographs in 59 patients with SLE demonstrated abnormalities in 34, most commonly periarticular calcification or swelling, acral sclerosis, malalignment, or soft tissue calcification.[48]

Vascular manifestations of lupus erythematosus are generally confined to the very small arteries, such as interlobular arteries of the kidney, or renal glomerular capillaries. Histologic changes may vary widely; mild abnormalities are characterized by deposition of fibrinoid material within the intima, generally accompanied by fibroblast proliferation. Progressive deposition of material leads to luminal compromise and destruction of wall muscle and elastic elements. In advanced disease, necrotizing arteritis can develop.[45] Digital arteriograms in two of my patients with SLE showed arterial occlusions, which in one were indistinguishable from those occurring in scleroderma (Fig. 16–13*B*). The other patient had normal digital arteries. Renal arteriograms in SLE reaffirm the predominantly small-vessel distribution of disease; most abnormality occurs within renal glomeruli, with loss of glomerular granularity on magnification renal arteriograms. Interlobular arteries are commonly narrowed, but not occluded.

Polyarteritis Nodosa

Polyarteritis nodosa (Figs. 16–13, and 16–14), along with the other collagen vascular diseases that have already been mentioned, frequently produces mild arthralgias and myalgias, but actual joint effusion is unusual. The predominant manifestation is a necrotizing arteritis that may affect arteries anywhere in the body. Arteriography of involved areas may demonstrate small aneurysms, a feature virtually pathognomonic of necrotizing arteritis. Aneurysms may not develop, or at least are not visible, in many cases. Once formed, they may also disappear, apparently as a result of healing.[38] Other features include arterial stenoses, occlusions, collateral circulation, marginal irregularities, and evidence of tissue infarction. Arteries in and around joints may be affected (Fig. 16–13*C*), but are rarely studied angiographically. Renal arteries are involved in a high percentage of cases, usually in patients with hypertension or hematuria, and renal arteriography may be the most effective method for reaching a diagnosis (Fig. 16–14*B*).

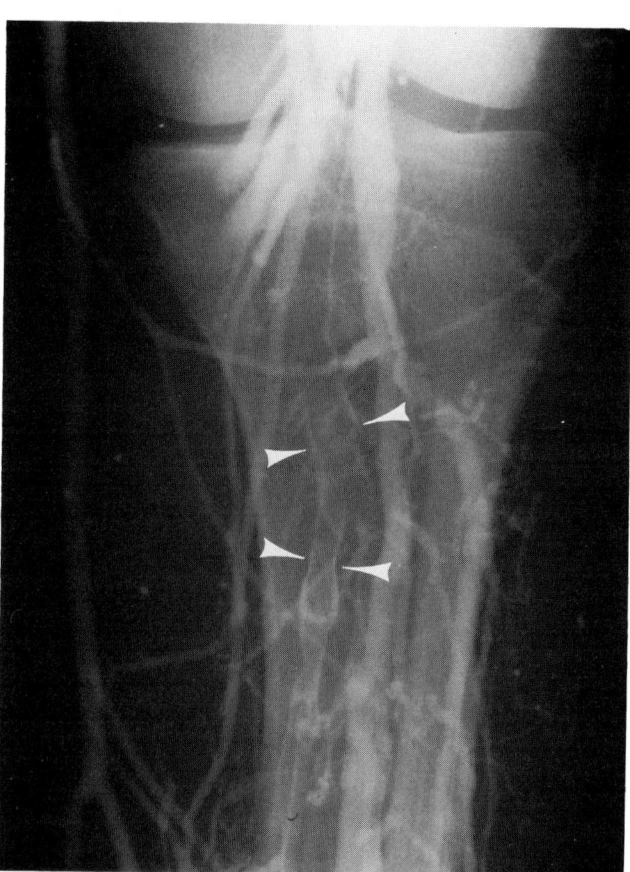

Figure 16–15. *Thrombophlebitis producing pain and swelling about the knee joint.*

Note the thin accumulation of contrast medium between the intraluminal thrombus and the vein wall, outlining the presence of thrombus (arrowheads).

VENOUS DISEASE

The swelling and tenderness of thrombophlebitis may sometimes simulate joint disease clinically. Venography is the most definitive diagnostic procedure. In the presence of thrombosis of lower extremity veins, intraluminal defects due to thrombi are almost always visualized (Fig. 16–15). Fresh thrombi largely fill the obstructed venous lumen, and commonly they demonstrate convex proximal and distal margins. A thin rim of contrast medium may be insinuated between the thrombus and the venous wall.

A popliteal cyst of the knee joint may simulate the swelling of thrombophlebitis.[11] Contrast arthrography, as well as venography, will permit a specific diagnosis to be made. Indeed, a popliteal cyst may coexist with venous obstruction, in view of the propensity of these cysts to obstruct the popliteal vein.

MISCELLANEOUS DISORDERS

Occupational Acro-osteolysis

This condition was described in 1967 by Wilson and co-workers.[50] The syndrome is characterized primarily by resorption of portions of distal phalangeal tufts, some digital tenderness, and Raynaud's phenomenon. It was observed in 31 of 3000 workers involved in the manufacture of polyvinylchloride. Arteriography in one patient demonstrated mild hypervascularity adjacent to areas of bone resorption (Fig. 16–16) and distal occlusion of the princeps pollicis artery.

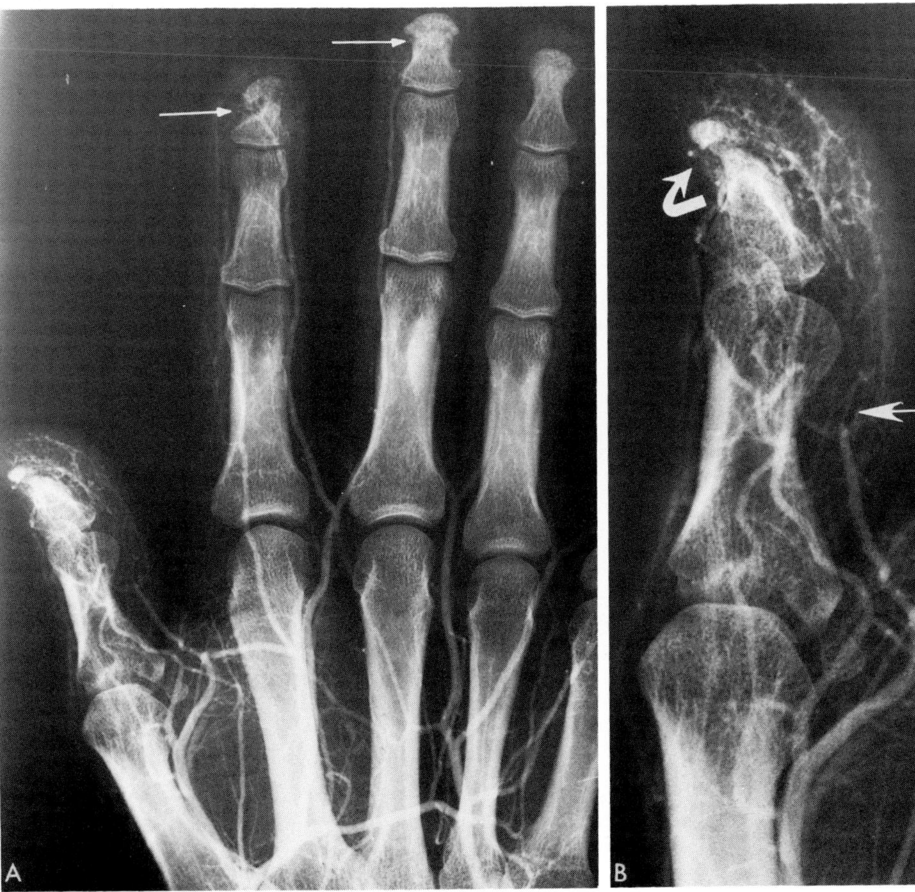

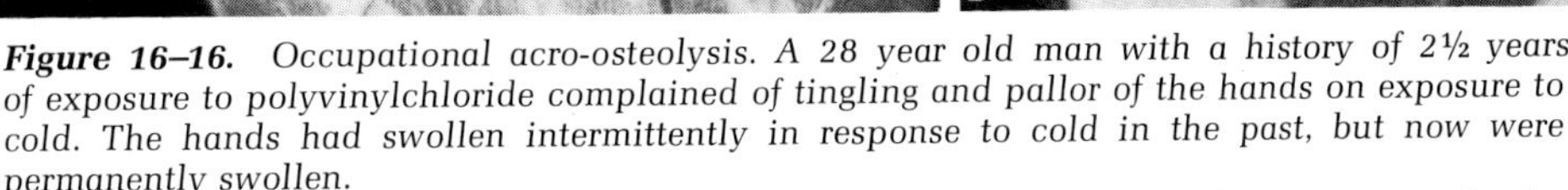
Figure 16–16. *Occupational acro-osteolysis. A 28 year old man with a history of 2½ years of exposure to polyvinylchloride complained of tingling and pallor of the hands on exposure to cold. The hands had swollen intermittently in response to cold in the past, but now were permanently swollen.*

A *Conventional arteriogram of the hand shows no major arterial occlusions, except for the thumb. There has been resorption of the distal phalanges producing transverse defects (arrows).*

B *Arteriogram of the thumb, performed on cardboard. Note the excellent detail that can be obtained with this technique. Straight arrow indicates the site of occlusion of the princeps pollicis artery. Curved arrow indicates the transverse line of bone resorption. (From Bookstein JJ: In AK Poznanski [Ed]: The Hand in Radiologic Diagnosis. Philadelphia, WB Saunders Co, 1974.)*

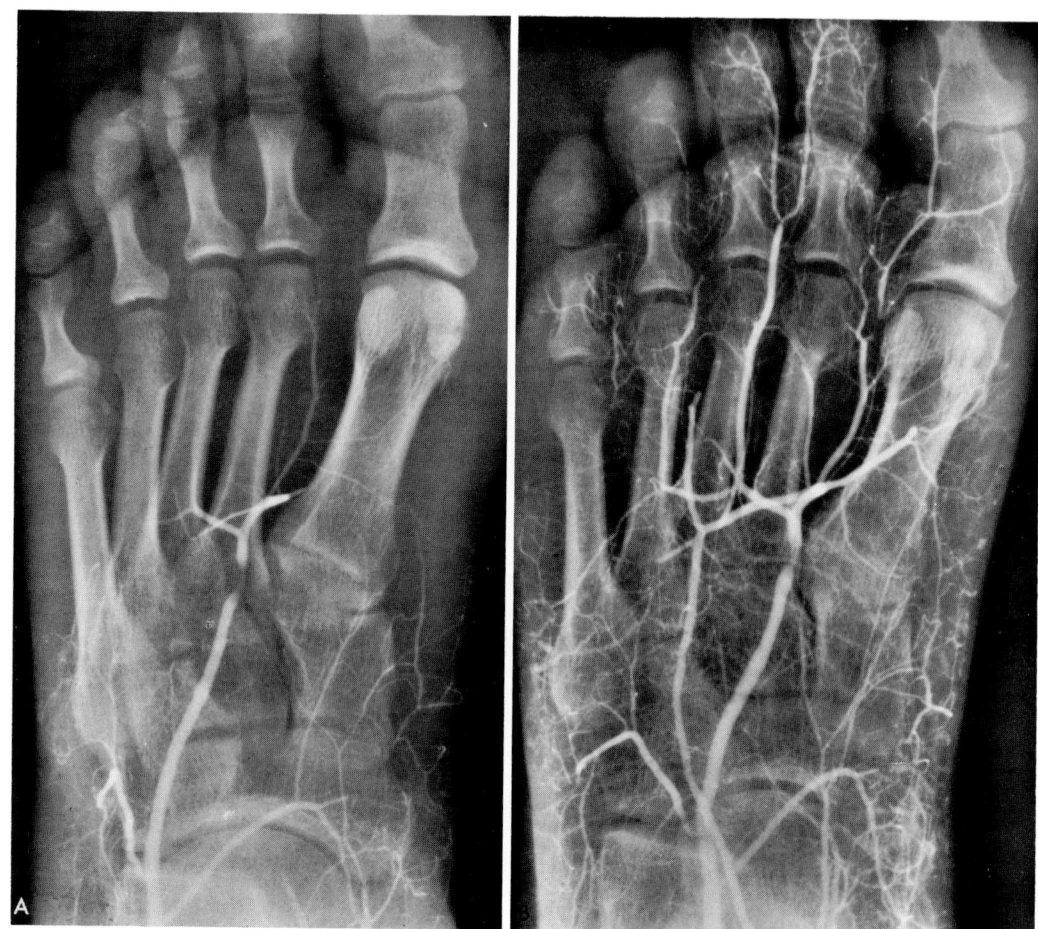

Figure 16–17. Frostbite. *A 30 year old man suffered pedal frostbite after becoming lost and walking in the snow for 36 hours.*

A *Angiography of the left foot 3 days after cold exposure showed slow flow with concentric tubular narrowing of the distal dorsalis pedis artery, severe spasm of the metatarsal arch, and lack of opacification of the digital arteries of the first, third, fourth, and fifth toes. Reserpine (0.5 mg) was injected into the left superficial femoral artery.*

B *Repeat angiography after 2 days demonstrates much less spasm. Portions of all toes are now perfused. The patient was discharged a few weeks later, after losing only a small amount of tissue from the large toe.*

(From Gralino BJ, et al: Radiology 119:301, 1976.)

Frostbite

The importance of vascular injury in the pathogenesis of frostbite is well recognized.[16, 33] Experimental studies have demonstrated that within minutes of thawing, capillaries and venules become occluded with thrombi. Several hours later, most of the blood flow is via peripheral precapillary shunts. Arteriography will demonstrate marked slowing of blood flow in sizeable branches, probably due to spasm and more distal obstruction (Fig. 16–17). As the condition improves, arterial flow improves, but residual occlusions may persist.

Osteonecrosis of the Hip

The ischemic origin of osteonecrosis of the hip has been assumed for many years. Recently, Theron[46] has demonstrated occlusion of the superior capsular arteries in such patients, using superselective arteriography of the medial and lateral circumflex, obturator, and superior and inferior gluteal arteries (Fig. 16–18). Normally, the femoral head is supplied primarily by arteries arising from the medial femoral circumflex artery. In patients with idiopathic osteonecrosis of the hip, occlusion of branches may be evident in the early phases. Later, the branches may recanalize. It remains to be determined, however, whether the arterial occlusion is the cause or the effect of the necrosis.

SUMMARY

The role of angiography in the diagnosis and treatment of a variety of musculoskeletal problems is described in this chapter. This role includes the

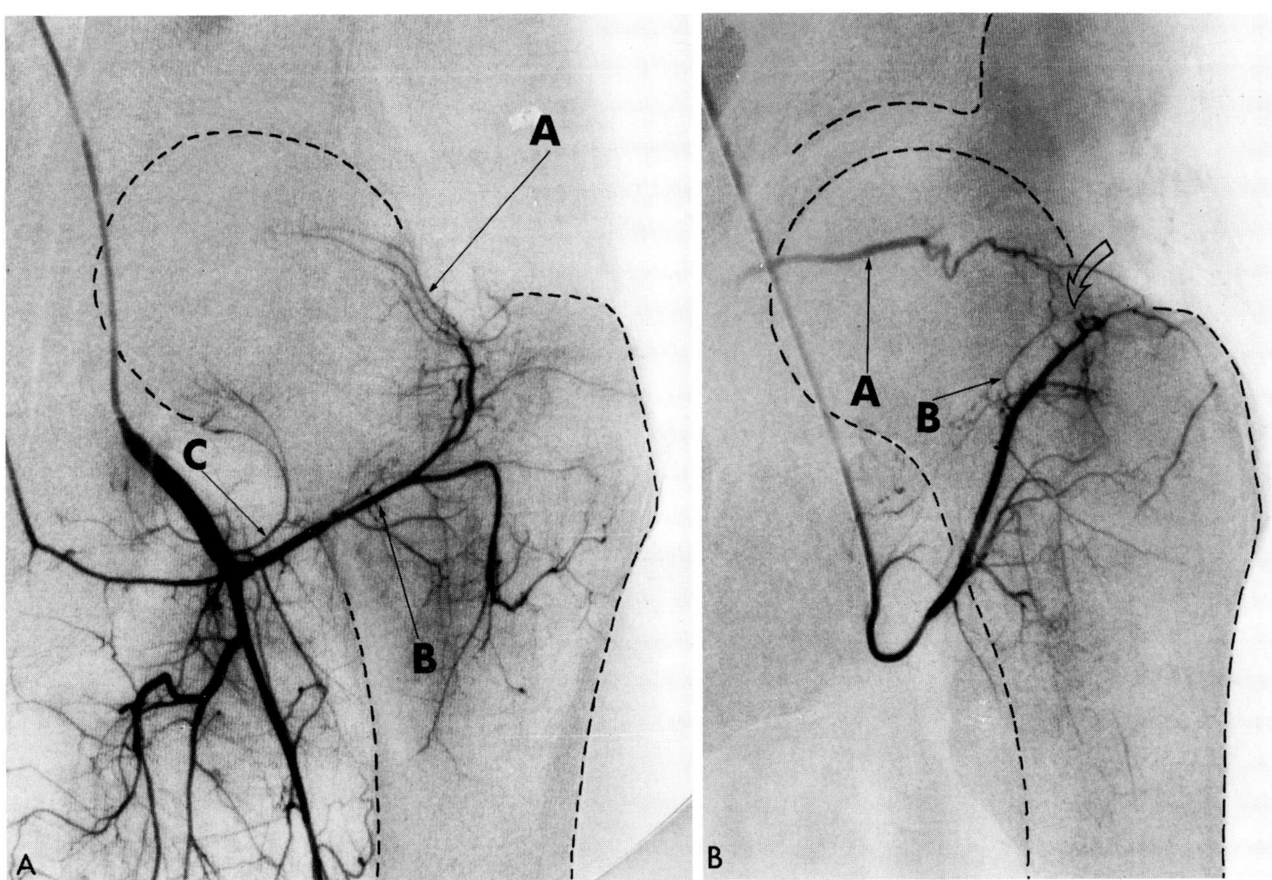

Figure 16–18. Superselective angiography in osteonecrosis of the hip.

A *Normal left hip for comparison. Superselective injection of the medial circumflex artery. A, Superior capsular branches; B, superior branch of the medial circumflex artery, which surrounds the femoral neck posteriorly; C, inferior capsular branch.*

B *Necrosis of the left femoral head. Mild depression of the femoral head was evident on plain lateral projection. Superselective injection of the superior branch of the medial circumflex artery showed obvious interruption of the superior capsular arteries and their stumps (open arrow). There is reflux of contrast material from a hypertrophied posterior branch of the femoral neck (B) into the inferior gluteal artery (A).*

(Modified after Theron J: Radiology 124:649, 1977.)

documentation of vascular injury following trauma, the control of hemorrhage, the visualization of a variety of primary arterial diseases, the evaluation of the nature and extent of soft tissue masses, the visualization of arteritis complicating collagen vascular disorders, and the detection of peripheral venous abnormalities, which may simulate articular or peri-articular disease.

REFERENCES

1. Bookstein JJ: Arteriography. *In* AK Poznanski (Ed): The Hand in Radiologic Diagnosis. Philadelphia, WB Saunders Co, 1974, p 65.
2. Bruk MI: Articular and vascular manifestations of polymyalgia rheumatica. Ann Rheum Dis *26*:103, 1967.
3. Budin J, Feldman F: Soft tissue calcifications in systemic lupus erythematosus. Am J Roentgenol *124*:358, 1975.
4. Cannon PJ, Hassar M, Case DB, et al: The relationship of hypertension and renal failure in scleroderma (progessive systemic sclerosis) to structural and functional abnormalities of the renal cortical circulation. Medicine *53*:1, 1974.
5. Clark WS, Kulka JP, Bauer W: Rheumatoid aortitis with aortic regurgitation. Am J Med *22*:580, 1957.
6. Conn J, Bergan JJ, Bell JL: Hypothenar hammer syndrome: Posttraumatic digital ischemia. Surgery *68*:1122, 1970.
7. Crossland, SG, Slovin AJ: The role of arteriography in diagnosing unsuspected vascular injuries. Am Surg *44*:98, 1978.
8. Cruickshank B: The arteritis of rheumatoid arthritis. Ann Rheum Dis *13*:136, 1954.
9. Dabich L, Bookstein JJ, Zweifler A, Zarafonetis C: Digital arteries in patients with scleroderma: Arteriographic and plethysmographic study. Arch Intern Med *130*:708, 1972.
10. DeLaurentis DA, Wolferth CC, Wolf FM, Naide D, Nedwich A: Mucinous adventitial cysts of the popliteal artery in an 11 year old girl. Surgery *74*:456, 1973.
11. Doppman JL: Baker's cyst and normal gastrocnemiosemimembranosus bursa. Am J Roentgenol *94*:646, 1965.
12. Ekelund L, Laurin S, Lunderquist A: Comparison of a vasoconstrictor and a vasodilator in pharmacoangiography of bone and soft tissue tumors. Radiology *122*:95, 1977.
13. Feldman F, Casarella WJ, Dick HM, Hollander BA: Selective intra-arterial embolization of bone tumors. Am J Roentgenol *123*:130, 1975.
14. Rouanet JP, Chalut J, Bacourt F, Gruner M, Goldlust D: Rare cause of arterial aneurysm: Exostosis. J Radiol Electrol Med Nucl *57*:171, 1976.
15. Friedman IA, Sickley JF, Poske RM, Black A, Bronsky D, Hartz WH Jr, Feldhake C, Reeder PS, Katz EM: The LE phenomenon in rheumatoid arthritis. Ann Intern Med *46*:1113, 1957.
16. Gralino BJ, Porter JM, Rösch J: Angiography in the diagnosis and therapy of frostbite. Radiology *119*:301, 1976.
17. Greenway G, Resnick D, Bookstein JJ: Popliteal pseudoaneurysm as a complication of adjacent osteochondroma: Angiographic diagnosis. Am J Roentgenol *132*:294, 1979.
18. Hudson TM, Haas G, Enneking WF, Hawkins IF: Angiography in management of musculoskeletal tumors. Surg Gynecol Obstet *141*:11, 1975.
19. Hunder GG, Allen GL: Giant cell arteritis : A review. Bull Rheum Dis *29*:980, 1978.
20. Hutcheson J, Klatte EC, Kremp R: The angiographic appearance of myositis ossificans circumscripta. Radiology *102*:57, 1972.
21. Inada K, Hirose M, Iwashima Y, Matsumoto K: Popliteal artery entrapment syndrome: A case report. Br J Surg *65*:613, 1978.
22. Insua JA, Young JR, Humphries AW: Popliteal artery entrapment syndrome. Arch Surg *101*:771, 1970.
23. Kindblom L-G, Merck C, Svendsen P: Myxofibrosarcoma: A pathologico-anatomical, microangiographic and angiographic correlative study of eight cases. Br J Radiol *50*:876, 1977.
24. Laws JW, Lillie JG, Scott JT: Arteriographic appearances in rheumatoid arthritis and other disorders. Br J Radiol *36*:477 1963.
25. Laws JW, Sallab RA, Scott JT: An arteriographic and histologic study of digital arteries. Br J Radiol *40*:740, 1967.
26. Levin DC, Gordon DH, McSweeney J: Arteriography of peripheral hemangiomas. Radiology *121*:625, 1976.
27. Levin DC, Watson RC, Baltaxe HA: Arteriography in diagnosis and management of acquired peripheral soft-tissue masses. Radiology *104*:53, 1972.
28. McDonald EJ, Goodman PC, Winestock DP: The clinical indications for arteriography in trauma to the extremity. Radiology *116*:45, 1975.
29. Natali J, Merland JJ: Superselective arteriography and therapeutic embolization for vascular malformations (angiodysplasias). J Cardiovas Surg *17*:465, 1976.
30. Olcott C, Newton TH, Stoney RJ, Ehrenfeld WK: Intra-arterial embolization in the management of arteriovenous malformations. Surgery *79*:3, 1976.
31. Ostberg G: On arteritis with special reference to polymyalgia arteritica. Acta Path Microbiol Scand (Suppl) *237*:1, 1973.
32. Prando A, deSantos LA, Wallace S, Murray JA: Angiography in giant-cell bone tumors. Radiology *130*:323, 1979.
33. Quintanilla R, Krusen FH, Esser HE: Studies on frostbite with special reference to treatment and the effect on minute blood vessels. Am J Physiol *149*:149, 1947.
34. Rabinowitz JG, Twersky J, Guttadauria M: Similar bone manifestations of scleroderma and rheumatoid arthritis. Am J Roentgenol *121*:35, 1974.
35. Resnick D, Greenway G, Vint VC, Robinson CA, Piper S: Selective involvement of the first carpometacarpal joint in scleroderma. Am J Roentgenol *131*:283, 1978.
36. Ring EJ, Athanasoulis C, Waltman AC, Margolies MN, Baum S: Arteriographic management of hemorrhage following pelvic fracture. Radiology *109*:65, 1973.
37. Ring EJ, Waltman AC, Athanasoulis C, Smith JC Jr, Baum S: Angiography in pelvic trauma. Surg Gynecol Obstet *139*:375, 1974.
38. Robins J, Bookstein JJ: Regressing aneurysms in periarteritis nodosa. Radiology *104*:39, 1972.
39. Rubin BE, Fortune WP, May MM: Therapeutic embolization for postoperative hemorrhage about the hip of a patient with Pseudomonas infection. J Bone Joint Surg *60A*:988, 1978.
40. Schlesinger A, Gottesman L: Cystic degeneration of the popliteal artery. Am J Roentgenol *127*:1043, 1976.
41. Smith DC, Hirst AE: Spontaneous aortic rupture associated with chronic steroid therapy for rheumatoid arthritis in two cases. Am J Roentgenol *132*:271, 1979.
42. Sokoloff L, Wilens SL, Bunim JJ: Arteritis of striated muscle in rheumatoid arthritis. Am J Pathol *27*:157, 1951.
43. Stanley RJ, Cubillo E: Nonsurgical treatment of arteriovenous malformations of the trunk and limb by transcatheter arterial embolization. Radiology *115*:609, 1975.
44. Svendler C-A, Sonderlundh S: Angiographic diagnosis in polymyalgia arteritica. Acta Radiol (Diagn) *18*:333, 1977.
45. Talbott JH: Collagen Vascular Diseases. New York, Grune & Stratton 1974, p. 1.
46. Théron J: Superselective angiography of the hip. Radiology *124*:649, 1977.
47. Wallace S: Personal communication.
48. Weissman BN, Rappoport AD, Sosman JL, Schur PH: Radiographic findings in the hands in patients with systemic lupus erythematosus. Radiology *126*:313, 1978.
49. Williams RC Jr: Rheumatoid Arthritis as a Systemic Disease. Philadelphia, WB Saunders Co, 1974, p 56.
50. Wilson R, McCormick W, Tatum C, Creech J: Occupational acroosteolysis. JAMA *201*:577, 1967.
51. Yaghmai I: Angiographic features of osteosarcoma. Am J Roentgenol *129*:1073, 1977.
52. Yaghmai I: Angiographic manifestations of soft-tissue and osseous hemangiopericytomas. Radiology *126*:653, 1978.
53. Ziff M: The agglutination reaction in rheumatoid arthritis. J Chronic Dis *5*:644, 1957.
54. Zvaifler NJ: Vasculitides: Classification and Pathogenesis. Aust NZ J Med *8*(Suppl 1):134, 1978.
55. deShazo RD: The spectrum of systemic vasculitis. Postgrad Med *58*:78, 1975.
56. van Urk H, Perlberger RR, Muller H: Selective arterial embolization for control of traumatic pelvic hemorrhage. Surgery *83*:133, 1978.

17

BONE IMAGING BY RADIONUCLIDE TECHNIQUES

by Naomi Alazraki, M.D.

The dynamic nature of bone provides the basic theme for interpretation of bone scans. The integrity of bone as a living tissue in constant activity is displayed by the scintillation camera or scanner on x-ray or Polaroid film images. In addition to its role as the structural support of the body, bone is important in the regulation of many elements in the body, including calcium, phosphate, and hydrogen ion, and therefore is an important indicator of many disease processes. Until the emergence of the bone scan as a clinical procedure in 1961, only radiography was available for imaging the skeletal system. As demonstrated by various investigations,[1] osseous destruction may not be seen on a radiograph until as much as 50 per cent or more of the bone in a vertebral body has been destroyed. With this recognition that radiography was a relatively insensitive technique for evaluating abnormalities of the bone, enthusiasm for a more sensitive imaging approach developed. In 1961, Fleming and co-workers[2] demonstrated localization of strontium-85 in normal bone with increased uptake of the radionuclide at sites of osseous abnormalities. Since that time, the high sensitivity of the bone scan, particularly following advances in radiopharmaceutical preparations and in imaging instrumentation, has been well established by many investigators.[3–8]

The use of radionuclides for evaluating the skeletal system has a history that long predates the advent of the strontium-85 bone scan. In addition, bone necrosis, osteomyelitis, and bone neoplasms were described in radium dial workers between 1917 and 1925.[9,10] Chronic ingestion of the radium by these workers resulted in deposition of the radioactive material in the bone. In 1935, Chiecwitz and Hevesy[11] studied phosphorus metabolism in rats and noted that ^{32}P was deposited in the bones of adult rats. In studying the metabolism of neoplasms of bone, Treadwell and associates[12] in 1942 used strontium-89, a beta ray emitter, as a tracer, and with autoradiographic studies identified deposition of the radioactive strontium in the osteogenic productive regions in normal bone as well as in osteogenic sarcomas. Following these observations, in 1958 Bauer and Ray[13] noted that strontium behaved biologically similarly to calcium. Between 1958 and 1961, several investigators,[14,15] using strontium-85 and a point-dash counting technique, studied patients with bone metastases, and finally the technique of the bone scan emerged in 1961.[16] Unfortunately, there is no isotope of calcium that emits gamma rays in energy ranges suitable for imaging with the instrumentation that is available today. Thus, strontium was utilized as the next best imitator of calcium.

In addition to the bone scan, other radioactive techniques that can be utilized to evaluate bone or mineral metabolism have included autoradiography, mineral absorption or photon densitometry, and neutron activation analysis for the determination of whole body calcium levels. Autoradiography is generally used as a research tool and involves the administration of a beta-emitting radionuclide to an animal. Following an appropriate time period during which incorporation of the radionuclide into the tissue to be studied (i.e., the bone) takes place, the animal is sacrificed. The tissue is sectioned, and a photographic emulsion is applied over the section. The tissue remains in contact with the emulsion for a sufficient period of time to allow exposure of the emulsion from the beta emissions of the radionuclide in the sectioned tissue. When the film is developed, the degree of darkening of the emulsion will be proportional to the number of beta emissions from the radionuclide in the tissue. The autoradiograph, therefore, serves as a way of visualizing the site of uptake of the radioisotope on a cellular level. In the case of radioactive phosphorus-32 or an isotope of calcium, quantitation of the amount of radionuclide in the section provides a basis for determining major mineral and organic metabolic patterns in bone and rates of bone turnover.[17]

Photon densitometry or absorptiometry was shown to be useful for measuring bone mineral mass in the early 1960s and today is utilized clinically to estimate the calcium mineral content of bone. The procedure involves scanning of a patient's wrist that is placed between an ^{125}I source and a sodium iodide detector.[18] The greater the mineral content of the bone, the fewer the number of photons that penetrate the bone to be detected by the sodium iodide crystal. Quantitation of bone density of the distal radius (or some other accessible defined point) can be accomplished at different invervals, allowing estimation of the patient's response to therapy and of the progression of various diseases, such as secondary hyperparathyroidism,[19] osteoporosis,[20] and other conditions that alter bone mineral content.[21]

In vivo neutron activation analysis has been utilized in some centers to determine total body calcium content. This procedure involves bombarding the subject with neutrons from a nuclear reactor or a particle accelerator. The neutrons are absorbed by the atomic nuclei in the tissue, producing isotopes of the bombarded elements. The radioactive isotopes can be measured and the amount of the stable element originally present in the subject can then be calculated, since for a given number of neutrons entering a sample, the quantity of the radioactive isotope that is produced will be closely proportional to the amount of the stable element originally present. In humans, small doses of neutrons are used to measure large quantities of material. For a few minutes, the patient is exposed to a uniform neutron flux and is then transferred to a whole body counter, in which gamma rays emitted by the produced radioactive isotopes can be measured. With a neutron dose of about 1 roentgen equivalent (rem), sodium, chlorine, and calcium can all be determined within a few per cent.[22–25] This procedure, however, is not utilized clinically for a number of reasons, including the limited availability of neutron fluxes and whole body counters, as well as the potentially high radiation exposure resulting from the production of radioactive isotopes in vivo that have varying physical half-lives. These radioisotopes continue to expose the patient to radiation long after the neutron flux bombardment has ceased. Despite these limitations in the procedure, various investigators have reported the feasibility of determining total body calcium by in vivo neutron activation analysis. Since more than 99 per cent of the body's calcium is located within the skeleton, the measurement of total body calcium reflects the state of bone mineralization.

In clinical practice, radionuclide imaging is the technique that is most widely used in the detection of bone abnormalities. Like most procedures in nuclear medicine, the bone scan is an extremely sensitive but relatively nonspecific modality. Any process that disturbs the normal balance of bone production and resorption can produce an abnormality on the bone scan. These abnormalities may be manifested as regions of increased or decreased activity. The large majority of lesions appear as focal areas of increased activity, since the usual response to an insult is osteogenesis. In normal images, there are areas in the skeleton that show greater and lesser concentration of the radionuclide. These differences in the degree of radionuclide concentration throughout the normal skeleton usually correspond to differences in bone turnover; for example, in children the epiphyses and metaphyseal growth plates (sites at which bone turnover is most rapid and active) appear as foci of intense tracer activity. In adults, metaphyses of tubular bones may show more activity than diaphyses.

The amount of radiopharmaceutical agent accumulated in any region of bone depends upon two major factors: the rate of bone turnover and the integrity of the blood supply. Of these two factors, the intactness of the vascular supply appears to have a more important influence on the bone scan; if there is an absence of blood perfusion to a localized region of bone, the radiopharmaceutical cannot be delivered to this area, and a photon-deficient, or "cold," region may be visualized on the scan.[26] Genant and associates[27] studied the rates of both blood flow and osteogenesis in experimental animal models and confirmed that the rate of blood flow in bone is the most important factor in determining the degree of radiopharmaceutical uptake on the bone scan. Studies that were performed earlier utilizing fluorine-18[28] also established the importance of bone perfusion in the production of the bone scan.[29] Recently, Siegel and co-workers[30] reported experimental data utilizing technetium-99m hydroxyethylene diphosphonate (^{99m}Tc-HEDP), which also suggested that bone blood flow is the major factor in determining the distribution of the radiopharmaceutical; following femoral artery ligation, a decrease in ^{99m}Tc-diphosphonate uptake in the bones of the affected limb was seen, even in the presence of healing fractures. Studies by Sagar and associates[132] in animals have uncovered a nonproportional relationship between increments in bone blood flow and augmentation of ^{99m}Tc-MDP (methylene diphosphonate) uptake. These investigators suggested a "diffusion-limited" phenomenon governing bone uptake of ^{99m}Tc-MDP in response to increased bone blood flow. They found that a fourfold increase in tibial blood flow produced only a 33 per cent augmentation of ^{99m}Tc-MDP tibial uptake. Following sectioning of tibial sympathetic nerve supply, the diffusion-limitation effect of enhanced ^{99m}Tc-MDP uptake in response to increased blood supply persisted, but at a higher flow rate level.

RADIOPHARMACEUTICALS

Over the years, a number of radiopharmaceuticals have been utilized for bone scanning. Strontium-85 was the first imageable radionuclide that was successful in identifying abnormalities within bone. The basis for its behavior is its ability to substitute biologically for calcium and be incorporated into the hydroxyapatite crystal of bone as a strontium-hydroxyapatite structure.[31] After reaching the bone via the bloodstream, the strontium is believed to freely diffuse across the capillary membrane. Strontium is rapidly incorporated into the bones; approximately 30 to 50 per cent of the administered dose is labeled to the bones within 1 hour following its administration. The remainder of the strontium-85 is excreted by the kidneys and the gastrointestinal tract. Superimposed activity by the gastrointestinal tract may interfere with bone imaging, which makes it advisable to perform the scan several days after injection of the strontium (usually 7 days).[16] Strontium-85 is a very poor radionuclide for clinical use because of its 65 day physical half-life and unfavorable gamma energy emission of 513 keV. In order to minimize the patient's radiation exposure, only small doses of 100 microcuries (μCi) can be used. At this dose, and with the added disadvantage of the sodium iodide crystal's inefficiency for detecting the high-energy gamma emission of the ^{85}Sr, a bone scan takes several hours to perform and results in images of relatively poor quality compared with the images that can be obtained with other agents. Strontium-87m is a more effective radiopharmaceutical than ^{85}Sr, as it has a 388 keV gamma ray emission and only a 2.8 hour physical half-life. Its disadvantages are that it is extremely expensive, as a generator produced agent ($^{85}Y \rightarrow {}^{87m}Sr$), and its short physical half-life requires that imaging be performed 2 to 3 hours after injection, at a time when plasma levels of ^{87m}Sr are still elevated enough to cause an unfavorable bone-to-blood background count ratio.

Fluorine-18 has a 1.9 hour physical half-life and is therefore not widely available; its use is limited to centers with rapid access to a cyclotron or reactor that produces radioiosotopes for medical use. Fluorine-18 is a positron emitter; the resulting 511 keV annihilation x-rays can be imaged by the conventional scintillation imaging systems that are available in most institutions. However, a 511 keV photon requires heavy collimation and is inefficiently imaged by the scintillation camera. In contrast to its physical limitations as a bone imaging agent, ^{18}F has superior biologic characteristics. Approximately 50 per cent of the administered dose is incorporated into the $Ca_{10}(PO_4)_6(OH)_2$ (calcium hydroxyapatite) crystal, probably by exchange for hydroxyl radicals, which are of similar physical size to the fluorine atom.[32, 33] The remaining 50 per cent of the injected ^{18}F is rapidly excreted by the kidneys so that blood clearance is faster for ^{18}F than it is for the other bone-seeking radiopharmaceuticals that have been used. Even when imaging is performed at 2 to 3 hours following intravenous or oral administration of ^{18}F, the bone-to-blood and bone-to–soft tissue background count ratios are very favorable.

In 1971, Subramanian and McAfee introduced technetium-99m polyphosphate as a bone imaging agent.[34] Subsequent work resulted in the discovery of other ^{99m}Tc-labeled phosphate compounds, such as HEDP (hydroxyethelenediphosphonate), PPi (pyrophosphate), and MDP (methylene diphosphonate),[35, 36] compounds that have dramatically improved the resolution of bone imaging, allowing definition of small osseous anatomic structures. Technetium-99m has a physical half-life of 6 hours and emits a 140 keV gamma ray, which is ideal for imaging with the available scintillation cameras and scanners. The low radiation exposure resulting from this agent permits the utilization of doses of 15 to 20 millicuries (mCi) for each bone scan. Thus, a whole body, head-to-toe image in an anterior or a posterior projection may be performed in 20 to 35 min, and approximately 1 hour is required to produce both posterior and anterior total body images of exceptionally high quality, depending upon instrumentation and biologic variables.

The ^{99m}Tc-phosphate compounds that are currently utilized for bone imaging can be categorized as condensed phosphates (inorganic compounds) and phosphonates (organic compounds). The first of the phosphate radiopharmaceuticals introduced for clinical imaging was polyphosphate as ^{99m}Tc-tripolyphosphate, an inorganic compound composed of chains of three phosphate residues. This compound was rapidly replaced by a longer chain polyphosphate containing approximately 46 phosphate residues.[37] Pyrophosphate, which contains only two phosphate residues, subsequently replaced the polyphosphates. The diphosphonates, which are organic analogues of pyrophosphate and are clinically more stable than the polyphosphates in that they are not susceptible to enzymatic hydrolysis in vivo, also gained clinical confidence. Two agents in this category that are widely used today are HEDP and MDP. Imidodiphosphonate, which contains a P-N-P bond,[38] is another category of polyphosphate compound which can be labeled with ^{99m}Tc and utilized for bone imaging. Other potential phosphate-containing bone imaging compounds include phosphonate analogues of chelating agents (DTPA, EDTA) and other variations on the methylene phosphonic acid structure.

Technetium-99m is the most widely used radioisotope in clinical nuclear medicine. Following binding to various pharmaceuticals, it is used for brain, liver, and lung scans, radionuclide angiographic studies, cardiac ejection fraction and gated cardiac blood pool wall motion studies, as well as bone and bone marrow scans. It is eluted from a molybdenum-99 generator in the form of pertechnetate ion ($^{99m}TcO_4^-$), which is a +7 valence state. Technetium-99 pertechnetate is utilized in its ionic sodium pertechnetate form for radionuclide angiographic studies, thyroid, salivary gland, gastric mucosal, or Meckel's diverticulum imaging. Following intravenous injection of ^{99m}Tc pertechnetate, it localizes throughout the extracellular fluids in the body. If ^{99m}Tc pertechnetate is mixed with a solution of one of the phosphate or phosphonate compounds and then injected intravenously, the distribution in vivo remains the same as for technetium pertechnetate alone, indicating a failure of the technetium to be bound to the phosphate or phosphonate. Technetium-99m must be in a chemically reduced form for binding or chelation to occur. Reduction of technetium from a +7 valence state (TcO_4^-) to a +4 valence state is easily accomplished by mixing the ^{99m}Tc pertechnetate following its elution from the generator with tin (Sn^{+2}) in the form of stannous chloride. Mixing the ^{99m}Tc pertechnetate, stannous chloride, and one of the phosphate compounds in a solution results in a technetium-tin-phosphate complex that preferentially localizes within bone when injected intravenously.[31]

Bone uptake localization half-times have been measured as 15 to 30 min, which is much more rapid than the half-time disappearance from the blood, which has been measured at about 1 hour. The technetium-phosphate complex that is not localized within bone is excreted into the urine via glomerular filtration. There are slight variations among the various phosphate compounds in the proportion of the administered dose that localizes in the bone and in the rate of excretion of the compound by the kidneys. At 1 hour after intravenous administration, 58 per cent of the administered MDP, 48 per cent of administered HEDP, and 47 per cent of administered PPi was found in the bones.[37] Studies of blood clearance and urinary excretion of the technetium-phosphate complexes,[37, 39] have shown that diphosphonate compounds are cleared more rapidly from the blood than either pyrophosphate or polyphosphate. MDP appears to be cleared from the blood more rapidly than HEDP, which enhances MDP's slight advantage in bone deposition and, therefore, its role as a radiopharmaceutical for bone imaging.

The phosphate compounds are bound to protein after intravenous injection. The degree of protein binding may influence the blood clearance and urinary excretion rates of these compounds. Another factor that contributes to differences in rates of blood clearance is the variable nature of the binding of the compounds to red blood cells. For example, 10 to 30 per cent of the whole blood ^{99m}Tc pyrophosphate activity is bound to red cells at 1 to 3 hours after injection.[40] Conversely, only a negligible amount of ^{99m}Tc-HEDP or ^{99m}Tc-MDP is bound to these cells. Six hour urine collections show that about 68 per cent of the administered technetium-labeled diphosphonate compounds is excreted, compared with 50 per cent of the technetium-labeled pyrophosphate and 46 per cent of the technetium-labeled polyphosphate.

All these phosphate compounds can inhibit both formation and dissolution of hydroxyapatite crystals in vitro and in vivo. In fact, these agents, particularly the diphosphonate, have been used in the management of patients with Paget's disease of bone[41] and of some patients with idiopathic calcinosis universalis. Pharmacologic doses of diphosphonate may retard bone growth and ectopic calcification in these patients. The mechanism of this action has been postulated to be the accretion of the diphosphonate onto the mineral surfaces of bone, resulting in a retardation of further build-up or loss of mineral ion. Inhibition of the conversion of noncrystalline calcium phosphate to hydroxyapatite crystal by diphosphonate has also been proposed.

The mechanism by which the ^{99m}Tc-labeled phosphate compounds are incorporated into bone is not entirely understood. Since the technetium-phosphate compounds do not carry significant ionic charge, they may be able to diffuse relatively freely across the bone capillary wall, similarly to the behavior of strontium and fluorine. Having arrived at the bone site, therefore, the phosphate compound may chemisorb (chemical and physical processes leading to adsorption) at kink and dislocation sites on the surface of the hydroxyapatite, resulting in a release of tin and ^{99m}Tc, which are hydrolyzed and deposited either separately or together as hydrated tin oxide and technetium dioxide.[30] Sites of rapid bone turnover, such as growth centers and reactive bone lesions, are associated with a large mineral surface that is available for exchange and chemisorption by the ^{99m}Tc-tin-phosphate complex. Although the hypothesis that the ^{99m}Tc-phosphate compounds bind at the bone crystal surface is the current dominant theory, it has also been proposed that such binding predominates at the organic matrix, particularly the immature collagen.[42, 43]

INSTRUMENTS

The most widely used instrument for imaging skeletal distribution of radionuclides is the scintillation camera, which may be equipped with a scanning mode for displaying the whole body distribution of the radiopharmaceutical on a single x-ray film. Scintillation cameras detect the distribution of radiopharmaceutical in vivo by externally recording the interactions of gamma rays emitted from the body with a sodium iodide crystal in the camera head. The scintillation camera detection system involves an array of photomultiplier tubes ranging in number from 37 to 61 in current models (one manufacturer markets a 91 tube camera), which process the scintillations that result from interactions of the gamma rays in the sodium iodide crystal such that each gamma ray interaction of the appropriate energy level is displayed on an XY axis corresponding in position to its origin in the body. This results in an image of the distribution of the radionuclide in vivo. The images are recorded on Polaroid film with a radioactive scintillation displayed as a white dot, or on x-ray film with a radioactive scintillation displayed as a black dot. The scintillation camera may be equipped with a 10 in diameter sodium iodide crystal, a 15 in diameter sodium iodide crystal, or a 20 in diameter sodium iodide crystal (marketed by one manufacturer as a "jumbo camera").

Lead collimators are needed in front of the sodium iodide crystal to minimize the number of scattered photons that can interact with the crystal. For bone and joint imaging, either high-resolution or all-purpose low-energy collimators are used. If stationary spot imaging is performed, 100,000 to 500,000 counts are obtained per image, the greater count rate resulting in a higher quality image, which of course takes longer to obtain. For spot images, it is advisable to utilize a pinhole or low-energy converging collimator to magnify small regions of interest and maximize the resolution of the image.

Equipping the scintillation camera with a scanning mode option consisting of either a moving table or a moving detector head will permit the obtaining of total body images, which can be displayed on a single 8 × 10 in x-ray film. A total body radionuclide bone image in the anterior or posterior projection obtained 2 hours following intravenous injection of 15 mCi of ^{99m}Tc-labeled phosphate compounds will generally take about 30 min. This time will vary, depending upon the collimator used, the degree of uptake of the radiopharmaceutical in the bones, the amount of renal excretion, the size and build of the patient, the number of millicuries injected, the time elapsed between injection and imaging, and the width of the window setting around the 140 keV photon energy peak of ^{99m}Tc. In most institutions, at least anterior and posterior total body views are obtained, supplemented with spot images of questionably abnormal regions. A 20 per cent window is usually utilized, limiting the recording of counts to those photons that fall within 20 per cent of the 140 keV peak of activity.

The rectilinear scanner is an older imaging instrument that has been phased out of production by most manufacturers. It has only one photomultiplier tube behind a single sodium iodide crystal of either 3 in, 5 in, or 8 in diameter that moves across and down the body, recording the radiation that is detected beneath it. The counts are displayed by blackening of an x-ray film on a point-by-point basis. These instruments are tomographic in that they utilize focusing collimators and preferentially record counts from a plane at a particular depth in the body.

More recently, tomographic imaging instruments capable of displaying multiple planes of selective activity from a single scan of the body have been perfected and are in clinical use. These instruments offer a potential similar to that of computed tomographic radiographic imaging devices. This approach can provide more detailed information, both qualitative and quantitative, on the localization of radiopharmaceuticals in bones and joints.

CLINICAL APPLICATIONS

Since the emergence of bone scanning in 1961, the clinical utility of this technique has continued to grow. Originally, the bone scan methodology gained clinical attention because of its ability to provide more sensitive detection than x-rays in the evaluation of metastatic disease. Certainly, radionuclide bone imaging is widely used in the detection of osseous metastasis in patients with primary neoplasms that frequently spread to the bone, e.g., carcinoma of the prostate and carcinoma of the breast. In addition to neoplasm, the bone scan is valuable in the early diagnosis of osteomyelitis and in evaluating the response of the infection to therapy. Radionuclide bone imaging has not yet achieved wide clinical use in metabolic diseases. Potentially, however, the bone imaging may be a sensitive indicator of metabolic alterations. It may also prove valuable in following the therapeutic responses in particular metabolic disorders. Vascular diseases such as aseptic necrosis lend themselves well to examination by bone scan, since radionuclide bone imaging is so sensitive to blood flow and to the reparative osteogenic processes that usually accompany vascular diseases of the bone. Following traumatic insults to bone, the radionuclide study may be particularly helpful clinically in processes in which the radiograph is not so sensitive — e.g., stress fractures. Articular diseases can also be well evaluated with scintigraphy. Thus, a partial list of indications for radionuclide bone imaging would include the following:

1. To screen for bone metastases.
2. To localize metastases for diagnostic biopsies.
3. To diagnose osteomyelitis before radiographic changes are evident; to follow the response to therapy in chronic osteomyelitis; to aid in differentiating cellulitis from osteomyelitis; and to aid in evaluating painful prostheses for infection and for loosening.
4. To detect and evaluate the extent of articular involvement in various forms of arthritis, including osteoarthritis, rheumatoid arthritis, and rheumatoid "variant" disorders.
5. To aid in the work-up and characterization of benign bone lesions, particularly those that are sometimes difficult to visualize by radiographic techniques because of their nature or location.
6. To aid in the work-up of compression fractures, particularly when there is a question of the age of the compression fracture, as may occur in medicolegal cases.
7. To evaluate bone pain of any etiology in the presence of normal roentgenograms.
8. To aid in diagnosis and management of aseptic necrosis of bone.
9. To aid in management of myositis ossificans.

NEOPLASM

Skeletal Metastasis

The axial skeleton is a major site of metastases; of all skeletal metastases, approximately 80 per cent localize in the axial skeleton, 10 per cent in the skull, and 10 per cent in the long bones.[44] Various studies have documented that approximately 10 to 40 per cent of patients with skeletal metastases have normal radiographs at a time when the bone scan is abnormal, and fewer than 5 per cent of bone scans are normal when radiographs show localized abnormalities.[16] It is not uncommon for the bone scan of a patient who is free of any bone pain and whose radiographs are entirely normal to show multiple foci of metastatic disease. Occasionally, a region may be painful and yet normal on radionuclide bone images. In these latter cases, evaluation by radiography may show a lytic lesion that apparently has not caused sufficient reactive bone formation on a histologic level to result in increased radiopharmaceutical

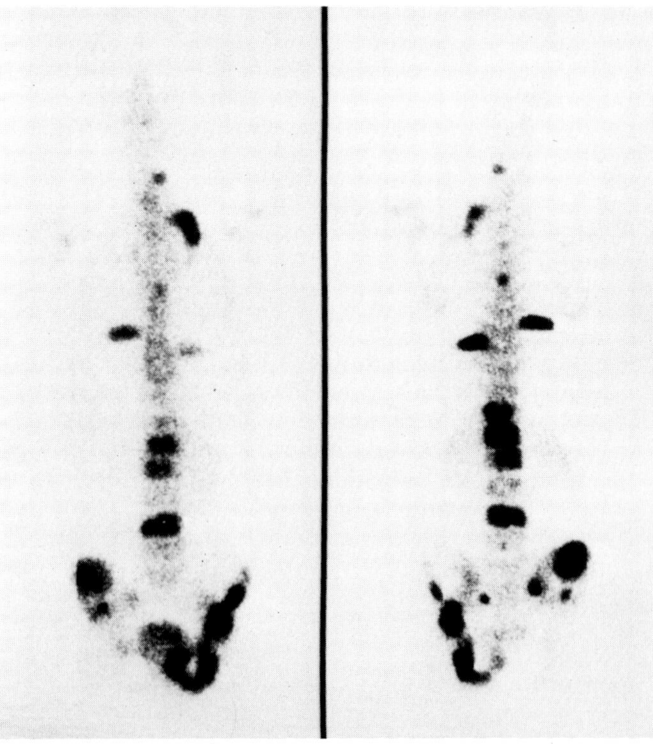

Figure 17–1. Metastatic bone disease. Anterior and posterior views from a ^{99m}Tc pyrophosphate bone scan in a patient with primary cancer of the prostate. There are multiple hot foci of increased uptake of the radiopharmaceutic agent, involving the spine, pelvis, and ribs. The lesions are concentrating the radiopharmaceutic agent so avidly that the blood background, kidneys, and normal bones are hardly visible.

accumulation on the bone scan. Anaplastic tumors and multiple myeloma are two major categories of malignant disease that characteristically may not stimulate sufficient osteoblastic reaction for an abnormal focus to be imaged on scan. Figure 17–1 demonstrates a radionuclide bone image in a patient with metastatic bone disease.

Lesions that are lytic radiographically are not necessarily purely lytic histologically. At a cellular level, both osteoblastic and osteoclastic activity may be increased. The radiographically evident lytic nature of a lesion simply reflects the fact that the resorption process is occurring at a more rapid rate than the osteogenic process. In these cases, the bone scan is usually positive because it reflects osteogenic activity in the lesion, which is usually increased above that in the normal adjacent bone. In approximately 5 per cent of metastases, the bone scan is indeed negative in the presence of a radiographically evident destructive lesion, indicating that the osteogenesis within the lesion or its blood supply is not greater than that in the normal surrounding bone.

The bone scan is frequently used to follow the response of neoplasm to irradiation, chemotherapy, or hormone therapy in patients with cancer and bone metastases. It is not uncommon to see dramatic changes in the bone scan following therapy, with resolution of previously abnormal areas throughout the skeleton, findings that are usually interpreted as a favorable therapeutic response. However, this response cannot necessarily be interpreted to mean that no viable tumor cells remain in a region that has converted to normal on the radionuclide images (Fig. 17–2). An individual lesion may also show apparent worsening on a bone scan obtained after completion of therapy. In some cases, this response has been identified as a transient process, which may represent repair and healing of the bone rather than progression of disease.

Another scintigraphic pattern that may be associated with widespread metastatic bone disease is the "superscan" seen on whole body imaging. When metastatic bone disease is far advanced, the skeletal system may avidly extract the radiopharmaceutical from the blood, resulting in greater than 50 per cent bone concentration of the radiopharmaceutical and leaving less available radiopharmaceutical for excretion by the kidneys. Consequently, on the image, the kidneys may not be visualized and the blood background may be markedly free of radioactivity, with the generalized bone-to-background ratio of counts being unusually high (Figs. 17–3 and 17–4). Conversely, one or more photon-deficient or cold areas can represent the scintigraphic response to skeletal metastases (Fig. 17–5).

In about 6 to 8 per cent of patients with skeletal metastases, only a single focal lesion may be seen on the scan. Since many solitary bone lesions are malignant, radiographic evaluation of the site of focal radionuclide abnormality must be performed. In contrast to radiographic characteristics that aid in the differentiation between benign and malignant

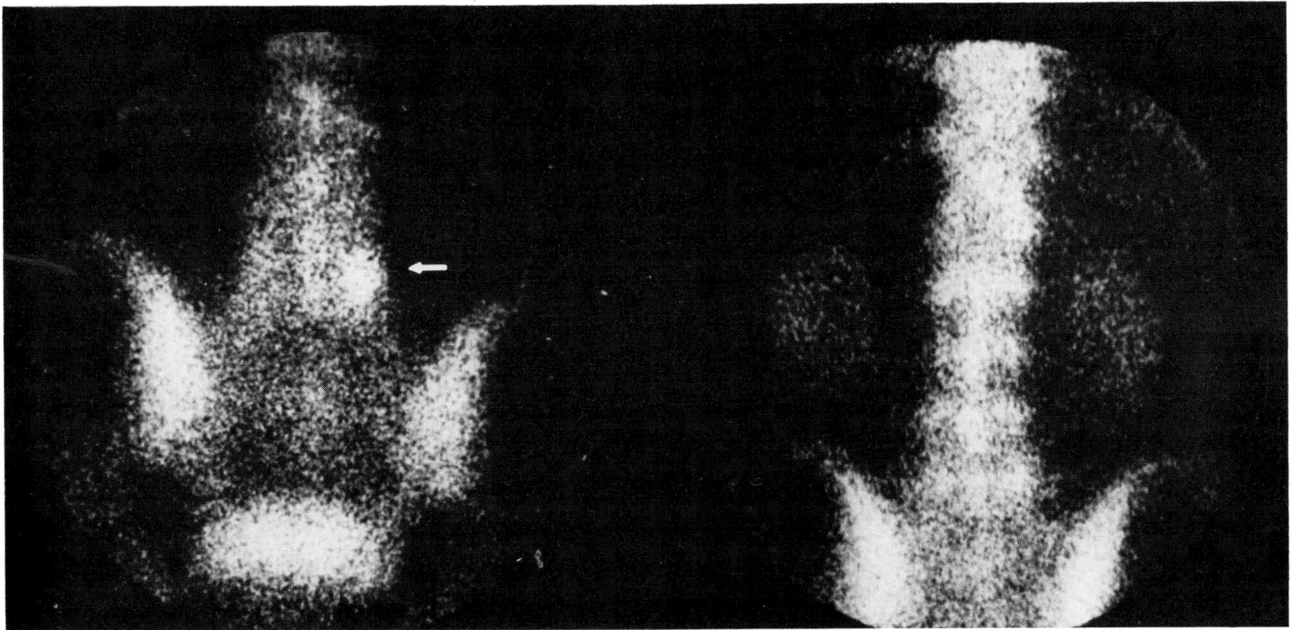

Figure 17–2. *Metastatic disease with response to chemotherapy. Scintillation camera views of the patient's lower spine following ^{99m}Tc pyrophosphate scans performed approximately 1 year apart in a patient with primary cancer of the prostate. On the image at left, a focus of increased activity is noted in the right side of the L5 vertebral body (arrow). One year later, the abnormal focus in L5 is no longer apparent. The patient had been treated with chemotherapy for prostate cancer and responded well.*

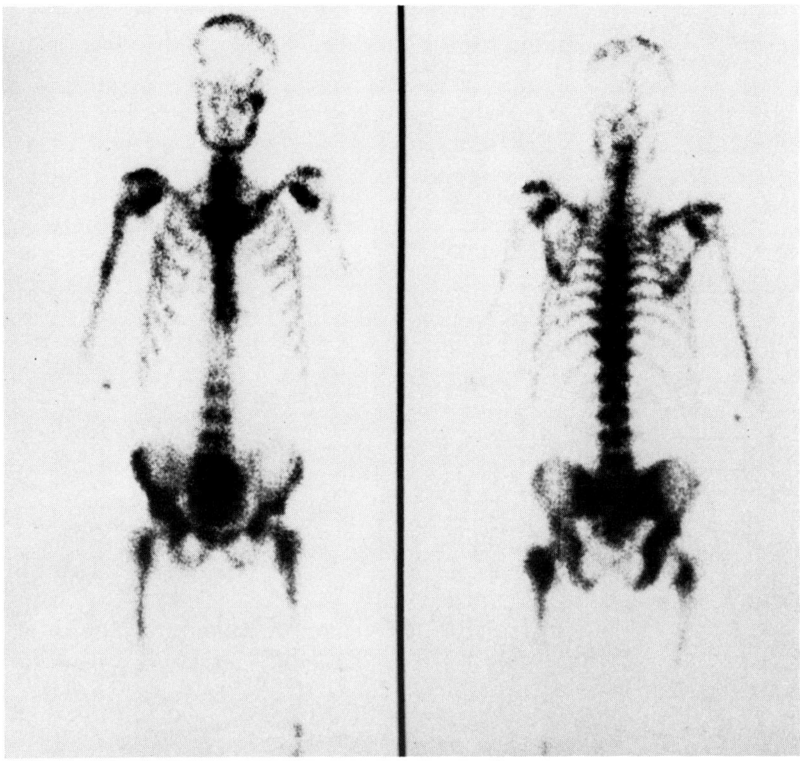

Figure 17–3. "Superscan" in metastatic disease. Anterior and posterior whole body images from a ^{99m}Tc pyrophosphate scan on a patient with primary cancer of the prostate. The "superscan" pattern shows absence of activity in the kidneys, low blood background activity, and generalized uniformly increased uptake by all the bones in the body. Some areas of greater and lesser uptake can be identified on closer examination, particularly in the right humerus, the left distal femur, the right posterior pelvis and iliac bone, the left mandible, the skull, and the ribs.

processes, scintigraphic abnormalities can give only a very general indication of the aggressiveness of the lesion. When a single lesion is found on the radiographs, the scan is helpful in confirming the solitary nature of the lesion, in identifying the presence of other bony lesions, and in characterizing the lesion as being "high grade" or "low grade" in radiopharmaceutical concentration. In general, malignant lesions are hyperemic and, therefore, "hotter" on the scintigraphic image than benign lesions (Fig. 17–6). Additionally, a radionuclide angiogram can be performed with the scintillation camera centered over the radiographically identified abnormality at the time of intravenous injection of the radiopharmaceutical; the degree of vascularity of the lesion can be surmised on sequential scintiphotos by comparing the vascularity at the site of abnormality with that of surrounding normal bone.

Attempts to define the best approach to the detection of skeletal metastases by combining radiography and nuclear imaging, with an eye to cost effectiveness, have been considered. In one study,[45] an analysis of examinations requested by clinicians without radiologic guidance in 141 patients being evaluated for tumor staging indicated that excessive studies were performed in 18 per cent of these individuals and that inadequate or inappropriate studies were performed in 27 per cent. In actuality, the necessary data for arriving at the optimum combined radiographic and nuclear imaging approach to the determination of skeletal metastasis in various neoplasms are still in the process of being gathered.

McNeil[44] has approached the problem by first examining the incidence of bone metastases at autopsy in several malignant diseases. A decision-making analysis for the use of bone scans in primary and secondary tumors is then based on data currently available on the yield of the abnormal bone scan in that disease relative to autopsy results, the assumed health benefits associated with information gained from the scan, and the financial costs. These analyses have been applied to breast cancer, lung cancer, prostate cancer, and primary bone tumors.

Breast Cancer. There is a large disparity between the incidence of bone metastases from breast cancer found at autopsy and that detected at the time of initial therapy and follow-up. Indications are that many individuals have occult bone metastases, undetected at the time of surgery and early follow-up. The incidence of bone metastases at autopsy in patients with primary breast cancer ranges from 50 to 85 per cent. The reported incidence of bone metastases in patients with primary breast cancer at the time of surgery and thereafter has varied considerably.[46-48] The incidence of positive bone scans for metastatic disease in patients with breast cancer at the stage 1 or 2 level has ranged from 2 to 38 per cent. Most studies indicate that the frequency of a true-positive bone scan in stage 1 or 2 disease is in the neighborhood of 2 per cent, whereas in stage 3 disease the incidence of true-positive bone scans increases to about 28 per cent. Investigators have found that bone metastasis becomes apparent on follow-up scans 3 to 4 years after surgery in about

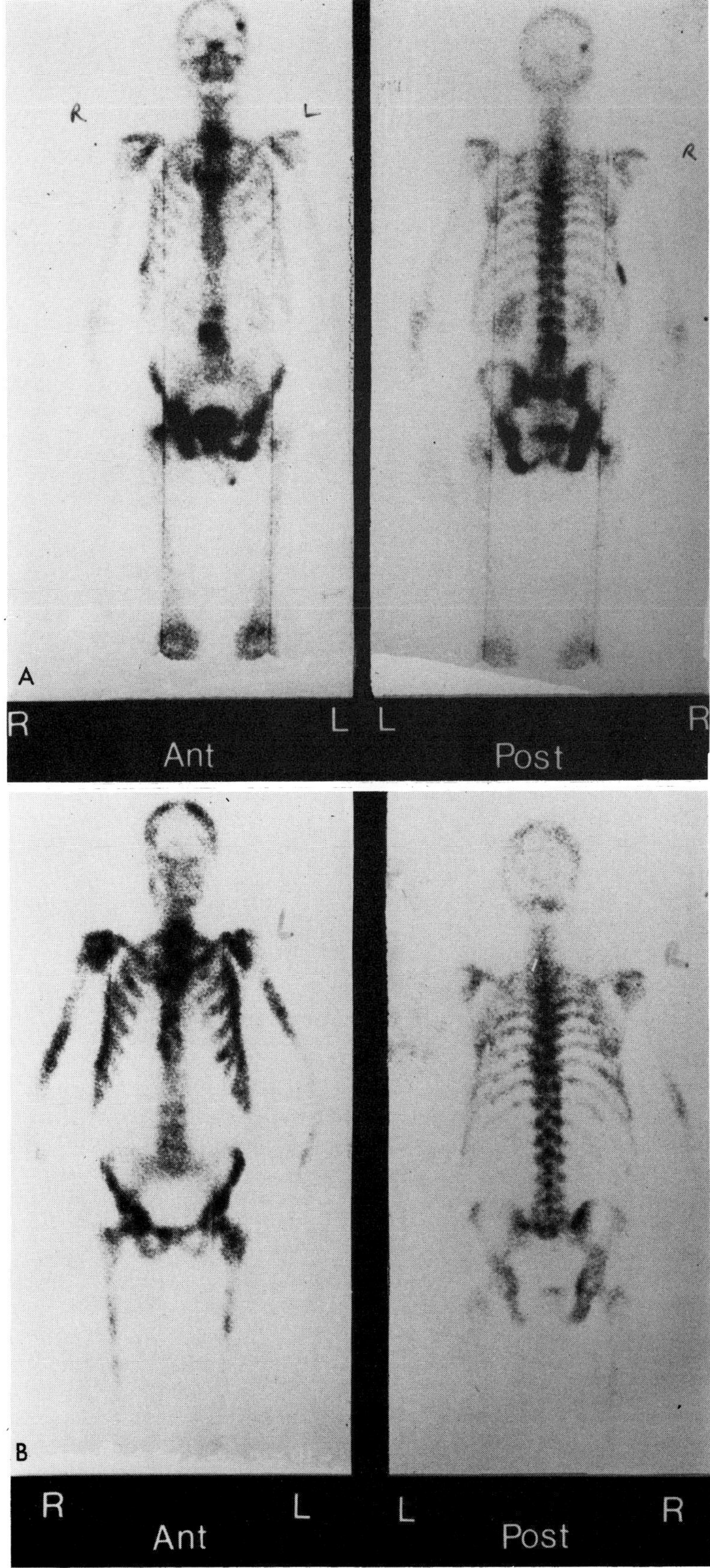

Figure 17–4. *Progression of metastatic bone disease. Anterior and posterior* ^{99m}*Tc methylene diphosphonate (MDP) whole body images in a patient with primary cancer of the prostate.* **A,** *On 1/19/78, there are multiple focal regions of increased activity in the pelvic bones, lumbar spine, ribs, and skull. The findings are suggestive of metastatic disease.* **B,** *The same patient was re-imaged approximately 1 year later. The patient's metastatic bone disease has progressed to the pattern of a "superscan," reflecting generalized involvement of almost every bone in the body. The pattern consists of poor visualization of the kidneys, very low blood background activity, and generalized increased bony activity with some irregularities noted on careful inspection, particularly in the humeri, femurs, skull, and ribs.*

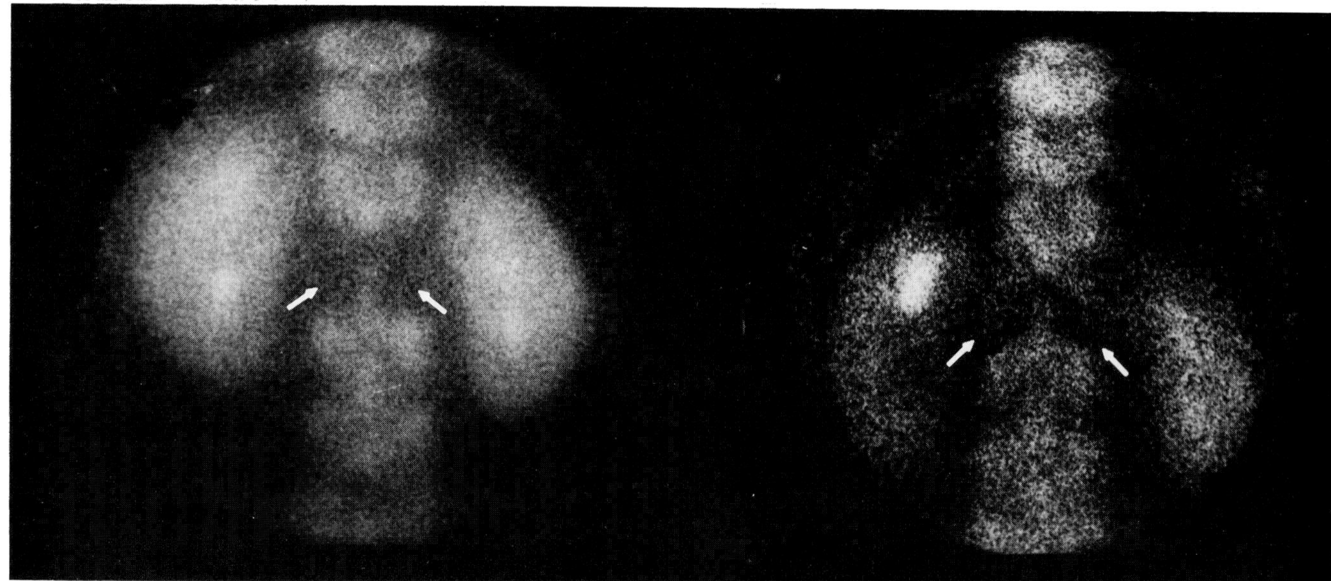

Figure 17–5. *Cold focus in metastatic disease. Single scintillation camera views of the upper lumbar spine in two patients; the patient on the left has primary lung cancer, whereas the patient on the right has primary breast cancer. Both patients have metastatic disease involving the bones. The photon-deficient or "cold" vertebral body shown in each of these scans is a reflection of metastatic disease in the lumbar vertebral bodies (arrows). Note that the spinous processes of the lumbar vertebrae in both cases appear to be intact. The cold region seen on the scan is postulated to be a secondary effect either of total interruption of blood supply to the vertebral body because of the presence of necrotic tumor that has outgrown its blood supply, or of total replacement of the bony structure by tumor leaving no viable osteoblasts to produce bone that can accrete the radiopharmaceutical. Incidentally noted is a dilated calix in the upper pole of the left kidney in the patient with breast cancer.*

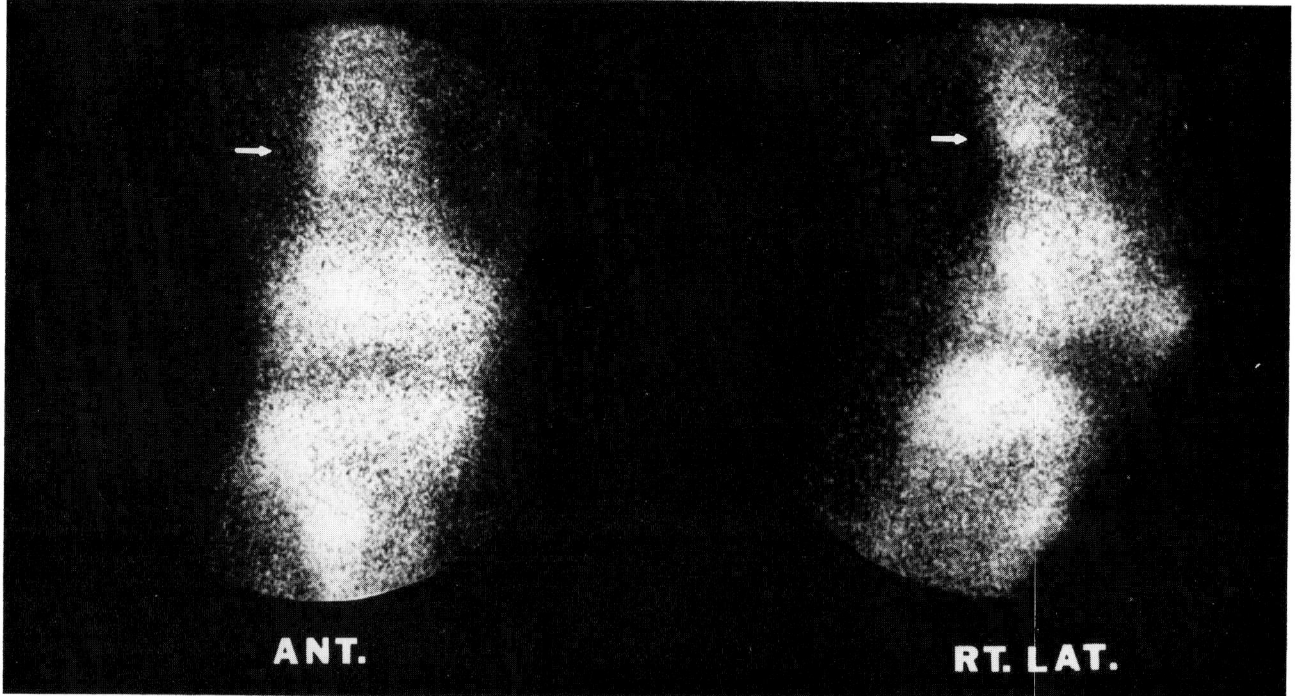

Figure 17–6. *Benign bone lesion. Scintillation camera images of the right knee for a ^{99m}Tc pyrophosphate bone scan. In both views, the distal diaphyis of the femur shows a focus of increased activity, which corresponds to a benign fibrous cortical defect (arrow). The degree of increased activity is much less than the normal activity in the metaphyses of this young adult.*

20 to 30 per cent of patients who had negative bone scans and no evidence of bone metastases at the time of surgery.[46-48] Fifty per cent of the patients in whom bone metastases were seen at 3 years after treatment had actually manifested their disease by 12 months after therapy and 75 per cent by 18 months after therapy. The increased sensitivity of the scan compared with the radiograph appears to give the scan a 6 to 18 month lead over the radiograph in converting to abnormal results. McNeil has concluded from these data that patients with clinical stage 3 breast carcinoma should have preoperative bone scans.[44] Patients with stage 1 and stage 2 disease should have baseline evaluations at the time of therapy and follow-up scans at 6, 12, 18, and 24 months to detect those who may have had occult metastatic disease, undetected at the time of initial therapy.

Lung Cancer. Two to 35 per cent of patients with stage 1 or 2 adenocarcinoma, epidermoid carcinoma, or large cell carcinoma of the lung reveal a true-positive yield for bone metastases on bone scan.[49, 50] At autopsy, the incidence of such metastases in patients with primary lung cancer ranges from 30 to 50 per cent. Comparative studies of the bone scan and radiograph in the detection of skeletal metastases in this neoplasm have not yet been accomplished. Since adequate data are lacking, it is difficult to conclude whether or not preoperative bone scans are warranted in the work-up of patients with lung cancer, although McNeil has suggested that even if the yield is low, the operative mortality rate in this disease may justify a preoperative bone scan.[44]

Prostate Cancer. The incidence of bone metastases at autopsy in patients with primary prostate carcinoma ranges from 50 to 70 per cent. A Veterans Administration cooperative study has shown that patients with stage 1 or 2 disease (stages A and B) showed a 7 per cent yield of positive bone scans, whereas in patients with more advanced, stage 3 disease, 18 per cent had positive bone scans.[44] Although no specific data are available, it is apparent that a large number of patients with primary prostate carcinoma develop positive bone scans on follow-up examinations. Characteristically, only 54 per cent of patients with bone metastases have pain at the time of their scan conversion from normal to abnormal, whereas 12 per cent of those without detectable bone metastases may have pain.[51] Thus, pain is apparently a symptom that is difficult to interpret as an indicator of the presence or absence of bone metastases. The high incidence of bone metastases detected in this disease even during early stages strongly supports the routine use of the bone scan in staging of the disease and follow-up of these patients.

Primary Malignant Bone Tumors. The incidence of skeletal metastases at autopsy in patients with primary osteosarcoma is about 25 per cent. Although pulmonary metastases are also frequent in these patients, Goldstein and co-workers[52] reported that about 15 per cent of patients developed bone metastases in the absence of or prior to lung metastases. These investigators also noted that approximately 25 per cent of all bone lesions were seen by 7 months, 50 per cent by 14 months, and 75 per cent by 24 months after clinical presentation. Thus, it seems reasonable that children who present with osteosarcoma should have a bone scan as a baseline study in order to verify the presence or absence of distant metastases. On the other hand, the question of whether or not the bone scan is more accurate than the radiograph in delineating the local extent of the primary tumor is unanswered, since general hyperperfusion of the involved extremity may account for a larger abnormality on the scan than on the radiograph without necessarily being indicative of tumor extension.

In Ewing's sarcoma, about 60 per cent of patients have bone metastases at autopsy.[44] At the time of clinical presentation, bone metastases were diagnosed in 12 per cent of children with Ewing's sarcoma, whereas 33 per cent of patients showed bone metastases on follow-up examinations.[53, 54] These skeletal metastases occurred prior to or in the absence of pulmonary metastases in more than half the patients who were studied. Thus, it would seem reasonable that children with Ewing's sarcoma should have a bone scan at the time of initial presentation and during follow-up periods of at least 2 years.

Neuroblastoma. Bone scanning has been recommended as the screening procedure of choice in children suspected of having skeletal metastases in neuroblastoma.[55] Gilday and associates found no false-negative bone scans in 30 cases of neuroblastoma and recommended that radiographs be obtained only if a lesion was evident on the nuclear image.[55] Other investigators[56] have reported false-negative bone scans in neuroblastoma. In one series, a total of 18 lesions were detected in 6 patients, of which 14 were demonstrated by radiography and only 4 were positive by radiography and scintigraphy. No lesions that were detected by scan alone were reported in this series. Skeletal foci of neuroblastoma show predilection for the metaphyseal regions of long bones, at which sites the abnormalities may be obscured by the avid uptake of radiopharmaceutical in adjacent epiphyses. This fact coupled with the small size and lytic nature of the lesion is cited as an explanation for the high rate of false-negative radionuclide examinations in patients with neuroblastoma.[56]

Benign Bone Tumors and Tumor-Like Lesions

In the evaluation of benign bone lesions, the scan may be clinically valuable, particularly in pa-

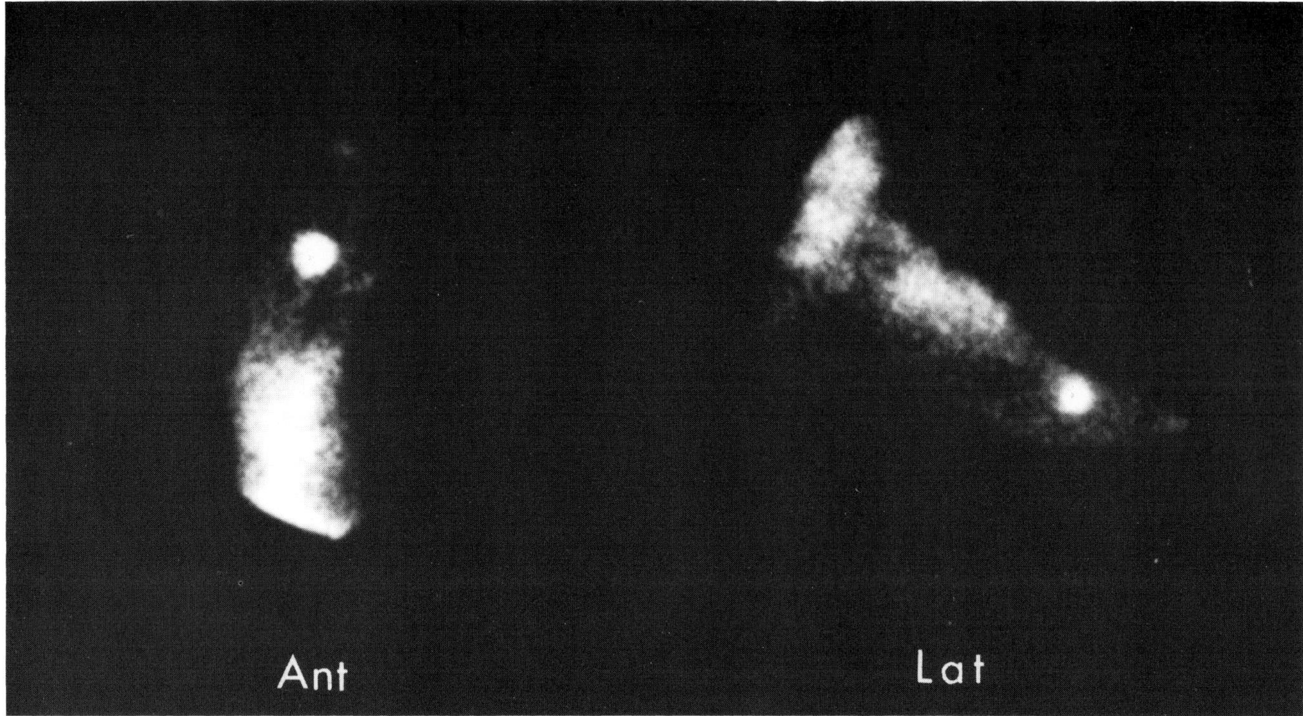

Figure 17–7. *Osteoid osteoma. Anterior and lateral views of the left foot from a ^{99m}Tc MDP bone scan from a patient complaining of pain in the left foot. A focal region of markedly increased uptake is identified and consistent with the diagnosis of osteoid osteoma.*

tients who present with pain and in whom radiographs fail to reveal a bone lesion. Not uncommonly, small lesions that are difficult to see on the roentgenogram because of their location may be quite apparent on the bone scan. An osteoid osteoma is a lesion that characteristically is quite "hot" on the bone scan and yet may be difficult to detect on a radiograph[57] (Fig. 17–7).

Several other benign bone lesions are frequently "hot" on the bone scan, including Paget's disease and fibrous dysplasia. The extent of radiopharmaceutical concentration in these lesions reflects the degree of hyperemia and osteogenesis.

Bone cysts show normal or slightly increased radiopharmaceutical concentration, and a central area of decreased counts may be present. When a fracture complicates a bone cyst, the scan will be "hot." In the absence of such a fracture, the radionuclide appearance may be useful in the distinction between a benign cyst and a malignant bone lesion.

In the skull, a mild degree of increased uptake in the frontal or parasagittal region will usually reflect the presence of hyperostosis frontalis internis. The mild nature of the augmented radionuclide activity and its characteristic anatomic distribution allow accurate diagnosis in these cases. In children, sutural sites may show increased activity, which regresses to normal following closure of the sutures. In infants, the bone scan may be of clinical value in examining patients with potential premature closure of sutures and in determining the necessity for surgical intervention.[58, 59]

Bone islands have a variable appearance on the bone scan. When larger than 3 cm in size, they may manifest as focal regions of increased activity on the bone scan. Generally, bone islands that are less than 3 cm in size show normal uptake of the radiopharmaceutical. The bone scan, when accompanied by a radionuclide angiogram performed at the time of intravenous injection of the radiopharmaceutical, may be helpful in differentiating a bone island from a more aggressive lesion, since an element of increased vascularity would make the diagnosis of bone island unlikely.

Other benign bone tumors and tumor-like lesions, including eosinophilic granuloma, fibrous cortical defect, enchondroma, and osteochondroma, will frequently show increased radiopharmaceutical uptake on the nuclear images. The scan may be clinically helpful in identifying multiple lesions in these diseases, as well as in their follow-up, particularly if malignant transformation is suspected.

INFECTION

The diagnosis of bone infection remains a major clinical problem, particularly since the radiograph is relatively insensitive to the early changes of osteomyelitis and frequently may not become positive until 10 to 14 days after the onset of the disease. The sensitivity of the bone scan is such that as early as 24 hours after the onset of symptoms, the scan may be positive and will usually remain positive until the lesion is completely healed.[60] The role of the radionuclide study in the evaluation of osseous inflammatory disease includes (1) early detection, (2) differentiation of osteomyelitis from cellulitis, and (3) identification of renewed activity in cases of chronic osteomyelitis. Regarding the first, the high degree of sensitivity of the bone scan for identifying and localizing the abnormality in the presence of normal radiographs makes the scan clinically important in the work-up of patients with possible osteomyelitis. Occasionally, very early in the course of osteomyelitis, the lesion will present on the scan as a "cold" or photon-deficient focus.[26, 61] This appearance probably can be explained by the pathophysiology of early osteomyelitis, specifically an interruption of bone blood supply secondary to sludging and thrombosis induced by the inflammatory infiltration of cells, which may originate in the marrow. Several such cases have been reported, particularly in neonates or young children. With time, the pattern of a focally increased region of activity will replace the photon-deficient area as bone reparation occurs and an infarctive process is replaced by a hyperemic response. Thus, the spectrum of the radionuclide pattern in osteomyelitis varies from areas that are photon-deficient to those that have augmented radionuclide activity (Fig. 17–8). Between these two points, of course, lies the range for a normal degree of uptake. If the patient is imaged during the transient normal period on this spectrum, a false-negative scan will result.

As a result of reports of occasional false-negative results early in the course of osteomyelitis, gallium-67 bone imaging has been utilized as an adjunct to technetium imaging. Gallium-67 citrate images are obtained 6 and 24 hours following the injection of 5 mCi for the diagnosis of osteomyelitis. Reports on the use of ^{67}Ga for imaging active osteomyelitis have uniformly revealed correct identification of infection in nearly all cases. In many patients, particularly children, the gallium images are more accurate in identifying focal lesions adjacent to growth plates that were masked by adjacent high-intensity uptake on bone scans. Figure 17–9*A* shows the bone scan and Figure 17–9*B* the gallium scan in a 21 year old man complaining of right hip pain. The bone scan failed to show a definite abnormality, and only in retrospect, following visualization of the abnormality in the right sacroiliac joint on the gallium study, can a faint degree of increased uptake on the technetium study be identified. Osteomyelitis was subsequently confirmed by blood cultures and radiography.

The differentiation between osteomyelitis and cellulitis may be a very difficult clinical problem in which sequential ^{99m}Tc-MDP and ^{67}Ga imaging may

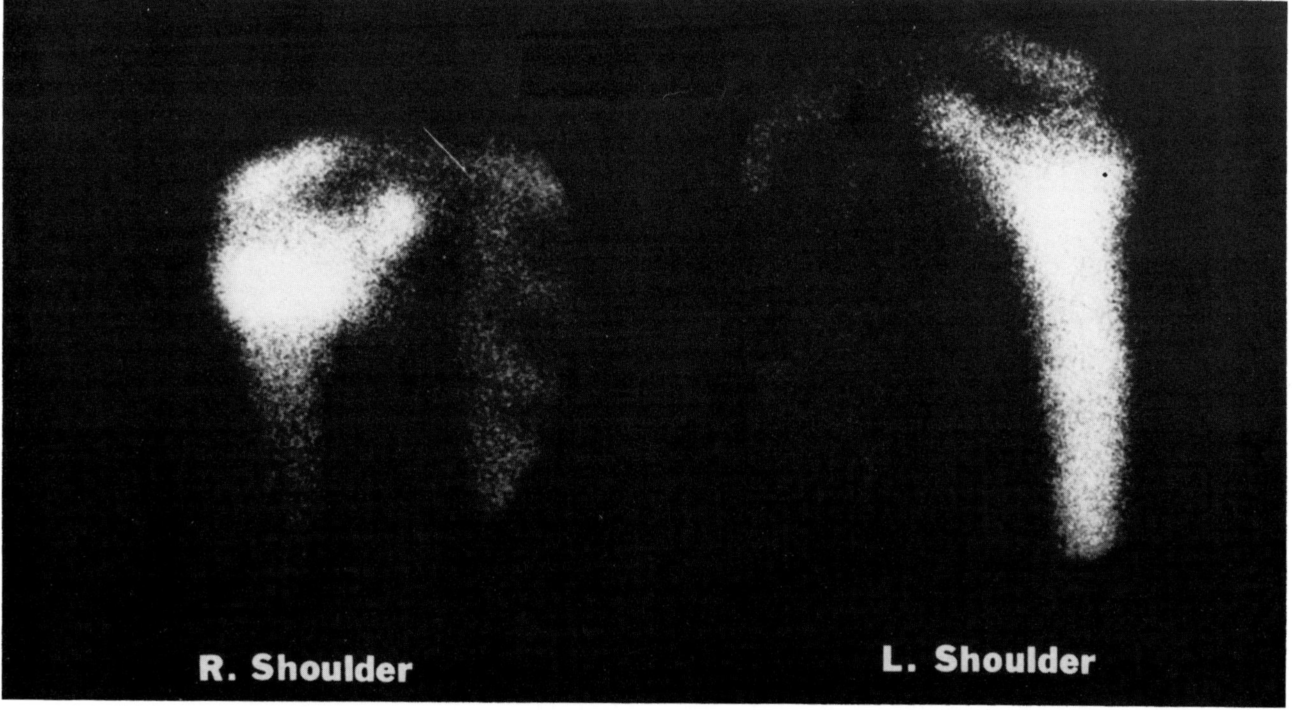

Figure 17–8. *Acute osteomyelitis. Scintillation camera views of the shoulders in a patient with osteomyelitis. The left shoulder view shows a markedly increased uptake involving the proximal humerus and extending to the level of midshaft. At a later time, radiographs of this region showed periosteal elevation and other findings consistent with the diagnosis of acute osteomyelitis. The right shoulder is normal.*

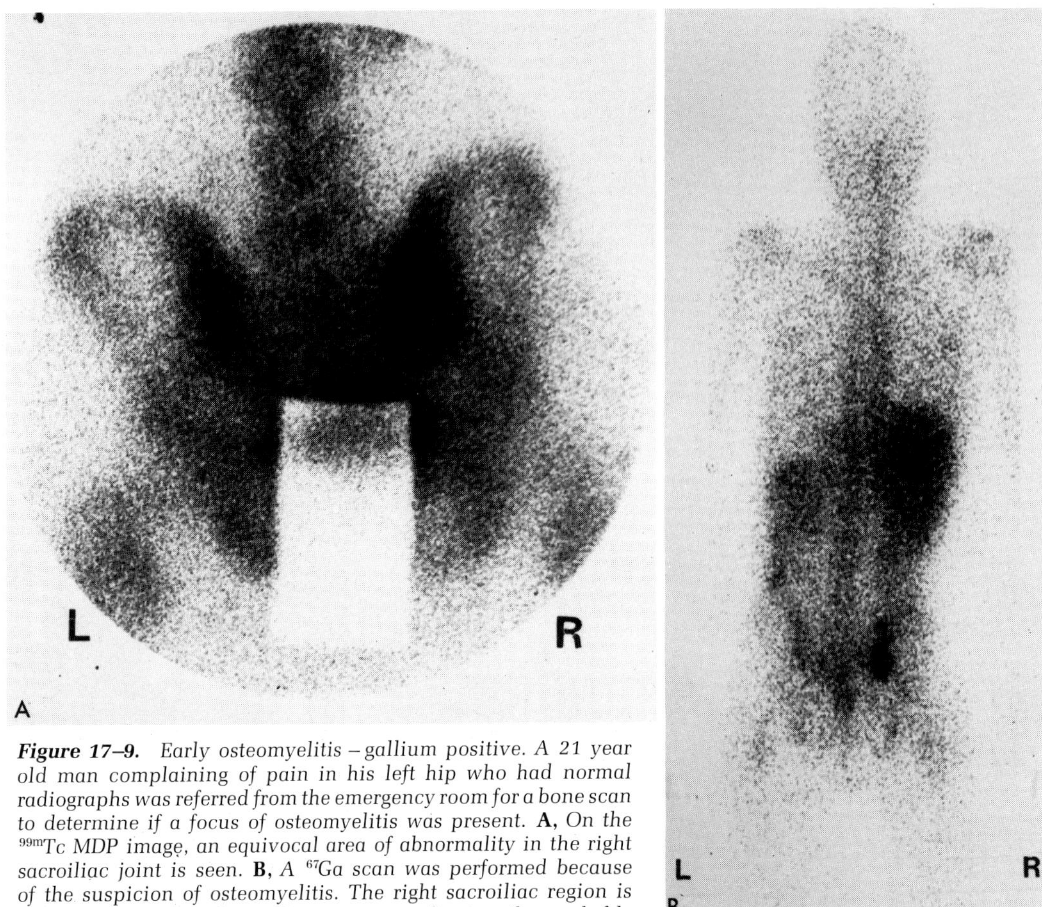

Figure 17–9. Early osteomyelitis – gallium positive. A 21 year old man complaining of pain in his left hip who had normal radiographs was referred from the emergency room for a bone scan to determine if a focus of osteomyelitis was present. **A,** *On the* ^{99m}*Tc MDP image, an equivocal area of abnormality in the right sacroiliac joint is seen.* **B,** *A* ^{67}*Ga scan was performed because of the suspicion of osteomyelitis. The right sacroiliac region is highly positive on the gallium scan, confirming the probable diagnosis of osteomyelitis. Blood cultures eventually revealed* Staphylococcus aureus *and radiographs became positive approximately 1 week later.*

be helpful.[62,63] For example, at the time of intravenous injection of ^{99m}Tc-MDP, sequential imaging with the scintillation camera centered over the bone in question produces a radionuclide angiogram that is followed by an immediate blood pool image, disclosing the degree of vascular abnormality of the involved bone. Generally, in either osteomyelitis or cellulitis, increased vascularity will be seen. Routinely, delayed images are obtained in several projections at about 2 hours following injection. In either osteomyelitis or cellulitis, focal increased activity may be seen on these images in the region in question. If a second set of delayed images is made at about 5 hours postinjection, the ratio of counts in the region being examined relative to the surrounding normal bone will have increased compared with the ratio at 2 hours in patients with osteomyelitis. In cellulitis, however, one would expect that the ratio of counts would slowly decrease over this time period, as most of the activity within the region is due to the hypervascular characteristics of the soft tissue inflammation. Although ^{67}Ga images may be abnormal in either osteomyelitis or cellulitis, generally, in osteomyelitis, images will show more focal increased activity over the bone, whereas in cellulitis, a less focal, less well defined increase in radioactivity is seen. This approach of combined radionuclide angiography, blood pool imaging, conventional and delayed nuclear bone imaging, and gallium imaging is demonstrated in Figures 17–10 and 17–11.

Gallium imaging has been shown to be extremely accurate in following the response to therapy in chronic osteomyelitis, as well as in indicating the presence of renewed activity of infection. In one study, 14 patients with chronic osteomyelitis were followed over a 2 year period by clinical, radiographic, and bone and gallium scans, which were performed approximately every 6 months.[63] The results indicated that although radiographic findings did not substantially change over the course of therapy, both the bone scan and the gallium scan revealed changes that accurately reflected the response to therapy. When there was poor response or no response, there was little or no change in the scans. Bone scans tended to remain positive for longer periods of time than did the gallium scans, probably because of continued bone remodeling and osteogenesis, even after the infectious process had subsided. The gallium scan, on the other hand, tended to remain positive only as long as an active

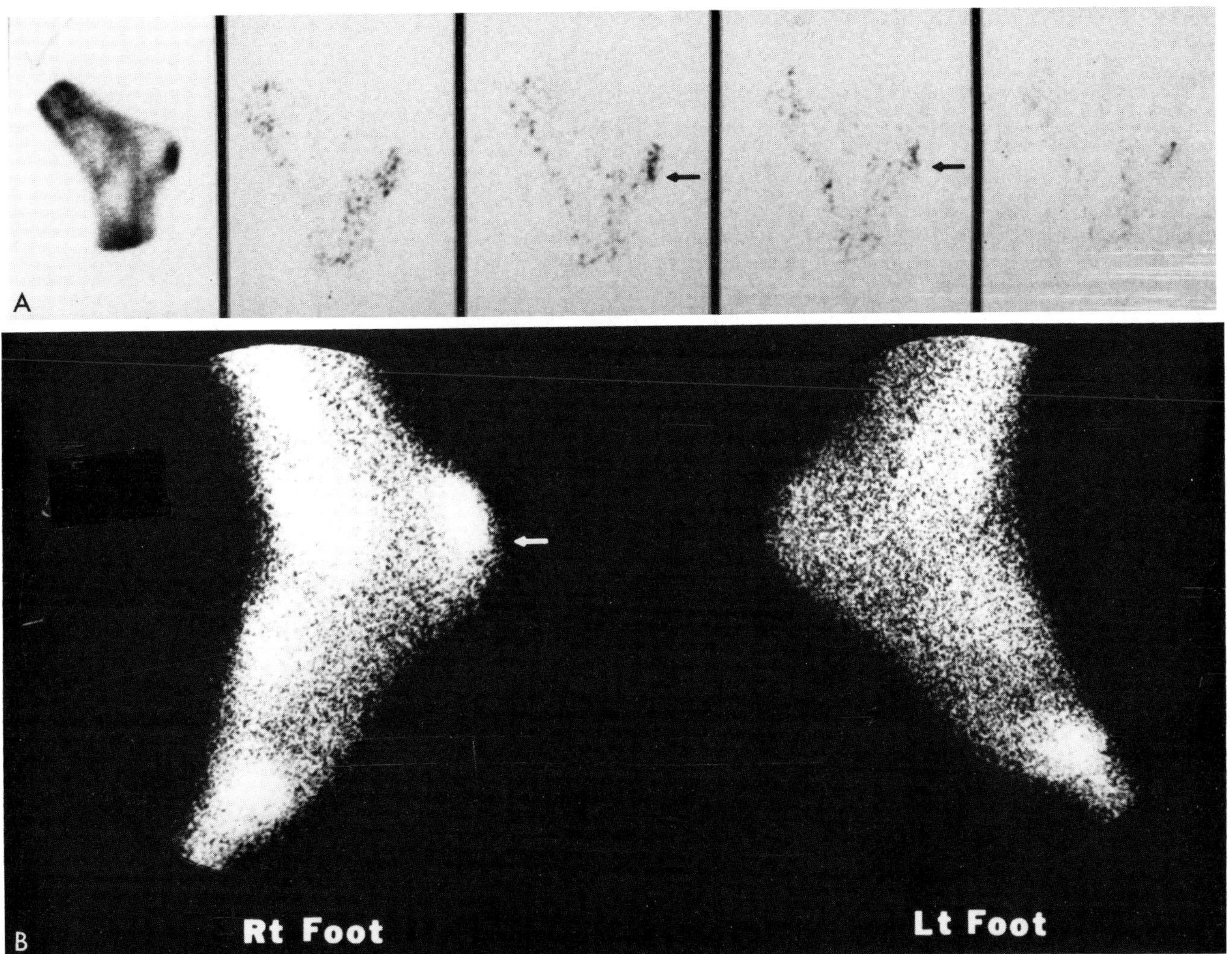

Figure 17–10. *Osteomyelitis versus cellulitis.* **A,** *Radionuclide angiogram of the foot in a patient with a diabetic ulcer of the heel. The sequential 1 second images (right to left) show a focus of increased activity in the region of the calcaneus, indicating hypervascularity to that area, consistent with either osteomyelitis or cellulitis (arrows).* **B,** *Delayed images of the ^{99m}Tc pyrophosphate bone scan of the feet show that the region of the calcaneus continues to be quite hot (arrow) compared with the normal left foot. The degree of increased uptake was interpreted as consistent with osteomyelitis. Note also that the other bones of the involved foot show generalized increased uptake as well, probably reflecting a hypervascular state of the entire inflamed foot.*

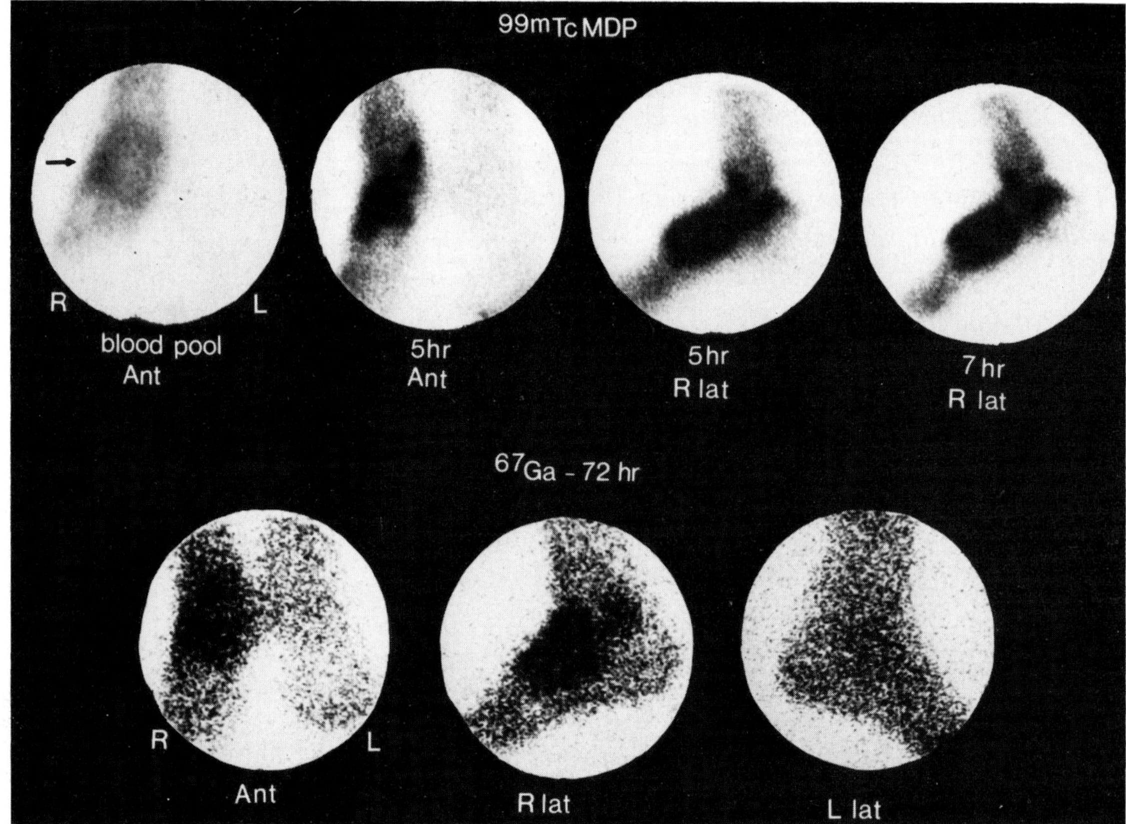

Figure 17–11. *Osteomyelitis versus cellulitis – bone and gallium scans. ^{99m}Tc-MDP immediate blood pool image, delayed ^{99m}Tc-MDP images, and ^{67}Ga scan images of the feet in a diabetic patient are shown. Note that the blood pool image shows markedly increased activity involving the right foot, particularly the region of the tarsal bones (arrow). Delayed images show persistence of increased activity in the region of the tarsal bones, with an increasing ratio of counts in the tarsal bone area relative to other bones at 7 hours. The ^{67}Ga scan confirms a high probability of osteomyelitis involving the tarsal bones because of the markedly increased uptake seen in the abnormal foot relative to the normal left side. Later radiographic studies confirmed the presence of osteomyelitis involving several of the tarsal bones.*

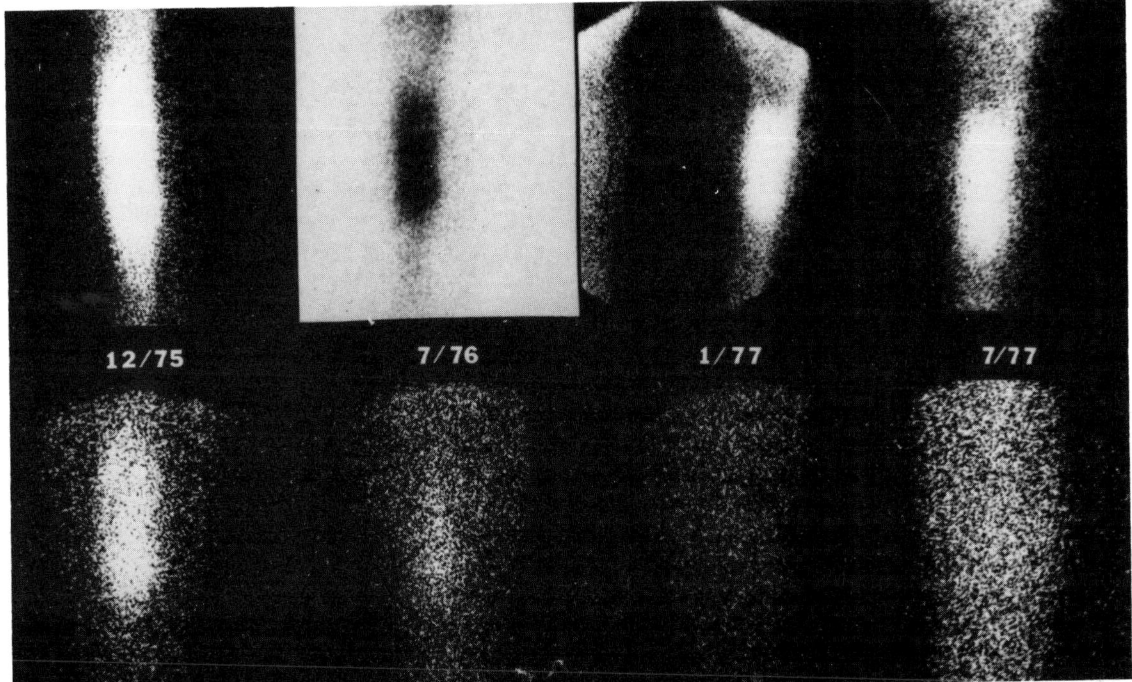

Figure 17–12. *Chronic osteomyelitis—clinical cure. The upper row shows a sequence over a 1 1/2 year period of ^{99m}Tc phosphate bone scans in a patient with chronic osteomyelitis. The bottom row shows the corresponding sequence of gallium scans. Note that the lesion on bone scan appears to improve slightly between 12/75 and 7/77. The gallium scan shows more dramatic resolution of the abnormal focus of activity between 12/75 and 7/76, with a return to normal on 1/77 and 7/77. Clinically, the patient responded well to antibiotic therapy. A possible explanation for the disparity between the results of the gallium and ^{99m}Tc phosphate images in this patient includes a continuing bone remodeling process preventing the ^{99m}Tc phosphate images from returning to normal, and a cure of the acute infectious process reflected by the return of the gallium images to normal.*

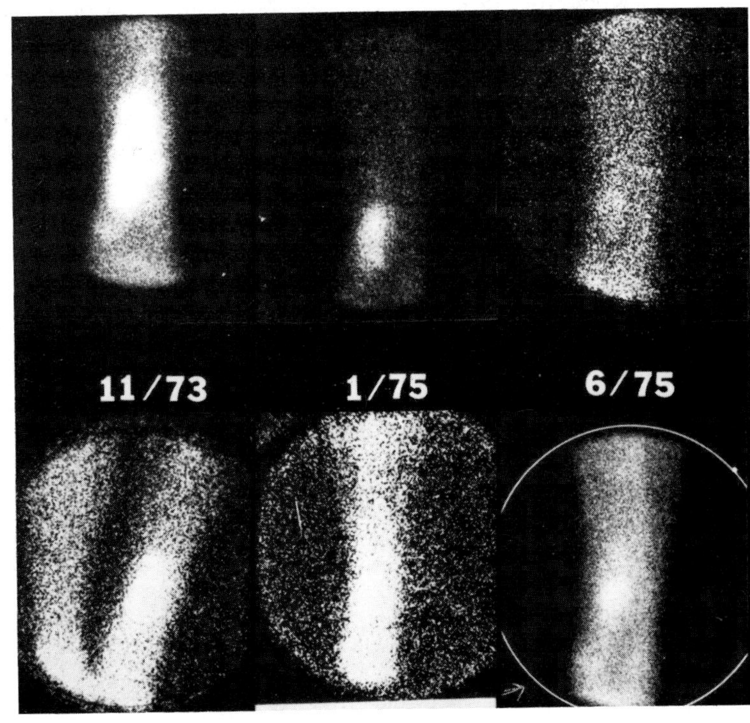

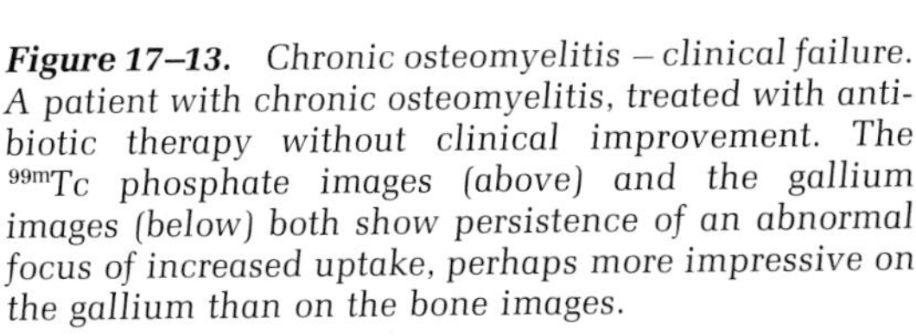

Figure 17–13. *Chronic osteomyelitis – clinical failure. A patient with chronic osteomyelitis, treated with antibiotic therapy without clinical improvement. The ^{99m}Tc phosphate images (above) and the gallium images (below) both show persistence of an abnormal focus of increased uptake, perhaps more impressive on the gallium than on the bone images.*

infectious process continued.[63] Figures 17–12 and 17–13 demonstrate follow-up studies of patients with bone and gallium scans over a 2 year period in cases of clinical cure and failure.

Patients with septic arthritis have also been studied by ^{99m}Tc-MDP and ^{67}Ga imaging. Generally, these patients also manifest positive bone and gallium scans. Lisbona and Rosenthall[64] documented in their series that changing activity of ^{67}Ga uptake paralleled the patient's clincial course more closely than did the ^{99m}Tc-MDP image in septic arthritis.

In acute osteomyelitis, bone and gallium scans have been used to follow the response to therapy and as a potential guide for determining when intravenous antibiotics should be discontinued.[65] Scans improved markedly within the first 2 to 4 weeks of treatment, but abnormalities persisted at 6 weeks in over 50 per cent of cases, despite clinical resolution of disease.

Pain following joint replacement may be caused by loosening of the prosthesis, infection, or both. Evaluation of ^{67}Ga or ^{99m}Tc-phosphate bone imaging for diagnosis of infection or loosening of prostheses has been performed. In one series of 26 patients with hip or knee prostheses who had bone and gallium scans and who underwent subsequent surgery, correlation of the scintigraphic and surgical results revealed a 75 per cent sensitivity for the diagnosis of infection by both gallium and bone scans, with a specificity of 73 per cent.[66] Scan evidence for presence or absence of loosening was in agreement with the surgical findings in 16 patients with loosening and in 2 patients without loosening. The sensitivity for detecting loosening by scan was 100 per cent, whereas the specificity was 40 per cent. The overall results of the radionuclide study in correctly classifying the prosthesis as diseased or nondiseased (loosening with or without infection) was 80 per cent. This study reported a 75 per cent sensitivity and 73 per cent specificity for the scan diagnosis of infection. There were several false-positive scans, many of which had been obtained in patients with rheumatoid arthritis. The radionuclide criteria that were used for the diagnosis of infection were moderate to severe focal increased uptake on both bone and gallium images. The diagnosis of loosening was based upon an abnormal bone scan, which varied in severity from very mild to severe alterations, and a gallium scan that was only mildly abnormal or even normal. Figures 17–14 to 17–16 demonstrate the bone and gallium scan results in patients with painful prostheses. Additional studies[67–71] have reported a high degree of accuracy in correlating implant loosening with scan results, whereas others[66] have reported a somewhat poorer ability of the scans to distinguish infection from loosening. Nonetheless, a

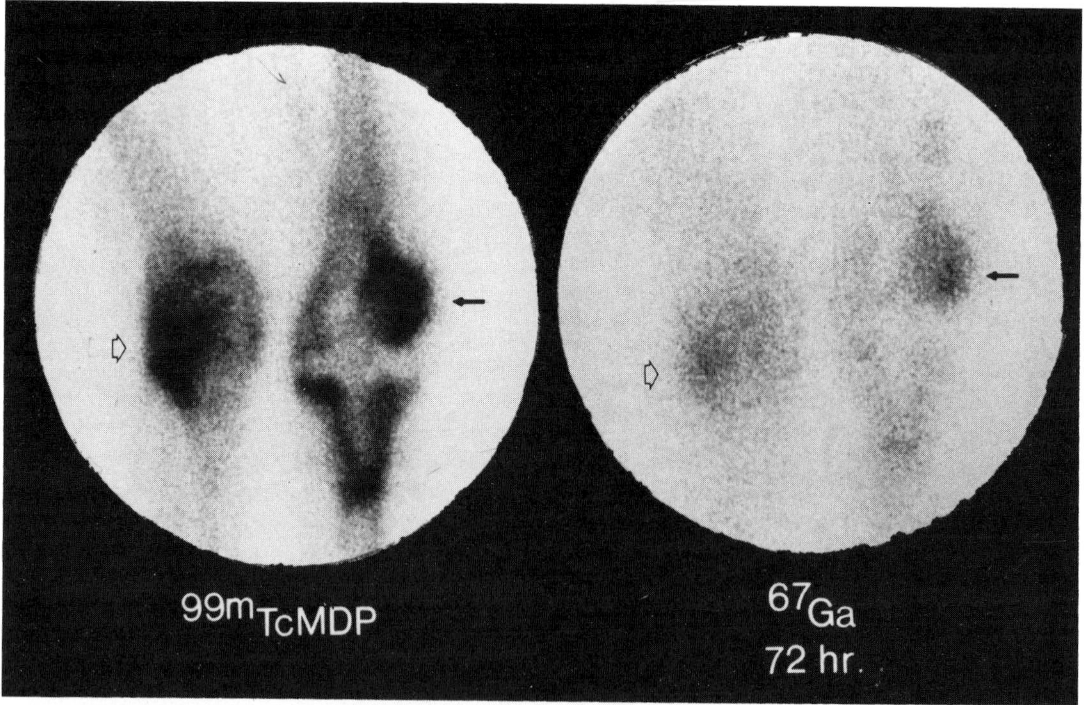

Figure 17–14. *Painful prosthesis – loosening versus infection. The ^{99m}Tc-MDP bone image and ^{67}Ga image of the knees in a patient with underlying rheumatoid arthritis and a painful left knee prosthesis are shown. The ^{99m}Tc MDP study shows increased uptake around the tibial portion of the prosthesis and a focus of increased uptake in the lateral femoral portion, which is matched by marked increased uptake on the gallium image in the same regions (solid arrows). The findings are consistent with osteomyelitis, which was confirmed at surgery. Note that there is increased uptake on bone and gallium images in the opposite knee affected by rheumatoid arthritis (open arrows).*

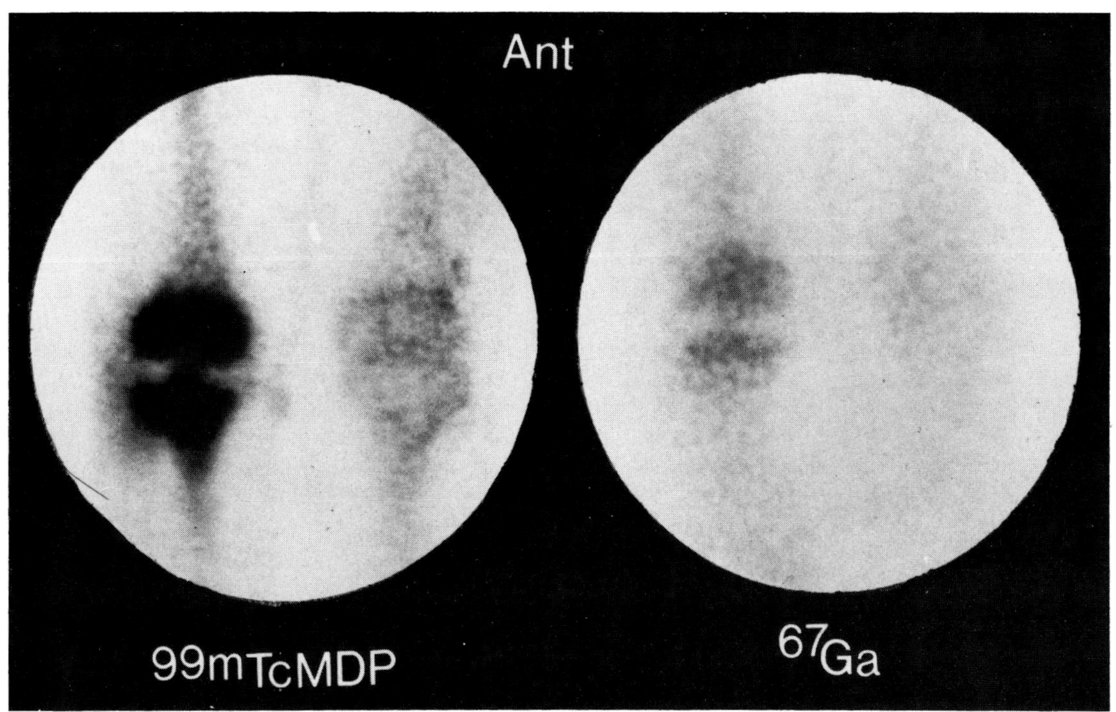

Figure 17–15. Painful prosthesis. Bone and gallium images of the knees in a patient with a painful prosthesis involving the right knee. Both bone and gallium studies show markedly increased uptake about both femoral and tibial components. At surgery, infection was confirmed.

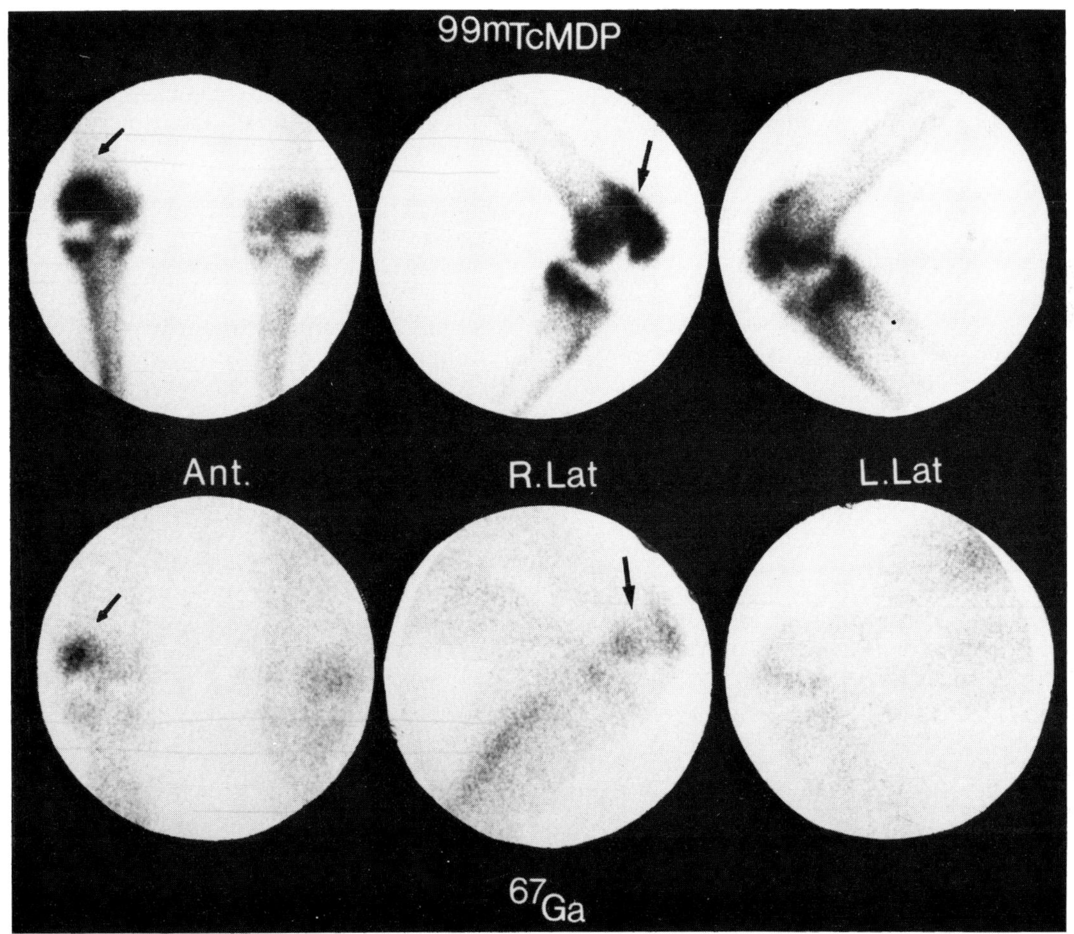

Figure 17–16. Painful prosthesis. Bone and gallium images in a patient with bilateral knee prostheses and a painful right knee. The right knee shows markedly increased uptake in the femoral component on both bone and gallium studies (arrows). At surgery, no infection was found; however, there was abundant granulation tissue and loosening of the prosthesis.

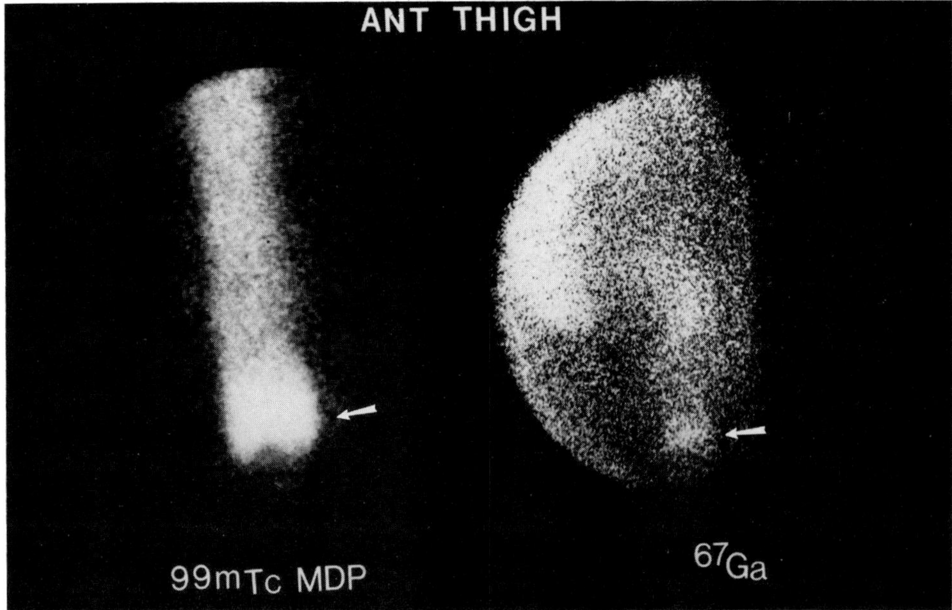

Figure 17–17. *Amputation: evaluation of stump for infection. ^{99m}Tc-MDP bone and ^{67}Ga images of the distal stump of an above-the-knee amputation being evaluated for possible osteomyelitis. Note that there is markedly increased uptake at the distal stump on the ^{99m}Tc MDP image, with a focus of increased uptake on the gallium image (arrows). The patient was treated for osteomyelitis.*

normal bone scan would appear to weigh heavily against the need for surgical intervention for loosening or infection of prostheses.

The radionuclide study can also be used in the assessment of osteomyelitis involving the stump of an amputated limb. Frequently, because of constant irritation to the bone produced by weight-bearing on the prosthesis, the radiograph will show osseous irregularities that make the diagnosis of early osteomyelitis very difficult. Likewise, the bone scan may show increased radionuclide uptake secondary to the continual trauma to the distal stump. However, markedly increased uptake, matched or exceeded by abnormal activity on a gallium image, should alert the physician to a high probability of osteomyelitis (Fig. 17–17).

TRAUMA

Conventional radiography has proved to be an extremely sensitive tool for detecting fractures and for following the healing response. However, some fractures are not readily detected by conventional radiography. A good example of such a fracture is the stress fracture. Stress fractures result from repetitive prolonged muscular action on a bone that is unaccustomed to such stress. Fatigue fractures and insufficiency fractures are two types of stress fractures. The fatigue fracture most commonly affects military recruits and athletes who impose repetitive, perhaps abnormal, muscular stress or torque on normal bones. The insufficiency fracture occurs as a result of normal physiologic stresses on abnormal bones having deficient elastic resistance. Conditions that predispose to insufficiency fractures include osteoporosis, osteomalacia, Paget's disease, osteopetrosis, rheumatoid arthritis, fibrous dysplasia, hyperparathyroidism, and irradiation.

The bone scan may be helpful in imaging either fatigue or insufficiency fractures, especially when radiographs are unrevealing. The high degree of sensitivity of the bone scan surpasses that of radiography in detecting stress fractures and other forms of periosteal injury without fracture. Wilcox and coworkers[72] reported an evaluation of bone scintigraphy in 34 patients with physical findings and histories suggestive of stress fracture of the lower extremity. Of the 34 individuals, 21 had abnormal studies, 11 involving the femoral neck, 9 involving the tibia, and 1 involving the femur. All the abnormal radionuclide studies were apparent prior to or at the time of appearance of radiographic changes. Of the 9 with abnormal tibial studies, radiographic changes never evolved in 3. No false-negative results were found among the 13 patients with normal scintigrams. Thus, the bone scan may be an effective screening examination for patients presenting with exercise related pain in the lower extremities[73] (Fig. 17–18).

Studies of the pathophysiology of fracture healing show that repair at the fracture site usually begins within 24 hours after the event. Bone scans may show focal abnormalities, perhaps as early as 24 hours after injury but usually by 3 days.[74] The degree of uptake on the bone scan increases, reaching a maximum at a few months[75] (Fig. 17–19). This phase is then followed by a decrease in uptake, eventually approaching normal levels. Matin[76] reported that 80 per cent of 204 patients with fractures had abnormal bone scans at 24 hours following injury, and 95 per cent had abnormal scans by 72 hours. Several investigators[76–78] have found that fractures can appear abnormal on scans obtained within a few hours of injury, although differences in the scintigraphic time pattern have been noted in older patients when

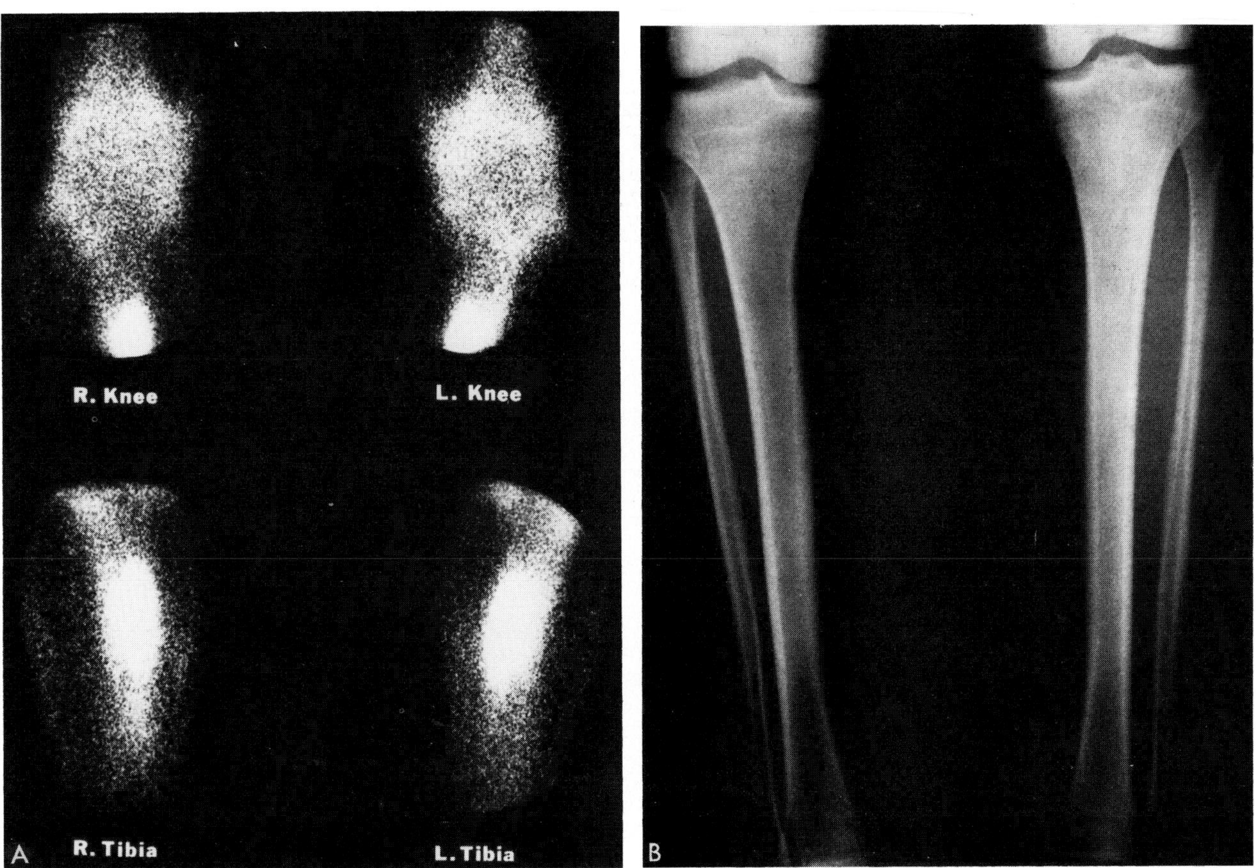

Figure 17–18. *Stress fractures.* **A,** *^{99m}Tc pyrophosphate bone images of both upper legs in a 21 year old military recruit complaining of pain in the shins. Markedly increased uptake is noted over both proximal tibia. The findings are consistent with stress fractures.* **B,** *Radiographs taken at the time of the bone scan were interpreted as completely normal.*

compared with that of persons under 65 years of age. Older patients reveal a lag in the appearance of augmented activity at the fracture site on the scan and in the rapidity with which the scan returns to normal.

Although there is some variability in the time of appearance of fractures on scan, even greater variability exists in the time periods necessary for return of the scan to normal. It is not uncommon to identify abnormal increased focal uptake at a fracture site that is several years old, even as much as 20 years old. Nonetheless, it may be possible to identify the approximate age of a fracture on the scan by the degree of increased uptake. Generally, recent fractures show intense increased uptake, while older fractures show normal or mild increased uptake. Since the radiograph may not be helpful in distinguishing between an acute compression fracture and one that has been present for years (if there are no prior radiographs for comparison), the bone scan may have a medicolegal impact in some cases.

Recent studies have examined the potential contribution of the bone scan in assessing the course of fracture healing and nonunion and in predicting which fractures might respond favorably to percutaneous electrical stimulation.[79, 80] In a study of pa-

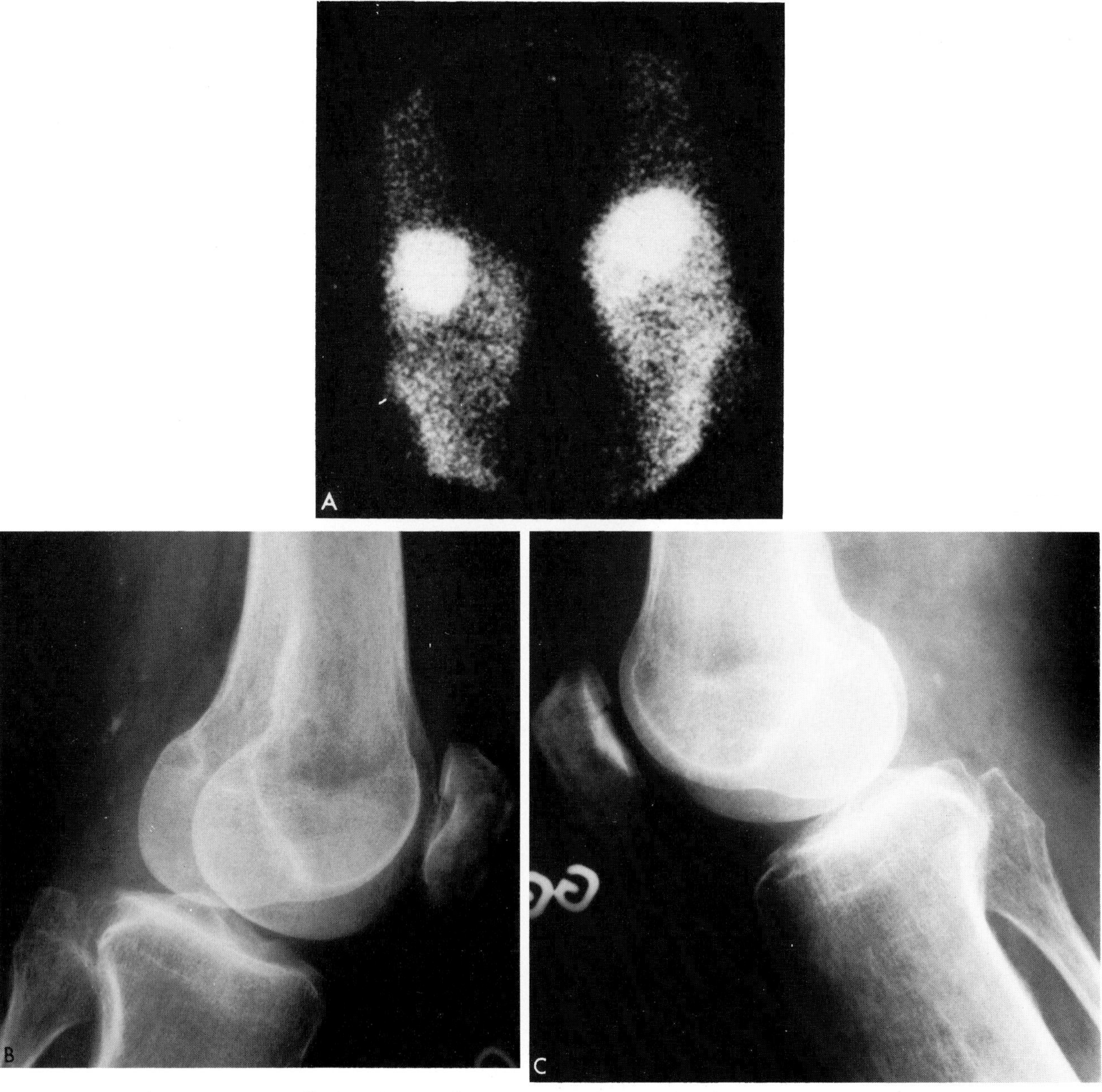

Figure 17–19. *Patella fractures.* **A,** *^{99m}Tc-MDP knee image shows bilateral hot patellae. The differential diagnosis for hot patellae includes chondromalacia, degenerative joint disease, fractures, and other conditions.* **B, C,** *Radiographs confirm the presence of bilateral patellar fractures.*

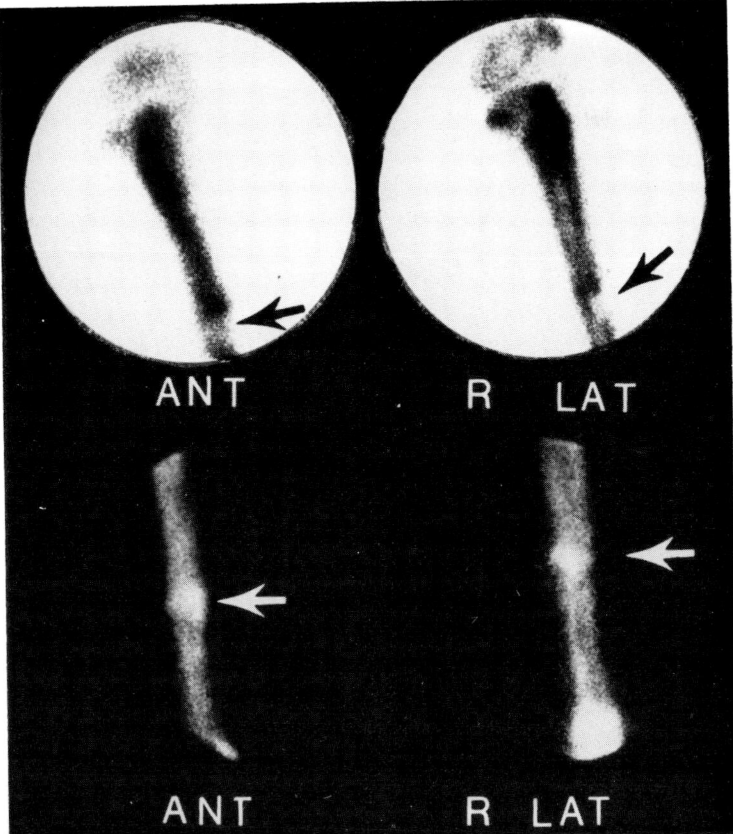

Figure 17–20. *Fracture nonunion. ^{99m}Tc-MDP bone images of a patient with nonunion of a fracture site in the tibia at the time when the upper row of images was obtained (black arrows). Several months later, follow-up ^{99m}Tc-MDP images show activity bridging the gap of the previously photon-deficient fracture site (white arrows). This indicates successful healing.*

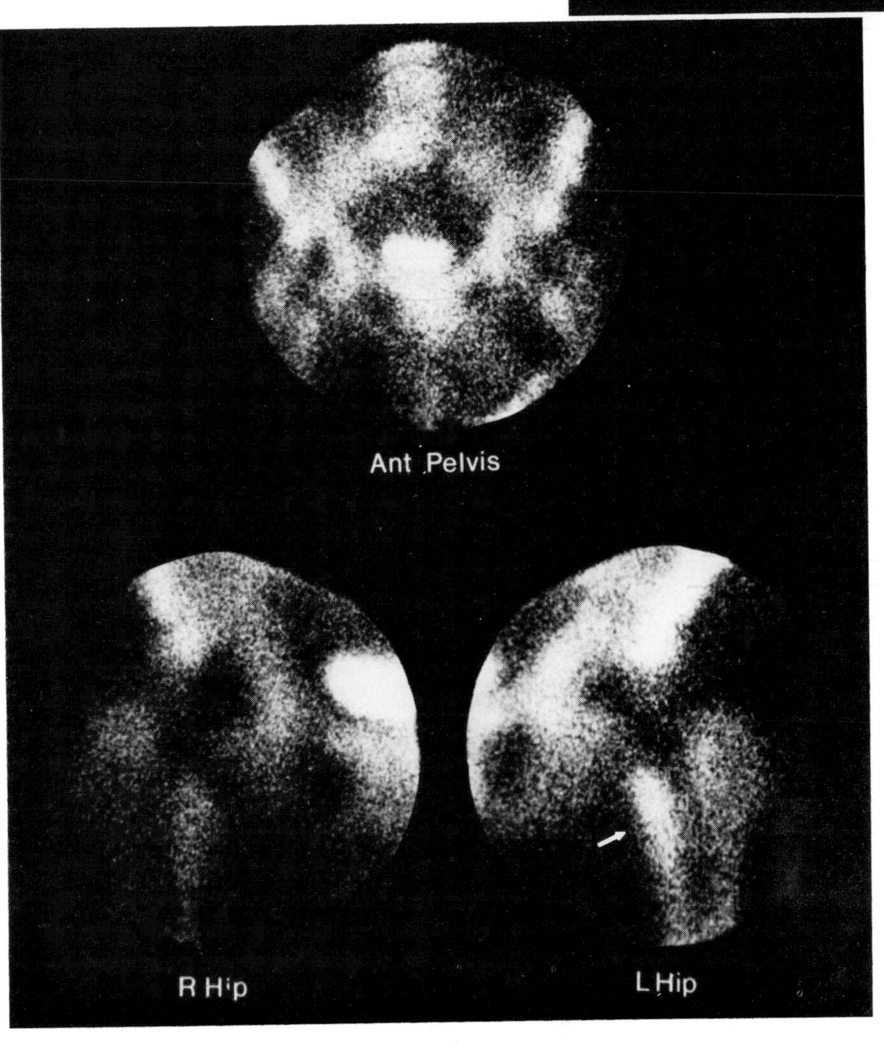

Figure 17–21. *Hip prostheses. ^{99m}Tc pyrophosphate bone images of the pelvis and both hips in a patient with bilateral hip prostheses that had been implanted more than 9 months previously. The right hip is normal and the left hip shows very mildly increased uptake over a medial portion of the femoral part of the prosthesis (arrow). The scan is considered to be normal.*

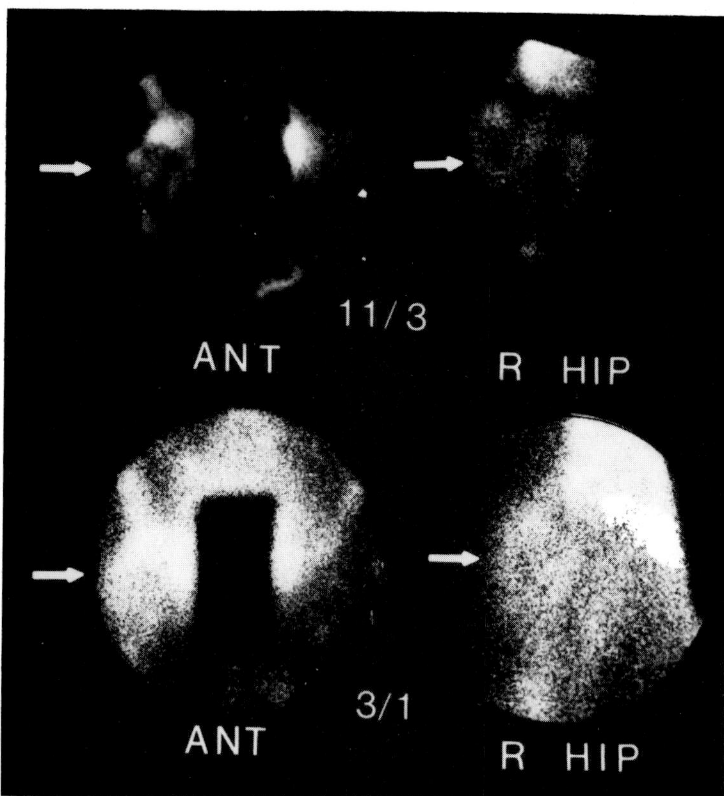

Figure 17–22. Hip prosthesis with heterotopic ossification. ^{99m}Tc pyrophosphate bone images of the pelvis and right hip in a patient with a right hip prosthesis and complicating heterotopic ossification. Uptake of the radiopharmaceutical can be seen extending around the prosthesis into the soft tissues, indicating heterotopic bone formation (arrows).

tients with fibrous union, bone scans showed two patterns of radionuclide concentration: (1) intense activity at the fracture site, which appeared quite homogeneous, and (2) a line of decreased activity (negative defect) at the fracture site surrounded by increased uptake on both sides.[80] Of 66 patients with intense radionuclide activity at the fracture site, 62 showed evidence of a good healing response with electrical stimulation. In nine patients with a negative radionuclide defect at the fracture site, eight did not respond to percutaneous electrical stimulation (Fig. 17–20).

Similarly, persistent radionuclide activity can be noted at sites of surgical trauma. This is not infrequent following craniotomy or prosthetic joint surgery. Typically, within 6 to 9 months following surgery, the bone scan should return to a relatively normal baseline level of uptake around a prosthesis (Fig. 17–21). Not infrequently, heterotopic ossification can appear about a joint prosthesis; radiopharmaceutical uptake in the heterotopic bone must not be mistaken for another process, such as infection or loosening (Fig. 17–22).

METABOLIC BONE DISEASE

A balance between the two continuous processes of cancellous and cortical bone resorption and production is necessary for maintaining normal calcium homeostasis and normal skeletal structural integrity. Specific imbalances in osseous resorption and production exist in many metabolic diseases, imbalances which, if sufficiently severe, become apparent on radionuclide studies. Generally, metabolic diseases affect all parts of the skeleton. However, in some specific entities, particular bones may be affected more than others, and it is the characteristic distribution of disease throughout the skeleton that provides the basis for accurate scintigraphic as well as radiographic diagnosis.

Until recently, the use of nuclear imaging in metabolic bone disease was extremely limited. Gradually, an increasing number of reports have addressed the role of bone imaging and quantitative radionuclide and photon densitometry studies in the evaluation of such disease. The sensitivity of bone scintigraphy in detecting focal abnormalities of bone has been documented in metabolic disorders.[81–83] For example, the insufficiency type of stress fracture (pseudofracture) that may appear in osteomalacia can be identified as a focal area of increased uptake on bone scans even when radiologic surveys are normal, although subsequent coned-down radiographs of areas of abnormalities may confirm the presence of these fractures.[81] Studies have indicated that the appearance of the bone scan in some patients with osteomalacia is sufficiently different from that in normal persons that the presence of a metabolic disorder can be identified. Generally, the mean bone-to–soft tissue uptake ratio of counts in the osteomalacia group has been significantly higher than in the control group. Fogelman and co-workers[81] reported a mean 24 hour ^{99m}Tc-HEDP retention of 41 per cent in osteomalacia patients compared with normal persons, who had a mean retention of about 20 per cent. In osteomalacia, the most consistent subjective abnormality on bone imaging was an increased uptake of tracer in the long bones, the wrists, the calvarium, and the mandible. These findings have also been noted in other metabolic disorders, such as hyperparathyroidism. Increased activity in the costochondral junctions and the appearance of a "tie sternum" have been cited as additional radionuclide characteristics of some metabolic disorders, as have focal regions of increased uptake at sites of pseudofractures and brown tumors in hyerparathyroidism.

The radiograph is a relatively insensitive tool for detecting the presence and the extent of bone disease in patients with primary hyperparathyroidism. Quantitative analysis of the radionuclide distribution has been examined as a means of diagnosing and evaluating the extent of this disease. Measurement of rates of disappearance from blood and urinary excretion of ^{99m}Tc-labeled phosphate were performed in normal individuals and in patients with primary hyperparathyroidism, pseudohypoparathyroidism, and postsurgical untreated hypoparathyroidism.[82] The blood disappearance curves of the labeled phosphate were identical in these three groups. However, significantly increased urinary excretion of labeled tracer was recorded in those individuals with hyperparathyroidism and pseudohypoparathyroidism. The bone scans were abnormal in 58 per cent of the hyperparathyroid patients, with focal abnormalities being evident in the distal extremities, the skull, and the mandible. About half of these patients showed radiographic abnormalities, including subperiosteal resorption and osteopenia. In other studies of patients with primary hyperparathyroidism, investigators have documented increased whole body retention of ^{99m}Tc-labeled phosphate.[83–86] Their findings suggest that monitoring of excretion and retention of labeled phosphate might be a more sensitive means of determining abnormalities that accompany certain metabolic bone diseases than is whole body imaging.

In renal osteodystrophy[85] bone scans usually reveal absence of renal images, reflecting poor renal function. Furthermore, focal abnormalities similar to those that are occasionally seen in scans of patients with primary hyperparathyroidism may be identified. Increased activity has been reported in the ends of the long bones and at the costochondral junctions in as many as 80 per cent of these patients when radiographic abnormalities were identified in only 48 per cent.[85] Quantitative monitoring shows markedly increased 24 hour retention of the labeled phosphate, as well as increased skeletal tracer accumulation relative to that in soft tissue.

In patients with osteomalacia, whole body monitoring also shows an increase in the 24 hour retention of the labeled phosphate. The images demonstrate increased bone-to–soft tissue activity ratios of varying degrees, probably rarely identifiable as a "superscan." The scans may also show focal areas of increased uptake in the axial skeleton, long bones, wrists, costochondral junctions, sternum, calvarium, mandible, and sites of pseudofractures.

Scintigraphic patterns in patients with osteoporosis apparently are quite variable; studies may be normal or reveal areas of increased or decreased radiopharmaceutical localization in bones. Whole body retention of labeled phosphates is usually normal.[84] Disuse bone atrophy results in osteoporosis, which by experimental and clinical studies has been found to be associated with a high rate of bone formation. Scans have shown increased radiopharmaceutical concentration in bones affected by disuse osteoporosis.[87] Increased regional bone blood flow has been postulated to explain the augmented concentration of radiopharmaceutical in bones of paralyzed limbs. However, patients with paraplegia of longer than 9 years' duration may not have increased technetium-phosphate localization in the paralyzed limbs. Radiocalcium balance and kinetic studies in disuse osteoporosis have shown that during the first several years of disuse, bone formation is increased up to twice normal and bone resorption is increased even more; the results of radionuclide studies in patients with long-standing paralysis are consistent with their having decreased osteogenesis as well as decreased bone resorption in the paralyzed limbs.[88]

Other entities that have been evaluated by bone scintigraphy include regional migratory osteoporosis and the reflex sympathetic dystrophy syndrome or Sudeck's atrophy. In regional migratory osteoporosis, focal abnormalities on bone scan may be seen even before roentgenographic changes become evident. In addition, the scan may remain positive even after clinical recovery. One report[89] describing the bone scan in this entity concluded that the diagnosis can be strongly suggested by the correlation of history, laboratory findings, physical examination, radiography, and bone scan, thereby sparing patients multiple invasive procedures, such as biopsy and angiography. In migratory osteoporosis, severe joint pain may be accompanied by scan findings of "migrating" increased periarticular uptake.[90] Increased osseous blood flow to the involved, osteoporotic areas has also been demonstrated by dynamic radionuclide angiographic studies.

PAGET'S DISEASE

In 1877, Sir James Paget described osteitis deformans in a patient whom he had followed for 20 years.[91] As radiography became established, the frequency of Paget's disease became increasingly evident as asymptomatic cases were detected. Autopsy studies show an incidence of Paget's disease of 3 per cent in patients older than 40 years.[92] The disease incidence increases with age and is most prevalent during the seventh decade of life, with men being more frequently affected than women. The pathophysiology of Paget's disease is characterized by increased bone resorption and increased formation of abnormally "soft" new bone that is highly cellular, containing numerous vascular spaces and a disorganized trabecular pattern. The abnormal bone that is produced is subject to deformity from normal weight-bearing. Pain is a common clinical complaint in pagetic patients. Complications include pathologic fracture, secondary degenerative joint disease, and sarcomatous degeneration to osteogenic sarcoma, chondrosarcoma, or fibrosarcoma. These complications occur in fewer than 3 per cent of patients with Paget's disease.[93]

Polyostotic involvement predominates in this disease. The bones that are most often involved include the pelvis, thoracolumbar vertebrae, femur, skull, scapula, tibia, and humerus in approximate order of descending frequency. Bone blood flow and osteogenesis are markedly increased, and therefore the bone scan shows characteristic intense increased activity in the affected areas. The deformity and the enlargement of the bones that are seen on radiographs are equally characteristic on the radionuclide images.

The markedly increased blood flow in affected bones suggests the possibility that arteriovenous fistulas are formed within the osseous tissue as part of the disease process. However, the presence of arteriovenous fistulas has not been documented by histology, arteriography, or radiolabeled microsphere techniques. In patients in whom as much as 35 per cent of the skeleton is involved by Paget's disease, high cardiac outputs have been reported due to the markedly increased blood flow to the affected bones.[94]

Radiographically, Paget's disease may become manifest as lytic or sclerotic foci. During the early osteoporotic or lytic phase, most typically seen in the cranial vault as osteoporosis circumscripta, the bone scan shows markedly increased activity, with greater activity at the advancing margins of the lesion and less increased activity in its central portion[95] (Fig. 17–23). As the disease progresses and the osteolytic and osteoblastic activities become equalized, the radiographs may show a mixed sclerotic and lytic pattern, which may then be followed by a predominantly osteoblastic radiologic appearance. In the later sclerotic phase of the disease, increased osteoblastic and osteoclastic activity may have ceased, and the healed lesions still radiographically apparent may appear normal on the scan. Thus, the bone scan may be useful in determining true activity of the disease process,[96, 97] as the radiograph will remain static in the sclerotic phase. In assessing response of pagetic bone to therapy with calcitonin, diphosphonate, or mithramycin, the bone scan may be particularly helpful, and the changing radionuclide pattern may even be quantitated with computer techniques (Fig. 17–24).

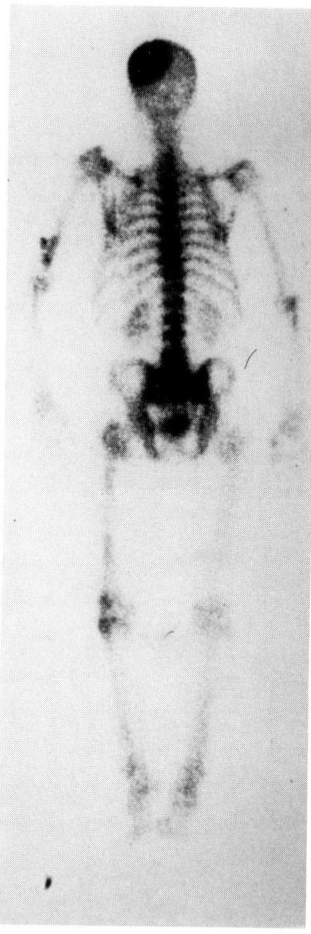

Figure 17–23. *Paget's disease – osteoporosis circumscripta. Total body ^{99m}Tc-MDP bone image in a patient with early Paget's disease involving the skull.*

VASCULAR DISEASE

The diagnosis and prognosis of aseptic necrosis of bone are major clinical problems that have not yet been well enough characterized by any available diagnostic technique to accurately guide clinical management. Interruption of blood supply to a bone may result from many pathologic processes, including trauma, hematologic problems, vasculitis, metabolic disorders, fat embolization, and corticosteroid therapy. Radiographically, detection of aseptic necrosis is very difficult, since the affected bone has a degree of radiodensity that is similar to that of normal bone. A true increase in the bone radiodensity follows, owing to compression of dead bone and

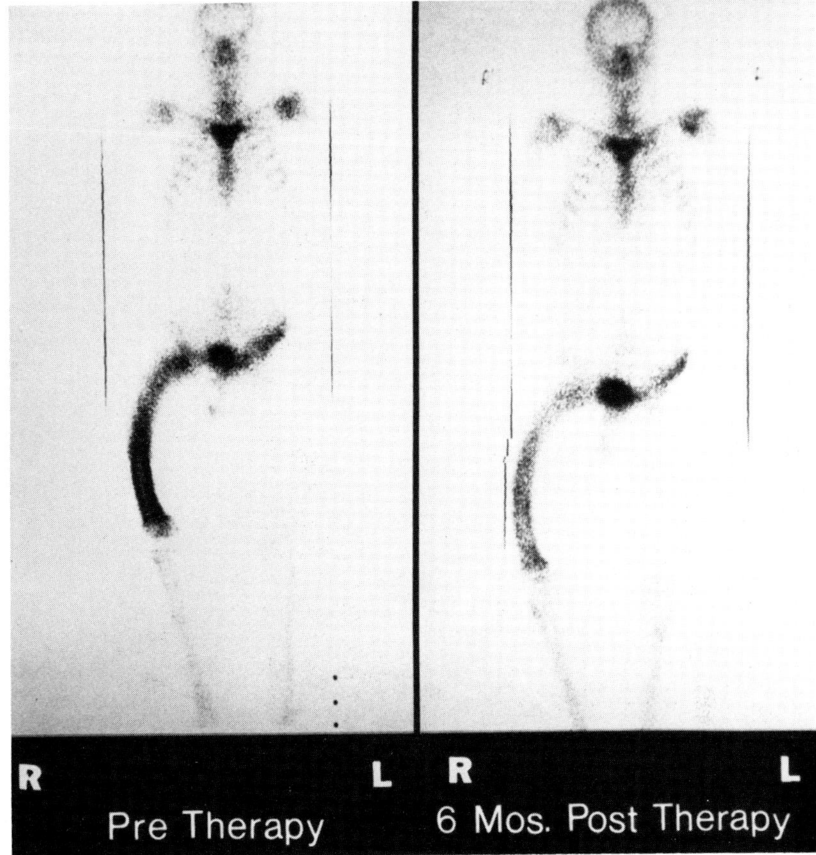

Figure 17–24. *Paget's disease – response to therapy. Two anterior view total body bone images performed 6 months apart following calcitonin therapy in a patient with Paget's disease. The images show a typical pagetic femoral deformity with markedly increased uptake and apparent enlargement and bowing of the osseous structure. Following therapy, the degree of increased uptake in the pagetic bone is greatly lessened.*

revascularization with an accompanying production of new bone. These changes, however, may not become radiographically apparent for several weeks or even months following the acute process. Initially, on the bone scan, if there has been a substantial interruption of blood supply, the radiopharmaceutical cannot reach the involved area and there may be decreased activity on the scan. As the bone reacts to the insult and attempts to repair the damage with revascularization and reossification, scintigraphy may show increased activity in the involved area. Later, secondary degenerative joint disease may appear, with a concomitant increase in radionuclide uptake about the joint.[98]

Thus, foci of aseptic necrosis of bone may appear on scintillation images as areas of either decreased or increased radiopharmaceutical uptake. Presumably, as the radionuclide pattern changes between these two states, there may be a period in which normal uptake is evident. It is therefore important to obtain high resolution images of the affected regions. Either converging or pinhole collimation will be helpful in the recognition of focal "cold" defects, especially if adjacent reactive changes with increased radiopharmaceutical uptake are already present. Figure 17–25 demonstrates the findings of increased uptake about a recent femoral neck fracture, accompanied by aseptic necrosis of the femoral head, which has resulted in a "cold" area on the image. The pinhole collimator markedly improves the interpreter's ability to identify the two distinct abnormalities.

Orthopedic surgeons who deal with problems of aseptic necrosis, particularly of the femoral heads, need to consider at an early disease stage, before radiographic flattening of the femoral head is evident, whether or not a total hip replacement is necessary. If aseptic necrosis of the femoral head has resulted in nonviable bone that has lost its ability to recover, it may be advisable to perform a femoral head replacement prior to the development of secondary degenerative changes of the hip. However, if the affected femoral head will revascularize and recover, a total hip arthroplasty may not be required. Although attempts to use the bone scan as a prognostic indicator in this clinical setting have not yet met with definitive success, bone marrow imaging may be useful in predicting the viability of bone in patients with aseptic necrosis.[99] In general, absence of radiocolloid uptake in the femoral neck on the bone marrow scan indicates vascular impairment, whereas presence of radiocolloid uptake indicates an intact vascular supply through the femoral neck marrow space.

In patients with sickle cell anemia, both bone and bone marrow imaging may be helpful in the diagnosis of infarction, revealing focal regions of decreased activity in acute bone infarcts.[100] With healing, the bone scan converts from a pattern of

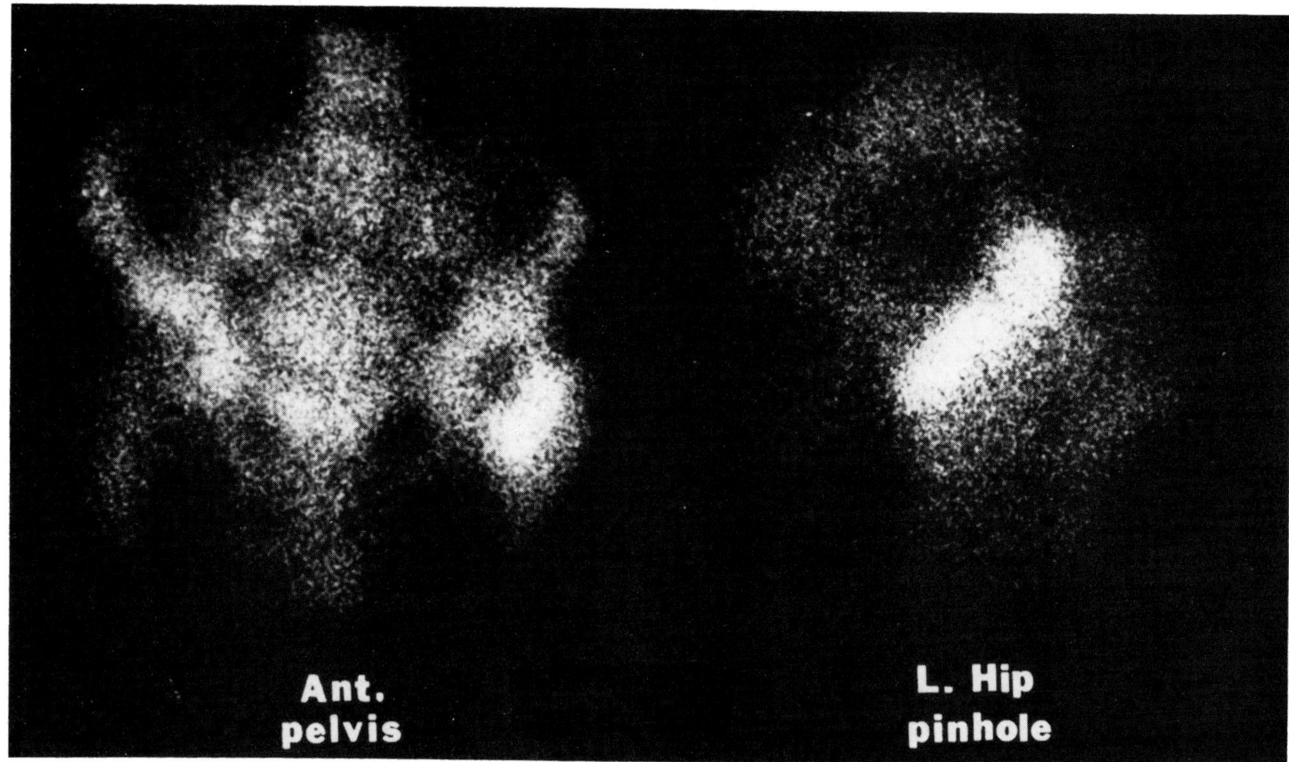

Figure 17–25. *Aseptic necrosis.* ^{99m}*Tc pyrophosphate bone images of the pelvis and left hip with pinhole collimator view in a patient with an acute fracture through the femoral neck and secondary aseptic necrosis of the left femoral head. The pinhole view shows that the femoral head is cold and that the linear fracture through the femoral neck is hot.*

decreased focal activity to one of increased focal activity in the affected region, whereas the bone marrow scan may show the return of reticuloendothelial radiocolloid concentration in the affected area.[101] However, differentiation between bone infarction and osteomyelitis in patients with sickle cell anemia who present with pain is difficult to obtain even with the use of bone, bone marrow, and gallium imaging. Although increased activity of gallium occurs in regions of osteomyelitis, this agent may also accumulate in regions of infarction. Likewise, there is an overlap of findings that are detected by bone marrow scan and bone scan in osteomyelitis and infarction. However, a bone marrow scan using ^{99m}Tc-labeled sulfur colloid may show abnormal regions of decreased uptake in osteomyelitis, whereas in septic arthritis, the bone marrow scan may remain normal. Thus, in the differentiation between osteomyelitis and septic arthritis, the bone marrow scan may be helpful.[102]

In the evaluation of Legg-Calvé-Perthes disease, the bone scan has been cited for its superior sensitivity compared with radiography. The necrosis of the femoral capital epiphyses that affects children 4 to 8 years of age, more frequently boys, is believed to be of vascular etiology. Characteristically, early in the course of this disease, radionuclide imaging shows a focal region of decreased radiopharmaceutical uptake in the anterolateral aspect of the proximal femoral epiphysis, although the entire epiphysis may be involved in some cases. Revascularization and healing are subsequently demonstrated on the scan as areas of increased activity in the femoral head and adjacent femoral neck.[103] In clinical practice, the problem of differentiation between Legg-Calvé-Perthes disease and synovitis or arthritis may arise. In the latter situation, the scan shows increased periarticular activity but no epiphyseal defect. In addition, the gallium scan may be helpful in the diagnosis of septic arthritis. The prognosis in Legg-Calvé-Perthes disease has been related to the degree of epiphyseal involvement.[104] A more accurate assessment of the extent of epiphyseal involvement can be obtained if pinhole imaging techniques are used to optimize the image details of small areas within hips of pediatric patients (Fig. 17–26).

Radiographically, it may be difficult at times to distinguish between bone infarcts and benign bone lesions such as enchondroma. The bone scan may be helpful since dynamic imaging with sequential exposures made at the time of injection of the radiopharamaceutical can characterize the degree of vascularity of the lesion. A bone infarct would be expected to show decreased vascularity, while an enchondroma or other benign lesion would most likely show some degree of vascularity.

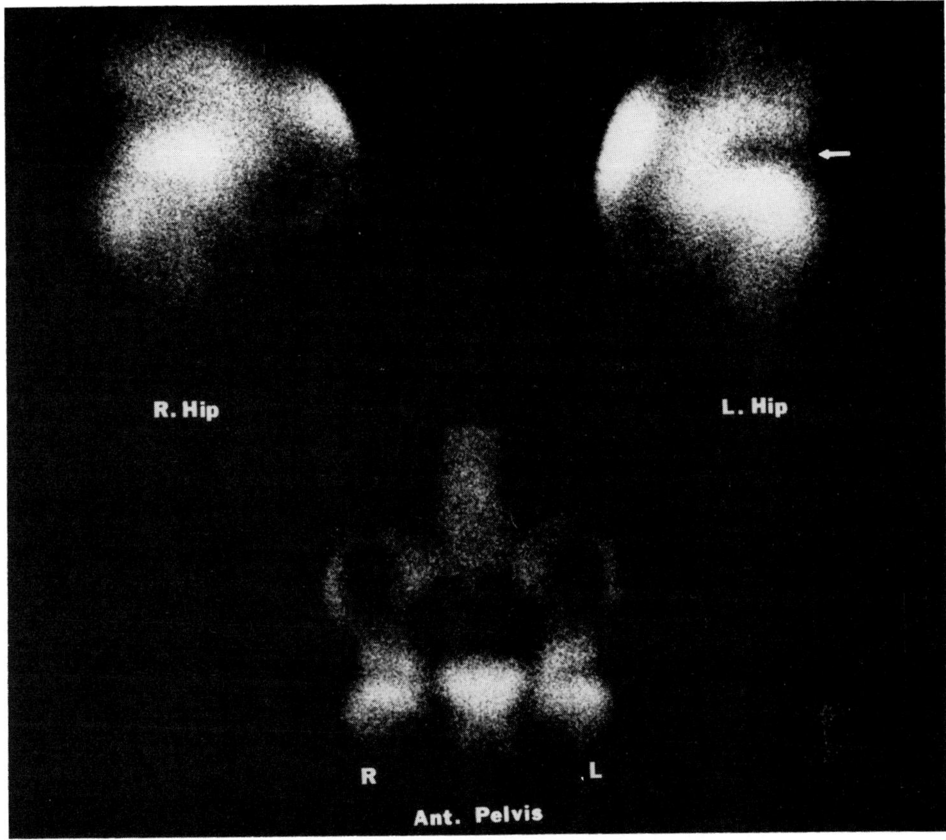

Figure 17–26. *Legg-Calvé-Perthes disease. ^{99m}Tc pyrophosphate bone images in a 6 year old child with a diagnosis of Legg-Calvé-Perthes disease. The left hip view shows a larger area of decreased counts in the region of the femoral growth plate (arrow), consistent with the diagnosis of Legg-Calvé-Perthes disease. The finding could easily be missed on the anterior pelvis view, but is seen on the pinhole collimator view.*

ARTICULAR DISEASE

The first radionuclide joint images were performed in 1965 with ^{131}I-labeled albumin,[105] with the rationale that joints involved in inflammatory disease would show increased tracer accumulation due to increased synovial blood flow and abnormal synovial capillary permeability. Iodine-131–labeled albumin, an intravascular label, therefore, seemed to be the appropriate agent. In 1967, technetium-99m pertechnetate, which localizes in the blood pool and the extracellular fluid compartments, was used for joint imaging.[106] These joint images were far superior to the ^{131}I-labeled albumin images because of the preferred physical characteristics of ^{99m}Tc for imaging with the scintillation camera or scanner compared to the 365 keV gamma emission of ^{131}I. Soon after the introduction of ^{99m}Tc-labeled phosphate compounds for bone imaging in 1971,[8] these agents were applied to joint imaging as well.[107] Since diseases affecting the joints also stimulate osteogenesis in the periarticular bone, it was thought that joints affected by arthritis would have abnormal uptake of the phosphate-labeled agents in the adjacent bone. Furthermore, there is an increase in synovial vascularity secondary to the joint disease, which also causes increased vascularity in the adjacent bone. The result on imaging, therefore, is focally increased tracer accumulation in the periarticular osseous structures. Comparisons of the ^{99m}Tc-labeled phosphate images with ^{99m}Tc pertechnetate images have indicated that the phosphate-labeled compounds are far more sensitive in detecting abnormal joints than the pertechnetate.[108]

In the presence of a joint effusion with increased synovial capillary permeability, these agents diffuse across the synovial membrane into the effusion. These tracers may also bind to proteins within the joint capsule or in the joint fluid. Additionally, with ^{99m}Tc-labeled phosphate compounds, the same principles that govern its uptake within bone also apply to its accumulation in articular diseases, i.e., chemical and physical processes resulting in adsorption onto hydroxyapatite crystals at bone surfaces, with close correlation to bone blood flow and bone surface–to-volume ratios. In the epiphyseal and metaphyseal bone, there is typically a higher bone surface–to-volume ratio and higher local blood flow than in other areas of bone.[109] In degenerative arthritis, destruction of articular cartilage also results in abnormal stress on the bone adjacent to the chondral surface. Thus, remodeling and sclerosis of bone occur and are accompanied by increased blood supply to the region.

In most institutions, ^{99m}Tc-labeled phosphate compounds for joint imaging are used in doses similar to those used for bone imaging, i.e., 15 to 20 mCi, with scintigraphy performed approximately 2 hours after the intravenous injection of the material. The patient is encouraged to drink fluids so as to optimize the renal excretion of the tracer from the blood background. Generally, a total body image will be obtained in anterior and posterior projections unless the examination is limited to specific joints. Alternatively, in a joint survey, scintillation camera images with a converging collimator may be used to evaluate each individual joint, accumulating approximately 250,000 counts per image for peripheral joints. If a whole body scan is performed, spot images utilizing the converging or pinhole collimator for abnormal joints may be performed selectively. For careful evaluation of any one joint, frontal and lateral views should be obtained, particularly in the knees, since increased activity related to the overlying patella and patellofemoral compartment may be misinterpreted as lateral femorotibial compartment disease on a frontal view. For the hips, anterior and posterior views are important and are performed routinely. In children, frog-leg and straight anteroposterior views of the hips may be helpful.

Normal Joints. Normal joints show symmetric activity, although the shoulder joint on the side of dominant handedness occasionally shows more activity than that in the opposite shoulder. Greatest activity is normally seen in the periarticular regions, with predictable variations in the degree of activity for different joints. For example, in the hand, activity around joints is normally greatest in the wrist and in the metacarpophalangeal joints, with uniform diminishing activity, which progresses from the first to the fifth digit. For each individual digit, the activity is greatest in the proximal joints and diminishes distally. The degree of activity in epiphyseal regions in children is much greater than the activity seen in periarticular structures in adults. For example, around the knee joint in an adult, the degree of increased activity is proportional to the mass of bony structures, e.g., the medial femoral condyle has slightly more activity than the lateral femoral condyle, and the normal degree of periarticular activity is only minimally elevated compared with that in other bony structures.

Degenerative Joint Disease. In the evaluation of osteoarthritis of the knee, Thomas and coworkers[110] demonstrated a practical application for radionuclide joint imaging in guiding the orthopedic surgeon in deciding on the necessity of surgery and in selecting a surgical approach. Fifty-six osteoarthritic knees in 52 men and 1 woman being considered for surgery were evaluated by history, physical examination, assessment of knee function, radiography with and without weight-bearing, double-contrast arthrography, and ^{99m}Tc polyphosphate bone imaging. All modalities were correlated finally with direct inspection by either arthroscopy or surgery. The radionuclide joint imaging correlated more closely than any of the other modalities with direct inspection. The results of the bone scan indicated the extent and the severity of the joint disease and affected the choice of surgery. High tibial valgus osteotomy is generally more successful in patients with varus deformity in whom the lateral femorotibial compartment has been preserved; if there is lateral compartmental disease, a high tibial valgus osteotomy will probably be unsuccessful, leaving unicompartmental replacement of the involved medial femorotibial compartment or total knee replacement as the surgical alternatives. On the basis of clinical examination and radiography with and without weight-bearing, 28 knees in this series had absent or mild lateral femorotibial compartmental disease. The radionuclide images in 15 knees and the arthrogram in 5 knees detected a higher level of disease in the lateral femorotibial compartment than was otherwise suspected. The radionuclide study confirmed absence of lateral tibial and femoral disease in 10 of the 28 cases and presence of mild disease in 3 cases. The surgical management plan was altered because of the detection of moderate lateral compartment abnormalties in 7 of the 28 patients. Long-term evaluation of these patients will be needed to establish the validity of this approach (Fig. 17–27).

Rheumatoid Arthritis and "Rheumatoid Variant" Diseases. Documentation of the sensitivity of the bone scan in detecting and estimating the extent of joint involvement in patients with rheumatoid arthritis or a "rheumatoid variant" disease such as psoriatic arthritis, ankylosing spondylitis, and Reiter's syndrome has been reported in several studies.[111–114] The bone scan is considered the most sensitive imaging indicator of active disease in these arthritides. The pattern of abnormal radionuclide activity in rheumatoid arthritis consisting of symmetric peripheral joint abnormalities may be distinguishable from that in the rheumatoid variant diseases, which tend to have more central skeletal involvement and asymmetric peripheral joint abnormalities. However, compared with the radiograph, the bone scan is less specific in its ability to distinguish among the clinical entities. Nonetheless, the scintigraphic abnormalties often appear before radiographic or clinical abnormalities. The bone scan shows greatest sensitivity in detecting abnormalities in the smaller peripheral joints. For the shoulder, hip, and knee joints, the incidence of clinical abnormality is equal to or slightly greater than the incidence of focal increased activity on the bone scan. In the axial skeleton of patients with rheumatoid arthritis, the results are less conclusive. Abnormalities of the sacroiliac joints as measured by increased radionuclide activity are found to be more common than abnormalities noted by clinical and radiographic examinations. Other studies using computer profiles of the distribution of radioactivity on images of the sacroiliac joints have also indicated

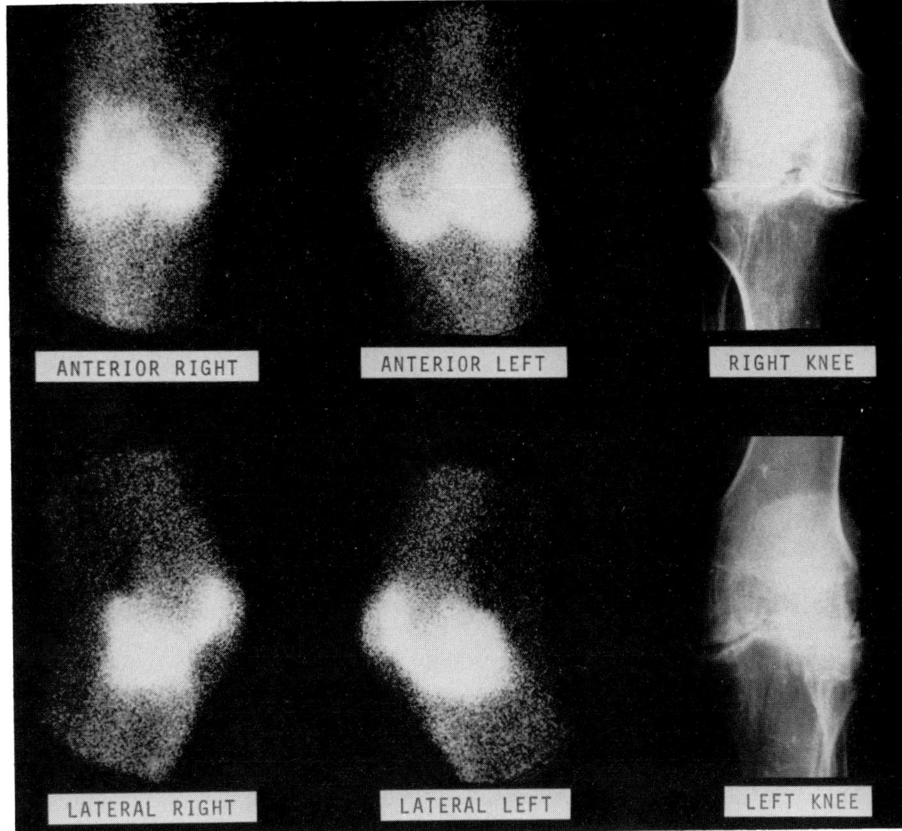

Figure 17–27. *Degenerative knee disease.* ^{99m}*Tc polyphosphate bone images of the knees in a patient with severe osteoarthritis showing marked tricompartment abnormalities on both sides.*

more frequent detection of increased activity than could be correlated with clinical or radiographic abnormalities.[114] These findings have supported a broad variation in the normal degree of radiopharmaceutical uptake in the sacroiliac joints. On radionuclide images of the spine, it may be difficult to distinguish between active and inactive disease and the presence or absence of coincident disorders, such as degenerative disease.

Studies of quantitative images of the sacroiliac joints using computer-generated ratios of activity over the sacroiliac regions compared with that in the central portion of the sacrum, or profile curves of the changes in uptake across the sacroiliac region, have suggested that separate ratios should be obtained for each sacroiliac joint and, perhaps, for the superior, middle, and inferior regions of each joint as well.[113, 114] This would indicate that disease can be so localized within the sacroiliac joint as to affect only one articulation or only one region of the articulation. The application of quantitative sacroiliac joint radionuclide examination may prove to be useful in following the course of patients with ankylosing spondylitis, sacroiliitis of psoriatic arthritis, or Reiter's syndrome, and in many HLA-B27 positive individuals without back pain or radiographic evidence of sacroiliac disease. Lentle and associates[113] observed an association between sacroiliitis and increased sacroiliac-to-sacrum count ratios in patients who were suspected clinically of having ankylosing spondylitis or Reiter's syndrome and who had the histocompatibility antigen B27. They also detected scan evidence of sacroiliitis in patients with psoriasis, uveitis, and Crohn's disease, some of whom had normal radiographs.

Weissberg and colleagues[112] reported that 23 joints of 640 joints examined in patients with rheumatoid variant disorders were noted to have radiographic changes of osteoarthritis, and 21 of those manifested no increased activity by bone scan. In addition, 10 of 14 patients with rheumatoid arthritis who had degenerative changes in the spine had normal radionuclide uptake in the spine on scan. Several reports have shown that patients with classic ankylosing spondylitis in whom there was ankylosis of sacroiliac joints on radiography showed normal or slightly decreased radionuclide activity in the sacroiliac joints on scintigraphy. This probably reflected the inactivity of disease at the time of the scan.[112–114, 116] Thus, it would appear that the radionuclide examination may offer a means of differentiating inflammatory from degenerative joint alterations and active from "burned-out" disease. Correlation of the radionuclide study with the radiograph is necessary for fuller understanding of the disease processes that are present.

In patients with rheumatoid arthritis, the characteristic pattern that is seen on bone scan consists of symmetric involvement of joints.[115] In the knees, there is usually symmetric medial and lateral femorotibial compartmental uptake with or without increased radionuclide accumulation in the patellofemoral compartment. In a few patients with classic rheumatoid arthritis, asymmetric involvement has been seen. This finding, which is more frequent in the initial stages of the disease, possibly reflects the localized distribution of stress forces and remodeling that can be seen very early in the inflammatory process. A pattern consisting of a dense band of increased activity at the epiphyseal-metaphyseal area about the small joints of the hands and the feet, which is often seen normally in young patients, has been noted in older patients with rheumatoid arthritis.

Follow-up bone scans in patients being treated for rheumatoid arthritis do not always correlate with the clinical course of the disease. Some investigators have noted that joints may actually show increased radionuclide activity in the face of clinical improvement. Nonetheless, the bone scan is considered to be an extremely sensitive indicator of activity in rheumatoid arthritis and rheumatoid variant diseases. Weissberg and associates[112] reported on a comparison between nuclear imaging utilizing ^{99m}Tc pyrophosphate and clinical or radiologic evaluation in over 1000 joints of patients with various articular disorders, especially arthritis. The results indicated agreement between the scan and the radiograph in 67 per cent of examined joints. Abnormal scan activity was seen in 20 per cent of the joints that had no radiographic abnormalities, whereas 13 per cent of the joints examined showed radiographic abnormality in the absence of bone scan abnormality (Figs. 17–28 to 17–34).

In addition to the arthritides that were discussed previously, the bone scan and the gallium scan are positive in septic arthritis (Fig. 17–35).

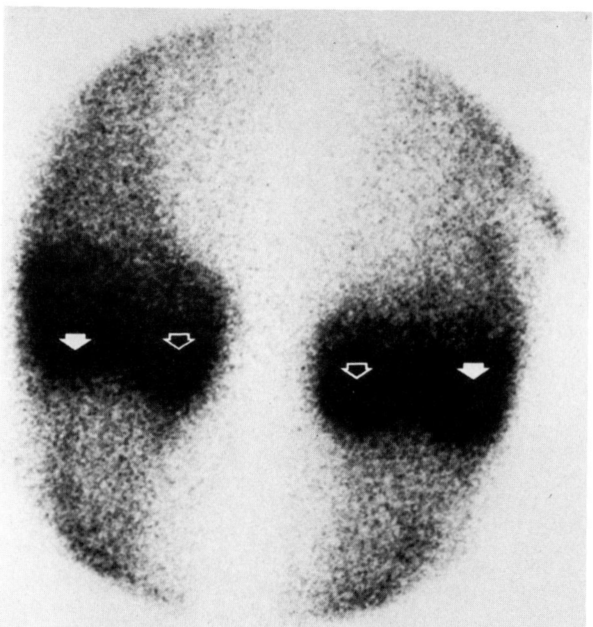

Figure 17–29. *Rheumatoid arthritis. Radionuclide bone images of both knees in a patient with rheumatoid arthritis. Images show symmetric distribution of abnormal activity in all femorotibial compartments, medially (open arrows) and laterally (solid arrows). (From Weissberg DL, et al: Am J Roentgenol 131:665, 1978. Copyright 1978, American Roentgen Ray Society.)*

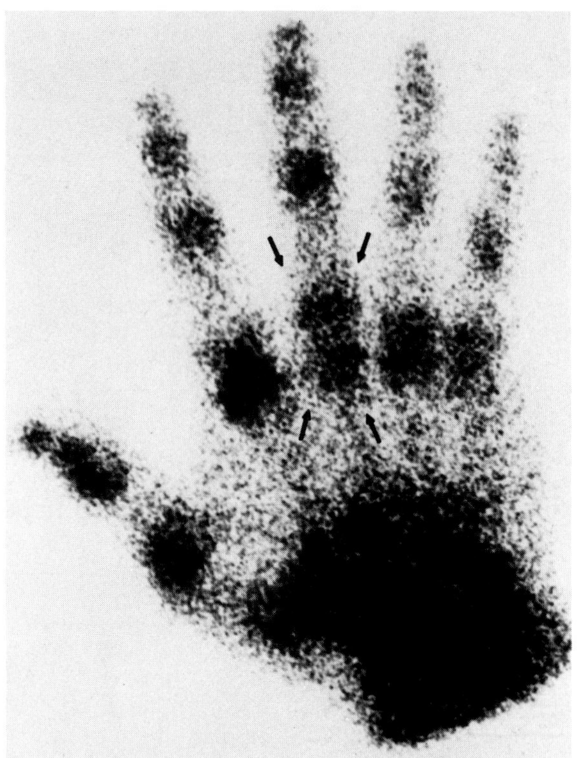

Figure 17–28. *Rheumatoid arthritis. Right hand image from a ^{99m}Tc pyrophosphate bone study in a patient with rheumatoid arthritis. Bands of activity at epiphyseal-metaphyseal areas (arrows) may normally be seen in young patients. In middle-aged individuals, they are abnormal. Multiple joints of the hand and wrist are involved in this patient. (From Weissberg DL, et al: Am J Roentgenol 131:665, 1978. Copyright 1978, American Roentgen Ray Society.)*

DISEASES OF SOFT TISSUE

A multitude of soft tissue lesions have been reported to concentrate bone-seeking radiopharmaceuticals[117–125] (Figs. 17–36 and 17–37). In identifying a cause for uptake of these agents by soft tissue, it is important to correlate the scan with a radiograph of the affected region, since soft tissue calcification or heterotopic ossification may be evident. However, even in the absence of any soft tissue densities on the roentgenogram, the presence of microscopic foci of calcification or heterotopic bone formation below the limits of resolution of the radiograph cannot be excluded. Bone- and calcium-forming tumors such as osteosarcoma, neuroblastoma, and colonic carcinoma metastases, myositis ossificans,

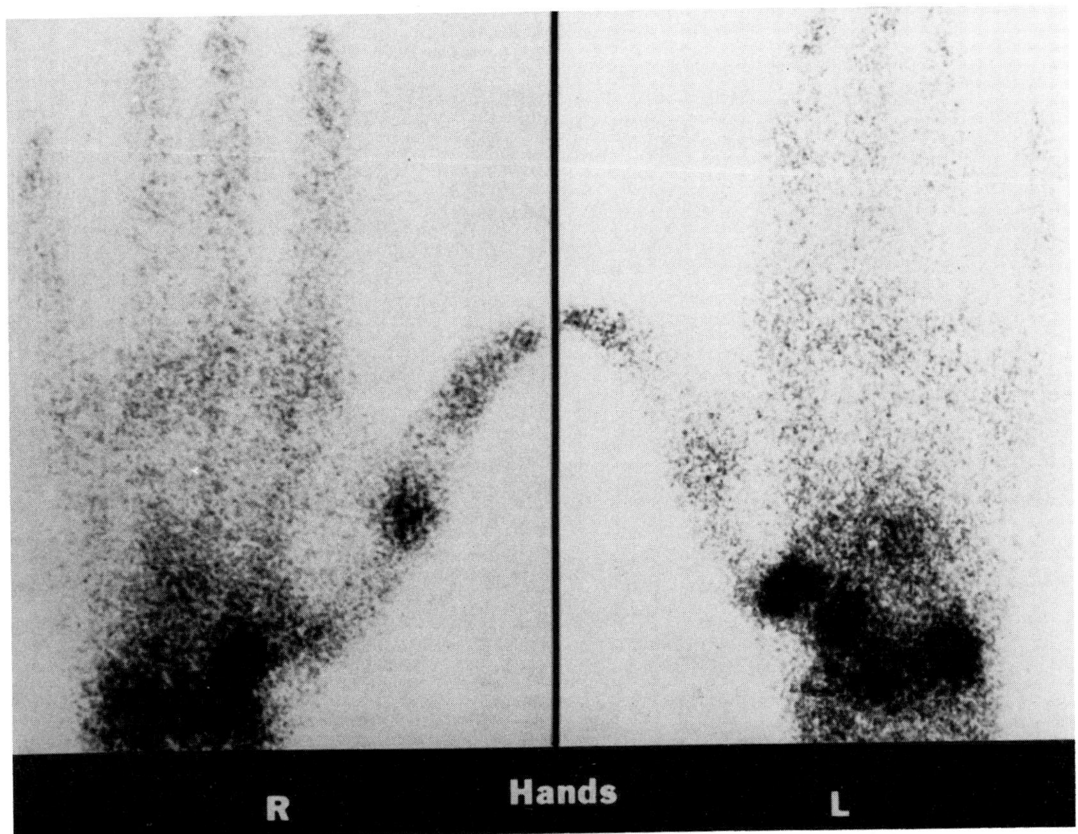

Figure 17–30. Rheumatoid arthritis. Images of both hands in a patient with very early rheumatoid arthritis and normal radiographs. Abnormalities are identified in both wrists and the metacarpophalangeal joint of the right thumb.

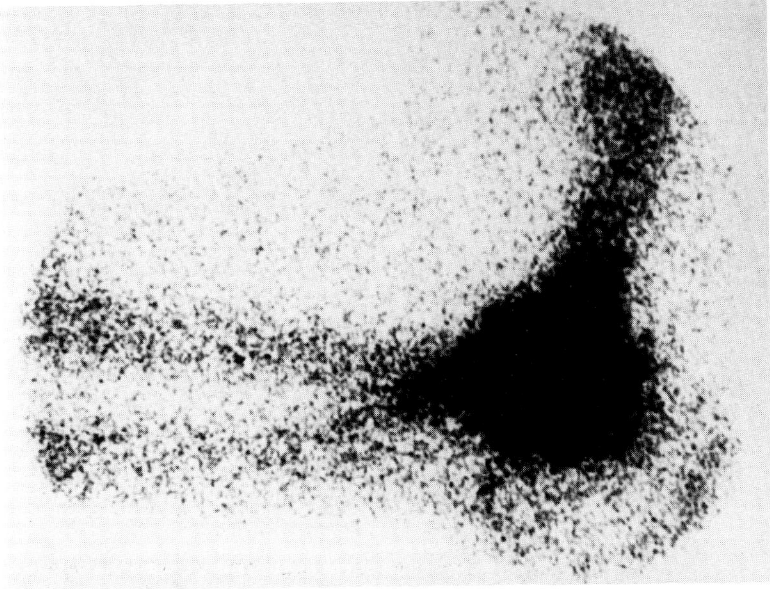

Figure 17–31. Rheumatoid arthritis. The right elbow of a patient with rheumatoid arthritis and with effusion of this joint. Increased activity in the joint and surrounding soft tissue confirms the presence of active disease.

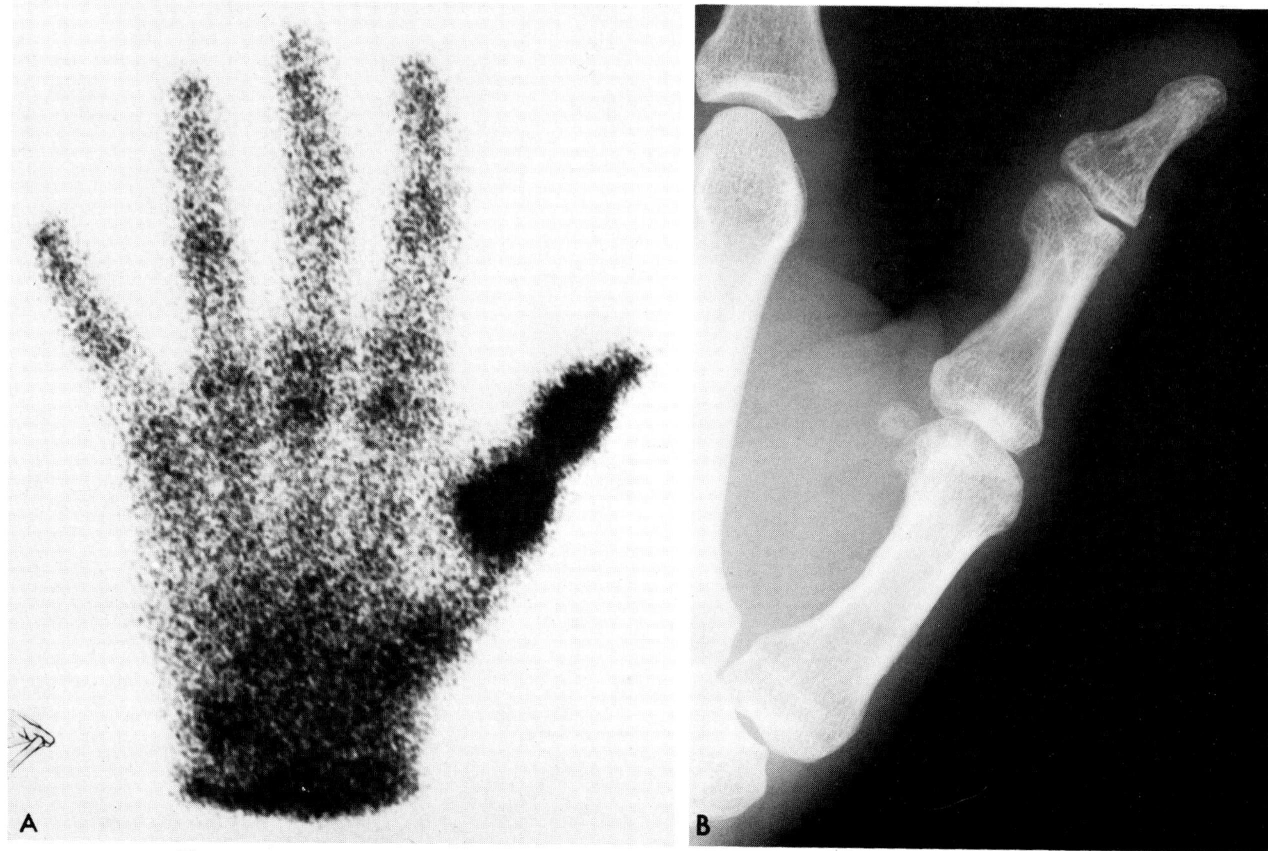

Figure 17–32. *Psoriatic arthritis.* **A,** *Radionuclide bone image shows foci of increased uptake in the interphalangeal and metacarpophalangeal joints of the thumb. Other joints are normal.* **B,** *Radiograph shows only minimal periarticular soft tissue swelling. Later radiographic and clinical abnormalities developed in these joints. (From Weissberg DL, et al: Am J Roentgenol 131:665, 1978. Copyright 1978, American Roentgen Ray Society.)*

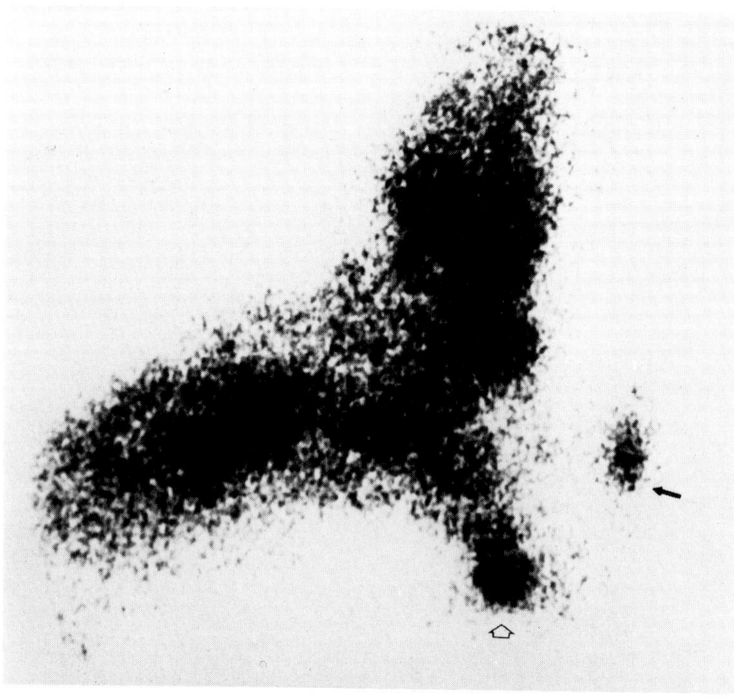

Figure 17–33. *Ankylosing spondylitis. Left foot and ankle on a* ^{99m}*Tc pyrophosphate bone study in a patient with ankylosing spondylitis. The focus at the inferior aspect of the calcaneus (open arrow) corresponds to a site of small cortical erosion and bone production seen on the radiograph, whereas the focus of increased activity in the superoposterior aspect of the calcaneus (solid arrow) corresponds to inflammatory changes in the retrocalcaneal bursa.*

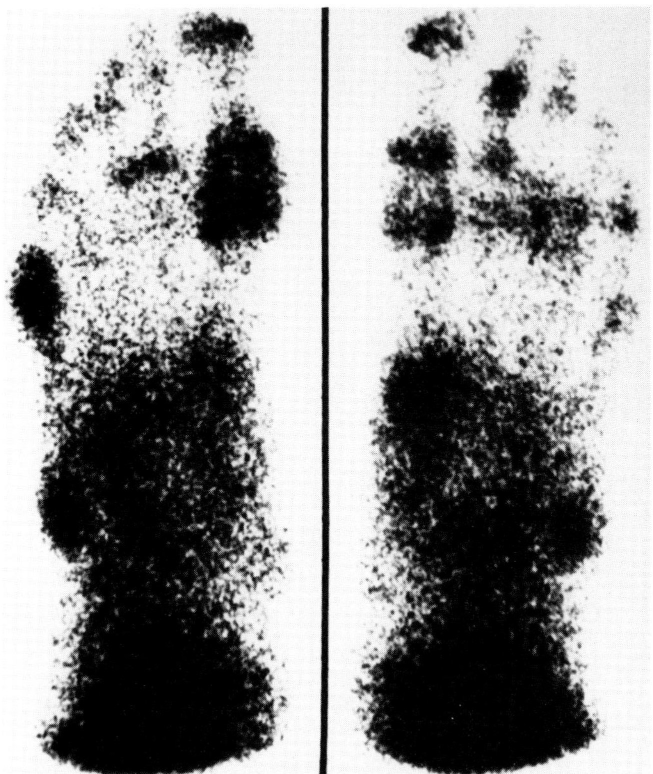

Figure 17–34. *Psoriatic arthritis. Images of both feet from a ^{99m}Tc pyrophosphate bone study in a patient with psoriatic arthritis. Note the asymmetric involvement of distal joints.*

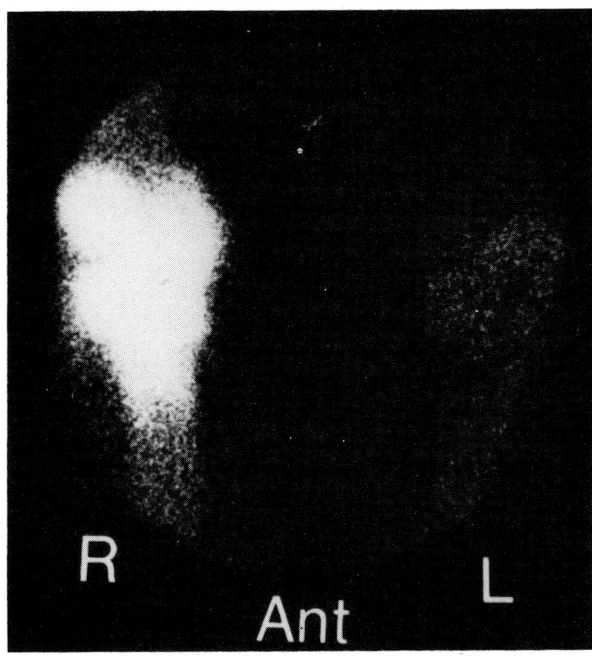

Figure 17–35. *Septic arthritis. ^{99m}Tc pyrophosphate knee images in a patient with septic arthritis involving the right knee.*

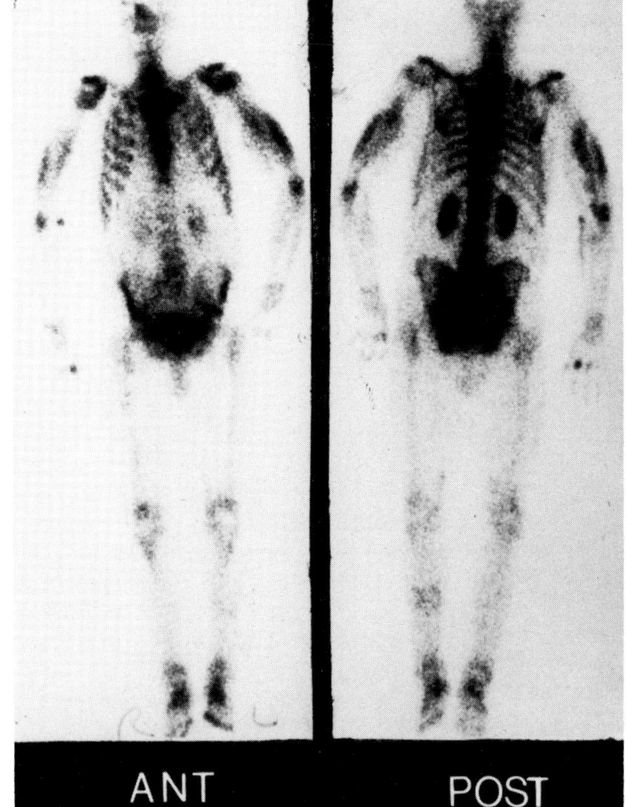

Figure 17–36. *Soft tissue disease. Anterior and posterior ^{99m}Tc pyrophosphate bone images in a patient with an inflammatory polymyositis. The bone-seeking radiopharmaceutical has accumulated in the skeletal muscles, particularly in the upper arms.*

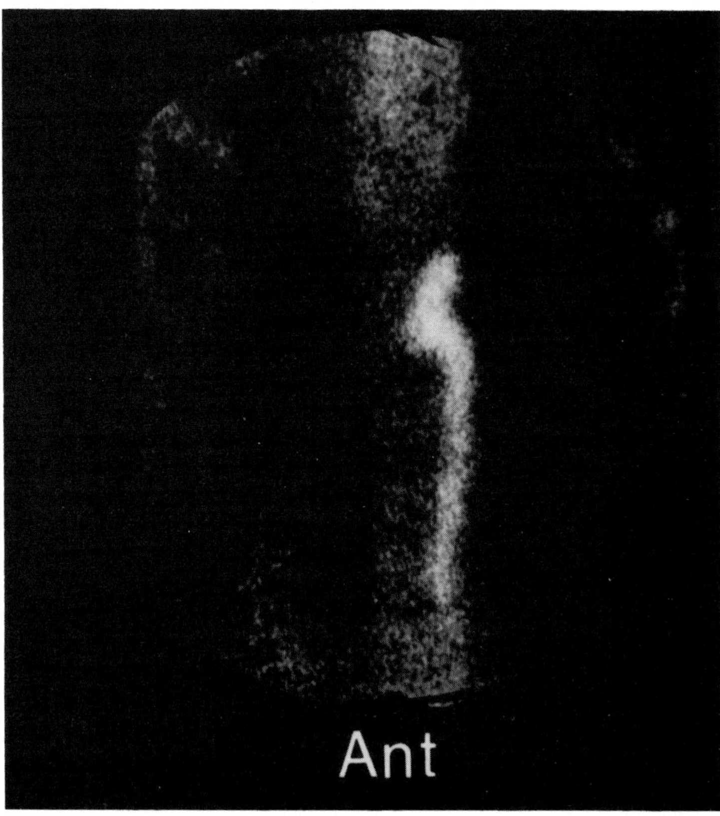

Figure 17–37. Soft tissue scar. Scintillation camera image shows increased uptake in a linear pattern over the abdomen in a patient 2 weeks following abdominal surgery. The uptake corresponds to the patient's abdominal scar.

dermatomyositis, diffuse interstitial pulmonary calcification associated with hyperparathyroidism or mitral stenosis, metastatic soft tissue calcification, and cardiac valvular calcifications are all examples of lesions with foci of calcification or ossification that may be positive on bone scans. In addition, certain lesions that do not typically show calcification may concentrate the bone-seeking radiopharmaceuticals, including various benign or malignant soft tissue tumors, myocardial and cerebral infarction, pyogenic and fungal soft tissue infections, noninfectious inflammatory diseases of the heart and skeletal muscle, amyloidosis, healing soft tissue wounds, intramuscular injection sites, and normal and diseased breast tissue.[123]

The factors that determine the localization of the ^{99m}Tc-labeled phosphate compounds in noncalcified or ossified soft tissue tumors are not well understood. Increased vascularity, altered capillary permeability or cellular calcium metabolism, presence of immature collagen, and atypical binding of the ^{99m}Tc-phosphate compound to phosphatase enzymes are among the factors that have been considered in attempts to explain the localization of the bone-seeking radiopharmaceuticals in the soft tissue lesions.[31, 124] In the cases in which calcification or ossification is present in the soft tissue lesion, the mechanism of ^{99m}Tc-phosphate compound uptake is presumed to be adsorption to the calcific focus similar to the adsorption of ^{99m}Tc-phosphate compound that occurs onto the hydroxyapatite crystal in normal bone. In fact, the composition of the pathologic calcifications in many of these lesions has been shown to be similar to that of calcium deposits found in normal bone on x-ray diffraction studies.

In cases of damaged muscle, e.g., myocardial infarcts, inflammatory myopathies, or ischemic injuries of skeletal muscle, the mechanism for concentration of the ^{99m}Tc-phosphate compounds is thought to be related to the abnormal movement of calcium from plasma into the damaged muscle cell. These compounds are able to move into the damaged cells through abnormally permeable sarcolemma and then to adsorb onto the intracellular calcium deposits.[124] Utilization of ^{99m}Tc-phosphate compounds for imaging acute myocardial infarcts has become common in clinical practice and is quite sensitive for detecting myocardial infarction between 24 hours and 7 days following the acute injury.[126] Prior to 24 hours and later than 7 days after the infarct, the sensitivity of concentration of the ^{99m}Tc-phosphate compounds within the infarcted myocardial muscle falls off precipitously, for reasons that are not well understood.

Paraosteoarthropathy, or ectopic ossification associated with neuromuscular disorders, develops in approximately 20 to 30 per cent of patients following spinal cord injury, and in some series in as many as 50 per cent of such patients.[127, 128] It is also associated with other forms of paraplegia and quadriplegia;

since it may lead to joint ankylosis, it is a serious complication. The etiology of such ossification is not known. Ectopic ossification associated with spinal cord injury most often begins 4 to 10 weeks following the injury and progresses for approximately 6 to 14 months, with the eventual formation of hard, bony masses that may be palpable in the soft tissues. Radiographs are often normal in the early stages, or may show soft tissue swelling within the first 3 weeks. By 2 or 3 months, bone may become apparent, after which a trabecular pattern may become evident. By 12 to 18 months, the mass of new bone becomes stable radiographically. The bone scan in these patients is commonly abnormal before radiographic changes are evident, and it shows an early increase in accumulation of ^{99m}Tc-phosphate in the involved region.[129, 130] Furthermore, bone and bone marrow scanning is effective in assessing the maturity of the ectopic bone. If surgical resection is planned to relieve flexion-extension deformity or limitation of motion, it is advisable to be certain that the ectopic bone has matured at the time of surgical intervention, since the likelihood of recurrence will then be minimized. Other laboratory tests, such as the measurement of serum alkaline phosphatase or urinary hydroxyproline excretion, have not been reliable predictors of the maturity of the ectopic bone. Serial bone scans show that the activity within the ectopic bone tends to decline, reaching a plateau level as the ossification reaches maturity. Bone marrow scanning utilizing ^{99m}Tc-labeled sulfur colloid, which is trapped in the reticuloendothelial cells of the marrow, reveals uptake in the ectopic bone only when bone marrow has been formed. Thus, the presence of

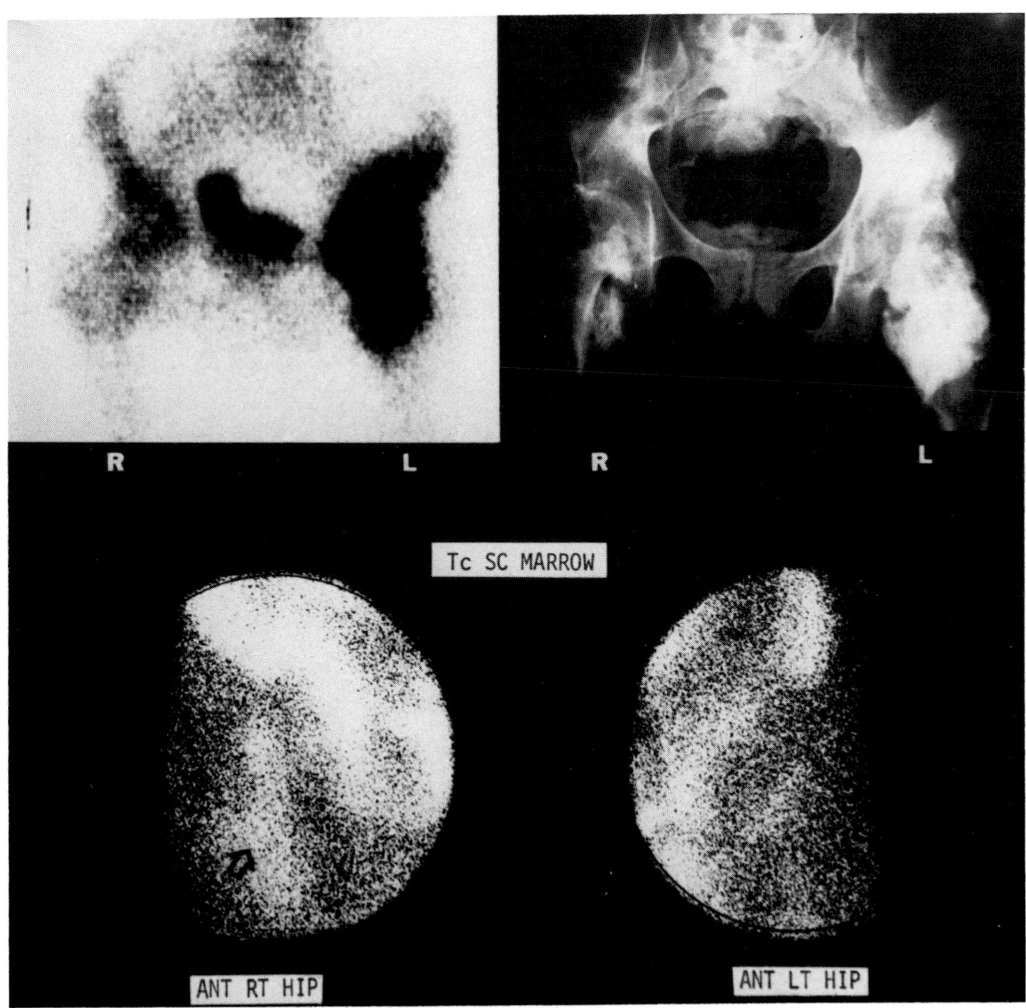

Figure 17–38. Heterotopic ossification. Radionuclide bone image and x-ray (above) in a patient with spinal cord injury and heterotopic bone formation surrounding both hip joints. ^{99m}Tc sulfur colloid bone marrow images (below) show uptake of radiopharmaceutical in the region of the heterotopic bone (arrow), particularly in the right hip. This indicates the presence of bone marrow formation in the maturing heterotopic bone.

bone marrow activity is another indicator of the maturity of the ectopic bone (Fig. 17–38).

IRRADIATION INJURY

Following irradiation, the bone scan usually shows decreased osseous uptake of the radiopharmaceutical relative to the level of uptake in the bone outside the therapy port. Occasionally, very shortly after radiation therapy, the bone scan will show increased uptake. These radionuclide changes can be explained by available histologic data. Initially, there is an increase in the remodeling of cortical bone, which peaks between 3 and 6 months following irradiation. Changes in bone vascularity accompany the bone remodeling,[131] and there is increased regional skeletal blood flow, presumably because of an inflammatory response to radiation. Subsequently the hypermia subsides, as does the increased tracer accumulation. Microvascular injury affecting the osteoblasts adds to a reduction in new bone formation, resulting in eventual decreased uptake on the bone scan. Since irradiation of normal bone is associated with extensive changes on the bone scan, the use of the radionuclide study to monitor the therapeutic response of a bone lesion to radiation therapy is questionable.

SUMMARY

During approximately 20 years of experience with bone scanning, we have witnessed broad expansions in the clinical impact of radionuclide imaging on disorders of bones, joints, and soft tissues. This increased impact had its groundwork laid by advances in radiopharmaceuticals and instruments that are utilized for bone imaging. The progression from strontium-85 to technetium-99m–labeled phosphate compounds, coupled with the advance from crude rectilinear scanning techniques to whole body scintillation imaging with large crystal cameras and sophisticated electronics, has encouraged utilization of radionuclide modalities in the evaluation of musculoskeletal diseases. Many clinical studies have documented the high degree of sensitivity of the bone scan compared with that of the radiograph in detecting osseous and articular abnormalities.

REFERENCES

1. Schmorl G, Junghanns H: The Human Spine in Health and Disease. 2nd American Ed. New York, Grune & Stratton, 1971, pp. 2, 158.
2. Fleming WH, McIlraith JD, King ER: Photoscanning of bone lesions utilizing strontium-85. Radiology *77*:635, 1961.
3. Charkes ND, Sklaroff DM: Early diagnosis of metastatic bone cancer by photoscanning with strontium-85. J Nucl Med *5*:168, 1964.
4. DeNardo GL, Volpe JA: Detection of bone lesions with the strontium-85 scintiscan. J Nucl Med *7*:219, 1966.
5. Harmer CL, Burns JE, Sams A, Spittle M: The value of fluorine-18 for scanning bone tumors. Clin Radiol *20*:204, 1969.
6. Galasko CSB: Detection of skeletal metastases from carcinoma of the breast. Surg Gynecol Obstet *132*:1019, 1971.
7. Blau M, Nagler W, Bender MA: Fluorine-18: A new isotope for bone scanning. J Nucl Med *3*:332, 1962.
8. Subramanian G, McAfee JG, O'Mara RE, et al: ^{99m}Tc-polyphosphate PP46: A new radiopharmaceutical for skeletal imaging (Abstr). J Nucl Med *12*:399, 1971.
9. Blum T: Osteomyelitis of the mandible and maxilla. J Am Dent Assoc *11*:802, 1924.
10. Looney WB: The initial medical and industrial use of radioactive materials (1915–1940). Am J Roentgenol *72*:838, 1954.
11. Chiewitz O, Hevesy G: Radioactive indicators in the study of phosphorus metabolism in rats. Nature (London) *136*:754, 1935.
12. Treadwell A de G, Low-Beer BV, Friedell HL, Lawrence JH: Metabolic studies on neoplasm of bone with the aid of radioactive strontium. Am J Med Sci *204*:521, 1942.
13. Bauer GCH, Ray RD: Kinetics of strontium metabolism in man. J Bone Joint Surg *40A*:171, 1958.
14. Bauer, GCH, Wendeberg B: External counting of ^{47}Ca and ^{85}Sr in studies of localized skeletal lesions in man. J Bone Joint Surg *41B*:558, 1959.
15. Gynning I, Langeland P, Lindberg S, Waldeskog B: Localization with ^{85}Sr of spinal metastases in mammary cancer and changes in uptake after hormone and roentgen therapy. Acta Radiol *55*:119, 1961.
16. DeNardo GL, Jacobson SJ, Raventos A: ^{85}Sr bone scan in neoplastic disease. Semin Nucl Med *2*:18, 1972.
17. Jowsey J, Riggs BL: Assessment of bone turnover by microradiography and autoradiography. Semin Nucl Med *2*:3, 1972.
18. Cameron JR, Sorenson J: Measurement of bone mineral in vivo: An improved method. Science *142*:230, 1963.
19. Griffiths HJL, Zimmerman RE, Bailey G, Snider R: The use of photon absorptiometry in the diagnosis of renal osteodystrophy. Radiology *109*:277, 1973.
20. Goldsmith NF, Johnston JO, Ury H, Vose G, Colbert C: Bone mineral estimation in normal and osteoporotic women. J Bone Joint Surg *53A*:83, 1971.
21. Mazess RB (Ed): Third International Conference on Bone Mineral Measurement. Am J Roentgenol *126*:1266, 1976.
22. Fremlin JH: Determination of whole-body calcium by neutron activation analysis in vivo. Semin Nucl Med *2*:86, 1972.
23. Cohn SH, Dombrowski CS: Measurement of total-body calcium, sodium, chlorine, nitrogen, and phosphorus in man by in vivo neutron activation analysis. J Nucl Med *12*:499, 1971.
24. Nelp WB, et al: Measurement of total body calcium (bone mass) in vivo with the use of total body neutron activation analysis. J Lab Clin Med *76*:151, 1971.
25. Chamberlain MJ, Fremlin JH, Peters DK, Philip H: Total-body calcium by whole body neutron activation: A new technique for study of bone disease. Br Med J *2*:581, 1968.
26. Goergen TG, Alazraki NP, Halpern SE, et al: "Cold" bone lesions: A newly recognized phenomenon of bone imaging. J Nucl Med *15*:1120, 1973.
27. Genant HK, Bautovich GJ, Singh M, et al: Bone-seeking radionuclides: An in vivo study of factors affecting skeletal uptake. Radiology *113*:373, 1974.
28. Van Dyke D, Anger HO, Yano Y, et al: Bone blood flow shown with ^{18}F and the positron camera. Am J Physiol *209*:65, 1965.
29. Charkes ND, Makler PT, Philips C: Studies of skeletal tracer kinetics. I. Digital-computer solution of a five compartment model of (^{18}F) fluoride kinetics in humans. J Nucl Med *19*:1301, 1978.
30. Siegel BA, Donovan RL, Alderson PO, et al: Skeletal uptake of ^{99m}Tc-diphosphonate in relation to local bone blood flow. Radiology *120*:121, 1976.
31. Jones AG, Francis MD, Davis MA: Bone scanning: Radionuclide reaction mechanisms. Semin Nucl Med *6*:3, 1976.
32. Blau M, Ganatra R, Bender MA: ^{18}F-fluoride for bone imaging. Semin Nucl Med *2*:31, 1972.
33. O'Mara RE, Subramanian G: Experimental agents for skeletal imaging. Semin Nucl Med *2*:38, 1972.
34. Subramanian G, McAfee JG: A new complex of ^{99m}Tc for skeletal imaging. Radiology *99*:192, 1971.
35. Thrall JH: Technetium-99m labeled agents for skeletal imaging. CRC Crit Rev Clin Radiol Nucl Med *8*:1, 1976.
36. Merrick MV: Bone scanning. Br J Radiol *48*:327, 1975.
37. Davis MA, Jones AG: Comparison of ^{99m}Tc-labeled phosphate and phosphonate agents for skeletal imaging. Sem Nucl Med *6*:19, 1976.

38. Subramanian G, McAfee JG, Blair RJ, Rosenstreich M, Coco M, Duxbury CE: Technetium-99m labeled stannous imidodiphosphate, a new radiodiagnostic agent for bone scanning: Comparison with other ^{99m}Tc complexes. J Nucl Med *16*:1137, 1975.
39. Krishnamurthy GT, Tubis M, Endow JS, Singhi V, Walsh C, Blahd WH: Clinical comparison of the kinetics of ^{99m}Tc labeled polyphosphate and diphosphonate. J Nucl Med *15*:848, 1974.
40. Subramanian G, McAfee JG, Blair RJ, Kallfelz FA, Thomas FD: Technetium-99m methylene diphosphonate — a superior agent for skeletal imaging: Comparison with other technetium complexes. J Nucl Med *16*:744, 1975.
41. Khairi MRA, Altman RD, DeRosa GP, Zimmermann J, Schenk RK, Johnston CC: Sodium etidronate in the treatment of Paget's disease of bone. A study of long-term results. Ann Intern Med *87*:656, 1977.
42. Rosenthall L, Kaye M: Observations in the mechanism of ^{99m}Tc-labeled phosphate complex uptake in metabolic bone disease. Semin Nucl Med *6*:59, 1976.
43. Kaye M, Silverton S, Rosenthall L: Technetium-99m-pyrophosphate: Studies in vivo and in vitro. J Nucl Med *16*:40, 1975.
44. McNeil BJ: Rationale for the use of bone scans in selected metastatic and primary bone tumors. Semin Nucl Med *8*:336, 1978.
45. Mall JC, Bekerman C, Hoffer PB, Gottschalk A: A unified radiological approach to the detection of skeletal metastases. Radiology *118*:323, 1976.
46. Citrin DL, Furnival CM, Bessent RG, Greig WR, Bell G, Blumgart LH: Radioactive technetium phosphate bone scanning in preoperative assessment and follow-up study of patients with primary cancer of the breast. Surg Gynecol Obstet *143*:360, 1976.
47. Gerber FH, Goodreau JJ, Kirchner PT: Tc-99m EHDP bone scanning in breast cancer. J Nucl Med *16*:529, 1975.
48. McNeil BJ, Pace PD, Gray EB, Adelstein SJ, Wilson RE: Preoperative and follow-up bone scans in patients with primary carcinoma of the breast. Surg Gynecol Obstet *147*:745, 1978.
49. Ramsdell JW, Peters RM, Taylor AT, Alazraki NP, Tisi GM: Multiorgan scans for staging lung cancer: Correlation with clinical evaluation. J Thorac Cardiovas Surg *73*:653, 1977.
50. Gutierrez AC, Vincent RG, Bakshi S, Takita H: Radioisotope scans in the evaluation of metastatic bronchogenic carcinoma. J Thorac Cardiovasc Surg *69*:934, 1975.
51. Schaffer DL, Pendergrass HP: Comparison of enzyme, clinical, radiographic, and radionuclide methods of detecting bone metastases from carcinoma of the prostate. Radiology *121*:431, 1976.
52. Goldstein H, McNeil BJ, Zufalle E, Jaffe N, Treves S: Changing indications for bone scintigraphy in patients with osteosarcoma. Radiology *135*:177, 1980.
53. Goldstein H, McNeil BJ, Zufalle E, Treves S: Is there still a place for bone scanning in Ewing's sarcoma? J Nucl Med *21*:10, 1980.
54. McNeil BJ, Cassady JR, Geiser CF, Jaffe N, Traggis D, Treves S: Fluorine-18 bone scintigraphy in children with osteosarcoma or Ewing's sarcoma. Radiology *109*:627, 1973.
55. Gilday DL, Ash JM, Reilly BJ: Radionuclide skeletal survey for pediatric neoplasms. Radiology *123*:399, 1977.
56. Kaufman RA, Thrall JH, Keyes JW Jr, Brown ML, Zakem JF: False-negative bone scans in neuroblastoma metastatic to the ends of long bones. Am J Roentgenol *130*:131, 1978.
57. Gilday DL, Ash JM: Benign bone tumors. Semin Nucl Med *6*:33, 1976.
58. Gates GF, Dore EK: Detection of craniosynostosis by bone scanning. Radiology *115*:665, 1976.
59. Sty JR, Boedecker RA, Babbitt DP: Skull scintigraphy in infantile hypophosphatasia. J Nucl Med *20*:305, 1979.
60. Handmaker H, Leonards R: The bone scan in inflammatory osseous disease. Semin Nucl Med *6*:95, 1976.
61. Teates CD, Williamson BRJ: "Hot and cold" bone lesion in acute osteomyelitis. Am J Roentgenol *129*:517, 1977.
62. Gilday DL, Paul DJ, Paterson J: Diagnosis of osteomyelitis in children by combined blood pool and bone imaging. Radiology *117*:331, 1975.
63. Alazraki NP, Fierer J, Resnick D: The role of gallium and bone scanning in monitoring response to therapy in chronic osteomyelitis (Abstr). J Nucl Med *19*:696, 1978.
64. Lisbona R, Rosenthall L: Observations on the sequential use of ^{99m}Tc-phosphate complex and ^{67}Ga imaging in osteomyelitis, cellulitis, and septic arthritis. Radiology *123*:123, 1977.
65. Kolyvas E, Rosenthall L, Ahronheim GA, Lisbona R, Marks M: Serial ^{67}Ga-citrate imaging during treatment of acute osteomyelitis in childhood. Clin Nucl Med *3*:461, 1978.
66. Alazraki NP, Minteer-Convery M, Convery FR: Accuracy of bone and gallium scanning in patients with painful prosthetic replacement. Proceedings of the Society for Nuclear Medicine, 4th Annual Western Regional Meeting, Monterey, California, 1979 (abstract).
67. Williamson BRJ, McLaughlin RE, Wang GJ, Miller CW, Teates CD, Bray ST: Radionuclide bone imaging as a means of differentiating loosening and infection in patients with a painful total hip prosthesis. Radiology *133*:723, 1979.
68. Rosenthall L, Lisbona R, Hernandez M, Hadjipavlou A: ^{99m}Tc-pp and ^{67}Ga imaging following insertion of orthopedic devices. Radiology *133*:717, 1979.
69. Reing CM, Richin PF, Kenmore PI: Differential bone scanning in the evaluation of a painful total joint replacement. J Bone Joint Surg *61A*:933, 1979.
70. Sakimura IT, Dorr L, Montgomery J, Siemsen J: Bone and gallium scan following total hip replacement to differentiate loosening from infection. Proceedings of the Society for Nuclear Medicine, 4th Annual Western Regional Meeting, 1979 (abstract).
71. Hattner RS, Hunter J, Genant HK, Murray W: Utility of skeletal scintigraphy in the detection of failed total knee arthroplasty. Proceeding Society for Nuclear Medicine, 4th Annual Western Regional Meeting, Monterey, California, 1979 (abstract).
72. Wilcox JR Jr, Moniot AL, Green JP: Bone scanning in evaluation of exercise related stress injuries. Radiology *123*:699, 1977.
73. Geslien GE, Thrall JH, Espinosa JL, Older RA: Early detection of stress fractures using ^{99m}Tc-polyphosphate. Radiology *121*:683, 1976.
74. Marty R, Denney J, McKamey MR, Rowley MJ: Bone trauma and related benign disease: Assessment by bone scanning. Semin Nucl Med *6*:107, 1976.
75. Wendeberg B: Mineral metabolism of fractures of the tibia in man studied with external counting of Sr^{85}. Acta Orthop Scand Suppl *52*:1, 1961.
76. Matin P: The appearance of bone scans following fractures, including immediate and long-term studies. J Nucl Med *20*:1227, 1979.
77. Rosenthall L, Hill RO, Chuang S: Observation on use of ^{99m}Tc-phosphate imaging in peripheral bone trauma. Radiology *119*:637, 1976.
78. Fordham EW, Ramachandran PC: Radionuclide imaging of osseous trauma. Semin Nucl Med *4*:411, 1974.
79. Stevenson JS, Bright RW, Dunson GL, Nelson FR: Technetium-99m phosphate bone imaging: A method for assessing bone graft healing Radiology *110*:391, 1974.
80. Alavi A, Desai A, Esterhai J, Brighton C, Dalinka M: Bone scanning in the evaluation of non-united fractures. J Nucl Med *20*:647, 1979.
81. Fogelman I, McKillop JH, Bessent RG, et al: The role of bone scanning in osteomalacia. J Nucl Med *19*:245–248, 1978.
82. Krishnamurthy GT, Brickman AS, Blahd WH: Technetium-99m-Sn-pyrophosphate pharmacokinetics and bone image changes in parathyroid disease. J Nucl Med *18*:236, 1977.
83. Sy WM: Bone scan in primary hyperparathyroidism. J Nucl Med *15*:1089, 1974.
84. Fogelman I, Bessent RG, Turner JG, et al: The use of whole-body retention of Tc-99m diphosphonate in the diagnosis of metabolic bone disease. J Nucl Med *19*:270, 1978.
85. Sy WM, Mittal AK: Bone scan in chronic dialysis patients with evidence of secondary hyperparathyroidism and renal osteodystrophy. Br J Radiol *48*:878, 1975.
86. Wiegmann T, Rosenthall L, Kaye M: Technetium-99m pyrophosphate bone scans in hyperparathyroidism. J Nucl Med *18*:231, 1977.
87. Prakash V, Kamel NJ, Lin MS, et al: Increased skeletal localization of ^{99m}Tc diphosphonate in paralyzed limbs. Clin Nucl Med *1*:48, 1976.
88. Rasmussen H, Bordier P: The Physiological and Cellular Basis of Metabolic Bone Disease. Baltimore, Williams & Wilkins Co, 1974.
89. Bray ST, Partain CL, Teates CD, Guilford WB, Williamson BRJ, McLaughlin RC: The value of the bone scan in idiopathic regional migratory osteoporosis. J Nucl Med *20*:1268, 1979.
90. Strashun A, Chayes Z: Migratory osteolysis. J Nucl Med *20*:129, 1979.
91. Paget J: On a form of chronic inflammation of bones (osteitis deformans). Med Chir Trans *60*:37, 1877.
92. Schmorl G: Uber Ostitis deformans Paget. Virchows Arch Pathol Anat Physiol *283*:694, 1932.
93. Serafini AN: Paget's disease of bone. Semin Nucl Med *6*:47, 1976.
94. Rhodes BA, Greyson ND, Hamilton CR Jr, White RI Jr, Giurgiana FA, Wagner HN Jr: Absence of arteriovenous shunts in Paget's disease of bone. N Engl J Med *287*:686, 1972.
95. Rausch JM, Resnick D, Goergen TG, Taylor A: Bone scanning in osteolytic Paget's disease: Case report. J Nucl Med *18*:699, 1976.
96. Wellman HN, Schauwecker D, Robb JA, et al: Skeletal scinti-imaging and radiography in the diagnosis and management of Paget's disease. Clin Orthop *127*:55, 1977.
97. Shirazi PH, Ryan WG, Fordham EW: Bone scanning in evaluation of Paget's disease of bone. CRC Crit Rev Clin Radiol Nucl Med *5*:523, 1974.
98. Alazraki NP: Aseptic necrosis discussion. *In* BA Siegel (Ed): Nuclear Radiology Syllabus. Chicago, American College of Radiology, 1978.
99. Meyers MH, Telfer N, Moore TM: Determination of the vascularity of the femoral head with technetium-99m sulphur colloid. J Bone Joint Surg *59A*:658, 1977.

100. Lutzker LG, Alavi A: Bone and marrow imaging in sickle cell disease: Diagnosis of infarction. Semin Nucl Med *6*:83, 1976.
101. Alavi A, Bond JP, Kuhl DE, Creech RH: Scan detection of bone marrow infarcts in sickle cell disorders. J Nucl Med *15*:1003, 1974.
102. Feigin DS, Strauss HW, James AE Jr: The bone marrow scan in experimental osteomyelitis. Skel Radiol *1*:103, 1976.
103. Danigelis JA: Pinhole imaging in Legg-Perthes' disease: Further observations. Semin Nucl Med *6*:69, 1976.
104. Catterall A: The natural history of Perthes' disease. J Bone Joint Surg *53B*:37, 1971.
105. Weiss TE, Maxfield WS, Murison PJ, et al: Iodinated human serum albumin (I-131) localization studies of rheumatoid arthritis joints by scintillation scanning. Arthritis Rheum *8*:976, 1965.
106. Alarcón-Segovia D, Trujegue M, Tovaz E, et al: Scintillation scanning of the joints with technetium-99m. Proceedings of the Annual Meeting of the American Rheumatism Association, New York, 1967.
107. Desaulniers M, Fuks A, Hawkins D, et al: Radiotechnetium polyphosphate joint imaging. J Nucl Med *15*:417, 1974.
108. Bekerman C, Genant HK, Hoffer PB, Kozin F, Ginsberg M: Radionuclide imaging of the bones and joints of the hand: A definition of normal and comparison of sensitivity using ^{99m}Tc-pertechnetate and ^{99m}Tc-diphosphonate. Radiology *118*:653, 1975.
109. Hoffer PB, Genant HK: Radionuclide joint imaging. Semin Nucl Med *6*:121, 1976.
110. Thomas RH, Resnick D, Alazraki NP, Daniel D, Greenfield R: Compartmental evaluation of osteoarthritis of the knee: A comparative study of available diagnostic modalities. Radiology *116*:585, 1975.
111. McCarty DJ, Polcyn RE, Collins PA: ^{99m}Technetium scintiphotography in arthritis. II. Its nonspecificity and clinical and roentgenographic correlations in rheumatoid arthritis. Arthritis Rheum *13*:21, 1970.
112. Weissberg DL, Resnick D, Taylor A, Becker M, Alazraki N: Rheumatoid arthritis and its variants: Analysis of scintiphotographic, radiographic, and clinical examinations. Am J Roentgenol *131*:665, 1978.
113. Lentle BC, Russell AS, Percy JS, Jackson FI: The scintigraphic investigation of sacroiliac disease. J Nucl Med *18*:529, 1977.
114. Goldberg RP, Genant HK, Shimshak R, Shames D: Applications and limitations of quantitative sacroiliac joint scintigraphy. Radiology *128*:683, 1978.
115. Sy WM, Bay R, Camera A: Hand images: Normal and abnormal. J Nucl Med *18*:419, 1977.
116. Russell AS, Lentle BC, Percy JS: Investigation of sacroiliac disease: Comparative evaluation of radiological and radionuclide techniques. J Rheumatol *2*:45, 1975.
117. Brown M, Swift TR, Spies SM: Radioisotope scanning in inflammatory muscle disease. Neurology *26*:517, 1976.
118. Rosenthal DI, Chandler HC, Azizi F: Uptake of bone imaging agents by diffuse pulmonary metastatic calcification. Am J Roentgenol *129*:871, 1977.
119. Buja LM, Tofe AJ, Kulkarni PV, Mukherjee A, Parkey RW, Francis MD, Bonte FJ, Willerson JT: Sites and mechanisms of localization of technetium-99m phosphorus radiopharmaceuticals in acute myocardial infarcts and other tissues. J Clin Invest *60*:724, 1977.
120. Byun HH, Rodman SG, Chung KE: Soft tissue concentration of ^{99m}Tc-phosphates associated with injections of iron dextran complex. J Nucl Med *17*:374, 1976.
121. Garcia AC, Yeh SDJ, Benua RS: Accumulation of bone-seeking radionuclides in liver metastasis from colon carcinoma. Clin Nucl Med *2*:265, 1977.
122. Rosenfield N, Treves S: Osseous and extraosseous uptake of fluorine-18 and technetium-99m polyphosphate in children with neuroblastoma. Radiology *111*:127, 1974.
123. Alazraki NP: Soft tissue localization of bone imaging radiopharmaceuticals. *In* BA Siegel (Ed): Nuclear Radiology Syllabus. Chicago, American College of Radiology, 1978.
124. Siegel BA, Engel WK, Derrer EC: Localization of technetium-99m diphosphonate in acutely injured muscle. Relationship to muscle calcium deposition. Neurology *27*:230, 1977.
125. Poulouse KP, Reha RC, Eckelman WC: Extra-osseous localization of Tc-99m-pyrophosphate. Br J Radiol *48*:724, 1975.
126. Berman DS, Amsterdam EA, Hines HH, Salel AF, Bailey GJ, DeNardo GL, Mason DT: New approach to interpretation of technetium-99m pyrophosphate scintigraphy in detection of acute myocardial infarction. Clinical assessment of diagnostic accuracy. Am J Cardiol *39*:341, 1977.
127. Silver JR: Heterotopic ossification: A clinical study of its possible relationship to trauma. Paraplegia *7*:220, 1969.
128. Alazraki NP: Myositis ossificans associated with spinal cord injury. *In* BA Siegel (Ed): Nuclear Radiology Syllabus. Chicago, American College of Radiology, 1978.
129. Tanaka T, Rossier AB, Hussey RW, Ahnberg DS, Treves S: Quantitative assessment of para-osteo-arthropathy and its maturation on serial radionuclide bone images. Radiology *123*:217, 1977.
130. Suzuki Y, Hisada K, Takeda M: Demonstration of myositis ossificans by ^{99m}Tc-pyrophosphate bone scanning. Radiology *111*:663, 1974.
131. King MA, Casarett GW, Weber DA: A study of irradiated bone. I. Histopathologic and physiologic changes. J Nucl Med *20*:1142, 1979.
132. Sagar VV, Piccone JM, Charkes ND: Studies of skeletal tracer kinetics. III. Tc-99m (Sn) methylenediphosphonate uptake in the canine tibia as a function of blood flow. J Nucl Med *20*:1257, 1979.

18

QUANTITATIVE BONE MINERAL ANALYSES

by Harry K. Genant, M.D.

Advances in the radiologic sciences in the past 15 to 20 years have permitted the development and application of a number of noninvasive techniques for quantitative bone mineral analyses. These techniques offer sensitive, precise, and accurate measurements for the detection and serial assessment of metabolic bone disease.

The requirements for a clinically useful measurement of bone mineral differ, depending upon the specific clinical problem under investigation. For serial determination in a given patient, precision — i.e., the ability to reproduce a measurement — is critical. On the other hand, as a diagnostic procedure to separate a patient from a normal population, accuracy is required. The various techniques available strive to accomplish one or both of these major goals.

The pattern and rate of bone loss in peripheral versus axial skeleton or compact versus cancellous bone may vary appreciably in different disease states. Therefore, the variations in sensitivity observed for different types of measurements made at different anatomic sites are not only a function of systematic errors found with each technique but are also complicated by the physiologic variation occurring naturally at different regions of the body. Additionally, a comparison of the sensitivity of techniques is complicated by the problem of clinically defining "normal" and "diseased" populations.

For example, by all methods of measurement of age-related bone loss, it is apparent that there is overlap between osteoporotic patients and age-matched controls, and, in general, the difference between the two groups is on the order of one standard deviation. This observation is true for peripheral or axial skeleton measurements and for compact or cancellous bone determinations.[54] Osteoporotic patients in this setting are generally defined as those individuals sustaining vertebral fractures, the so-called "vertebral crush" syndrome. But it is clear that some osteoporotic patients do not suffer fractures of the spine, whereas others with relatively normal mineralization may do so. Additionally, there is evidence that patients with femoral neck fractures may differ in some respects from those with vertebral fractures, although both patients are frequently osteoporotic. Thus, these biologic discrepancies in combination with technical errors lessen the discriminative capability or diagnostic potential of any given technique.

QUANTITATIVE HISTOMORPHOMETRIC ANALYSIS

Quantitative histomorphometric analyses of transiliac bone biopsies are quite useful in the diagnosis of metabolic bone disease. These techniques, when used with double tetracycline labeling,[25] provide information on both cortical and trabecular bone dynamics. This method and calcium tracer kinetics are the only two procedures that can measure rates of bone turnover and are extremely useful from that standpoint. Static biopsy measurements are not as useful; however, they can be used to obtain parameters such as trabecular bone volume (TBV) and relative osteoid volume.[59]

Some investigators use TBV as an index of bone mass. For diagnostic purposes, this may have some validity; however, for serial studies the imprecision of this measurement argues against its use. The use of quantitative iliac histomorphometry for bone mass in serial studies has several disadvantages: (1) It is invasive, therefore necessitating long intervals between successive biopsies for patient tolerance and iliac remodeling,[25] (2) it is imprecise, with differences of up to 20 per cent between right and left sides of the iliac crest at the same time,[83] (3) although perhaps a better site than the radius, the iliac crest is not necessarily representative of the spine or femoral neck, and (4) the necessary techniques for proper quantitative work are not widely available.

RADIOGRAMMETRY

The simple measurement of cortical thickness is easy to perform with a caliper, or with a hand lens having a reticle. It is reproducible within 5 to 10 per cent depending upon the site measured, and is backed by a large body of normative data.[20, 28, 60, 82] Simple cortical measurements may be represented in several ways: One is simply the summation of both cortices as an index of bone mass; another is the combined cortical thickness divided by total bone width as a measure of density; finally, a circular cross section of bone may be assumed with the bone width and cortical thickness measurements converted to cortical areas, which more closely parallel actual physical mass (Fig. 18–1).

Systematic errors ranging from 1 to 40 per cent are introduced by variation in soft tissue thickness and in radiographic geometry.[70] As a consequence of these inaccuracies and the imprecision in the measurement, the compact bone areas by radiogrammetry at different skeletal locations are only moderately

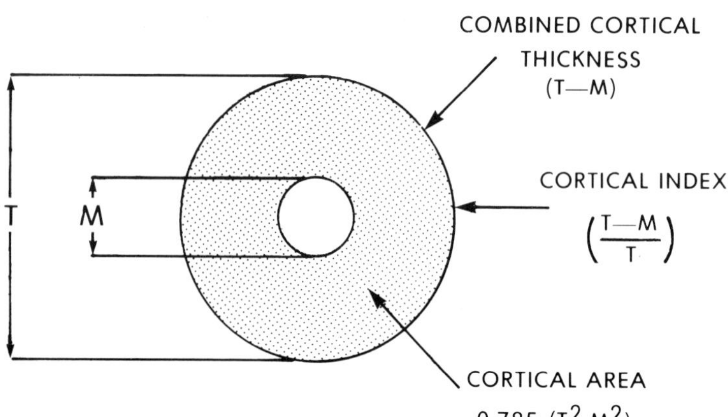

Figure 18–1. Schematic representation of a cross section of a tubular bone, showing several parameters determined by radiogrammetry.

intercorrelated (r = 0.5 to 0.7), whereas biologic intercorrelation is high (r > 0.9). Additionally, such measurements are only moderately correlated with other quantitative methods, such as photon absorptiometry and total body calcium determinations.[54]

Despite these deficiencies, simple cortical measurements, particularly when obtained at several anatomic sites, provide some useful information, either as an individual diagnostic study or as a serial determination. The results of radiogrammetry may be applied in patient management or clinical research. For example, extensive data on metacarpal changes in populations[21, 26, 27, 29, 70] show an aging loss in compact bone area of 6 to 7 per cent per decade in women and 3 per cent per decade in men. In a study of patients with primary hyperparathyroidism,[31, 32] 80 per cent of men and 84 per cent of women were found to have cortical thickness measurements less than the mean values of respective controls (Fig. 18–2).

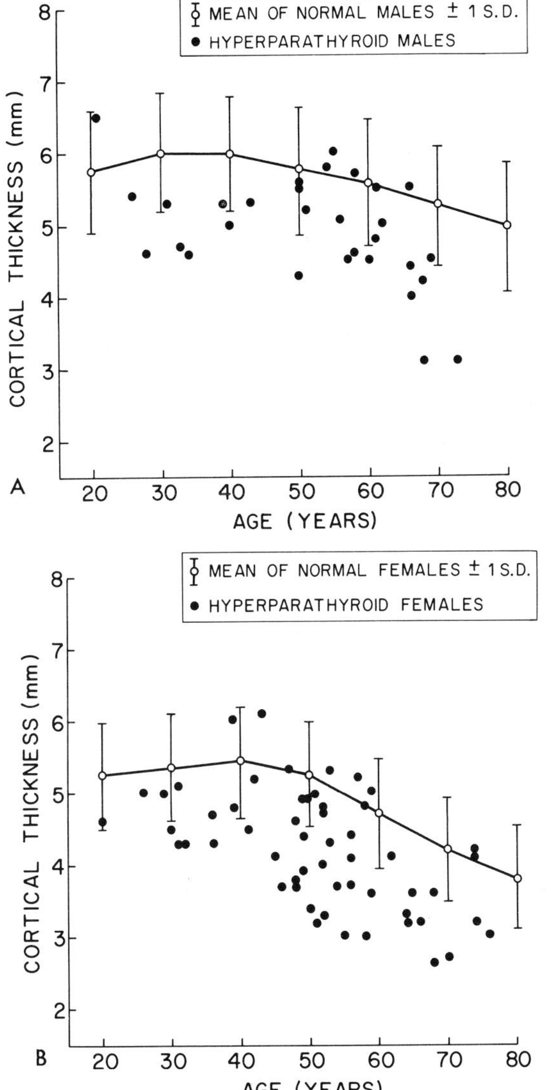

Figure 18–2. The combined cortical thickness of the second metacarpal is plotted versus age for normal (Garn) and hyperparathyroid males **(A)** and females **(B)**. (From Genant HK, et al: In RB Mazess [Ed]: Proceedings of International Conference on Bone Mineral Measurement. Washington, DC, National Institute of Arthritis, Metabolism and Digestive Diseases, 1974, p 177.)

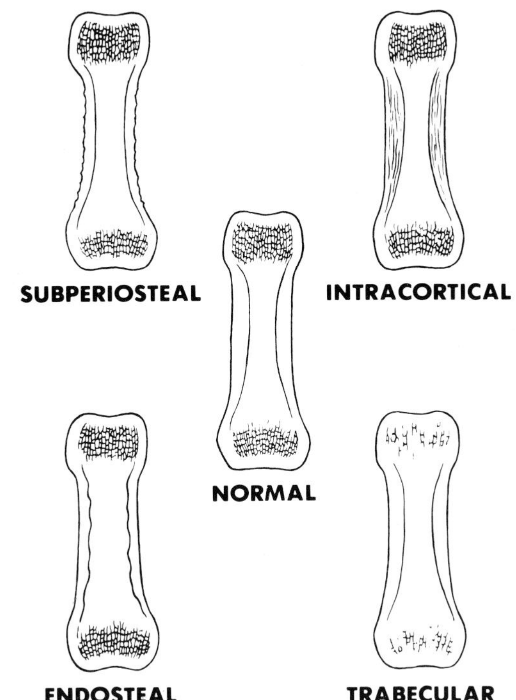

Figure 18–3. Schematic representation of four forms of bone resorption. Intracortical resorption and trabecular bone resorption are not measured by radiogrammetry.

The potential insensitivity of radiogrammetry relates to the failure to measure intracortical resorption or porosity and irregular endosteal scalloping or erosion. Intracortical resorption and trabecular bone resorption (Fig. 18–3) are important determinants of high bone turnover states and are not measured by this technique.[23, 32, 33, 37, 58, 81]

PHOTODENSITOMETRY

Photodensitometry[18, 22, 51, 58] is a technique that employs an x-ray source, radiographic film, and a known standard wedge. It has proved reproducible in experienced hands and is possibly more sensitive than simple cortical measurement. Complicated technical requirements have limited the clinical scope of this technique, however.

It has been known for many years that the photographic density on a film is roughly proportional to the mass of bone in the beam. By mere visual examination of radiographs, however, relatively large changes in bone mineral (25 to 50 per cent) must occur before differences can be determined. In an effort to quantitate bone mass, certain investigators[4, 7, 49, 50, 56, 65, 76] have measured the optical density of radiographs that have been exposed with the anatomic part and a reference wedge simultaneously. Multiple technical problems arise, however, including nonuniformity of the x-ray intensity, beam hardening due to the polychromatic radiation source, and variation in film sensitivity related to processing. Although the precision and accuracy of photodensitometry generally are on the order of 5 to 10 per cent for the peripheral skeleton, some laboratories have reported considerably better results.[18, 22, 51, 57]

SINGLE ENERGY PHOTON ABSORPTIOMETRY

Photon absorptiometry[2, 11, 48, 78] was introduced by Cameron and Sorenson[10] and Lanzl and Strandjord[48] in the early 1960s. The Lanzl-Strandjord method[48] consists of measuring the transmission through a finger of a narrow collimated beam of radiation emanating from an iodine (^{125}I) source (Fig. 18–4). The diaphysis of the middle phalanx of the third digit of the left hand is used, and detection is by means of a sodium iodide scintillation crystal connected to a photomultiplier, discriminator, and scaler. The result is adjusted for bone width and is expressed as the linear absorption coefficient, μ_B, in cm^{-1}. The coefficient is a measure of the mineral content of overall phalangeal bone (cortical and medullary).

Many similar devices have been used, but the most widely accepted and clinically applied today is the Norland-Cameron,[11] which measures the radial shaft using an ^{125}I source interfaced with a sodium iodide scintillation detector (Fig. 18–5).

In the Cameron technique, the forearm is surrounded by a water bag so that the path thickness is kept constant, and a baseline measurement is obtained in the region of the interosseous membrane. The source and detector translate across the tubular bone, and the changes in beam intensity are proportional to the bone mass. The transmitted beam is electronically processed to give a measurement of bone mineral content in grams for a 1 cm wide path in the longitudinal axis, i.e., gm/cm. In addition, the bone width is automatically determined, based on an edge discrimination function, which permits a calculation of bone mineral content per area scanned, i.e., gm/cm^2.

Since a highly collimated beam is utilized, errors due to scatter are minimized, and the nearly monoenergetic radiation source reduces the errors due to beam hardening. Another reason for the improved accuracy and precision for this technique compared to x-ray photodensitometry is the use of electronic equipment that counts each detected photon, eliminating the imprecision related to unknown processing errors in a film system.[11, 54] Considerable normative data are available, and many clinical studies have supported its usefulness.[40, 78] A reproducibility of 2 per cent and an accuracy of approximately 6 per cent have been demonstrated.[11] Radiation exposure for this technique is low (less than 10 mrem) and the inherent precision is high, which supports its usefulness in serial measurements.

The measurement obtained is primarily an integral of cortical bone, since the diaphysis, where measurements are generally made, contains little cancellous bone. The metaphysis, which contains proportionally more trabecular bone (up to 25 to 40 per cent of total integral bone[75]) is more difficult to measure as a result of repositioning errors and the consequent poor precision (~5 per cent). The impetus for measuring a region having greater cancellous bone such as the metaphysis is that it has a greater surface to volume ratio than a region of compact bone and shows alteration earlier and more dramatically in many metabolic bone disorders.[20, 37, 40, 71, 81] In this instance, however, the loss of precision with the Nor-

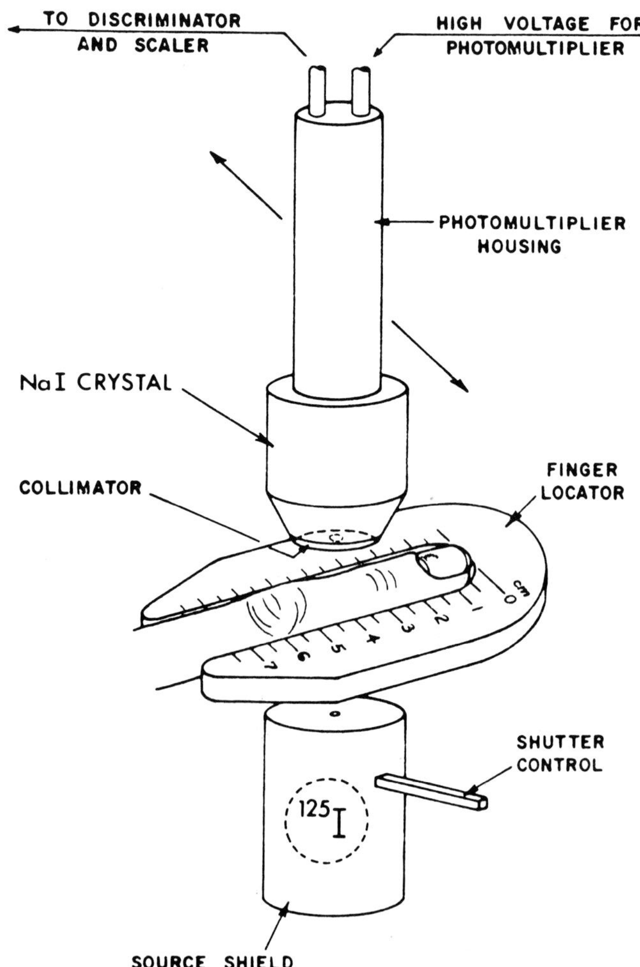

Figure 18–4. *Schematic representation of the Lanzl method of photon absorptiometry. (From Lanzl LH, Strandjord N: In Proceedings of Symposium on Low Energy X- and Gamma Sources and Applications. Chicago, Illinois Institute of Technology Research Institute, October 30, 1964.)*

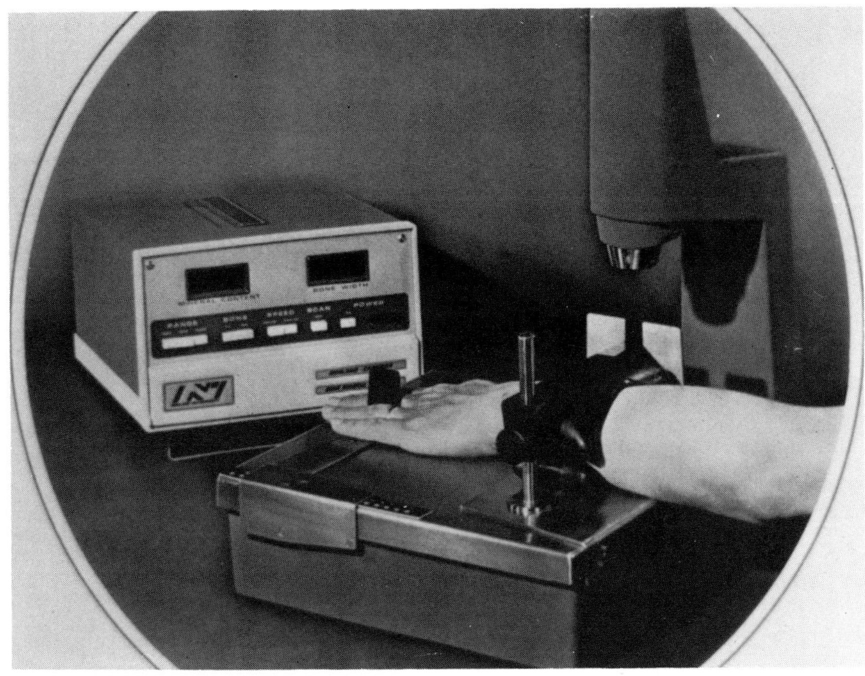

Figure 18–5. *The commercially available Norland-Cameron densitometer is shown.*

land-Cameron determination at the metaphyseal site outweighs any potential gain in sensitivity.[54]

In order to maximize sensitivity for calcium with photon absorptiometry of peripheral bones, a relatively low-energy isotope source is generally utilized such as ^{125}I with a mean energy of 27 keV. In general, the linear attenuation coefficient of any substance will depend upon the photon energy being used. The attenuation coefficient of substances such as bone mineral that have a high atomic number (z) is accentuated at low energies relative to substances with low z values, such as soft tissue. This results from the fact that the photoelectric absorption coefficient is proportional to z^3, and at low energies, it predominates over Compton scattering, which is proportional to z and is less energy dependent.[43, 54] Thus, the choice of photon energy affects greatly the accuracy and sensitivity of bone mineral content (BMC) measurements. This fact is shown schematically in Figure 18–6, which demonstrates the far greater energy dependence of the linear attenuation coefficient of bone than that of soft tissue or fat. Unfortunately, because of dosimetric and statistical considerations, the low-energy source ^{125}I cannot be used for thicker body parts.

The measurements obtained by photon absorptiometry are highly correlated with weight of bone, mass at other scan sites, weight of other long bones, total skeletal weight, and total body calcium.[54] Wilson[87] has shown measurements of the radius and ulnar shafts which are highly correlated ($r = 0.85$) with bone mineral content of the femoral neck and less highly correlated ($r = 0.7$) with bone mineral content in the spine.

Studies of BMC in normal and osteoporotic persons[17, 37, 77, 79, 84] show that people with osteoporosis fall about one standard deviation (15 per cent) below levels of age-matched controls and two

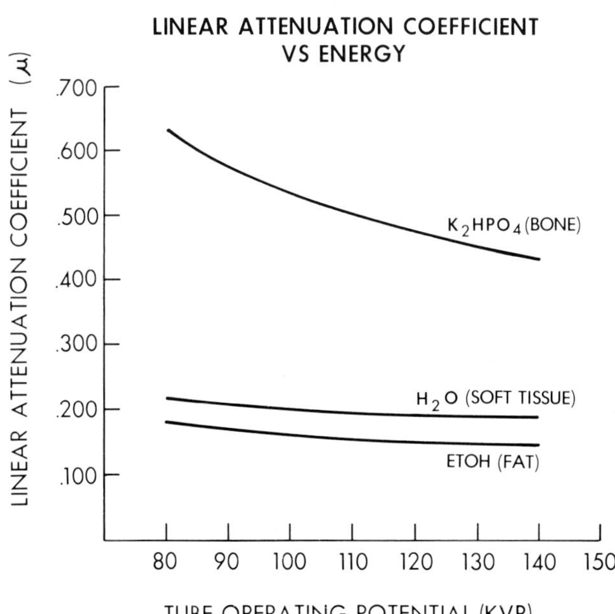

Figure 18–6. *Linear attenuation coefficients of bone equivalent (K_2HPO_4), soft tissue equivalent (H_2O), and fat (ethyl alcohol) are shown as a function of photon energy. Note the greater energy dependence for the mineral equivalent.*

standard deviations (30 per cent) below levels of young adults. These results indicate considerable overlap between osteoporotic patients and controls, but they are similar to those obtained by iliac crest biopsy and trabecular bone volume determination.[54] In a study[31, 32] of patients with primary hyperparathyroidism using photon absorptiometry of the phalanx, 80 per cent of men and 83 per cent of women had values below the expected means for age and sex (Fig. 18–7). In addition, in this same study, serial assessment by absorptiometry following parathyroidectomy revealed remineralization in a majority of cases (Fig. 18–8).

A major limitation of the photon absorptiometry techniques is that they reflect the status of peripheral tubular bones and measure primarily the cortex. These measurements may not reflect the overall skeletal status for an individual patient in many metabolic diseases and, therefore, may be of restricted diagnostic value.[19] There is accumulating evidence to suggest that metabolic processes occur more rapidly in cancellous bone.[20, 24, 38, 52, 64]

In metabolic conditions causing rapid flux in skeletal mass, such as immobilization,[72] or in the treatment of osteoporotic patients with calcium fluoride and vitamin D,[41] substantial changes may appear in spinal mineral content while only minimal changes appear in the peripheral skeleton. Thus, the spine may be more responsive to hypermetabolic states, making it more sensitive for measurement.

DUAL ENERGY PHOTON ABSORPTIOMETRY

The single energy photon absorptiometry methods assume that the projection path consists only of bone mineral and soft tissue and that the path length is constant. Either but not both assumptions may be removed by using a dual energy projection technique. In most investigations, the constant path length assumption has been removed to provide the capability for quantitative measurements of the axial skeleton, in particular the spine.[19, 43, 37, 69] In the technique reported by Wilson and Madsen,[88] a high-purity, high-activity gadolinium (^{153}Gd) source, which has photons of predominantly 44 keV and 100 keV, is used as the transmission source. The scans are performed on a modified whole body rectilinear scanner. The precision of measurement in humans is 2 to 3 per cent (coefficient of variation) and the

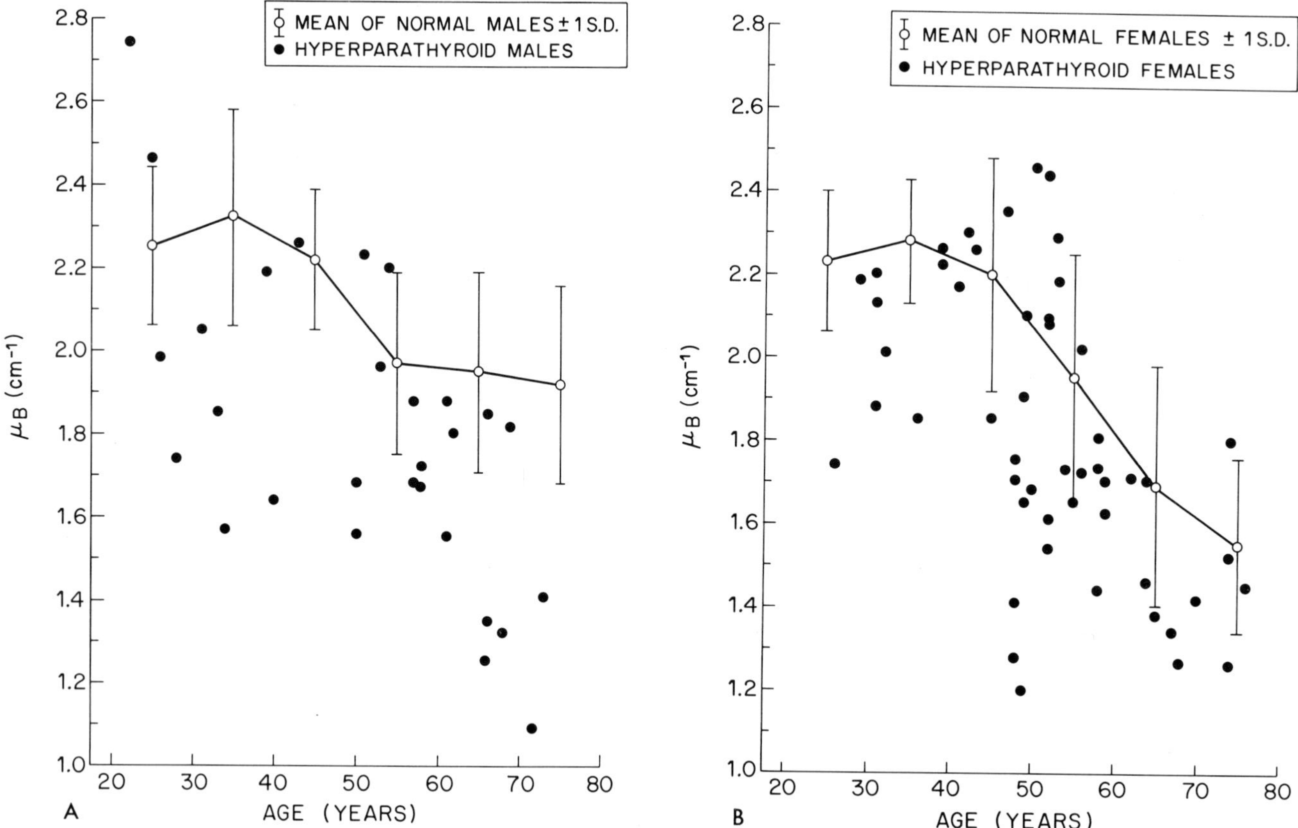

Figure 18–7. *The linear absorption coefficient of bone versus age for normal and hyperparathyroid males* **(A)** *and females* **(B)** *is shown. (From Genant HK, et al: In RB Mazess [Ed]: Proceedings of International Conference on Bone Mineral Measurement. Washington DC, National Institute of Arthritis, Metabolism and Digestive Diseases, 1977, p 177.)*

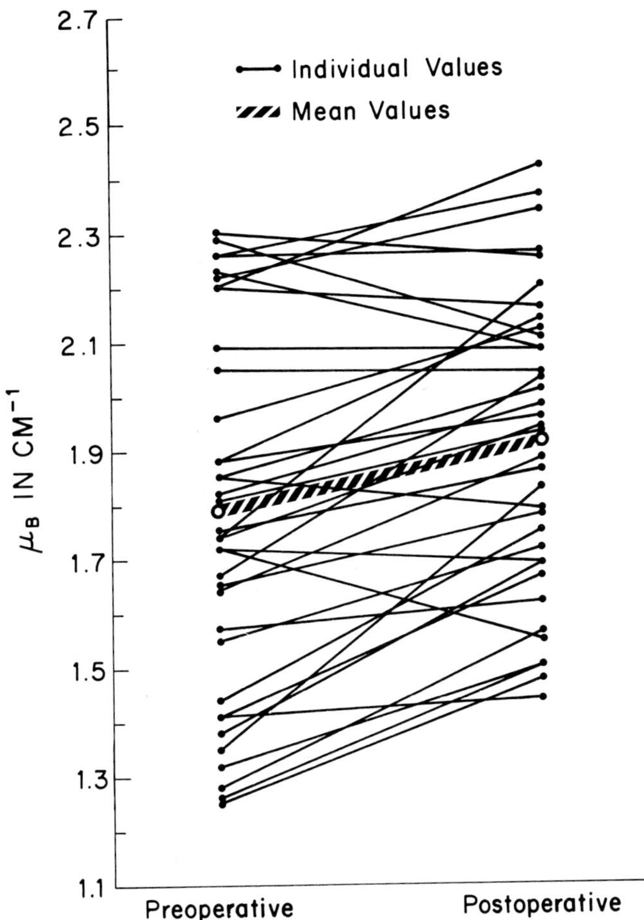

Figure 18–8. The linear attenuation coefficient of phalangeal bone is shown for hyperparathyroid patients prior to parathyroidectomy and 1 to 3 years postoperatively. Most patients show remineralization following parathyroidectomy. (From Genant HK, et al: Radiology 109:513, 1973.)

accuracy in phantoms with dipotassium hydrogen phosphate solutions is 1 to 2 per cent (standard error of estimate).

X-ray spectrophotometry, devised by Jacobson[43] is a variant of the dual energy photon absorptiometry of Wilson. This system uses an x-ray tube that is electronically switched between two different kilovoltages, and that functions by adjusting the thickness of a "soft tissue" wedge and a "bone mineral" wedge in the beam automatically to maintain constant intensity. Thus, the wedge thicknesses provide direct readout of mineral and soft tissue components. A large body of clinical results using x-ray spectrophotometry has been reported by Dalen and Jacobson[19] and Roos.[72]

NEUTRON ACTIVATION ANALYSIS

In vivo neutron activation analyses (NAA) have been under investigation at several centers for the past decade.[13, 15, 16, 63] In this method, neutrons bombard a small fraction of the total ^{48}Ca in the body producing ^{49}Ca (half-life of 8.8 min), which is then counted externally. The neutrons (with energies of 1 to 15 MeV) are derived from accelerators, reactors or alpha neutron sources. The technique provides an estimate of bone mineral content since, at least in the skeleton, calcium makes up a constant fraction (0.395) of the mineral. Radiation dose for such measures range from 200 to 3000 mrem, depending on the neutron energy and the detector efficiency. Recent studies suggest a precision and accuracy on the order of 2 to 5 per cent.[86]

A total body calcium measurement by NAA reflects primarily compact bone, which constitutes approximately 85 per cent of the total skeletal mass and, therefore, correlates closely with other measurements of cortical bone.[54] Studies have been performed in which total body calcium measurements by neutron activation have been compared with results obtained by peripheral photon absorptiometry; correlation coefficients on the order of 0.9 were obtained.[3, 17, 53] Processes occurring initially or predominantly in cancellous bone may not be as readily detected with this technique. For example, in osteoporotic patients, the correlation between peripheral measurements by photon absorptiometry and total body neutron activation is not ideal. Heterotopic calcification, such as vascular and costochondral calcification, or heterotopic ossification, such as osteophytosis and myositis ossificans, will cause inaccuracies in the estimation of skeletal calcium by NAA.

In an attempt to measure predominantly cancellous bone, methods have been developed[55] for partial body neutron activation in which areas of the trunk (i.e., pelvis, spine, and rib cage) are measured. Precision and dosages for these local measurements are comparable to those obtained with the total body activation techniques. Although normalization of spinal calcium results has improved discrimination, substantial overlap between normal controls and osteoporotic patients still is seen.

Complicated technical requirements and the expensive equipment used confine the availability of this technique to several large research centers. The dual energy photon absorptiometry technique[88] would appear to give similar information to that of the partial body activation at a substantially lower — i.e., several orders of magnitude less — level of radiation exposure. In addition, it utilizes equipment that is less expensive and far more readily available.[54, 88]

COMPTON SCATTERING

Compton scattering techniques have been used to estimate the density of selected volumes of bone.[14, 30, 45, 61, 68, 85] These methods depend upon the

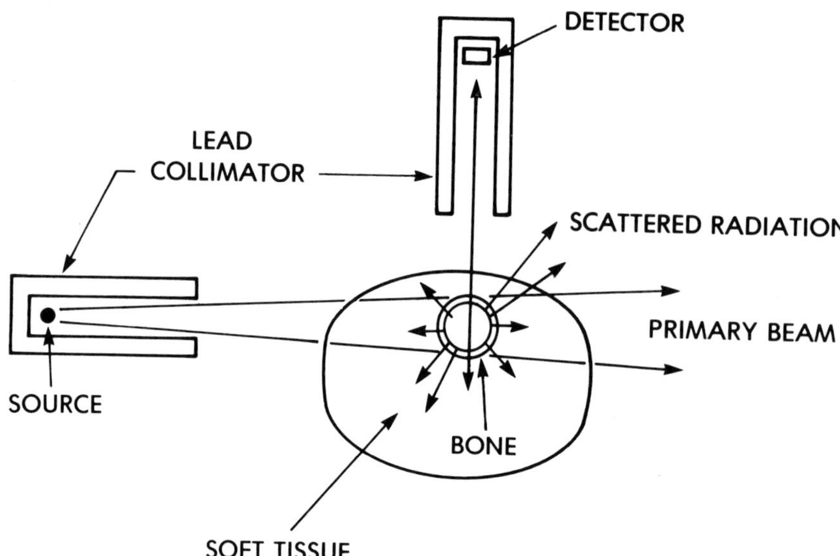

Figure 18–9. Schematic representation of the source and detector for Compton scatter densitometry. (After Joseph PH: In F Feldman [Ed]: Radiology, Pathology and Immunology of Bones and Joints. New York, Appleton-Century-Crofts, 1978, p 175.)

information extracted primarily from the scattered beam, not from the transmitted beam. The electron density of a tissue volume is estimated by the extent of Compton scattering produced by incident radiation. The incident radiation is generally a relatively high photon energy, on the order of 100 to 500 keV, emanating from a monoenergetic isotope source. A highly collimated gamma ray source and a highly collimated detector are positioned such that their "sensitive areas" project pathways that intersect perpendicular to each other within the object and that define the volume to be measured (Fig. 18–9). The technique measures a composite of all the medullary components producing the scatter, not simply the density of bone mineral. The detected scatter is proportional to the electron density, independent of atomic number z. For this reason, the method is somewhat less sensitive to calcium level than is the photon absorptiometry applied at low energies.[61] The precision of the method is on the order of 3 to 5 per cent, and the radiation dose varies from 200 to 2000 mrem. The accuracy is affected by photon attenuation in tissues outside of the region of interest and multiple scattering of photons within the region of interest. The use of high photon energy diminishes these problems but at the expense of increased radiation dose.[5, 6, 46] The method remains largely a research tool at the moment, and extensive clinical evaluation has not yet been reported.

A variant of the above scattered photon technique is *coherent scattering* as proposed by Puumalainen.[66] With this method, both Compton and coherent scattering of photons are determined in a volume of interest, such as cancellous bone. This is made possible by the use of a solid state detector, which provides good discrimination. Coherent scattering, like photoelectric absorption, depends upon the atomic number cubed (z^3), and thus the ratio of coherent to Compton scattered photons is a measure of effective atomic number, independent of density. A decreased ratio therefore may be observed in osteopenic diseases. Likewise, the ratio is unaffected by scatter outside the region of interest, so that complicated corrections for this inaccuracy are not necessary.

COMPUTED TOMOGRAPHY (CT)

The recent development of computed tomography (CT) for diagnostic imaging provides a new modality for quantitative skeletal mineral determination. The theoretic advantages of the computed tomographic technique[8, 9, 34, 67, 74] over other modalities for bone mineral determination include the following: (1) transaxial display of data, which permits identification of the anatomy and separate determination of cortical, cancellous, or integral bone; (2) capability of determining linear absorption coefficient for a readily defined volume of bone; and (3) in the dual energy mode, the ability to determine mineral content in the presence of variable fat and soft tissue content.

A study recently reported by Reich and associates[67] utilized a Delta CT scanner and correlated the results with those obtained using the Norland-Cameron densitometer, both techniques measuring an integral of bone in the radial shaft. A fairly high correlation ($r = 0.72$) was obtained. In addition, the accuracy was determined by measuring tubular bones devoid of soft tissue and placed in a water bath. The CT results correlated well ($r = 0.97$) with subsequent calcium determination in specimens, indicating that a high degree of accuracy is achievable in vitro. Precision was not determined, and there was no attempt to determine separately the mineral content of cortical and cancellous bone, nor the mineral content in the presence of variable soft tissue components.

Similar results were reported by Posner and Griffiths[64] on dog long bones scanned in vitro and by Bradley and co-workers[9] on cadaveric lumbar vertebrae scanned in vitro. Ischerwood and associates[42] have reported preliminary results on scanning the forearm of human subjects. Repositioning introduced the most significant error. Five scans obtained over a period of 7 days on a volunteer showed a reproducibility of about 2 per cent for integral bone mineral estimation. Orphanoudakis and co-workers[62] reported promising results with the use of a commercial scanner combined with a hollow cylindric calibration phantom into which the forearm is placed for measurement.

A specially devised CT instrument for bone mineral analysis was recently reported by Ruegsegger and colleagues,[74] which uses an ^{125}I source and computer-assisted reconstruction. It showed excellent capability for separate determination of cortical and cancellous bone in the radius and provided an approximately 2 per cent precision rate. Accuracy was not determined. However, it should be noted that the error due to unknown fat content depends greatly upon the beam energy as well as on the relative amount of fat.[80] Thus, with a low energy source such as ^{125}I (mean energy, 27 keV), the attenuation of mineral is accentuated relative to fat and soft tissue due to the z dependence of the photoelectric attenuation process, which predominates at the low photon energy. At this low energy, the error in determining bone mineral content due to variable amounts of fat in the marrow space of the radius has been estimated to be less than 3 per cent.[43] Moreover, beam hardening error, which can be considerable with a low-energy polychromatic source, is reduced by the nearly monochromatic ^{125}I photon spectrum. It is apparent, therefore, that the technique of CT reconstruction using a ^{125}I source may be superior to that achievable with commercially available CT scanners for peripheral small bones.

The several methods that have been discussed for measurement of spinal mineral content, including dual-energy linear photon absorptiometry and neutron activation analysis, have the potential disadvantage that they measure integral vertebral bone. For the lumbar vertebrae, this bone consists of 50 to 60 per cent dense compact bone in the cortex, pedicles, and processes, with the remainder being cancellous bone in the vertebral body. Less than half of the total bone measured may be "high-turnover" bone. The usefulness of computed tomography for measurement of bone mineral in the vertebrae lies in its abilities to quantitatively image a thin transverse slice through the abdomen and to spatially separate compact and cancellous bone. Thus, we now have the potential ability to measure changes serially in bone mineral content (1) noninvasively, (2) in cancellous bone, in which measurement of changes is more sensitive than in cortical bone, and (3) at the site of clinical involvement, in the vertebrae. In addition, as this technique is developed, the widespread availability of whole body CT scanners will make vertebral mineral determination a clinically useful tool to a large number of medical facilities.

The Basis of CT Bone Mineral Estimation

Bone mineral determination using computed tomography is dependent upon the ability of CT to image a thin transverse slice through the body and to evaluate the attenuation of any region of interest. The method is based on the relationship between the linear attenuation coefficient of a mixture of compounds as a function of energy, $\mu(E)$, and the attenuation coefficients and concentrations of each of the pure compounds. The dimensionless "CT number," H, calculated by most scanners is a function of the linear attenuation coefficient of the mixture relative to those of water and of air.

The single energy method for bone mineral estimation assumes that the bone mixture consists of water-equivalent soft tissue and bone mineral. One can calculate the concentration of bone mineral (c_b) in the mixture using the relationship

$$c_b = \frac{\rho_b}{H_b(V) - H_s(V)} [H(V) - H_s(V)]$$

where $H_b(V)$ is the CT number of pure bone mineral at tube potential V, $H_s(V)$ is the CT number of water equivalent soft tissue, $H(V)$ is the (measured) CT number of the bone mixture, and ρ_b is the density of pure bone mineral. In practice, $H_b(V)$ and $H_s(V)$ are determined using a phantom containing "mineral equivalent" and "soft tissue equivalent" components — normally K_2HPO_4 and water — scanned at the same time as the patient. Results are then expressed as a function of this mineral equivalent (i.e., in milligrams of K_2HPO_4).

It is known that there is a substantial and variable fat content in bone mixture. Ignoring this fat may cause substantial error in the calculated concentration of bone.[80] The dual energy CT method involves measuring the CT number of a bone mixture in a particular area of interest at two kilovolt peak (kVp) values. The linear set of mixture rule equations, containing the fat contributions, generated at the two different kVps, are then solved simultaneously for c_b.

Spinal Bone Mineral Determinations by CT

Work at our center in the last 5 years[1, 12, 31–35, 73] has addressed many of the problems of vertebral mineral determination by CT. The technical problems of this method can be divided into two main categories — those problems primarily affecting precision and those affecting accuracy of bone mineral measurement.

In order to develop CT techniques for clinical

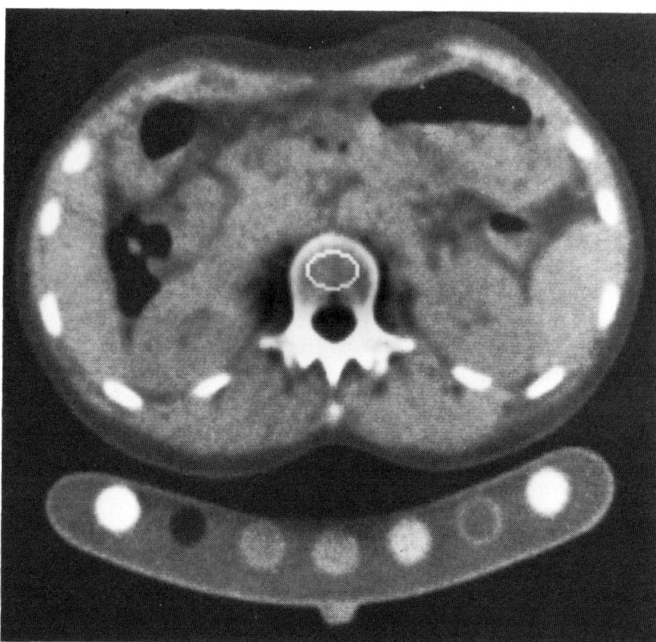

Figure 18–10. *CT scan at the level of the midbody of L1, showing the oval region of interest and the crescent-shaped phantom containing standard solutions.*

utility in serial studies, phantom studies were done to define the potential problems.[1] Two main sources of error were identified: time-related drift in the scanner and patient repositioning between studies. Long-term drift in the effective energy of the scanner beam, related to software and hardware modifications by the manufacturer, were found to cause variations of 30 to 40 Hounsfield (H) units over 3 months in the range of values found for vertebral mineral. Day to day variation was ± 8 H units, representing ± 4 per cent in mineral content. To compensate for these variations, phantoms were developed that are scanned simultaneously with the patient (Fig. 18–10). Vertebral mineral determina-

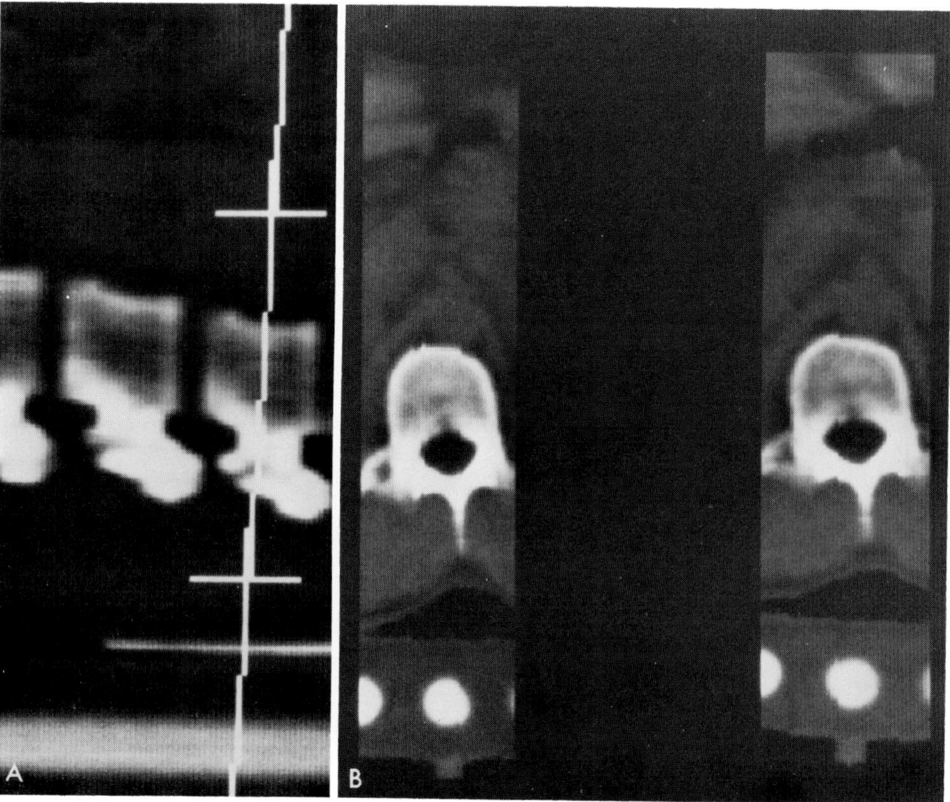

Figure 18–11. *Sagittal reconstruction of the upper lumbar spine demonstrating the method of localizing the midportion of the vertebral body* **(A)**. *Reconstructed cross-sectional slices 7 pixels thick are shown for the L1 vertebral body of a patient who had two examinations separated by 3 months* **(B)**.

tions are calibrated to both mineral equivalent (K_2HPO_4) and soft tissue equivalent (water, glycerol) materials present in the phantom, to compensate for both x-ray tube output and effective energy variations.

Precise repositioning of patients in serial studies is necessary because of the large change in CT number with only a 3 to 4 mm variation in position along the Z axis. Even with relatively thin slices (5 mm), small changes in positioning can cause errors of up to 10 per cent in the measured mineral content.

Recent developments using volume reconstruction of the vertebrae from multiple axial slices have significantly reduced these repositioning errors. Multiple contiguous nonoverlapping 5 mm thick slices are obtained through L1 and L2. A volume containing the vertebral column is reconstructed by linear interpolation. A plane is passed through the midportion of each vertebral body, as determined by the vertebral end-plates and disc spaces (Fig. 18–11*A*). Once this midplane is determined (to ± 1.3 mm), a 10 mm thick axial slice is reconstructed (Fig. 18–11*B*), encompassing most of the plateau region in the vertebra and averaging the inhomogeneities within the cancellous bone. The average CT number in a 4 cu cm volume element is determined using an oval region of interest (see Fig. 18–10) and is normalized to mineral and soft tissue equivalent solutions in a phantom scanned simultaneously. Precision for mineral determination in fresh excised vertebral specimens placed in torso phantoms, using these positioning and normalization techniques, is 2.8 per cent (SD).

Our experience in developing these methods has shown that, whereas the accuracy of CT for spinal mineral determination may not yet be sufficient for diagnostic capability, the precision for serial measurements in a clinical setting now is high enough that a change of 5 to 6 per cent in vertebral mineral will be detected. Preliminary results of serial CT spinal mineral determination in a group of oophorectomized women taking variable doses of estrogen are shown in Figure 18–12 and are compared with results of peripheral bone mineral measurements. The greater sensitivity of spinal CT for monitoring osteoporosis is suggested.

The question of how to improve the accuracy of CT mineral determinations in the spine has not yet been satisfactorily answered. The effective beam energy used in any scan must be known to accurately determine the linear attenuation coefficient of the bone mixture. First order corrections for beam hardening incorporated into scanner software reduce the error from this problem, and further work is being done to eliminate this effect. The use of single energy CT may introduce inaccuracies of 5 to 20 per cent in the measurement of vertebral mineral concentration due to the variable fat content in the spinal marrow.[36] Dual energy CT techniques can reduce this inaccuracy, but precision in the measurement is less than with single energy determinations.

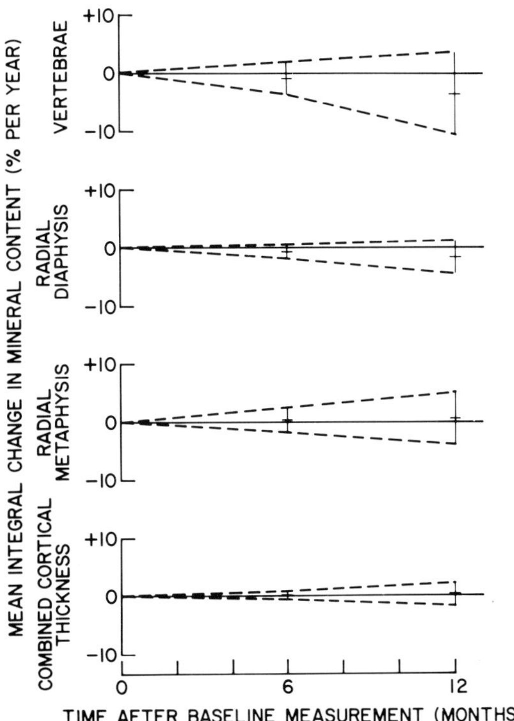

Figure 18–12. *A comparison of vertebral CT determination and three methods of peripheral measurement is shown for a group of 17 oophorectomized women who are placed on placebo or variable doses of estrogen. There is a suggestion of greater loss of mineral from the spine than from the peripheral sites. (From Genant HK, et al, 1980.[34])*

As the precision of single energy measurements has improved, however, so has that of dual energy methods. Nevertheless, for serial studies in patients, the single energy CT determinations of vertebral density will continue to be the method of choice. For diagnostic purposes, the use of dual energy CT appears promising but further developmental work must be done before it will be clinically useful as a discriminator for osteoporosis.

SUMMARY

A variety of methods exists for quantitative bone mineral analysis, each with its own limitations. The recent development of computed tomography has provided a new and exciting modality for such analysis. Further development and experimentation with this latter technique must be accomplished before its widespread clinical application will be realized.

REFERENCES

1. Abols Y, Rosenfeld D, Genant HK: Spinal bone mineral determination using computerized tomography in patients, controls and phantoms. Proceedings of the 4th International Conference on Bone Measurement. Washington DC, US Government Printing Office, 1979.
2. Aitken JM, Smith CB, Horton PW, Clark DL, Boyd JF, Smith DA: The interrelationships between bone mineral at different skeletal sites in male and female cadavera. J Bone Joint Surg *56B*:370, 1974.
3. Aloia JF, Vaswani A, Atkins H, Zanzi I, Ellis K, Cohn SH: Radiographic morphometry and osteopenia in spinal osteoporosis. J Nucl Med *18*:425, 1977.
4. Anderson JB, Shimmins J, Smith DA: A new technique for measurement of metacarpal density. Br J Radiol *39*:443, 1966.
5. Battista JJ, Santon LW, Bronskill MJ: Compton scatter imaging of transverse sections: Corrections for multiple scatter and attenuations. Phys Med Biol *22*:229, 1977.
6. Battista JJ, Bronskill MJ: Compton-scatter tissue densitometry: Calculation of single and multiple scatter photon fluences. Phys Med Biol *23*:1, 1978.
7. Baylink DJ, Vose GP, Dotter WE, Hurxthal LM: Two new methods for the study of osteoporosis and other metabolic bone diseases. II. Vertical bone densitometry. Lahey Clin Bull *13*:217, 1964.
8. Boyd DP, Genant HK, Korobkin MT: Improving the accuracy of CT body scanning as applies to bone mineral quantitation (Abstr.) Annual Sessions of the Radiological Society of North America, Chicago, November 1976.
9. Bradley JG, Huang HK, Ledley RS: Evaluation of calcium concentration in bones from CT scans. (Prepublication copy: HK Huang, Georgetown University Medical Center, 3900 Reservoir Rd, NW, Washington, DC 20007.)
10. Cameron JR, Sorenson JA: Measurement of bone mineral in vivo: An improved method. Science *142*:230, 1963.
11. Cameron JR, Mazess RB, Sorenson JA: Precision and accuracy of bone mineral determination by direct photon absorptiometry. Invest Radiol *3*:141, May-June, 1968.
12. Cann CE, Genant HK: Precise measurement of vertebral mineral content using computed tomography. J Comput Assist Tomogr (In press).
13. Chamberlain MJ, Fremlin JH, Holloway I, Peters DK: Use of the cyclotron for whole body neutron activation analysis: Theoretical and practical considerations. Int J Appl Radiat Isot *21*:725, 1970.
14. Clarke RL, Van Dyk G: A new method for measurement of bone mineral content using both transmitted and scattered beams of gamma-rays. Phys Med Biol *18*:532, 1973.
15. Cohn SH, Dombrowski CS, Fairchild RG: In vivo neutron activation analysis of calcium in man. Int J Appl Radiat Isot *21*:127, 1970.
16. Cohn SH, Shukla KK, Dombrowski CS, Fairchild RG: Design and calibration of a "broad-beam" ^{238}Pu, Be neutron source for total-body neutron activation analysis. J Nucl Med *13*:487, 1972.
17. Cohn SH, Ellis KJ, Wallach S, Zanzi I, Atkins HL, Aloia JF: Absolute and relative deficit in total-skeletal calcium and radial bone mineral in osteoporosis. J Nucl Med *15*:428, 1974.
18. Colbert C, Mazess RB, Schmidt PB: Bone mineral determination in vitro by radiographic photodensitometry and direct photon absorptiometry. Invest Radiol *5*:336, 1970.
19. Dalen N, Jacobson B: Bone mineral assay: Choice of measuring sites. Invest Radiol *9*:174, 1976.
20. Dequeker J: Bone and aging. Ann Rheum Dis *34*:100, 1975.
21. Dequeker J: Bone Loss in Normal and Pathological Conditions. Leuven, Belgium, Leuven University Press, 1972.
22. Doyle FH: Some quantitative radiological observations in primary and secondary hyperparathyroidism. Br J Radiol *39*:161, 1966.
23. Duncan H: Cortical porosis: A morphological evaluation. *In* ZFG Jaworski (Ed): Proceedings of the First Workshop on Bone Morphometry. Ottawa, Ontario, University of Ottawa Press, 1976, p. 78.
24. Ein-Gal M, Rosenfeld D, Macovski A: The consistency of the shadow: An approach to preprocessing in computerized tomography. Digest of Papers, OSA Meeting on Image Processing for Reconstruction from Projections, Stanford, CA, 1975.
25. Frost HM: Tetracycline based histological analysis of bone remodeling. Calcif Tissue Res *3*:211, 1969.
26. Garn SM: Earlier Gain and the Later Loss of Cortical Bone: In Nutritional Perspective. Springfield, Ill, Charles C Thomas, 1970.
27. Garn SM, Rohmann CG, Wagner B: Bone loss as a general phenomenon in man. Fed Proc *26*:1729, 1967.
28. Garn SM, Poznanski AK, Nagy JM: Bone measurement in the differential diagnosis of osteopenia and osteoporosis. Radiology *100*:509, 1971.
29. Garn SM, Poznanski AK, Larson K: Metacarpal lengths, cortical diameters and areas from the 10-state nutrition survey, including: estimated skeletal weights, weight, and stature for whites, blacks, and Mexican-Americans. *In* ZFG Jaworski (Ed): Proceedings of the First Workshop of Bone Morphometry. Ottawa, Ontario, University of Ottawa Press, 1976, p. 367.
30. Garnett ES, Kennett TJ, Kenyon DB, Webber CE: A photon scattering technique for the measurement of absolute bone density in man. Radiology *106*:209, 1973.
31. Genant HK, Vander Horst J, Lanzl LH, Mall JC, Doi K: Skeletal demineralization in primary hyperparathyroidism. *In* RB Mazess (Ed): Proceedings of International Conference on Bone Mineral Measurement, Washington DC, National Institute of Arthritis, Metabolism and Digestive Diseases, 1974, p 177.
32. Genant HK, Heck LL, Lanzl LH, et al: Primary hyperparathyroidism. A comprehensive study of clinical, biochemical and radiographic manifestations. Radiology *109*:513, 1973.
33. Genant HK, Kozin F, Bekerman C, et al: The reflex sympathetic dystrophy syndrome. A comprehensive analysis using fine-detail radiography, photon absorptiometry, and bone and joint scintigraphy. Radiology *117*:21, 1975.
34. Genant HK, Cann CE, Ettinger B, Gordan GS: Bone mineral determination in the axial and appendicular skeleton of oophorectomized women (Abstr). Endocrine Society Meeting, Washington DC, June 18–20, 1980.
35. Genant HK, Boyd DP: Quantitative bone mineral analysis using dual energy computed tomography. Invest Radiol *12*:545, 1977.
36. Genant HK, Boyd DP, Rosenfeld D, Abols Y, Cann CE: Quantitative bone mineral analysis using computed tomography. *In* S Cohen (Ed): Non-Invasive Measurements of Bone and Their Clinical Applications. CRC Press, West Palm Beach, Florida, 1980.
37. Goldsmith NF, Johnston JO, Ury H, Vose G, Colbert C: Bone mineral estimation in normal and osteoporotic women. J Bone Joint Surg *53A*:83, 1971.
38. Gordan GS, Vaughan C: Clinical Management of the Osteoporoses. Acton, Mass, Publishing Sciences Group, Inc, 1976.
39. Gustafsson L, Jacobson B, Kusoffsky L: X-ray spectrophotometry for bone mineral determinations. Med Biol Eng *12*:113, 1974.
40. Hahn TJ, Boisseau VC, Avioli LV: Effect of chronic corticosteroid administration on diaphyseal and metaphyseal bone mass. J Clin Endocrinol Metab *39*:274, 1974.
41. Hansson T, Roos B: Effect of combined therapy with sodium fluoride, calcium, and vitamin D on the lumbar spine in osteoporosis. Am J Roentgenol *126*:1294, 1976.
42. Ischerwood I, Rutherford RA, Pullan BR, Adams PH: Bone-mineral estimation by computer-assisted transverse axial tomography. Lancet *2*:712, 1976.
43. Jacobson B: Bone salt determination by x-ray spectrophotometry. *In* JR Cameron (Ed): Proceedings of Bone Measurement Conference. US Atomic Energy Commission Conference 700515, 1970, p. 237.
44. Joseph PM: Bone mineral determination: Methods and techniques to date. *In* F Feldman (Ed): Radiology, Pathology and Immunology of Bones and Joints. New York, Appleton-Century-Crofts, 1978, p 175.
45. Kennett TJ, Garnett ES, Webber CE: An in vivo measurement of absolute bone density. J Can Assoc Radiol *23*:168, 1972.
46. Kennett TJ, Webber CE: Bone density measured by photon scattering. II. Inherent sources of error. Phys Med Biol *21*:770, 1976.
47. Krokowski E: Quantitative analysis of calcium in the spine using x-rays of different energy qualities. Symposium on Bone Mineral Determinations, Stockholm/Studsvik, May 1974.
48. Lanzl LH, Strandjord N: Radioisotope device for measuring bone mineral. Proceedings of Symposium on Low-Energy X- and Gamma Sources and Applications. Chicago, Illinois Institute of Technology Research Institute, October 30, 1964.
49. Mack PB, O'Brien AT, Smith JM, Bauman AW: A method for estimating the degree of mineralization of bones from tracings of roentgenograms. Science *89*:467, 1939.
50. Mack, PB, Brown WN, Trapp HD: The quantitative evaluation of bone density. Am J Roentgenol *61*:808, 1949.
51. Mack PB: Radiographic bone densitometry. Washington DC, National Aeronautics and Space Administration, March 25, 1965, p 31.
52. Madsen M, Peppler W, Mazess RB: Vertebral and total body bone mineral content by dual photon absorptiometry. Proceedings of the Eleventh European Symposium on Calcified Tissues, 1975.
53. Manzke E, Chesnut CH, Wergedal JE, Baylink DJ, Nelp WB: Relationship between local and total bone mass in osteoporosis. Metabolism *24*:605, 1975.
54. Mazess RB: Non-invasive measurement of bone. *In* US Barzel (Ed): Osteoporosis. Vol II. New York, Grune & Stratton, 1979, p 5.
55. McNeill KG, Thomas BJ, Sturtridge WC, Harrison JE: In vivo neutron activation analysis for calcium in man. J Nucl Med *14*:502, 1973.
56. Meema HE, Bunker ML, Meema S: Loss of Compact bone due to menopause. Obstet Gynecol *26*:333, 1965.
57. Meema HE, Meema S: Cortical bone mineral density versus cortical thickness in the diagnosis of osteoporosis: a roentgenologic-densitometric study. J Am Geriat Soc *17*:120, 1969.
58. Meema HE, Meema S: Comparison of microradioscopic and morphometric findings in the hand bones with densitometric findings in the proximal

radius in thyrotoxicosis and in renal osteodystrophy. Invest Radiol *7*:88, 1972.

59. Minaire P, Meunier P, Edouard C, Bernard J, Courpron P, Bourret J: Quantitative histological data on disuse osteoporosis. Calcif Tissue Res *17*:57, 1974.
60. Rao PS, Gregg EC: Attenuation of monoenergetic gamma rays in tissues. Am J Roentgenol *123*:631, 1975.
61. Olkkonen H, Karjalainen P: A ^{170}Tm gamma scattering technique for the determination of absolute bone density. Br J Radiol *48*:594, 1975.
62. Orphanoudakis SC, Jensen PS, Rauschkolb EN, Lang R, Rasmussen H: Bone mineral analysis using single-energy computed tomography. Invest Radiol *14*:122, 1979.
63. Palmer HE, Nelp WB, Murano R, Rich C: The feasibility of in vivo neutron activation analysis of total body calcium and other elements of body composition. Phys Med Biol *13*:269, 1968.
64. Posner I, Griffiths HJ: Comparison of CT scanning with photon absorptiometric measurement of bone mineral content in the appendicular skeleton. Invest Radiol *12*:542, 1977.
65. Pridie RB: The diagnosis of senile osteoporosis using a new bone density index. Br J Radiol *40*:251, 1967.
66. Puumalainen P, Uimarihuhta A, Alhava EM, Olkkonen H: A new photon scattering method for bone mineral density measurements. Radiology *120*:723, 1976.
67. Reich NE, Seidelmann FE, Tubbs RR, MacIntyre WJ, Meaney TF, Alfidi RJ, Pepe RG: Determination of bone mineral content using CT scanning. Am J Roentgenol *127*:593, 1976.
68. Reiss KH, Steinle B: Medical application of the Compton effect. Siemens Forsch-u Enwicklungsber *2*:16, 1973.
69. Reiss KH, Killig K, Schuster W: Dual photon x-ray beam applications. *In* RB Mazess (Ed): Proceedings of the International Conference on Bone Mineral Measurement, Washington DC, National Institute of Arthritis, Metabolism, and Digestive Diseases, 1974, p 80.
70. Roh YS: Evaluation of Bone Mass and Bone Remodeling in Vivo and Its Clinical Application in Osteoarthrosis and Osteoporosis. PhD Thesis, Catholic University of Louvain, Belgium, 1973.
71. Roos B, Rosengren B, Skoldborn H: Determination of bone mineral content in lumbar vertebrae by a double gamma-ray technique. *In* JR Cameron (Ed): Proceedings of the Bone Measurement Conference US Atomic Energy Commission Conference 700515, 1970, p 243.
72. Roos B: Dual Photon Absorptiometry in Lumbar Vertebrae. Goteborg, Akademisk Avahling, 1974.
73. Rosenfeld D, Abols Y, Genant HK: Analysis of multiple energy computed tomography techniques for the measurement of bone mineral content. Proceedings of the 4th International Conference on Bone Measurement. Washington DC, US Government Printing Office, 1979.
74. Ruegsegger P, Elsasser U, Anliker M, Gnehm H, Kind H, Prader A: Quantification of bone mineralization using computed tomography. Radiology *121*:93, 1976.
75. Schlenker RA, VonSeggen WW: The distribution of cortical and trabecular bone mass along the lengths of the radius and ulna and the implication for in vivo bone mass measurements. Calif Tissue Res *20*:41, 1976.
76. Schraer H, Schraer R, Trostle HG, D'Alfonso A: The validity of measuring bone density from roentgenograms by means of a bone density computing apparatus. Arch Biochem Biophys *83*:486, 1959.
77. Shapiro JR, Moore WT, Jorgenson H, Reid J, Epps CH, Whedon D: Osteoporosis: Evaluation of diagnosis and therapy. Arch Intern Med *135*:563, 1975.
78. Smith DM, Johnston C Jr, Yu P-L: In vivo measurement of bone mass. JAMA *219*:325, 1972.
79. Smith DM, Khairi MRA, Johnston CC Jr: The loss of bone mineral with aging and its relationship to risk of fracture. J Clin Invest *56*:311, 1975.
80. Sorenson JA, Mazess RB: Effects of fat on bone mineral measurements. *In* JR Cameron (Ed): Proceedings of Bone Measurement Conference. US Atomic Energy Commission Conference 700515, 1970, p 255.
81. Steinbach HL: The roentgen appearance of osteoporosis. Radiol Clin North Am *2*:191, 1964.
82. Virtama P, Helela T: Radiographic measurements of cortical bone. Acta Radiol(Suppl) (Stockholm) *293*:7, 1969.
83. Visser WJ, Niermans HJ, Roelofs JMM, Raymakers JA, Duursma SA: Comparative morphometry of bone biopsies obtained by two different methods from the right and left iliac crest. *In* PJ Meunier (Ed): Bone Histomorphometry. Paris, Armour-Montagu, 1977, p 79.
84. Wahner H, Riggs BL, Beabout JW: Diagnosis of osteoporosis: Usefulness of photon absorptiometry at the radius. J Nucl Med *18*:432, 1977.
85. Webber CE, Kennett TJ: Bone density measured by photon scattering. I. A system for clinical use. Phys Med Biol *21*:760, 1976.
86. Williams ED, Boddy K, Harvey I, Haywood JK: Calibration and evaluation of a system for total body in vivo activation analysis using 14 MeV neutrons. Phys Med Biol *23*:405, 1978.
87. Wilson CR: Prediction of femoral neck and spine bone mineral content from the BMC of the radius or ulna and the relationship between bone strength and BMC. *In* RB Mazess (Ed): Proceedings of the International Conference on Bone Mineral Measurement. Washington DC, National Institute of Arthritis, Metabolism, and Digestive Diseases, 1974, p. 51.
88. Wilson CR, Madsen M: Dichromatic absorptiometry of vertebral bone mineral content. Invest Radiol *12*:180, 1977.

19

NEEDLE BIOPSY OF BONE

by Donald Resnick, M.D.

Open biopsy is an accepted surgical procedure in the diagnosis of a variety of skeletal disorders, including neoplastic, inflammatory, and metabolic conditions. Because this procedure requires considerable time and expense, operating room space, and personnel, as well as utilization of general anesthesia in most cases, repeated attempts have been made in the past to devise special instruments for percutaneous needle biopsy of bone.[1–13] More recently, advances in radiology, including image intensification, biplane videofluoroscopy, and high resolution radionuclide bone scanning, have underscored the fact that radiologists are in a unique position to perform such closed needle biopsies.[14–16]

The bone specimen can be obtained in one of two ways: an aspiration by needle or a core by trephine. Tissue obtained by needle aspiration is small in quantity and distorted, with loss of cellular configuration; tissue obtained by trephine biopsy is greater in quantity and intact, although this technique requires larger needle size. Needle aspiration is most useful for tissue culture to exclude infection, although some investigators report the value of needle aspiration in establishing a wide variety of clinical diagnoses[17, 18, 28]; trephine biopsy is a better technique for histologic diagnosis.[19, 29, 30]

ADVANTAGES AND DISADVANTAGES

Some of the advantages of closed needle biopsy of bone over open biopsy are obvious:

1. The method is relatively simple and the instruments are not technically complicated. The physician can gain expertise in the procedure in a short period of time. Closed needle biopsy can be accomplished quickly, usually within 45 minutes.
2. The patient is not submitted to any great risk. General anesthesia is not required and, in fact, the technique can be applied as an outpatient procedure, although we recommend that the patient be observed in the hospital for 24 hours following biopsy. Local complications such as infection are infrequent, and damage to internal organs does not occur if the procedure is accomplished carefully. The patient is not subjected to a major operative procedure even if a deep area of the skeleton must be biopsied.
3. Utilization of modern fluoroscopic equipment facilitates accurate needle placement and the site of such needle placement can be permanently recorded with spot film or overhead radiographs prior to biopsy.

The major disadvantages of closed needle biopsy are the following:

1. A relatively small amount of material is withdrawn. This is particularly true with fine needle biopsies in which meager cytologic material may not be representative of the entire lesion, leading to an inaccurate pathologic diagnosis. This disadvantage is not so apparent with trephine biopsy, as a larger quantity of tissue is removed. In certain situations, repeat closed or open biopsy is necessary.
2. The biopsy procedure is relatively "blind" in nature so that the ideal area of the lesion may not be biopsied. Utilization of high-quality fluoroscopic control minimizes this disadvantage.
3. The success of this procedure requires an experienced pathologist who cooperates closely with the radiologist. However, for open biopsies a similar situation exists, in which cooperation among a capable orthopedic surgeon, radiologist, and pathologist is required.
4. Although theoretically one could maintain that closed biopsy of a tumor may lead to its dissemination in neighboring and distant tissues, this is not a realistic complication of the procedure.

INDICATIONS AND CONTRAINDICATIONS

Although the indications for needle biopsy of bone will vary from one institution to another, certain guidelines do exist. General indications for this procedure include the following:

Neoplastic Disease

The procedure is indicated in the evaluation of patients with widespread osteolytic or osteoblastic lesions in whom the most probable diagnosis is metastatic disease. This indication could be expanded to include tumors, such as reticulum cell sarcoma, for which the anticipated modes of therapy would be chemotherapy or radiation therapy rather than surgery. The diagnosis of multiple myeloma should be documented by appropriate laboratory examination rather than by closed bone biopsy. After this diagnosis has been established, sternal or iliac crest marrow aspiration is a more appropriate examination. Occasionally closed biopsy techniques may be useful in a patient with solitary plasmacytoma.

The closed biopsy technique is also useful in evaluating debilitated patients with bone lesions that are not readily accessible to open biopsy in whom a long surgical procedure would not be well tolerated.

Surgical intervention and open biopsy are much more useful than closed biopsy in establishing a diagnosis of primary bone neoplasm.

Metabolic Disease

In order to accurately establish the presence and type of metabolic disease, open wedge resection or percutaneous biopsy of the iliac crest should be accomplished, as it is necessary to obtain a full-thickness bone sample with both cortices and medulla.[20] Large-core biopsy needles are utilized for this procedure, providing adequate material for histologic preparation.[32]

Infectious Disease

Closed needle biopsy or aspiration can be useful in establishing a diagnosis of osteomyelitis and septic arthritis. Material should be obtained both for histologic diagnosis and appropriate tissue culture.

Articular Disease

Although closed bone biopsy is not usually necessary in the diagnosis of articular disorders, it may be utilized to evaluate patients with subchondral cystic lesions in whom the exact diagnosis is in doubt. In this fashion, the presence of osteonecrosis, infection, degenerative disease, rheumatoid arthritis, or intraosseous ganglia may be substantiated.

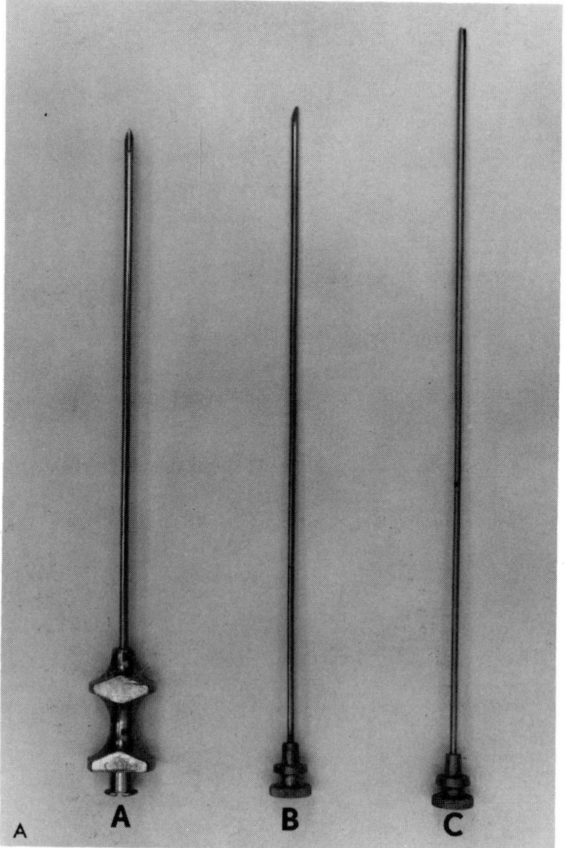

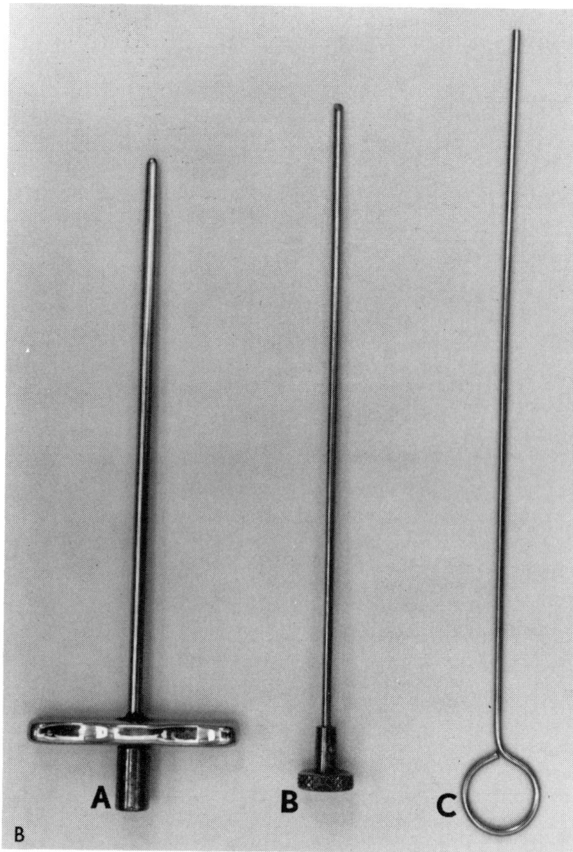

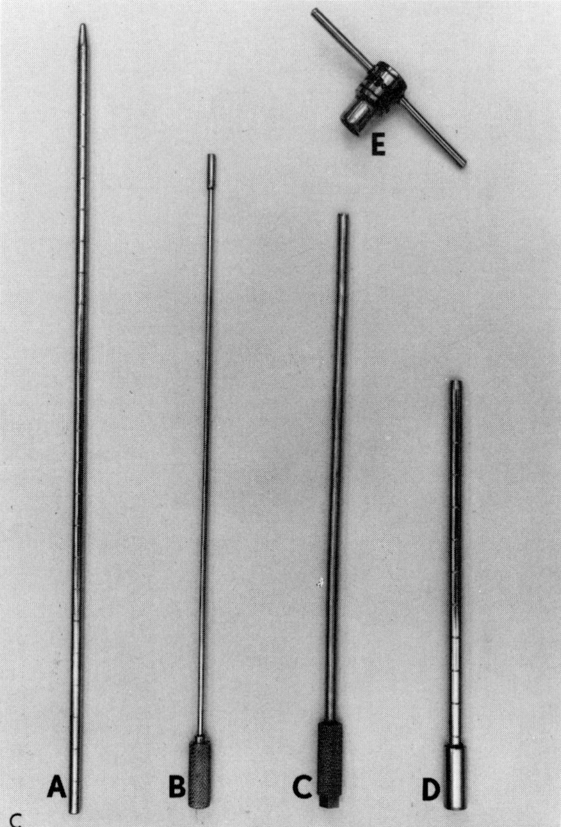

Figure 19–1. *Types of trephine needles.*

A *Vim-Silverman needle: Parts consist of an outer needle (A), obturator (B), and inner blades (C). The outer needle and obturator are inserted together. The obturator is then removed and the inner needle is inserted beyond the tip of the outer needle, engaging the biopsy tissue.*

B *Kormed needle: Parts consist of an outer needle (A), obturator (B), and probe (C). The outer needle and obturator are inserted together. The obturator is removed and the needle is advanced into the bone with a to-and-fro motion. After the needle is removed, the probe can be used to remove the biopsy tissue.*

C *Craig needle: Parts consist of a guide (A), probe (B), cutting needle (C), cannula (D), and handle (E). The guide is inserted into the biopsy site and the cannula is placed over the guide and held firmly against the bone. After the guide is removed, the cutting needle is inserted through the cannula. The handle is placed on the needle and the needle is advanced, utilizing a to-and-fro motion. After the needle is removed, the probe can be used to dislodge the specimen.*

Illustration continued on the opposite page

Miscellaneous Disorders

Closed bone biopsies can provide information in a wide variety of additional diseases, including Paget's disease, fibrous dysplasia, eosinophilic granuloma, and sarcoidosis.

Caution should be employed in obtaining biopsy material from a vertebral lesion with extensive destruction because of the possibility of causing considerable hemorrhage and spinal instability. Furthermore, one should utilize a right-sided approach to vertebral lesions whenever possible because of the presence of the aorta on the left side.

Metastatic deposits from certain primary neoplasms such as thyroid and renal carcinoma may be extremely vascular. It is not uncommon to note excessive bleeding during closed biopsy of these lesions, although the hemorrhage is generally controlled.

BIOPSY SITES

The utilization of radionuclide studies in the localization of appropriate biopsy sites should be emphasized. Scintigraphy may identify additional lesions that are more accessible to closed needle biopsy than the initially detected abnormality. Closed biopsy of radiographically and scintigraphically positive lesions is more successful than biopsy of lesions that are apparent only on radionuclide scans, although definite diagnoses may be established in the latter situation as well.[16, 31]

The preferred biopsy site is a prominent area of a non–weight-bearing bone. Additional accessible areas for biopsy are the pelvis and extremities. Biopsy of the lumbar spine is more easily performed than biopsy of the thoracic spine. Biopsy of the cranial vault and ribs should be undertaken with appropriate caution to ensure that the needle is not

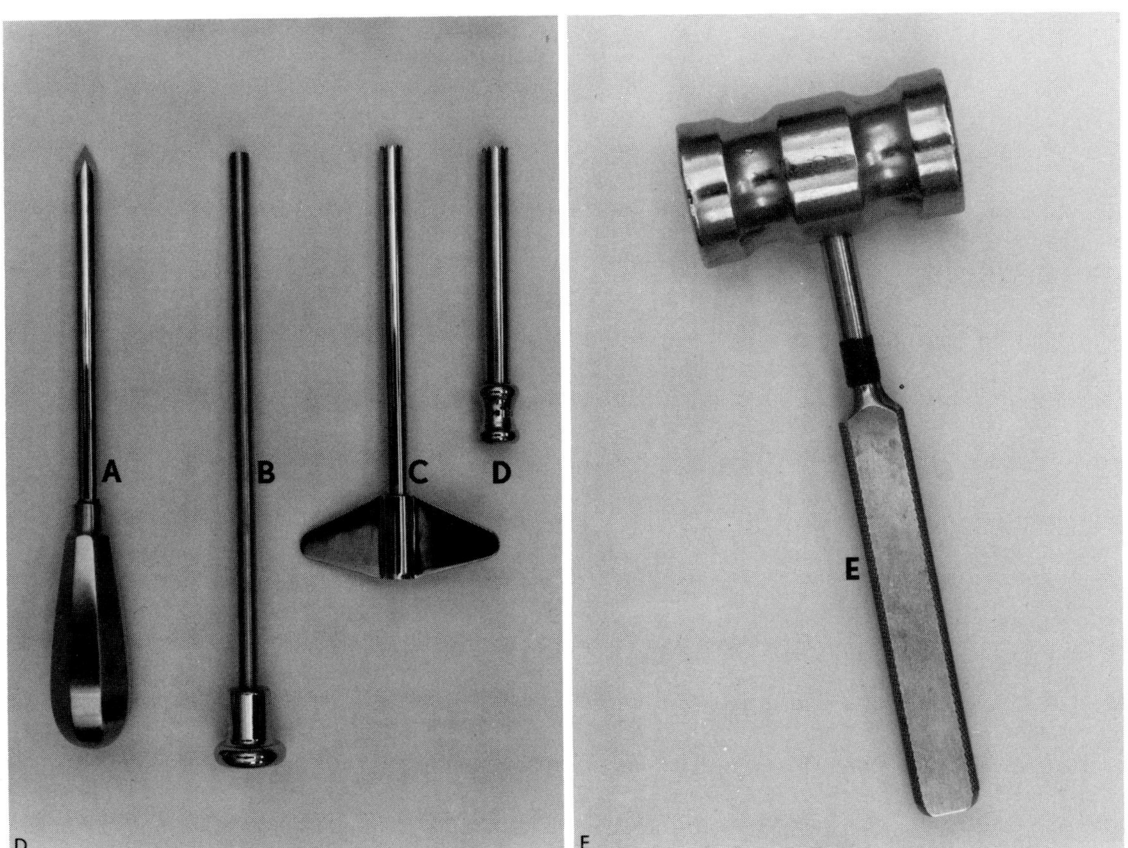

Figure 19–1. Continued

D, E *Meunier needle: Pertinent parts are guides (A, B), inner needle (C), outer needle (D), and hammer (E). Prior to biopsy, local anesthesia should be administered. A spinal needle is inserted through the skin and directed against the bone. A tap with the hammer (E), allows the needle to enter the bone marrow. A small amount of lidocaine can be administered directly into the marrow. The guide (B) and outer needle can be inserted down to the biopsy site. The guide is removed and the outer needle is advanced into the bone. The inner needle is inserted through the outer needle and extended into the bone with a twisting motion. The caliber of this needle allows a large specimen to be removed.*

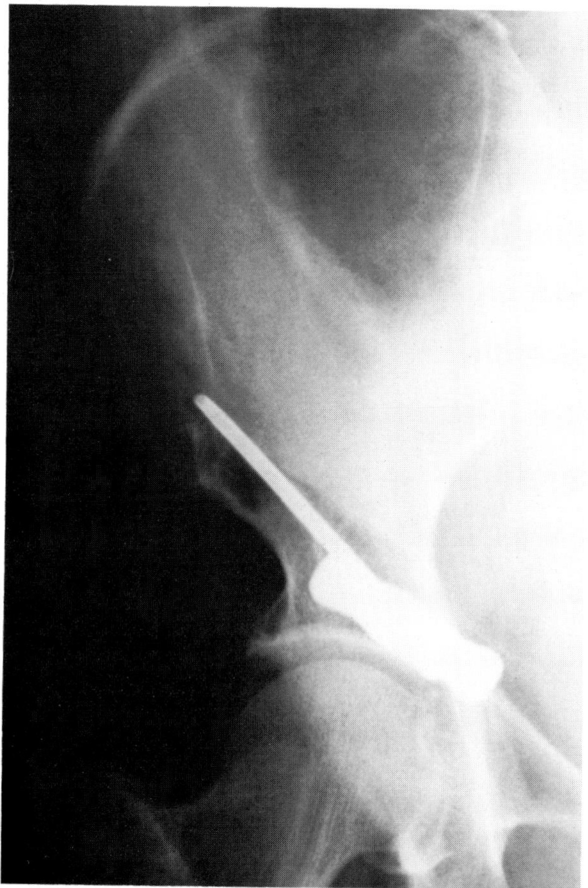

Figure 19–2. Iliac biopsy with Kormed needle: Skeletal metastasis. Observe that the outer needle has engaged a segment of abnormal bone.

inserted too deeply. Some investigators suggest that solitary lesions of the ribs that are demonstrable by radionuclide examination but not by radiographic examination should not be biopsied.[19]

NEEDLES: TYPES AND TECHNIQUES

A variety of needles are available for both trephine and aspiration biopsy. Trephine needles are of two basic types[19] (Fig. 19–1): some needles such as the Vim-Silverman (Fig. 19–1*A*) and Westerman-Jensen needles contain narrow, paired cutting blades that engage the tissue[21, 22]; other needles, such as the Kormed (Fig. 19–1*B*), Craig (Fig. 19–1*C*), Turkel, Ackermann, and Meunier (Fig. 19–1*D, E*) needles consist of round tubes with serrated edges that cut the tissue.[10, 23]

In our experience, the Kormed and Craig needles have been used most extensively (Figs. 19–2 to 19–4). The procedure for utilizing the Craig needle is simple. Following administration of local anesthesia into the skin, subcutaneous tissue, and periosteum, a blunt guide is inserted through the skin down to the biopsy site and its position is checked with fluoroscopy. A cannula is placed over the guide and held firmly against the bone. The guide is removed, and the cutting needle is then inserted through the cannula. This needle is approximately 2.5 cm longer than the cannula, this distance representing the depth of the biopsy specimen to be taken. With a to-and-fro twisting motion utilizing a variable amount of pressure, the cutting needle is driven into the bone and its position is again checked with fluoroscopy. A radiograph is obtained for documentation of accurate needle placement. While at its full depth, the needle is moved back and forth to dislodge the specimen from surrounding osseous tissue. The cutting needle is then removed, and the cannula is left in place. The cannula can subsequently be moved to a different location if a second biopsy specimen is required. The tissue is removed from the cutting needle with a long, thin probe and placed in an appropriate specimen container.

Minor differences exist between the Craig and both the Turkel and Ackermann needles.[19] With these latter instruments, the guide and cannula are inserted together. The cutting and removing of the specimen are accomplished in a fashion similar to that employed with the Craig needle. Of these three needles, the Ackermann needle is preferred for obtaining biopsy specimens of vascular lesions. The Turkel needle is more useful for evaluating sclerotic lesions because it contains stronger teeeth on its cutting surface.

The Westerman-Jensen and Vim-Silverman needles are particularly useful for biopsies of soft tissues and weakened bone. These needles contain three basic parts: an outer needle, an obturator, and inner blades. Initially, the obturator and outer needle are inserted through the skin into the bone or soft tissue. The obturator is then removed and the inner needle with its engaging blades is inserted beyond the tip of the outer needle, grasping the osseous or soft tissues. The outer needle is then advanced further, enclosing the inner needle, and both needles are removed together.

Aspiration needles of different sizes are available.[7, 12, 14, 17, 18, 24, 25] For evaluating many lesions, an 18 or 20 gauge needle may be sufficient. The needle with stylet is guided into the lesion with gentle pressure under fluoroscopic control. The stylet is removed and a syringe is utilized for tissue aspiration. It has been suggested that rotation of the syringe will allow more adequate biopsy samples. The material is placed on appropriate slides for cytology and, if required, in laboratory containers for culture and bacteriologic identification.

ADDITIONAL TECHNIQUES OF NEEDLE BIOPSY

The patient should not eat on the morning of the examination and is given both a mild sedative and pain medication. An intravenous catheter is placed

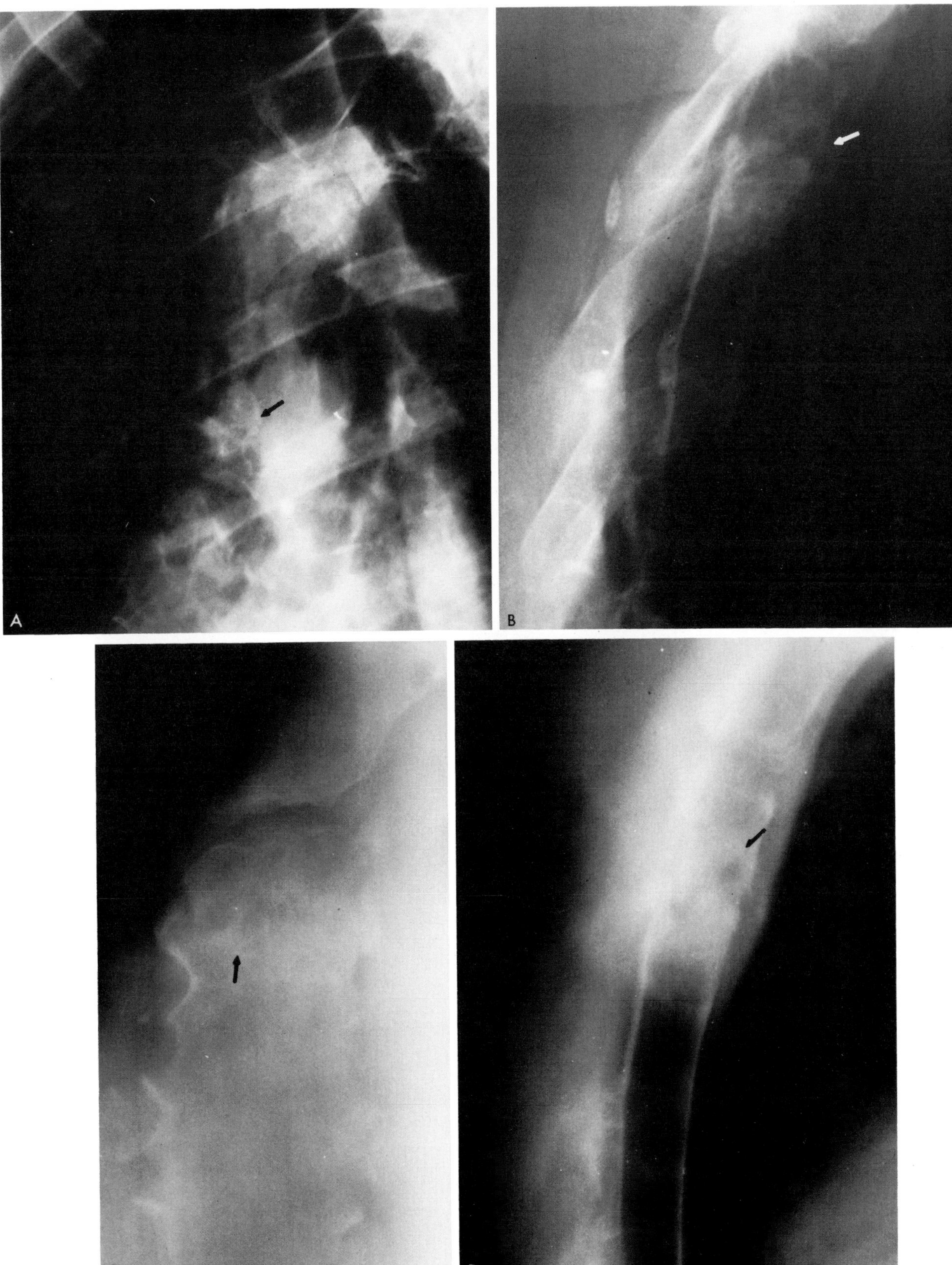

Figure 19–3. *Sternal biopsy with Kormed needle: Healing fracture.*

A, B *Oblique and lateral radiographs demonstrate a fracture of the body of the sternum (arrow).*

C, D *Frontal and lateral tomograms better delineate the fracture (arrow) and surrounding bony eburnation and soft tissue mass. Because the patient denied trauma and the lesion was associated with extensive sclerosis, a biopsy was recommended to exclude neoplasm.*

Illustration continued on the following page

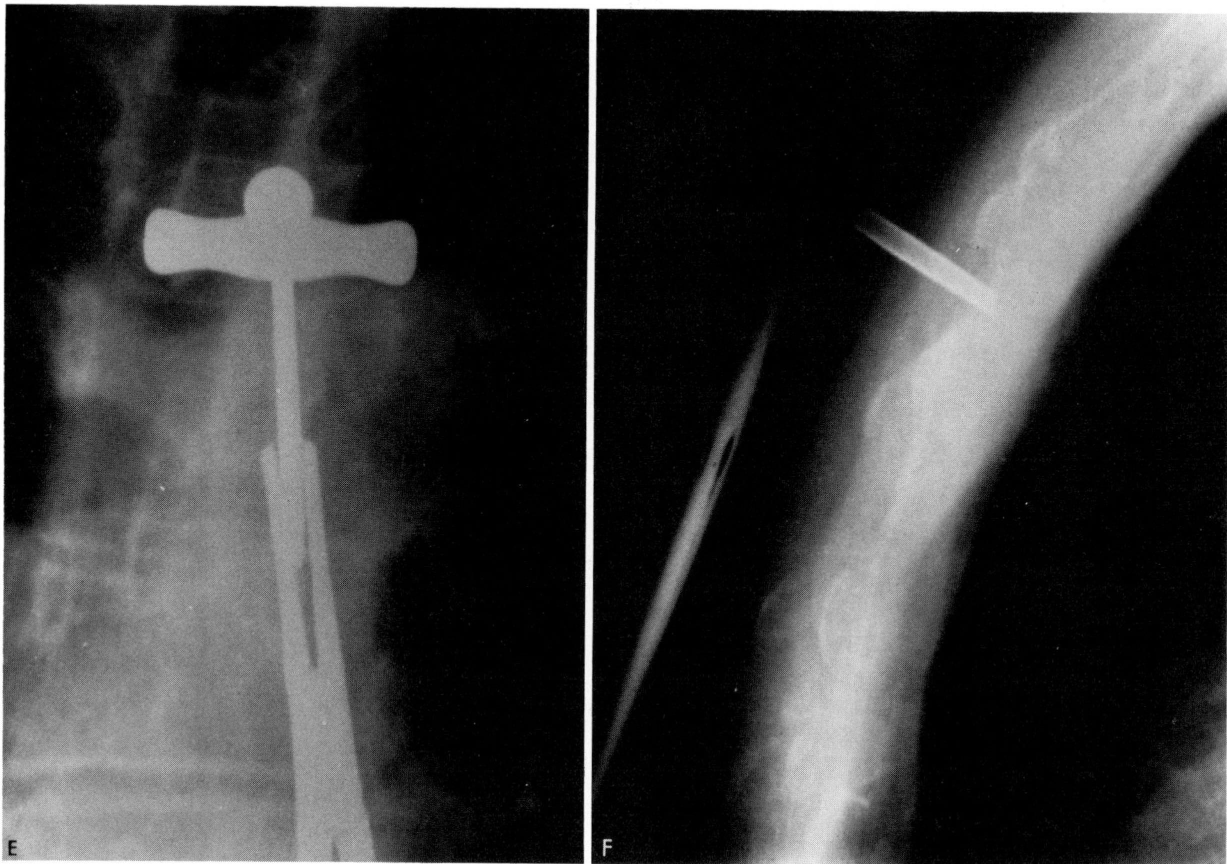

Figure 19–3. Continued
E, F *The outer needle is anchored in the lesion. The clamp is used to eliminate the possibility of inserting the needle too deeply.*

in the arm and saline solution is administered to keep the line open. All pertinent radiographs and radionuclide examinations are reviewed prior to the study. The examination is performed utilizing single plane or biplane fluoroscopy. The latter method is particularly useful when a vertebral body is being biopsied. Ample local anesthesia is infiltrated into the skin, subcutaneous tissue, and periosteum at the biopsy site. Fluoroscopic guidance during the procedure is employed. Bed rest and a mild analgesic agent may be required for 24 hours following the procedure. Following rib biopsy, chest radiographs should be obtained to exclude the presence of a pneumothorax.

Biopsy techniques for vertebral bodies have been well outlined.[13] These techniques vary, depending upon the level of the vertebral lesion. If possible, a right-sided approach should be employed.

Biopsy of the Tenth Through Twelfth Thoracic Vertebrae and the Lumbar Vertebrae (Fig. 19–5*A*)

The patient is placed in the prone position on the table. The point of needle entrance is 6.5 cm from the spinous process of the vertebra to be biopsied. A 20 gauge spinal needle is inserted at an angle of 145 degrees to the horizontal and passed slowly down to the bone. Inserting the needle at a greater angle may allow the dura to be entered; inserting the needle at a lesser angle may result in the vertebral body not being encountered. The angle of 145 degrees is ideal for biopsy of the vertebral body; it must be altered slightly if the posterior elements are to be biopsied. After checking the needle position under fluoroscopy and administering appropriate anesthesia, the physician inserts the biopsy needle in the same fashion.

Biopsy of the First Through Ninth Thoracic Vertebrae (Fig. 19–5*B*)

The patient is placed prone on the table. The point of entrance of the spinal needle is 4 cm from the spinous process of the vertebra to be biopsied. The needle is inserted at an angle of 120 to 125 degrees from the horizontal, passing over the superior aspect of the adjacent rib. The needle position is monitored several times with fluoroscopy as the needle is passed down to the bone. Appropriate anesthesia is administered, and the biopsy needle is inserted in the same fashion. Penetration of either needle should not exceed 7 cm.

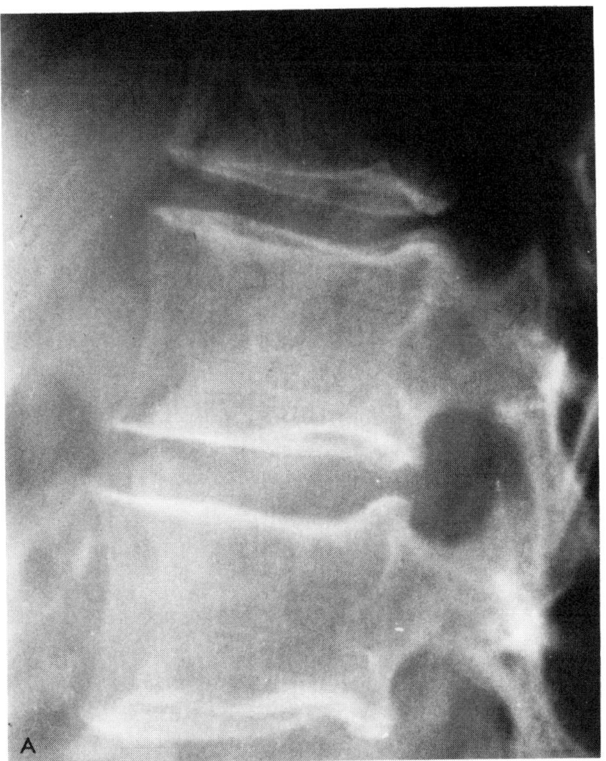

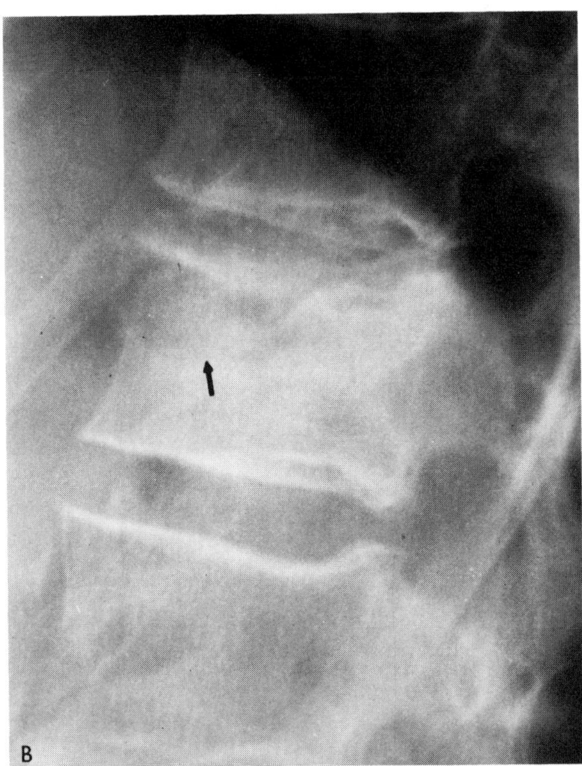

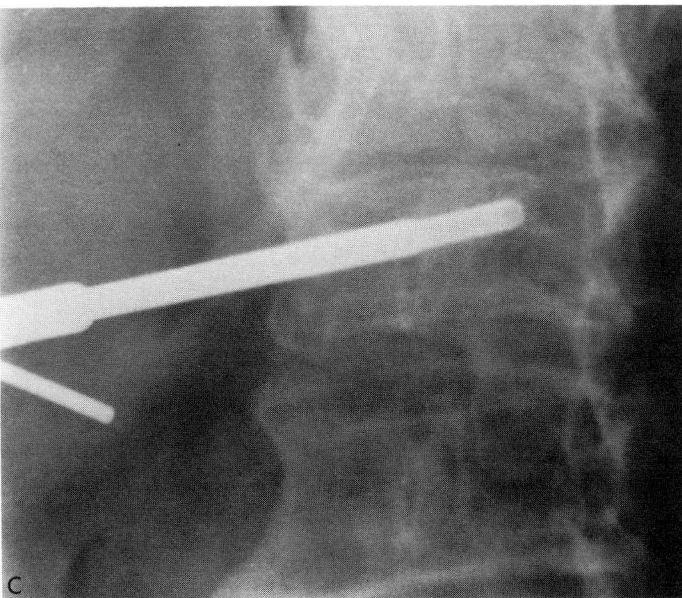

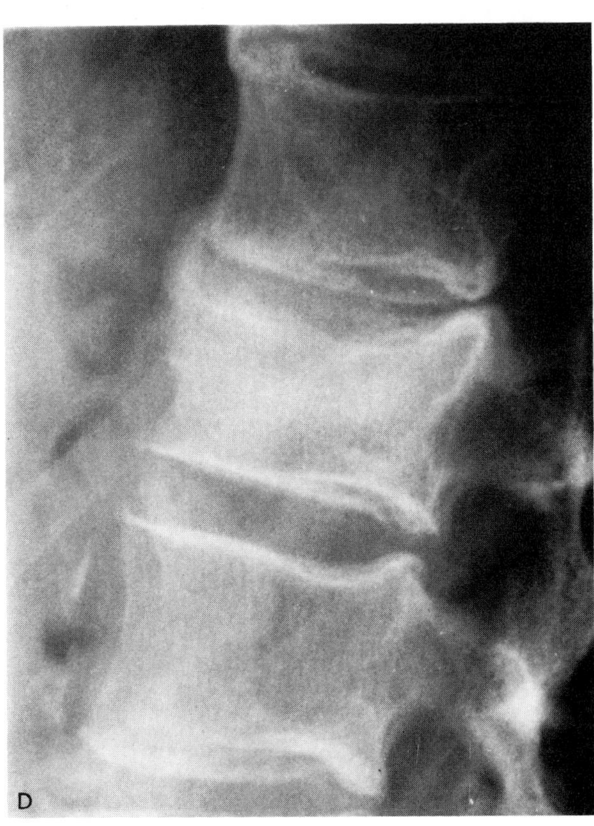

Figure 19–4. *Lumbar vertebral body biopsy with Craig needle: Healing fracture.*

A *Initial radiograph reveals normal vertebral body.*

B *One year later, collapse of the superior aspect of the lumbar vertebral body with adjacent lysis and sclerosis is apparent (arrow). The patient denied trauma.*

C *The cutting needle is anchored into the vertebral body. Biopsy revealed healing fracture without tumor.*

D *One year following biopsy, healing of the fracture with an adjacent osteophyte can be seen.*

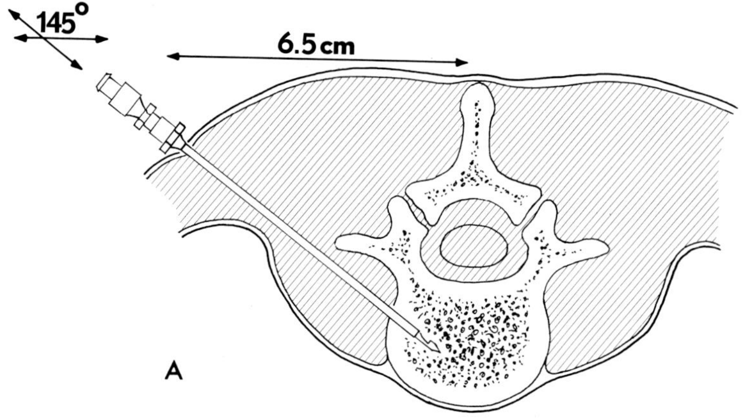

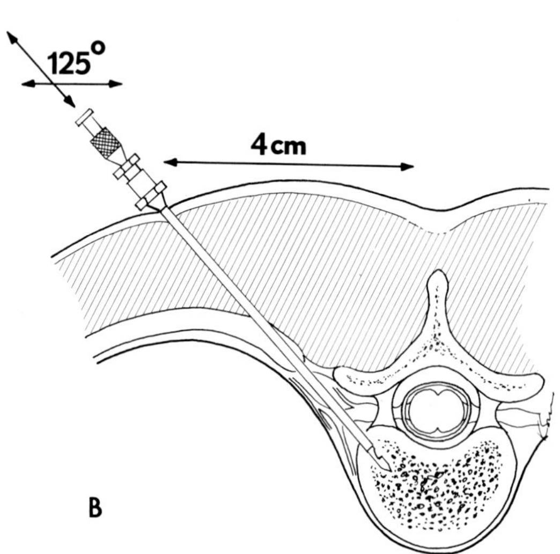

Figure 19–5. *Technique of spinal biopsy.*
A *Lower thoracic and lumbar vertebrae: The needle is inserted 6.5 cm from the spinous process at an angle of 145 degrees from the horizontal.*
B *Upper thoracic vertebrae: The needle is inserted 4 cm from the spinous process, over the rib at an angle of 125 degrees from the horizontal.*

RESULTS OF NEEDLE BIOPSY

Most observers believe that trephine biopsy is superior to aspiration biopsy in establishing a histologic diagnosis because of the larger sample of tissue obtained. The accuracy of trephine biopsy, however, depends in large part on the expertise of the pathologist as well as on the adequacy of the specimen. Debnam and Staple reported than an accurate diagnosis was made or disease was excluded in 81 per cent of patients or 74 per cent of biopsy sites,[19] which was a higher accuracy rate than had previously been recorded.[11, 26, 27] They attributed their relative success to careful selection of patients and biopsy site, the use of bone scanning, detailed radiographic study of involved sites, and careful biopsy technique under fluoroscopic control. Although there is apparent variability in the success rate of this procedure, needle biopsy of bone, when carefully performed and interpreted, can be an accurate procedure. It is expected that computed tomography will aid in this procedure.[33]

COMPLICATIONS

The procedure is usually performed without significant complication. Mild pain and discomfort are common. Hemorrhage can result when biopsies are obtained from patients with vascular tumors or when a venous or arterial structure is injured, particularly in biopsies of the spine. Acute paraplegia has been occasionally reported after spinal biopsy.[27] Pneumothorax may complicate rib biopsy, and fistulae rarely may appear after biopsy of a superficial infectious lesion. In selected patients, needle biopsy of bone is a safe procedure, which can be readily accomplished in the Radiology Department.

REFERENCES

1. Siffert R, Arkin AM: Trephine biopsy of bone with special reference to lumbar vertebral bodies. J Bone Joint Surg *31A*:146, 1949.
2. Ackermann W: Vertebral trephine biopsy. Ann Surg *143*:373, 1956.
3. Kendall PH: Needle biopsy of vertebral bodies. Ann Phys Med *5*:236, 1960.
4. Valls J, Ottolenghi CE, Schajowicz F: Aspiration biopsy in the diagnosis of lesions of vertebral bodies. JAMA *136*:376, 1948.
5. Martin HE, Stewart FW: Advantages and limitations of aspiration biopsy. Am J Roentgenol *35*:245, 1936.
6. Hyman G: Comparison of bone-marrow aspiration and skeletal roentgenograms in diagnosis of metastatic carcinoma. Cancer *8*:576, 1955.
7. Ottolenghi CE: Diagnosis of orthopedic lesions by aspiration biopsy. Results of 1061 punctures. J Bone Joint Surg *37A*:443, 1955.
8. Hoffman WJ: New technique and instruments for obtaining biopsy specimens. Am J Cancer *15*:212, 1931.
9. Robertson RC, Ball RP: Destructive spine lesions: Diagnosis by needle biopsy. J Bone Joint Surg *17*:749, 1935.
10. Turkel H, Bethell FH: Biopsy of bone marrow performed by new and simple instrument. J Lab Clin Med *28*:1246, 1943.
11. Ackermann W: Application of the trephine for bone biopsy. Results in 635 cases. JAMA *184*:11, 1963.
12. Schajowicz F, Derqui JC: Puncture biopsy in lesions of the locomotor system. Review of results in 4050 cases, including 941 vertebral punctures. Cancer *21*:531, 1968.
13. Ottolenghi CE: Aspiration biopsy of the spine. J Bone Joint Surg *51A*:1531, 1969.
14. Lalli AF: Roentgen-guided aspiration biopsies of skeletal lesions. J Can Assoc Radiol *21*:71, 1970.
15. Rabinov K, Goldman H, Rosbash H, Simon M: The role of aspiration biopsy of focal lesions in lung and bone by simple needle and fluoroscopy. Am J Roentgenol *101*:932, 1967.
16. Debnam JW, Staple TW: Needle biopsy of bone. Radiol Clin North Am *13*:157, 1975.
17. Thommesen P, Frederiksen P: Fine needle aspiration biopsy of bone lesions: Clinical value. Arch Orthop Scand *47*:137, 1976.
18. Akerman M, Berg NO, Persson BM: Fine needle aspiration biopsy in the evaluation of tumor-like lesions of bone. Acta Orthop Scand *47*:129, 1976.
19. Debnam JW, Staple TW: Trephine bone biopsy by radiologists. Results of 73 procedures. Radiology *116*:607, 1975.
20. Johnson KA, Kelly PJ, Jowsey J: Percutaneous biopsy of the iliac crest. Clin Orthop Rel Res *123*:34, 1977.
21. Tenopyr J, Silverman I: The importance of biopsy in tumor diagnosis. Radiology *36*:57, 1941.
22. Ellis LD, Jensen WN, Westerman MP: Needle biopsy of bone and marrow. Arch Intern Med *114*:213, 1964.
23. Craig FS: Vertebral body biopsy. J Bone Joint Surg *38A*:93, 1956.
24. Hajdu SI, Melamed MR: Needle biopsy of primary malignant bone tumors. Surg Gynecol Obstet *133*:829, 1971.
25. Schajowicz F: Aspiration biopsy in bone lesions. J Bone Joint Surg *37A*:465, 1955.
26. Cramer LE, Kuhn C III, Stein AH Jr: Needle biopsy of bone. Surg Gynecol Obstet *118*:1253, 1964.
27. Stahl DC, Jacobs B: Diagnosis of obscure lesions of the skeleton. Evaluation of biopsy methods. JAMA *201*:229, 1967.
28. Adler O, Rosenberger A: Fine needle aspiration biopsy of osteolytic metastatic lesions. Am J Roentgenol *133*:15, 1979.
29. Moore TM, Meyers MH, Patzakis MJ, Terry R, Harvey JP Jr: Closed biopsy of musculoskeletal lesions. J Bone Joint Surg *61A*:375, 1979.
30. DeSantos LA, Murray JA, Ayala AG: The value of percutaneous needle biopsy in the management of primary bone tumors. Cancer *43*:735, 1979.
31. Collins JD, Bassett L, Main GD: Kagan C: Percutaneous biopsy following positive bone scans. Radiology *132*:439, 1979.
32. Meunier P, Courpron P, Giroux JM, Edouard C, Bernard J, Vignon G: Bone histomorphometry as applied to research on osteoporosis and to the diagnosis of hyperosteoidosis states. *In* SP Nielsen, E Hjorting-Hansen (Eds): Calcified Tissues 1975: Proceedings of the Eleventh European Symposium on Calcified Tissues. Copenhagen, Denmark, FADL Publishing Co, 1976, p 354.
33. Hardy DC, Murphy WA, Gilula LA: Computed tomography in planning percutaneous bone biopsy. Radiology *134*:447, 1980.

SECTION III

NORMAL VARIANTS AND ARTIFACTS

20

NORMAL ANATOMIC VARIANTS AND ARTIFACTS THAT MAY SIMULATE DISEASE

by Theodore E. Keats, M.D.

The diagnostician must be familiar with normal variation if he is not to give his patients diseases which they do not have.

John Caffey

The roentgenographic examination represents a major contribution to the diagnosis and differential diagnosis of skeletal disorders. This is particularly true in view of the fact that the identification of the disease process and its differentiation from other disorders is often still a difficult process by clinical and laboratory examination. It is, therefore, of great importance that the physician be aware of the many anatomic variants and roentgenographic pitfalls that may mislead in the assessment of the patient with skeletal complaints.

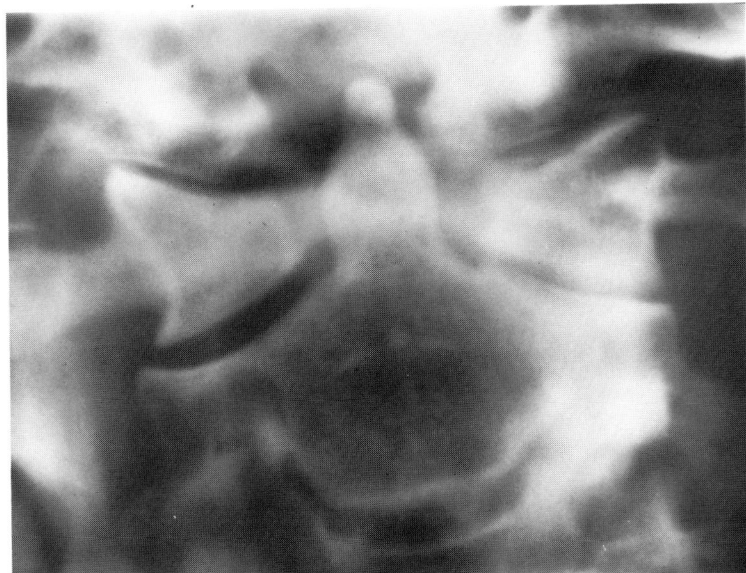

Figure 20–1. *Normal pointed configuration of the odontoid tip.*

Nature has supplied us with a myriad of anatomic variations that complicate the roentgenographic examination. Many of these are simply the changes of growth, others are variations in individual development, and still others are positional artifacts, but all of these are potentially misleading.

Because of the limitation of space, I have chosen from a large amount of material a number of entities which to my mind are often confused with true disease, or which have potential for harm if they are misinterpreted. This survey is by no means exhaustive, and the interested reader is urged to consult the more comprehensive works on the subject of normal anatomic variation for help with problems that are not presented here.[11, 14]

CERVICAL SPINE

Erosion and destruction of the odontoid process is a well recognized characteristic of a number of the inflammatory arthritides and one should not confuse minor variations of configuration with manifestations of this inflammatory process (Figs. 20–1 and 20–2). Similarly, in the search for involvement of the

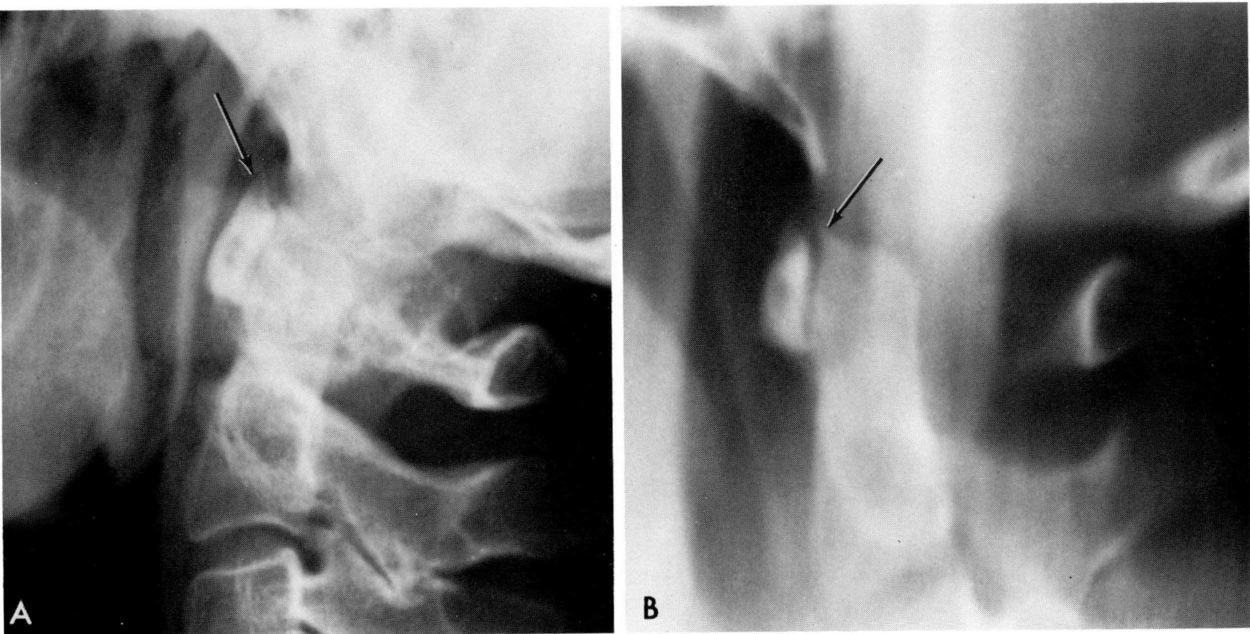

Figure 20–2. *Pointed configuration of the superior aspect of the anterior arch of C1 and the tip of the odontoid process (arrow), which should not be mistaken for an erosive alteration.* **A,** *Plain film;* **B,** *laminogram.*

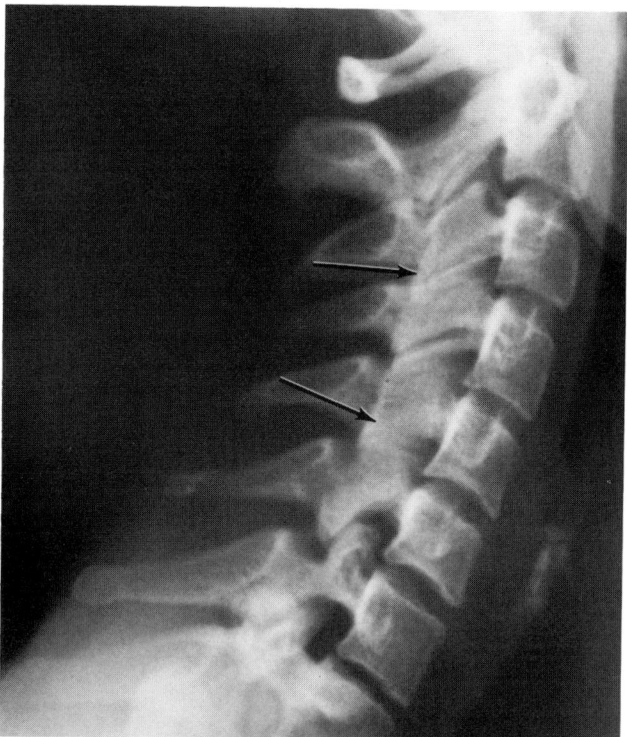

Figure 20–3. Simulated fusion of the posterior cervical elements produced by projection (arrows).

apophyseal joints of the cervical spine, these joints in the midcervical spine may not be well seen and give the appearance of fusion owing to positioning of the spine and the direction of the x-ray beam (Fig. 20–3). This matter is easily resolved by obtaining oblique projections that will show well-defined articular surfaces in the normal individual.

Another apparent abnormality, which may be produced by faulty positioning, is factitial calcification of the posterior spinal ligament as the result of slight rotation of the spine at the time of filming, so that two posterior aspects of the vertebral bodies are seen (Fig. 20–4). This situation, too, will be resolved by repetition of the examination with correct positioning of the spine.

The superior articular surfaces of the fifth to seventh cervical vertebrae in some normal individuals may show a groove or depression, which should not be mistaken for an erosive process or traumatic alteration[20] (Fig. 20–5).

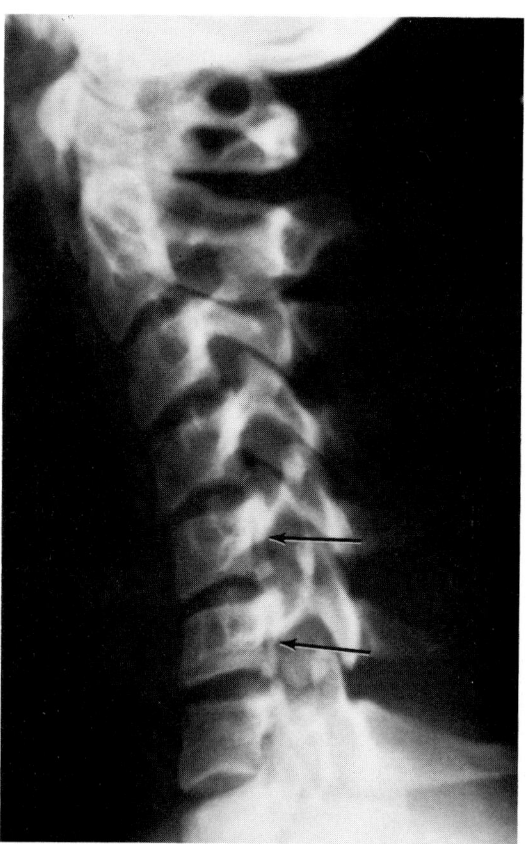

Figure 20–4. Simulated posterior spinal ligament calcification (arrows) produced by rotation of the neck at the time of filming.

CLAVICLE AND RIBS

The point of insertion of the rhomboid ligament at the inferior aspect of the medial portion of the clavicle in some individuals is reflected as a deep and, at times, irregular fossa (Fig. 20–6*A*). These fossae are not always present bilaterally, nor are they

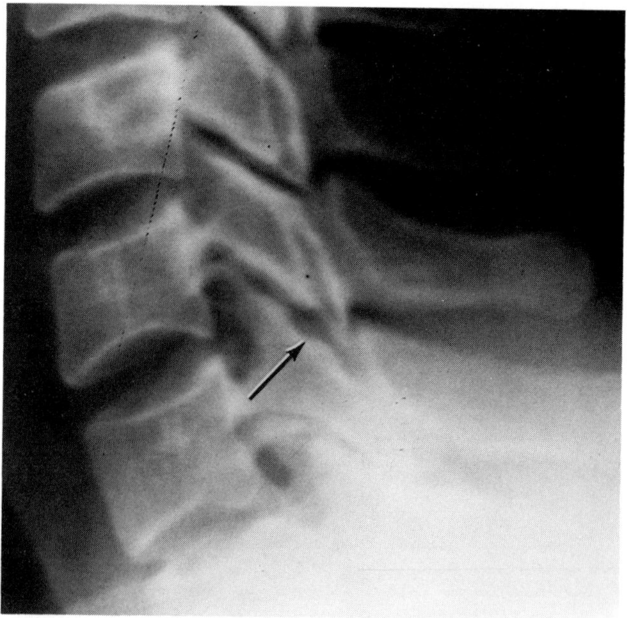

Figure 20–5. Insignificant irregularities of the joint surface of the articular process of the sixth cervical vertebra (arrow).

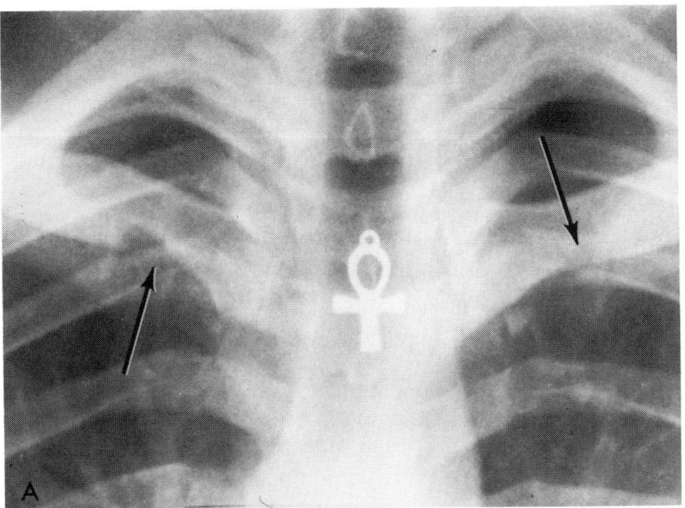

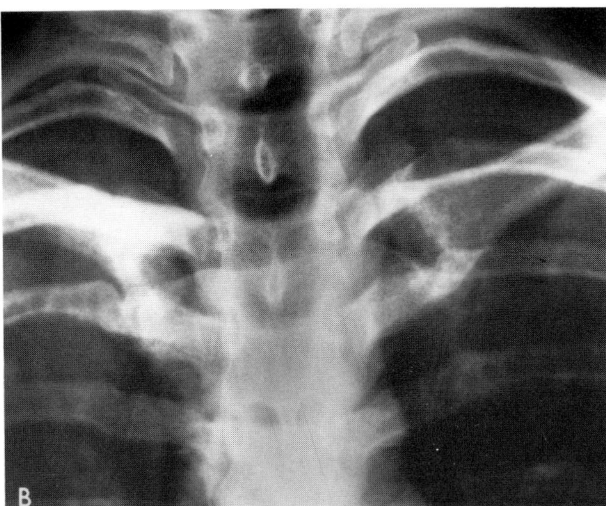

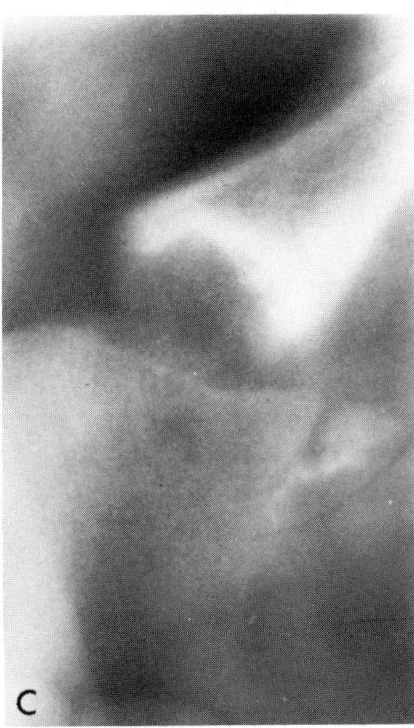

Figure 20–6. **A,** *Rhomboid fossae, the insertion points of the rhomboid ligament (arrows).* **B,** *Plain film, and* **C,** *laminogram, of normal irregularity of the medial ends of the clavicles of an adolescent before development of the secondary ossification centers.*

symmetric in configuration if they occur bilaterally. They are, at times, sufficiently striking to be confused with a destructive process.

A potential pitfall in the radiologic search for evidence of arthritis is the appearance of the medial ends of the clavicles in adolescence (Fig. 20–6*B*, *C*). Before the secondary centers appear at approximately the age of 17 years, the medial ends of the clavicles appear cupped and irregular, and this appearance might be mistaken for an inflammatory arthritis or as evidence of a metabolic bone disorder.

Loss of the cephalic margins of the posterior aspects of the upper ribs is a recognized phenomenon that occurs in a variety of diseases, including the collagen vascular disorders. It is seen most commonly in rheumatoid arthritis and in hyperparathyroidism. However, it may also be seen in the elderly as a manifestation of the restrictive lung disease of the aged (Fig. 20–7). The common denominator in all the conditions in which it has been described is probably disuse.[13]

UPPER EXTREMITY

Marginal irregularities of the edges of the glenoid fossa, a common finding in pubertal children, may simulate marginal joint destruction of arthritis (Fig. 20–8). Such irregularities are particularly marked at the superior margin. These irregularities disappear by the time the secondary centers of ossification become evident.

One should be careful not to interpret the density produced by the superimposed shadows of the

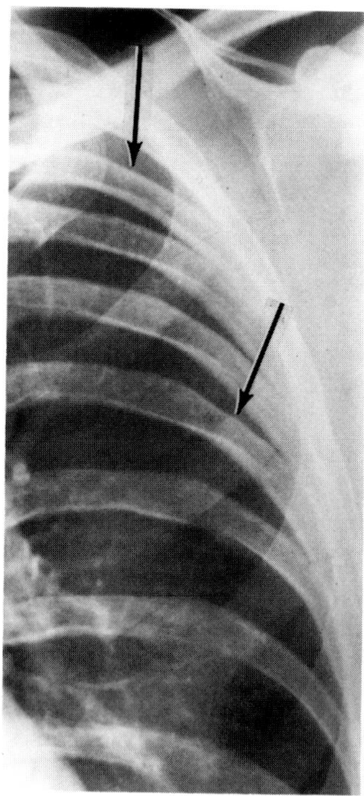

Figure 20–7. Simulated erosion of the upper rib margins in an asymptomatic elderly man (arrows).

humeral head and the scapula as evidence of aseptic necrosis of the humeral head (Fig. 20–9).

Notches or shallow grooves in the medial cortex of the metaphysis of the proximal end of the humerus are seen as a normal variant in children between the ages of 10 and 16 years (Fig. 20–10). These are asymptomatic and apparently represent a transient event in the growth period. These cortical alterations may be unilateral or bilateral and are of concern only in that they may be mistaken for an inflammatory or neoplastic alteration.[18]

The greater tuberosity of the humerus in some individuals contains a large amount of cancellous bone, which then projects in the radiograph as a circumscribed area of radiolucency that may simulate a destructive lesion (Fig. 20–11).

The thin flange of bone that constitutes the lateral cortical margin of the distal portion of the humerus is often projected in a fashion that simulates periosteal proliferation (Fig. 20–12). This is misinterpreted as evidence of reactive new bone formation. Similarly, the thin flanges of bone that serve as the attachment of the interosseous membrane in the forearm may likewise be mistaken as abnormal periostitis (Fig. 20–13).

Patients in whom the ulna is relatively short in comparison with the radius often show a rather deep fossa at the site of the inferior radioulnar articulation, which may stimulate an inflammatory arthritic process (Fig. 20–14).

The triangular cartilage of the wrist just distal to the end of the ulna is frequently a site of abnormal calcification. One should keep in mind that there is an accessory bone, the os triangulare, that may be found in this position as well (Fig. 20–15), and it often occurs bilaterally.

Congenital fusions of the carpal bones are often a familial trait. These fusions most commonly involve the lunate and triquetral bones (Fig. 20–16) but may involve others, such as the scaphoid and trapezium (Fig. 20–17).

The pisiform is a sesamoid bone and ossifies in

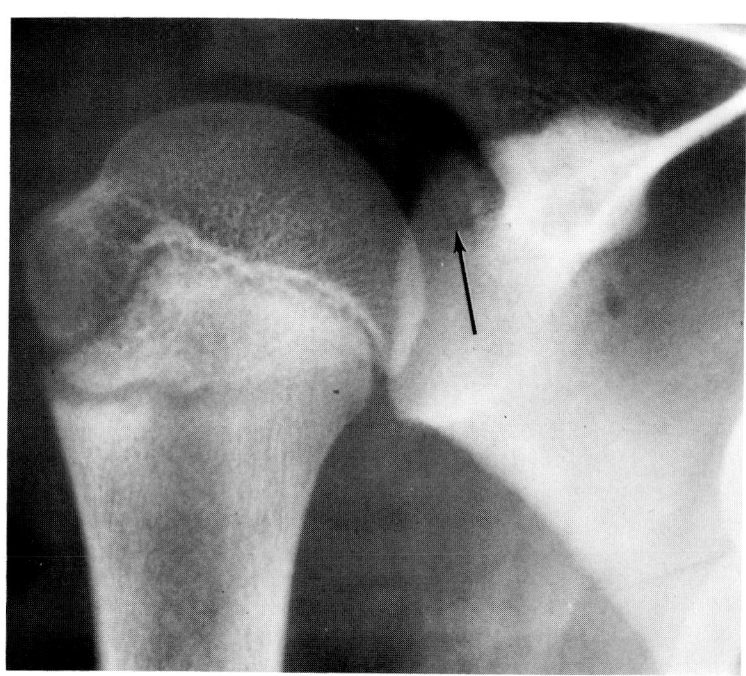

Figure 20–8. Normal developmental irregularity of the glenoid fossa in a 14 year old boy (arrow).

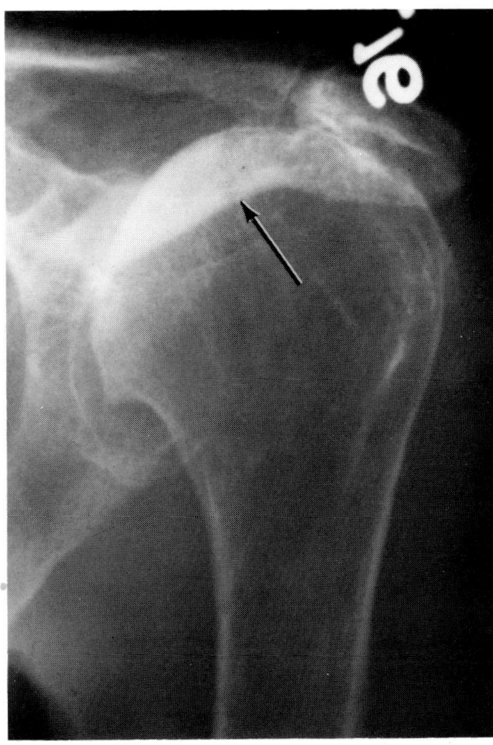

Figure 20–9. Overlapping shadows of the humerus and scapula (arrow) simulating aseptic necrosis of the humeral head in a patient with a rotator cuff tear.

an irregular fashion, best seen in the lateral projection. Such irregularity should not be confused with a pathologic process in young children (Fig. 20–18).

Narrow medullary cavities of the metacarpals are normal variations in development and are without pathologic significance (Fig. 20–19).

Spur-like extensions of the medial aspects of the epiphyses of the distal ends of the metacarpals represent a transient event in the ossification of this end of the bone (Fig. 20–20). In some individuals, after completion of growth, a spur-like extension of the radial side of the metaphysis of the distal ends of the metacarpals may be seen in the oblique projection (Fig. 20–21).

Common sources of confusion in the early diagnosis of rheumatoid arthritis are apparent small defects in the bases of the proximal phalanges (Fig. 20–22). These can be disregarded if there are no associated erosions in the metacarpal heads or disturbances in joint architecture.[7]

The nutrient canals of the distal ends of the proximal phalanges may be quite prominent and cast shadows that simulate areas of intraosseous bony destruction (Fig. 20–23).

The bony ridges and projections seen in the proximal phalanges, which represent areas of insertion of muscles, should not be confused with reactive new bone formation (Fig. 20–24).

Ivory epiphyses in the hands of healthy children

Text continued on page 716

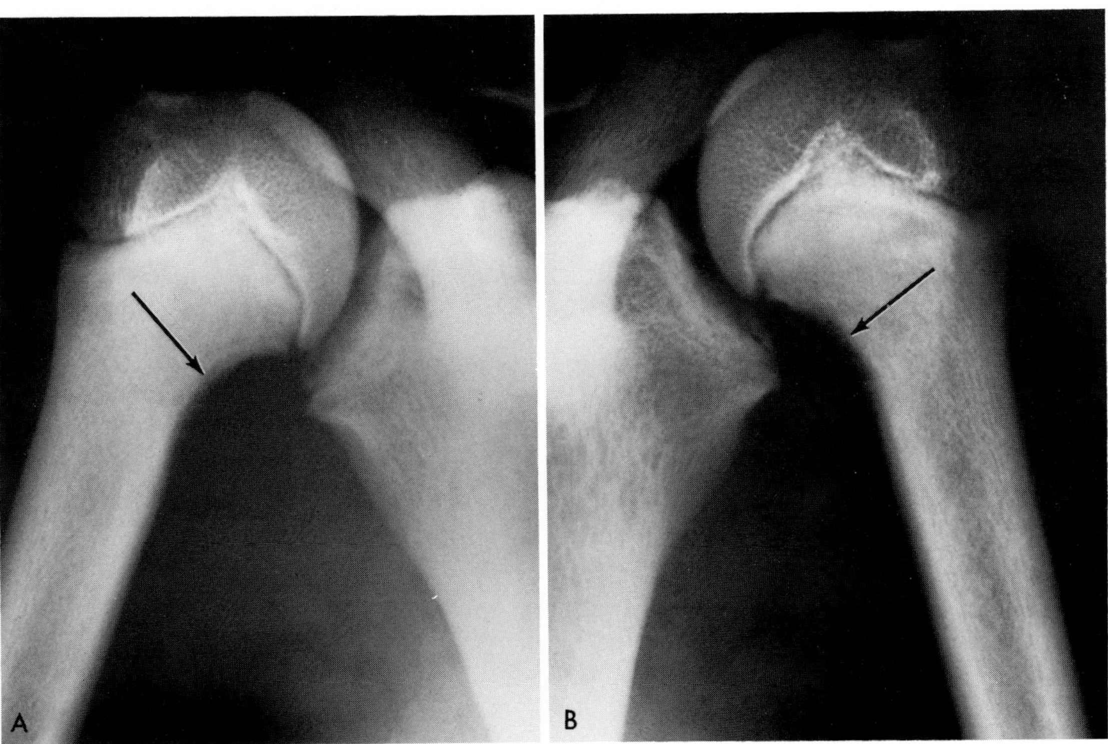

Figure 20–10. The cortical defects in the medial humeral metaphyses (arrow) of this 10 year old girl are normal variations of growth.

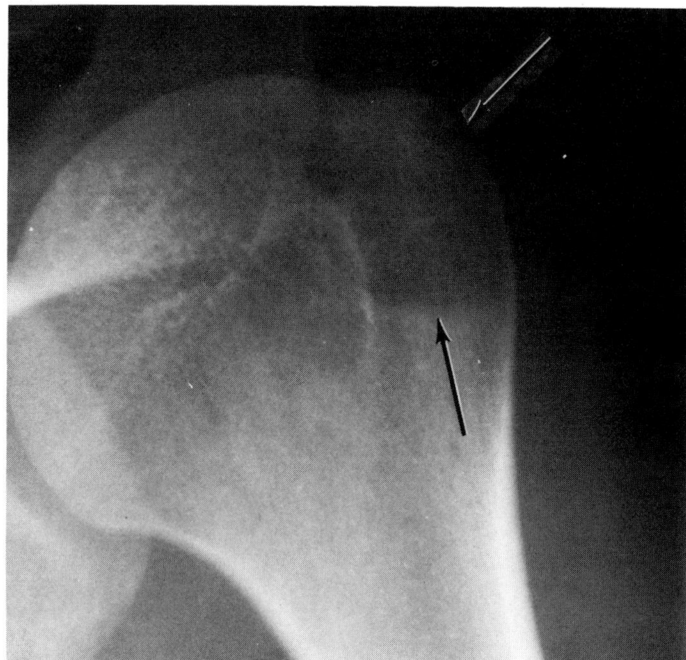

Figure 20–11. *Simulated destructive lesion of the humerus produced by the cancellous bone of the greater tuberosity (arrows).*

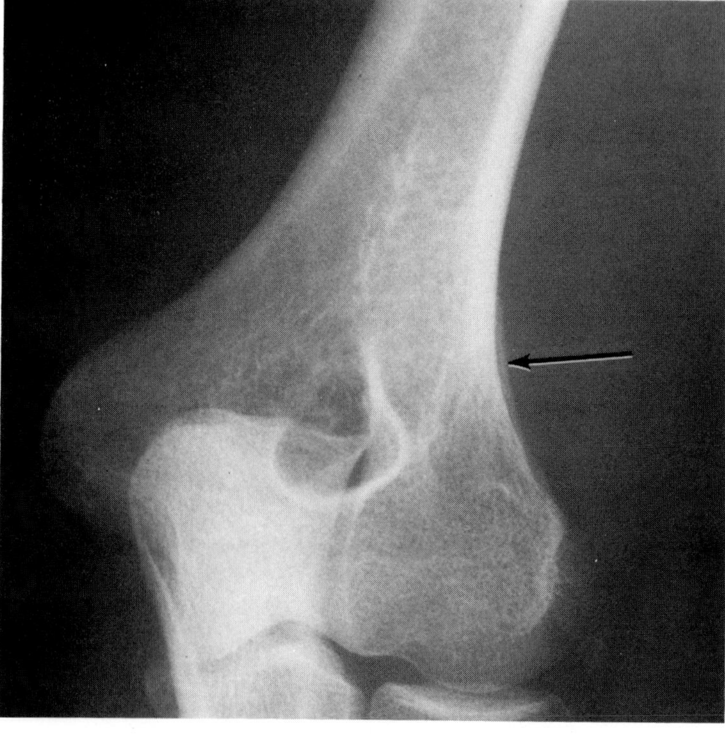

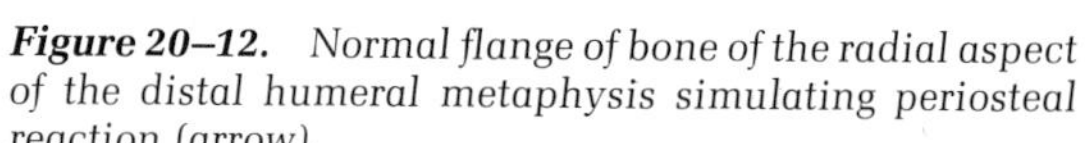

Figure 20–12. *Normal flange of bone of the radial aspect of the distal humeral metaphysis simulating periosteal reaction (arrow).*

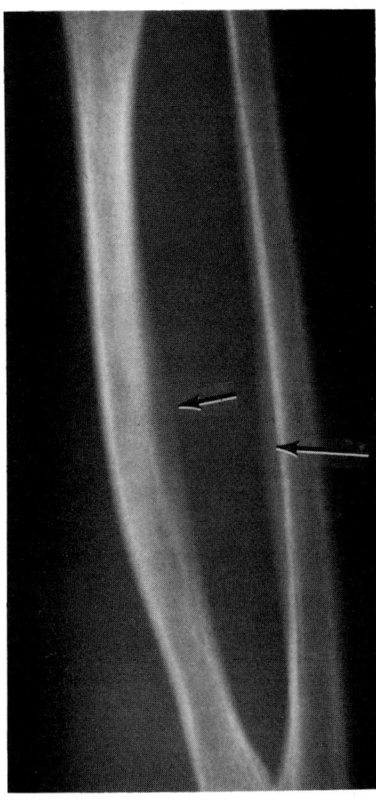

Figure 20–13. Normal bony flanges for the insertion of the interosseous membrane that may simulate new bone formation (arrows).

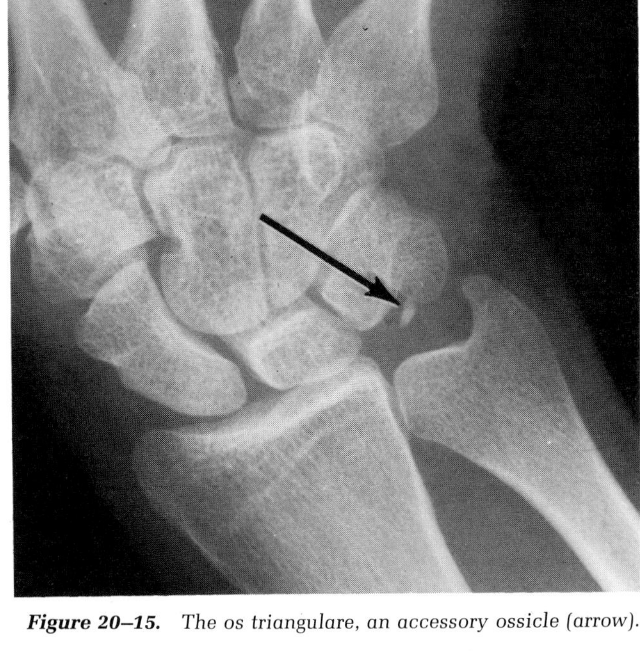

Figure 20–15. The os triangulare, an accessory ossicle (arrow).

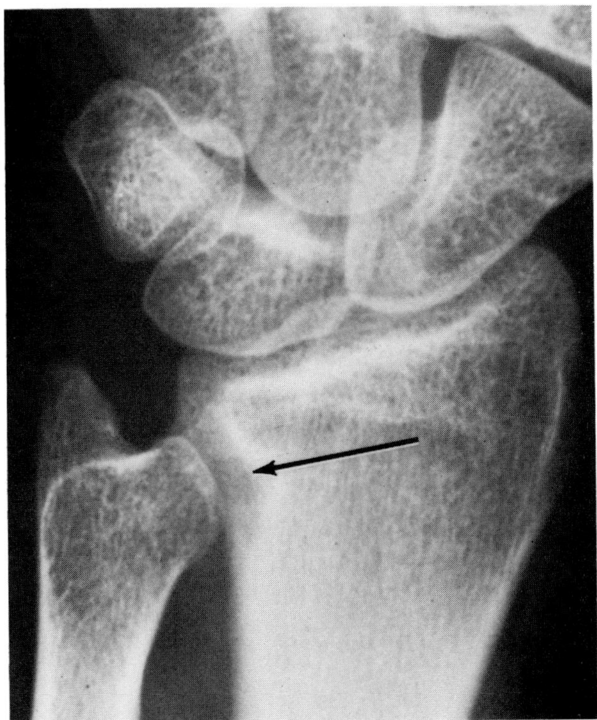

Figure 20–14. In patients who have a relatively short ulna, the fossa at the inferior radioulnar articulation should not be mistaken for a destructive or arthritic process (arrow).

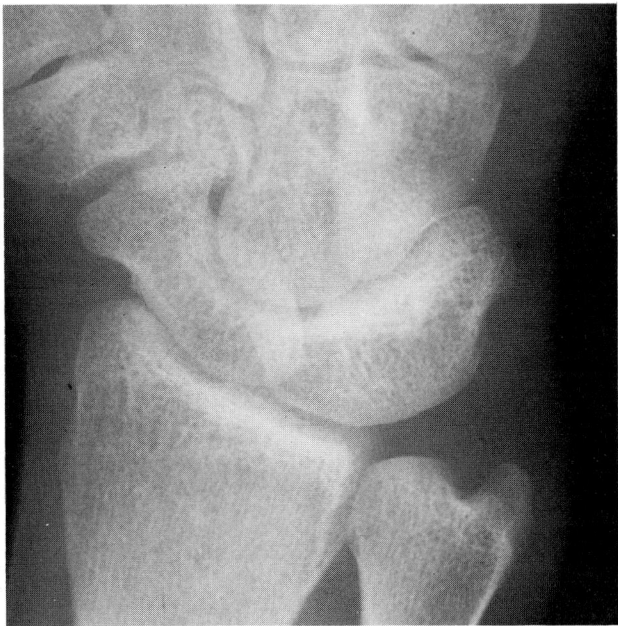

Figure 20–16. Congenital fusion of the lunate and triquetral bones.

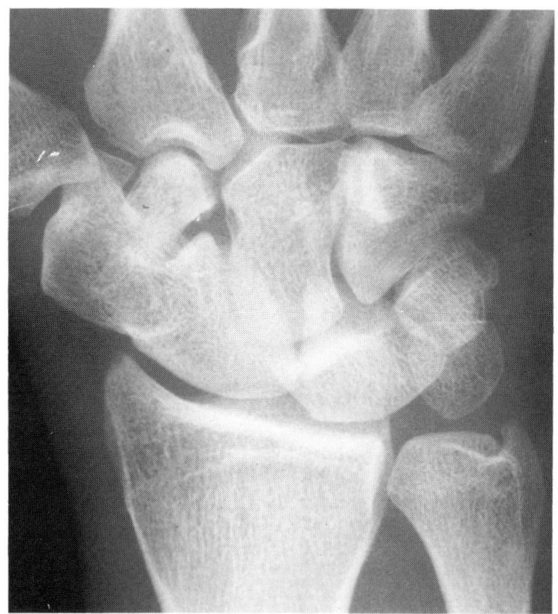

Figure 20–17. *Congenital fusion of the scaphoid and trapezium.*

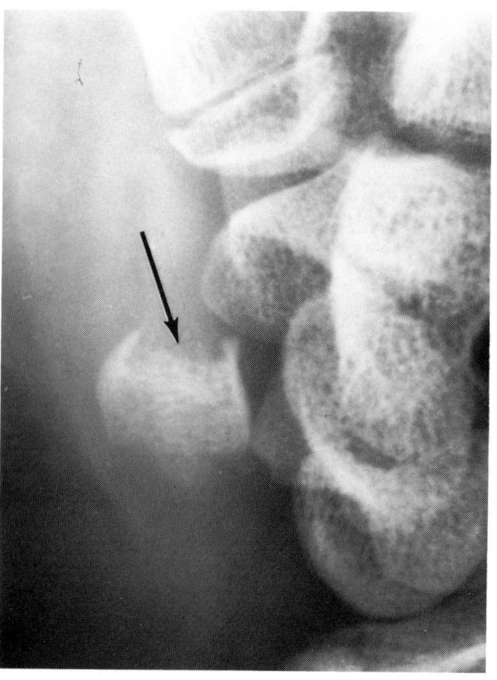

Figure 20–18. *Normal irregularity of the pisiform bone in an 11 year old boy (arrow).*

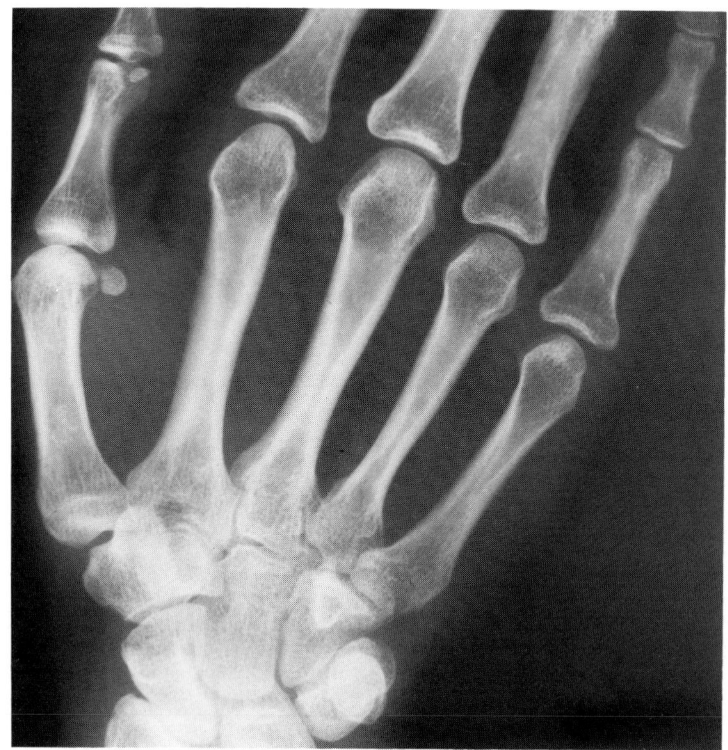

Figure 20–19. *Narrowing of the medullary cavities of the metacarpals, a normal variant.*

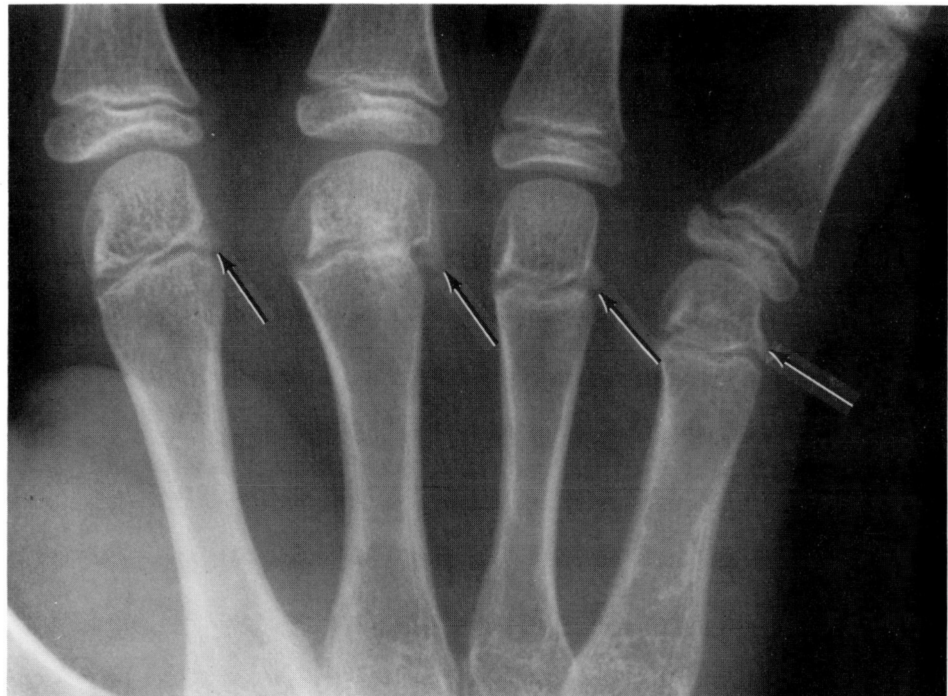

Figure 20–20. *Developmental spurs (arrows) of the metacarpal heads in a normal 13 year old boy.*

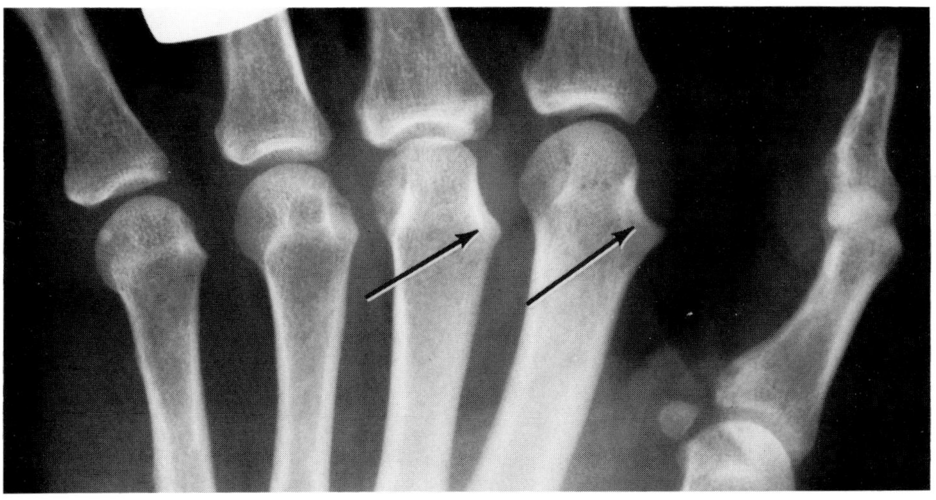

Figure 20–21. *Normal spur-like metacarpal heads (arrows).*

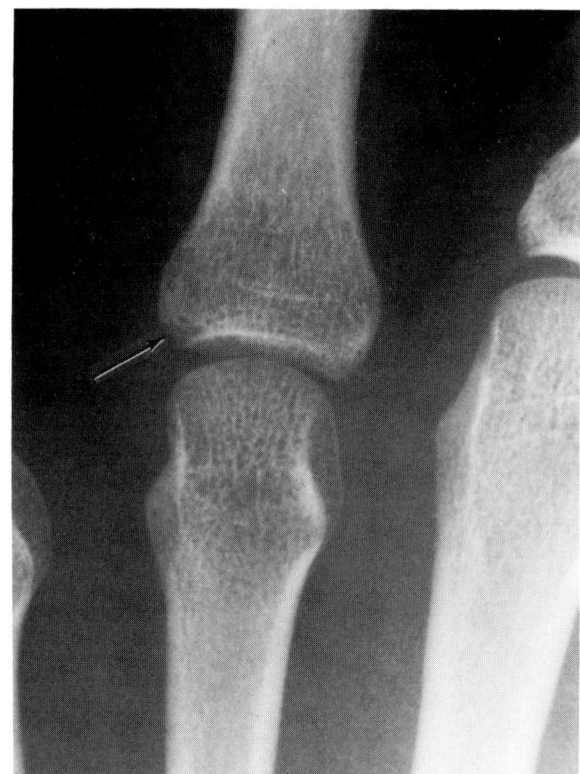

Figure 20–22. *Normal minor irregularity of the base of the proximal phalanx of the fourth finger (arrow). These minor irregularities should not be mistaken for the erosions of early rheumatoid arthritis.*

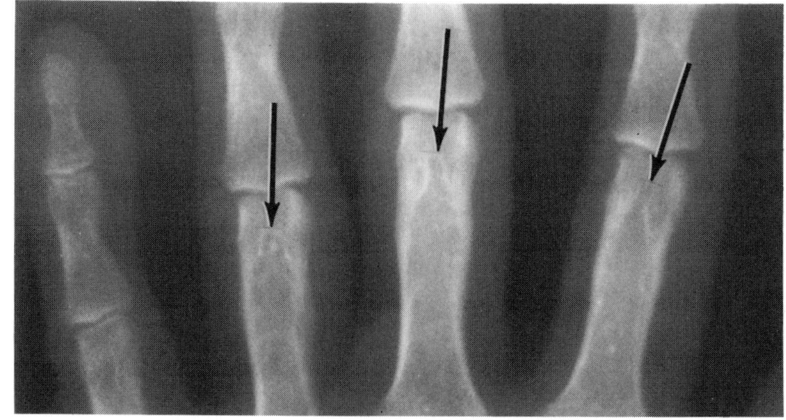

Figure 20–23. *Nutrient canals in the heads of the proximal phalanges (arrows).*

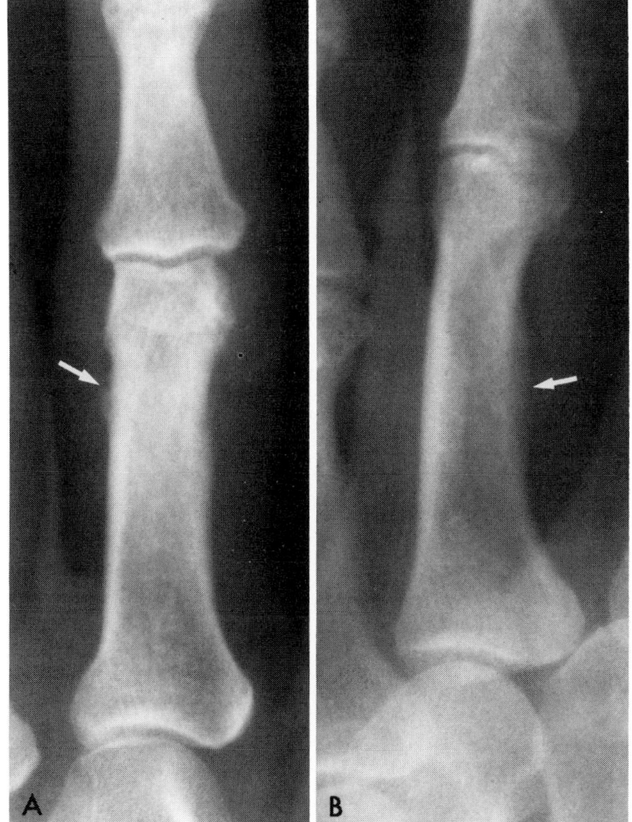

Figure 20–24. Normal ridges and projections on the phalanges associated with muscular insertions, not to be mistaken for periosteal new bone (arrow).

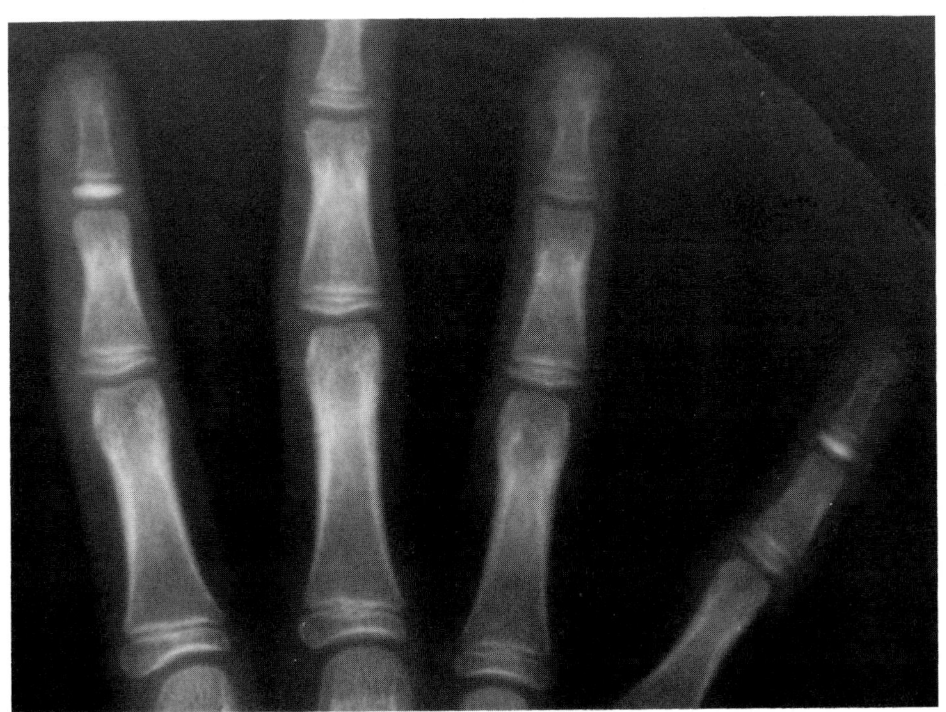

Figure 20–25. Ivory epiphyses of the bases of the distal phalanges of the second and fifth fingers in a normal 12 year old girl.

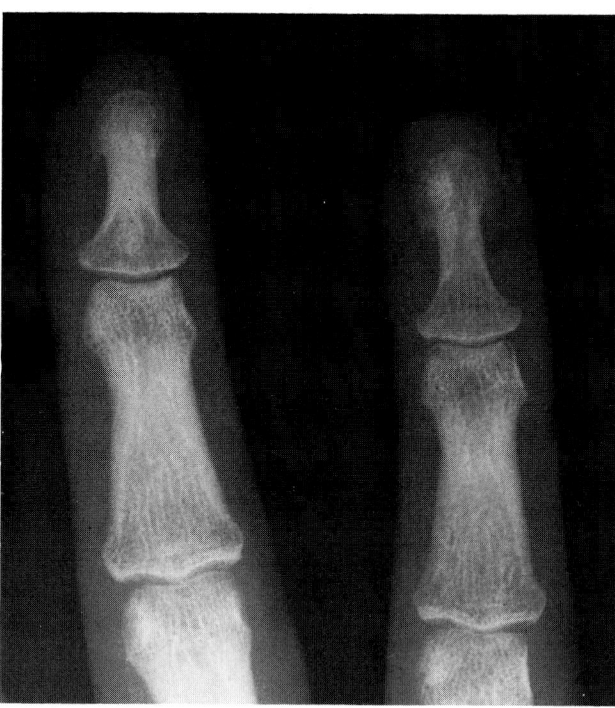

Figure 20–26. *Sclerosis of the terminal phalanges in a patient with no associated disease.*

may be seen as an anatomic variant (Fig. 20–25). There may, at times, be an associated delay in maturation of the hand, particularly the phalanges. There is apparently no association with aseptic necrosis of these ossification centers.[15] Similarly, sclerosis of the terminal phalanges may be seen in healthy adults, particularly in women over the age of 40 years[8] (Fig. 20–26).

PELVIS

The appearance of the sacroiliac joints in adolescents bears a distinct resemblance to the changes of ankylosing spondylitis (Fig. 20–27). It is well to bear in mind that, in youngsters, the joint spaces are wide, with irregular and often dense joint margins.

Obliquity of the pelvis at the time of filming may simulate obliteration of one sacroiliac joint (Fig. 20–28*A*). Improved positioning or sacroiliac views will reveal the true state of affairs (Fig. 20–28*B*).

The paraglenoidal sulci are anatomic variants evident as fossae in the ilia adjacent to the inferior margins of the sacroiliac joint (Fig. 20–29). They are seen only in women and should not be confused with areas of bone destruction.

Cephalad angulation of the x-ray beam will produce a double contour of the superior margins of the pubic bones that simulates periosteal new bone formation (Fig. 20–30). This effect is not seen when the beam is directed perpendicularly to the film.

In the aged, the bone of the brim of the pelvis often appears laminated and thickened, an appearance that may be confused with Paget's disease (Fig. 20–31).

The normal pubertal symphysis pubis is wide, with irregular joint margins (Fig. 20–32). This appearance may mimic a destructive arthritis.

Alterations in the symphysis pubis occur after parturition (Fig. 20–33*A*). With passage of time, the density of the bone regresses and cyst-like areas of radiolucency remain as permanent stigmata (Fig. 20–33*B*).

The normal ischiopubic synchondroses are a source of confusion, since they often appear as swollen radiolucent areas in young children (Fig. 20–34*A*). This is a normal phenomenon of growth and not evidence of disease. It is important to remember that these synchondroses do not always close synchronously (Fig. 20–34*B*) and, at times, may reappear after initial closure.

The inferior aspects of the ischia may be markedly irregular in adolescent children. This phenomenon is thought to be the result of strong muscular pull at the sites of insertion and is self-limited (Fig. 20–35). These irregularities disappear with completion of growth and are not of clinical significance. A similar alteration may also be seen at the anterior inferior iliac spine at the point of insertion of the rectus femoris muscle[17] (Fig. 20–36).

HIP

The capital femoral epiphysis may ossify from multiple centers rather than from a single center (Fig. 20–37). This appearance in an ossification center should not be taken as a manifestation of disease, such as aseptic necrosis. In like fashion, the roofs of the acetabula in young children are often grossly irregular, representing areas of ossification in the cartilaginous matrix (Fig. 20–38).

Protrusio acetabuli is a normal phenomenon in children from approximately 4 to 12 years of age and is not a reflection of acetabular abnormality (Fig. 20–39).[1]

The fossae for the nutrient vessels in the acetabulum may be mistaken for a destructive lesion in the femoral head if they are fully superimposed upon the head (Fig. 20–40). In addition, the fovea capitis of the femoral head should not be confused with an erosion of the articular surface (Fig. 20–41). Additional spurious shadows in the acetabulum may be produced by an undulation in the anterior margin of the acetabulum coupled with superimposition of the shadow of the ischium (Fig. 20–42) or by superimposition of bony shadows of the posterior wall of the acetabulum projected through the femoral head (Fig. 20–43). Similar overlapping shadows of the acetabulum may produce an area of double

Text continued on page 724

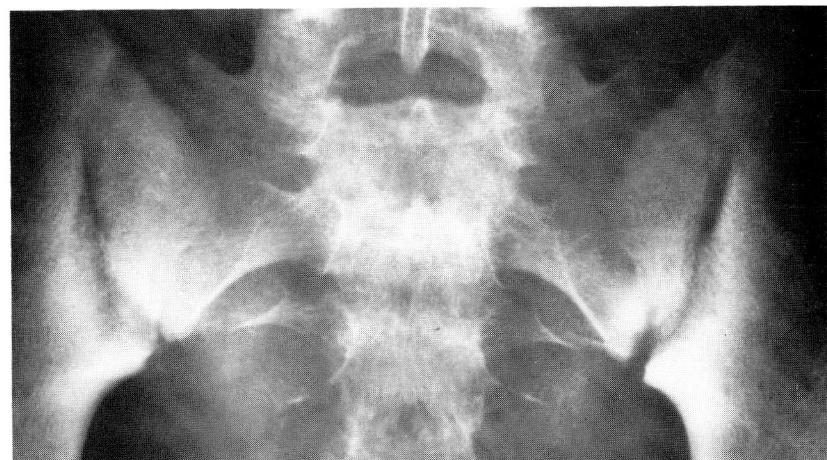

Figure 20–27. *Normal appearance of the adolescent sacroiliac joints, which may simulate the changes of ankylosing spondylitis.*

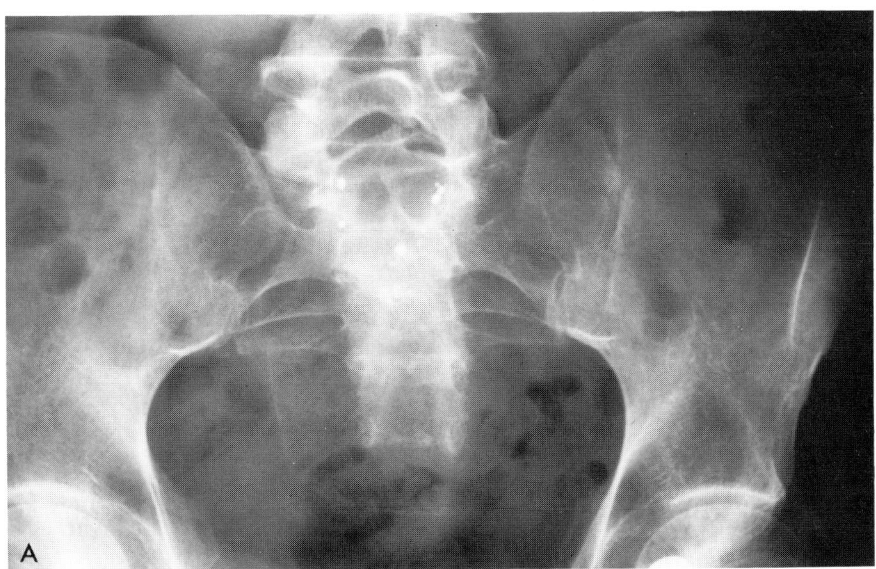

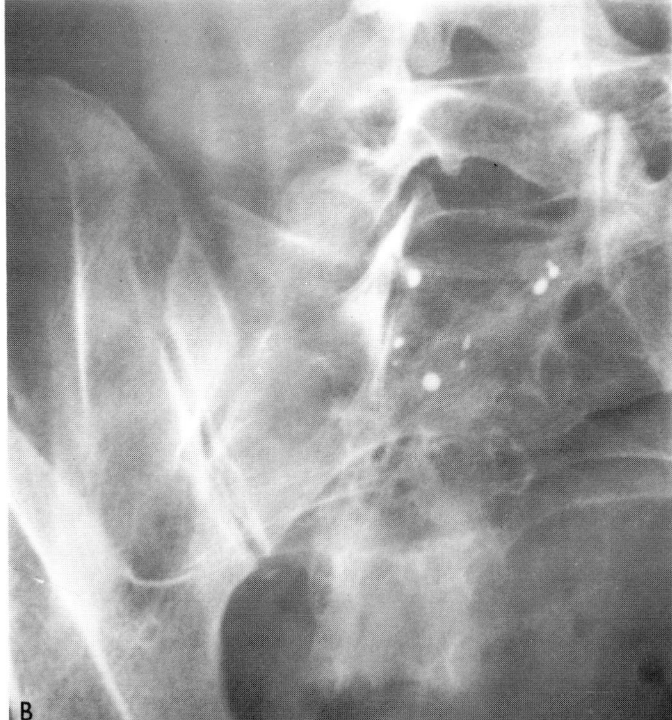

Figure 20–28. **A,** *Simulated obliteration of the right sacroiliac joint produced by rotation of the pelvis.* **B,** *Oblique sacroiliac view shows normal joint.*

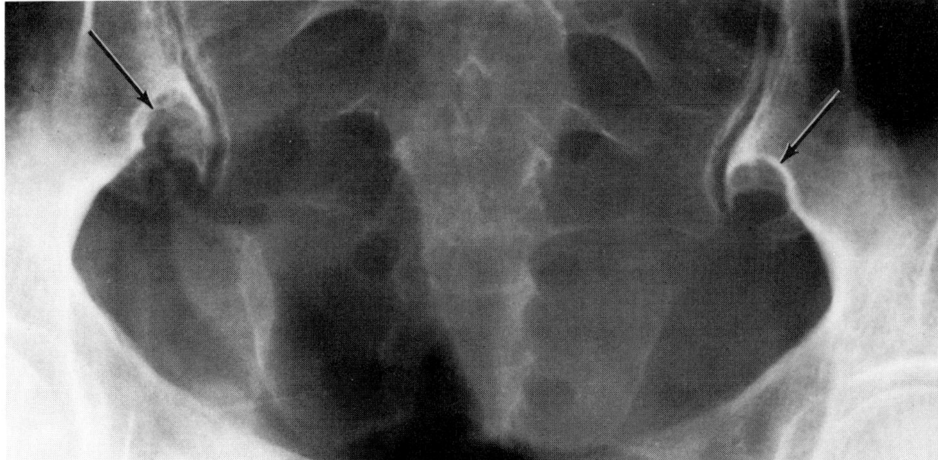

Figure 20–29. *Paraglenoidal sulci, an anatomic variant (arrows).*

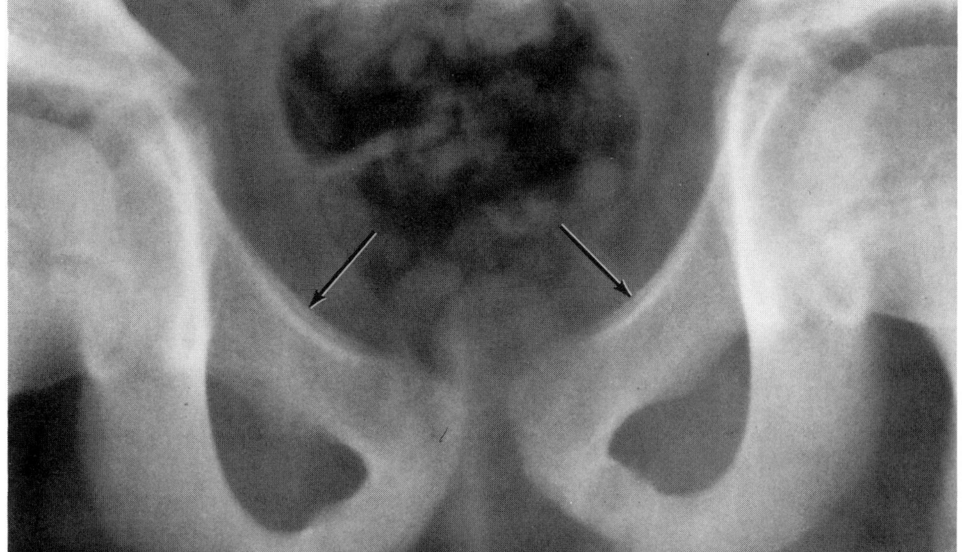

Figure 20–30. *Simulated periosteal proliferation of bone of the superior margins of the pubic bones (arrows) due to cephalad angulation of the x-ray beam.*

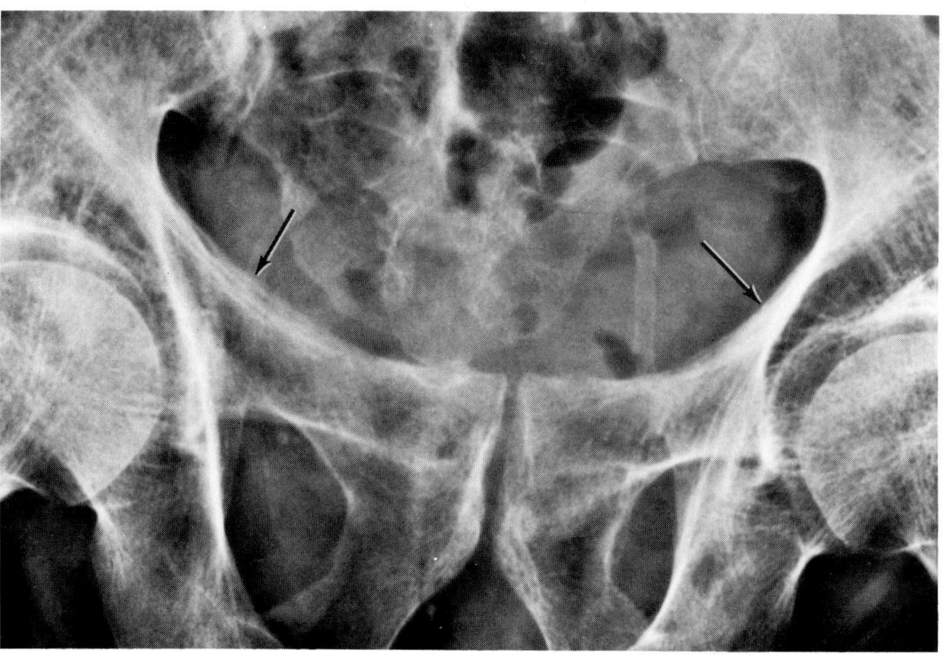

Figure 20–31. *Aging changes in the iliopectineal line, which may simulate Paget's disease (arrows).*

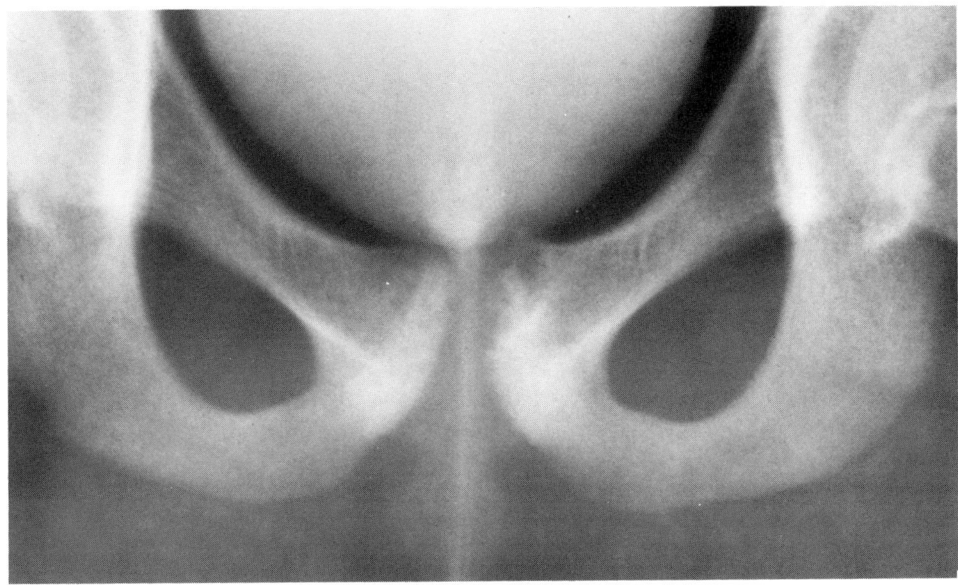

Figure 20–32. *Normal developmental irregularity of the symphysis pubis in a 12 year old boy. Incidentally noted is contrast material in the bladder.*

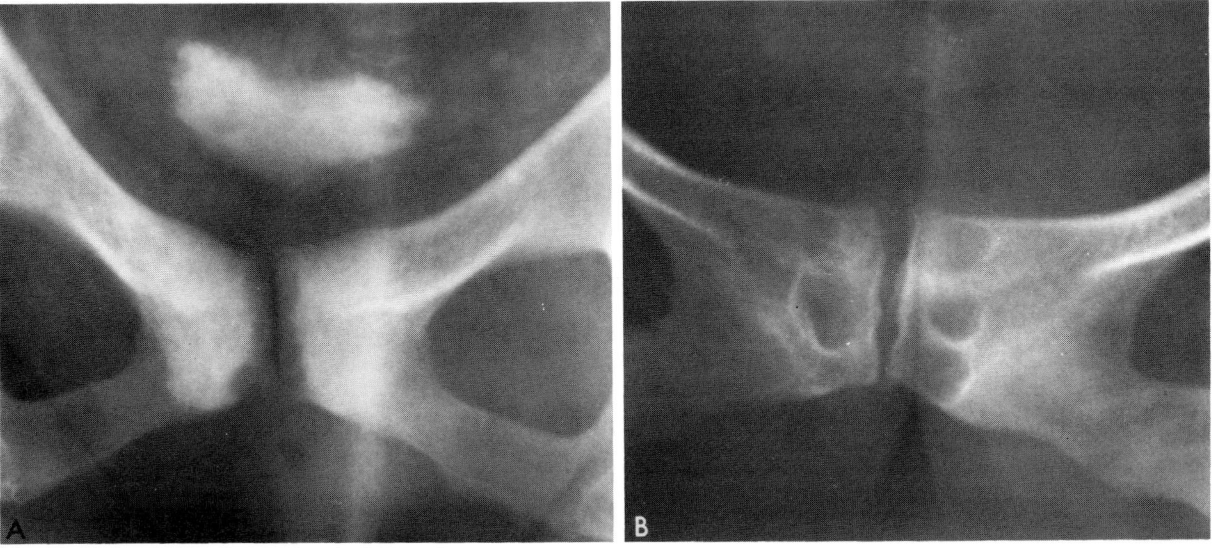

Figure 20–33. *Postpartum changes in the symphysis pubis.* **A,** *Recent changes.* **B,** *Old changes.*

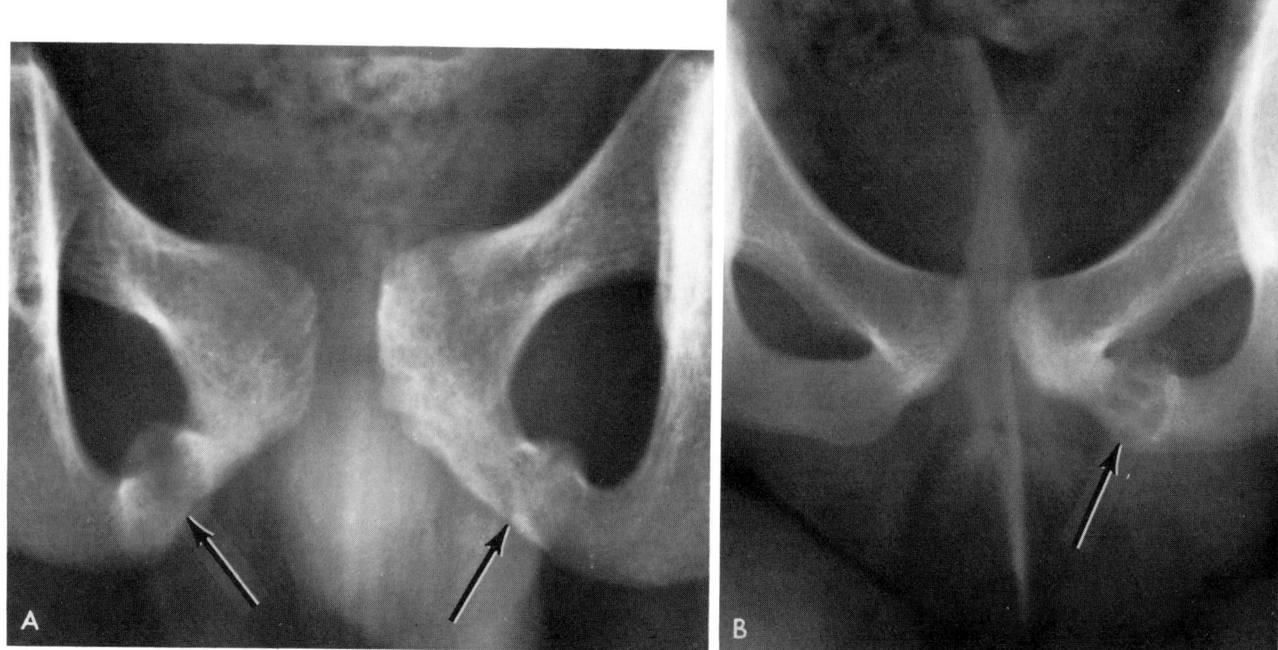

Figure 20–34. **A,** Normal ischiopubic synchondroses in a 4 year old boy (arrows). **B,** Normal asymmetric closure of the ischiopubic synchondroses in a 12 year old boy (arrow).

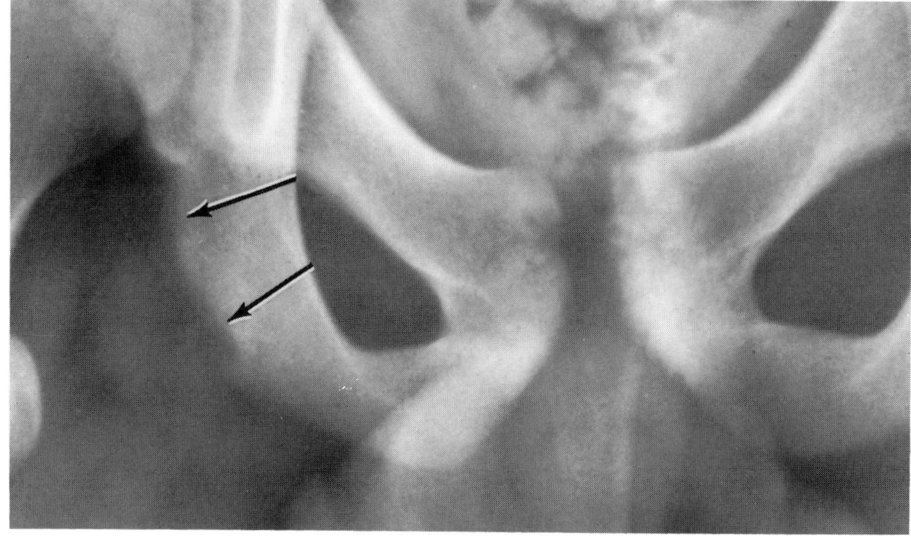

Figure 20–35. Developmental irregularity of the ischium in a 16 year old boy (arrows). Note also wide irregular appearance of the normal symphysis pubis.

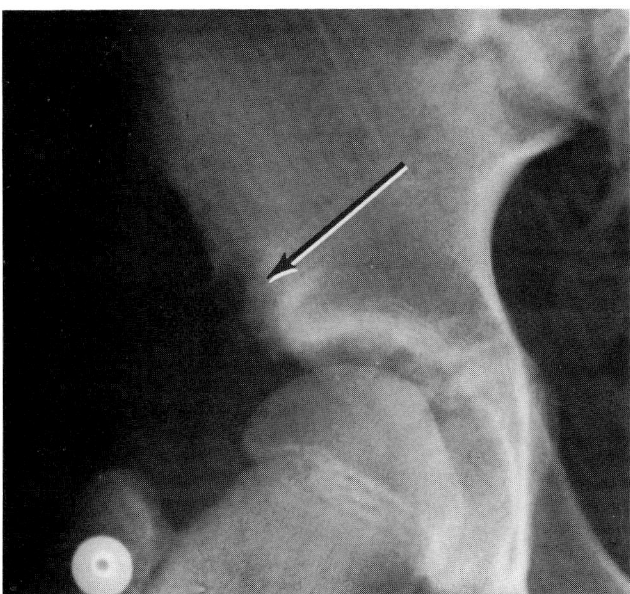

Figure 20–36. *Developmental irregularity of the area of the anterior inferior iliac spine in a young boy (arrow).*

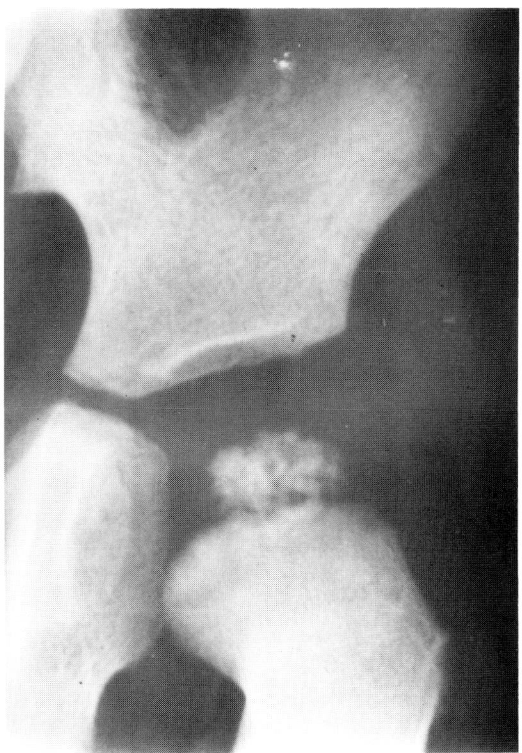

Figure 20–37. *Normal irregular ossification of the capital femoral epiphysis of the left hip in a young child. This appearance in a single center does not necessarily indicate the presence of disease.*

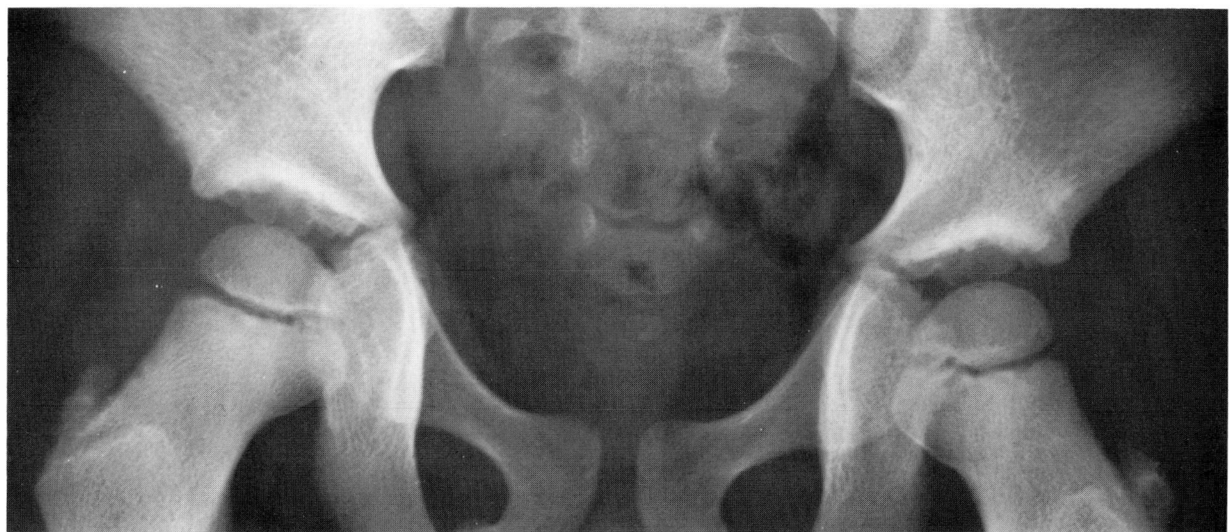

Figure 20–38. *Normal irregularity of the acetabular roofs in a 5½ year old child.*

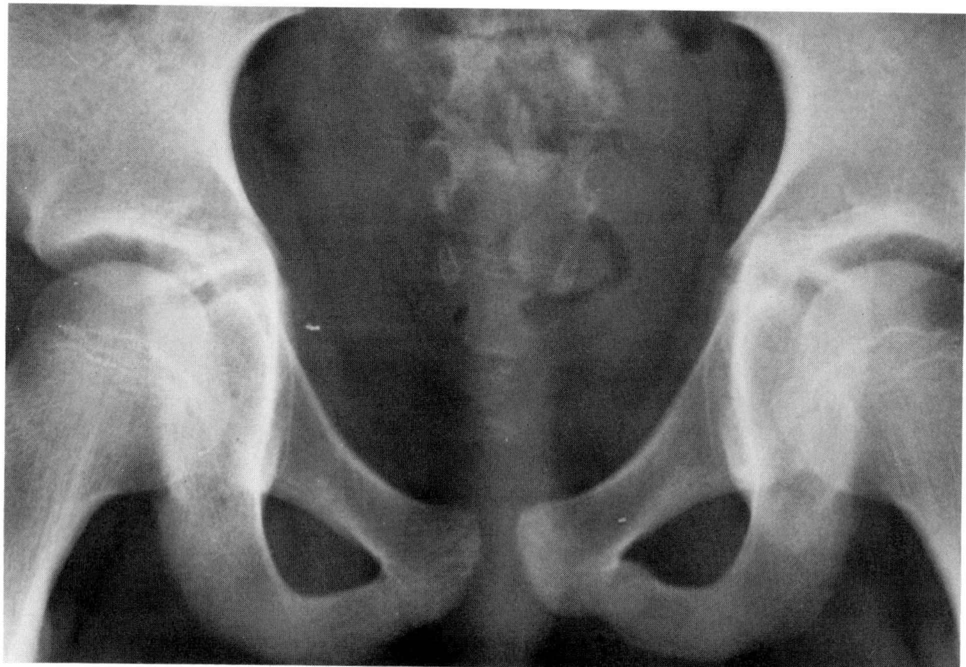

Figure 20–39. *Normal intrapelvic protrusion of the acetabula in a 9½ year old girl.*

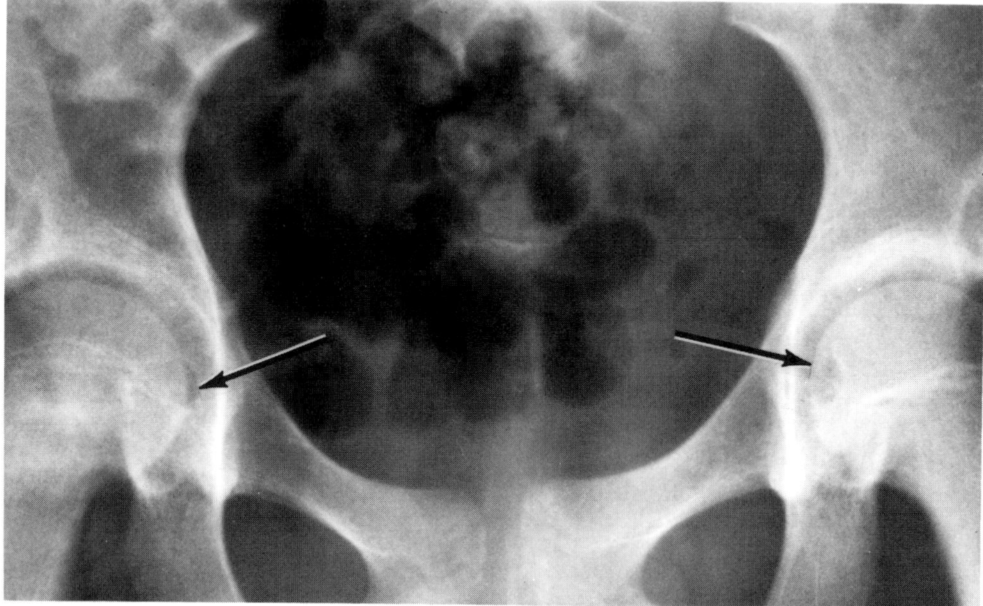

Figure 20–40. *Fossa for nutrient vessel of the acetabulum (arrows) simulating a destructive lesion in the left femoral head owing to overlap of osseous structures.*

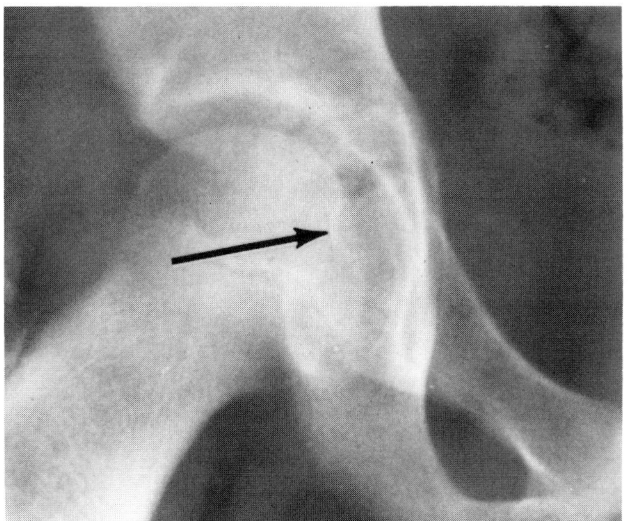

Figure 20–41. *The normal fovea capitis (arrow).*

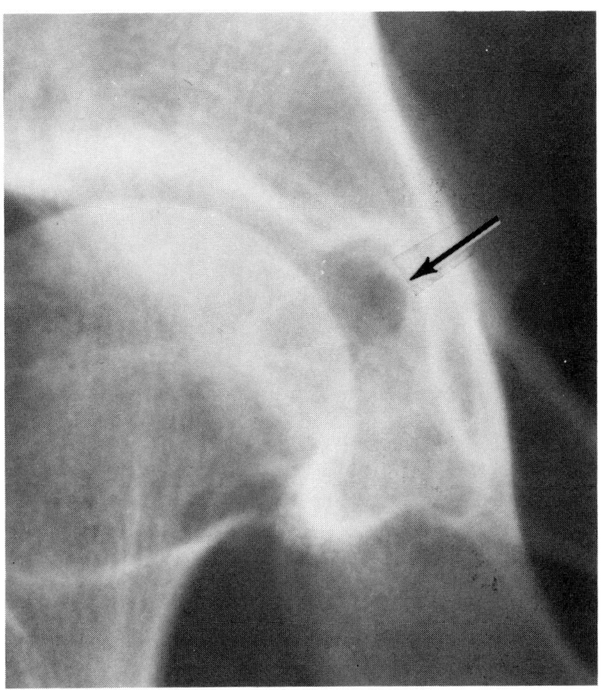

Figure 20–42. *Pseudocyst of the acetabulum.*

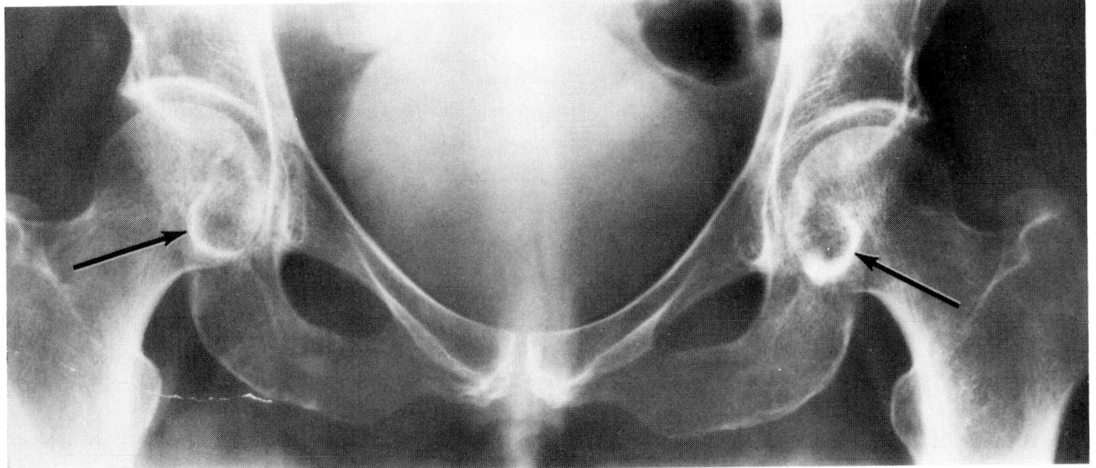

Figure 20–43. *Simulated destructive lesions of the femoral heads produced by a bony strut in the posterior wall of the acetabulum projected through the femoral heads (arrows).*

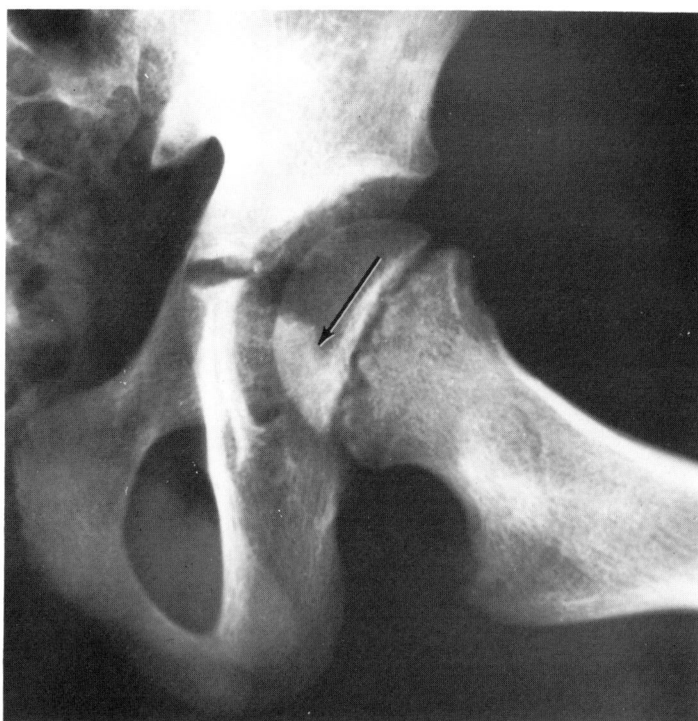

Figure 20–44. Overlapping shadows of the femoral head and acetabulum simulating aseptic necrosis (arrow).

density that may be confused with aseptic necrosis of the femoral head (Fig. 20–44).

It has been shown by Brown[4] that apparent bulging of the "capsular" shadow of the hip can be produced by filming the hip in abduction and external rotation, producing an appearance suggesting fluid in the joint (Fig. 20–45). Comparison of the soft tissue shadows about the hip from side to side requires that both hips be in neutral position to obtain useful information.

The secondary ossification centers for the posterior margin of the acetabulum are often multiple and

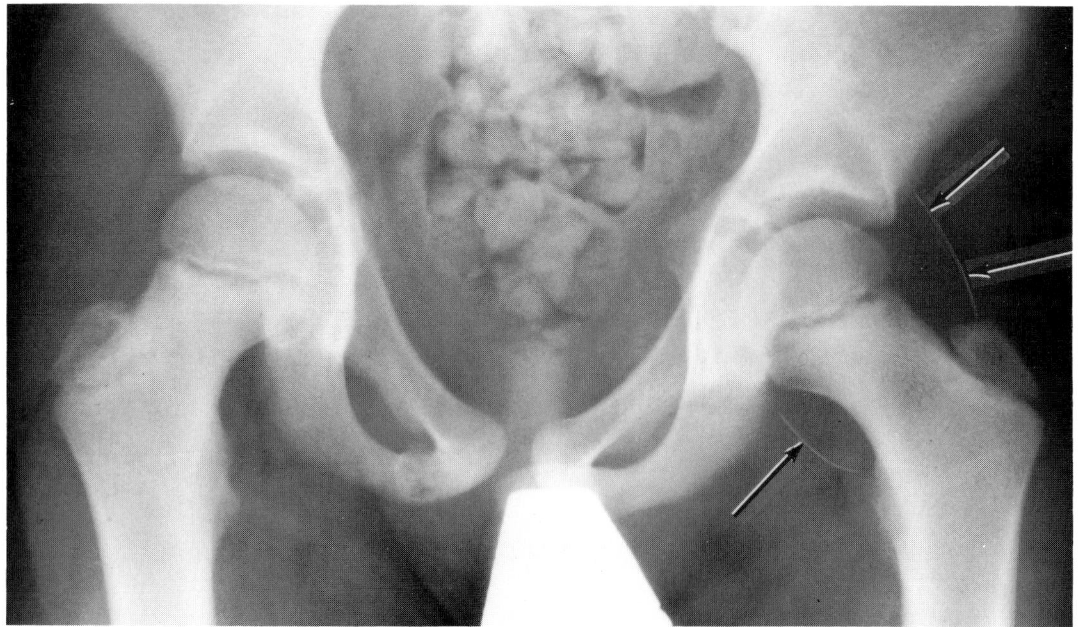

Figure 20–45. Apparent bulging of the "joint capsule" of the left hip in a 9 year old boy (arrows) due to malpositioning of the hip at the time of filming. Compare with shadows of the opposite side. (Illustration has been altered to accentuate the findings.)

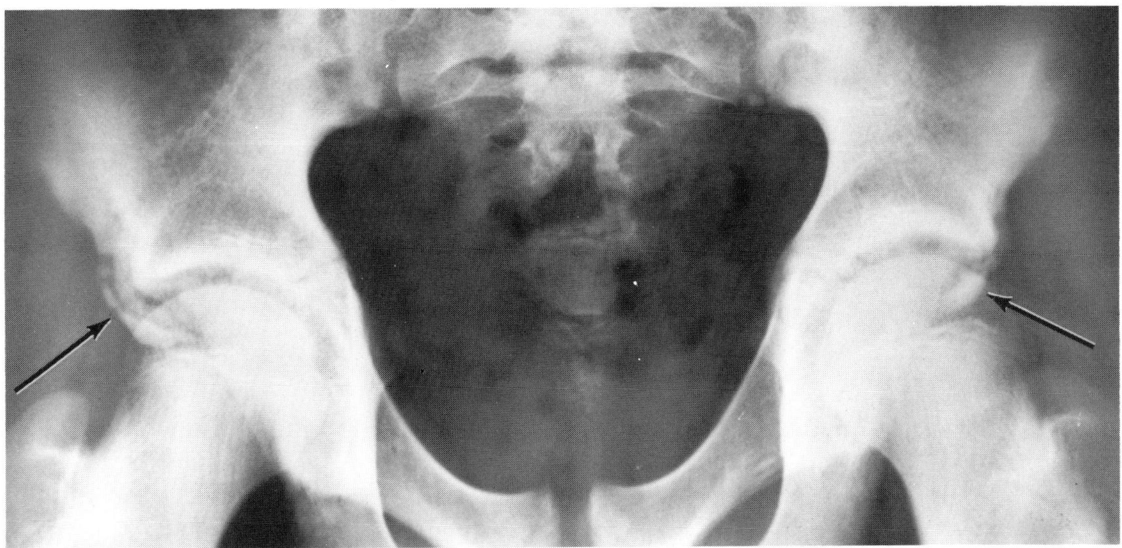

Figure 20–46. *Secondary ossification centers of the acetabular margins in a 14 year old girl (arrows).*

not necessarily symmetric bilaterally (Fig. 20–46). Remnants of these ossification centers may be confused with fractures.

LOWER EXTREMITY

The superior margins of the femoral necks are ill defined in young children and, at times, may have an appearance which suggests new bone formation. This is particularly prominent at about the ages of 4 to 5 years (Fig. 20–47). In older children, similar growth irregularities may be seen in the greater trochanter (Fig. 20–48).

There are several rather striking cortical irregularities seen in the distal femoral metaphysis in adolescent children which may lead to needless concern and investigation. One of these is seen in the lateral projection in the anterior cortex[12] and the others in the posterior cortex on the medial side[2] (Fig. 20–49). The posterior irregularity is larger and, therefore, its etiology has been the subject of considerable debate. It has been considered to be a fibrous

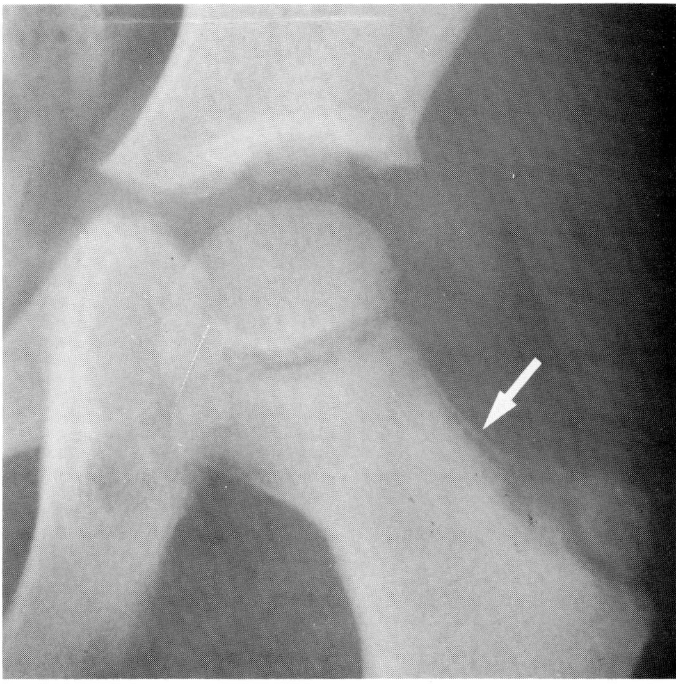

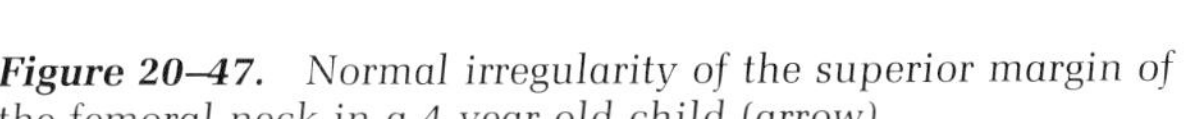

Figure 20–47. *Normal irregularity of the superior margin of the femoral neck in a 4 year old child (arrow).*

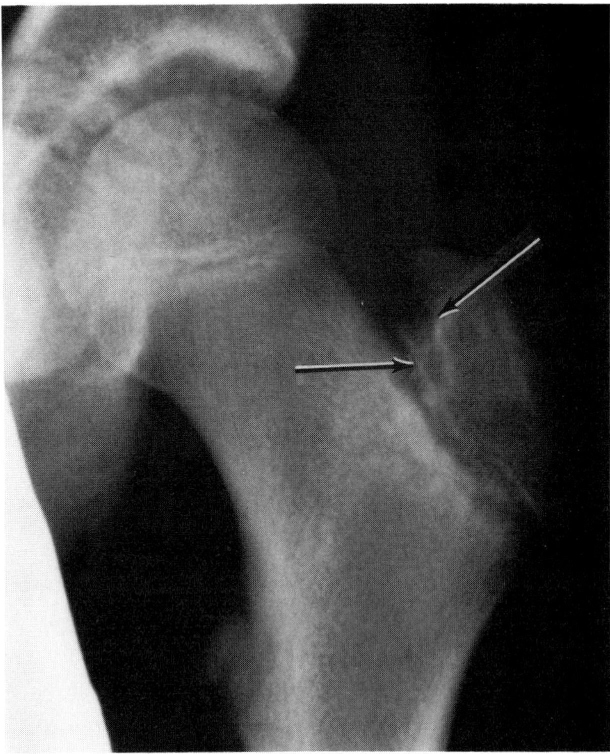

Figure 20–48. Normal irregularities of ossification of the greater trochanter in a 12 year old boy (arrows).

cortical defect[3] as well as an avulsive lesion.[5] In any case, the irregularity is commonly seen posteriorly, as well as posteromedially (Fig. 20–50) and should not be mistaken for an inflammatory or neoplastic lesion. It is sufficiently characteristic radiographically to obviate the need for biopsy.[21] One can often find evidence of this same process in the adult manifested as a fossa in the cortex (Fig. 20–51).

The nutrient foramen at the distal end of the femur is intra-articular and is seen as one or several discrete areas of radiolucency, which may be mistaken for a destructive lesion in the intercondylar area (Fig. 20–52). Conversely, in some normal individuals, this same region may be occupied by an area of sclerosis that has been misinterpreted as various significant lesions (Fig. 20–53).

The distal articular surface of the femur in young children is radiologically grossly irregular, representing islands of ossification in the cartilaginous epiphysis (Fig. 20–54). These irregularities are best seen from the ages of 6 to 12 years and are confused with osteochondritis dissecans. They are well delineated in the tunnel projection (Fig. 20–54*A*) and are most evident in the posterior aspects of either or both condyles (Fig. 20–54*B*). They can be differentiated from osteochondritis dissecans by their occurrence in a younger age group and by their appearance in areas of the condyles that are not usually involved in osteochondritis dissecans.

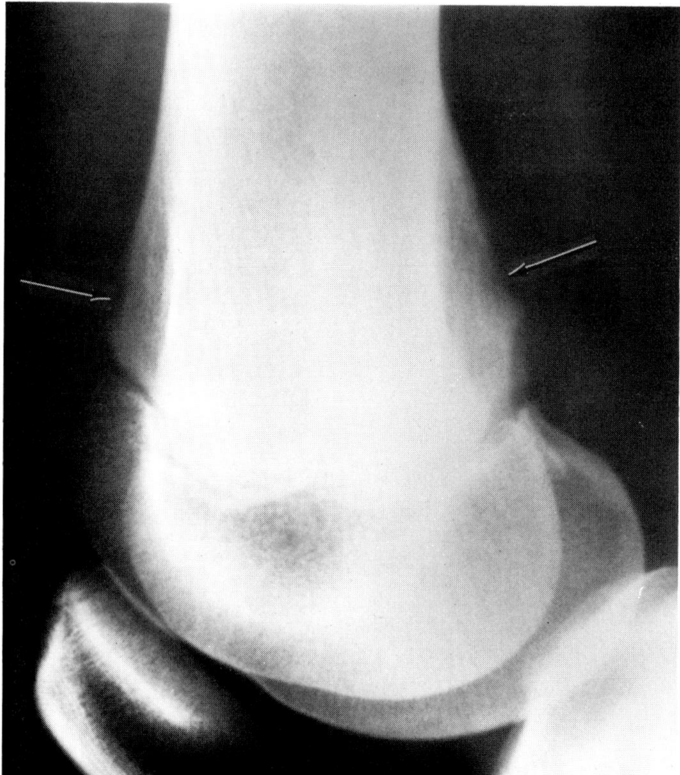

Figure 20–49. Normal cortical irregularities on the anterior and posterior aspects of the distal femur in a 15 year old boy (arrows).

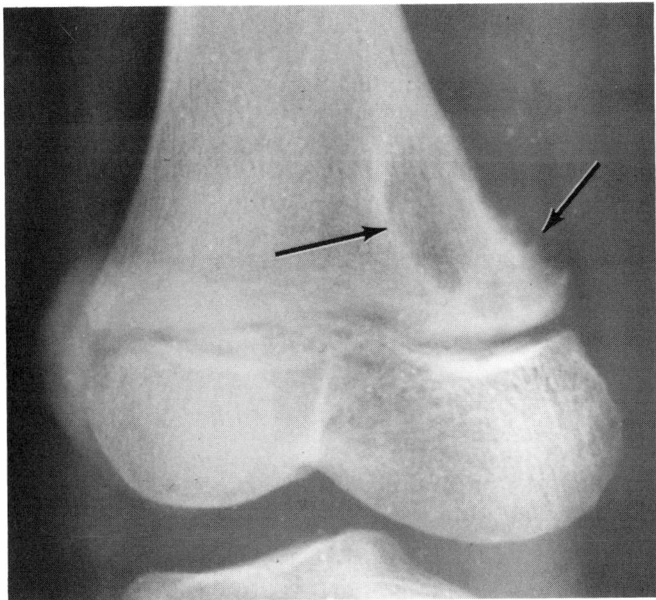

Figure 20–50. Normal irregularity of cortex of medial and posterior aspects of the medial femoral condyle in a 12 year old girl (arrows).

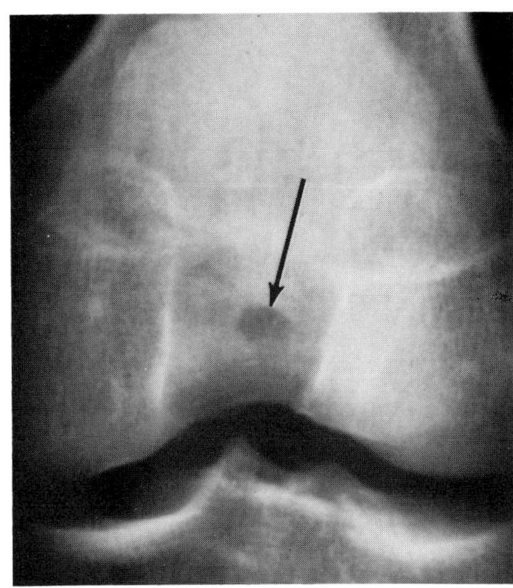

Figure 20–52. The nutrient foramen of the distal end of the femur (arrow).

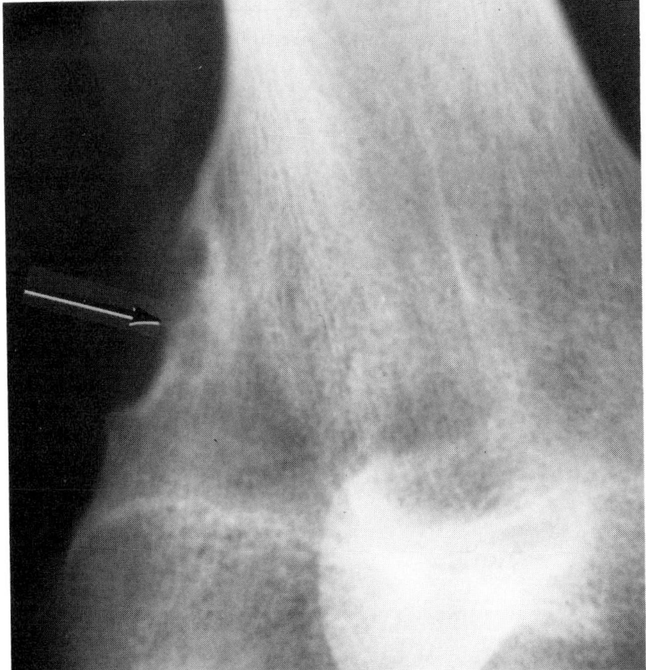

Figure 20–51. Remnants of the posterior femoral cortical irregularity in a 21 year old man (arrow).

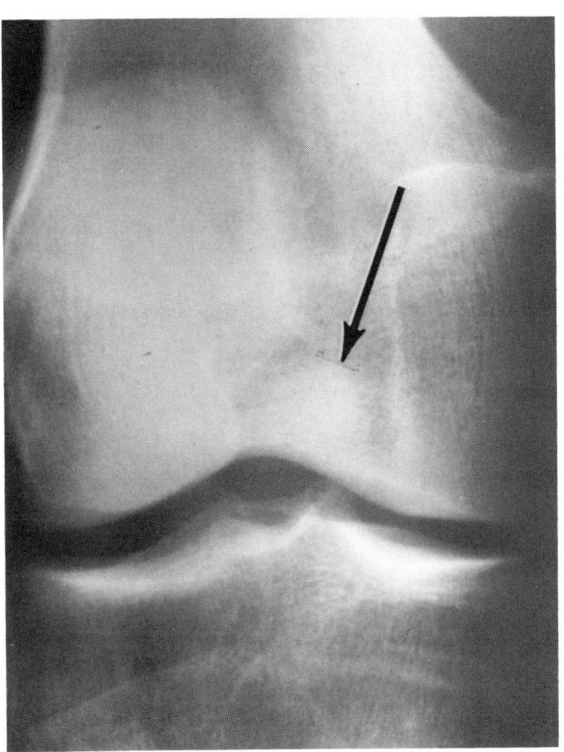

Figure 20–53. Normal area of bony density in the intercondylar fossa (arrow).

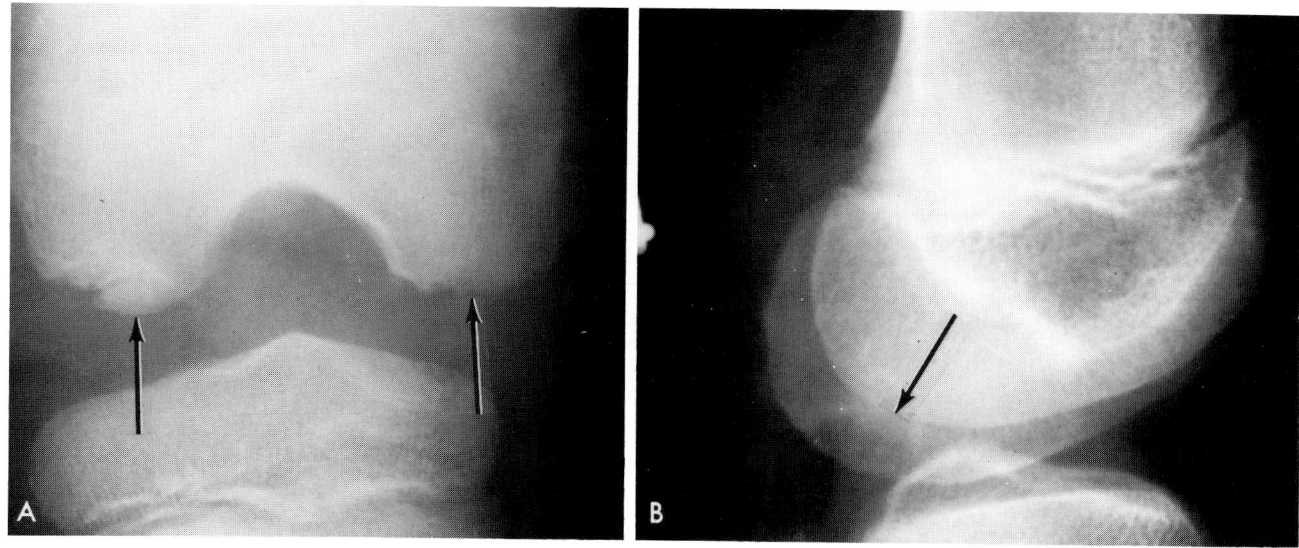

Figure 20–54. **A,** *Normal irregularity of ossification of the articular surfaces of the distal femur in a 10 year old boy, simulating osteochondritis dissecans (arrows).* **B,** *These irregularities are located posteriorly, as illustrated in a 12 year old boy (arrow).*

In adults, grooves may be seen in the articular surface of the medial condyle in tangential patellar views and are a source of misinterpretation[9] (Fig. 20–55). These grooves may be evident in the lateral projection as well (Fig. 20–56).

The ossification of the distal femoral epiphysis may be quite irregular in children, particularly in its lateral aspect, and this results in areas of relative radiolucency that may be quite alarming[6] (Fig. 20–57).

A circumscribed radiolucent defect may be seen in the dorsal aspect of the patella in young people, usually as an incidental finding (Fig. 20–58). The defect is self-limited and apparently represents a variant in ossification. It is not a manifestation of osteochondritis dissecans of the patella.[10]

The tibial tubercle is notoriously irregular in its ossification, and this irregularity in itself is not necessarily a reflection of traumatic avulsion or "osteochondrosis" (Fig. 20–59). Furthermore, the lateral aspect of the tibial tubercle in the adult may be seen in the frontal projection as a laminated-appearing mass on the lateral aspect of the tibia and may be confused with a lesion producing new bone

Text continued on page 735

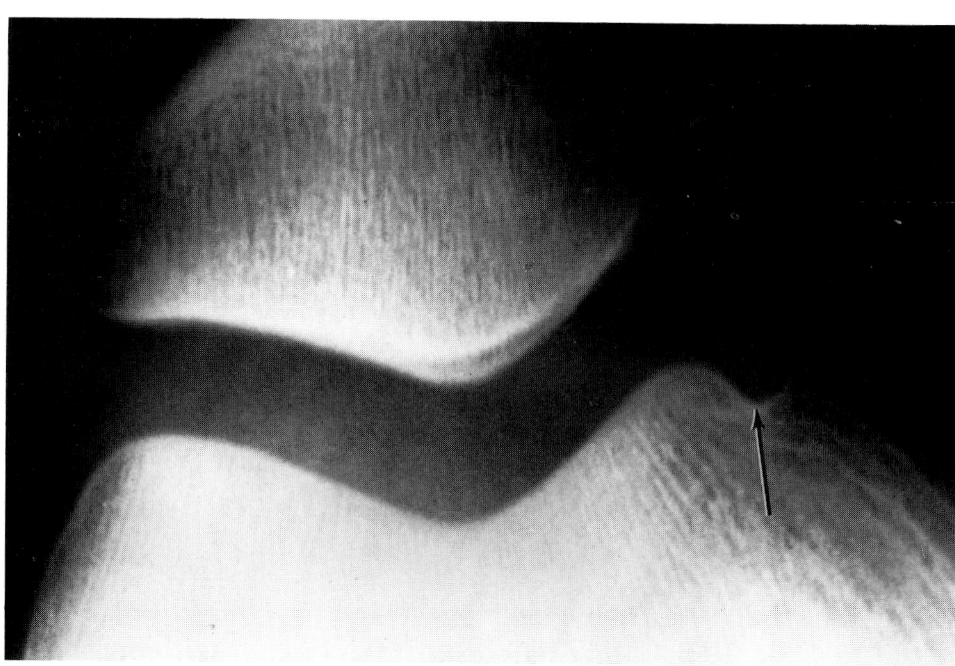

Figure 20–55. *Normal grooves in the articular surface of the medial condyle of the femur, seen in a tangential patellar view (arrow).*

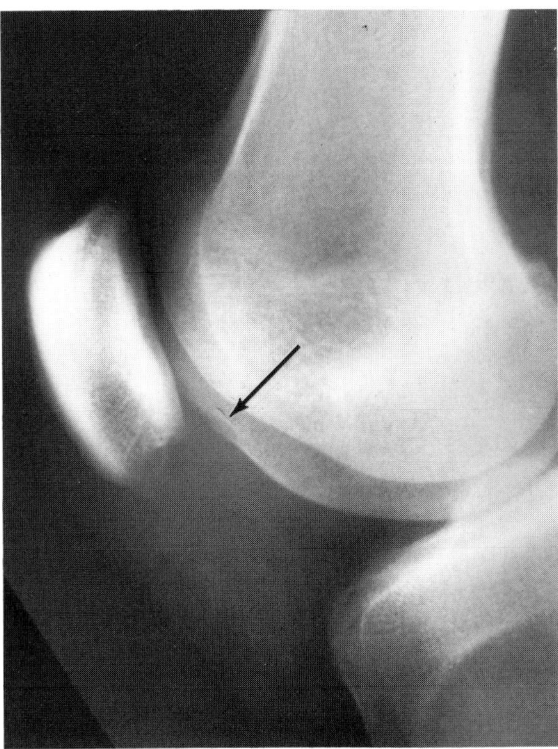

Figure 20–56. *Normal depression of the articular surface of the medial condyle of the femur (arrow).*

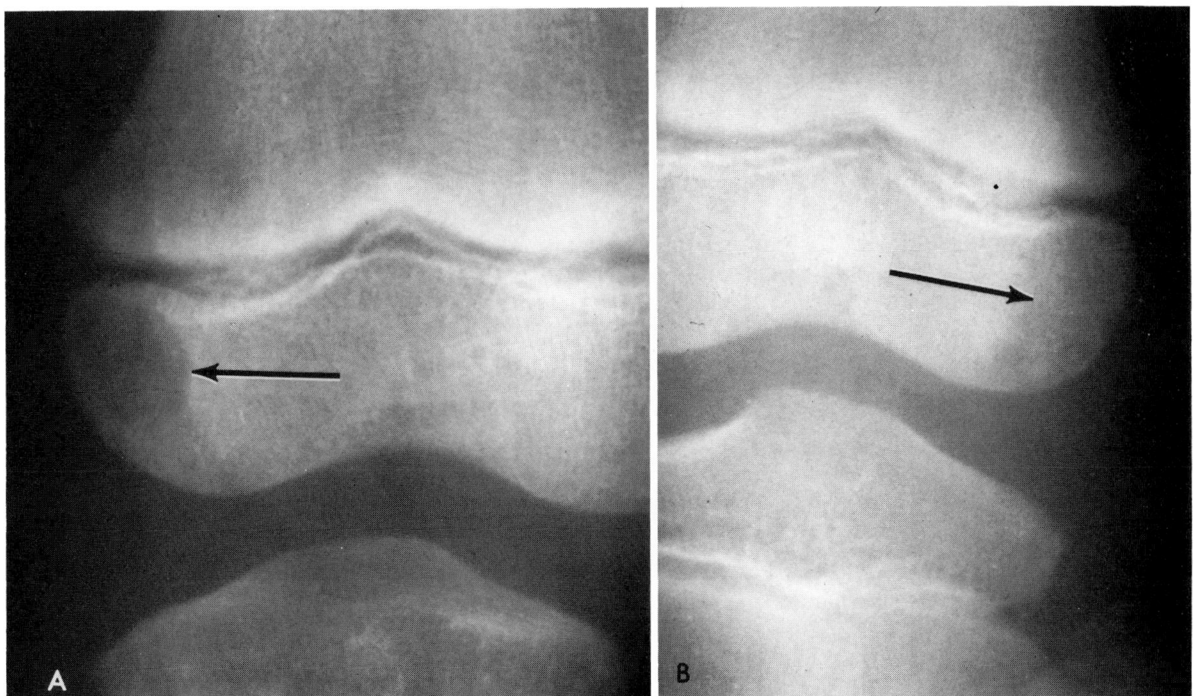

Figure 20–57. *Normal developmental areas of radiolucency in the lateral aspects of the distal femoral epiphyses in a 6 year old boy (arrow).*

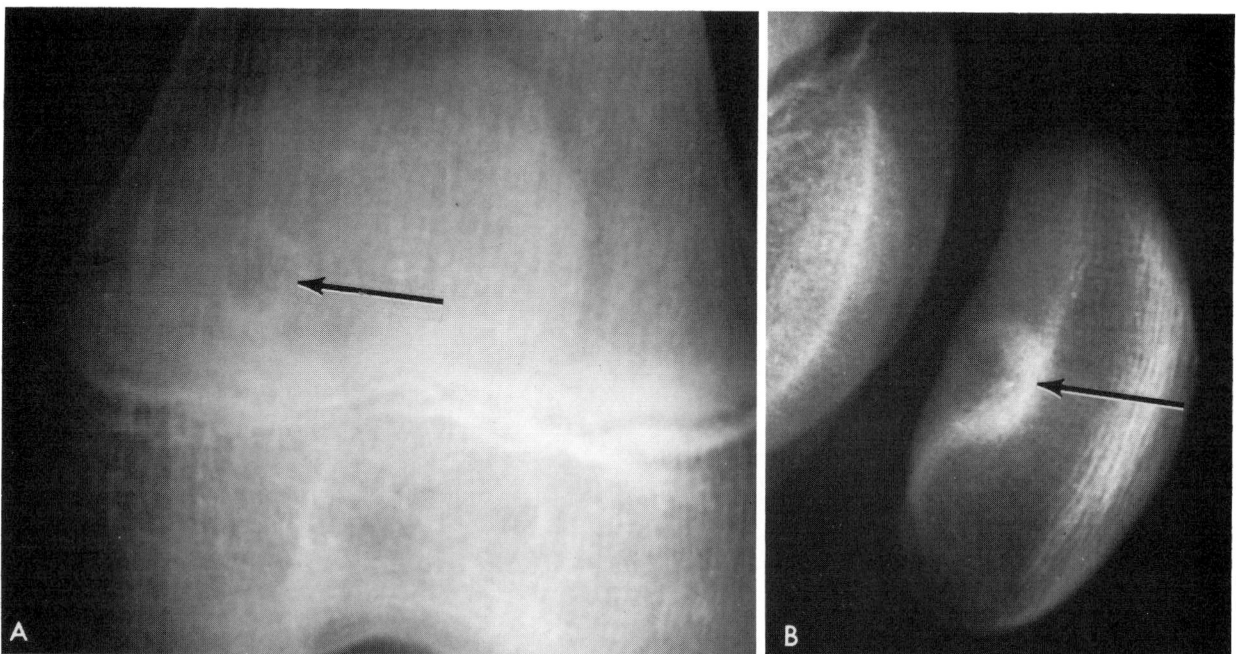

Figure 20–58. The dorsal patellar defect (arrow) in an adolescent boy. Two year follow-up radiograph (not shown) showed its complete disappearance.

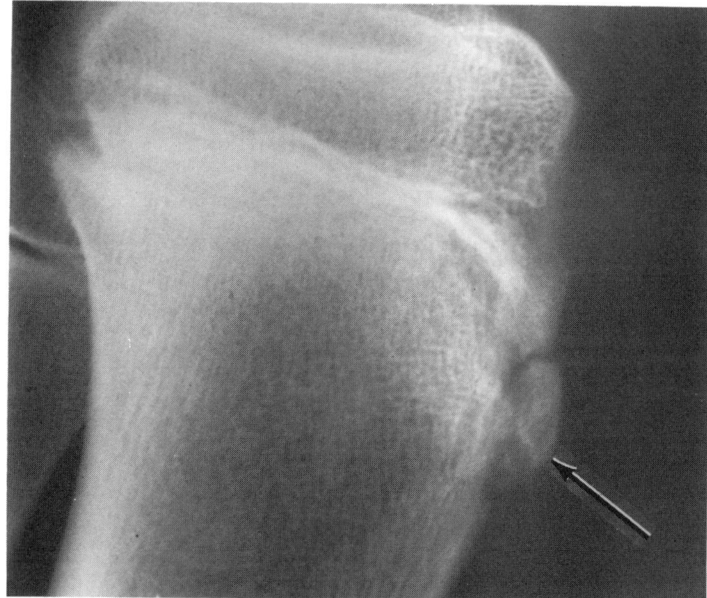

Figure 20–59. Normal variation in appearance of the ossification center of the tibial tubercle in an adolescent (arrow).

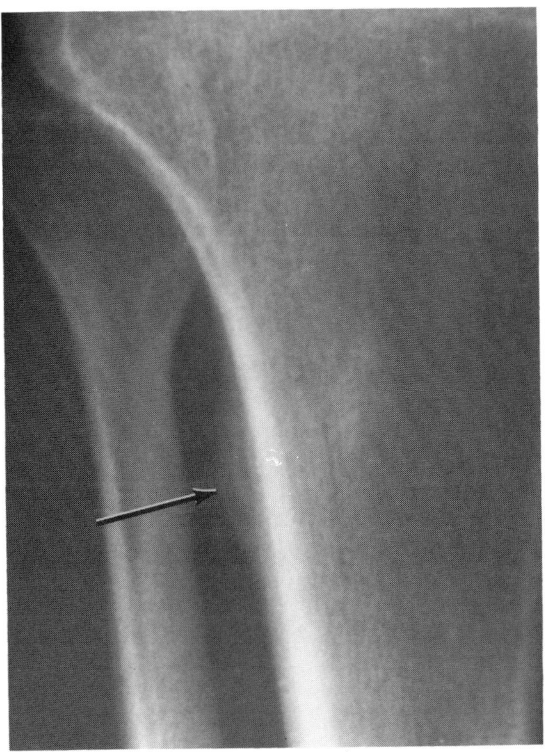

Figure 20–60. The tibial tubercle simulating laminated periostitis (arrow).

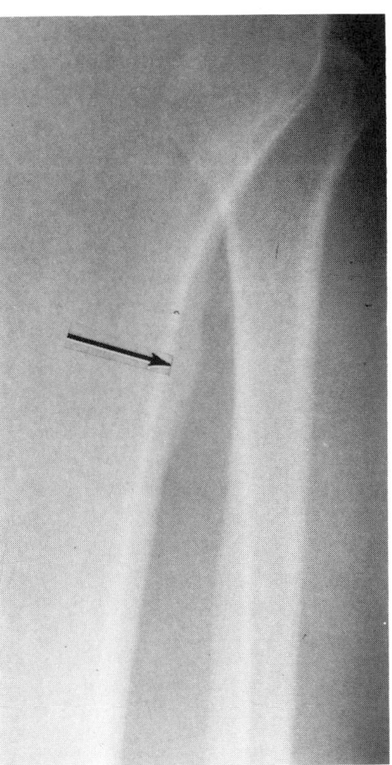

Figure 20–61. Pseudoperiostitis of the tibia, simulated by the tibial tuberosity (arrow). Note also the spurious thickening of the lateral cortex of the tibia and the medial cortex of the fibula due to slight external rotation of the leg.

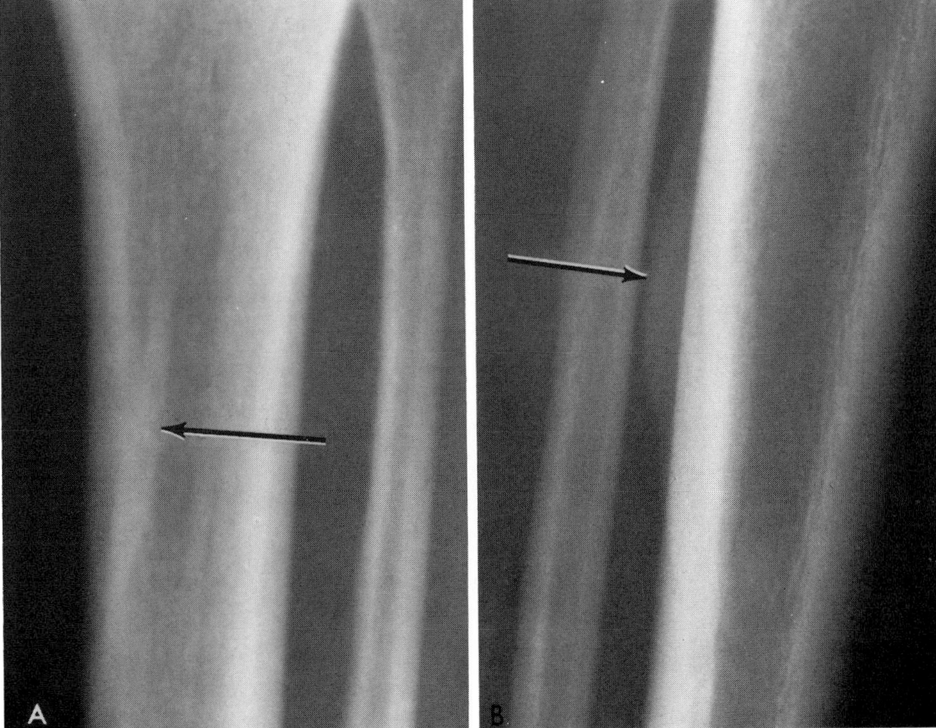

Figure 20–62. The soleal line, which may be mistaken for periosteal new bone (arrow).

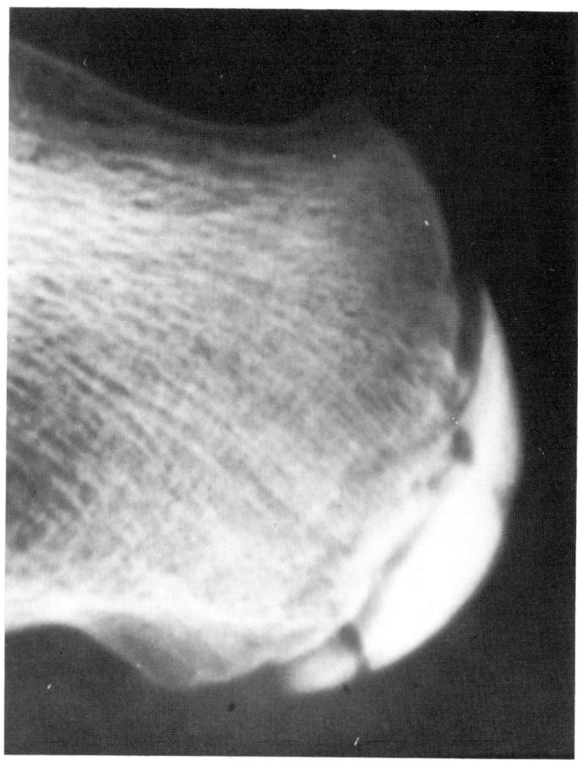

Figure 20–63. *Normal density and "fragmentation" of the calcaneal apophysis.*

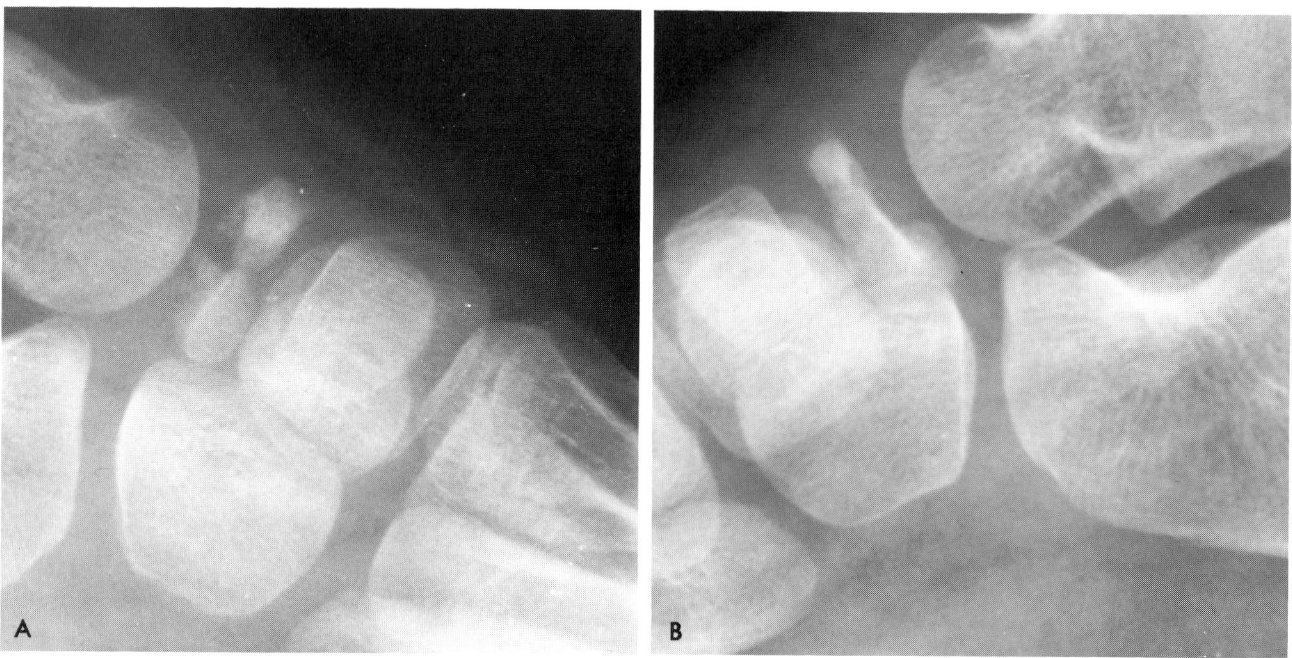

Figure 20–64. *Normal developmental irregularity of the tarsal navicular bones in a 6 year old boy.*

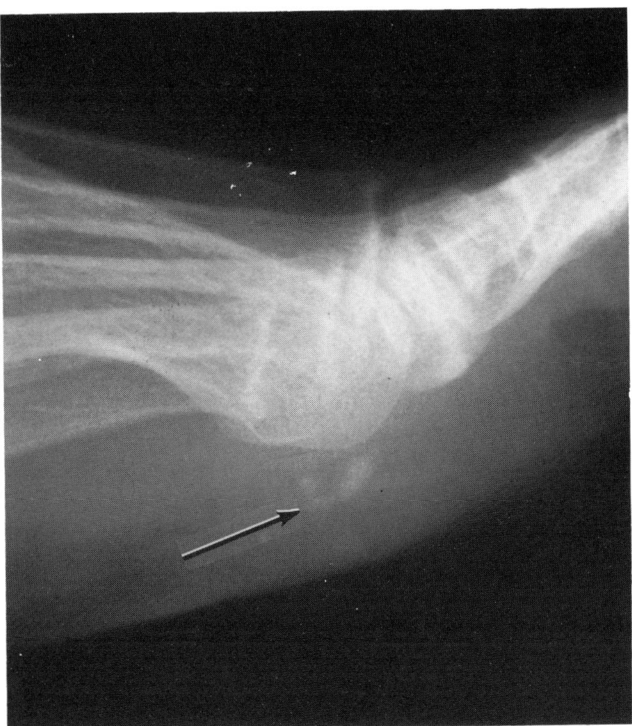

Figure 20–65. The normal irregular appearace of the ossifying sesamoid bones in the foot of a 12 year old boy (arrow).

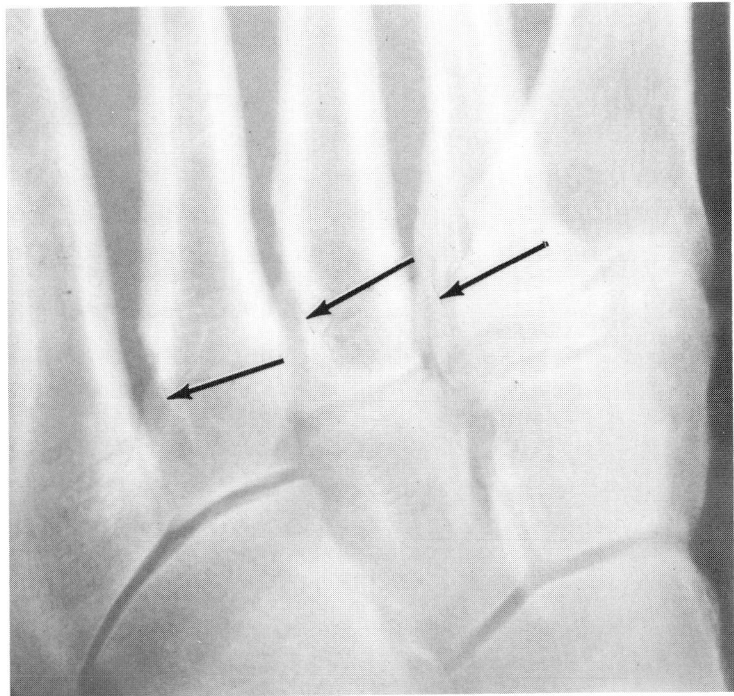

Figure 20–66. Normal irregularities of the bases of the metatarsals seen in the oblique projection (arrows).

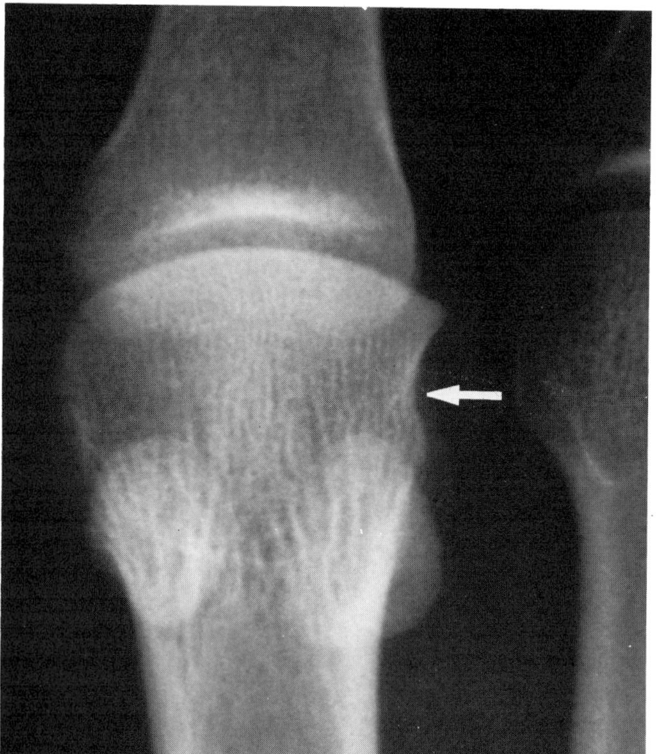

Figure 20–67. Normal fossa at the lateral aspect of the head of the first metatarsal (arrow).

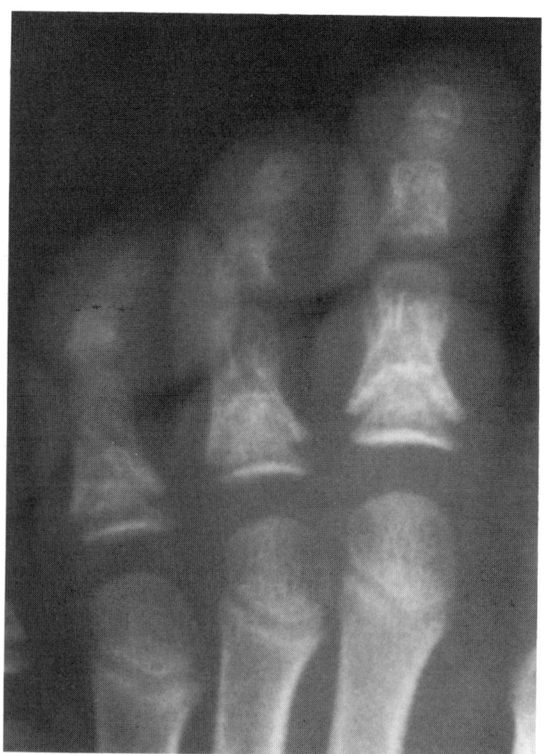

Figure 20–69. Cone-shaped epiphyses at the bases of the proximal phalanges may occur in normal children and are unrelated to any skeletal dysplasia or arthropathy.

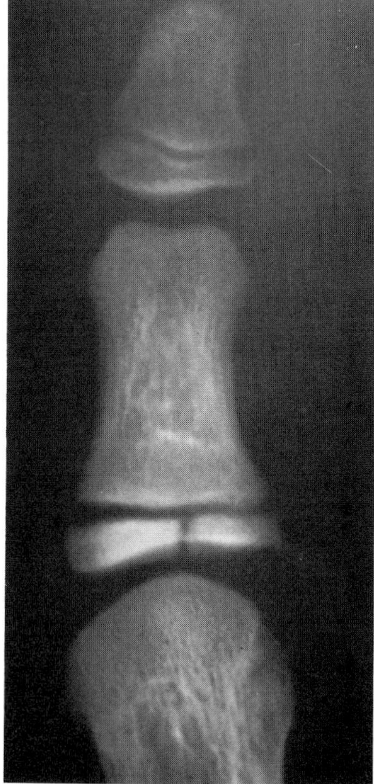

Figure 20–68. A dense ossification center at the base of the proximal phalanx of the great toe with or without its midline cleft is a normal variation of growth.

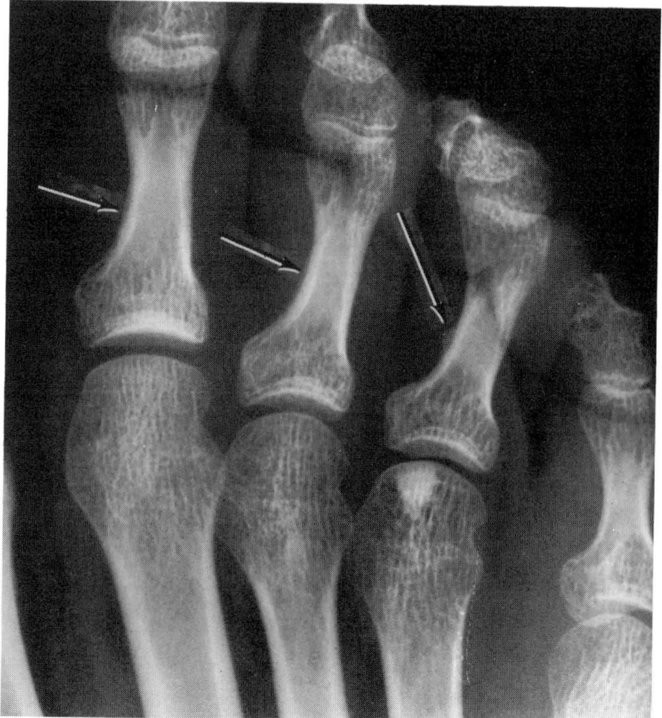

Figure 20–70. Normal bony excrescences on toes (arrows), not to be mistaken for periosteal proliferation.

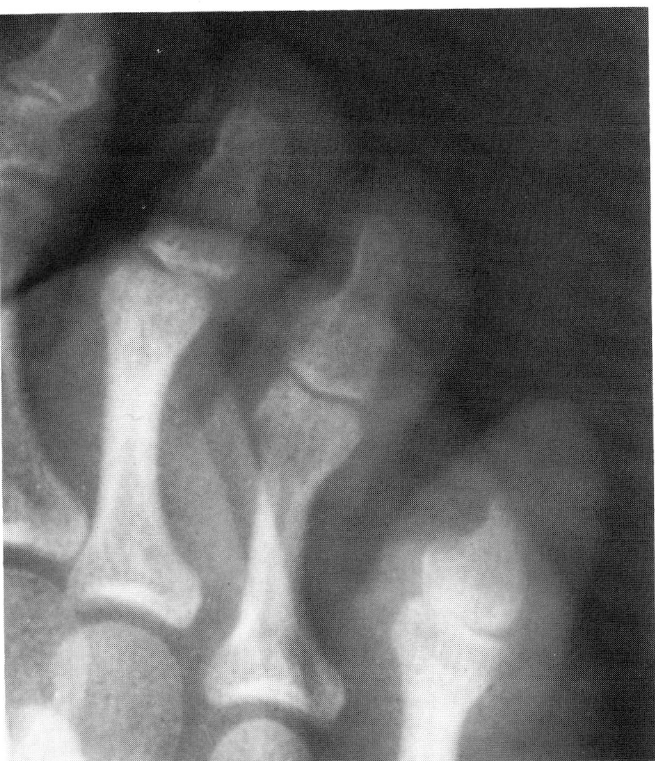

Figure 20–71. *Nonsegmented middle and distal phalanges in the third, fourth, and fifth toes.*

(Fig. 20–60). Similar spurious thickening of the lateral cortex of the tibia and the medial cortex of the fibula may be produced by slight external rotation of the leg (Fig. 20–61).

A recently reported source of misinterpretation is the soleal line of the tibia, which is a cause of tibial pseudoperiostitis.[16] The origin of the soleus muscle may result in a prominent osseous crest, which mimics a large area of periostitis in the posterior aspect of the proximal portion of the shaft of the tibia (Fig. 20–62). It is always associated with normal, undisturbed architecture of the underlying bone.

The ossification of the calcaneal apophysis is associated with two troublesome radiologic aspects. It is normally dense in children who walk, and it also may develop from multiple centers (Fig. 20–63). Neither of these findings should be confused with aseptic necrosis or osteochondritis. Similar irregularities in ossification without increased density may be seen in the tarsal navicular bones (Fig. 20–64). These centers invariably unite and form a single bone. In the stage of irregular ossification, the lack of sclerosis will differentiate this normal finding from osteochondritis (Köhler's disease).

In children with painful feet, the irregular ossification of the developing sesamoid bones should not be mistaken for pathologic calcification in the plantar soft tissues (Fig. 20–65).

The bases of the metatarsals are normally irregular, particularly as seen in the oblique projection (Fig. 20–66). The lateral aspect of the head of the first metatarsal often shows a deep fossa, which should not be mistaken for an erosion (Fig. 20–67).

The ossification center of the base of the proximal phalanx of the great toe is similar to the calcaneal apophysis in that it is usually dense and may occasionally be bifid. Both alterations are normal variants of growth (Fig. 20–68).

Cone-shaped epiphyses are seen in the proximal phalanges in many normal children and are not necessarily expressions of generalized or local disease (Fig. 20–69).

In the search for early periostitis of the phalanges as an expression of inflammatory arthritis one should not mistake the normal osseous excrescences of the proximal phalanges as periostitis (Fig. 20–70).

Many normal individuals do not develop distal interphalangeal joints in their toes. This is most commonly seen in the fifth toe but may also occur in the third and fourth toes. This condition, therefore, is not a manifestation of ankylosis (Fig. 20–71).

The ungual tufts of the toes may not be seen in children and some adults, resulting in a pointed configuration of the distal phalanx. This does not represent a resorptive phenomenon (Fig. 20–72).

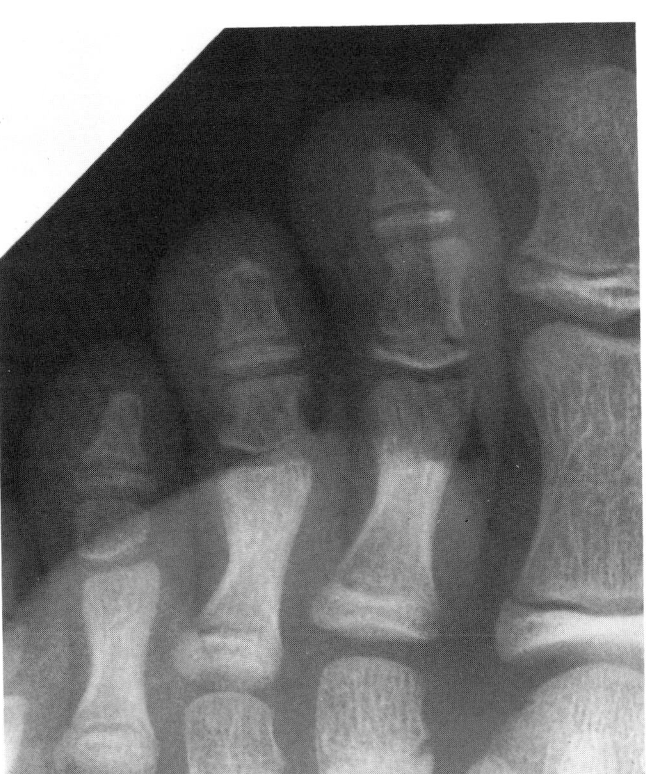

Figure 20–72. *Pointed terminal phalanges without tufts may be seen as a normal variant in young children and are unrelated to disease. In this patient, note also the variations in growth of the middle phalanges.*

SUMMARY

The examples of variation in development described in this chapter are only a few of the problems that beset any physician who uses the roentgenographic method in the study of skeletal disease. It is obvious that a broad appreciation of the alterations that are part of the normal growth of the skeleton, as well as a knowledge of many of the normal variations of the adult skeleton that may mimic significant disease, is necessary in order to avoid errors of commission.

I wish to express my appreciation to the Year Book Medical Publishers for permission to reproduce material from my book, An Atlas of Normal Roentgen Variants that may Simulate Disease.

REFERENCES

1. Alexander C: The aetiology of primary protrusio acetabuli. Br J Radiol *38*:567, 1965.
2. Barnes GR, Gwin JL: Distal irregularities of the femur simulating malignancy. Am J Roentgenol *122*:180, 1974.
3. Brower A, et al: Histological nature of the cortical irregularity of the medial posterior distal femoral metaphysis in children. Radiology *99*:389, 1971.
4. Brown I: A study of the "capsular" shadow in disorders of the hip in children. J Bone Joint Surg *57B*:175, 1975.
5. Bufkin WJ: The avulsive cortical irregularity. Am J Roentgenol *112*:487, 1971.
6. Caffey J: Pediatric X-Ray Diagnosis. 6th Ed. Chicago, Year Book Medical Publishers, 1972.
7. Dihlmann W: Practical significance and problems of early radiologic symptoms demonstrated by Norgaard sign of chronic rheumatoid polyarthritis. Fortschr Geb Rontgenstr Nuklearmed *112*:247, 1970.
8. Goodman N: The significance of terminal phalangeal osteosclerosis. Radiology *89*:709, 1967.
9. Harrison RB et al: The grooves of the distal articular surface of the femur — a normal variant. Am J Roentgenol *126*:751, 1976.
10. Haswell DM, Berne AS, Graham CB: The dorsal defect of the patella. Pediatr Radiol *4*:238, 1976.
11. Keats TE: An Atlas of Normal Roentgen Variants that may Simulate Disease. 2nd Ed. Chicago, Year Book Medical Publishers, 1979.
12. Keats TE: The distal anterior femoral metaphyseal defect: An anatomic variant that may simulate disease. Am J Roentgenol *121*:101, 1974.
13. Keats TE: Superior marginal rib defects in restrictive lung disease. Am J Roentgenol *124*:449, 1975.
14. Köhler A, Zimmer EA: Borderlands of the Normal and Early Pathologic in Skeletal Roentgenology. 11th Ed. New York, Grune & Stratton, 1968.
15. Kuhns LR, et al: Ivory epiphyses of the hands. Radiology *109*:643, 1973.
16. Levine AH, et al: The soleal line: A cause of tibial pseudoperiostitis. Radiology *119*:79, 1976.
17. Murray RO, Jacobson HG: The Radiology of Skeletal Disorders. 2nd Ed. New York, Churchill Livingstone, 1977.
18. Ozonoff MB, Ziter FMH Jr: The upper humeral notch. Radiology *113*:699, 1974.
19. Shopfner CE: Periosteal bone growth in normal infants. Am J Roentgenol *97*:154, 1966.
20. Smith, GR, Abel MS: Anatomical variations in the articular masses of the seventh cervical vertebra simulating fracture. Clin Radiol *28*:181, 1977.
21. Dunham WK, Marcus NW, Enneking WF, Haun C: Developmental defects of the distal femoral metaphysis. J Bone Joint Surg *62A*:801, 1980.

SECTION IV

CLASSIFICATION OF ARTICULAR DISEASE

21

CLASSIFICATION OF ARTICULAR DISEASE

by Donald Resnick, M.D.

There are many different types of articular disorders. The cause of some of these diseases is known; the etiology of others is unknown. Various schemes have been utilized to classify these disorders[1, 2]; however, each year further elucidation of recognized disorders and identification of previously unrecognized diseases necessitate the modification of existing schemes. Multiplicity of terms also contributes to difficulty in classification of articular disease.[3]

Classification of rheumatic diseases might be attempted on the basis of clinical, pathologic, or radiographic findings. The division of arthritis into categories based upon patterns of clinical presentation is difficult. In some diseases, these clinical patterns vary widely; a disorder may begin as an acute arthritis and subsequently pass into subacute and chronic stages. Other diseases frequently are asymptomatic. Categorization of articular disease based upon pathologic aberration may seem more ideal, but reports of nonspecific pathologic findings in some diseases and fragmentary descriptions of pathologic changes in others make this type of classification less than optimal. Classification of articular disease on the basis of radiographic change presents additional difficulties. Radiographic findings relate to the way in which bone and soft tissue react to insult; these tissues can react in only a limited number of ways, resulting in similarity of roentgenographic alterations in many diseases. Classification systems based upon roentgenographic changes are, therefore, difficult to apply and certainly not ideal.

Despite this apparent hardship in arriving at an optimal scheme, investigators have demonstrated continued interest in dividing articular disorders into appropriate categories. A general classification of joint disease into five major groups has been suggested. These groups included definite infectious disease, possible infectious disease, degenerative disease, traumatic disease, and metabolic disease. A

Table 21–1
NOMENCLATURE AND CLASSIFICATION OF ARTHRITIDES AND OTHER RHEUMATIC DISORDERS*
(Tentatively Adopted by International League Against Rheumatism, 1957)

I. Diseases and Disorders of Connective Tissue Accepted as Rheumatic
  A. Articular
    1. Inflammatory
      a. Idiopathic
        (1) Rheumatic fever
        (2) Rheumatoid arthritis
        (3) Atypical forms
          (a) Arthritis with psoriasis—psoriatic arthropathy
          (b) Juvenile rheumatoid arthritis (Still-Chauffard disease)
          (c) Rheumatoid arthritis with hypersplenism (Felty's syndrome)
          (d) Polyarthritis with keratoconjunctivitis sicca (Sjögren's syndrome)
        (4) Special forms
          (a) Ankylosing spondylitis (rheumatoid spondylitis)
          (b) Intermittent hydrarthrosis
          (c) Palindromic rheumatism
      b. Infectional—Arthritis due to specific infection
    2. Degenerative
      a. Osteoarthritis, degenerative joint disease (osteoarthrosis)
      b. Osteochondrosis
      c. Intervertebral disc syndromes
  B. Nonarticular
    1. Bursitis
    2. Fasciitis
    3. Fibrositis
    4. Myositis, myalgia
    5. Neuritis, neuropathy, neuralgia
    6. Periarthritis
    7. Tendinitis, peritendinitis
    8. Tenosynovitis, tenovaginitis
    9. Disorders of fatty tissue (panniculitis)

II. Diseases and Disorders with Rheumatic Features
  1. Inflammatory, idiopathic (diffuse collagen diseases)
    a. Dermatomyositis
    b. Polyarteritis nodosa, diffuse arteritis
    c. Systemic lupus erythematosus
    d. Scleroderma
  2. Hypersensitivity states with musculoarticular reactions to serum, drugs, etc.
  3. Traumatic
    a. Postural syndromes
    b. Traumatic arthropathy
  4. Associated with:
    a. Cutaneous or mucosal features
      (1) Erythema multiforme
      (2) Erythema nodosum
      (3) Purpura (various types), purpura rheumatica
      (4) Polyarthritis with urethritis and conjunctivitis (Reiter's disease)
    b. Metabolic disturbances
      (1) Alcaptonuria
      (2) Gout
    c. Endocrine disturbances
      (1) Acromegaly
      (2) Hyperparathyroidism
      (3) Myxedema, etc.
      (4) Menopause
      (5) Osteoporosis: Menopausal, senile, and others
    d. Blood diseases: Hemophilia, Leukemia, etc.
    e. Pulmonary diseases: Hypertrophic pulmonary osteoarthropathy, sarcoidosis, etc.
    f. Nervous system disease: Neuroarthropathy, reflex dystrophy
    g. Psychiatric states and psychologic syndromes
    h. Neoplastic diseases of articular or periarticular tissues
    i. Osteochondrodystrophies

*From Hollander JL, McCarty DJ Jr: Arthritis and Allied Conditions. 8th Ed. Philadelphia, Lea & Febiger, 1972.

Table 21–2
CLASSIFICATION OF ARTICULAR DISORDERS*

I. Polyarthritis of Unknown Etiology
- A. Rheumatoid arthritis
- B. Juvenile rheumatoid arthritis (including Still's disease)
- C. Ankylosing spondylitis
- D. Psoriatic arthritis
- E. Reiter's syndrome
- F. Others

II. "Connective Tissue" Disorders (Acquired)
- A. Systemic lupus erythematosus
- B. Progressive systemic sclerosis (scleroderma)
- C. Polymyositis and dermatomyositis
- D. Necrotizing arteritis and other forms of vasculitis
  1. Polyarteritis nodosa
  2. Hypersensitivity angiitis
  3. Wegener's granulomatosis
  4. Takayasu's (pulseless) disease
  5. Cogan's syndrome
  6. Giant cell arteritis (including polymyalgia rheumatica)
- E. Amlyoidosis
- F. Other (see also Rheumatoid arthritis; Sjögren's syndrome)

III. Rheumatic Fever

IV. Degenerative Joint Disease (Osteoarthritis, Osteoarthrosis)
- A. Primary
- B. Secondary

V. Nonarticular Rheumatism
- A. Fibrositis
- B. Intervertebral disc and low back syndromes
- C. Myositis and myalgia
- D. Tendinitis and peritendinitis (bursitis)
- E. Tenosynovitis
- F. Fasciitis
- G. Carpal tunnel syndrome
- H. Other (see also Shoulder-hand syndrome)

VI. Diseases with Which Arthritis Is Frequently Associated
- A. Sarcoidosis
- B. Relapsing polychondritis
- C. Schönlein-Henoch purpura
- D. Ulcerative colitis
- E. Regional enteritis
- F. Whipple's disease
- G. Sjögren's syndrome
- H. Familial Mediterranean fever
- I. Other (see also Psoriatic arthritis)

VII. Arthritis Associated with Known Infectious Agents
- A. Bacterial
  1. Gonococcus
  2. Meningococcus
  3. Pneumococcus
  4. Streptococcus
  5. Staphylococcus
  6. Salmonella
  7. Brucella
  8. *Streptobacillus moniliformis* (Haverhill fever)
  9. *Mycobacterium tuberculosis*
  10. *Treponema pallidum* (syphilis)
  11. *Treponema pertenue* (yaws)
  12. Other (see also Rheumatic fever)
- B. Rickettsial
- C. Viral
  1. Rubella
  2. Mumps
  3. Viral hepatitis
  4. Other
- D. Fungal
- E. Parasitic

VIII. Traumatic and/or Neurogenic Disorders
- A. Traumatic arthritis (the result of direct trauma)
- B. Neuropathic arthropathy (Charcot joints)
  1. Syphilis (tabes dorsalis)
  2. Diabetes mellitus (diabetic neuropathy)
  3. Syringomyelia
  4. Myelomeningocele
  5. Congenital insensitivity to pain (including familial dysautonomia)
  6. Other
- C. Shoulder-hand syndrome
- D. Mechanical derangement of joints
- E. Other (see also Degenerative joint disease; Carpal tunnel syndrome)

IX. Arthropathy Associated with Known or Strongly Suspected Biochemical or Endocrine Abnormalities
- A. Gout
- B. Chondrocalcinosis articularis ("pseudogout")
- C. Alkaptonuria (ochronosis)
- D. Hemophilia
- E. Sickle cell disease and other hemoglobinopathies
- F. Agammaglobulinemia (hypogammaglobulinemia)
- G. Gaucher's disease
- H. Hyperparathyroidism
- I. Acromegaly
- J. Thyroid acropachy
- K. Hypothyroidism
- L. Scurvy (hypovitaminosis C)
- M. Hyperlipoproteinemia type II (xanthoma tuberosum and xanthoma tendinosum)
- N. Fabry's disease (angiokeratoma corporis diffusum or glycolipid lipidosis)
- O. Hemochromatosis
- P. Other (see also Inherited and Congenital Disorders)

X. Neoplasms
- A. Synovioma
- B. Primary juxta-articular bone tumors
- C. Metastatic malignant tumors
- D. Leukemia
- E. Multiple myeloma
- F. Benign tumors of articular tissue
- G. Other (see also Hypertrophic osteoarthropathy)

XI. Allergy and Drug Reactions
- A. Arthritis due to specific allergens (e.g., serum sickness)
- B. Arthritis due to drugs
- C. Other (see also Systemic lupus erythematosus [drug-induced lupus-like syndromes—e.g., hydralazine and procainamide syndromes]; Hypersensitivity angiitis)

XII. Inherited and Congenital Disorders
- A. Marfan's syndrome
- B. Homocystinuria
- C. Ehlers-Danlos syndrome
- D. Osteogenesis imperfecta
- E. Pseudoxanthoma elasticum
- F. Cutis laxa
- G. Mucopolysaccharidoses (including Hurler's syndrome)
- H. Arthrogryposis multiplex congenita
- I. Hypermobility syndromes
- J. Myositis (or fibrodysplasia) ossificans progressiva
- K. Tumoral calcinosis
- L. Werner's syndrome
- M. Congenital dysplasia of the hip
- N. Other (see also Arthropathy Associated with Known or Strongly Suspected Biochemical or Endocrine Abnormalities)

XIII. Miscellaneous Disorders
- A. Pigmented villonodular synovitis and tenosynovitis
- B. Behçet's syndrome
- C. Erythema nodosum
- D. Relapsing panniculitis (Weber-Christian disease)
- E. Avascular necrosis of bone
- F. Juvenile osteochondritis
- G. Osteochondritis dissecans
- H. Erythema multiforme (Stevens-Johnson syndrome)
- I. Hypertrophic osteoarthropathy
- J. Multicentric reticulohistiocytosis
- K. Disseminated lipogranulomatosis (Farber's disease)
- L. Familial lipochrome pigmentary arthritis
- M. Tietze's syndrome
- N. Thrombotic thrombocytopenic purpura
- O. Other

*From Primer on the Rheumatic Diseases. Section 4, Classification of Rheumatic Disease. 7th Ed. JAMA *224* (Suppl 5):16, 1973. Copyright 1973, American Medical Association.

more extensive classification system was introduced by the International League Against Rheumatism in 1957 (Table 21–1). In 1963, the American Rheumatism Association adopted a classification system,[4] which has subsequently been expanded[5] (Table 21–2).

The organization of this book follows in some part the classification scheme in Table 21–2. Certain deletions and additions are utilized where more recent evidence has suggested that modifications in this scheme might be appropriate. The authors recognize that the discussion of certain disorders in more than one location in the book creates redundancy, although this type of repetition is not without value. In no way do we believe that our table of contents represents an ideal method for classifying articular disorders.

REFERENCES

1. Hollander JL: Introduction to arthritis and the rheumatic diseases. *In* JL Hollander, DJ McCarty Jr (Eds): Arthritis and Allied Conditions. A Textbook of Rheumatology. 8th Ed. Philadelphia, Lea & Febiger, 1972, p 3.
2. Wood PHN: Nomenclature and classification in rheumatology. *In* JT Scott (Ed): Copeman's Textbook of the Rheumatic Diseases. 5th Ed. Edinburgh, Churchill Livingstone, 1978, p 14.
3. Ruhl MJ, Sokoloff L: A thesaurus of rheumatology. Arthritis Rheum *8*:97, 1965.
4. Blumberg B, Bunim JJ, Calkins E, Pirani CL, Zvaifler NJ: ARA nomenclature and classification of arthritis and rheumatism (tentative). Arthritis Rheum *7*:93, 1964.
5. Primer on the Rheumatic Diseases. Section 4: Classification of Rheumatic Disease. 7th Ed. New York, The Arthritis Foundation, p 16 (reprinted in JAMA *224* [Suppl 5], 1973).

SECTION V

MEDICAL AND SURGICAL EVALUATION OF ARTICULAR DISEASE

SYMPTOMS AND SIGNS OF ARTICULAR DISEASE

by Rodney Bluestone, M.B., F.R.C.P.

22

Rheumatology is a very clinically oriented subspecialty of internal medicine. The symptoms and signs of rheumatic disease may be very revealing and often suggest a probable diagnosis at the time of initial clinical presentation. In large measure this diagnostic process depends on detecting the true pattern of distribution of the arthropathy. In the case of an established chronic rheumatic disease, the pattern of distribution is even more diagnostic. The radiographs contribute largely, first by demonstrating the true distribution of the arthropathy (including involvement of relatively asymptomatic or clinically inaccessible joints), and second by providing a diagnostic "bonus" by revealing radiographic changes that themselves may be characteristic of a specific rheumatic disease process.

The osteoarticular system, together with its supporting soft tissue structures, is a fairly homogeneous anatomic structure and, like so many other organ systems within the body, is capable of generating only a limited number of symptoms and signs. One should remember, however, that some rheumatic diseases are systemic in nature, and in these situations there is considerable scope for the development of extraskeletal involvement, which may dominate the clinical presentation.

By applying these general principles, the clinical evaluation of patients with arthritis frequently becomes a finite diagnostic exercise. One may elicit the symptoms and signs of osteoarticular disease, paying particular attention to their clinical (nonradiographic) distribution. If the disease has already progressed to any degree of chronicity, the radiographic changes detected in both symptomatic and asymptomatic regions of the skeleton will result in a more accurate definition of this distribution. In addition, the radiographic changes themselves may include some features characteristic of a specific arthropathy. The physician will also note the presence or absence of certain extraskeletal symptoms and signs. Following the completion of this exercise, the nature of the rheumatic disease is obvious in most cases. This clinical assessment is aided by the fact that many of the common rheumatic diseases tend to

Table 22–1
THE SYMPTOMS AND SIGNS OF RHEUMATIC DISEASE

Symptoms	Signs
Pain	Swelling
Stiffness	Tenderness
Swelling	Limited range of motion
Dysfunction	Painful range of motion
Systemic complaints	Muscle wasting
	Instability and subluxations
	Deformities
	Extraskeletal (systemic) signs

favor victims of a certain sex or age group. Thus, symptoms and signs suggestive of a particular clinical syndrome elicited in a patient known to be more vulnerable to that disease by virtue of sex or age increase the index of suspicion and favor an early diagnosis. Moreover, the clinical profiles of the major rheumatic diseases tend to retain a great degree of uniformity from one patient to another. Therefore, the type of patient presenting with osteoarticular symptoms, in combination with the clincal features of the pathologic process, usually is helpful in making an accurate diagnosis.

Only in relatively few patients are laboratory tests necessary to confirm or refute the clinical diagnostic impression. In a few instances, these laboratory tests may indeed be crucial, and such tests will be discussed in order of priority in Chapter 23. Nevertheless, many laboratory tests are deemed helpful even in the presence of a fairly firm clinical diagnosis, since they aid in the assessment of disease activity and may then be used to help monitor the effectiveness of subsequent therapeutic efforts.

This chapter will not attempt to reproduce the detailed material available in several rheumatology texts.[1–4] Hence, the large number of various diseases that may affect the musculoskeletal system will not be covered exhaustively; nor will undue attention be given to the unending possibilities for theoretic differential diagnoses that may exist in many clinical situations. Rather, this chapter will deal with the *clinical approach* to the patient presenting with musculoskeletal symptoms. Such an approach will enable the reader to better appreciate other sections of this textbook so that the wide array of morphologic and radiographic changes illustrated throughout can be seen to result in a relatively restricted class of symptoms and signs (Table 22–1).

SYMPTOMS

Pain

Pain is the most conspicuous symptom arising from osteoarticular disease. The site of the pain frequently reflects its origin and is therefore of key concern to the physician. Most diseases that affect joints or periarticular tissues give rise to pain at a site where the area of maximum intensity accurately reflects the site of the pathologic process. Thus, a swollen and inflamed peripheral synovial joint is diffusely painful all over that joint; and inflammation within many of the small joints of the spine usually manifests itself as diffuse midline pain felt up and down the back. However, the physician must be prepared to recognize radiating pain syndromes in patients with rheumatic disease, and these radiating patterns may sometimes lead the clinician away from the true source of the symptom. Examples of this are pain due to sacroiliitis presenting as a sciatica-like syndrome felt in the buttock and down the back of the thigh; hip joint disease presenting as pain down the anterior and medial aspects of the thigh into the knee; an inflamed trochanteric bursa presenting as a burning pain down the upper lateral aspect of the thigh; and an inflamed or irritated anserine bursa resulting in an intense burning discomfort felt down the anteromedial aspect of the shin.

Moreover, any disease of the spine that carries the potential for compression or irritation of the spinal nerve roots may present with a neuralgic syndrome. This is very obvious in patients with cervical spondylosis, presenting with brachial neuralgia, and in those with degenerative joint disease of the lumbosacral spine (with or without a clear-cut episode suggesting a prolapsed disc), presenting with sciatica.

The actual mechanisms of rheumatic disease pain are undoubtedly complex and not always understood. Some mechanisms seem fairly obvious. A newly inflamed or hemorrhagic synovial joint that becomes full of exudative fluid or blood readily triggers the agonizing pain of acute articular distention, presumably due to stretching of the usually tight fibrous capsule abundantly supplied with nerve endings. Indeed, it is not uncommon to see this type of pain abating in patients with chronic synovitis as their joint capsules become chronically stretched and relatively less sensitive. Pain from an acutely ruptured joint can be very sudden and intense. In this situation the intra-articular pressure rises so much that the hitherto unstretched capsule ruptures, permitting escape of the synovial fluid into the soft tissue planes, where it is capable of generating a massive sterile inflammatory response. This situation is exemplified by a ruptured popliteal bursa with dissection down into the calf muscles ("pseudophlebitis syndrome") or by a ruptured elbow joint with dissection into the antecubital fossa. Capsular pain appears to be very important in some forms of chronically immobilized joints. This mechanism is particularly prominent following any form of traumatic or inflammatory insult within or around the shoulder joint, with or without direct involvement of the capsule. Once the capsule has been inflamed or torn, it undergoes a fibrous shrinkage so that movement of the joint in any direction results in stretching of the contracted capsule and intense pain. A similar shrinkage of the capsule is thought to follow prolonged immobilization, even in the absence of a primary capsular lesion. This situation is presumably one source of pain arising from contractured joints, with similar components originating from the foreshortened ligaments and tendons. Active disease of the vascular subchondral bone or adjacent periostitis appears to be another potent cause of arthropathic pain and may differ somewhat in its character from that due to simple synovial distention. Often the patient describes a deeper and more sustained type of pain, which may sometimes be related to periarticular bone formation as part of the healing process. Other rheumatic syndromes are characterized by pain that cannot readily be ascribed to any known mechanism. This is particularly seen in many of the soft tissue rheumatism syndromes, in which localized pain and tenderness may be ascribed to bursitis or focal areas of muscle spasm, yet very little data exist on the precise pathologic process. Many of the soft tissue rheumatism syndromes affecting the torso, especially on the posterior trunk, may well be due to referred pain from minor degrees of subluxation, ligamentous tearing, and hematoma formation in the deep vertebral and perispinal structures. Indeed, direct needling of the vertebral ligaments may evoke pain localized to discrete areas on the anterior or posterior torso, and these sites of referred pain may then become involved by areas of focal muscle spasm that themselves become tender and the source of more pain. This particular mode of musculoskeletal pain could conceivably account for some of the more generalized symptoms of inflammatory or degenerative rheumatic disease.

Some pain syndromes due to rheumatic disease are characterized by identifiable aggravating or relieving factors. It would be expected that the pain of inflammatory peripheral joint disease would be aggravated following use of the involved joint, and this is frequently the case. If the inflammatory process is acute or severe, pain is even felt at rest. Contrariwise, the pain of degenerative joint disease is nearly always greatly exacerbated by use, especially when the process involves weight-bearing regions. However, in patients with osteoarthrosis of the hip a stage is sometimes reached in the clinical evolution of the syndrome at which severe nocturnal pain may be a significant component of the patient's history. Interestingly, inflammatory disease of the spine due to ankylosing spondylitis is usually aggravated by rest, especially when sitting or lying for prolonged periods of time. This pain is usually relieved by physical activity, although the associated secondary perispinal muscle spasm may itself make such activity painful.

Stiffness

Generalized stiffness is a peculiar symptom of unknown origin, but one that is very prevalent among patients with various types of rheumatic disease. Every patient has his or her own definition of stiffness, but in general the symptom implies a sensation that the entire skeleton feels relatively immobile and difficult or painful to move.[5] This is a very conspicuous symptom in patients with widespread inflammatory joint disease, best characterized by rheumatoid arthritis. In that disease the stiffness is presumed to arise from the universal synovitis that frequently prevails in the disorder. It is usually most apparent after a period of rest and is therefore most conspicuous in the early morning on arising. Early morning stiffness, therefore, forms a rather valuable diagnostic clue to the diagnosis of even early rheumatoid arthritis, in addition to providing one subjective monitor for assessing the efficacy of therapy. More localized stiffness is usually recounted by patients to describe a loss of range of motion within a specified joint. When due to an active inflammatory process, local stiffness is always accompanied by obvious pain. However, in joints that have been inflamed in the more distant past or in which there is a very low grade inflammatory process, progressive loss of range of motion may be a prominent symptom of the rheumatic disease. Interestingly, the early morning stiffness accompanying both rheumatoid arthritis and ankylosing spondylitis is usually relieved by hot showers or baths taken immediately on arising. This phenomenon has no doubt contributed to the traditional popularity of spa centers for the treatment of rheumatic diseases, where a soak in a soothing hot tub of mineralized water frequently evokes dramatic, if somewhat temporary, symptomatic relief.

Swelling

Swelling of a joint is a critical physical sign. Unfortunately, a history of a swollen joint is rarely dependable. Many patients may interpret a sensation as swelling and dutifully report it to their physician. Sometimes a patient may notice swelling around a joint, but rarely are patients able to discern true synovial distention from the soft tissue swelling within the periarticular tissues. Thus, although the history of a swollen joint or joints is important, it must never be accepted as firm evidence of arthritis unless accompanied by objective signs. Nevertheless, in some forms of rheumatic disease such as crystal-induced synovitis (gout and pseudogout) the previous episodes of localized painful swelling of a single joint may be so dramatic and clear-cut as to leave little doubt that it did actually occur. Even so, diagnosing acute gout or pseudogout on the basis of the patient's history alone becomes a hazardous exercise. Indeed, one of the special skills of clinical rheumatology is to persuade patients to remain under observation long enough that the physician may personally witness the episodes of joint swelling that have led them to seek a medical opinion.

Dysfunction

Depending on the severity and extent of target tissue involvement, disease of the osteoarticular structures may result in mild, moderate, or profound dysfunction. This dysfunction may be strictly localized, such as loss of use of a single inflamed joint. However, even such local involvement, if severe enough in degree, may be so profound as to result in total disability. This is typically seen in patients with acute monoarticular arthritis due to sepsis or crystal-induced inflammation, or in the flitting arthropathy of acute rheumatic fever, in which the involved joints are so painful that the patient is rendered totally immobile. If the arthropathic process is local and chronic, regional dysfunction is a natural consequence. This dysfunction may result from irreversible joint contracture, local skeletal deformities following long-standing inflammation (notably in the growing child), or even disruption of periarticular tissues, such as is seen in the complete severence of the long head of the biceps tendon or a torn supraspinatus rotator cuff. Some common forms of chronic rheumatic disease result in a widespread joint inflammation or degeneration, with destruction and deformity. When this process is universal, dysfunction may be noticed as a loss of many of the usual abilities required for the activities of daily living. This gradual disability is something that patients invariably notice but may not volunteer unless directly asked. Thus, in the assessment of the diagnosis, functional consequences, and therapeutic responsiveness of any patient with rheumatic disease, the subject should be keenly questioned about his or her lifestyle and the impact of the symptoms on daily activities. General activities such as ambulation, ability to work, sleeping patterns, recreational pastimes, and sexual intercourse may all provide a broad index of the functional impact of the patient's rheumatic disease. If the functional history indicates areas of gross impairment, the physician can concentrate on the specific reasons for the handicap. Common examples of dysfunctional symptoms include loss of manual dexterity; loss of grip strength; shoulder pain on raising the arms above the head (e.g., for attention to the hair); difficulty in getting up from and sitting down on a chair or the toilet seat; difficulty in putting on shoes and stockings or socks in the mornings; and the inability to abduct the legs for sexual intercourse. Historical data relating to musculoskeletal function are unique to the field of rheumatic diseases, and the importance of such data is not widely enough appreciated by practicing physicians. Yet the information tells the clinician more about the distribution, severity, and consequences of a rheumatic disease process than any other single historical fact and should never be overlooked as an integral part of the history of a patient presenting with any form of acute or chronic rheumatic disease at any stage in its natural history.

Extraskeletal Manifestations

Although some rheumatic diseases affect osteoarticular structures primarily, with only secondary effects on periarticular soft tissues, there are some diseases that although primarily rheumatic also involve other target-organ systems. Thus, the physician must always be aware of extraskeletal rheumatic syndromes generating symptoms such as generalized malaise, fever, undue fatigue, and various other constitutional complaints. In some instances the extraarticular features may be very distinctive and in themselves rather suggestive of a specific pathologic process. Thus, the dry, sore eyes and dry mouth of sicca syndrome may be more conspicuous than the arthropathic component in a patient with Sjögren's syndrome. The middle-aged man with rheumatoid arthritis may have more prominent symptoms from the pleuropulmonary involvement than from the articular disease. Clearly, it is impossible to practice the art of clinical rheumatology without being prepared to focus on all other symptoms and signs of more widespread target-organ involvement.

PHYSICAL SIGNS

Articular Swelling

It cannot be stressed too much that a distended joint is the only dependable physical sign of an inflamed joint. Most inflammatory rheumatic diseases are characterized by the production of an exudative synovial fluid, which distends the capsule and causes an enlargement and bulging of the entire joint outline. This production of excess synovial fluid may result from acute or chronic inflammation of the synovial membrane, the release of intrasynovial joint space crystals able to evoke a brisk phlogistic response, acute mechanical derangements of intra- or periarticular structures, active disease of the adjacent subchondral bone, or the introduction of foreign bodies or bacteria into the synovial space. All result in joint swelling detectable as the cardinal physical sign of synovitis. In the absence of joint distention one can never diagnose any type of inflammatory arthritis with certainty, although one must realize that a previous inflammatory episode may well have resolved by the time the patient seeks a consultation. However, chronic inflammation of a joint can never be diagnosed without demonstration of overt swelling. The physical sign of joint distention is best elicited by a combination of inspection and palpation, with due consideration to the regional anatomy of the joints under scrutiny. Clearly, most of the peripheral (synovial) joints are readily inspected and palpated.[6] A distended peripheral joint is usually evident on careful inspection, especially when compared directly with a normal contralateral region. Gentle palpation should reveal a sensation of intra-articular fluid either by direct ballottement (e.g., patellar tap) or by the sensation of an evoked fluid wave felt between two fingers or two hands. In the case of the knee joint, a bulge sign indicative of even a tiny effusion can often be better visualized than palpated. There is no exception to this rule, so that swelling in a toe, finger, knee, or elbow joint should be demonstrable no matter how small the volume of the intra-articular exudate. Remember that many patients present to the physician with persistent arthralgias, and the firm demonstration of the *absence* of joint distention usually permits a strong reassurance as to the innocent nature of the symptoms. Nevertheless, it should be realized that there are numerous articulations within the human skeleton that are relatively inaccessible to the examiner's eyes and hands. These include most of the spinal joints, the sacroiliac articulations, and to some degree the shoulder and hip joints. Unfortunately, inflammation in any of these sites may result in pain without demonstrable or dramatic physical signs. It is in these inaccessible sites that the demonstration of a painfully limited range of motion then assumes a more important diagnostic role as an indicator of possible inflammatory arthritis.

Technically speaking, joint swelling may be due to para-articular bony enlargement. Proliferative osteophytes around the margins of joints may result in a visible and palpable bone-hard expansion of the joint contour. This form of enlargement, although important, does not carry the diagnostic implications of swelling due to synovial distention. Nevertheless, it is a valuable sign of bony remodeling, usually indicative of a primary or secondary degenerative intra-articular process. In addition, bony proliferation around joints is seen in many clinical states, including following trauma and in patients with various metabolic and endocrine disorders.

Tenderness

Osteoarticular tenderness is one of the most difficult physical signs for the physician to interpret. A great deal of elicited tenderness is under subjective control, so that many normal individuals have rather sensitive tissues, particularly at those regions of the skeleton characterized by superficial ligamentous-bony junctions or costochondral articulations. An obviously distended, inflamed joint may well be tender; but the primary physical sign is so dramatic and important that the additional sign of tenderness is relatively insignificant. On the other hand, deeply palpated tenderness over otherwise inaccessible joints such as the sacroiliac regions or spine may be an important indicator of an underlying disease process. Perhaps the most important example of the detection of local tenderness is in the field of soft tissue rheumatism syndromes. In these various syndromes, local and focal pain and tenderness, with faithful reproduction of the pain following firm pressure over the tender area, is an important physical sign. In fact, some of the classic tissue rheumatism syndromes, such as tennis elbow, subacromial bursitis, and trochanteric bursitis, depend for their diagnosis on the clear-cut and reproducible tenderness and pain on heavy palpation over a superficial specific anatomic site.

Range of Joint Motion

A diseased joint inevitably loses some range of motion. The more severe and acute the articular disease, the quicker and more permanent the loss of range of motion. Thus, persistent inflammatory or destructive joint disease will result in more loss of movement than episodic arthritis or a low-grade degenerative arthropathy. Nevertheless, no matter what degree of recovery may follow, once a joint has been persistently inflamed, there is inevitable loss of mobility. Therefore, the clinical demonstration of loss of range of motion becomes an important sign for several reasons. First, combined with the symptom of pain and the physical sign of distention, it may confirm the presence of a disease process within that joint. Second, as a sign by itself even painless loss of range of motion may be a strong indicator of a previous inflammatory arthritis, which has long since resolved. This is particularly well seen in large hinge joints (wrists, elbows, and knees), in which loss of range of motion may be an early and sensitive sign of prior arthritis. It is to be hoped that the historical facts would indicate whether the original articular insult was most likely degenerative, traumatic, or inflammatory. If the arthropathy is still active, and especially if it is inflammatory in nature, the loss of range of motion is frequently painful. This sign is very clearly demonstrated in chronic inflammatory diseases of the wrist and knee, in which painful loss of range of motion is usually indicative of an active synovitis and therefore is a rather valuable diagnostic clue to the presence of diseases such as rheumatoid arthritis. In the relatively inaccessible joints of the spine and hip, a painless or painful loss of range of motion assumes even greater importance as indicating osteoarticular disease within those deeper parts of the skeleton. Thus, the clinician must be prepared to test the range of motion in various regions of the spine and to move the hip joint through the entire complex range of motions permitted by ball-and-socket articulations. Limitation of motion in these areas may be a fairly reliable indicator of rheumatic disease. If this evoked limitation is painful, the physician may more likely consider the presence of an active disease process, although this association is not as reliable as in the more peripheral joints. Indeed, osteoarthrosis of the hip or spine may lead to a very painful limitation of motion even though the underlying pathologic process is noninflammatory in nature.

Stability

It is important for the physician to be familiar with the normal at-rest postures of the peripheral joints as well as with the upper limits of normal for the range of articular motion. Joint stability depends to a great extent on the integrity of the periarticular tissues — notably the capsule, ligaments, and muscle surrounding the joint. If there has been gross intra-articular destruction completely altering the normal architecture of the joint, that articulation may well become unstable. However, even lesser degrees of intra-articular disease, such as a chronic rheumatoid type of synovitis with persistent capsular distention, often lead to joint instability. This develops partly as a result of the chronic distended state resulting in capsular weakness and partly because of the "sympathetic" periarticular atrophy and wasting of the soft tissues. In this way persistent inflammation of even a mild kind may eventually lead to joint instability. The instability may be evident at rest, as shown by the abnormal posture of a peripheral joint, digit, or limb, or it may be evoked on passive or active movement of the joint when it becomes apparent that the normal range of motion is either excessive or inappropriate in its range. In assessing the dysfunctional aspects of chronic joint disease, articular laxity or subluxation is a very important mechanicophysical sign. Not only may it be of diagnostic importance but in addition it may actually determine specific therapeutic strategies designed to lessen the impact of the insecure skeletal component.

It is not widely realized that some normal individuals have naturally hypermobile joints. Idiopathic and benign hypermobility is especially seen in otherwise normal young women who are considered to be "double-jointed." This hypermobility may be demonstrated by forced hyperextension of the thumb toward the radial margin of the forearm; hyperextension of the outstretched elbow well beyond 180 degrees; remarkable ease in touching the floor in a straight leg forward bending position; and voluntary hyperextension of the middle and terminal phalanges of the fingers. Recognition of hypermobility may be important since it frequently explains the totally innocent and nonspecific arthralgias sometimes experienced by such individuals.[7] Moreover, there is a whole group of metabolic and congenital diseases that are also characterized by musculoskeletal hypermobility. Usually these underlying disorders are obvious enough, but the patient may occasionally present to the physician with the mild arthralgias related to his secondary hypermobility syndrome.

Deformities

It is easy to understand how disease affecting the bones, joints, and periarticular structures can lead to temporary and then permanent deformities of digits, parts of limbs, or even entire extremities. The mechanisms leading to deformity in rheumatic disease are multiple and much more complex than is initially apparent. Destruction of joint architecture can clearly lead to a malalignment of the articulating bones. However, there appear to be more subtle influences at work to account for many of the deformities seen in chronic inflammatory joint disease of the type typified by rheumatoid arthritis. In that situation, inappropriate and unbalanced muscular pull across inflamed joints may result in deformities all out of proportion to the degree of articular destruction. It is important for the physician to gauge the reversibility of such deformities. Many therapeutic and surgical measures designed to lessen the deformities of inflammatory joint disease are dependent on the degree of demonstrable reversibility. Equally important, but sometimes less spectacular, are the deformities of the axial skeleton and chest wall. Congenital or acquired deformities affecting the spine are easily overlooked. Yet, these may be potent clinical clues to the cause of backache or may reflect a current pathologic process, in which involvement of the spinal and costovertebral joints is a major diagnostic clue.

A precise measurement of the range of motion of affected joints may be necessary to detect and follow the development of functionally important contractures and deformities throughout the skeleton. Moreover, the recognition of certain types of deformity can be of considerable diagnostic help. Examples of this are seen in the characteristic early ulnar deviation of the hands due to chronic rheumatoid arthritis; the typical boutonnière and swan-neck deformities of chronic inflammatory joint disease affecting the finger joints; hallux valgus of an osteoarthritic great toe joint; and the exaggerated cervical lordosis–thoracic kyphosis with loss of the lumbar lordosis seen in patients with ankylosing spondylitis.

The recognition of deformities is also very important when looking for physical signs that might account for the historical evidence of functional disabilities previously outlined by the patient. Frequently, the physical limitations affecting arthritic patients can be readily explained by such deformities. In an age in which reconstructive orthopedic surgery recognizes few limits, documentation of deformities is an essential part of the assessment of patients with all forms of rheumatic disease prior to planning a definitive therapeutic program, which might well include surgical measures.

Muscle Wasting

Articular disease of any chronicity is quickly followed by a secondary reflex wasting of surrounding muscles. The secondary muscular atrophy may itself become an important component contributing to the chronicity and sequelae of the intra-articular pathologic process. This is particularly well seen in joints such as the knees, in which wasting of the quadriceps muscle adds further to the instability of an inflamed joint. Moreover, there are some rheumatic diseases in which the pathologic process may actually involve muscle as a direct target tissue. Clearly, muscle inflammation and wasting itself may then result in symptoms and would certainly add to the burden of any associated arthropathic process. The major physical signs of muscle disease are wasting and weakness. Periarticular wasting is a valuable clue to the presence of chronic arthropathy and is best detected by careful inspection, especially if one can compare an involved site with a normal contralateral region. Muscle strength is an important semiobjective observation that can be assessed in all the major muscle groups, particularly the large flexor and extensor muscles of the shoulder and pelvic girdles as well as the more peripheral parts. The physical sign of generalized muscle weakness is very important since one can hardly diagnose a primary myopathic disease without it. However, there is a potentially large subjective element in assessing muscle strength, so that considerable skill is required for this part of the examination. Moreover, patients with painful joints may well have an apparent muscle weakness as a result of pain being aggravated by movement. This secondary inhibition of muscle use may then resemble true weakness. In particular, patients with widespread inflammatory joint disease such as rheumatoid arthritis may present with widespread and symmetric muscle wasting and weakness. In some instances this clinical picture may be due to a low-grade myositis, but in most cases it is due to profound muscle atrophy secondary to the primary arthropathy.[8] Likewise, muscle tenderness is a common nonspecific physical sign. Relatively few diseases of muscle are associated with severe or sustained tenderness, so that most patients with moderately tender musculature show no evidence of an underlying myopathic process.

Extra-Articular Signs

Just as rheumatic disease affecting extra-articular tissues may manifest itself by symptoms of a versatile and generalized nature, so may the physical signs reflect extension of the disease process outside of the skeleton and supporting tissues. Thus, important diagnostic clues may be gleaned from the detection of lymphadenopathy, hepatosplenomegaly, pericarditis, pleurisy, sicca syndrome, and so forth. Some relatively early extra-articular signs are particularly noticeable in patients with rheumatoid arthritis and may initially dominate the clinical picture. These include carpal tunnel syndrome due to compression of the median nerve within the anterior compartment of the wrist; the presence of subcutaneous nodules, which may be seen very early in some forms of rheumatoid disease; and the demonstration of keratoconjunctivitis sicca in patients with Sjögren's syndrome in whom the arthropathic component of their illness may be relatively inconspicuous.

CLINICAL PATTERNS OF OSTEOARTICULAR INVOLVEMENT

The clinical rheumatologist is keenly aware that the total distribution of an arthropathy throughout the entire skeleton frequently provides the most important clue to a definitive diagnosis. That is to say, certain rheumatic diseases are characterized by fairly predictable patterns of skeletal involvement.[9] The pattern may be established and evident early in the course of the disease or may only become well defined after the arthritis has progressed into a chronic or relapsing pattern. Just as the distribution of a rash or lesion is of key diagnostic importance in dermatology diagnosis and analysis of the second heart sound is the key in cardiac auscultation, so the *distribution* of the arthropathy is a potent diagnostic guide applicable to most patients with rheumatic disease. In addition, many rheumatic diseases are more commonly seen in patients of a certain age or sex than in others. Although this is only a broad generalization, it is nevertheless a valid clue aiding the diagnostic process. Knowledge of the age and sex of the patient presenting with arthritis together with the total distribution of the arthropathy can frequently yield a tentative diagnosis. Clearly, the radiographs play a key role in establishing the true distribution of the articular disease especially once the pathologic process is established and becomes chronic. These principles will be emphasized when considering the main rheumatic diseases seen in clinical practice. In each category of rheumatic disease discussed below diagnosis is frequently possible by carefully noting the patient's symptoms, methodically eliciting the physical signs of articular or periarticular disease, assessing the total distribution of the arthropathy, including the radiographic distribution, and then considering the presence or absence of specific extra-articular features. On occasion, additional information gleaned from laboratory testing may be necessary or desirable; this will be discussed in detail in Chapter 23.

Soft Tissue Rheumatic Syndromes

These syndromes are best described as local and focal areas of periarticular pain and tenderness usually detectable with no other form of true rheumatic disease. They are an extremely common affliction of mankind and, depending on the region involved, are described with a large variety of popular semimedical terminologies.[10, 11, 12, 13] Included in these entities are syndromes such as carpal tunnel syndrome, tennis elbow, golfer's elbow, deQuervain's tenosynovitis, subacromial bursitis, bicipital tendinitis, rotator cuff tendinitis, shoulder joint capsulitis, subscapular bursitis, trapezius muscle spasm, costochondritis, trigger spots on the posterior torso (often referred to as localized areas of fibrositis or fibromyositis), subgluteal bursitis, trochanteric bursitis, anserine bursitis, subachilles bursitis, plantar fasciitis, and metatarsalgia. These syndromes affect patients of all ages and both sexes but are particularly seen in older age groups and in younger individuals who undergo vigorous physical activity.

If one scrutinizes this large array of local and focal pain syndromes, certain potential pathologic processes become evident. First, some of the syndromes are undoubtedly due to local irritation or inflammation within a bursa. The recognition of the various anatomic bursae permits a ready understanding of how an inflammatory process in such a potential sac can result in pain and tenderness felt close to a joint margin and therefore be able to superficially mimic articular disease. Frequently a bursitis may arise as a posttraumatic or idiopathic event and bear no relation to any systemic form of rheumatic disease. Once developed it may become a very chronic process and persist, with symptoms lasting for months or even years. A surprising amount of dysfunction may be attributable to a chronic bursitis. For instance, it is not uncommon for elderly individuals to suffer insomnia over many months as a secondary effect of a low-grade trochanteric bursitis. Similarly, a chronic subacromial bursitis can result in pain and stiffness of the shoulder joint lasting many months before the true primary lesion is recognized. Second, some of the soft tissue syndomes would appear to be due to local inflammation within or around a tendon sheath. Local tenosynovitis can become chronic and stenosing and result in persistent pain and tenderness, especially when the involved muscle is put to use. Some of these syndromes appear to result from referred pain from presumed deeper (often perispinal) subluxations, hematomas, or ligamentous and capsular tears, in which the symptoms of the lesion are referred to a more superficial site on the torso. Under these circumstances, the site of referral may itself become involved by local areas of painful and tender muscle spasm, resulting in the classical "trigger point." Finally, some forms of soft tissue rheumatism syndrome appear to be due to actual tears in a fibrous aponeurosis or at a ligamentous bony junction. This is best seen in some forms of tennis elbow, in which the tendinous insertion of the forearm extensor apparatus at the lateral condyle of the humerus may be traumatized or actually torn away from the periosteum of the humerus. Similar lesions in the capsule or tendinous insertions around the shoulder joint account for many soft tissue rheumatism syndromes in that area.

Since by definition a soft tissue rheumatism syndrome is characterized by a local and focal symptom-sign complex, the diagnosis should be readily apparent if one is aware of the common sites of involvement. In general, there is no true arthropathy, so that a swollen or limited joint should never be detected other than by that loss of range of motion secondary to a chronic capsulitis. Thus, the only true physical sign should be extreme local tenderness, which usually reproduces the patient's spontaneous pain. Some of the soft tissue rheumatism syndromes are characterized by radiating pain. This is notably the case with tennis elbow, in which the pain frequently radiates down the forearm; with a shoulder joint capsulitis, in which the pain radiates over the lateral aspect of the upper arm; and with a trochanteric bursitis, in which pain radiates down the lateral aspect of the thigh. Radiographic changes should not be apparent in these syndromes, with the exception of occasional ectopic calcification within the damaged or inflamed tendon or joint capsule. This is classically seen in the temporary supraspinatus calcification of calcific tendinitis of that site. Occasionally, a distended periarticular bursae (such as the subachilles space) may be apparent radiographically.

Because of the localized nature of the syndromes one should not expect to find other evidence of extraskeletal systemic disease. Occasionally, however, patients may present with multiple soft tissue syndromes. This is particularly the case in some elderly individuals, in whom the clinical picture may then more closely mimic an arthropathy or even suggest the clinical profile of polymyalgia rheumatica or metabolic bone disease. However, even under these circumstances careful attention to the precise symptoms and signs of musculoskeletal pain and tenderness usually reveals the true nature of the disorder.

Table 22–2
GENERALIZED OSTEOARTHROSIS: FAVORED JOINTS FOR INVOLVEMENT

Peripheral	Central
Distal interphalangeal	Lower cervical spine
First carpometacarpal	Lumbosacral spine
Knees	Hips
First metatarsophalangeal	(Temporomandibular joints as a solitary lesion)

Osteoarthritis (Degenerative Joint Disease)

Although osteoarthritis may present with one area of regional involvment, if the patient is carefully scrutinized the pathologic process is usually found to be a more generalized disease. The arthropathic wear-and-tear process then displays a typical pattern of distribution (Table 22–2). This pattern includes the distal interphalangeal joints of the hands; the joints at the base of the thumb (first carpometacarpal joint in particular); the lower cervical spine; the intervertebral and zygoapophyseal joints of the lumbosacral spine; the large weight-bearing joints (notably the hips and knees); and the first metatarsophalangeal joints. Thus, the patient presenting with symptomatic osteoarthritis at one of these sites frequently has evidence of the same pathologic process within some or all of the other regions mentioned. In addition and unrelated to this pattern of distribution, osteoarthritic changes are very common in the temporomandibular joint and may actually present as an isolated arthropathic disorder in relatively young individuals.

The predominant symptom of osteoarthritis is pain, and this is usually most noticed on weight-bearing and is relieved by rest. Occasionally, however, the presumed subchondral reactive sclerosis results in enough nocturnal pain so that symptoms continue even when at rest. Even so, the situation is usually exacerbated by weight-bearing. The main physical sign of osteoarthritis is usually a moderately painful limitation of range of motion of the involved joint or skeletal region. When the process involves the lower cervical spine, additional symptoms of brachial neuralgia may be apparent or induced on movement of the neck. Similarly, involvement of the lumbosacral spine may also include a significant element of disc herniation, with compression of lumbosacral nerve roots and resultant sciatica. Detectable joint swelling is usually due to bony expansion resulting from osteophytic development at the joint margins (Fig. 22–1). Occasionally, truly distended joints are encountered, but the synovitis should never be dramatic, persistent, or widespread. Indeed, the presence of considerable synovial distention should make one seriously question a primary osteoarthritis as the sole pathologic process. There are several circumstances, however, under which a primary osteoarthritic joint may become acutely swollen. These include associated chondrocalcinosis with recurrent acute or chronic pseudogout syndrome; fragmentation of articular cartilage with an intrasynovial foreign body effect; or a grossly unstable articulation that undergoes repeated traumatic subluxation. In addition, a distinctive form of osteoarthritis affecting the small joints of the hands may display a component of synovitis, leading to

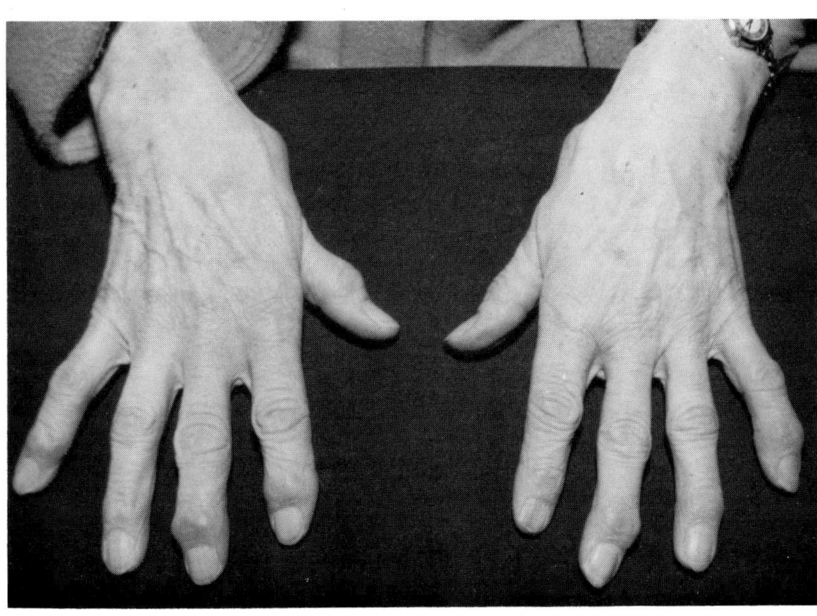

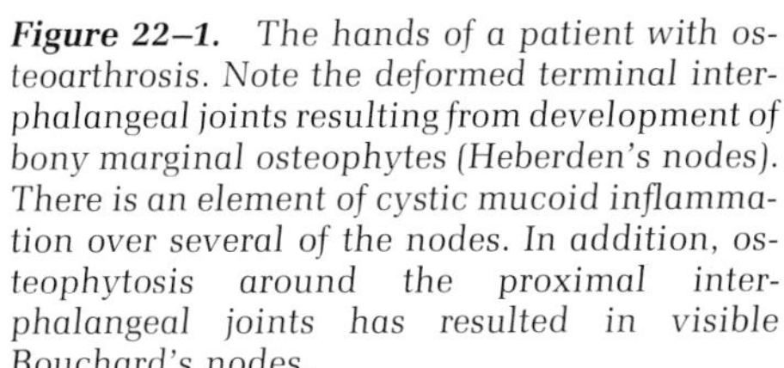

Figure 22–1. *The hands of a patient with osteoarthrosis. Note the deformed terminal interphalangeal joints resulting from development of bony marginal osteophytes (Heberden's nodes). There is an element of cystic mucoid inflammation over several of the nodes. In addition, osteophytosis around the proximal interphalangeal joints has resulted in visible Bouchard's nodes.*

erosion and undue deformity.[14] This erosive osteoarthritis may result in distention of small joints over a relatively prolonged period of time.

Depending on the degree of cartilage destruction, the painful and limited range of motion may be accompanied by undue crepitus. Once gross articular degeneration has developed, subluxation of hinge joints (notably the knee) is not unusual.

Since osteoarthritis is primarily a disease of cartilage, the pathologic process is largely confined to the joint. Thus, one would not expect to find directly related extra-articular manifestations of this disease. However, the pathologic process afflicts an older population of patients, so that unrelated disease in other organ systems is not uncommon.

Chronic Nonspecific Inflammatory Disease Typified by Rheumatoid Arthritis

Rheumatoid arthritis may affect patients of either sex and any age group. However, it shows a predilection for young and middle-aged women.[15] It likewise has a favored pattern of articular involvement that frequently becomes evident as the disease process becomes established (Table 22–3). This pattern includes the symmetric involvement of the proximal interphalangeal and metacarpophalangeal joints of the hands; the metatarsophalangeal joints of the feet; the hinge joints, typified by the wrists, elbows, ankles, and knees; and, to a slightly lesser extent, the shoulders, subacromial bursae, and hips. In addition, it may affect the upper cervical spine at the atlanto-axial junction in afflicted patients of any age group but can also involve the neurocentral and apophyseal joints of the entire neck, particularly in children and elderly patients.

Table 22–3
RHEUMATOID ARTHRITIS – THE TYPICAL ARTICULAR DISTRIBUTION OF DISEASE

Peripheral	Central
Proximal interphalangeal	Shoulders
Metacarpophalangeal	Hips
Metatarsophalangeal	Upper cervical spine
Wrists	
Elbows	
Knees	
Ankles	

The major symptoms of rheumatoid arthritis are pain and stiffness. The pain may be severe, and the earlier the disease the more noticeable it is. This is presumably because most of the initial pain of rheumatoid arthritis is due to acute or subacute articular distention by the inflammatory intrasynovial exudate. Indeed, under some circumstances the intra-articular pressure may become so high that acute rupture of the joint may occur. This is most often seen in patients with active synovitis of the knee joint when the inflammatory process presents in the popliteal space as an enlarging bursa, which may rupture into the calf.[16] The synovial distention may become a less potent source of pain as the disease progresses and becomes chronic, but the pannus-mediated articular destruction itself appears to be a painful process. Thus, even patients with very chronic and established rheumatoid arthritis usually feel pain, and this pain may be exacerbated on using the joint, especially when such motion results in closer apposition of the eroded bone surfaces. Gener-

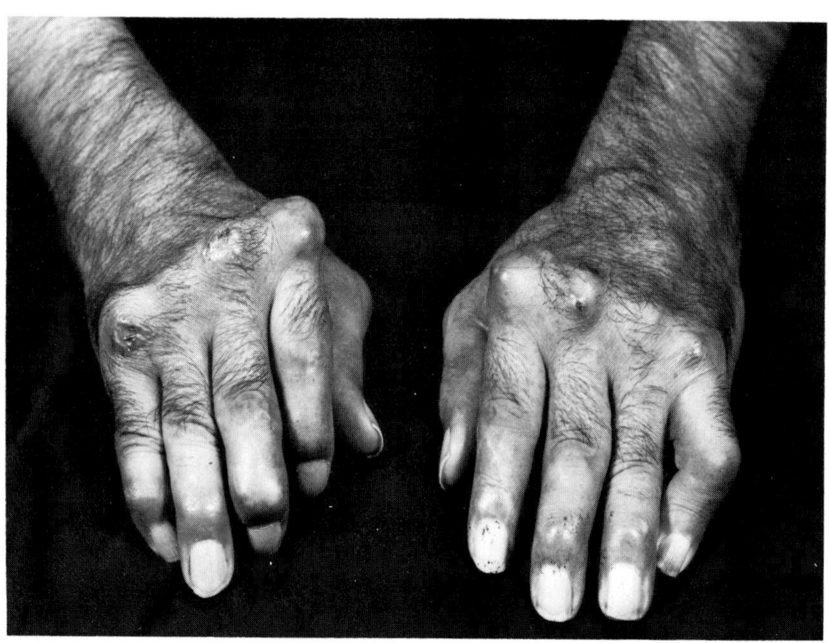

Figure 22–2. *The hands of a patient with advanced rheumatoid arthritis. Note the uniform swelling of the metacarpophalangeal joints together with the swelling of several proximal interphalangeal joints. The wrists are also involved, together with obvious extensor tendon sheath synovitis on the dorsum of the left hand. The deformities include moderate ulnar deviation of the fingers and early flexion contractures of several digits, due partly to arthritis of the proximal interphalangeal joints and partly to a stenosing tenosynovitis of the flexor tendon apparatus. There are multiple small rheumatoid nodules directly overlying the metacarpophalangeal joints and some of these have ulcerated.*

alized early-morning stiffness is a very typical feature of rheumatoid arthritis and may be more striking in extent and severity than the accompanying articular pain. Indeed, it may be so impressive as a symptom as to provide a valuable diagnostic clue and can then be used as an indicator of future therapeutic response. Moreover, the extent of the joint stiffness frequently suggests probable areas of rheumatoid synovitis that are not evident to the patient or physician as articular pain or swelling.

The cardinal physical sign of rheumatoid arthritis is joint swelling due to synovial distention. It is virtually impossible to diagnose rheumatoid arthritis unless the physician actually observes a persistently swollen joint. Widespread chronic articular swelling detected in the distribution outlined above is almost pathognomonic for rheumatoid disease (Figs. 22–2 and 22–3). Moreover, even mildly severe but persistent synovitis invariably leads to a permanent loss of range of motion, eventually evident after the inflammatory process has subsided. Therefore, a combination of joint distention in some regions and a painful loss of range of motion in others may add up to evidence of a prior widespread and symmetric polyarthritis of the rheumatoid type. In addition, the development of a newly restricted and painful joint in a patient with well-established rheumatoid disease can be taken as reasonable evidence of disease extension to that area. Thus, one may frequently suspect rheumatoid involvement of a hip or shoulder joint even though one cannot demonstrate the distended joint capsule. Because rheumatoid arthritis is a chronic inflammatory and destructive disease, there are significant periarticular sequelae. These sequelae themselves may provide valuable physical signs helpful in reaching a correct diagnosis. Notably, periarticular muscle wasting, tenosynovitis with boggy and chronically distended tendon sheaths, attenuated tendons with rupture and subsequent loss of muscle belly movement, and various subluxations and reversible or irreversible deformities may all result from the chronic rheumatoid process. Although no single deformity is absolutely diagnostic of rheumatoid arthritis, an obvious synovitis in the typical pattern of distribution for the disease combined with the development of ulnar deviation of the hands, stenosing tenosynovitis of the digital flexor sheaths, boutonnière and swan-neck deformities of the digits, and plantar subluxation of the metatarsal heads may all facilitate an immediate recognition of the underlying or previous arthropathy.

The recognition that many patients with rheumatoid arthritis display a uniform constellation of clinical, radiographic, and laboratory signs has permitted the development of widely accepted diagnostic criteria for the disease. It is important to realize, however, that rheumatoid arthritis may be fairly atypical in its initial presentation and even in its subsequent development. The clinician must be aware of these atypical rheumatoid arthritis syndromes and be prepared to diagnose the disease in the absence of the more usual widespread destructive arthropathy described previously (Table 22–4). An example of atypical rheumatoid arthritis is very early or subclinical rheumatoid disease in which the pain and stiffness are out of proportion to objective joint swelling. Under such circumstances a careful

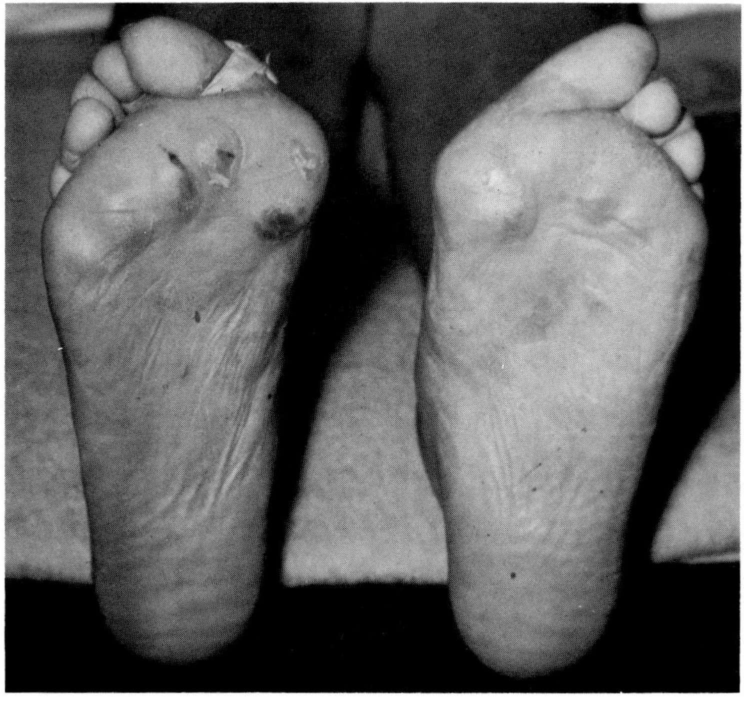

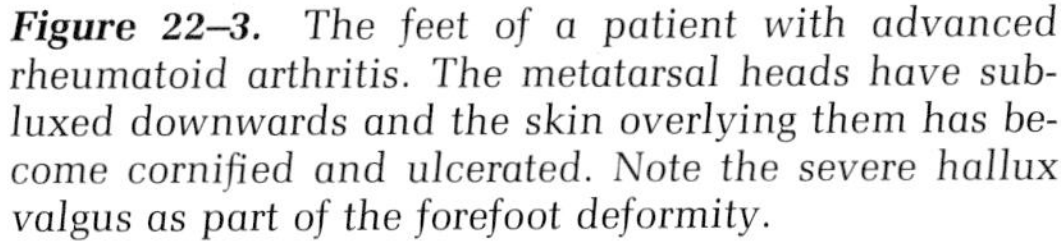

Figure 22–3. The feet of a patient with advanced rheumatoid arthritis. The metatarsal heads have subluxed downwards and the skin overlying them has become cornified and ulcerated. Note the severe hallux valgus as part of the forefoot deformity.

Table 22–4
ATYPICAL RHEUMATOID ARTHRITIS SYNDROMES

Very early (preclinical) disease
Juvenile disease
Rheumatoid disease beginning in old age
Chronic monoarticular arthritis
Dominant extraskeletal manifestations
Palindromic onset

and prolonged observation of the patient usually results in detection of the cardinal physical signs as they eventually appear. It is in this type of patient that the newer diagnostic techniques of scintigraphy and thermography may be helpful in detecting "preclinical" synovitis.

Juvenile rheumatoid arthritis (JRA) may appear in several diverse but well-characterized forms.[17] Careful longitudinal studies of children with juvenile chronic polyarthritis suggest that juvenile rheumatoid arthritis is seen primarily as three major symptom complexes. About 20 per cent of children with JRA present with an acute systemic disease, notably toddlers and infants below the age of 3 years; this form is characterized by high fevers, a spectacular polymorphonuclear leukocytosis, a serious anemia, hepatosplenomegaly, lymphadenopathy, and a widespread polyarthritis. These children are invariably negative for rheumatoid factor and frequently respond to salicylate therapy. However, about one fourth of them develop chronic articular disease, and all appear to be at risk for future relapses even after many years of complete recovery. A second group of children with JRA (constituting about 35 per cent of the total) presents with a pauciarticular arthritis, particularly affecting girls up to about 8 years of age, in whom the clinical picture is of two or three chronically swollen joints. In these individuals the arthritis is rarely severe, but the important extra-articular manifestation is a chronic iridocyclitis (detectable in about one fourth of patients), which may be symptomless and yet devastating in its effects. The iridocyclitis of pauciarticular JRA is at present a potent cause of blindness acquired in childhood. Interestingly, although these children are usually seronegative for rheumatoid factor, those who have chronic iridocyclitis frequently display serum antinuclear antibodies. Finally, about 45 per cent of children with JRA present with polyarticular synovitis displaying the adult type of symmetric and widespread distribution. Most of these are older children and are negative for serum rheumatoid factor; they carry a very good prognosis but may still eventually suffer isolated gross deformities subsequent to persistent inflammation involving an epiphysis. However, a small proportion of children with polyarticular JRA are seropositive and display the classic extra-articular feature of subcutaneous nodules. They frequently develop eroded joints, so that not only do they have the problems of growth defects due to local inflammation, but also they may actually undergo destruction of articular structures. This group of seropositive, polyarticular JRA patients is confined predominantly to teenage girls in whom the prognosis appears to match that seen in equally seriously involved adults with rheumatoid arthritis.

The onset of rheumatoid arthritis in an elderly individual may result in a very difficult clinical presentation. Even though the rheumatoid arthritis itself may be quite typical in its distribution and resultant symptoms and signs, the tolerance level in an elderly person already suffering from inevitable osteoarthritis may be such as to result in an inordinate amount of disability. Since old people may quickly become totally disabled and retreat to bed, the initial presentation can rapidly be masked by an extreme debility, emaciation, the rapid development of contractures, gross muscle weakness, and all the systemic complications of total immobilization.

Rheumatoid arthritis may present as a chronic monoarticular arthritis. This is a very challenging clinical picture.[18] Indeed, it is virtually a diagnosis of exclusion since one must go through the process of looking for other causes of a sharply localized and chronic articular inflammation. Nevertheless, in looking at a large series of patients with chronic monoarticular arthritis one can identify individuals with likely rheumatoid arthritis by virtue of the presence of rheumatoid factor, nodules, other subtle symptoms, and the later development of typical polyarticular disease. However, some individuals appear to have nonspecific rheumatoid arthritis–like synovitis confined to a single joint for many years; most of these individuals do not go on to develop polyarticular disease, although a few may.

Sometimes the extra-articular manifestations of rheumatoid arthritis are present early in the disease or may be so severe as to dominate the clinical presenting picture.[19] In either case their recognition facilitates a correct diagnosis. Subcutaneous or tendon sheath rheumatoid nodules, carpal tunnel syndrome, and keratoconjunctivitis sicca may all be evident almost at the onset of the arthritis. In addition, it is not uncommon for middle-aged men with seropositive rheumatoid arthritis to present to the physician with severe peripheral neuropathy, myositis, cutaneous vasculitis, fibrosing alveolitis, pleurisy, pericarditis, or uveitis. At the time of their presentation, the underlying rheumatoid arthritis is usually fairly obvious. However, the symptoms and signs of the articular process may be barely apparent or may be deemphasized by both the patient and the clinician in the face of obvious extraskeletal pathology, so that the true nature of the disease process is not appreciated. Nearly always, however, the rheumatoid process within the joints makes its presence known, although the prognosis and management of these patients may continue to be dominated by the extraarticular features.

Finally, rheumatoid arthritis may display a palindromic onset.[20] That is to say, patients may develop episodic attacks of rheumatoid arthritis which then disappear, leaving no intercurrent evidence of synovial inflammation. Thus, the concept of palindromic rheumatism implies episodic and nondestructive, but true, inflammatory arthritis. Many of these individuals are young to middle-aged women, and frequently the disease process evolves to become more permanent and established, with the eventual development of the pattern of distribution and serologic stigmata characteristic of rheumatoid arthritis. Clearly, however, many other chronic rheumatic diseases may begin in a palindromic fashion, and only long-term observation and careful examination for extra-articular features will help the physician decide whether the episodic onset is, in fact, a manifestation of diseases such as systemic lupus erythematosus, psoriatic arthritis, colitic arthritis, or various other relapsing syndromes.

Chronic Nonspecific Spondyloarthritis Typified by Ankylosing Spondylitis

This form of rheumatic disease is perhaps best considered as a prototype for a whole group of disorders referred to as the seronegative spondyloarthropathies (Table 22–5).[21] Ankylosing spondylitis is particularly evident in adolescent and young adult men but may be equally prevalent in women although not so clinically apparent. The pattern of skeletal distribution for the disease process is strikingly different from that of the other arthropathies discussed thus far. Ankylosing spondylitis particularly affects the cartilaginous joints, notably the intervertebral joints of the spine, the central joints of the anterior chest wall, and the symphysis pubis. Thus, it has a strikingly axial distribution. Moreover, when it does involve synovial joints, these too are most likely to be within the spine. Thus, sacroiliac, costovertebral, and apophyseal joint involvement is commonly seen. However, other synovial joints may be involved but with a predilection for the large proximal synovial joints of the upper and lower girdles, notably the hips, shoulders, and knees, in that order.

Table 22–5
THE SERONEGATIVE SPONDYLOARTHROPATHIES

Ankylosing Spondylitis
In adults
In children
With colitis
Some Postinfectious Arthropathies
Reiter's disease
Salmonella arthritis
Yersinia arthritis
Psoriatic Arthritis

The predominant symptom is one of pain, and in view of the pattern of involvement most of this pain presents as backache. Since pain originating from the sacroiliac joint may be referred to the region of the buttock or down the back of the thigh, the initial symptom may simulate an attack of sciatica. Unlike the pain of rheumatoid arthritis, the pain of ankylosing spondylitis is frequently aggravated by rest, especially in a recumbent position. Indeed, most patients with ankylosing spondylitis notice that if they keep active and mobile, their pain is eased. Similarly, stiffness is a marked symptom of this disease but again it is largely confined to the spine and proximal limb joints. The stiffness, like the pain, is seriously aggravated by prolonged periods of rest, either sitting or lying, and is relieved by physical activity. The physical signs are usually less overt than those seen in patients with rheumatoid arthritis. Most of the target areas in ankylosing spondylitis are not readily accessible to the examiner's eyes and hands. Moreover, much of the primary inflammatory process lies within articular cartilage, subchondral bone, articular capsules, and ligaments, with less synovitis than previously was realized. Thus, even involved joints may not necessarily be very distended, and even an obviously swollen articulation is often the result of a chronic and progressive subchondral, chondral, or capsular inflammatory process. Hence, it is frequently possible to detect swollen and tender cartilaginous joints on the anterior chest wall or at the symphysis pubis. However, the evidence of multiple spinal joint involvement is usually apparent only by the presence of a painful stiffness and limitation of range of motion within the entire axial skeleton. This is elicited by a series of classic clinical maneuvers designed to test the overall mobility of the entire spine, of the hip joints, of the costovertebral junctions, and of the sacroiliac articulations.[22] Although these tests of axial mobility are relatively nonspecific, a widespread and painful limitation of range of motion in a young adult man complaining of pain in the back is a very suggestive clinical profile for ankylosing spondylitis. The pattern of skeletal involvement combined with the tendency for the inflammatory lesion of ankylosing spondylitis to resolve by fibrosis, calcification, and ossification accounts for the well-recognized deformities associated with this disease. Even in the relatively early stages of the disorder the physician may observe an increase in the cervical and thoracic kyphosis and loss of the lumbar lordosis (Fig. 22–4). In patients with more advanced disease the increased tendency to forward stoop becomes more exaggerated, and the cervical kyphosis may be extreme. A flexion contracture of the hips and knees may also develop, so that the patient with classic end-stage disease is depicted as a middle-aged man who walks with a severe forward stoop, knees and hips slightly bent, his eyes transfixed to the ground. Clearly, detection of the earlier

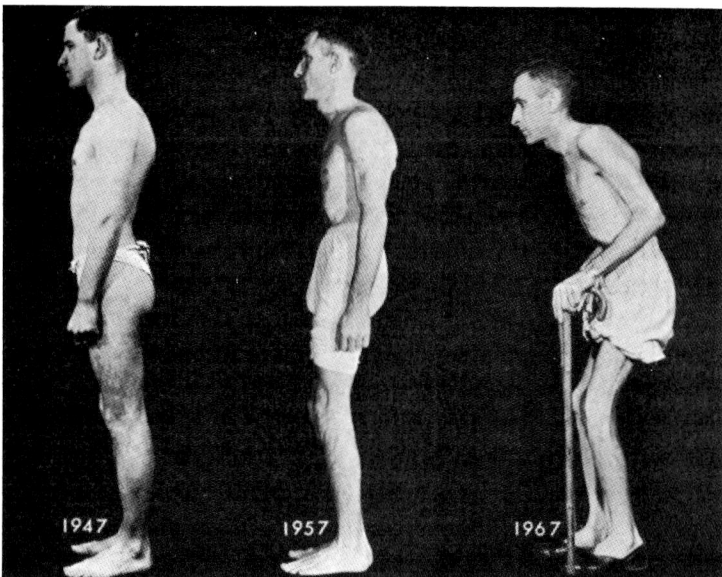

Figure 22–4. The progressive changes in posture of a patient with chronic ankylosing spondylitis. Note the tendency to a stooping position with progressive immobility of the neck, back, hips, and knees. The severe deformities should be preventable with appropriate therapy. (From Ogryzlo, MA, et al: Postgrad Med 45:182, 1969.)

postural changes is important for diagnosis; the end-stage gross deformities barely entertain a need for a differential diagnosis.

Occasionally, severe involvement of more peripheral joints, such as the wrists, knees, or ankles, will include a frank synovitis, thereby resulting in the typical signs of a distended and painfully restricted articulation. Although this is usually seen in the presence of a more obvious axial involvement, peripheral joint disease may dominate the clinical picture or precede and overshadow the spinal symptoms and signs. Under these circumstances, the diagnosis of ankylosing spondylitis is more difficult. Nevertheless, the clinical and radiographic features of ankylosing spondylitis are uniform enough to justify a widely accepted set of diagnostic criteria, which focus almost exclusively on the spondylitis and sacroiliitis characteristic of the disease.

The extra-articular features of ankylosing spondylitis are not as extensive, severe, or common as those associated with rheumatoid arthritis. About 25 per cent of patients with ankylosing spondylitis at some time or other develop an acute nongranulomatous and potentially recurrent iritis. This may be evident at the time of clinical presentation, or its past presence may be implied by the detection of an irregularly scarred and depigmented pupil. Patients with end-stage, severe disease may occasionally manifest aortic regurgitation, bilateral apical pulmonary fibrosis, or dural cysts presenting as a cauda equina syndrome. Although it is very important for the clinician to detect these rare complications of the disease, they are hardly worth considering as early diagnostic features. There are several atypical forms of ankylosing spondylitis, however, that the clinician must bear in mind.[23] These include the definite association between chronic inflammatory bowel disease and ankylosing spondylitis, so that the two disorders occur together more often than they would be expected to. Hence, in patients presenting with spondyloarthropathy there might be detected some additional evidence of subclinical or overt bloody diarrhea. Contrariwise, patients presenting with the symptoms and signs of ulcerative colitis or Crohn's disease may also exhibit or develop symptoms and signs of ankylosing spondylitis. It is now also recognized that ankylosing spondylitis can present in childhood, in which it may rather closely mimic the pauciarticular form of juvenile rheumatoid arthritis. It may affect young boys over the age of 8 years and manifest itself as persistent knee or ankle joint swelling with little back pain. However, these children do not develop chronic iridocyclitis or a positive test for antinuclear antibody but may suffer recurrent attacks of acute iritis. Eventually, they begin to complain of backache, and if their rheumatic disease progresses, they develop ankylosing spondylitis in adolescence.

Chronic Nonspecific Spondyloarthritis Typified by Psoriatic Arthritis

A certain percentage of patients with psoriatic skin and nail disease develops a seronegative spondyloarthropathy.[24] That is to say, in consort with their skin disease, but sometimes preceding or overshadowing it, there develops a chronic inflammatory process affecting peripheral joints or the spine, or both. Psoriatic arthropathy can affect patients of either sex and at any age. Anyone who is susceptible to developing psoriasis can also develop psoriatic arthritis. The categorization of psoriatic spondy-

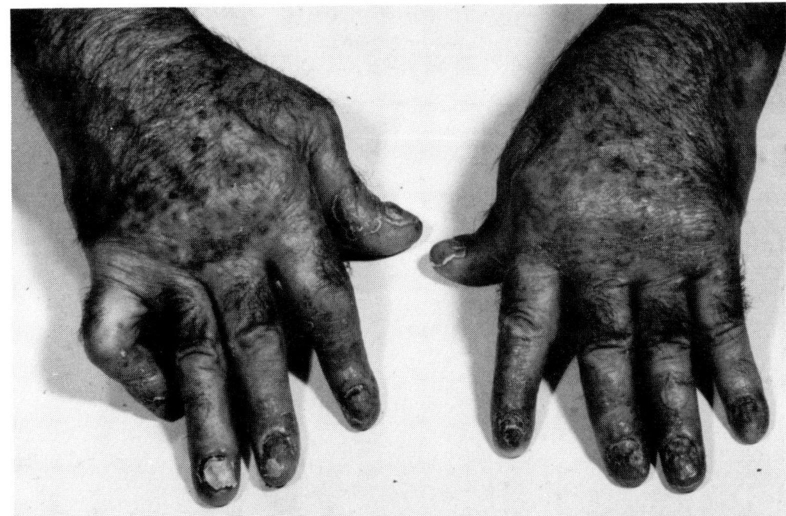

Figure 22–5. The hands of a patient with severe psoriatic arthropathy. There is obvious psoriatic involvement of the skin and fingernails. An asymmetric destructive arthritis has affected many of the hand joints, especially the metacarpophalangeal and wrist areas. The flexion contracture of the right fifth finger is due to a postinflammatory bony fusion of the proximal interphalangeal joint.

loarthropathy is less clear-cut than that of the other typical rheumatic disease profiles discussed previously. However, certain clinical patterns of osteoarticular involvement are recognized, including erosive destruction of the distal interphalangeal joints (nearly always associated with psoriasis of the adjacent fingernail) (Fig. 22–5); an asymmetric oligoarthritis of peripheral small or large synovial joints; a widespread and symmetric destructive arthropathy of many peripheral joints resulting in serious deformities and subluxations ("arthritis mutilans"); predominant sacroiliitis or spondylitis, or both, with a regional distribution of involvement resembling that seen in asymmetric ankylosing spondylitis; and patients with any combination of these patterns. Clearly, the precise symptoms and signs would depend upon the extent and severity of osteoarticular involvement present in the individual patient. They will, therefore, vary from occasional acutely painful swelling of one or two small peripheral joints (e.g., "sausage digits") to severe and generalized pain, stiffness, and deformity affecting most of the joints of the body. The presence of psoriatic skin or nail disease is an obvious clue to the underlying nature of the arthropathy. However, the skin disease may develop long after the arthropathy becomes clinically evident or may be so limited in extent as to be overlooked by even the most discerning clinician. The absence of the common extra-articular features of rheumatoid arthritis should help deter the physician from misdiagnosing rheumatoid disease in a patient with widespread and symmetric psoriatic arthritis. However, this distinction is one of the hardest differential diagnoses to make in rheumatology, especially since some psoriatic patients may also demonstrate positive test results for rheumatoid factor. Nevertheless, as discussed in the relevant sections of this book, the morphoradiographic changes of psoriatic joint disease are usually quite distinctive from those of typical rheumatoid arthritis.

Acute Nonspecific Spondyloarthritis of the Postinfectious Type

There is a group of rather dramatic and fairly acute rheumatic diseases seen particularly in young, previously healthy individuals that are clearly postinfectious in origin. Although the amount of pathologic and epidemiologic data is scant, the clinical features strongly suggest a clinical pattern of involvement similar to that seen in other nonspecific spondyloarthropathies of a more chronic kind (e.g., ankylosing spondylitis and some forms of psoriatic arthritis). Moreover, some of these acute postinfectious spondyloarthropathies may then show persistent inflammatory activity over the years and evolve in such a way as to more closely resemble asymmetric forms of the chronic spondyloarthropathies. More rarely, patients with ankylosing spondylitis or psoriatic arthritis may at times demonstrate some of the extra-articular features seen in these more acute postinfectious forms of spondyloarthropathy.

The most classic clinical presentation in this category is Reiter's disease. The acute onset of a large or small joint oligoarthritis in a previously healthy and sexually active young adult man is the characteristic feature of this syndrome.[25] The arthritis may be so acute and severe as to result in a clinical picture resembling acute septic arthritis. Involvement of the small joints of the hands or feet may even present as a dactylitis. Many such patients probably have a wider distribution of inflammatory foci within ligaments and tendons, especially around the axial skeleton, since they frequently have a mild backache and perispinal or pelvic brim tenderness largely overshadowed by the more dramatic peripheral joint manifestations. The symptoms and signs are usually those of an obviously acutely inflamed peripheral joint or joints, with all of the attendant systemic malaise and disability expected to accompany a very serious acute inflammatory process anywhere in the body. The extra-articular features are very characteristic and provide the most potent diagnostic clues. They include the major features of sterile conjunctivitis or iritis and nonspecific urethritis in men or trigonitis and cervicitis in women. These extra-articular features may dominate the clinical presentation, precede the arthropathy, follow the arthropathy, or not be noticed at all. Thus, the diagnosis is difficult in patients failing to demonstrate two or three characteristics of the classic triad of conjunctivitis, urethritis, and arthritis with an obvious temporal relationship. Other minor criteria of diagnostic help include mucocutaneous lesions with the skin rash of keratoderma blennorrhagicum (which histologically strongly resembles pustular psoriasis), a similar lesion on the glans penis (circinate balanitis), and painless superficial ulceration of the palate and tongue (Fig. 22–6). One frequent target area for the inflammatory arthritis in patients with Reiter's dis-

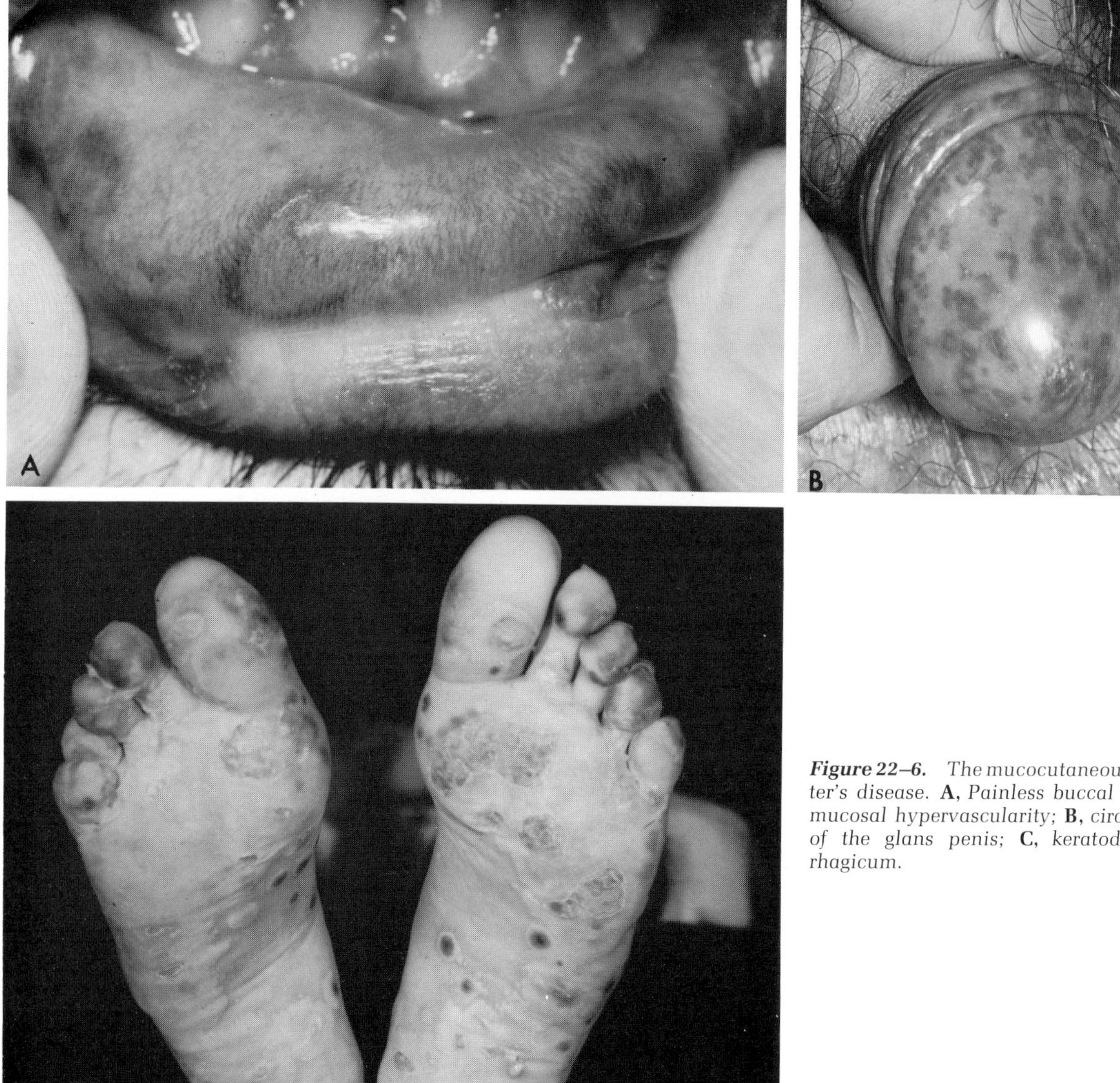

Figure 22–6. *The mucocutaneous lesions of Reiter's disease.* **A,** *Painless buccal ulceration and mucosal hypervascularity;* **B,** *circinate balanitis of the glans penis;* **C,** *keratoderma blennorrhagicum.*

ease is the ankle and hindfoot. This is especially the case when the attack becomes chronic and prolonged or relapsing in nature. Under these circumstances the disease may be characterized by a chronic inflammatory and destructive arthritis of the joints in the hindfoot together with an accompanying plantar fasciitis in complete absence of other extra-articular signs. If the patient presents to the physician for the first time at this stage of the disease, the preceding episode of urethritis and arthritis (combined with the typical radiographic changes outlined elsewhere in this textbook) evident in a sexually active young adult man should still suggest the diagnostic possibility of incomplete chronic Reiter's disease.[26]

Another more recently recognized form of a postinfectious spondyloarthritis is that seen following an attack of yersiniosis.[27] The term "yersiniosis" refers to an acute infectious disease due to the enteropathic organism *Yersinia enterocolitica*. A mild gastroenteritis and mesenteric adenitis are usual. Although most individuals recover from this form of endemic diarrhea without sequelae, a few victims later develop fever, a sterile large joint polyarthritis, skin lesions characterized as erythema nodosum or erythema multiforme, first degree heart block, and a low incidence of iritis or conjunctivitis. Thus, the clinical picture appears to resemble a "halfway house" between Reiter's disease and acute rheumatic fever. However, the profile of a previously healthy young person with a recent history of gastroenteritis, together with certain specific laboratory features (see Chapter 23), should suggest the correct diagnosis. Patients with this syndrome may also go on to develop a chronic spondyloarthropathy resembling chronic Reiter's disease and maturing to exhibit the radiographic and clinical features of an asymmetric ankylosing spondylitis.

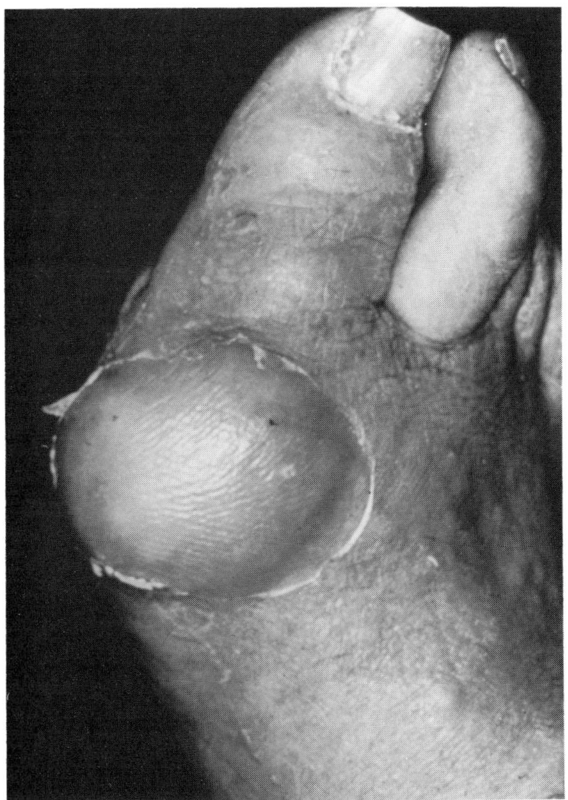

Figure 22–7. *Great toe of patient suffering from acute gouty arthritis. There is massive swelling and erythema of the involved area. The inflammatory process is several days old, as indicated by desquamation of the overlying skin.*

A similar sterile, acute, usually large joint asymmetric polyarthritis may be seen following systemic salmonellosis. Most patients with salmonellosis develop overt diarrhea and dehydration and then recover from their illness. A few individuals, especially those with compromised host defense systems, may develop septicemia and a salmonella pyoarthrosis with clear evidence of joint sepsis due to invasion of the synovial space by the offending organism. Still other patients may have an overt or silent salmonella septicemia and several weeks later develop a sterile arthritis, which appears to be clinically identical to the other types of postinfectious arthropathies described previously. Since salmonella gastroenteritis is one recognized cause of postdysenteric Reiter's disease, it is perhaps not surprising that a salmonella septicemia should also be able to induce a similar type of arthropathy.

Acute Monoarticular Syndromes Due to Crystals

There is a group of very acute monoarticular arthropathies that we now recognize are due to the intensely phlogistic potential of intra-articular crystal deposits. Thus far, three types of crystals have been shown to play a pathogenic role in eliciting this type of acute inflammatory joint disease. They include sodium urate, which produces typical gout attacks; calcium pyrophosphate, which causes attacks of pseudogout; and microspherules of calcium hydroxyapatite, which are now thought to be able to incite an acute inflammatory response within certain tissues.

The most typical and best-recognized form of crystal-induced inflammation is, of course, sodium urate gout.[28] In this condition the patient is nearly always a middle-aged or elderly man (although occasionally the disease is seen in postmenopausal or castrated women) in whom there is often a strong family history of the disorder. The symptoms and signs are those of a hyperacute and serious inflammation of a single joint, which classically is the great toe but may on occasion be a larger hinge joint — notably the ankle, tarsus, wrist, knee, or elbow — or the olecranon bursa. In this setting the development of an obviously red, swollen, and agonizingly painful joint over the course of 24 hours provides a very characteristic picture (Fig. 22–7). On occasion, the disease has become recurrent and chronic by the time the patient presents to the physician, and the few extra-articular manifestations of this disorder may then be apparent. These include gouty tophi in soft tissues around joints, over tendon sheaths, or in the helix of the ear, and the presence of a low-grade interstitial nephritis, usually evident as mild proteinuria. The renal consequences of hyperuricemia and gout may sometimes be evident as a past or present history of recurrent uric acid calculi, but this may not be noted at the time the acute arthritis occurs. Although gout is a disease peculiarly limited to the connective tissues of the skeleton and the interstitium of the kidney, the individual with gout frequently displays certain other features. These include a moderate degree of obesity and non–insulin-dependent diabetes mellitus, a history of dietary and alcoholic indiscretion, obvious hypertension, and hyperlipidemia, usually characterized as a carbohydrate responsive hypertriglyceridemia. This overall profile of a susceptible individual can be an impressive clinical aid if the diagnosis of recurrent gouty arthritis is in doubt. Only if the patient has experienced severe recurrent attacks of uncontrolled acute gouty arthritis would one expect to find evidence of articular deformity resulting from tophaceous destruction of subchondral bone and periarticular structures (Fig. 22–8). Not uncommonly, a patient may have a polyfocal attack of urate gout and present to the clinician with two, three, or even four skeletal areas of intense inflammation. This presentation may be atypical enough to suggest various other hyperacute polyarticular syndromes, but the clinical appearance of each affected joint still looks totally compatible with urate gout; consequently, subsequent investigations or therapeutic responsiveness should leave little room for differential diagnosis.

The diagnostic entity of acute pseudogout due to the intrasynovial deposition of calcium pyrophosphate crystals is now widely recognized.[29] Although the clinical picture may appear very similar to acute urate gout, it should be remembered that pyrophosphate crystal deposition disease is seen in elderly individuals of both sexes with a somewhat different pattern of distribution from that seen in urate gout. Individuals with acute pseudogout frequently have inflammatory episodes in the knees, wrists, and shoulders, in that order of frequency, with a greater tendency for polyarticular attacks than is seen in urate gout. Patients with acute pseudogout should reveal little in the way of extra-articular manifestations. Of course, they invariably are older individuals, so that other, unrelated organ system disease may be present. Some individuals with widespread chondrocalcinosis suffer a chronic or relapsing low-grade pseudogout syndrome with subsequent continuing painful destruction of their articular surfaces. The clinical picture may then be one of a more persistent large joint polyarthritis, with a great deal of pain, limitation of range of motion, and disability.

Since the underlying metabolic abnormality leading to acute pseudogout is marked by chondrocalcinosis, it is important for the physician to realize that an increased incidence of cartilage calcification

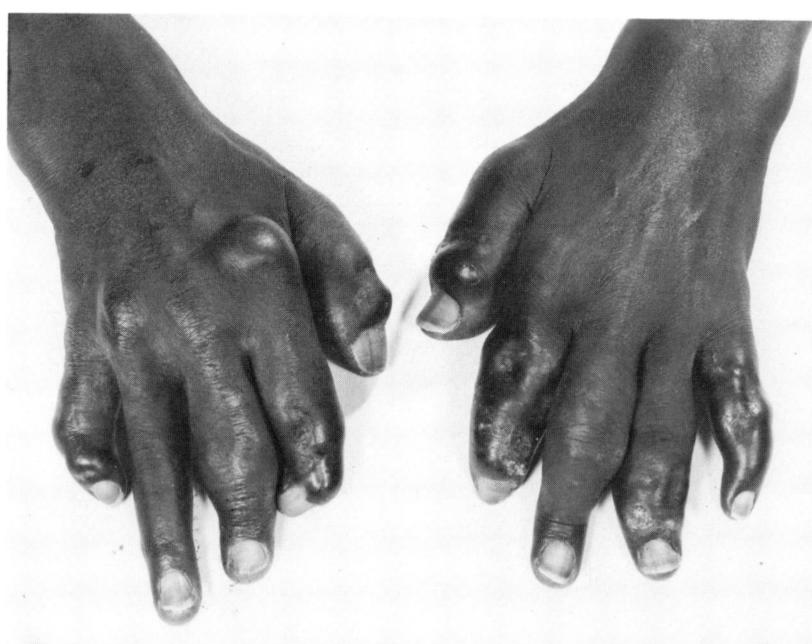

Figure 22–8. *The hands of a patient with chronic tophaceous gout. The extensive tophus formation and associated pandactylitis have resulted in destruction of many digital bones and joints.*

is associated with a variety of endocrine and metabolic disorders. Thus, a patient presenting with recurrent attacks of acute pseudogout should be screened clinically for the presence of one of these associated diseases. The associated states include hemochromatosis, hyperparathyroidism, acromegaly, and perhaps diabetes mellitus. Finally, there may be an increased association between urate gout and pyrophosphate gout. Therefore, it is not uncommon to find patients suffering from acute crystal-induced inflammation in which two phlogistic elements may be identified, and the attack can then be ascribed to both urate and pyrophosphate gout occurring simultaneously.

Finally, one recently recognized form of crystal-induced arthritis and periarthritis is now ascribed to calcium hydroxyapatite deposits. These microspherular crystalline forms may be found within the amorphous calcium deposits of periarticular soft tissues, as well as in the calcium deposits of degenerating cartilage in close physical association with calcium pyrophosphate. The acute inflammatory response incited by this form of crystal may well account for the occasional episodes of acute periarticular inflammation seen in patients with radiographic evidence of calcific tendinitis or capsulitis.[30] There are no discrete clinical profiles suggestive of this form of inflammatory joint disease, although the local inflammatory lesion overlying a deposit of soft tissue calcification in an otherwise healthy individual may suggest the diagnosis. Calcium hydroxyapatite-induced synovitis may be virtually indistinguishable from that due to the frequently associated calcium pyrophosphate crystal deposition disease. There is one clinical situation in which recurrent calcium hydroxyapatite inflammation of soft tissues appears to be rather prominent. In patients with chronic renal failure undergoing hemodialysis in whom there is a protracted increase in the serum calcium:phosphorus ratio, extensive ectopic calcification may develop. These patients frequently demonstrate attacks of pericalcific inflammation mimicking acute gout or pseudogout. Awareness of this syndrome should, however, rapidly lead to the correct diagnosis.

Acute Monoarticular Syndromes Due to Synovial Bacterial Infections

Acute septic arthritis may be induced by an enormous variety of microbial organisms.[31] There is no typical pattern of articular involvement, although certain contemporary clinical profiles have emerged, and no doubt others will continue to emerge from time to time. Thus, acute gonococcal arthritis frequently presents with a large joint and tendon sheath oligoarthritis in sexually active individuals[32]; acute gram-negative bacterial discitis of the spine frequently presents as one or two localized areas of abscess formation in the vertebral column of drug abusers; acute or chronic atypical tuberculosis of the hip may be seen in immunosuppressed individuals; and acute septic arthritis of the sternoclavicular and sternomanubrial joints has been reported in a group of heroin addicts. Clearly, in an immunologically compromised individual or in a patient suffering from any form of septicemia, virtually no articular space is immune to becoming a target site of metastatic infection.

The symptoms and signs of an acute septic joint are virtually identical to those seen in crystal-induced synovitis. There is acute pain and swelling of the involved joint with total dysfunction, which may extend to the entire extremity and even to the entire body. Occasionally, the physical signs reveal an obvious site of entry, such as a skin wound, or infection of the urethra, cervix, rectum, or throat. Additionally, the extra-articular signs may include those of a generalized septicemia, with evidence that the infectious process has affected other target tissues. Examples of this would include the signs of bacterial endocarditis in the heart; skin petechiae or purpura; the characteristically sparse and scattered necrotic pustules of gonococcal septicemia; dramatic fevers and sweating; and even widespread peripheral vascular occlusion or gangrene. Obviously, since an acutely septic joint may be but one manifestation of many serious systemic diseases, there is no limit to the potential complexity of the associated symptoms and signs that might be evident.

Acute infection of a joint may become a more chronic and less spectacular process. This is particularly seen in certain forms of bacterial arthritis, such as tuberculous disease and also fungal joint infections, especially in those areas endemic for coccidioidomycosis or blastomycosis. Under these circumstances, the clinical picture is usually of a chronic monoarticular arthritis with or without a preceding history of more acute inflammatory features. Since this sort of process may equally arise in the spine, the physical signs may be restricted to tenderness over the painful area on the back, although even here gross deformity may develop if the inflammatory process continues unabated for very long. One might expect the extra-articular evidence to include clues to the underlying nature of the infectious process. However, isolated tubercular or fungal joint and bone disease is becoming increasingly recognized in patients who otherwise appear to be perfectly healthy.[33] Alternatively, there may be historical evidence of a previous systemic infection, but by the time the process becomes localized in the osteoarticular tissues all signs of prior dissemination may be gone. It therefore becomes axiomatic that patients presenting with a chronic monoarticular arthritis must be presumed to have an infective process until proved otherwise.

Acute Oligo- or Polyarthritis Due to Viral Infections

Many viruses are known to be potentially arthritogenic. Therefore, the onset of a fairly acute but self-limiting oligo- or polyarthritis affecting many small or large synovial joints in a young individual with a recent history of varicella, mumps, rubella, or infectious mononucleosis may suggest the possibility of a viral arthritis. However, this is a very difficult entity to prove, and even the long-delayed serum viral antibody titer determinations may not provide an adequate screening for the virus in question. Nevertheless, the appearance of a sterile, mild to moderately severe oligo- or polyarthritis in a young individual exposed to a known viral infectious disease should alert the physician to the possible diagnosis. The extra-articular features might include those other manifestations of the particular viral disease, and since the natural history of the entire syndrome should be one of gradual but complete remission, the subsequent turn of events may serve to confirm the clinical impression. Certain contemporary trends are also apparent for this form of infectious arthritis. Notably, a preicteric hepatitis B infection may manifest itself as a symmetric small joint polyarthritis lasting several weeks before the jaundice appears and the condition of the joints improves.[34] Similarly, widespread use of certain batches of rubella vaccine has resulted in a high frequency of rubella arthritis among young female vaccinees. Interestingly, rubella arthritis may appear as late as 60 days after immunization and last for 60 days thereafter before spontaneously resolving.

Acute Monoarticular Arthritis Due to Trauma or Hemarthrosis

Patients may suffer severe, acute, painful swelling of joints and periarticular tissues as a result of traumatic derangement or of posttraumatic or spontaneous hemarthrosis. The former event should be associated with a clear-cut history of the traumatic episode, and it is particularly prone to occur in the large weight-bearing joints, notably knees and ankles. Although small microfractures of the subchondral bone may be important in this form of traumatic arthritis, it is recognized that soft tissue derangement can also evoke a large synovial effusion, leading to a painfully distended joint. Spontaneous hemarthrosis is one dreaded complication seen in patients with hereditary or acquired coagulation defects and is most typically seen in young boys with hemophilia. In these patients the early hemarthrosis is characterized by mild to moderate arthralgias, which may become very severe over a 24 to 48 hour period. Physical examination usually reveals a single joint that appears tense and acutely inflamed. Even in this disease there is a characteristic pattern, with involvement of the knees, elbows, ankles, and hips, in that order.[35] The extra-articular signs of a traumatized or blood-filled joint will depend on whether or not there have been other manifestations of trauma or of the bleeding diathesis. It should be recognized, however, that some children with hemophilic arthropathy manifest no other signs of serious bleeding since, for reasons that are unclear, the synovial cavity appears to be a peculiarly vulnerable site for vascular leakage. Certain patients with repeated episodes of posttraumatic synovitis or hemarthrosis may go on to develop persistent and destructive chronic synovitis, which results in a progressively abnormal articulation. The reasons for this are not clear, but synovectomy has been performed in many athletes with this form of chronic posttraumatic synovitis. More readily understood are the chronic articular changes seen in patients with classical hemophilia. In this condition the recurrent bleeding episodes in and around the joint may be the cause not only of chronic distention but also of progressive subluxation, which may present to the clinician as irreversible contractures and deformities.

Transient, Relapsing, and Nondeforming Arthritis

Many diseases that were considered the province of internal medicine are now thought to be associated with episodic or persistent circulating immune complexes.[36] One peripheral manifestation of the circulating immune complex state appears to be a transient, nonerosive, and nondeforming synovial joint arthritis (Fig. 22–9). The pattern of articular involvement for this type of arthropathy frequently includes the large hinge joints of the limbs (elbows, wrists, knees, and ankles); there is also a tendency for concomitant acute tenosynovitis in the more distal parts of the upper and lower limbs. Examples of diseases that may manifest with this form of transient arthropathy include chronic inflammatory bowel disease; subacute bacterial endocarditis; Henoch-Schönlein purpura; postrenal transplant rejection syndrome; chronic active hepatitis; acute rheumatic fever; and ileojejunal bypass arthropathies. In addition, doubtlessly numerous other syndromes will become better recognized as assays for circulating immune complexes become more refined. Since this form of arthropathy is usually a short-lived affair, joint destruction or deformities should not occur. Occasionally, however, the episodes of arthritis may become so frequent and serious that minor destructive changes are seen.

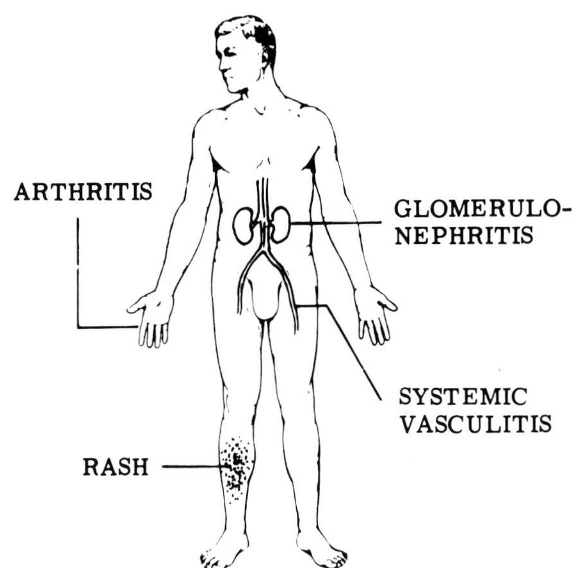

Figure 22–9. *A schematic representation of human immune complex disease. The constellation of arthritis, cutaneous or systemic vasculitis, and glomerulonephritis suggests this pathogenetic mechanism of disease.*

Even in the absence of destruction, persistent joint capsule distention may itself lead to chronic deforming changes in the absence of frank destruction. This is best seen in the Jaccoud's type of arthropathy, which follows recurrent rheumatic fever synovitis of the metacarpophalangeal joints;[37] a similar process appears to account for some of the nonerosive deformities seen occasionally in patients with persistent systemic lupus erythematosus arthritis. The intermittent nature of the arthropathy in association with a well-characterized underlying systemic disease should lead to an accurate diagnosis.

Collagen-Vascular Diseases

The collagen-vascular diseases include such disorders as systemic lupus erythematosus, systemic sclerosis, dermatomyositis, and the vasculitic syndromes. Many of the diseases covered by this broad categorization are, in fact, unrelated and display considerable diversity in pathogenesis, clinical expression, and complications. However, some of the disease manifestations are evident in the musculoskeletal system and therefore sometimes demand diagnostic considerations relevant to the other rheumatic diseases discussed previously.

Patients with systemic lupus erythematosus may have a fairly widespread and troublesome small and large peripheral joint polyarthritis.[38] Indeed, the lupus arthritis may dominate the illness for several years. However, sooner or later the myriad extra-articular manifestations of this multisystem disorder usually prevail and overshadow the articular pathology. In patients with chronic lupus arthropathy, deformities of the Jaccoud's type may occur, in which case the differential diagnosis from rheumatoid arthritis becomes a little more difficult. However, careful review of the symptoms and signs usually reveals evidence of the collagen-vascular disease, confirmed by abundant serologic abnormalities as are detailed in Chapter 23.

Similarly, patients with systemic sclerosis may have a transient or even persistent low-grade synovitis affecting a few peripheral joints or periarticular tendon sheaths.[39] Because of the nature of the underlying lesion, an early loss of range of motion may develop and be accompanied by a noisy crepitant sensation over the surface of the joint. Nearly always, however, the more dramatic cutaneous and organ-system signs of systemic sclerosis are apparent, so that although joint contractures may become an important part of the total clinical picture they rarely result in a confusion of diagnosis.

Rarely, patients with dermatomyositis or polyarteritis may manifest an inflammatory arthropathy of one or two (usually large) joints. However, in nearly every case the more obviously involved tissues become clinically significant, and the treatment demanded for the more important manifestations quickly suppresses the low-grade and nondestructive arthropathy of these rarer collagen-vascular disorders.

SUMMARY

The pathologic process leading to the rheumatic diseases outlined in this textbook can result in a rather restricted number of symptoms and signs. The type of patient (age, sex, sexual habits), the degree of acuteness or chronicity, and the total skeletal distribution of the arthropathic process provide the most potent clues to clinical diagnosis of rheumatic disease. In addition, the presence or absence of associated extra-articular manifestations is of great diagnostic importance. Clearly, an assessment of the true distribution of the joint disease frequently requires the use of selective radiographs, especially once the arthropathy has become chronic or relapsing. Finally, the selective use of a few laboratory tests, which will be outlined in Chapter 23, should provide the clinician with the final data required for those relatively few patients in whom a purely clinical diagnosis is still elusive. The diagnosis of most rheumatic diseases is thereby facilitated, with some well-recognized pitfalls and deviations mentioned above. This is the clinical approach to rheumatology; understanding it will permit the readers of this textbook to more readily comprehend how the numerous morphoradiographic processes described herein may be manifested in the individual patient.

REFERENCES

1. Hollander JL, McCarty DJ (Eds): Arthritis and Allied Conditions. 9th Ed. Philadelphia, Lea & Febiger, 1979.
2. Katz W: Rheumatic Diseases: Diagnosis and Management, Philadelphia JB Lippincott Co, 1977.
3. Copeman W: Textbook of Rheumatic Diseases. 3rd Ed. Edinburgh, E & S Livingstone, 1964.
4. Kelley WN, Harris ED Jr, Ruddy S, Sledge CB (Eds): Textbook of Rheumatology. Philadelphia, WB Saunders (in press).
5. Steinberg AD: On morning stiffness. J Rheumatol *5*:3, 1978.
6. Bluestone R: Practical Rheumatology (videorecording). Chicago, AMA Council on Continuing Physician Education, 1978.
7. Kirk JA, Ansell BM, Bywaters EGL: The hypermobility syndrome. Musculoskeletal complaints associated with generalized joint hypermobility. Ann Rheum Dis *26*:419, 1967.
8. Reza MJ, Verity MA: Neuromuscular manifestations of rheumatoid arthritis: A clinical and histomorphological analysis. Clin Rheum Dis *3*:565, 1977.
9. Bluestone R: Radiographs in the diagnosis of rheumatic disease. Postgrad Med *65*:64, 1979.
10. Calliet R: Low Back Pain Syndrome. 2nd Ed. Philadelphia, FA Davis Co, 1968.
11. Cailliet R: Shoulder Pain. Philadelphia, FA Davis Co, 1966.
12. Cailliet R: Neck and Arm Pain. Philadelphia, FA Davis Co, 1964.
13. Cailliet R: Knee Pain and Disability. Philadelphia, FA Davis Co, 1973.
14. Peter JB: Erosive osteoarthritis of the hands: Its distinction from rheumatoid arthritis and osteoarthritis. West Med *8*:183, 1967.
15. Williams R Jr: Rheumatoid Arthritis as a Systemic Disease. Philadelphia, WB Saunders Co, 1974.
16. Katz RS, Zizic TM, Arnold WP, Stevens MB: The pseudothrombophlebitis syndrome. Medicine *56*:151, 1977.
17. Schaller J, Hanson V (Eds): Proceedings of the first ARA Conference on the Rheumatic Diseases of Childhood. Arthritis Rheum (Suppl) *20*:145, 1977.
18. Fletcher MR, Scott JT: Chronic monoarticular synovitis. Diagnostic and prognostic features. Ann Rheum Dis *34*:171, 1975.
19. Bluestone R, Bacon P (Eds): Extra-articular manifestations of rheumatoid arthritis. Clin Rheum Dis *3*:385–606, 1977.
20. Wajed MA, Brown DL, Currey HL: Palindromic rheumatism. Ann Rheum Dis *36*:56, 1977.
21. Moll JMH, Haslock I, Macrae IF, Wright V: Associations between ankylosing spondylitis, psoriatic arthritis, Reiter's disease, the intestinal arthropathies, and Behçet's syndrome. Medicine *53*:343, 1974.
22. Neustadt DH: Symposium, ankylosing spondylitis. Postgrad Med *61*:124, 1977.
23. Ogryzlo MA: Ankylosing spondylitis. *In* JL Hollander, DJ McCarty (Eds): Arthritis and Allied Conditions. 8th Ed. Philadelphia, Lea & Febiger, 1972.
24. Moll JMH, Wright V: Familial occurrence of psoriatic arthritis. Ann Rheum Dis *32*:181, 1973.
25. Weinberger HW, Ropes MW, Kulka JP, Bauer W: Reiter's syndrome, clinical and pathological observations. Medicine *41*:35, 1961.
26. Bluestone R, Pearson CM: Ankylosing spondylitis and Reiter's syndrome: Their interrelationship and association with HLA B27. Adv Intern Med *22*:1, 1977.
27. Laitinen O, Leirisalo M, Skylv G: Relation between HLA-B27 and clinical features in patients with Yersinia arthritis. Arthritis Rheum *20*:1121, 1977.
28. Klinenberg J (Ed): Proceedings of the Second Conference on Gout and Purine Metabolism. Arthritis Rheum (Suppl) *18*:659, 1975.
29. McCarty DJ (Ed): Proceedings of the Conference on Pseudogout and Pyrophosphate Metabolism. Arthritis Rheum (Suppl) *19*:275, 1976.
30. Dieppe PA, Crocker P, Huskisson EC, Willoughby DA: Apatite deposition disease. A new arthropathy. Lancet *1*:266, 1976.
31. Goldenberg DL, Cohen AS: Acute infectious arthritis. A review of patients with nongonococcal joint infections (with emphasis on therapy and prognosis). Am J Med *60*:369, 1976.
32. Holmes KK, Counts GW, Beaty HN: Disseminated gonococcal infection. Ann Intern Med *74*:979, 1971.
33. Davidson PT, Horowitz I: Skeletal tuberculosis; a review with patient presentations and discussion. Am J Med *48*:77, 1970.
34. Duffy J, Lidsky MD, Sharp JT, Davis JS, Person DA, Hollinger FB, Min K-W: Polyarthritis, polyarteritis, and hepatitis B. Medicine *55*:19, 1976.
35. Aronstam A, Arblaster PG, Rainsford SG, Turk P, Slattery M, Alderson MR, Hall DE, Kirk PJ: Prophylaxis in haemophilia: A double-blind controlled trial. Br J Haematol *33*:81, 1976.
36. McCluskey RT, Hall CL, Colvin RB: Immune complex mediated diseases. Hum Pathol *9*:71, 1978.
37. Bywaters EGL: Jaccoud's syndrome. A sequel to the joint involvement of systemic lupus erythematosus. Clin Rheum Dis *1*:125, 1975.
38. Dubois EL (Ed): Lupus Erythematosus: A Review of the Current Status of Discoid and Systemic Lupus Erythematosus and Their Variants. 2nd Ed. Los Angeles, University of Southern California Press, 1974.
39. Schumacher HR Jr: Joint involvement in progressive systemic sclerosis (scleroderma): A light and electron microscopic study of synovial membrane and fluid. Am J Clin Pathol *60*:593, 1973.

23

LABORATORY SIGNS OF ARTICULAR DISEASE

by Rodney Bluestone, M.B., F.R.C.P.

As discussed in Chapter 22, most of the diagnostic process in rheumatology depends largely on a clinical analysis of the patients' symptoms and physical signs. There are relatively few really important laboratory tests deemed necessary for the differential diagnosis. Thus, although there is an abundant array of laboratory procedures that may be applied to the characterization of patients with articular disease, there are very few absolutely crucial diagnostic tests available to the practicing physician. Nevertheless, many nonessential laboratory tests are useful as confirmatory or supportive aids in considering a specific clinical diagnosis. Moreover, some laboratory signs serve as useful indices for the activity and extent of a rheumatic disease process, including one potential parameter by which to gauge a patient's response to therapeutic efforts. Finally, certain laboratory signs have helped to broaden the vistas of clinical rheumatology and have permitted a more helpful and complete categorization of some classes of rheumatic disease. In this chapter the major laboratory signs of articular disease will be discussed by category, and the discussion will include the principles of the test system, their interpretation, and their potential role (or lack of one) in the clinical diagnosis of rheumatic disease.

CRUCIAL LABORATORY SIGNS

The few crucial tests in rheumatology all involve direct examination of aspirated synovial fluid or synovial membrane for the presence of pathologic material.[1] Therefore, in order to proceed with these tests, the physician must be prepared to aspirate a distended joint.[2] In most instances the best site for synovial aspiration is at the point of maximal distention. This is particularly the case in the knee joint, where a bulging synovial cavity readily presents on either side of the patella or in the popliteal fossa. Similarly, in the wrist or ankle joint, the point of maximal distention is usually obvious. For some deeply located joints, however, aspiration may be more difficult and require a detailed knowledge of surface anatomy. Hence, rather more skill is necessary to aspirate a shoulder or hip joint successfully. Even very small peripheral joints sometimes have to be aspirated, and for this purpose fine hypodermic needles are used in order to enter the joint space. However, since invariably an inflammatory focus is involved, there is a good chance of aspirating the exudate even if the tip of the needle is not precisely within the synovial cavity. Thus, even a swollen great toe joint can nearly always be successfully aspirated so as to yield the vitally important exudative fluid. Unfortunately, the joints of the spine are almost impossible to aspirate without using a large needle under direct radiographic control. This is a procedure that in most institutions would be performed by a radiologist with special knowledge of spinal anatomy.

Articular aspiration requires a strictly aseptic technique with adequate preparation of the overlying skin. Local anesthesia is well worth performing and can rarely be achieved adequately by surface anesthetics except in a patient with a grossly and acutely distended joint that is agonizingly painful and very close to the surface. In nearly every other instance it is desirable to use a local anesthetic from the level of the dermis down to the joint capsule before introducing a larger needle for the actual aspiration. As one advances the larger needle, the sudden "give" indicating entry into the synovial cavity is accompanied by the ability to withdraw synovial fluid into the syringe. This synovial fluid may vary from a few drops of exsanguineous exudate to 200 ml of fluid under high pressure flowing rapidly into the syringe. The aspirated fluid should be handled according to the information being sought. Anticoagulated specimens are required for accurate cell counts; unprocessed specimens are suitable for the macroscopic assessment of viscosity (i.e., the string test) and the mucin clot test; and measurement of complement concentrations requires immediate processing and frozen storage within an hour of aspiration for later assay. Smears of the fluid can be made immediately for bacteriologic examination, and some of the exudate can be plated on the appropriate media for culture and sensitivity studies. Examination for microcrystals is usually performed on an aliquot from the entire aspirated sample, but if the fluid is abundant in amount and the crystals are sparse it is useful to lightly centrifuge the exudate and then examine the harvested sediment for cell debris and crystals. Following completion of aspiration, the intra-articular needle is deliberately and rapidly withdrawn, and the minute puncture mark in the skin covered with a simple dressing.

Crystals

Synovial fluid examination for crystal identification is the only certain way to diagnose crystal-induced synovitis (acute gout or pseudogout). The clinical characteristics of these syndromes are described in Chapter 22, but the only certain way of making the diagnosis is to detect the appropriate crystal form in the exudate aspirated from within or around the inflamed joint, bursa, or tendon sheath. Crystals within synovial fluid can occasionally be delineated using regular light microscopy with or without phase contrast.[3] However, the only dependable way to detect them is by the use of polarizing microscopy. By virtue of its biophysical nature, crystalline material is birefringent when viewed under polarized light and appears as discrete, bright-glowing forms viewed against a completely black background.

With this method, even tiny amounts of synovial fluid can be examined microscopically for abundant or occasional crystalline forms. Depending on the relationship between the long axis of a crystal and the axis of slow vibration of polarized light, a crystalline form can be delineated as either positively or negatively birefringent. Furthermore, by including a first order red compensator into the polarizing system, the birefringence can be reflected as a distinct color (yellow or blue). A urate crystal is best recognized as a relatively long, needle-shaped structure that is intensely negatively birefringent (and appears bright yellow when its long axis is parallel to the axis of slow vibrations of light in the compensator) (Fig. 23–1). A calcium pyrophosphate crystal can be identified as a shorter, more oblong, and blunter structure that is weakly positively birefringent (and appears a weak blue when its long axis is parallel to the light source) (Fig. 23–2). In addi-

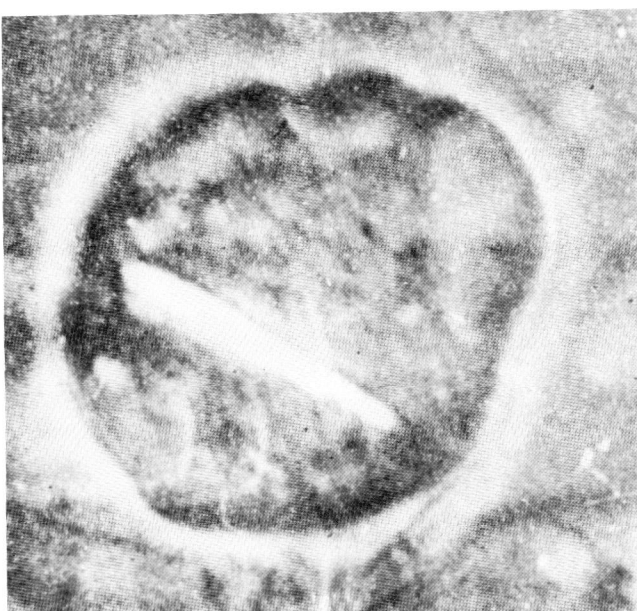

Figure 23–1. A monosodium urate crystal lying within a synovial fluid leukocyte viewed under polarizing microscopy. The specimen was aspirated from a gouty joint. (Courtesy of Dr. D. McCarty, Milwaukee, Wisconsin.)

tion, calcium pyrophosphate can occur as a triclinic or plate form, but even so it retains its characteristic polarizing properties.[4] Even a regular light microscope can readily be converted into a crude polarizing system by incorporating two cross Polaroid filters (analyzer and polarizer) inserted between the light source and objectives. A piece of cellophane tape adherent to a glass microscope slide can then serve as a first order red compensator.

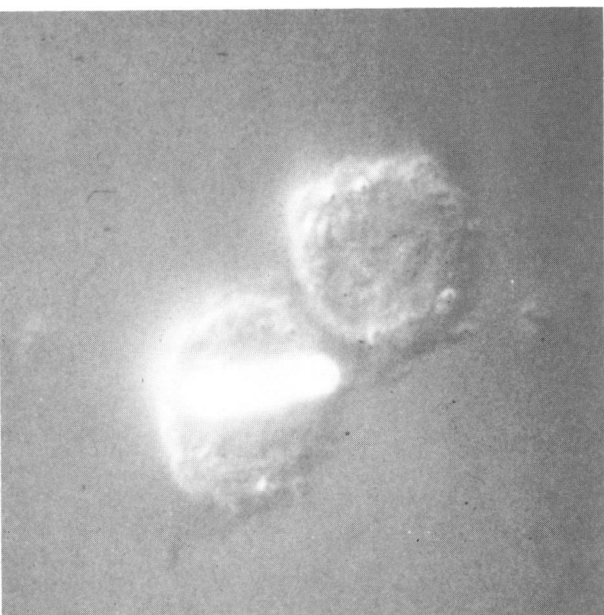

Figure 23–2. A calcium pyrophosphate crystal lying within a synovial fluid leukocyte viewed under polarizing microscopy. Note that the crystal form is blunt and oblong in comparison to a typical urate crystal. The specimen was aspirated from the joint of a patient suffering from acute pseudogout.

A vigorous pursuit to identify microcrystalline forms within aspirated synovial fluid is of great importance for correct diagnosis in patients presenting with a clinical syndrome compatible with acute gout or pseudogout. Frequently, attacks of crystal-induced synovitis are atypical, polyfocal, or clinically indistinct.[5] Moreover, the more recent recognition of a chronic pseudogout syndrome indicates that the crystal-induced inflammation may present as a low-grade and potentially destructive inflammatory polyarthritis. Thus, 30 minutes spent at a polarizing microscope with a recently aspirated specimen of joint fluid can yield one of the most accurate and definitive laboratory signs in the whole spectrum of rheumatology. The examiner should be prepared to recognize the presence of a mixed crystal population, since patients may suffer from attacks of acute arthritis due to both urate and pyrophosphate crystals. Middle-aged and elderly patients with septic arthritis may shed calcium pyrophosphate crystals from their cartilaginous deposits into the joint space, and these too can be microscopically detected side by side with the invading bacteria. Centrifuging the aspirated synovial fluid may enhance the sensitivity of polarizing microscopy, although it may eliminate the definitive sign of crystals engulfed by polymorphonuclear leukocytes. For reasons that are unclear, pseudogout is more frequently associated with large numbers of extracellular crystals, although the phlogistic mechanisms within the joint cavity are presumed to be similar to those for urate gout. Clearly, the longer the synovial fluid has been standing, the more chance is there that any partially ingested crystals will have been shed and fragmented, thereby making their detection within neutrophils less likely. Furthermore, it may be necessary to aspirate several inflamed joints repeatedly before finding the single crystal that provides a solution to a diagnostic problem. This is especially so in patients with recurrent attacks of acute-on-chronic pseudogout, in which it is not uncommon to require three or four separate synovial aspirations, each examined by careful polarizing microscopy, before the true nature of the inciting agent becomes evident.

It is not possible to identify calcium hydroxyapatite crystals readily with simple polarizing microscopy. However, a greater phlogistic role for this crystal form is now being considered. Other synovial fluid material may sometimes appear as birefringent or crystalline forms. False positive birefringence may be evoked by dust or silica particles, but the complete absence of any of the morphologic characteristics of biologic crystals is usually obvious. Recent injections of intra-articular steriods using some of the long-acting preparations that tend to crystallize within the joint space may result in detectable synovial steroid crystals and might explain the post-injection flare of synovitis sometimes observed. Prednisone crystals, however, are quite different in appearance from urate or pyrophosphate crystals, and a recent history of the intra-articular procedure is usually forthcoming. Finally, cholesterol crystals can be seen in many chronic effusions, but their flat, plate-like rectangular appearance with a corner "missing" is absolutely characteristic of this material. Aside from denoting chronicity, they are not thought to play any significant role in promoting an intra-articular inflammatory response.

Having emphasized that the detection of intrasynovial urate crystals is the only certain way to diagnose typical gout, it is now appropriate to consider the diagnostic role of serum urate concentrations in such patients. The amount of uric acid in the blood is the result of a constant homeostatic mechanism reflecting a balance between de novo purine synthesis together with dietary intake of preformed purines and the disposition of uric acid, mainly through renal excretion (with a lesser degradative component resulting from intestinal uricolysis). Thus, numerous potential causes of hyperuricemia may prevail in any individual patient.[6] By studying large populations of asymptomatic people, accepted normal ranges for serum urate concentrations have been established. For men, the upper limit of normal is approximately 7 mg per deciliter (dl) and for premenopausal women, the value is set somewhat lower at 6 mg per dl. One should remember, however, that these figures reflect a wide physiologic range of serum urate concentrations. Moreover, since there are many potential mechanisms that may induce transient hyperuricemia and many of these are not associated with disease states, day-to-day fluctuation in the serum urate concentration may be ascribed to alterations in dietary purine intake, an increased or decreased amount of endogenous nucleic acid turnover, or alterations in the renal tubular handling of urate. The latter mechanism of hyperuricemia is a frequent result of many commonly used drugs, including low-dose salicylates and thiazide diuretics. Nevertheless, a substantial number of people can be recognized who have persistent hyperuricemia unexplained by identifiable exogenous factors. Many of these individuals have an increased endogenous de novo production of purines or a relative underexcretion of urinary uric acid, or both. This does not necessarily imply that they have renal disease, but their glomerular clearance of uric acid appears to require a comparably higher serum urate concentration than normal.[7] It is also now well recognized that many people, especially men, may be persistently hyperuricemic and yet show no evidence of target organ disease. Whether or not asymptomatic hyperuricemia is potentially injurious to the kidneys is as yet an unanswered question, although short-term observations suggest little or no risk attached to the metabolic aberration. However, a small percentage of hyperuricemic subjects may develop urate deposition disease, manifested as intrasynovial crystallization of sodium urate (i.e., acute gout), tophus formation, renal stones, and chronic interstitial nephritis. Thus, most patients who present with acute urate gout are or have recently been hyperuricemic. Indeed, it is somewhat unusual (but not impossible) to develop acute gouty arthritis without evidence of significant hyperuricemia. Therefore, the accurate diagnosis of acute gout requires a demonstration of intrasynovial urate crystals, and the patient is usually hyperuricemic. It should be stressed that the demonstration of significant hyperuricemia does not mean a diagnosis of gout but merely a underlying metabolic aberration, which in some individuals is complicated by recurrent gouty attacks. Clearly, then, the measurement of the serum urate concentration is no more than a supportive biochemical test in a patient in whom other circumstances strongly suggest gouty episodes. However, the prevention of future attacks of gout largely depends on the effective lowering of the serum urate concentration. Consequently, serial measurement of the serum urate concentration is a highly effective way of monitoring hypouricemic drug therapy and provides the physician with a fairly accurate prognostic indicator for future gout attacks. By contrast, most patients with chondrocalcinosis and recurrent attacks of pseudogout are normouricemic unless they happen to be suffering from the combined form of crystal-induced disease. Most patients with chondrocalcinosis and recurrent pseudogout have no known associated biochemical aberration. However, since there is an increased association of chondrocalcinosis with certain endocrine and metabolic diseases, patients with recurrent pseudogout attacks should certainly be screened for biochemical evidence of overt hyperparathyroidism or hemochromatosis.[8]

Microorganisms

Synovial aspiration with appropriate examination of the exudate is the only certain way to diagnose septic arthritis.[9] This is true whether it is an acute or chronic septic arthritis, but in the latter instance the appropriate bacteriologic testing of the inflamed synovial membrane may be required. In particular, the demonstration of acid-fast bacilli or various fungal forms may not be possible in the synovial exudate but may actually require direct microscopy and culture of small pieces of excised or needle-biopsied synovium. Indeed, the procedure of open or closed synovial biopsy is mandatory in any patient with a chronic monoarticular arthritis, since this is the only way to exclude the possibility of a granulomatous synovitis, especially that due to tuberculous or fungal infection.

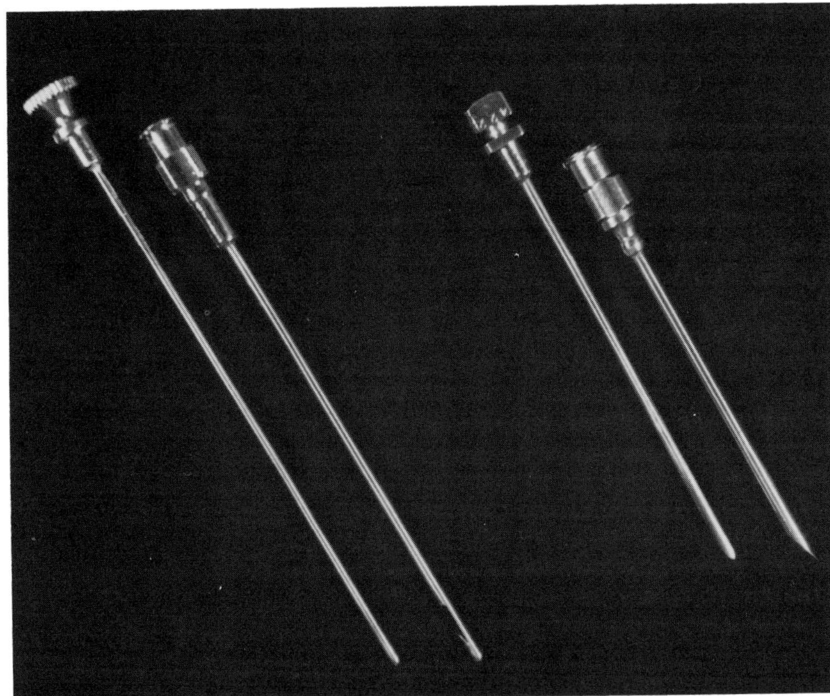

Figure 23–3. A synovial biopsy needle. Left, A 15 gauge aspirating needle closed at the tip and notched to create a hood and matching stylet. Right, A 14 gauge needle and matching stylet.

Although the technique for closed synovial biopsy is identical to that for aspiration of fluid, the biopsy needle is significantly larger and usually requires a small scalpel cut of the skin to satisfactorily introduce the trocar (Fig. 23–3). Small pieces of synovial membrane can usually be obtained from any large and distended synovial hinge joint, although the amount of synovial exudate present may not distend the joint adequately for the procedure. Under these circumstances, sterile saline solution can be injected into the articular cavity, thereby causing adequate distention. Closed biopsy of a child's joint or of an adult's small joint may be much more difficult, and open biopsy is usually preferred. The tiny pieces of biopsied tissue should normally be fixed in formalin for microscopy, including staining and histologic examination for bacteria and fungi. In addition, a piece can be sent for direct bacteriologic culture. If the diagnosis of chronic crystal-induced arthritis is being entertained, a small specimen should be preserved in absolute alcohol to permit polarizing microscopy of the cut sections. In some clinical situations, microscopic examination and culture of aspirated synovial fluid or membrane would probably accompany a parallel examination of other biologic fluids. Thus, the diagnosis of gonococcal arthritis or tenosynovitis might depend on the typical clinical profile together with a positive smear or culture obtained from any of the sites likely to be involved including the joint or tendon sheath space, the cervix, rectum, pharynx, or aspirated/incised necrotic skin pustule. Likewise, even in the presence of an obviously septic joint with positive culture results, the clinican is frequently concerned about the possibility of a generalized septicemia, so that concomitant blood cultures may be indicated.

Thus, the diagnosis of septic arthritis strongly depends upon the demonstration of the infectious agent within or around the joint space. In most instances this is an essential laboratory sign of articular disease, without which the diagnosis cannot be confirmed. In exceptional circumstances, such as a young adult with clinically characteristic gonococcal septicemia, the presence of the organism within another site can often be assumed to be the causative factor of the arthritis seen in that clinical context. Finally, the diagnosis of a chronic septic arthritis, especially that due to acid-fast bacilli or fungi, requires equally stringent criteria but may necessitate examination of articular tissue as well as synovial fluid in order to demonstrate the offending organism (Fig. 23–4).

Other Cardinal Tests

There are a few other rare examples in which examination of aspirated synovial fluid provides an absolutely diagnostic appearance. Occasionally, patients with a paraproteinemia associated amyloidosis develop extensive amyloid deposits within and around articular structures. Some of these deposits may be found within the articular cartilage, and fragments of amyloid-containing cartilage may on occasion be aspirated from the bulky, enlarged joints.[10] The microscopic characteristics of amyloid

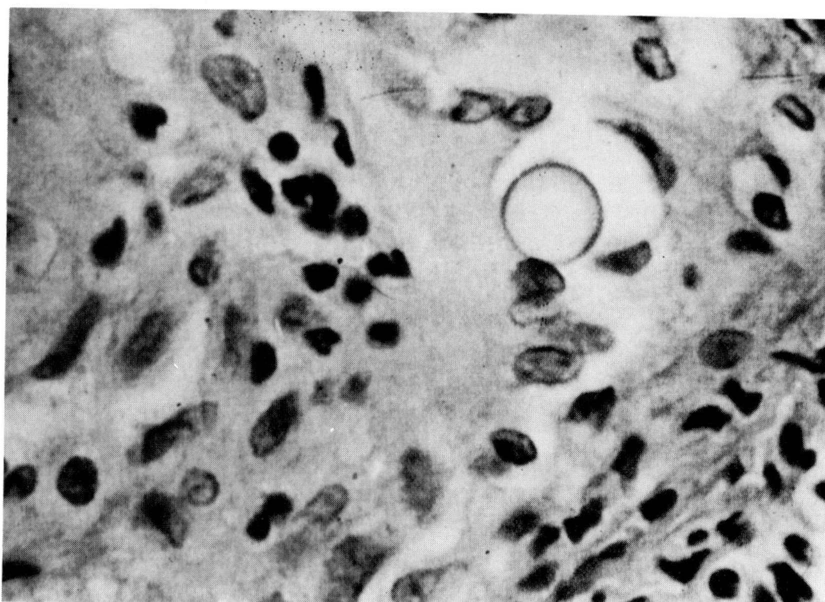

Figure 23–4. Synovial biopsy specimen from a patient with chronic monoarticular arthritis. Histologic examination revealed a typical cyst form of coccidioidomycosis. (Courtesy of The Arthritis Foundation.)

material can then be demonstrated using Congo red stains and polarizing microscopy, so that the identification of intrasynovial amyloid fragments is considered to be absolutely diagnostic for the rare syndrome of amyloid arthropathy. In nearly every case, however, the clinical diagnosis is evident as an overt or latent dysproteinemia. Similarly, the occasional patient with a hairline fracture extending through the subchondral bone into the joint space may leak marrow elements into the synovial cavity, as well as manifest a low-grade posttraumatic effusion. Examination of the synovial fluid might then reveal free-floating marrow cells or numerous fat globules, identified either by pure light microscopy or after use of appropriate stains to show the ectopic cell forms.[11] This laboratory sign may be evident in the absence of a radiographically visible bony fracture and then provides a valid way of diagnosing a posttraumatic effusion involving a minor fracture. On rare occasions an ochronotic joint may present with a small effusion, and the aspirated synovial fluid then reveals a "salt-and-pepper" appearance due to the suspension of minute ochronotic cartilage fragments.

NONSPECIFIC LABORATORY TESTS ON SYNOVIAL FLUID

The various other tests that are commonly performed on synovial fluid are all relatively nonspe-

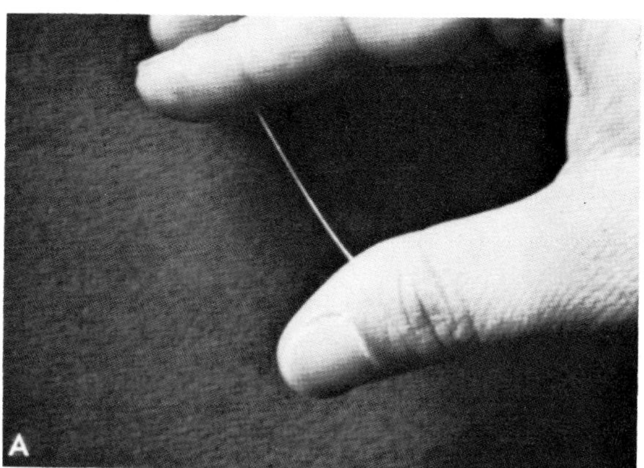

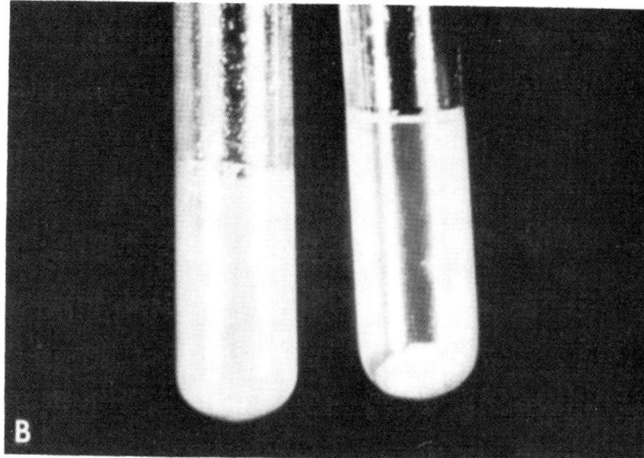

Figure 23–5. **A,** *A string test to demonstrate the viscosity of synovial fluid. Inflammatory synovial fluid is less viscous and demonstrates little or no stringing. (From Germain BF: Synovial Fluid Analysis in the Diagnosis of Diseases of the Joints. A Scope Publication, The Upjohn Company, Kalamazoo, Michigan, 1976.)* **B,** *The mucin clot test to demonstrate synovial fluid viscosity. A drop of synovial fluid is added to dilute acidic acid. Inflammatory fluid readily fragments and disperses within the acid (on left); good quality synovial fluid forms a tight clot and remains separate from the surrounding acid (on right).*

cific and do not carry the diagnostic weight attached to the crucial tests described above. Nevertheless, the general characterization of aspirated synovial fluid is a valid and valuable adjunct to the clinical profile and may serve to modify the diagnostic impression. The biophysical qualities of the synovial fluid may reflect the chronicity or nature of the pathologic process causing the effusion.[12] Normal synovial fluid is a clear, acellular, and highly viscous material containing large amounts of hyaluronic acid, and these physical characteristics become progressively lost in the presence of chronic inflammation. Thus, synovial fluid aspirated from a noninflamed or a very recently inflamed joint might display quite good viscosity (which can be gauged subjectively by a simple string test) and should also possess adequate hyaluronic acid (which can be assessed semiquantitatively by a mucin clot test). The principle of the mucin clot test is that synovial fluid with an adequate hyaluronate content will retract and form a tight clot when dropped into dilute (2 per cent) acetic acid. Inflammatory synovial fluid with its degraded hyaluronate will not form any such clot and quickly disperses within the acid to form a shower of disrupted particles (Fig. 23–5). Thus, the small amount of synovial fluid sometimes obtainable from an osteoarthrotic joint frequently has good viscosity and displays an intact mucin clot test. Conversely, the inflammatory synovial fluid obtained from patients with a chronic synovitis is usually highly mobile and possesses very poor clot retraction. The opposite situation (i.e., a greatly increased hyaluronate content and hyperviscosity) is seen in patients with hypothyroid arthropathy. In this syndrome, a low-grade synovial distention of the knee and tendon sheaths around the wrist may be detected. Interestingly, the aspirated synovial fluid may demonstrate an enormously long string test, presumably due to the greatly increased amounts of collagen and hyaluronate (Fig. 23–6). The clinical picture, combined with these extraordinary characteristics, provides a very clear and definitive diagnostic profile.[13]

The closer the synovial fluid protein concentration is to the serum values, the more likely it is that a significant chronic inflammation with massive hypervascularity of the subsynovial stroma has occurred. It should be remembered that some of the exuded plasma proteins are those involved in the normal coagulation process. Therefore, synovial fluid from very inflamed joints with a high plasma protein content may quickly clot following aspiration. This phenomenon may then interfere with the further characterization of the fluid, particularly the obtaining of an accurate differential white cell count. For this reason it is sometimes desirable to apportion some of the aspirated fluid into a container for anticoagulation studies pending hematologic examination. Since the synovial fluid plasma proteins leaking from the hypervascular tissue will also include antibodies, it should be possible to detect specific antibodies within the aspirate. In particular, it might prove helpful to be able to demonstrate rheumatoid factor in the early rheumatoid joint even before the autoantibody is apparent in the circulation. Unfortunately, however, technical problems in handling the fluid render this form of assay too difficult for routine use. Nevertheless, it is sometimes possible to adequately digest the synovial fluid by adding hyaluronidase and thereby reveal the presence of antiglobulins in patients with very early or monoarticular rheumatoid arthritis, even in the absence of serum rheumatoid factor. One should be aware that a prozone phenomenon is not unusual, so that a positive titer within the synovial fluid may become apparent only after dilution.[14]

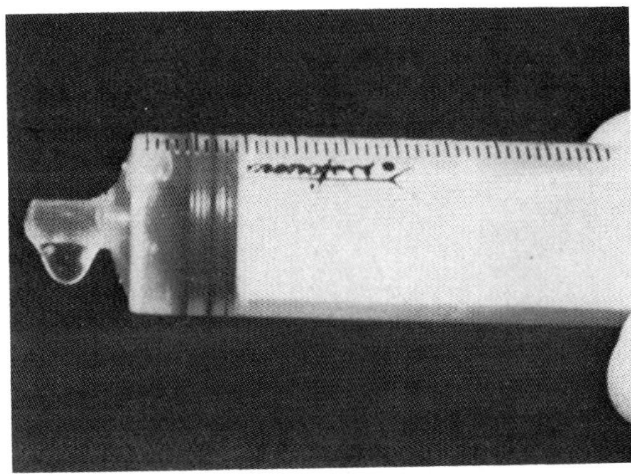

Figure 23–6. *Semigelatinous synovial fluid from myxedematous patients often requires several seconds to begin vertical fall from syringe, even with greater than usual pressure on plunger. If allowed to "string out" vertically from a Pasteur pipette, unbroken streams of greater than 45 cm occur in these fluids. (From Dorwart B, Schumacher HR: Am J Med 59:780, 1975.)*

Synovial fluid complement concentrations provide an index of intra-articular complement consumption. That is to say, certain rheumatic diseases may involve the formation of intrasynovial immune complexes (discussed later in this chapter) and these complexes appear to consume complement, resulting in a selective decrease of this exuded plasma protein.[15] Thus, many patients with rheumatoid arthritis demonstrate a selective depletion of synovial fluid complement compared to concomitant serum values. Conversely, patients with active systemic lupus erythematosus tend to demonstrate lowered serum complement concentrations, and when they have a chronic effusion assayed in this way, their synovial fluid complement concentration matches the lowered serum values. Interestingly, the synovial fluid from patients with one of the seronegative spondyloarthropathies usually possesses a normal or even relatively high concentration of complement. Since complement estimations demand careful handling and storage of the biologic specimens, they are not recommended for routine use. Nevertheless, a selective depletion of synovial fluid complement can provide one useful laboratory sign of early or atypical rheumatoid arthritis.

The cell content of synovial fluid is also a rough indicator of the type of pathologic process leading to the effusion. A severe posttraumatic effusion or hemarthrosis is naturally characterized by the appearance of almost pure blood, although the hematocrit value of the aspirated fluid is rarely more than two thirds that of the peripheral blood taken at the same time. The presence of frank blood within the synovial space acts as an irritant, quickly leading to further synovial fluid formation, thereby diluting the hematogenous material. Similarly, a very traumatic synovial aspiration may itself result in ruptured blood vessels and brisk intrasynovial bleeding. Under these circumstances, however, continued aspiration of the joint cavity should show some clearing of the red cells, and the final specimen of synovial fluid may then be characterized. A considerable degree of attention has been paid to the total and differential white blood cell counts within the synovial fluid in various arthropathies. In general, it can be stated that the more acute and infective the articular disease, the higher the synovial fluid total white blood cell count becomes and the greater the percentage of polymorphonuclear leukocytes. Thus, patients with acute septic arthritis may have spectacular synovial fluid white blood cell counts in excess of 100,000 per cu mm, the vast majority of which may be polymorphonuclear forms. Similarly, patients with crystal-induced synovitis may likewise reveal spectacularly high counts. However, it should be firmly emphasized that patients with septic arthritis or crystal-induced synovitis may display synovial fluid cell counts considerably lower than these extreme values; counts have been frequently documented at 15,000 to 20,000 cells per cu mm despite the obvious presence of bacteria or crystals. Moreover, a predominantly polymorphonuclear cell count well above 60,000 cells per cu mm is not unusual in the acute synovitis of Reiter's disease. Clearly, then, the actual

Table 23–1
SYNOVIAL FLUID FINDINGS IN HEALTH AND IN DISEASE AFFECTING THE JOINTS*

Condition	Appearance	Viscosity	Mucin Clot	WBCs Per Cu Mm	Polymorphonuclear Leukocytes (Per Cent)	Special Findings
Normal	Clear, yellow	High	Firm	100 to 200	10	Scanty fluid; no debris
Traumatic arthritis	Red-tinged to bloody	High	Firm	2000+	<20	Few cartilage fragments; many RBCs
Osteoarthritis	Clear, yellow	High	Firm	1000 to 3000	<20	Few to many cartilage fragments; debris
Systemic lupus erythematosus	Slightly cloudy	Slightly decreased	Firm	3000 to 5000	<30	LE cells on Wright's stained smear
Rheumatic fever	Slightly cloudy	Decreased	Firm	7000 to 10,000	<50	Few inclusion bodies among WBCs
Reiter's syndrome	Cloudy	Decreased	Friable	15,000	60+	Hemolytic complement increased; polymorphonuclear leukocytes in macrophages
Pseudogout	Slightly cloudy to cloudy	Decreased	Fairly firm	10,000+	60+	Rhomboid positively birefringent crystals in WBCs or cartilage fragments
Gouty arthritis	Cloudy to milky	Decreased	Fairly firm	15,000+	75+	Needle-like negatively birefringent crystals in WBCs or free
Rheumatoid arthritis (active)	Cloudy, greenish	Low	Friable	10,000 to 30,000	80+	Many WBCs containing cytoplasmic inclusions; hemolytic complement low; latex fixation test positive
Tuberculous arthritis	Cloudy	Low	Friable	25,000	50	Acid-fast bacilli may be found on smear; culture may be positive; glucose level lower than that in blood
Septic arthritis (acute)	Turbid to purulent	Low	Friable	Over 75,000	90+	Glucose level much lower than that in blood; culture positive; hemolytic complement low

*From Hollander JL: Postgrad Med 64:50, 1978.

synovial fluid white blood cell count is not an absolute diagnostic aid but serves only as a rough guide to the possibility that intrasynovial phlogistic material is present. Patients with rheumatoid arthritis may have a variable and changeable synovial fluid white blood cell count. The disease is said to be characterized by a predominantly lymphocytic exudate during the first few weeks of its evolution, but this is a very difficult phenomenon to document, since the patient probably does not present to the clinician until this phase is past. By the time the diagnostic tests are under way, most synovial fluids in rheumatoid diseases are characterized by moderately elevated total white blood cell counts with a predominance of polymorphonuclear leukocytes. Counts as high as 40,000 to 60,000 cells per cu mm are not unusual, although the extraordinarily high counts associated with the presence of bacteria or crystals are rarely seen. Contrariwise, it is unusual for patients with osteoarthritis or a simple posttraumatic effusion to demonstrate synovial fluid counts higher than 5000 to 10,000 cells per cu mm. In these instances the differential count more accurately reflects the situation in the peripheral blood although here, too, neutrophils may predominate. On occasion, some forms of proved or presumed viral arthritis are characterized by synovial fluid of the type seen in slight inflammation, in which the modestly increased cell count is largely due to an ingress of mononuclear cells.

A crude classification of synovial fluid (classes I, II, and III) may thereby be devised and can be used to broadly characterize the aspirated exudate in a semistandardized fashion (Table 23–1). To some extent the absolute number of white blood cells in the aspirated fluid contributes to the turbidity of the exudate. It is therefore possible to guess from the gross appearance of the fluid whether or not there are a high protein concentration and a high white blood cell content. Sterile posttraumatic or osteoarthritic effusions show the clearest fluids (classes I and II); septic or chronic inflammatory joints yield the most turbid samples (classes II and III). More refined studies on the synovial fluid cell ultrastructure have been pursued by various investigators. However, the morphologic changes described and ascribed to various rheumatic disease syndromes probably lack specificity and require considerable expertise in their detection and interpretation. Thus, such studies do not as yet provide a reasonable laboratory sign for the diagnosis and characterization of rheumatic disease.

Finally, the aspirated synovial fluid can be examined for several biochemical characteristics. The glucose concentration is usually found to be greatly diminished compared to normal serum values in patients with septic arthritis. However, this is not a specific finding, and relatively low synovial fluid glucose values may also be detected in some patients with chronic nonspecific synovitis of the rheumatoid type. Greater specificity appears to reside in the detection of elevated lactate concentrations in the synovial fluid of patients with nongonococcal septic arthritis.[16] The increased amounts of lactate broadly parallel the high white blood cell counts and decreased glucose concentrations typical of bacterial synovitis. The ready availability of a Mono-Test lactate kit may well facilitate the bedside diagnosis of this form of acute monoarticular arthritis. Once a synovial effusion becomes chronic, it is common for cholesterol to accumulate within the joint cavity. This may be seen macroscopically as obviously hyperlipemic synovial fluid with a deep straw-yellow color and may be reflected biochemically by the presence of a high concentration of measured cholesterol. However, aside from indicating chronicity, this has no diagnostic specificity.

HEMOGRAM

The quality, appearance, and cellular components of the peripheral blood may reflect a diverse group of acute and chronic rheumatic disease. As with any chronic disease state, a chronic rheumatic disease may be accompanied by a low-grade hypochromic anemia. This anemia may result in decreased hemoglobin concentrations of 9 to 10 gm per dl and is thought to be due to the inability of the reticuloendothelial system to release the stored iron (obtained from effete red blood cells) for reutilization in new red blood cell formation.[17] Thus, although the patient with chronic rheumatic disease may not technically be iron deficient, there is an internal "starvation in the midst of the plenty," with abundant marrow iron stores trapped within macrophages and not available for normoblast development. Under such circumstances the serum iron concentration and the total iron-binding capacity are decreased in concert so that the iron-binding index may remain within normal limits. The anemia of chronic disease is totally unresponsive to hematinic supplements. Improvement is only seen if the underlying inflammatory process abates, so that following the hemoglobin level in patients with chronic rheumatic disease is a fairly useful indicator of therapeutic response or increased disease activity. However, it is not unusual to detect an additional element of iron deficiency superimposed upon the recalcitrant form of chronic anemia. This is particularly the case in patients who have taken nonsteroidal anti-inflammatory drugs. All of the currently used nonsteroidal anti-inflammatory agents are capable of causing any degree of gastritis or gastric erosion. This side effect may lead to an acute-on-chronic gastrointestinal blood loss, which may be readily detectable but remains clinically insignificant in the majority of individuals. Not infrequently, however, the bleeding assumes greater proportions and may not be compensated for in the patient's dietary iron intake. Therefore, a falling hematocrit value with definite hypochromic indices and an undersaturated serum iron binding capacity should alert the physician to the superadded element of iron deficiency anemia. The source of the blood loss is often suggested by a history of dyspepsia following the use of oral anti-inflammatory drugs; examination of the stool for occult blood usually confirms the diagnostic suspicions. In some instances, patients with severe chronic rheumatic disease (usually in the form of rheumatoid arthritis) may develop a megaloblastic anemia due to folate deficiency. This is seen mainly in communities in which victims of crippling arthritis have been left to fend for themselves and thereby forced to exist on a frugal diet deficient in folate and vitamin C. The anemia may be suspected when the peripheral blood picture reveals typical megaloblastic features supported by the appropriate changes within the bone marrow. Measurement of the serum folate concentration is not a good guide to this form of anemia, since the serum folate level appears to be nonspecifically decreased in chronic rheumatoid arthritis. The more difficult, specific assay of red blood cell folate concentration may therefore be required to confirm the diagnosis.

The peripheral total and differential white blood cell count may aid in the diagnosis and assessment of rheumatic disease. Patients with very active inflammatory polyarthritis may have a modest and sustained polymorphonuclear leukocytosis. Patients with the acute systemic form of juvenile rheumatoid arthritis (Still's disease in a child or its adult equivalent) characteristically display strikingly elevated peripheral white blood cell counts,[18] and patients with an acute septic arthritis would likewise be expected to have leukocytosis as a reflection of their systemic toxicity. A leukopenia is an important hematologic laboratory sign in some rheumatic diseases or may reflect the iatrogenic consequences of drug therapy directed at the arthropathy. Patients with Felty's syndrome (rheumatoid arthritis, hepatosplenomegaly, and neutropenia) may be profoundly leukopenic, with total white blood cell counts sustained at less than 2000 per cu mm for prolonged periods of time. Since the most deficient cell is the polymorphonuclear leukocyte, the absolute degree of neutropenia may be even more serious, although there appears to be a rather imprecise correlation between the absolute neutrophil count and the incidence of systemic infections. A milder leukopenia may be seen as one manifestation of systemic lupus erythematosus. In this disease, there may also be a relative lymphopenia, which presumably reflects one of the numerous immunologic aberrations underlying the disease.[19] An absolute increase in the number of peripheral blood eosinophils may be one important laboratory sign in patients with certain types of vasculitis. Eosinophilia is often detected in middle-aged men with polyarteritis nodosa and in some patients with hypersensitivity angiitis.[20] It may be an important harbinger of gold toxicity in patients receiving this form of therapy for rheumatoid arthritis. An intense and peculiar subcutaneous tissue and peripheral blood eosinophilia is a hallmark of a rare syndrome known as eosinophilic fasciitis (Fig. 23–7), which clinically mimics localized areas of acute scleroderma.[21]

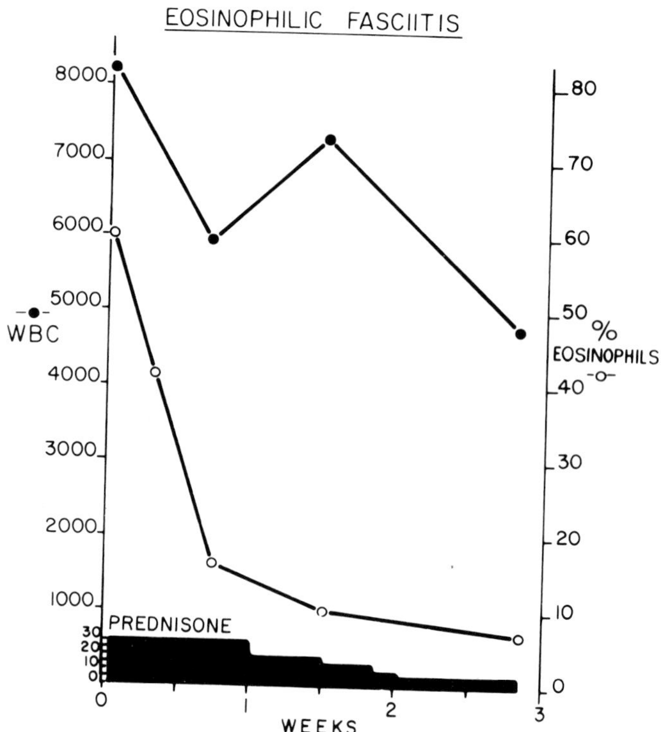

Figure 23–7. *Graph displaying the profound peripheral blood eosinophilia in a patient with eosinophilic fasciitis. The patient's lesion was steroid responsive.*

The peripheral blood platelets may provide a clue to the nature of the underlying rheumatic disease. Clearly, patients presenting with an acute hemarthrosis may have thrombocytopenia as the mechanism for their rheumatic disease. Although patients with profound thrombocytopenia do indeed bleed into their tissues, true hemarthrosis appears to be a rather uncommon complication of this primary hematologic disorder. However, patients with systemic lupus erythematosus may become severely thrombocytopenic, presumably due to circulating antiplatelet antibodies. This thrombocytopenic state may become the most threatening aspect of the patient's illness at any stage of the natural history of the disease.[22] Conversely, many patients with chronic rheumatic disease (typified by rheumatoid arthritis) appear to have a relative thrombocytosis with platelet counts of up to 600,000 per cu mm recorded. This "reactive" thrombocytosis does not appear to be physiologically important, and there is firm evidence for an increased incidence of venous thrombosis in patients with chronic rheumatic disease manifesting this altered hematologic state.[23]

PLASMA PROTEINS

Just as is the case with the blood cellular elements, plasma protein concentrations may provide laboratory signs pointing to the nature of a rheumatic disease. Some patients with severe chronic inflammatory rheumatic disease may become so debilitated that part of their clinical picture includes anorexia and weight loss, with their relative malnutrition reflected by a low serum albumin concentration. Similarly, some rheumatic diseases such as systemic lupus erythematosus are complicated by renal involvement. Many forms of renal disease may induce prolonged albuminuria leading to nephrosis, and as part of the nephrotic syndrome, a lowered serum albumin concentration often prevails. Rheumatologists are particularly interested in the detection and measurement of excess acute phase proteins in the patient's serum. These acute phase proteins are usually evident as increased amounts of alpha-1 and alpha-2 globulins apparent on plasma protein electrophoresis and include such individual components as fibrinogen, haptoglobin, and C reactive protein. Quantitation of these individual plasma protein components has been advocated as one way of assessing the severity and extent of the total inflammatory process in patients with chronic polyarthritis. Furthermore, they may be used to monitor the effectiveness of anti-inflammatory drugs in which, like hemoglobin concentration, they may reflect therapeutic responsiveness. For most purposes, however, the acute phase proteins are probably best measured in a single composite form as the erythrocyte sedimentation rate. Measurement of the erythrocyte sedimentation rate in patients with acute or chronic inflammatory disease most closely correlates with the serum fibrinogen concentration but also reflects many of the other acute phase proteins.[24] For reasons that are unclear, the uncorrected Westergren erythrocyte sedimentation rate is of particular use in assessing the extent and severity of inflammatory joint disease as well as its subsequent progression or response to treatment. Very high sedimentation rates are the rule in patients with polymyalgia rheumatica, some types of vasculitis, and acute or severe rheumatoid arthritis. An elevated sedimentation rate is nearly always seen in patients presenting with early ankylosing spondylitis. In this disease, however, the sedimentation rate appears to be a rather unreliable indicator of continuing chronic disease activity. Nevertheless, the demonstration of a completely normal erythrocyte sedimentation rate in a patient complaining of persistent arthralgias is a rather reassuring laboratory sign, sometimes reinforcing the clinician's doubts about the likelihood of the patient's having true rheumatic disease.

Qualitative and quantitative assessments of the plasma gamma globulins are of keen interest to the physician treating patients with rheumatic disease. Many of the chronic inflammatory rheumatic diseases are characterized by a diffuse and nonspecific hypergammaglobulinemia, which may be detected most readily as an increased "hump" in the gamma globulin portion of a plasma protein electrophoresis strip. Indeed, the hypergammaglobulinemia may be so pronounced as to result in the production of excess but normal free light chains, which may then be detectable in the urine. However, under those circumstances the urinary free light chains are dissimilar from true Bence Jones proteinuria since they are polyclonal and are not associated with an underlying paraproteinemia.[25] Nevertheless, in patients with an uncharacterized arthropathy and profound hypergammaglobulinemia, the physician must be careful not to overlook the possibility of a monoclonal plasma protein dyscrasia complicated by systemic amyloidosis, including an amyloid arthropathy.[26] In this illness plasma protein electrophoresis should reveal an obvious monoclonal spike. If this spike is small in amount and "buried" within a more diffuse hypergammaglobulinemia, examination of the concentrated urine by immunoelectrophoresis for monoclonal light chains becomes an important additive investigation.

There seems little reason for precisely quantitating the increased amounts of otherwise normal gamma globulins in patients with rheumatic disorders. However, there are several varieties of rheumatic disease associated with the hypogammaglobulinemic state. First, about 25 per cent of children with X-linked (Bruton's) hypogammaglobulinemia develop a chronic inflammatory arthropathy.[27] The arthropathy resembles rheumatoid disease in its clinical appearance, although it does not appear to be a very destructive form of inflammation. Clearly, these patients should demonstrate complete or near absence of serum IgG, IgA, and IgM (Fig. 23–8). Similarly, individuals with a selective deficiency of serum IgA appear to run an increased risk of developing various autoimmune diseases, including juvenile rheumatoid arthritis.[28] Thus, in patients with juvenile rheumatoid arthritis with a strong family history of arthritis or other forms of autoimmune disease, an estimation of the serum immunoglobulin concentrations may be a useful clue to the pathogenesis of the disease.

A specific hypergammaglobulinemia is perhaps of even greater interest in the field of contemporary rheumatology. Namely, the detection of a specific humoral antibody response directed against a known arthritogenic organism may be of considerable diagnostic help in certain selected clinical situations. A prime instance of this is the detection of

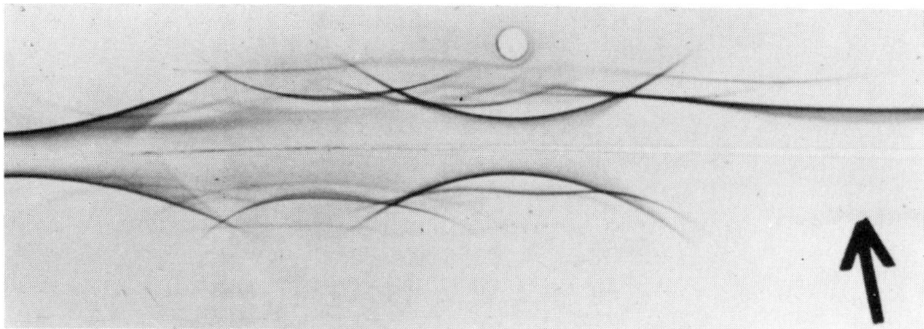

Figure 23–8. Serum immunoelectrophoresis in a patient with Bruton's congenital hypogammaglobulinemia. Patient's serum was placed in the lower well and a sample of normal serum in the upper well. The central trough contained antiserum to human plasma proteins. Note the absence of IgG, IgA, and IgM arcs indicated by the arrow.

antibodies to streptococcal antigens in the diagnosis of acute rheumatic fever.[29] The streptococcus possesses numerous intracellular toxins that are potent but short-acting antigens. Therefore, systemic invasion by the hemolytic streptococcus should evoke a brisk antibody response to one or another of these toxins. The most widely recognized antibody response is the antistreptolysin O titer which can be measured serially and should demonstrate either a rising titer or a fall from an initial high titer as necessary evidence to incriminate streptococcus-induced systemic disease. However, about 20 per cent of patients with acute rheumatic fever appear to demonstrate a restricted antibody response to the bacterial antigens, and in those patients detection of antideoxyribonuclease B or antihyaluronidase may be the only serologic clue to the recent streptococcal invasion. Fortunately, modern commercial tests incorporate a particle containing all the common streptococcal antigens (Streptozyme test) so that agglutination of this particle by the patient's serum can be depended on to reliably reflect the full range of potential antibody responses in patients with acute rheumatic fever. In addition, it is helpful to realize that patients with acute rheumatic fever polyarthritis nearly always demonstrate a very high antistreptolysin O titer. However, it is important to exclude a false-positive high titer due to the presence of altered lipoprotein molecules, which can be neutralized by dextran sulfate or a polyene antibiotic.[30] More recently, the clinical syndrome of yersiniosis has been better recognized. Infection with *Yersinia enterocolitica* usually produces endemic gastroenteritis with or without a mild septicemia.[31] However, some patients may then develop an acute nonspecific seronegative spondyloarthropathy with clinical features resembling those of acute Reiter's disease or acute rheumatic fever. The demonstration of serum antibodies to *Yersinia enterocolitica* is a very important laboratory sign in the diagnosis of this syndrome, and a negative titer may be essential in diagnosing an atypical attack of acute rheumatic fever in parts of the world where both diseases are endemic. The detection of an antibody response to meningococcus is helpful in recognizing postmeningococcal polyarthritis. This syndrome appears to be characterized by serious meningococcal meningitis followed by an acute "reactive" sterile polyarthritis developing during the convalescent phase. Demonstration of a high antibody titer to the organism in the patient's serum and joint fluid, in the appropriate setting, then suggests the correct diagnosis. Finally, several common viral syndromes may be complicated by a viral arthritis. These include infectious diseases such as rubella, mumps, varicella, hepatitis B, and infectious mononucleosis. Although the underlying viral infection may have been clinically apparent, the initial symptoms are sometimes mild and the arthropathy may be divorced from the prodromal illness by weeks or even months. Under such circumstances, the demonstration of a high and falling specific antiviral antibody titer may provide a comforting prognostic indicator of the inevitable recovery from the distressing arthritis. In the case of hepatitis B arthritis, detection of the circulating viral surface antigen may point to the etiology several weeks before the liver disease becomes overt.[32]

Finally, laboratory determination of plasma protein levels is sometimes best directed at the coagulation cascade. This is notably the case in patients with hemophilia, in whom the frequency and severity of acute hemarthrosis directly correlates with the circulating factor VIII level. Rarely, patients with drug-induced excess anticoagulation activity may develop intra-articular bleeding. Clearly, the estimation of the prothrombin and partial thromboplastin times provides the clinician with an immediate diagnostic laboratory sign.

AUTOANTIBODIES

A great deal of modern rheumatology has derived from the recognition of autoantibodies and their potential pathogenetic and diagnostic roles in patients with certain types of rheumatic disease. Autoantibodies may be regarded as circulating antibodies that appear to possess specificity for various antigens of the host's own body. Since this reaction would seem to be biologically inappropriate (one should not evoke an immune response against one's own tissues), their detection has spurred a great deal of research into the basic immunopathologic mechanisms underlying many forms of chronic rheumatic disease. Some autoantibodies appear to be organ-specific, reacting only with a tissue substrate located in one or several organ systems. Others, however, appear to be non–organ-specific, reacting with antigenic components of the body found in diverse tissues and organs.

One of the most important autoantibodies in the laboratory diagnosis of rheumatic disease is rheumatoid factor.[33] Rheumatoid factor is an antibody that reacts with the Fc portion of immunoglobulin G. It is therefore an antibody directed against an antigenic site on another antibody molecule, hence the synonym "antiglobulin." The antigen is available within the host as the patient's own serum IgG molecules, but rheumatoid factor usually reacts with IgG antigen originating from other individuals and even other species. The mechanism for the induction and continued production of rheumatoid factor is unknown, and its potential pathogenic role in initiating or perpetuating rheumatic disease is similarly conjectural. However, it appears to be one important mechanism for the production of immune complexes in vivo, which might be able to incite immune-mediated inflammatory disease. Most rheumatoid factor that we detect in our clinical laboratory tests consists of IgM agglutinating antibodies, but we should recognize the existence of other populations of antiglobulins, including IgG and IgA molecules. This may be a very important concept, since a patient who has negative conventional test results for rheumatoid factor may still indeed possess important antiglobulins that are undetectable in routine assays. Moreover, IgG antiglobulins appear to be potent components of in vivo immune complex formation. Thus, IgG antibody–IgG antigen complexes may play an important pathogenetic role in some of the extra-articular manifestations of rheumatoid disease, especially the vasculitis of middle-aged men with strongly seropositive arthritis.[34]

Numerous assays have been developed to detect rheumatoid factor, and most of the commercially available test systems are based on the reactivity of serum agglutinating IgM antiglobulins with either human or rabbit IgG antigen (Table 23–2). In most test systems, the antigen is coated onto a carrier particle so that reactivity with the serum antibody

Table 23–2
COMMONLY USED ASSAYS FOR RHEUMATOID FACTOR

Assay*	Sensitivity†	False Positives	Positive in Other Rheumatic Diseases	Positive in Nonrheumatic Disease States	Comments
FII Latex Fixation ≥ 1:320 Latex particles coated with heated human IgG	80%	5%	25%	30%	Easy; no absorption required; very sensitive; relatively nonspecific
FII Bentonite Flocculation 2+ or greater Similar to FII Latex Fixation	Similar to FII Latex Fixation				
Sensitized Sheep Cell Agglutination ≥ 1:28 Sheep red blood cells coated with rabbit gamma globulin	70%	<5%	20%	<5%	Heterophil antibodies must be absorbed or corrected for; relatively specific for rheumatoid arthritis but less sensitive
Rheumaton Sensitized sheep cells stabilized with aldehyde; presence of agglutination considered positive	Similar to Sensitized Sheep Cell Agglutination				Rapid and easy slide test; no dilution or inactivation; can be applied to synovial fluid
Rabbit IgG coated latex particles ≥ 1.4 slide method	80%	<5%	15%	Very low	Sensitive; very specific compared to other sensitive tests
Rabbit IgG coated latex particles ≥ 1:10 Tube dilution method	65%	0%	5%	Very low	Very specific for rheumatoid disease; somewhat less sensitive

*Positive titer or result indicated.
†Per cent positivity in patients with rheumatoid arthritis.

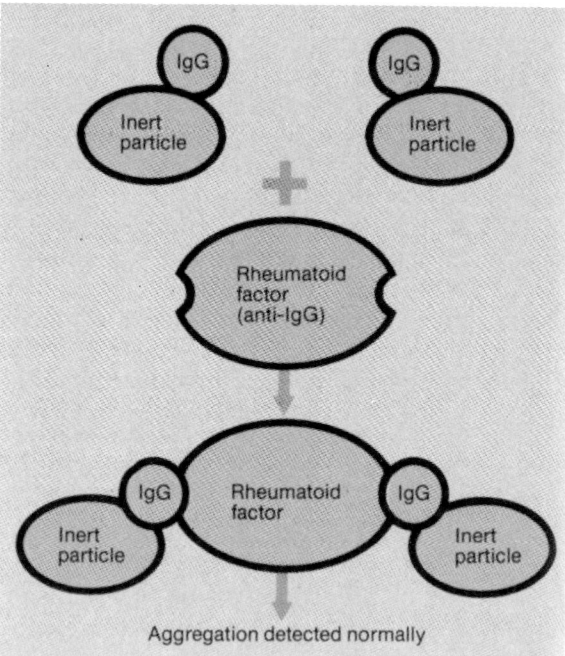

Figure 23–9. *The principle of the various rheumatoid factor tests. The sensitivity and specificity of any particular assay system is governed by the nature of the inert particle and source of the IgG antigen. (From Bluestone, R: Postgrad Med 65:64, 1979.)*

(rheumatoid factor) results in macroscopic agglutination of the particles (Fig. 23–9). By testing the patient's serum at increasing dilutions, the highest dilution still agglutinating the particles can be read as the end-point rheumatoid factor titer. The most commonly utilized assay system uses inert latex or bentonite particles coated with human IgG. The IgG is somewhat denatured during prior preparation, thus rendering it particularly antigenic. This is the basis of the latex or bentonite flocculation or fixation tests and provides a very sensitive indicator of serum antiglobulin levels. In fact, the test is so sensitive that a substantial proportion of normal people have a positive latex fixation test, at least at a low serum dilution (e.g., at less than 1:40 serum dilution). In particular, many elderly normal individuals are latex-positive for rheumatoid factor. Consequently, the vast majority of patients with rheumatoid arthritis would be expected to be positive in this type of antiglobulin assay, but the test is wanting in specificity. A more specific but less sensitive assay for rheumatoid factor is one in which the carrier particle is a sheep red blood cell coated by rabbit IgG that has been induced and harvested as an active nonagglutinating antibody to the red cell envelope. Reactivity of the IgG coating with serum rheumatoid factor will then result in agglutination of the sheep cells, and this forms the basis of the Rose-Waaler or sheep cell agglutination test for rheumatoid factor. Relatively few normal individuals have a positive rheumatoid factor test by this assay, but unfortunately many patients with early or mild rheumatoid arthritis may also show a negative sheep cell agglutination test (i.e., at less than 1:4 serum dilution). However, the demonstration of a high titer positive sheep cell agglutination test for antiglobulins is unusual other than in patients with established rheumatoid arthritis or occasional patients with collagen-vascular disease and universal autoantibody formation. More recently, the sheep cell agglutination test has been modified technically to enhance its sensitivity. The Rheumaton test is a modified sensitized sheep cell agglutination test for detecting antiglobulins.[35] In this assay system, the sheep erythrocytes sensitized with rabbit gamma globulin are mixed with various dilutions of serum on a glass slide. The highest dilution causing cell agglutination is then reported. Titers greater than 1:10 dilution indicate a positive test. This assay is nearly as sensitive as latex agglutination but is reputed to be more specific. As with other sensitized sheep cell tests, heterophil antibodies may give false-positive titers. Numerous other variations of rheumatoid factor tests appear to be feasible and have been developed but are not in widespread use. The precise assay used is less important than the reproducibility of the test system within the individual laboratory and the knowledge of what percentage of normal individuals without rheumatoid arthritis would be expected to show a positive test at a certain defined serum dilution.

The clinical implications of the presence or absence of rheumatoid factor may be important in the diagnosis of articular disease. Certainly most patients with rheumatoid arthritis sooner or later are seropositive. Seronegative rheumatoid arthritis may be suspected as a clinical entity, but this diagnosis invites further categorization into other, hitherto unrecognized rheumatic disease states. The diagnosis of classic rheumatoid arthritis does not demand the presence of rheumatoid factor, but its detection is a reassuring confirmatory laboratory sign for the physician. Moreover, in general, the higher the titer of rheumatoid factor present at the onset of rheumatoid disease, the worse the ultimate prognosis. This fact is apparent in studying large numbers of patients with rheumatoid arthritis but may not, of course, apply to an individual victim of the disease. Nevertheless, the detection of a high titer of rheumatoid factor early in the disease might render the physician somewhat cautious in assessing the overall prognosis for future complications and dysfunction. Among the important prognostic features for rheumatoid arthritis are the numerous extra-articular manifestations of the disease (see Chapter 22). Many of these complications are now recognized to be associated with circulating immune complexes incorporating antiglobulins.[36] Thus, many of the extra-articular manifestations, which may largely govern the ultimate prognosis of rheumatoid arthritis, are more liable to occur in patients who are strongly seropositive. The detection of the antiglobulins therefore becomes very important in diagnosing rheumatoid disease affecting nonarticular organ systems, the more so in those rare patients in whom the articular manifestations are mild or even totally inapparent. Similarly, rheumatoid disease affecting a solitary body cavity—whether it be a joint, pleural, or pericardial lining—may occasionally be manifested by the production of antiglobulins found exclusively in the localized exudate and not necessarily detectable in the circulation. Eventually, however, the patient should become generally seropositive, with abundant rheumatoid factor present in the serum as well as in the synovial, pericardial, or pleural fluid. Another very important application of rheumatoid factor tests is in the diagnosis of the seronegative spondyloarthropathies (i.e., ankylosing spondylitis and its related disorders). In these patients, the very absence of IgM-agglutinating rheumatoid factor is an important laboratory sign supporting a clinical diagnosis.[37] Indeed, the presence of IgM antiglobulins in a patient with a spondyloarthropathy constitutes one of the most difficult diagnostic situations confronting the rheumatologist. The difficulty may be typified by patients with psoriasis and severe destructive peripheral joint arthritis who are seropositive for rheumatoid factor. Investigative data demonstrating nonagglutinating IgG antiglobulins in some patients with spondyloarthropathy are very interesting but have not found their way into practical usage. Thus, for practical purposes, the spondyloarthropathies are still regarded as being classically seronegative, and this feature forms an integral part in defining that class of rheumatic diseases.

Another important serologic marker in the diagnosis of rheumatic disease is referred to as antinuclear antibody (ANA). In fact, this term may be interpreted as meaning a heterogeneous population of serum antibodies, all of which show in vitro reactivity with various components of human cell nuclei and cross reactivity with nucleic acid components from numerous other species. The pathogenetic implications of antinuclear antibody are unclear, and the immunochemical and in vitro reactivity of this autoantibody is under current intensive investigation. The various assays to measure antinuclear antibody probably all detect a heterogeneous population of immunoglobin molecules reactive against more than one type of nucleic acid antigen. However, newer assays are being developed that may well be more specific in terms of the actual antigen-antibody system concerned. This greater specificity may one day permit a more detailed pathogenetic and clinical classification of diseases such as systemic lupus erythematosus and other collagen-vascular disorders based on a combined clinico-laboratory profile.[38]

The oldest and traditional method of detecting antinuclear antibody is the LE cell test.[39] In this assay, serum antinuclear antibody is permitted to react with the nucleic acid antigens contained within nuclei of autologous and slightly damaged white blood cells. The subsequent formation of an immune complex (hematoxyphil body) invites autodigestion by other intact polymorphonuclear cells. With appropriate staining, the intact polymorphonuclear leukocyte containing a characteristic hematoxyphil body can be readily identified as an LE cell (Fig. 23–10). Certain technical factors, however, render this test somewhat undependable. The assay system must contain adequate, healthy neutrophils to phagocytose the immune complexes formed in vitro; yet enough cell fragmentation must be induced to expose nuclear antigens to the serum antinuclear antibody. Moreover, a long period of time must sometimes be spent at the microscope to detect even

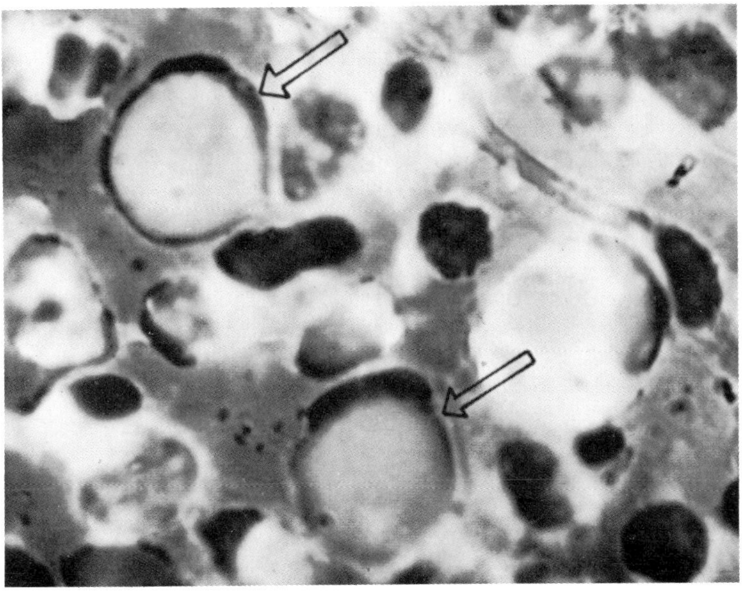

Figure 23–10. *Positive LE cell preparation (1800×). Two typical LE cells are shown (arrows). Using Wright's stain, the cells appear to be almost filled by pale, purple-pink homogeneous masses. The dark intact nuclei are compressed and flattened to the cell margins. (From Bluestone, R: In G Taylor (ed): Immunology in Medical Practice. Philadelphia, WB Saunders Co, 1975.)*

a single LE cell and to distinguish it from fragmented neutrophils, which may superficially resemble cells with ingested complexes (tart cells). In addition, the amount of antinuclear antibody present in the serum must be substantial in order to readily invoke this in vitro phenomenon. Furthermore, if a patient is taking mild to moderate doses of corticosteroid agents, the species of antinuclear antibody responsible for the LE cell phenomenon (mainly antideoxyribonucleoprotein) is readily suppressed, leading to a false-negative result. Thus, although a strongly positive LE cell test result is highly indicative of the presence of antinuclear antibodies, a negative test does not exclude the possibility that the patient has this immune aberration. Nevertheless, the discovery of LE cells within an aspirated pleural or peritoneal exudate has occasionally been of serendipitous diagnostic value.[40]

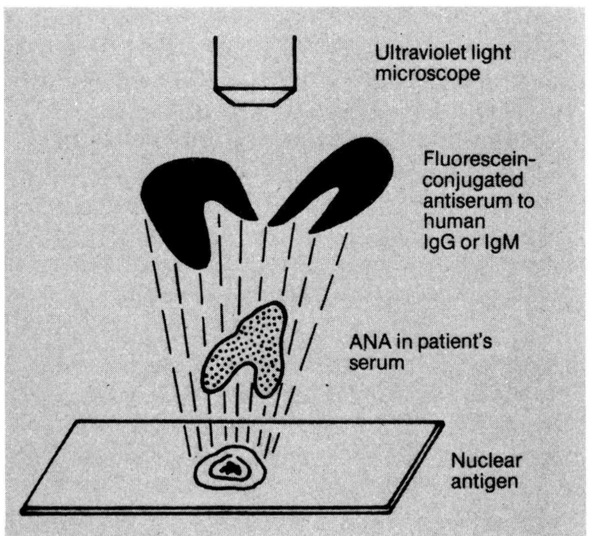

Figure 23–11. The principle of the indirect immunofluorescent test for antinuclear antibody. A negative result from this very sensitive assay would cast serious doubt upon a clinical diagnosis of systemic lupus erythematosus. (From Bluestone, R: Postgrad Med 65:64, 1979.)

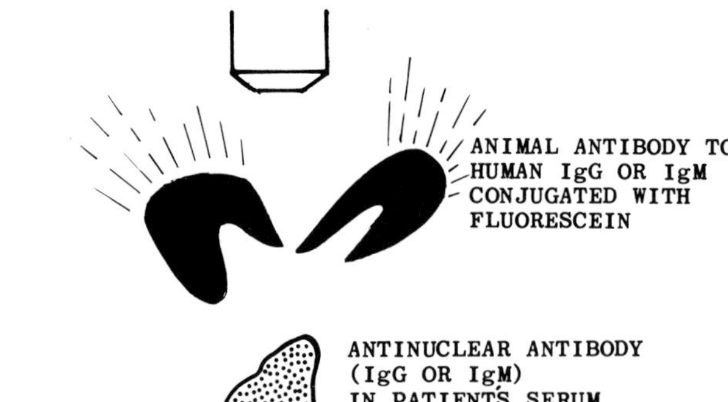

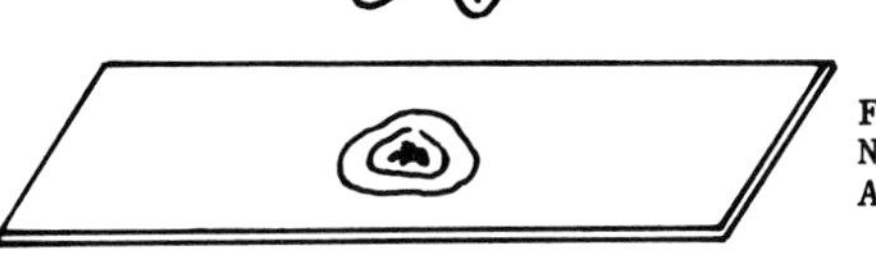

Figure 23–12. Schematic representation of antinuclear antibody detected by indirect immunofluorescence. The source of nuclear antigen may be human polymorphonuclear leukocytes in a blood smear, or cryostat-cut sections of rat or mouse liver, or a fibroblast monolayer. The antibody (IgG or IgM) in the patient's serum fixes to the nuclear antigens. After washing, the fixed antibody is demonstrated by a fluorescein-conjugated antiserum monospecific for human IgG or IgM viewed by ultraviolet microscopy. (From Bluestone R: In G Taylor (Ed): Immunology in Medical Practice. Philadelphia, WB Saunders Co, 1975.)

The more recent universal application of indirect immunofluorescence to detect antinuclear antibody has rendered the LE test somewhat outmoded as a worthwhile laboratory procedure (Fig. 23–11). The immunofluorescent assay usually incorporates a prepared substrate consisting of mammalian cells in which the harvesting and fixation readily facilitate exposure of the nuclear antigens.[41] Suitable antigenic preparations include human buffy coat cells smeared onto glass or monolayers of human or rat fibroblasts usually derived from long-term cultures or organ explants. If a patient's serum contains antinuclear antibody, the antibody will react with the various nuclear antigens for which it has specificity, and this reaction can then be detected by adding a commercial antiserum to human immunoglobulin conjugated with a fluorescein dye. Examination by ultraviolet light microscopy will reveal areas of positive fluoresence directly over the sites where the fluoresceinated antibody has attached to its antigen. If these sites correspond to nuclear substance, the positive fluorescence indicates the presence of antinuclear antibody within the original layer of test serum, which has become fixed to the nuclear antigens (Fig. 23–12). By using conjugated antisera to human IgG and IgM, most human antinuclear antibodies are thereby readily detected. Again, by testing a serum in serial dilutions, the titer of antinuclear antibody can be determined as the greatest dilution of serum giving positive immunofluorescent staining. With the current reliability of mammalian substrates for nuclear antigens and a ready availability of commercial antisera to human immunoglobulins adequately tagged with fluoresceinated dyes, this method has become a very dependable and reproducible laboratory test for antinuclear antibody. It is, however, a very sensitive assay, so that a significant number of normal individuals will yield positive fluorescent test results when their sera are used in an undiluted form. Therefore, clinical laboratories are obliged to predetermine the concentration at which most samples of normal sera fail to give a positive immunofluorescent test result for antinuclear antibody. Only positive titers above that dilution would then be considered significantly abnormal. Even so, false-positive results are not infrequent, but the converse is hardly true. Indeed, it is almost impossible to diagnose a patient as having systemic lupus erythematosus without a positive test for antinuclear antibody using the immunofluorescent method.

A great deal has been written on the specific pattern of immunofluorescence evoked by reacting sera containing antinuclear antibodies from various patients with the antigenic substrates. The immunofluorescent staining thereby obtained may appear in a variety of ways: as a homogeneous pattern, concentrated at the rim of the cell nucleus, speckled throughout the nucleus, or largely restricted to the nucleoli. For a time it was thought that the pattern of immunofluorescence might provide a degree of specificity regarding the form of collagen-vascular disorder from which the patient suffered. However, technical factors of the immunofluorescence procedure can provide far simpler explanations for varied staining patterns.[42] In particular, the actual concentration of serum tested may itself determine the pattern of nuclear fluorescence. Nevertheless, it is thought that antinuclear antibody detected by immunofluorescence revealing a speckled pattern in high titer is rarely found in the serum of healthy individuals and frequently indicates the presence of a collagen-vascular disease such as systemic lupus erythematosus or systemic sclerosis. Homogeneous staining is thought to be due to antibody to deoxyribonucleoprotein and correlates best with the LE cell factor. Nucleolar staining is reputed to be more common in patients with systemic sclerosis and severe Raynaud's phenomena, although this observation has been refuted. Presumably, the various staining patterns obtainable are yet another expression of the heterogeneous species of antinuclear antibodies that exist in various human disease states. Recently it has been found that some patients with a high titer of antinuclear antibody forming a speckled pattern by immunofluorescence tend to also possess antibodies that react with saline-extractable nuclear antigens. One of these antigens has been identified as ribonucleoprotein, and antibodies to ribonucleoprotein can be demonstrated using a red cell hemagglutination technique. Although the high titer antibodies thus demonstrated are not specific for any disease entity, they are invariably found in patients with the so-called mixed connective tissue disease syndrome in which the clinical features resemble a "halfway house" between systemic lupus erythematosus and systemic sclerosis. Contrariwise, antinuclear antibody with specificity for ribonuclease-resistant extractable nuclear antigen appears to be highly specific for patients with systemic lupus erythematosus. Clearly, new assays detecting different species of antinuclear antibodies will continue to evolve and might lead to further subcategorization of the various collagen-vascular diseases.

Another promising advance in the laboratory techniques available for aiding the recognition of rheumatic disease is the DNA binding assay.[43] The object of this assay is to detect the amount of serum material that is capable of binding radioactive DNA added in vitro (Fig. 23–13). By implication, this binding material corresponds to serum antibody to DNA and should include at least some of those same antibodies that show reactivity within the other tests mentioned previously. In addition, however, in vitro DNA binding probably reflects the presence of unique forms of antinuclear antibodies that might otherwise not be detected. It is now apparent that if extremely pure preparations of labeled mammalian DNA are available (e.g., double-stranded or undenatured DNA), a raised index of DNA binding is a valuable laboratory sign for the presence of pathogenic antinuclear antibodies. Indeed, under these circumstances it has been postulated that a raised DNA binding index is almost specific for systemic lupus erythematosus and is not found in other diseases characterized by a positive antinuclear antibody test result utilizing immunofluorescence. Of even more importance is the reputed normality of the DNA binding index in patients with drug-induced lupus syndromes when compared with patients who have the spontaneous form of the disease. Unfortunately, however, even a modest degree of DNA denaturation immediately reduces the specificity of DNA binding as a laboratory sign of systemic lupus erythematosus. Consequently, considerable interest is being shown in the kinetoplast of *Crithidia luciliae*, which may provide an ideal double-stranded DNA substrate for the detection of specific antideoxyribonucleic acid antibodies of systemic lupus erythematosus by indirect immunofluoresence.[44]

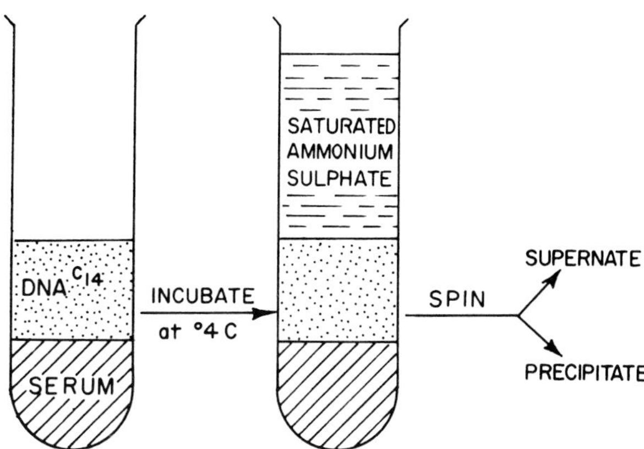

Figure 23–13. *Method for measuring DNA-binding activity. A radioactive form of native DNA is added to the test serum. Any DNA-antiDNA complexes are then precipitated with ammonium sulfate. The percentage binding activity of the serum is expressed as*

$$\frac{\textit{radioactive counts per minute (cpm) of precipitate}}{\textit{cpm of supernate + cpm of precipitate}} \times 100$$

(From Bluestone R: In G Taylor (Ed): Immunology in Medical Practice. Philadelphia, WB Saunders Co, 1975.)

The sensitive tests available for detecting antinuclear antibodies by immunofluorescence and by DNA binding also provide a useful index for following a patient's progress on treatment. Having diagnosed systemic lupus erythematosus with the aid of these laboratory tests, the physician can expect a prompt reduction in the ANA titer and DNA binding index following appropriate corticosteriod therapy. Indeed, it has been claimed that the results of these assays, together with the estimation of the serum complement concentrations (discussed later in this chapter), provide the clinician with a reliable prognostic indicator of imminent clinical relapse.[45] Thus, the clinical progress of most patients with systemic lupus is best reflected by their symptoms and signs or absence of them; but even in an apparently stable patient, a sudden rise in the ANA titer, an increase in the DNA binding index, and a decrease in the serum complement concentration may well portend that a stormy course is about to ensue.

Finally, it should be stressed that many patients with a wide variety of nonrheumatic autoimmune or chronic infectious diseases may display positive serologic test results for both antiglobulins and antinuclear antibodies. Furthermore, there is a recognized incidence of low-titer positive ANA test results in apparently normal individuals. Just as with the tests for antiglobulins, this innocent positivity is especially seen in a small proportion of elderly subjects. Many patients with other forms of autoimmune diseases, such as chronic active hepatitis, primary biliary cirrhosis, and autoimmune thyroiditis, may reveal strongly positive test results for antinuclear antibody. Thus, a positive result for an antinuclear antibody test is not specific for systemic lupus erythematosus but is virtually essential for the diagnosis of this rheumatic disease.

There are several other organ-specific autoantibodies of potential value in the diagnosis or exclusion of certain rheumatic disease states. About 50 per cent of patients with primary sicca syndrome (keratoconjunctivitis sicca), and probably a greater percentage of patients with the full Sjögren's syndrome (keratoconjunctivitis sicca plus rheumatoid arthritis or some other form of collagen-vascular disease), display a positive test for antibody to salivary duct epithelium.[46] This is usually detected by indirect immunofluorescence using human pancreatic duct as substrate and demonstrating that the patient's serum contains IgG or IgM antibodies able to react with the ductal antigens. Similarly, by using rat or rabbit uterine muscle as substrate, human antibodies to smooth muscle can be detected in a large variety of diseases, but most notably in patients with chronic active hepatitis.[47] Patients with this autoimmune liver disease may present with the peripheral manifestations of circulating immune complexes, including inflammatory polyarthritis. Although the underlying liver disease may be obvious, this is not always the case. The detection of smooth muscle antibodies in high titer may then be helpful in directing the clinician to the primary hepatic disorder. More recently, the relative lack of specificity of anti–smooth muscle antibodies has been emphasized. They have been found in patients with various postinfectious, neoplastic, and viral states, as well as in a significant number of patients with Reiter's disease.[48] The vast majority of patients with primary biliary cirrhosis possesses antimitochondrial antibodies.[49] These can be demonstrated by indirect immunofluorescence using sections of rat or rabbit renal tubules as substrate, to which the tubular cell mitochondria may be shown to be reactive with the patients' serum antibodies. Not infrequently, middle-aged women with primary biliary cirrhosis may display only latent liver disease and present to the physician with fatigue, malaise, arthralgias, and arthritis. The subsequent detection of a significantly elevated serum IgM concentration, and increased serum alkaline phosphatase concentration, and high titer of antimitochondrial antibodies then provides a valuable composite laboratory profile pointing to the autoimmune hepatic disease mimicking a primary rheumatic disorder.

Among the array of autoantibodies produced by patients with systemic lupus erythematosus are reaginic molecules able to react with cell membrane lipid. This explains the fact that some patients with the disease develop a positive Venereal Disease Research Laboratory (VDRL) test as an early laboratory sign (the VDRL test incorporates cardiolipin as a substrate).[50] Indeed, a significant number of biologic false-positive reactions to one or more of the standard laboratory tests for syphilis occur in patients with "preclinical" systemic lupus erythematosus.[51] Similar antibodies are probably responsible for the circulating anticoagulants demonstrated in a small proportion of patients with systemic lupus erythematosus.[52] In this situation the lipid-bearing prothrombin activator complex is inhibited by the patient's autoantibody. Even the usually reliable fluorescent treponemal antibody absorption (FTA-ABS) test for syphilis may yield a false-positive result in patients with collagen-vascular disease and high antinuclear antibody titers. The Reiter's treponeme used for the test system may permit antinuclear antibody to cross its damaged membrane, leading to a false-positive beaded pattern of fluorescence.[53] A similar mechanism probably accounts for the false-positive *Treponema pallidum* immobilization (TPI) test results that have been recorded in a few children with systemic lupus erythematosus. Similarly, the FTA-ABS test for *Toxoplasma gondii* may falsely be read as strongly positive in the presence of serum antinuclear antibody.[54] Finally, the production of autoantibodies to the red blood cell membrane is a common feature of systemic lupus erythematosus and can be recognized as a positive Coombs' test result (direct or indirect) demonstrating IgG or complement on the red blood cells. If the process is active enough, a hemolytic anemia ensues, with its characteristic hemogram including a significant reticulocytosis.

DETECTION OF IMMUNE COMPLEXES

Many pathogenetic mechanisms appear to be operative in the induction and perpetuation of the rheumatic diseases. One potential mechanism appears to be that of circulating immune complexes of a critical molecular size, which are able to lodge in or near the basement membrane of various capillaries and therein induce an inflammatory response resulting in damage to autologous tissue.[55] This is thought to be an important pathogenetic mechanism operative in many of the clinical manifestations of systemic lupus erythematosus, in the intra-articular inflammation of rheumatoid arthritis, and in a large variety of transient nondeforming arthropathies that seem to wax and wane in concert with an underlying systemic disease (see Chapter 22). Clearly, the clinician would be better able to diagnose and follow such events if circulating immune complexes in the patient's serum could be measured directly. Unfortunately, however, the clinical concepts are considerably further advanced than the harsher scientific realities. There are various methods in vogue for detecting immune complexes in vitro but no universally available and thoroughly dependable single assay exists (Table 23–3). The various assays developed may all be dependable in the hands of a few, and probably all truly detect immune complexes, although they obviously overlap in their sensitivities and specificities for the actual species of complexes measured. However, it seems quite likely that in the coming few years several dependable assays will be developed to permit the detection of immune complexes and will become widely available. One likely candidate for such an assay is the radioactive C1q binding test, which exploits the fact that immune complexes bind with this early complement component, and this binding can be quantitated if the C1q is adequately purified and appropriately radiolabeled (Fig. 23–14). Unfortunately, C1q is also highly

Table 23–3
THE VARIOUS ASSAYS USED TO DETECT CIRCULATING IMMUNE COMPLEXES*

Assay	Principle	Disadvantages and Possible Interfering Substances	Advantages	Sensitivity†
Raji Cell	B lymphoblastoid cells bind immune complexes (IC) through their complement receptors	Requires continuous cell cultivation. Only detects complexes that bind complement	Quantitative and reproducible; frozen sera can be used. Good for complexes formed near Ag-Ab equivalence	Varies with size of complex >35S: 6 11S–19S: 50
C1q				
Polyethylene Glycol (PEG)	IC have different precipitating properties from Ig in low concentrations of PEG	Detects only complexes that activate classical complement pathway	Better than Raji cell for IC with Ag excess	10
Deviation	C1q binding to Ig may be displaced by test sera	Polyanionic substances including DNA and endotoxin bind C1q	Ready availability of radiolabeled C1q	4
Rheumatoid Factor (RF) (Fc)				
Monoclonal	RF has high affinity for aggregated or complexed IgG	RF will interact with IC via recognition of Fc portion of Ig	Detects IgG-containing complexes	0.5–15
Polyclonal	Monoclonal RF is more efficient than polyclonal			1–10
Platelet Aggregation	IC cause platelets to aggregate	False positives with aggregated IgG, Ab to platelets and RF		4
Macrophage Uptake	IC inhibit macrophage function	RF and other factors		20–30

*Derived from McCluskey RT et al: Hum Pathol 9:71, 1978.
†Expressed as μg/ml of aggregated IgG detected.

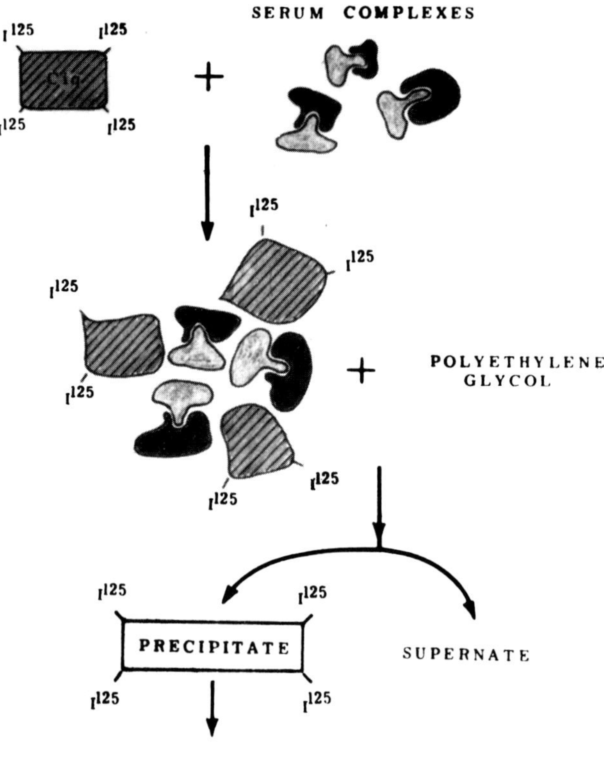

Figure 23–14. Schematic representation of the C1q binding assay for circulating serum immune complexes. The test system is based on the in vitro reactivity of radiolabeled C1q with preformed complexes. Polyethylene glycol precipitates complexes of a certain size, and the degree of radioactivity in the precipitate is an indirect measure of the preformed complexes.

reactive with endotoxin and other bacterial cell wall products, and this causes loss of specificity. Nevertheless, a great deal of attention has been directed to this field as more and more human diseases related to circulating immune complexes are being postulated and recognized.

The clinical laboratory is able to offer some indirect assays of immune complex–mediated disease, and these have particular application in the diagnosis and assessment of certain rheumatic disease states. One such approach is the measurement of the serum complement concentration. Conceivably, once excess circulating immune complexes become fixed in the tissues they are able to consume complement as part of the evoked phlogistic process. If the production of serum complement by the liver is not dramatically increased, the complement fixation may be reflected by depletion of serum levels. It is now very easy to measure serum complement either as the total hemolytic complement or as its predominant single plasma constituent, C3. Provided that the biologic specimen has been appropriately handled (not allowed to stand at room temperature for more than 30 or 40 minutes), the assay systems are quite reproducible. A marked reduction in total hemolytic complement or the third component of complement or both, may then be interpreted as indirect evidence of in vivo immune complex formation and tissue fixation of complement. In addition, one may also measure the complement concentrations in pleural, pericardial, and synovial fluid for evidence of a similar mechanism operative at these local sites. Interestingly, in certain diseases, such as rheumatoid arthritis, there is a selective depletion of complement within the joint space compared to the serum level, so that aspirated synovial fluid and concomitantly withdrawn blood can be assayed simultaneously for complement, permitting direct comparison with a correction factor applied for total protein content. It is important to remember, however, that a normal serum complement concentration does not exclude the possibility of immune complex disease. If a patient's liver is able to match the increased catabolic rate of the plasma protein by an increased synthesis, the serum concentration may be maintained at normal levels.[56] Under these circumstances, the best evidence of the increased complement consumption might be the detection of complement degradation products within the serum. Unfortunately, the techniques for this sort of assay are at present restricted to a few specialized laboratories.

In the clinical management of patients with systemic lupus erythematosus, a normal DNA binding index and C3 concentration would in general predict a quiescent disease course. Anti-deoxyribonucleic acid activity or decreased serum C3 concentrations or both, may be predictive of an impending clinical exacerbation, but the variation in time until this exacerbation occurs is of such magnitude that it makes abnormal test results of little clinical usefulness. In general, a patient with a high DNA binding index or a low serum C3 concentration would be followed more closely, but no therapeutic modulation would necessarily result. Clearly, as with any serologic test, the tremendous day-to-day variability of the assay system must be taken into account before interpreting the results.

Another important reason for serum complement estimations lies in the fact that hereditary deficiencies of the various complement components have now been recognized.[57] For reasons that are unclear, patients with some types of complement component deficiency are more prone than normal persons to develop certain rheumatic diseases, including systemic lupus erythematosus and probably juvenile rheumatoid arthritis. Most complement deficiencies can be detected by screening for total hemolytic complement and C3 concentrations, and if either of the assays reveals complete absence, more specialized studies to detect the precise complement deficiency can be initiated.

A useful but somewhat crude in vitro indicator of circulating immune complexes is the demonstration of serum cryoglobulins. Cryoglobulins are gamma globulins that become insoluble and precipitate at cold temperatures. This appears to be a peculiar biophysical property of some plasma immunoglobulins, especially when they are present in excess amount. It is a particularly common phenomenon in patients with paraproteinemia, in which a certain percentage of the monoclonal plasma protein appears to be cryoprecipitable. However, in some rheumatic diseases (notably in the blood of patients with systemic lupus erythematosus or essential cryoglobulinemia and in the synovial fluid of patients with rheumatoid arthritis) a cryoprecipitate may be detected and shown to consist of the antigenic and antibody components of an immune complex.[58] Detection and measurement of the plasma cryoglobulin therefore imply the presence of similar but soluble complexes circulating in the serum and perhaps related to the clinical expression of the patient's disease. In the rare disease termed essential cryoglobulinemia the cryoglobulins appear to accurately reflect the in vivo state, since clinical relapse and remission can be closely monitored by the absolute cryocrit value measured in such patients. Therefore, therapeutic efforts to control this disease can be guided by regular quantitation of the cryoglobulin concentrations. This is optimally performed by taking the patient's blood with a warm syringe, separating and centrifuging the plasma at warm temperatures, and then placing the cell-free plasma in an ice slurry for at least 48 hours. The resulting precipitate can be expressed as a volumetric percentage of the plasma sample (cryocrit).

Another way to detect immune complexes is by the direct immunohistologic demonstration of their presence in biopsied tissue. Thus, if a piece of human tissue contains immune complexes, it should be possible to demonstrate their presence by treating the tissue with specific antisera against human IgG or complement conjugated with a fluorescein label. This method of direct immunofluorescence on carefully prepared biopsied material has proved of great value in the diagnosis of lupus nephritis.[59] In this disease, the lumpy-bumpy deposition of IgG and complement along the renal glomerular basement membranes is of considerable diagnostic help and can often be correlated with the electron microscopic appearance of subepithelial and subendothelial electron-dense deposits (Fig. 23–15). This sort of diagnostic approach has revealed a whole series of renal diseases related to antibody- or immune complex–induced glomerular and tubular damage. A similar technique has been applied to various dermatologic diseases, including the cutaneous lesions of some rheumatic syndromes. Thus, immune deposits can be demonstrated at the dermoepidermal junction of most patients with discoid lupus erythematosus within the clinically involved skin.[60] In most patients with active systemic lupus erythematosus these deposits are also demonstrable, not only within the obvious lesions but frequently also in clinically uninvolved skin. Indeed, the demonstration of dermoepidermal junction immune deposits in the skin of patients known to suffer from systemic lupus erythematosus is thought to correlate quite well with a similar process taking place in the kidneys and has been suggested as one way of following the prognosis and response to therapy of patients with lupus nephritis.

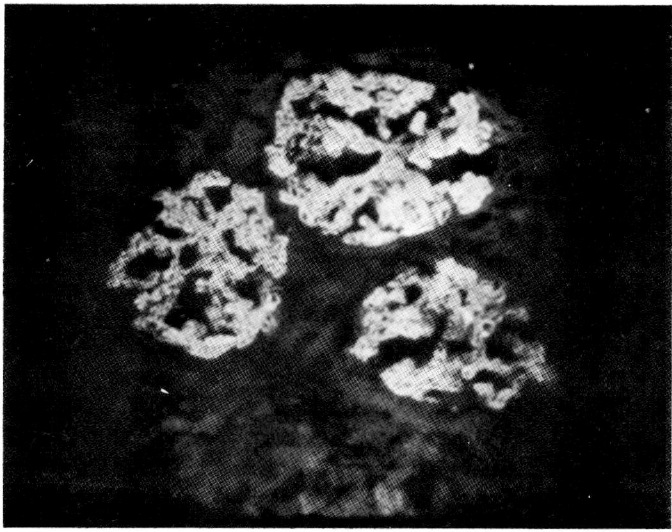

A

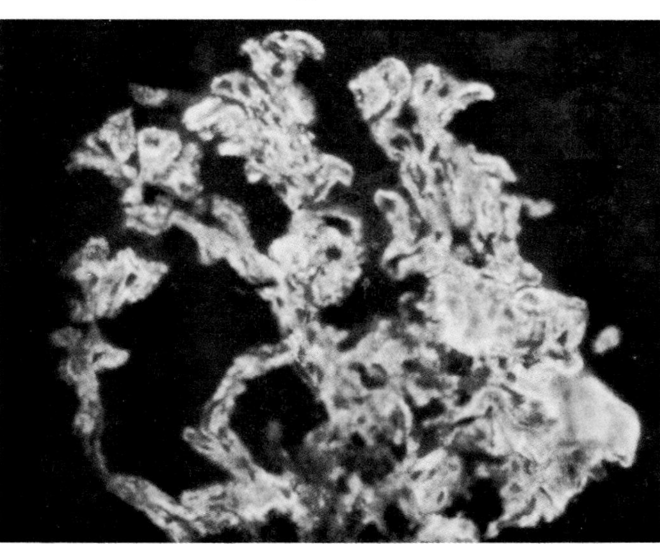

B

Figure 23–15. *Renal biopsy specimen from a patient with systemic lupus erythematosus (SLE), stained with fluorescein-conjugated antiserum to human C3 (125×)* **(A)**, *and human IgG (500×)* **(B)**. *Note the widespread and irregular deposition of complement within all the glomeruli and the "lumpy-bumpy" appearance of IgG deposition on the glomerular basement membrane. (From Bluestone R: In G Taylor [Ed]: Immunology in Medical Practice. Philadelphia, WB Saunders Co, 1975.)*

CELLULAR STUDIES

Recent years have seen an enormous increase in the recognition that cellular immune mechanisms are operative in the pathogenesis of many forms of rheumatic disease. Most of these studies have emerged from investigational laboratories and have provided overwhelming evidence that cellular immune mechanisms are indeed crucial in the initiation or perpetuation of diseases such as systemic lupus erythematosus, rheumatoid arthritis, and related syndromes.[61] In contrast to the hard experimental evidence is the notable lack of clinical laboratory tests available to the practicing physician for assessing and following the cellular immune status of patients with these diseases. Most in vitro tests of cellular immune function are simply too demanding for widespread clinical application. Despite a decade of startling advances in cellular immunology, the only readily available assay by which we can measure cellular immune function involves detection of delayed hypersensitivity to various skin test antigens. However, this crude assay, if properly performed, appears to be a reasonable way to assess grossly the integrity of the cellular immune system. The development of anergy, as shown by uniformly negative skin test results to common and universal antigens, is sometimes demonstrable in patients with systemic lupus erythematosus and may be seen in any patient undergoing long-term, high-dose corticosteroid or immunosuppressive therapy. Some laboratories are able to crudely assess overall lymphocyte function by measuring DNA synthesis following thymidine incorporation by lymphocytes stimulated with nonspecific mitogens. However, the interpretation of this assay is very difficult and may only serve to indicate selective anergy within certain subpopulations of immunocytes.

A new assay requiring the in vitro testing of viable white blood cells for detecting HLA antigens (tissue typing) is now broadly applied to the practice of clinical rheumatology.[62] This has arisen following the observation that the vast majority of Caucasian patients with ankylosing spondylitis and Reiter's disease possess the B locus gene HLA B27 on chromosome number 6. Thus, tissue typing of such patients should usually reveal positive test results for HLA B27 antigen. About 6 to 8 per cent of normal Caucasians are positive for this gene/antigen compared to 90 per cent positivity in Caucasians with ankylosing spondylitis or Reiter's disease. This association holds even when the rheumatic disease develops in childhood or is associated with chronic inflammatory bowel disease, especially ulcerative colitis. About 4 per cent of normal Afro-Americans are positive for the antigen, and in this population 50 per cent of patients with ankylosing spondylitis or Reiter's disease are HLA B27-positive. A similarly dramatic association between this genetically controlled cell surface antigen and rheumatic disease is seen in patients with certain forms of "reactive" sterile arthritis seen following infection with *Yersinia enterocolitica* or Salmonella. Finally, about 30 per cent of Caucasians with psoriatic spondylitis are positive for the antigen, so that in this disease the association is less valuable as a diagnostic laboratory sign. Clearly, the diagnosis of seronegative spondyloarthropathy in most patients is largely based upon a combined clinical and radiographic profile. However, in certain atypical patients or in the "forme fruste" syndromes, the detection of HLA B27 combined with negative test results for serum rheumatoid factor provides a valuable laboratory clue. Examples of this have been seen in the wider recognition of Reiter's disease in children and women; the differentiation of incomplete Reiter's disease from culture-negative gonococcal arthritis; the exclusion of ankylosing spondylitis in HLA B27-negative individuals with a strong family history of that disease; and the tentative diagnosis of ankylosing spondylitis in patients with typical symptoms of the disease during their preradiographic and even prescintigraphic phases.

Initially, the test for detecting HLA B27 was restricted to those few laboratories with expertise in the tissue-typing technique. However, with the wider availability of the appropriate antiserum and recognition of the potential application of this assay, the test has become more widely utilized. Nevertheless, the test still requires delivery of the patient's anticoagulated blood within 36 to 48 hours after venipuncture, since the assay system utilizes viable leukocytes (Fig. 23–16). More recently it has been recognized that some individuals with a well-defined seronegative spondyloarthropathy of the ankylosing spondylitis or Reiter's type may be negative for HLA B27 but positive for other B series antigens that are serologically cross reactive with B27. That is to say, some antisera reactive with HLA B27 may also react with HLA B7, BW22, and BW42. Clearly, detection of these B series antigens in certain select clinical situations may be of diagnostic value but requires considerable technical expertise.

BIOCHEMICAL STUDIES

There are very few biochemical tests with relative or absolute specificity for any of the rheumatic diseases. However, since many arthropathies are associated with a general systemic disorder, they may be reflected in the patient's biochemical indices.

Serum urate concentrations are of direct relevance in the recognition of the hyperuricemic state underlying recurrent gouty attacks and for monitoring the efficacy of hypouricemic therapy (discussed previously). It is important to remember that most

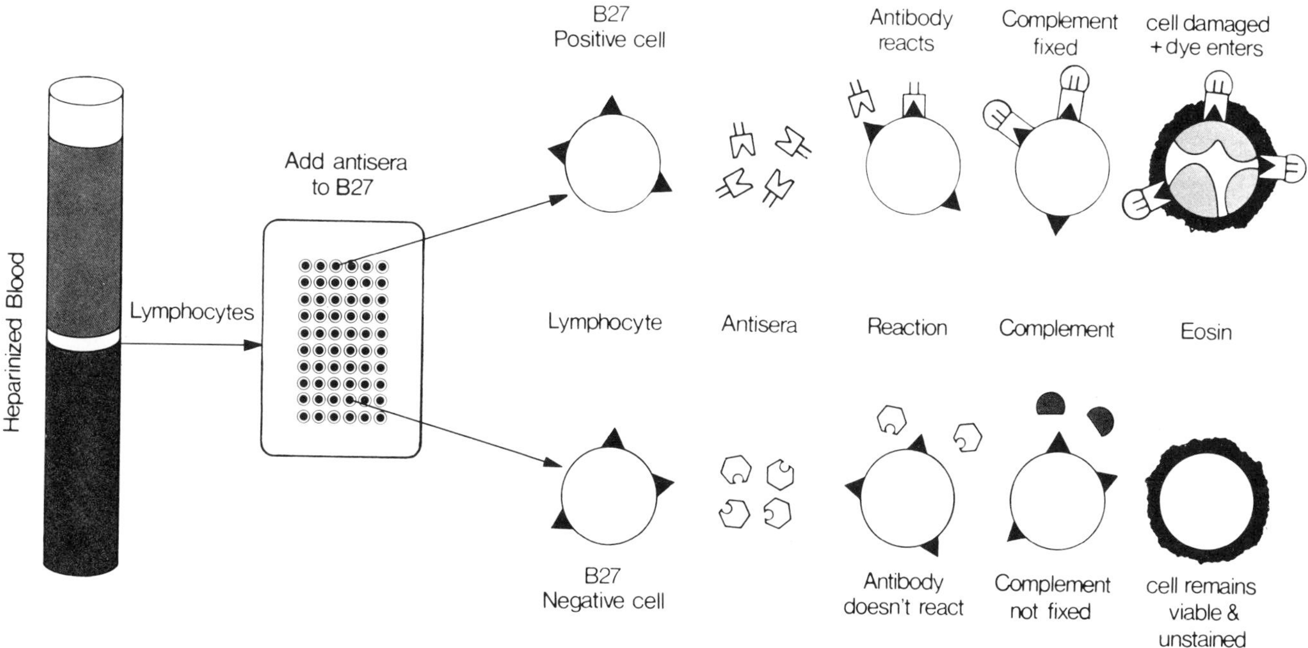

Figure 23–16. *HLA tissue typing. The blood is separated so as to harvest the buffy coat layer of leukocytes, which usually separates at the top of the interface between the sedimented red cells and the clear serum above. The leukocytes are then put into the test system to see whether they react with a panel of various antisera, which recognize the known histocompatibility antigens. The B27 positive cell reacts, whereas the B27 negative cell does not. (From Bluestone R, Pearson C: In HLA-B27: A New Diagnostic Tool for Ankylosing Spondylitis. Reproduced by special permission of copyright owner Merck &Co, Inc, Copyright 1977.)*

serum urate concentrations are measured by autoanalyzer, so that false-positive high values may be readily obtained, owing to the presence of serum chromogens other than uric acid. Thus, slightly elevated concentrations are frequently detected in normal individuals so that true hyperuricemia need not be considered unless the value is in excees of 9 mg per dl. There is no known harm resulting from sustained asymptomatic hyperuricemia, although tentative epidemiologic data suggest that the higher the serum urate concentration, the greater the future risk of developing gouty arthritis and renal stones. Nevertheless, the decision whether or not to treat asymptomatic hyperuricemia remains a thorny one, lacking reliable guidelines.

It should also be remembered that about one third of gouty subjects reveal a serum lipid profile of Type IV hyperlipoproteinemia characterized by a raised serum triglyceride concentration[63] (Fig. 23–17). Moreover, patients with essential Type IV hyperlipoproteinemia may frequently develop secondary hyperuricemia, sometimes complicated by gout. Thus, in some clinical circumstances it is almost impossible to distinguish between primary gout and associated hypertriglyceridemia versus the situation of essential type IV hyperlipoproteinemia complicated by hyperuricemia and gout.[64] In both instances the patient may demonstrate markedly elevated serum triglyceride concentrations, normal cholesterol levels, marked hyperuricemia, and gouty tophi with recurrent arthritis, and have a strong family history. In both circumstances the hyperlipoproteinemia appears to be responsive to carbohydrate restriction with or without lipid-lowering agents. What is not clear, however, is whether treating hyperuricemia necessarily benefits the hyperlipemic state. Complicating matters is the fact that some patients with Type IV hyperlipoproteinemia also demonstrate a nonspecific recurrent arthropathy, which has not been adequately characterized but appears to present as febrile low-grade recurrent arthritis or tenosynovitis with disproportionately severe arthralgias. In addition, patients with familial homozygous Type II hyperlipoproteinemia characterized by severe hypercholesterolemia may also develop a series of rheumatic complaints. These include the development of widespread tendinous xanthomas, which may present as periarticular and intratendinous nodules; the rare development of xanthomas replacing articular surfaces of joints and leading to their destruction; a flitting nonspecific and low-grade recurrent synovitis of unknown etiology originally described by Khachadurian and clinically mimicking an attack of acute rheumatic fever;[65] and finally, a problem of iatrogenic secondary hyperuricemia with or without gout if treatment is begun with nicotinic acid. In summary,

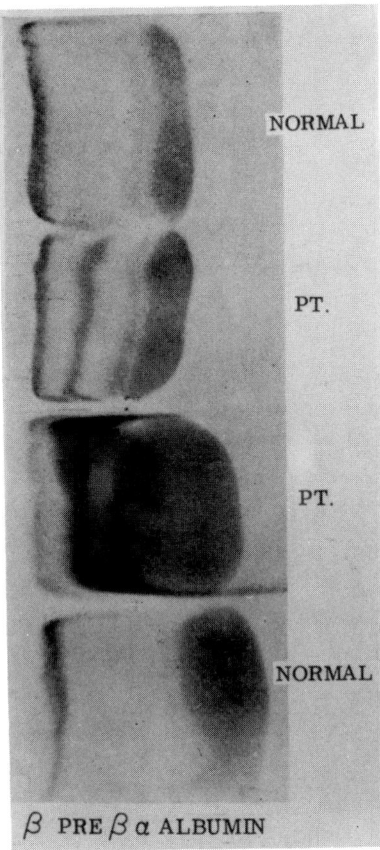

Figure 23–17. *Lipoprotein electrophoresis on cellulose acetate (oil red O stain) of fasting serum from two normal subjects and two patients, each of whom suffered from gout. Note that one patient (upper) displays moderately increased pre-β and the other (lower) patient displays a gross increase in this lipoprotein. Both patients were hypertriglyceridemic. (From Bluestone R, et al: Ann Rheum Dis 30:134, 1971.)*

several forms of hyperlipoproteinemia are associated with a variety of symptoms and signs manifesting in the musculoskeletal system.

Liver function tests can be helpful in the diagnosis and monitoring of several rheumatic diseases. In the first place, several primary autoimmune liver diseases, such as chronic active hepatitis and primary biliary cirrhosis, may be complicated by arthralgias and arthritis. Second, occasionally patients with collagen-vascular disease may exhibit direct involvement of the hepatic vasculature or parenchyma manifested as perturbed liver function tests. More important, however, is the now well-recognized and not infrequent problem of aspirin hepatotoxicity, most evident in young women or children given full therapeutic doses of the drug.[66] This is usually manifested as an asymptomatic rise in serum liver enzyme concentrations but may be associated with systemic symptoms and preclude further treatment with the drug.

Tests of renal function have great significance in patients suffering from those rheumatic diseases that may affect the kidneys. This is particularly seen in patients with systemic lupus erythematosus, in which the renal glomerulus is a primary target tissue of the disease process. It is also seen in any chronic rheumatic disease when that disease becomes complicated by systemic amyloidosis. Thus, serum creatinine concentration and creatinine clearance studies all help to characterize this complication. In addition, some iatrogenic problems in rheumatology focus on the kidneys. Gold toxicity is a rare but well-recognized complication of chrysotherapy, and more recently the widespread use of penicillamine has provoked a significant increase in penicillamine-induced nephropathy.[67, 68] Chronic phenacetin abuse, usually in the form of proprietary compound analgesic and anti-inflammatory drug combinations, is a well-known cause of renal papillary necrosis, which may progress so severely as to present with end-stage renal failure. In all of these clinical circumstances, the essential role of urinalysis cannot be overstressed. An examination of freshly voided urine for protein, sugar, and an abnormal sediment is often the only way of detecting the early renal lesion of systemic lupus erythematosus or drug-induced nephropathy. Finally, the revelation of excess urinary homogentisic acid reactive with NaOH is pathognomonic of alkaptonuria (ochronosis).

Although many drugs are used in the management of patients with rheumatic disease, few of them can be measured in the serum. The notable exception to this is with aspirin therapy, in which the serum salicylate concentration can be assayed accurately and inexpensively. This has facilitated a much more scientific and effective approach to the use of salicylate therapy, and it is now recognized that the optimal therapeutic blood concentration is between 20 and 30 mg per dl, which in most individuals should also be uricosuric.[69] Hence, most patients with a therapeutic blood level of salicylate should also demonstrate relative hypouricemia (i.e., serum urate concentration of less than 2 mg per dl) (Fig. 23–18). Serum salicylate concentrations have become a very important aspect of monitoring rheumatic disease treatment, especially when the therapeutic measures appear to be unmatched by an appropriate clinical response.

It is almost impossible to diagnose inflammatory myositis with certainty in the absence of elevated concentrations of serum muscle enzymes.[70] The most sensitive and best indicators of inflammatory muscle disease are the serum creatinine phosphokinase and aldolase concentrations, in that order. The other muscle enzymes present in serum are also released from the liver and are much less specific for muscle damage. It seems that a raised concentration of serum creatine phosphokinase is a reliable indicator of continuing muscle inflammation, destruction, and release of intrafibrillar enzymes. Therefore, when treating patients with inflammatory muscle disease, the physician has at hand a rather precise guide to the adequacy of steroid therapy. Further-

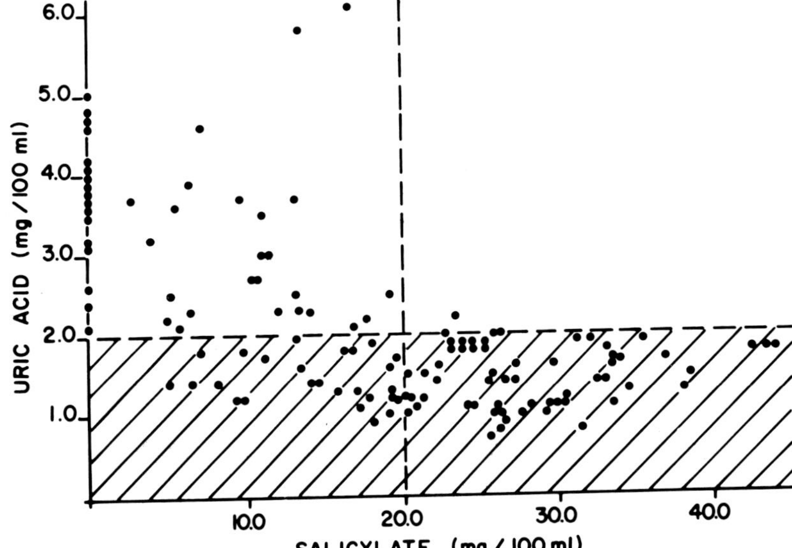

Figure 23–18. The relationship between serum urate and salicylate concentration. As serum salicylate concentrations increased, serum urate values decreased. Thus, at a serum salicylate concentration of 20 mg/ml or greater, the associated serum urate concentration was nearly always less than 2 mg. per dl. (From Emori W, et al: Arthritis Rheum 17:1058, 1974.)

more, it is important to realize that changes in the serum enzyme concentration may precede clinical response or relapse by many weeks.

Several rheumatic diseases indirectly affect subchondral bone. More importantly, several forms of metabolic bone disease may closely mimic an arthropathy in their clinical presentation. Therefore, some of the biochemical tests that serve as a broad indicator of bone metabolism are useful in the laboratory diagnosis of rheumatic diseases. In particular, measurement of the serum phosphorus, calcium, and alkaline phosphatase concentrations may well be useful in this regard. Many children with inflammatory polyarthritis display a moderately elevated serum alkaline phosphatase concentration, and a large percentage of adult patients with ankylosing spondylitis appear to have enough focal osteitis to provoke similar elevations. In patients with widespread chondrocalcinosis it is important to exclude hyperparathyroidism. Contrariwise, it is important to realize that patients with this form of hormone excess may manifest several different forms of rheumatic disease. Finally, the localization of symptoms as true bone pain may well be matched by biochemical evidence of osteomalacia or Paget's disease.

There are several well-known forms of endocrine arthropathy.[71] These include the peculiar degenerative joint disease of acromegaly; the unusual low-grade inflammatory polyarthritis of myxedema; the various forms of bone and joint disease of hyperparathyroidism, including a peculiar type of osteogenic synovitis; and the various periarticular soft tissue syndromes and neuropathic joints seen in patients with diabetes mellitus. Clearly, in all of these instances the rheumatic disease should follow the more obvious manifestations of the underlying endocrinopathy. However, this may not always be the case, so that the patient may present to the physician with dominant osteoarticular symptoms as the first indicator of the endocrine disease. In all these situations it is important for the clinician to be able to obtain the appropriate tests of endocrine function that will lead to a disclosure of the underlying systemic disease.

TISSUE STUDIES (BIOPSIES)

There are relatively few specific histopathologic features that indicate a single rheumatic disease. Some of the more helpful immunohistopathologic findings have been mentioned earlier in this chapter. There are, in addition, some useful biopsy procedures that may be indicated in certain patients presenting with symptoms and signs in their osteoarticular system. The most useful and relatively most specific of these will be detailed here. Indications for tissue biopsy, however, usually follow a careful clinical and laboratory evaluation, following which the detection of a discrete tissue lesion may make the diagnosis obvious, so that there is no longer an indication for biopsy. Nevertheless, it is difficult to be certain of dermatomyositis or polymyositis without seeing histologically abnormal muscle. Since the treatment of this disease frequently includes the use of very potent therapeutic agents, it is very comforting to the physician to be absolutely certain of the pathologic process before initiating a therapeutic strategy.

Rheumatoid nodules usually develop in patients with obvious and overt rheumatoid arthritis (Fig. 23–19). It is therefore important to recognize their existence, but excision is rarely necessary and frequently undesirable because there may be impaired skin healing over the excised nodule, and the

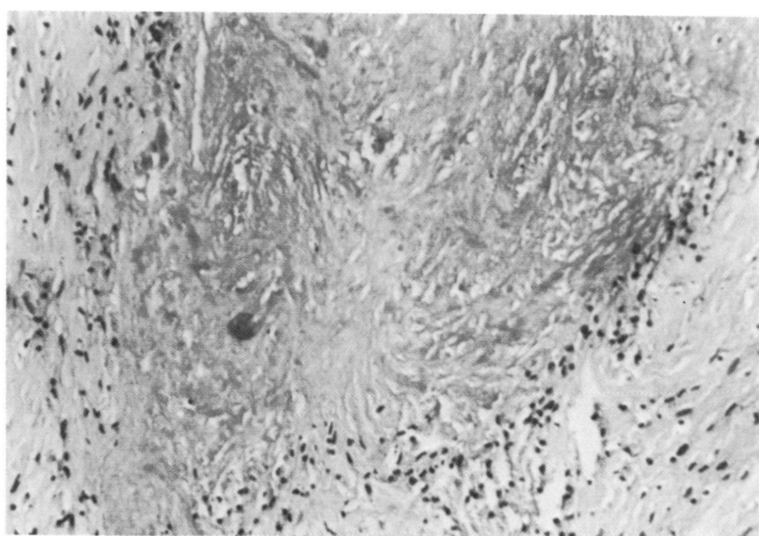

Figure 23–19. Subcutaneous nodule typical of rheumatoid arthritis. Note central necrosis surrounded by a cellular palisade. 150×. (From Ansell B, Loewi G: Clin Rheum Dis 3:387, 1977.)

nodules have a tendency to recur. Occasionally, however, rheumatoid arthritis may present with relatively little arthropathy or with an atypical distribution of the articular lesion. Under these circumstances excision biopsy of a nodule may be quite useful. Nodules may more rarely be detected both in patients with acute rheumatic fever and in those with systemic lupus erythematosus. It is unusual for the clinical and laboratory picture in these three diseases (rheumatoid arthritis, rheumatic fever, and systemic lupus erythematosus) to closely mimic each other, but some diagnostic difficulty may be encountered in the early stages of the illness. The histologic appearance of the nodules of rheumatic fever and systemic lupus erythematosus may be quite similar to those seen in rheumatoid arthritis, but subtle differences do exist and can usually be recognized by an experienced pathologist. Finally, the identification of rheumatoid nodules excised from visceral organs such as the pleural membrane or lung parenchyma may be an essential part of the diagnostic process in patients presenting with widespread extra-articular and systemic rheumatoid disease. A spectrum of other nodular lesions may be seen in patients with various rheumatic diseases, and these nodules may occasionally need to be excised for diagnostic purposes.[72] These include the peculiar lipid-filled lesions of multicentric reticulohistiocytosis, solitary xanthomas, and subcutaneous gouty tophi. In the latter instance, needle aspiration of the tophaceous material followed by polarizing microscopic examination of the aspirate rapidly reveals the true nature of the lesion.

Many rheumatic diseases are characterized by either a primary or a secondary alteration of the synovial membrane. Most of the more common rheumatic diseases, such as rheumatoid arthritis and the seronegative spondyloarthropathies, feature a nonspecific histopathologic change of the synovium that is of relatively little absolute diagnostic value. However, diseases such as tuberculosis, sarcoidosis, pigmented villonodular synovitis, fungal synovitis, synovial chondromatosis. and synovial sarcomas may all be diagnosed following recognition of their specific histopathology.[73] Clearly, excision biopsy of this type of lesion is essential to the diagnostic process, especially in those patients presenting with a chronic monoarticular joint or tendon sheath disease.

Secondary amyloidosis is a significant cause of death following many years of chronic inflammatory rheumatic disease in various geographic regions of the world. When a patient with long-standing rheumatoid arthritis or ankylosing spondylitis presents with proteinuria, the physician is obliged to consider secondary amyloidosis as one potential mechanism for the new clinical feature. The diagnosis of amyloidosis depends on recognition of the extraneous deposits within affected tissues. This recognition is best facilitated by rectal biopsy, since perivascular deposits of amyloid in the submucosal layers of the rectum are a very dependable hallmark of the disease. In fact, the sensitivity of rectal biopsy has rendered renal biopsy virtually unnecessary for this particular diagnostic consideration.[74]

A similar distinct pathologic process is seen in sicca syndrome (keratoconjunctivitis sicca) occurring either on its own or associated with a rheumatic or collagen-vascular disease. It is now recognized that the minor salivary glands of the lip and buccal mucosa tend to mirror the pathologic process present in the major salivary glands, so that lip biopsy in such patients would be expected to reveal periductal lymphocyte infiltration and secondary acinar atrophy.[75] Here again, the pathologic picture is so specific at this site as to render it virtually diagnostic for this autoimmune disease of salivary glands (Fig. 23–20).

Virtually all forms of vasculitic syndromes depend for their diagnosis on the demonstration of inflamed blood vessels.[76] This is the case whether

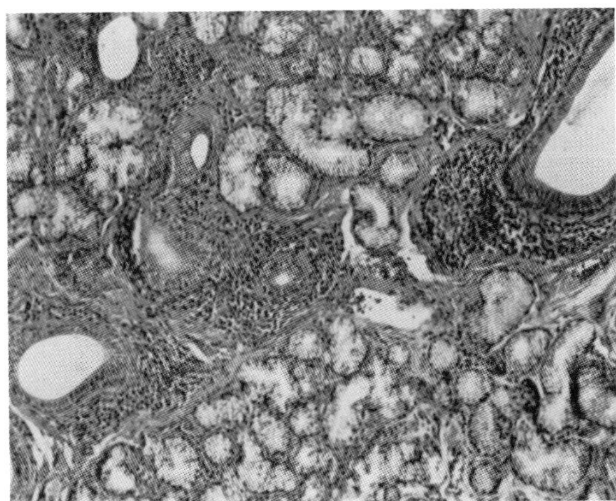

Figure 23–20. *Section of a labial biopsy showing lymphocytic infiltrates around the ducts and minor salivary glands. (Hematoxylin and eosin stain, 100×.) This histologic picture is highly characteristic of sicca syndrome. The involved acini have not yet undergone serious atrophy. (From Tarpley T Jr, et al: Oral Surg 37:64, 1974.)*

the vasculopathy affects large muscular arteries, small arterioles, or even capillaries and postcapillary venules. Occasionally this may involve postsurgical examination of necrotic or dysfunctioning visceral tissue but more usually implies the recognition of vasculitis or perivasculitis in biopsied dermal or subdermal tissue. Some of the deeper forms of dermal vasculitis (e.g., erythema nodosum, chronic relapsing nodular vasculitis, or Weber-Christian disease) can be diagnosed reliably in this fashion. In these disorders, the appearance of a panniculitis particularly affecting the septum is quite characteristic. Although the infiltrate may at first be largely neutrophilic, it rapidly becomes lymphocytic in nature, with or without a focal perivascular aggregation of the inflammatory cells. One rare form of vasculitic disease, relapsing polychondritis, classically involves cartilaginous inflammation as a direct and dominant manifestation.[77] In this disorder, a firm diagnosis may necessitate cartilage biopsy from a clinically involved site in order to demonstrate the cardinal pathologic lesion.

SUMMARY

There are many laboratory signs of articular disease and more tests become available year by year. It is important to stress, however, that in most instances a clinical diagnosis is readily achieved by carefully studying the patient's symptoms, signs, and radiographic features and noting the overall distribution of the arthropathy and the presence or absence of certain characteristic extra-articular manifestations. On occasion, a laboratory test is absolutely crucial to the diagnostic process, as in patients with septic or crystal-induced synovitis. In most situations, however, the laboratory tests help only to confirm or refute a suspected diagnosis or indicate to the clinician the severity, extent, and therapeutic response of the rheumatic disease. These considerations demand that the broad spectrum of tests discussed in this chapter be used in a highly selective fashion. They should never preempt a skilled clinical approach to the individual patient, whose physical appearance usually provides a most faithful mirror of the underlying disease process. Finally, it is noteworthy that several areas of laboratory testing have themselves contributed to a better clinicopathogenetic categorization of the rheumatic diseases, as well as led to more precise and scientific therapeutic regimens.

REFERENCES

1. Jessar RA: The study of synovial fluid. *In* JL Hollander, DJ McCarty (Eds): Arthritis and Allied Conditions. 8th Ed. Philadelphia, Lea & Febiger, 1972, p 67.
2. Intrasynovial Injection Technique. A Scope Publication. Kalamazoo, Michigan, The Upjohn Company, 1976.
3. Hughes GRV: Appendix B. Laboratory investigations. *In* M Mason, HLF Currey (Eds): An Introduction to Clinical Rheumatology. 2nd Ed. Philadelphia, JB Lippincott Company, 1975, p 315.
4. Germain BF: Synovial Fluid Analysis in the Diagnosis of Disease of the Joints. A Scope Publication. Kalamazoo, Michigan, The Upjohn Company, 1976.
5. Talbott J: Symposium Introduction: Gout. Postgrad Med *63*(5):132, 1978.
6. Klinenberg JR (Ed): Gout and purine metabolism. Proceedings of the Second Conference on Gout and Purine Metabolism. Arthritis Rheum (Suppl) *18*:659, 1975.
7. Klinenberg JR: Role of the kidneys in the pathogenesis of gout. Postgrad Med *63*:145, 1978.
8. Hamilton EB: Diseases associated with CPPD deposition disease. Arthritis Rheum (Suppl) *19*:353, 1976.
9. Bayer AS, Chow AW, Louie JS, Nies KM, Guze LB: Gram-negative bacillary septic arthritis: Clinical, radiographic, therapeutic and prognostic features. Semin Arthritis Rheum *7*:123, 1977.
10. Gordon D, Pruzanski W, Ogryzlo MA, Little HA: Amyloid arthritis simulating rheumatoid disease in five patients with multiple myeloma. Am J Med *55*:142, 1973.
11. Lawrence C, Seife B: Bone marrow in joint fluid: A clue to fracture. Ann Intern Med *74*:740, 1971.
12. Hollander JL: Painful joints: Clues to early diagnosis. Postgrad Med *64*:50, 1978.
13. Dorwart BB, Schumacher HR: Joint effusions, chondrocalcinosis, and other rheumatic manifestations in hypoparathyroidism. A clinicopathologic study. Am J Med *59*:780, 1975.
14. Bluestone R: Immunology of connective tissue diseases. *In* G Taylor (Ed): Immunology in Medical Practice. Philadelphia, WB Saunders Co, 1975, p. 91.
15. Bunch TW, Hunder GG, McDuffie FC, O'Brien PC, Markowitz H: Synovial fluid complement determination as a diagnostic aid in inflammatory joint disease. Mayo Clin Proc *49*:715, 1974.
16. Brook I, Reza MJ, Bricknell KS, Bluestone R, Finegold SM: Synovial fluid lactic acid: A diagnostic aid in septic arthritis. Arthritis Rheum *21*:774, 1978.
17. Bennett R:Haematological changes in rheumatoid disease. Clin Rheum Dis *3*:433, 1977.
18. Ansell BM: Heberton Oration 1977: Chronic arthritis in childhood. Ann Rheum Dis *37*:107, 1978.

19. Rivero SJ, Diaz-Jouanen E, and Alarcón-Segovia D: Lymphopenia in systemic lupus erythematosus: Clinical, diagnostic, and prognostic significance. Arthritis Rheum *21*:295, 1978.
20. Alarcón-Segovia D: The necrotizing vasculitides: A new pathogenetic classification. Med Clin North Am *61*:241, 1977.
21. Shulman L: Diffuse fasciitis with hypergammaglobulinemia and eosinophilia. A new syndrome (abstr). J Rheumatol (Suppl. 1)*1*:46, 1974.
22. Hughes GRV: Connective Tissue Diseases. Oxford, Blackwell, 1977.
23. Ehrenfeld M, Penchas S, Eliakim M: Thrombocytosis in rheumatoid arthritis. Recurrent arterial thromboembolism and death. Ann Rheum Dis *36*:579, 1977.
24. McConkey B, Crockson RA, Crockson AP: The assessment of rheumatoid arthritis. A study based on measurements of the serum acute phase reactants. Q J Med *41*:115, 1972.
25. Cooper A, Bluestone R: Free immunoglobulin light chains in connective tissue disease. Ann Rheum Dis *27*:537, 1968.
26. Katz GA, Peter JB, Pearson C, Adams WS: The shoulder-pad sign — a diagnostic feature of amyloid arthropathy. N Engl J Med *288*:354, 1973.
27. Good RA, Rötstein J, Mazzitello WF: The simultaneous occurrence of rheumatoid arthritis and agammaglobulinemia. J Lab Clin Med *49*:343, 1957.
28. Cassidy JT, Burt A: Isolated IgA deficiency in juvenile rheumatoid arthritis. Arthritis Rheum *10*:272, 1967.
29. Bisno AL, Pearce IA, Stollerman GH: Streptococcal infections that fail to cause recurrences of rheumatic fever. J Infect Dis *136*:278, 1977.
30. Watson KC, Kerr EJC: Polyene antibiotics in assessing significance of antistreptolysin O activity. J Clin Pathol *31*:230, 1978.
31. Laitinen O, Leirisalo M, Skylv G: Relation between HLA-B27 and clinical features in patients with yersinia arthritis. Arthritis Rheum *20*:1121, 1977.
32. Duffy J, Lidsky MD, Sharp JT, Davis JS, Person DA, Hollinger FB, Min K-W: Polyarthritis, polyarteritis, and hepatitis B. Medicine *55*:19, 1976.
33. Plotz CM, Singer JM: The latex fixation test. Results in rheumatoid arthritis. Am J Med *21*:893, 1956.
34. McDuffie FC: Immune complexes in the rheumatic diseases. J Allergy Clin Immunol *62*:37, 1978.
35. Lloyd KN, Withey JI: An evaluation of a new haemagglutination test for rheumatoid factors. Rheumatol Rehab *13*:37, 1974.
36. Mongan ES, Cass RM, Jacox RF, Vaughan JH: A study of the relation of seronegative and seropositive rheumatoid arthritis to each other and to necrotizing vasculitis. Am J Med *47*:23, 1969.
37. Moll JMH, Haslock I, Macrae I, Wright V: Associations between ankylosing spondylitis, psoriatic arthritis, Reiter's disease, the intestinal arthropathies and Behçet's syndrome. Medicine *53*:343, 1974.
38. Notman DD, Kurata N, Tan EM: Profiles of antinuclear antibodies in systemic rheumatic diseases. Ann Intern Med *83*:464, 1975.
39. Hargraves MM: Discovery of the LE cell and its morphology. Mayo Clin Proc *44*:579, 1969.
40. Carel RS, Shapiro MS, Shoham D, Gutman A: Lupus erythematosus cells in pleural effusion. The initial manifestation of procainamide-induced lupus erythematosus. Chest *72*:670, 1977.
41. Holborow EJ, Weir DM, Johnson GD: A serum factor in lupus erythematosus with affinity for tissue nuclei. Br Med J *2*:732, 1957.
42. Bickel YB, Barnett EV, Pearson CM: Immunofluorescent patterns and specificity of human antinuclear antibodies. Clin Exp Immunol *3*:641, 1968.
43. Pincus T, Schur PH, Rose JA, Decker JL, Talal N: Measurement of serum DNA-binding activity in systemic lupus erythematosus. New Engl J Med *281*:701, 1969.
44. Sontheimer RD, Gilliam JN: An immunofluorescence assay for double-stranded DNA antibodies using the *Crithidia luciliae* kinetoplast as a double-stranded DNA substrate. J Lab Clin Med *91*:550, 1978.
45. Urman JD, Rothfield NF: Corticosteroid treatment in systemic lupus erythematosus. Survival studies. JAMA *238*:2272, 1977.
46. Shearn M: Sjögren's Syndrome. Philadelphia, WB Saunders Co, 1971.
47. Sherlock S: Progress report: Chronic hepatitis. Gut *15*:581, 1974.
48. Bluestone R, Goldberg LS, Weisbart RH, Morris RI, Holborow EJ: Aberrant immunity in (HL-A) W27-positive rheumatic disease. Ann Rheum Dis (Suppl 1) *34*:46, 1975.
49. Schaffner F: Primary biliary cirrhosis. Clin Gastroenterol *4*:351, 1975.
50. Kraus SJ, Haserick JR, Lantz MA: Atypical FTA-ABS test fluorescence in lupus erythematosus patients. JAMA *211*:2140, 1970.
51. Beal RW, Merry DJ: The VDRL test in a blood transfusion service. J Clin Pathol *28*:854, 1975.
52. Lee SL, Miotti AB: Disorders of hemostatic function in patients with systemic lupus erythematosus. Semin Arthritis Rheum *4*:241, 1975.
53. Kraus SJ, Haserick JR, Logan LC, Bullard JC: Atypical fluorescence in the fluorescent treponemal-antibody-absorption (FTS-ABS) test related to deoxyribonucleic acid (DNA) antibodies. J Immunol *106*:1665, 1971.
54. Araujo FG, Barnett EV, Gentry LO, Remington JS: False-positive anti-toxoplasma fluorescent-antibody tests in patients with antinuclear antibodies. Appl Microbiol *22*:270, 1971.
55. McCluskey RT, Hall CL, Colvin RB: Immune complex mediated diseases. Hum Pathol *9*:71, 1978.
56. Weinstein A, Peters K, Brown D, Bluestone R: Metabolism of the third component of complement (C3) in patients with rheumatoid arthritis. Arthritis Rheum *15*:49, 1972.
57. Ruddy S: Complement, rheumatic diseases, and the major histocompatibility complex. Clin Rheum Dis *3*:215, 1977.
58. Barnett EV, Bluestone R, Cracchiolo A, Goldberg LS, Kantor G, McIntosh RM: Cryoglobulinaemia and disease. Ann Intern Med *73*:95, 1970.
59. Baldwin DS, Gluck MC, Lowenstein J, Gallo GR: Lupus nephritis. Clinical course as related to morphologic forms and their transitions. Am J Med *62*:12, 1977.
60. Uses for IF Tests/Cooperative Study: Uses for immunofluorescence tests of skin and sera. Utilization of immunofluorescence in the diagnosis of bullous diseases, lupus erythematosus, and certain other dermatoses. Arch Dermatol *111*:371, 1975.
61. Yu DT, Peter JB: Cellular immunological aspects of rheumatoid arthritis. Semin Arthritis Rheum *4*:25, 1974.
62. Bluestone R: Histocompatibility antigens and rheumatic diseases. A Scope Publication. Kalamazoo, Michigan, The Upjohn Company, 1978.
63. Bluestone R, Lewis B, Mervant I: Hyperlipoproteinemia in gout. Ann Rheum Dis *30*:134, 1971.
64. Bluestone R: Hyperlipoproteinemia and arthritis (two cases). Proc R Soc Med *64*:669, 1971.
65. Khachadurian AK: Migratory polyarthritis in familial hypercholesterolemia (type II hyperlipoproteinemia). Arthritis Rheum *11*:385, 1968.
66. O'Gorman T, Koff RS: Salicylate hepatitis. Gastroenterology *72*:726, 1977.
67. Samuels B, Lee JC, Engleman EP, Hopper J Jr: Membranous nephropathy in patients with rheumatoid arthritis: Relationship to gold therapy. Medicine *57*:319, 1978.
68. Bacon PA, Tribe CR, MacKenzie JC, Jones JV, Cumming RH, Amer B: Penicillamine nephropathy in rheumatoid arthritis. A clinical, pathological and immunological study. Q J Med *45*:661, 1976.
69. Emori HW, Champion GD, Bluestone R, Paulus HE: Serum uric acid determination. Arthritis Rheum *17*:1058, 1974.
70. Bohan A, Peter JB: Polymyositis and dermatomyositis. N Engl J Med *292*:344, 1975.
71. Bluestone R: Arthropathies associated with endocrine disorders. *In* WN Kelley, et al (Eds): Textbook of Rheumatology. Philadelphia, WB Saunders Co, 1980.
72. Moore CP, Wilkens RF: The subcutaneous nodule: Its significance in the diagnosis of rheumatic disease. Semin Arthritis Rheum *7*:63, 1977.
73. Goldenberg DL, Cohen AS: Synovial membrane histopathology in the differential diagnosis of rheumatoid arthritis, gout, pseudogout, systemic lupus erythematosus, infectious arthritis, and degenerative joint disease. Medicine *57*:239, 1978.
74. Gafni J, Sohar E: Rectal biopsy for the diagnosis of amyloidosis. Am J Med Sci *240*:332, 1960.
75. Chisholm DM, Mason DK: Labial salivary gland biopsy in Sjögren's disease. J Clin Pathol *21*:656, 1968.
76. Zeek PM: Periarteritis nodosa. A critical review. Am J Clin Pathol *22*:777, 1952.
77. McAdam LP, O'Hanlan MA, Bluestone R, Pearson CM: Relapsing polychondritis: Prospective study of 23 patients and a review of the literature. Medicine *55*:193, 1976.

24

ORTHOPEDIC INTERVENTION IN ARTICULAR DISEASE

by Clement B. Sledge, M.D.

The various forms of arthritis produce similar clinical consequences in the involved joints: pain, loss of function, progressive damage, and deformity. Reconstructive surgery may be indicated to *relieve* any or all of these disabilities. In selected situations, surgery may be indicated to *prevent* these consequences.

Although the general consequences of arthritic damage to the joint are similar, there are significant differences between osteoarthritis and rheumatoid arthritis; indeed, there are unique surgical aspects to many of the "rheumatoid variant" disorders. In some instances these unique features place the patient at risk from surgery, and in others they jeopardize the eventual result. These features will be discussed under the heading "Preoperative Evaluation" in order to emphasize two philosophic points: The surgeon who operates on arthritic patients, especially those with rheumatoid arthritis, should be familiar with the special technical aspects necessitated by the unusual requirements of the patient with multiple joint involvement, and the surgeon should be part of a team, composed of rheumatologists, nurses, therapists, social workers, and — most importantly — the patient. At first glance it may seem foolish to list the patient as part of the team. Doing so emphasizes the fact that the surgical patient with rheumatoid arthritis is frequently weak and discouraged, and must look forward to a series of operations before reasonable functional independence is achieved. Often the patient has excessive expectations regarding the outcome of surgery.[1] By participating in the planning and staging of the surgical events, the patient can better understand the duration of treatment, the necessity for prolonged physical therapy, and the ultimate realistic goal of the procedure or procedures.

Since relief of pain is the most consistent result of reconstructive surgery, pain is the primary indication for operative intervention. Restoration of motion and function, distinct from relief of pain, is less predictable and requires careful assessment of each patient's disability before improvement can be anticipated. Some surgical procedures in rheumatoid arthritis are as much prophylactic as they are therapeutic (synovectomy, fusion of the first and second cervical vertebrae, fusion of the base of the thumb, and so forth). The patient should understand the preventive aspects so that he or she will not be disappointed when the therapeutic result does not seem to justify the pain and the inconvenience of surgery.

Finally, the socioeconomic factors must be considered. The surgical patient with rheumatoid arthritis has an average length of hospitalization of about 18 days and may require two to six or more major procedures. The economic costs are considerable even when everything proceeds without complication. If a deep infection occurs after a joint replacement, the costs may be as high as $100,000 for the infected hip replacement. Many patients undergoing replacement of multiple joints either have left the work force because of disability, have not been gainfully employed, or have postponed surgery until they are ready for retirement. The majority are women who have not worked outside the home. These factors make calculation of a cost/benefit ratio difficult. Without putting a dollar value on "the quality of life," can such extensive procedures be justified by society? One recent study of 16 patients undergoing bilateral hip and knee replacement showed that none of those patients returned to work after this expensive series of operations involving an average of 3 months of hospitalization.[2] Precise data are not yet available, but preliminary studies strongly suggest that society does benefit in terms of the patient's decreased need for home help, home modifications, and hospitalization or confinement to an institution because of loss of independent functional capacity. The spouse can thus be relieved from his or her helping role and can return to the working force.[3, 4] For many individual patients, however, the goal must be relief of pain, restoration of functional independence, and a qualitative improvement in their existence without the hope of purely economic justification.

Certainly the major single advance in the care of patients with arthritis was the development of the concept of total joint replacement by Charnley nearly 20 years ago.[5] The concepts initially involved in replacement of the arthritic hip have now been expanded to apply to surgical intervention in the other joints. In patients with osteoarthritis, there are numerous alternatives to joint replacement, many of which are preferable, especially in younger patients. In patients with rheumatoid arthritis, procedures such as arthrodesis, synovectomy, repair of ruptured tendons, and other "nonprosthetic" procedures still play an important role. For predictable relief of pain and restoration in function, however, joint replacement surgery has revolutionized the outlook for patients with multiple joint involvement. Subsequent sections of this chapter will therefore emphasize joint replacement surgery in patients with rheumatoid arthritis and its variants, but when appropriate, alternative procedures will be mentioned, as will certain features pertinent to the patient with osteoarthritis.

PREOPERATIVE EVALUATION

The first consideration is whether a painful joint in a patient with rheumatoid arthritis requires surgery or not. If synovitis is the cause of the patient's pain and disability, continued medical management with drugs and physical modalities is appropriate. If it can be determined that structural damage to the joint is the problem, then it is unrealistic to expect that medication will be sufficient. A trial of anti-inflammatory medication and physical therapy is appropriate, particularly for the weight-bearing joints, for which the use of crutches may allow the acute disabling symptoms to subside to an acceptable level, even when there has been structural damage. If these measures fail and structural damage can be demonstrated on physical or radiographic examination, arthrodesis or arthroplasty can be considered. It is better to perform surgery on each joint as it becomes structurally destroyed rather than to wait until the patient has many destroyed joints requiring prolonged hospitalization, multiple anesthetics, and a series of debilitating surgical procedures. General operative risk should be assessed, especially from the point of view of the systemic manifestations of the rheumatic diseases. The patient should be in optimal medical condition and, when on steroid therapy, should be on the lowest possible maintenance dose. Obvious sources of infection should be identified and eradicated to prevent postoperative hematogenous seeding of the operative site. Carious teeth should be extracted or otherwise attended to before joint surgery, and urinary tract infections should be identified and treated. Many female patients have asymptomatic bacteriuria, and urine culture before surgery is an absolute requirement. In men, prostatic hypertrophy, if severe, should be treated before surgery to avoid postoperative catheterization with its attendant risk of infection and bacterial seeding. It is useful to determine if the patient is able to void in the supine position. Frequently, practicing voiding in the supine position preoperatively will facilitate this activity in the postoperative period. Most difficult to evaluate is the patient's motivation and ability to participate meaningfully in the postoperative program. Patients should be evaluated by physical and occupational therapists, both to assess their abilities to participate in the program and to determine what special requirements might be present in the postoperative period. Instruction in crutch ambulation before surgery shortens the postoperative learning period. If multiple procedures are envisioned, it is often useful to perform a simple procedure first so that the ability of the patient to follow the postoperative program can be assessed. If both hips and knees require surgery, the hip can be used for this assessment. The relief of pain and improvement in function following hip arthroplasty are essentially independent of the patient's cooperation. The postoperative period is characterized by minimal pain. If the patient is unable to cooperate with a therapy program following hip replacement, it is unlikely that he or she will be able to participate in the postoperative program following a more painful arthroplasty that requires maximal patient cooperation.

The patient with rheumatoid arthritis or its variants poses certain special problems that bear on the risks and results of surgery. The patient with rheumatoid arthritis frequently has multiple joints involved (Fig. 24–1), each interfering with the function of the others. The rheumatoid arthritic patient undergoing surgery is, on the average, 10 years younger than the typical patient with osteoarthritis undergoing similar procedures[6] and therefore has longer to live with the prosthetic joint than does the osteoarthritic patient. This means that there will be more time for the appearance of complications such as delayed infection or loosening and wear of the component parts. Much has been written of the increased susceptibility to infection in patients with rheumatoid arthritis,[7, 8] and we have recently documented that the patient with rheumatoid arthritis undergoing total hip replacement does have a significantly increased risk of late hematogenous seeding of the prosthetic joint.[9, 72] Approximately 10

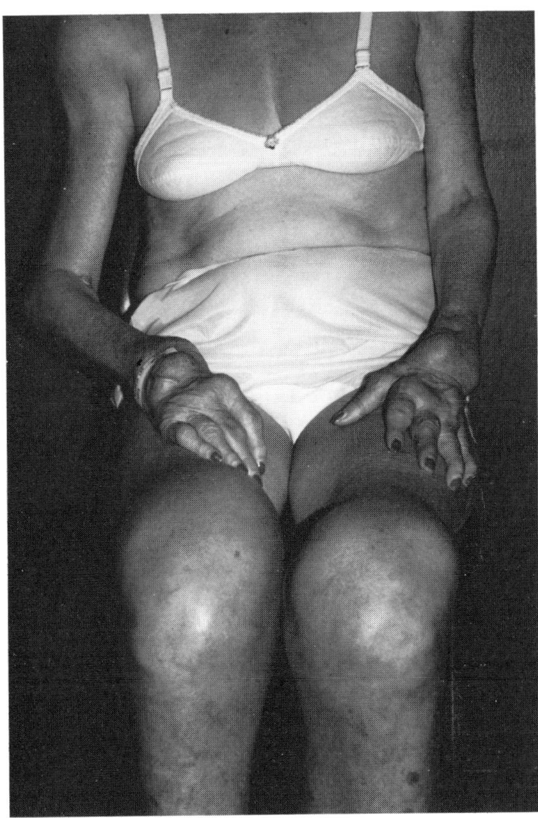

Figure 24–1. *The patient with rheumatoid arthritis often presents with involvement of several major joints. In this patient, both shoulders, wrists, hands, hips, and knees were involved. Prolonged hospitalization and multiple surgical procedures are necessary to restore such patients to a comfortable, functional status.*

per cent of patients coming to surgery at our institution are on maintenance steroids, and this has been shown in some studies to increase the risk of infection.[10] Aspirin, used by almost all patients, may predispose to intraoperative and postoperative bleeding. Careful assessment of bleeding and clotting time is useful, and platelet transfusions are occasionally required. Some patients are on chronic immunosuppressive treatment, and the effect of these drugs on postoperative infection must be considered.[11, 12] Although there is controversy regarding the relationship between penicillamine treatment and wound healing,[13-15] it is the opinion of most surgeons with experience in this field that there is a definite delay in wound healing in patients on penicillamine therapy. This may delay the postoperative rehabilitation program until satisfactory wound healing is achieved.

There is both clinical and laboratory evidence to suggest that the rheumatoid process is perpetuated in a given joint by retention of articular cartilage. Whether this is because of sequestered antigen-antibody complexes,[16, 17] the continued release of cartilage breakdown products producing synovial inflammation,[18, 19] or undiscovered factors is unknown. It has been a frequent observation, however, that patients undergoing total knee replacement in whom the patellar cartilage is retained will have involvement of the prosthetic joint during systemic "flare-ups," whereas patients in whom all cartilage has been removed will not experience involvement of the prosthetic knee in such flare-ups. The quality of bone in patients with rheumatoid arthritis frequently is poor. This may be related to direct involvement of the subchondral trabecular bone by granulation tissue in patients with rheumatoid arthritis, the anabolic effects of chronic steroid use, the bone resorption resulting from excessive production of prostaglandins by the synovium in rheumatoid arthritis,[20] or a proposed parathyroid hormone excess in these patients.[21, 22] Regardless of the cause, the quality of bone is of great concern with regard to the long-term fixation of prosthetic components to bone. Many prosthetic devices transfer the enormous joint reactive forces directly to the bone-cement interface, which may be unable to withstand these forces over a long period of time. For this reason, it is desirable to use prosthetic devices that are minimally constrained in order to transfer forces away from the bone-cement interface into the more compliant soft tissues.

The patient with juvenile rheumatoid arthritis (juvenile chronic arthritis) presents certain unique features that bear directly upon the expected results following surgical intervention.[23] As in ankylosing spondylitis, there appears to be a much greater involvement of the soft tissues surrounding the joint in juvenile rheumatoid arthritis, with the result that the ultimate range of motion achieved after joint arthroplasty is less than would be predicted from the range achieved at surgery.[24] Following arthroplasty, there is a progressive loss of motion in these patients, and the effect of this loss on ultimate functional capacity must be anticipated. The young age at which patients with juvenile rheumatoid arthritis undergo arthroplasty exposes their prosthetic joints both to greater functional demands and to longer periods of risk of developing late complications, such as infection and loosening.[25] In addition, these patients often have severe micrognathia, which may make intubation difficult or produce postoperative respiratory problems.[26] (Fig. 24–2). Careful preoperative analysis by the anesthesiologist will prevent difficulties with intubation and respiration following extubation, and fiberoptic intubation will minimize trauma and postoperative laryngeal edema.

The patient with ankylosing spondylitis has diminished chest excursion and is therefore at greater risk for postoperative pulmonary problems; he or she requires chest physical therapy to minimize these problems. Because of the rigidity of the cervical spine, intubation is extremely difficult, sometimes requiring preoperative tracheostomy before an anesthetic agent can be delivered. Ossifica-

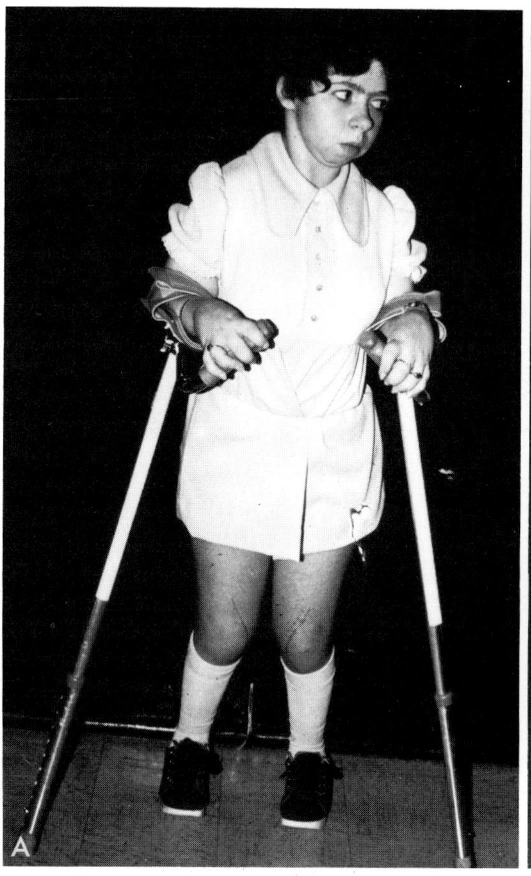

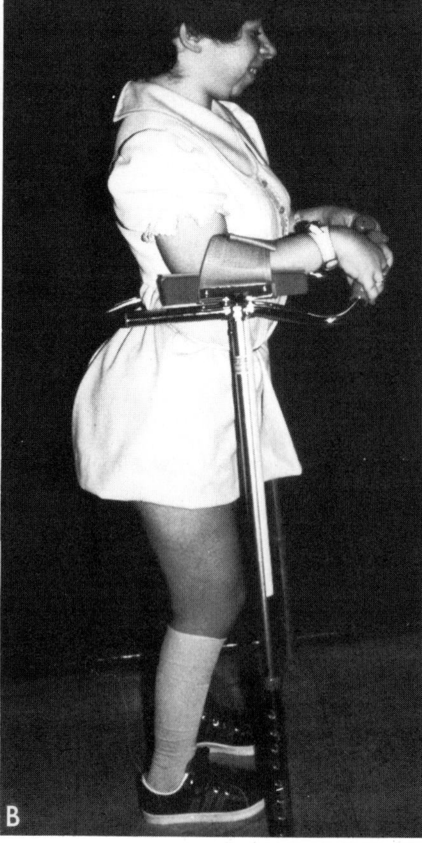

Figure 24–2. *The patient with juvenile rheumatoid arthritis (juvenile chronic arthritis) often has involvement of the temporomandibular joint and shortening of the ramus of the mandible (micrognathia) in addition to involvement of the joints of the extremities.*

tion in the spinal ligaments can produce great difficulty in performing spinal anesthesia; careful assessment of the patient by the anesthesiologist is useful in choosing the appropriate type and route of anesthetic agent and in anticipating difficulties. Following total hip replacement, the patient with ankylosing spondylitis frequently fails to achieve the same range of motion that patients with rheumatoid arthritis or osteoarthritis achieve.[27] This is due not only to the increased involvement of the periarticular soft tissues seen in this disease but to an increased incidence of heterotopic ossification in the muscles and capsules surrounding the hip joint.[28] A similar postoperative problem may develop in patients with osteoarthritis who reveal exuberant osteophytosis (Fig. 24–3). Although the range of mo-

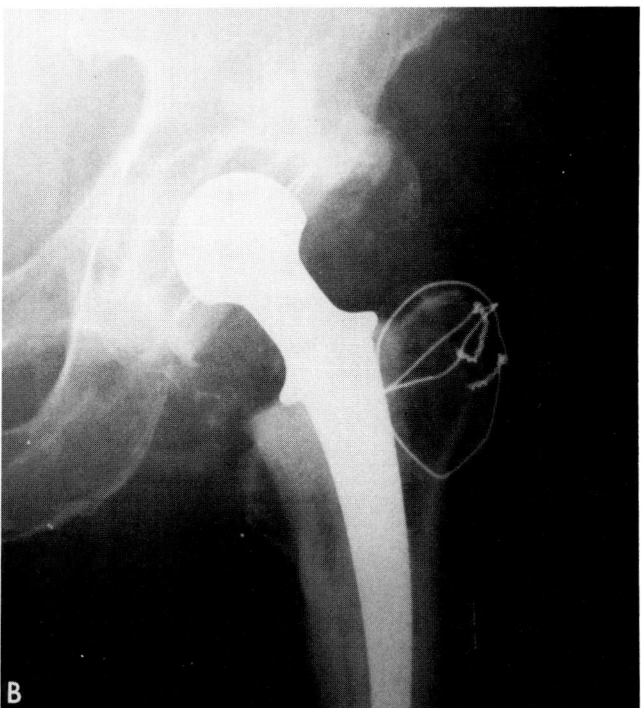

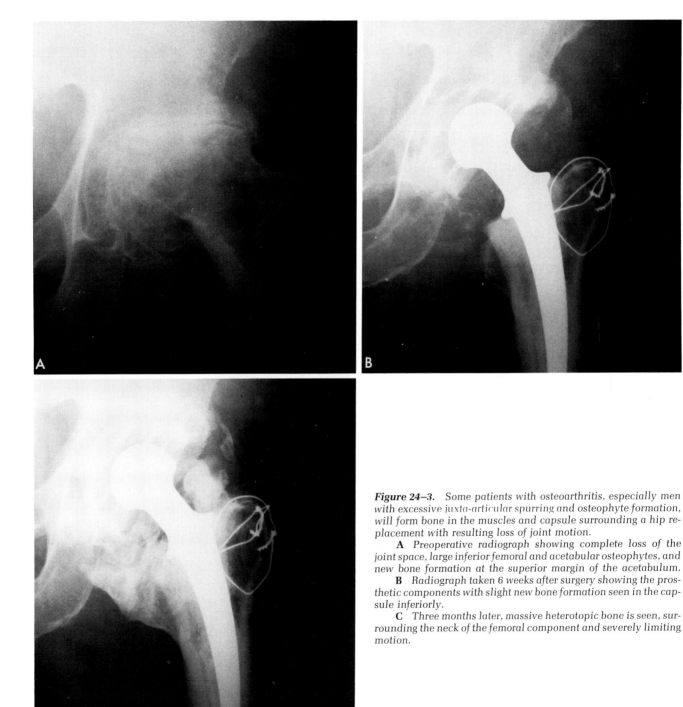

Figure 24–3. *Some patients with osteoarthritis, especially men with excessive juxta-articular spurring and osteophyte formation, will form bone in the muscles and capsule surrounding a hip replacement with resulting loss of joint motion.*

A *Preoperative radiograph showing complete loss of the joint space, large inferior femoral and acetabular osteophytes, and new bone formation at the superior margin of the acetabulum.*

B *Radiograph taken 6 weeks after surgery showing the prosthetic components with slight new bone formation seen in the capsule inferiorly.*

C *Three months later, massive heterotopic bone is seen, surrounding the neck of the femoral component and severely limiting motion.*

tion achieved may only be 65 degrees of hip flexion, this often allows a significant improvement in the patient's function and independence.[29] If warned of this preoperatively, the patient can make a more informed decision regarding the desirability of surgery and is less likely to experience disappointment in the postoperative period.

Patients with gout often experience painful postoperative "flares" that require skillful management as these postsurgical attacks of gouty arthritis are more difficult to treat than the usual spontaneous gouty attack.

Patients with psoriatic arthritis sometimes have involvement of the skin in the area of the proposed surgical incision. Several papers[30-32] report the frequent contamination of psoriatic skin with microorganisms and suggest an increased risk of infection following incision through such skin. Although our patients have not experienced this complication, it is desirable to clear up the skin in the operative site by appropriate local therapy before surgery.

The arthropathies related to inflammatory bowel disease pose a special threat of postoperative infection, due both to late hematogenous seeding from a focus of infection in the bowel and to the occasional source of contamination from a colostomy in proximity to the incision for hip replacement.

Systemic lupus erythematosus presents a very difficult problem for both the patient and the physician. The patient is often young and taking large doses of steroids, and may have a near-normal life expectancy. To implant a prosthetic joint in a young patient invites the long-term failures related to wear and loosening; to do so in a patient on chronic steroid treatment adds the further risk of infection. The presence of renal involvement in these patients may have implications with regard to their life expectancy. In the young patient with a limited life expectancy, prosthetic replacement may well be justified to relieve pain and improve the quality of life for the remaining years. On the other hand, in the patient with a normal life expectancy, there will almost certainly be late problems following joint replacement in the third and fourth decades of life. These patients often present with avascular necrosis (osteonecrosis) of a femoral condyle, with pain, deformity, and functional loss.[33] (Fig. 24–4). It may be better to accept the lesser result produced by a

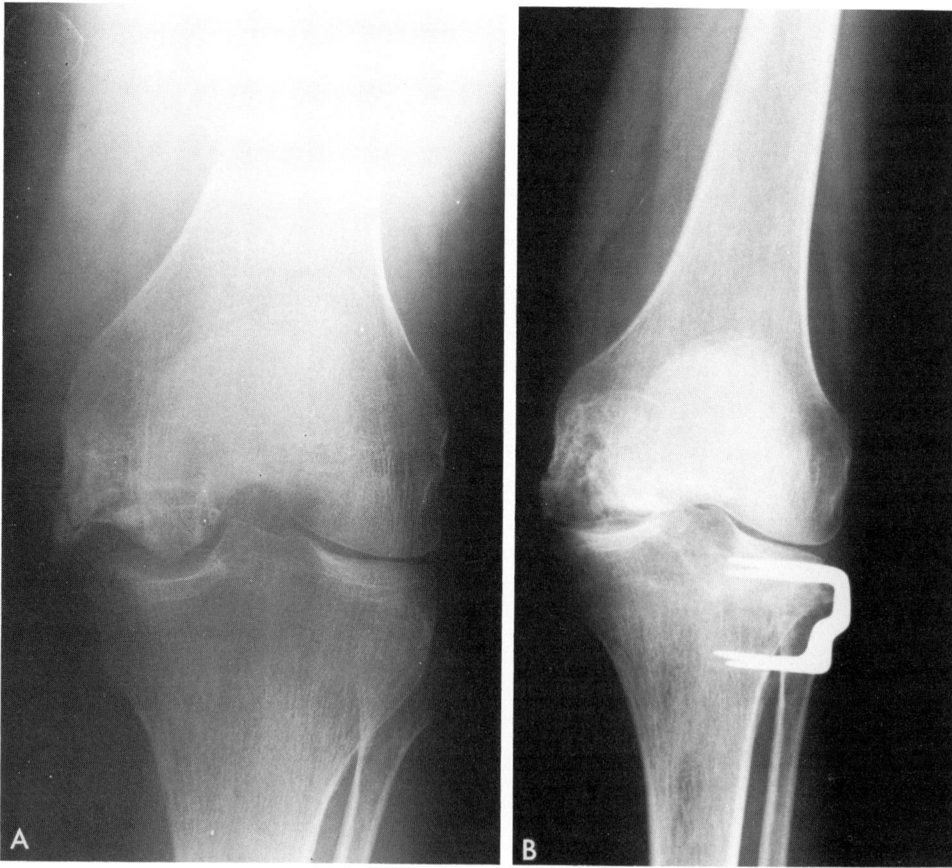

Figure 24–4. *Osteonecrosis in systemic lupus erythematosus.*

A *Avascular necrosis (osteonecrosis) of the medial femoral condyle with severe varus deformity and pain in a patient with systemic lupus erythematosus.*

B *Postoperative radiograph following high tibial osteotomy, placing the tibia in more valgus and transferring load to the lateral femorotibial compartment of the knee. Early radiographic evidence of healing of the lesion in the medial femoral condyle is seen and the patient was relieved of pain.*

high tibial osteotomy than to carry out joint replacement surgery with the high probability of eventual complication.

Patients with Reiter's syndrome as well as those with ankylosing spondylitis have a significant incidence of cardiac involvement. Careful preoperative cardiac assessment should be carried out in such patients.

In addition to the systemic problems encountered in patients with rheumatoid arthritis, the involvement of multiple joints presents special problems. Since the patient will require crutches after lower extremity surgery, it is essential to evaluate preoperatively the ability of the patient to use crutches. If there is extensive involvement of the shoulder, elbow or wrist, axillary crutches may not be appropriate. Forearm crutches will sometimes be a suitable alternative, particularly if involvement of the wrist or elbow makes the use of axillary crutches painful. Occasionally it will be necessary to carry out arthrodesis of the wrist before performing surgery on the lower extremities so that the patient will be able to use forearm crutches in the postoperative period. In addition, patients who do not have 110 degrees of knee flexion find it difficult to arise from a seated position without applying major force to the upper extremity[2] (Fig. 24–5). If the upper extremities are unable to cope with these forces, special attention must be directed to obtaining maximal hip and knee flexion after surgery in order to minimize the need for upper extremity assistance.

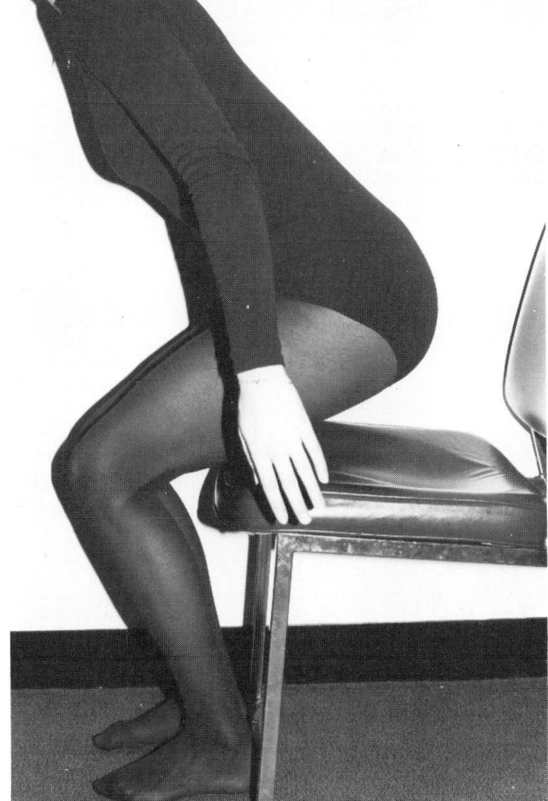

Figure 24–5. *Arising from a chair requires more than 90 degrees of knee flexion so that the foot can be placed under the center of mass, enabling the patient to arise with minimal use of the upper extremities.*

Patients with rheumatoid arthritis usually have involvement of both hips even though only one may require arthroplasty. Involvement of the contralateral hip will handicap the patient's postoperative recovery and may diminish the ultimate range of motion achieved in the operated hip. If it is obvious that both hips will require arthroplasty, it is preferable to carry out both during the same hospitalization to facilitate functional recovery. Except under unusual circumstances, such as extremely difficult and hazardous intubation, it is probably not justifiable to carry out bilateral total hip replacements during the same anesthetic period.

Patients undergoing hip or knee arthroplasty are sometimes disappointed to find that painful foot deformities prevent comfortable ambulation after their extensive surgical procedures. In addition, the plantar surface of the feet and the dorsum of the toes are subject to skin breakdown because of rheumatoid deformities. These may become sites of bacterial contamination following arthroplasty on more proximal joints. Areas of skin breakdown should be treated and healed before initiating surgery on proximal joints to prevent centripetal spread of infection. This can often be achieved by satisfactory shoe modifications and protective foot wear but may require surgical correction. Such surgery should be carried out before hip and knee arthroplasty so that problems of skin breakdown and infection, frequent after foot surgery, will not compromise the results of arthroplasties of the proximal joints.

The cervical spine is significantly involved in 30 to 40 per cent of patients with rheumatoid arthritis.[34-36] Usually this involvement is asymptomatic and unknown by the patient but should be sought in the preoperative evaluation to avoid the potentially disastrous consequences of excessive manipulation of the neck during intubation. The patient with marked atlanto-axial instability may sustain damage to the medullary respiratory center and long spinal tracts during such neck manipulation. While spinal anesthesia is being performed, the patient is often asked to "curl up" to facilitate insertion of the spinal needle. Flexion of the cervical spine in the presence of atlanto-axial instability should be avoided during this maneuver.

In addition to these general considerations, there are specific interactions between adjacent joints that may jeopardize the technical aspects of surgery. For example, involvement of the ipsilateral hip and knee usually leads to the performance of hip arthroplasty as the initial procedure. The position of the flexed knee is used as a guide for insertion of the femoral component during the hip arthroplasty. In the presence of severe knee instability or valgus deformity, proper placement of the hip component will be compromised.[37] If the component is placed in retroversion, postoperative dislocation of the hip becomes more frequent. Similarly, if the hip has been the site of an arthrodesis, the position of the knee components must be suitably altered, depending upon the degree of abduction or adduction of the arthrodesed hip.

CHOICE OF PROCEDURE

Operative Versus Nonoperative Treatment

In some instances, advanced age, increased risk factors, lack of patient motivation, or relatively minor pain will suggest that the patient should accept limited function rather than undergo a complex and potentially dangerous surgical procedure. In the upper extremity, the wrist in rheumatoid arthritis is a good example of this dilemma in choosing the appropriate therapeutic modality. Three options are available: splinting, arthrodesis, or arthroplasty. Arthrodesis provides a stable, painless wrist but jeopardizes function to some extent, particularly in the performance of personal hygienic chores.[38] For that reason, patients with bilateral involvement are often advised to have a wrist arthroplasty using some form of prosthetic implant.[39] Such prostheses carry the obvious risks of breakage, loosening, and infection. For some patients prostheses or fusion is indicated, but others would be better served by the use of a wrist splint, worn at night and during work but removed when flexibility is required.[40, 41] Similarly, in the lower extremity, painful foot and ankle deformities are often best managed by special shoes and inserts to minimize pressure points or an orthosis to splint the ankle and correct heel valgus.

Osteotomy

Osteotomy has limited usefulness in the treatment of patients with rheumatoid arthritis because of the usual massive destruction of the joint and limitation of motion. Some elderly patients in whom pain is the primary problem will benefit from osteotomies on both sides of the joint,[42] but for most, arthroplasty is preferable. In young patients with systemic lupus erythematosus who have a normal life expectancy, high tibial osteotomy is sometimes indicated for avascular necrosis (osteonecrosis) with

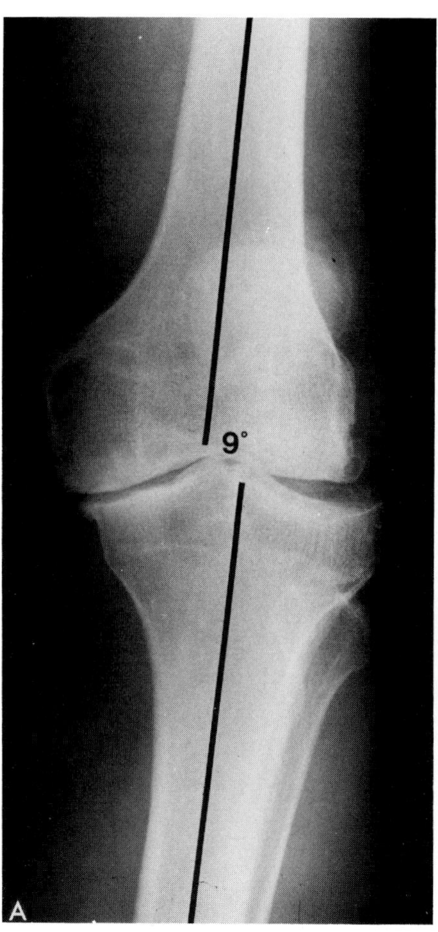

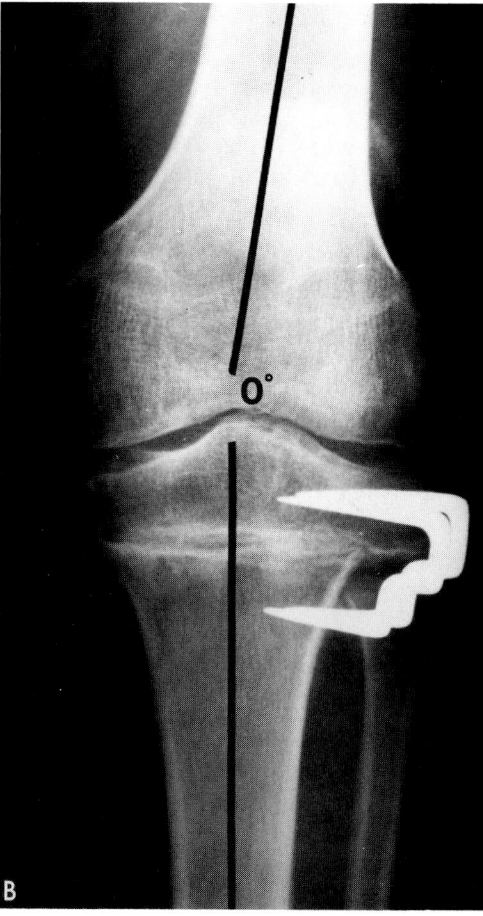

Figure 24–6. This patient had osteoarthritis of the medial femorotibial compartment of the knee with varus deformity and severe pain.

A The preoperative radiograph shows loss of articular cartilage in the medial femorotibial compartment with relative preservation of anatomy in the lateral femorotibial compartment, and a 9 degree varus deformity.

B Following resection of a laterally based wedge from the upper tibia, the varus deformity is corrected to slight knee valgus, weight-bearing forces are now transferred through the lateral femorotibial compartment, and pain is relieved.

involvement of one femoral condyle. In patients with ankylosing spondylitis and disabling spinal deformity, osteotomy of either the cervical or lumbar spine is occasionally necessary to correct the deformity.[43] The major usefulness of osteotomy is in patients with osteoarthritis in whom there is often sparing of a portion of the joint because of the mechanical nature of the disease process. In the knee there is commonly severe involvement of the medial femorotibial compartment, with loss of articular cartilage on both the tibial and femoral sides of the articulation but with relative sparing of the lateral femorotibial compartment (Fig. 24–6). In such instances, high tibial osteotomy will provide retention of motion and satisfactory diminution of pain in about 85 per cent of patients.[44, 45]

Because of the monoarticular nature of the osteoarthritic process, patients undergoing hip replacement will usually subject the prosthetic joint to excessive physical demands following restoration of function and abolition of pain. That, coupled with the 15 to 20 per cent incidence of loosening of the femoral component in 20 year follow-up evaluations of patients with total hip replacement, suggests that osteotomy of the hip should be considered in young active patients with osteoarthritis.[46]

Arthrodesis

As developments in total joint replacement have resulted in improved prostheses and surgical techniques, the usefulness of arthrodesis, with its attendant loss of joint function, has diminished. There remain, however, certain situations in which arthrodesis holds a clear-cut advantage over other procedures. Posttraumatic osteoarthritis of the ankle is best managed by arthrodesis. In addition to the reliability and long-term success of the procedure, a recent study has indicated that there is a clear functional advantage of arthrodesis over ankle replacement[47] (Fig. 24–7). Because ankle arthroplasty is still in an evolutionary phase with no consensus as to design or technique of procedure, arthrodesis remains an excellent choice, particularly in the patient with monoarticular involvement. Indeed, many patients with rheumatoid arthritis of the ankle are suitable candidates for arthrodesis if the subtalar and midtarsal joints are only minimally involved. However, later involvement of the subtalar and midtarsal joints, following arthrodesis of the ankle, may produce a stiff hindfoot and an abnormal gait, with transferring of excessive forces to the metatarsal heads and plantar aspect of the foot. Total joint replacement may then be advisable in patients in whom preoperative evaluation delineates hindfoot and midfoot involvement (Fig. 24–8). Occasionally, disabling foot pain may occur in patients with rheumatoid arthritis who have selective involvement of the talonavicular joint. Such patients often present with "ankle pain" but on careful clinical and radiographic examination will be found to have destruction of the talonavicular joint with relative sparing of the other joints of the hindfoot. In such patients, if conservative orthotic procedures fail, arthrodesis of the talonavicular joint is a highly satisfactory procedure, restoring alignment, preventing further deformity, and relieving pain[48] (Fig. 24–9).

In rheumatoid arthritis involving the wrist, particularly if involvement is primarily unilateral, arthrodesis remains the safest and most predictable

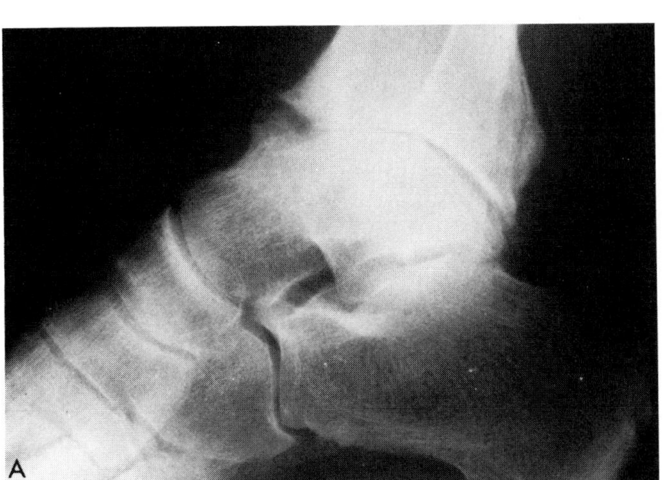

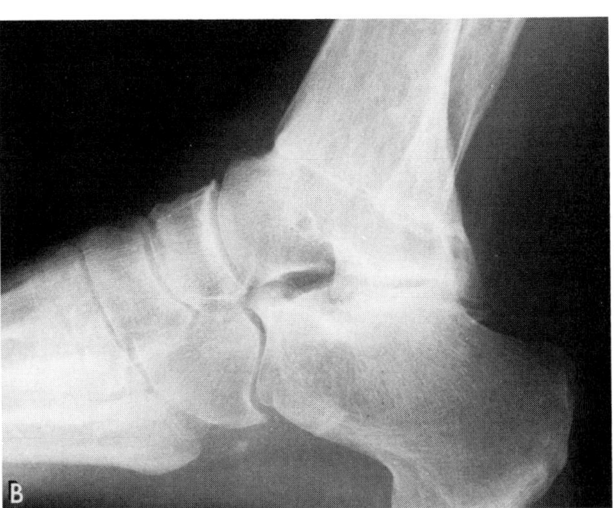

Figure 24–7. *This patient developed osteoarthritis of the ankle following an intra-articular fracture 12 years earlier.*

A *Preoperative lateral radiograph shows loss of articular cartilage and juxta-articular osteophyte formation in the ankle with preservation of normal joint structure in the remainder of the foot.*

B *Following arthrodesis of the ankle, pain was relieved and the patient resumed normal activities. Compensatory motion is provided by the midtarsal and subtalar joints with minimal functional deficit.*

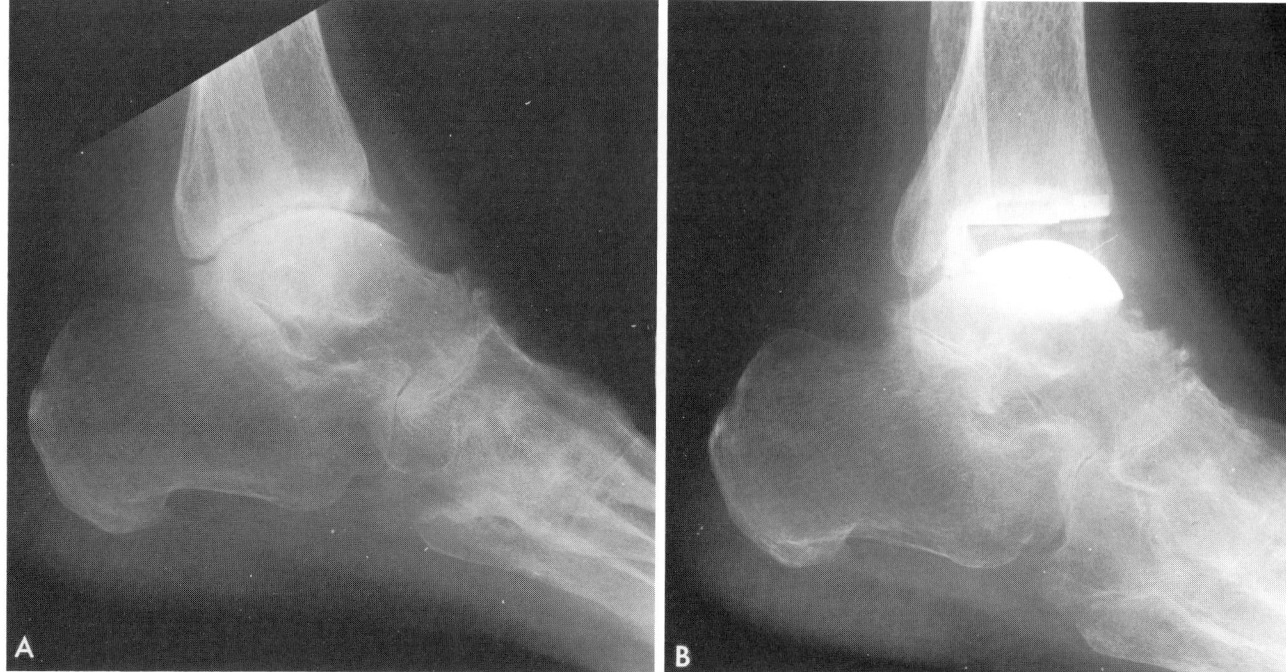

Figure 24–8. This patient with rheumatoid arthritis had involvement of the ankle joint as well as the subtalar and midtarsal joints. Ankle arthrodesis would have resulted in a stiff foot and ankle. Total joint replacement was therefore carried out.

A Preoperative radiograph showing involvement of the talonavicular and subtalar joints as well as the ankle itself.

B Postoperative radiograph showing implantation of a high-density polyethylene replacement for the tibial articular surface and a metallic prosthesis for the dome of the talus.

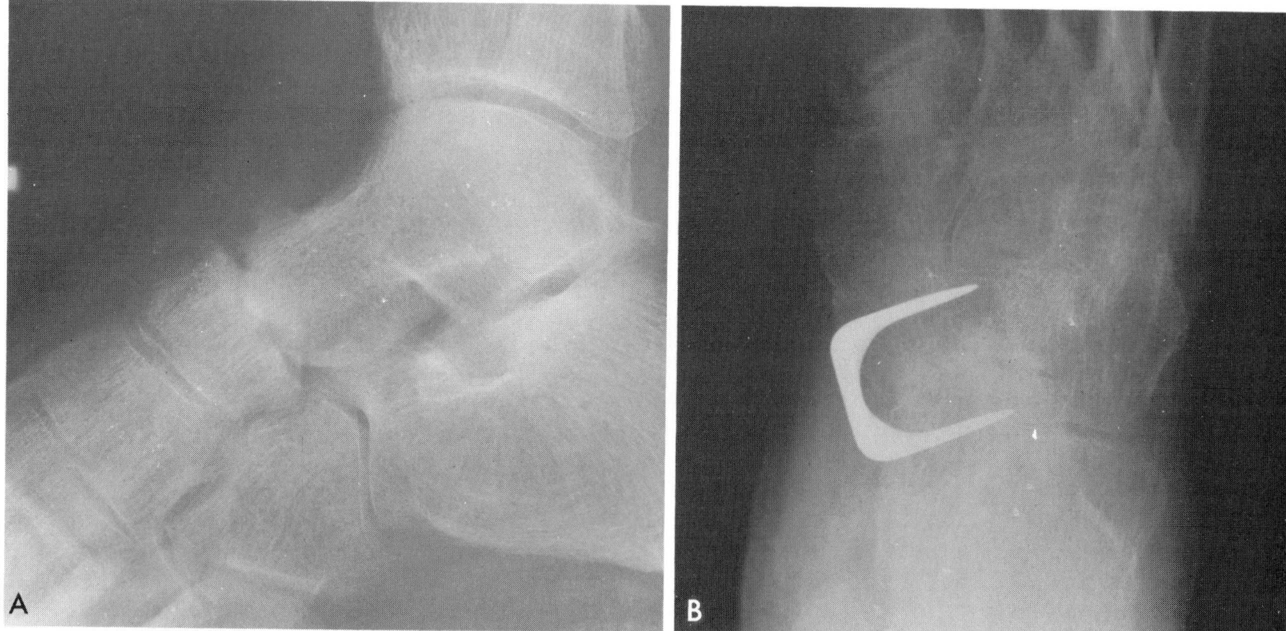

Figure 24–9. This patient with rheumatoid arthritis had isolated involvement of the talonavicular joint with loss of joint space, sclerosis, and pain.

A Preoperative radiograph.

B Postoperative radiograph following arthrodesis of the talonavicular joint using a metallic staple to secure fixation until the arthrodesis is solid.

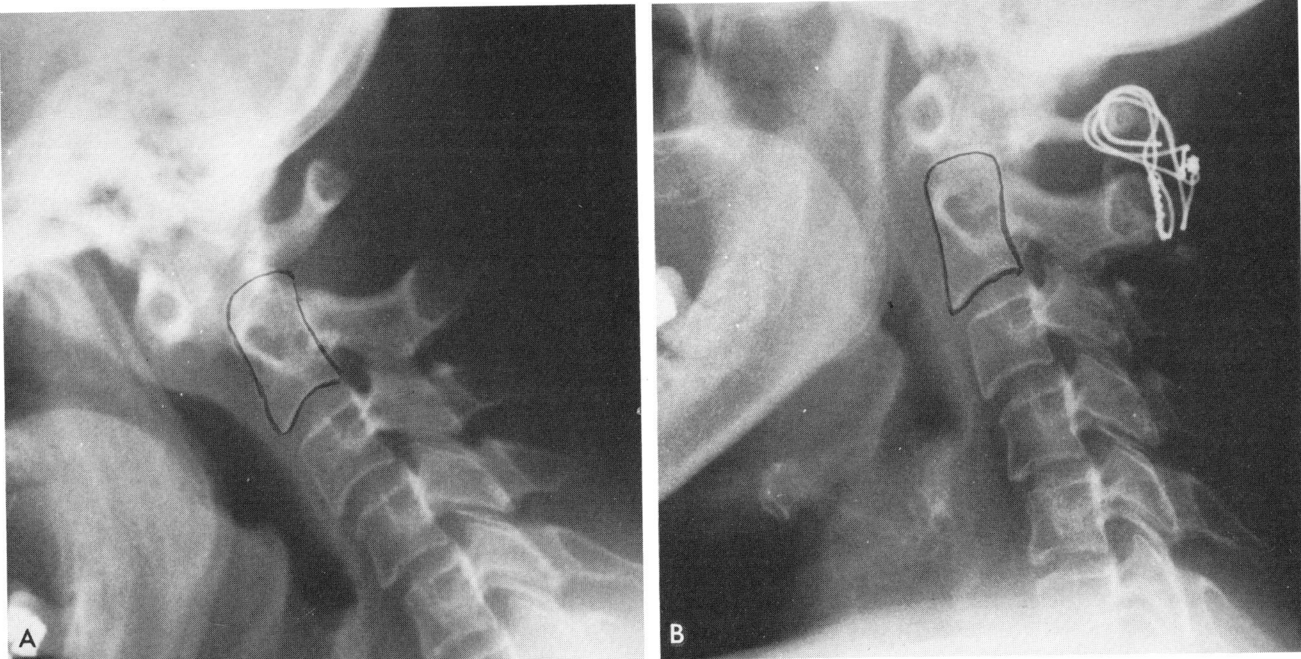

Figure 24–10. *Cervical spine involvement in rheumatoid arthritis.*

A *Flexion view of a patient with rheumatoid arthritis involving the atlanto-axial articulation with forward subluxation of the atlas jeopardizing the spinal cord and producing long tract signs, including paresthesias, weakness of the lower extremities, and bladder dysfunction. The odontoid process has been severely eroded with a pathologic fracture.*

B *Following reduction of the atlanto-axial subluxation, the spinous processes are wired together to achieve fixation while bone grafts are placed between the laminae of the atlas and axis to produce solid bony arthrodesis.*

procedure.[38] With extensive involvement of both hands and upper extremities, arthroplasty on one side may provide the range of wrist flexion for personal hygiene. The other universally accepted role for arthrodesis in patients with rheumatoid arthritis is in severe instability of the cervical spine. With involvement of the atlanto-axial articulation producing long-tract neurologic signs and chronic unremitting pain, posterior fusion of the first and second vertebrae is a dependable procedure, albeit one with significant morbidity[36, 49] (Fig. 24–10). Because of this morbidity, it is not our practice to carry out such fusion based on radiographic findings of instability but to reserve this procedure for patients with clear-cut long-tract signs, including weakness and loss of position sense in the lower extremities or bladder dysfunction. Occasionally patients will have such severe unremitting pain, in the absence of long-tract signs, that arthrodesis is indicated. The lower cervical spine may similarly require arthrodesis to relieve pain or neurologic loss.

Arthroplasty

Hemiarthroplasty, replacement of one articular surface of a joint, was an important developmental stage in the surgery of rheumatoid arthritis. In the past, mold arthroplasty of the hip (cup arthroplasty) provided relief of pain and satisfactory improvement of function in many patients with rheumatoid arthritis and ankylosing spondylitis.[50] The frequent need for revision surgery, coupled with the incomplete relief of pain or improvement in function, has caused this procedure to give way to total hip replacement.[51] There remain a few instances, however, in which it still may be indicated. In a young patient with monoarticular involvement of the hip, if arthrodesis is unacceptable, cup arthroplasty may be appropriate. In patients with septic arthritis of one hip, total hip arthroplasty carries an unacceptably high risk of infection, and cup arthroplasty may be preferable in this situation. Hemiarthroplasty of the knee, utilizing McKeever, McIntosh, or other tibial implants,[52, 53] is rarely carried out today since total knee replacement gives more predictable and more complete relief of pain and functional improvement.[54] As with cup arthroplasty of the hip, however, occasionally young patients or patients with a history of knee infection may still be appropriately considered for metallic hemiarthroplasty. Unicompartmental arthroplasty of the knee is a controversial procedure. It has been recommended for those patients with osteoarthritis involving one femorotibial compartment of the knee in whom the preoperative range of motion is unsatisfactory for consideration of

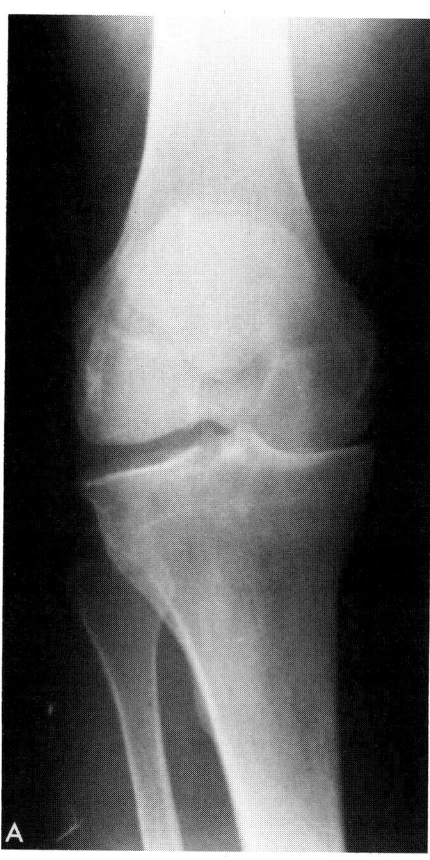

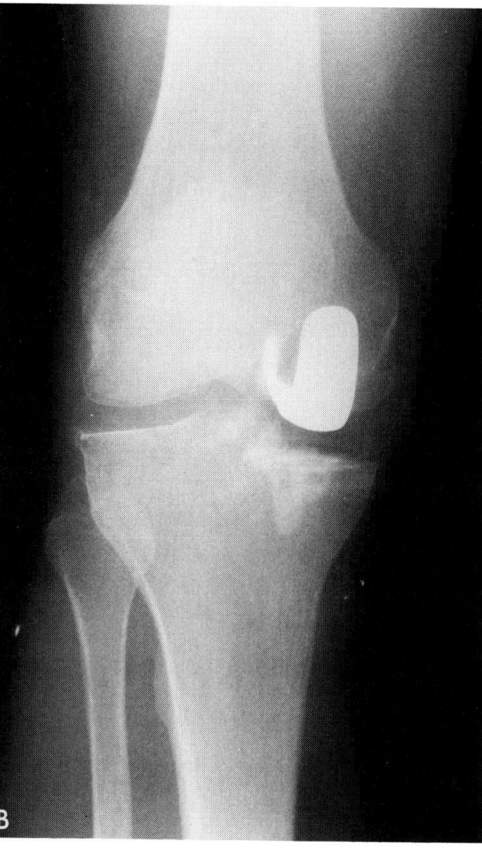

Figure 24–11. *An alternative to tibial osteotomy in patients with unicompartmental disease of the knee is prosthetic replacement.*

A *Preoperative radiograph of a patient with osteoarthritis showing narrowing of the medial femorotibial compartment with loss of articular cartilage and preservation of nearly normal anatomy in the lateral femorotibial compartment.*

B *Postoperative radiograph showing correction of the varus deformity by the implantation of a metallic femoral surface component and plastic tibial component.*

a tibial osteotomy or in whom the lateral, rather than the medial, femorotibial compartment is involved. All reported series of high tibial osteotomies point out that the results following correction of valgus deformity in patients with lateral femorotibial compartment involvement are less satisfactory than are the results of correction for medial femorotibial compartment involvement.[55] For this reason, prosthetic replacement of the damaged femoral and tibial surfaces in the medial femorotibial compartment is now widely performed (Fig. 24–11). Although there are few reports in the literature, presentations of large series suggest that the results are excellent in more than 90 per cent of the patients on short-term follow-up examination.[56] Whether or not the presence of artificial components in one compartment of the knee will lead to premature degeneration in the less involved compartment is unknown, but the possibility suggests caution in the application of this principle.[57]

Arthroplasties may be conveniently divided into two groups: anatomic and substitution arthroplasties. *Anatomic arthroplasty* is an attempt to duplicate the normal contours and functions of the joint. In the hip, a ball-and-socket joint, anatomic replacement is mechanically simple. The acetabulum is replaced with a cup of high density polyethylene while the femoral head is replaced with a metallic ball affixed to an intramedullary stem (Fig. 24–12). In recent years, analysis of long-term failures suggests that the intramedullary stem may be the site of late loosening by virtue of its bypassing the usual cortical support in the proximal femur.[58] For this reason, recent developments have suggested that "surface replacement" may have some advantages[59, 73] (Fig. 24–13). In this procedure, the head of the femur is replaced with a metallic cup cemented onto the cancellous bone of the femoral head. The neck is retained, and forces are transferred from the prosthetic joint along the normal cancellous structure to the cortex of the proximal femur. Theoretically, this should provide two long-term advantages: Retention of the normal route of load-bearing in the proximal femur should diminish the incidence of late loosening seen in devices with intramedullary stems, and, in the case of failure, more bone stock will remain for a revision procedure. Whether or not these theoretic advantages will be realized remains to be seen. Early series of surface replacements have demonstrated a 20 to 30 per cent incidence of loosening of the femoral component, which later technical refinements may diminish, but patients with inflammatory arthritis demonstrate prosthetic loosening more frequently than patients with degenerative arthritis and, in addition, sustain fractures of the femoral neck more frequently.[60, 61] In addition, technical con-

Text continued on page 811

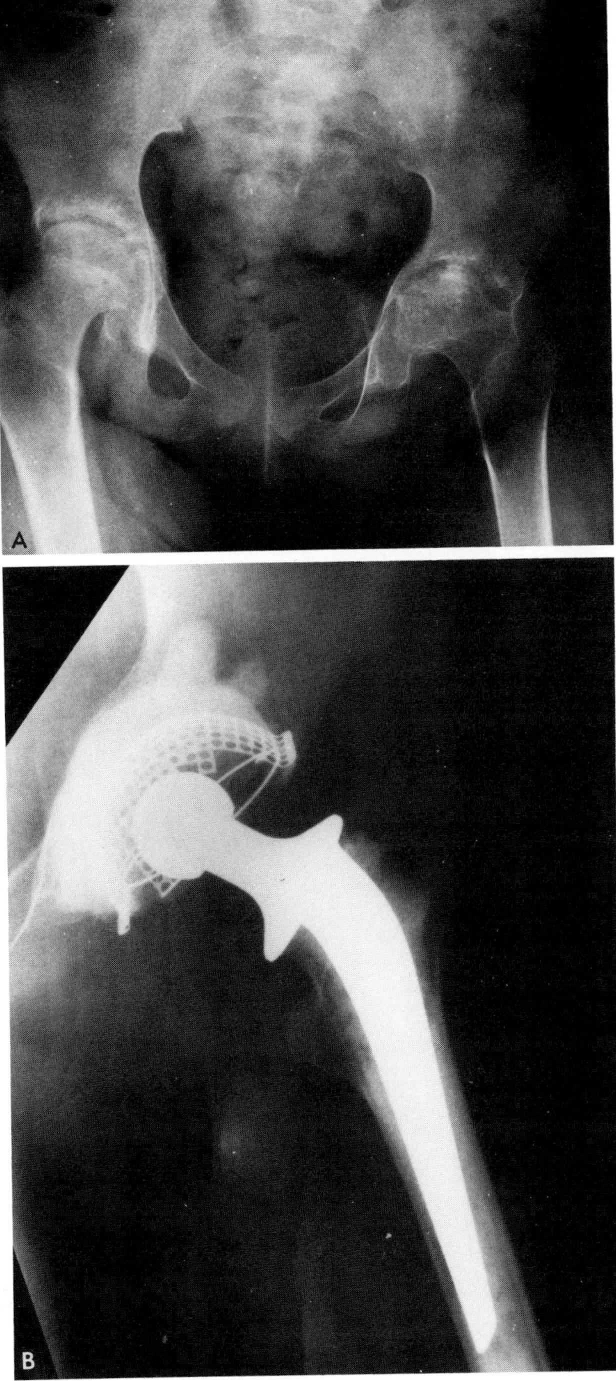

Figure 24–12. *This patient with juvenile rheumatoid arthritis (juvenile chronic arthritis) had achieved skeletal maturity but was severely incapacitated by pain and lack of hip motion.*

A *Preoperative radiograph showing destruction of the normal architecture of the left hip with the development of a protrusio acetabuli deformity. The right hip is also affected.*

B *Postoperative radiograph showing replacement of the left hip as well as correction of the protrusio acetabuli with the use of a metallic mesh to exteriorize the acetabular component to a normal position. Pain was relieved and function was greatly improved.*

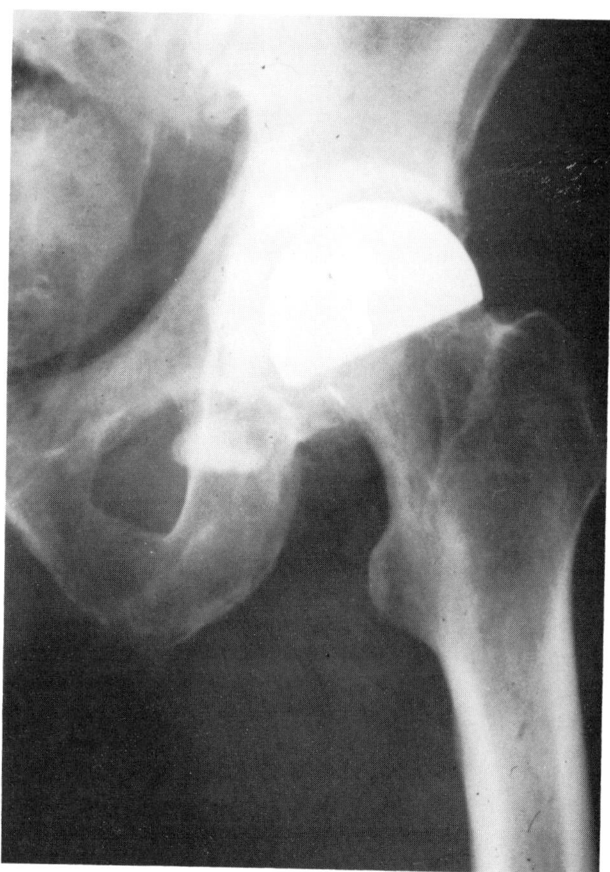

Figure 24–13. In younger patients, there are some theoretic advantages to preserving the femoral head and neck at the time of arthroplasty. This patient underwent "surface replacement" utilizing a plastic acetabular replacement and a metal cup cemented onto the prepared femoral head.

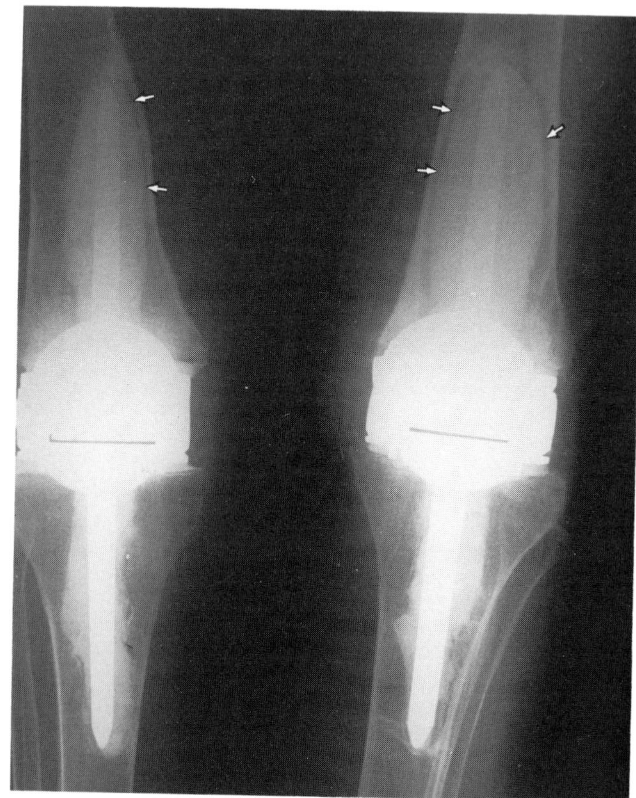

Figure 24–14. Metallic hinges, previously used to replace the knee, provided inadequate freedom of motion and transferred excessive stresses to the bone-cement interface, producing loosening. In this postoperative radiograph taken 2 years after hinge replacement of both knees, wide radiolucent zones (marked by arrows) are seen. Stress views demonstrated motion of the prosthesis-cement complex, and the patient had pain on weight-bearing.

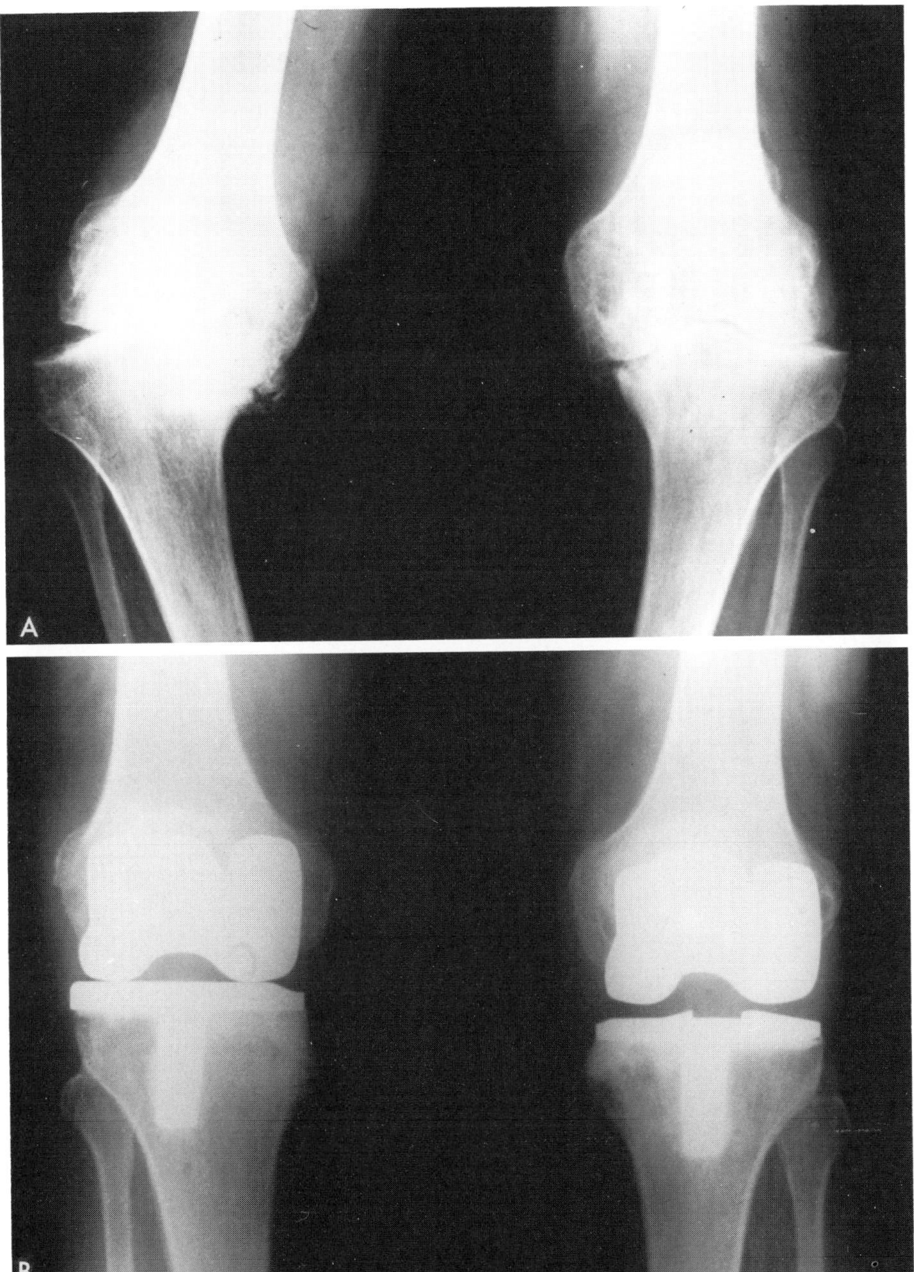

Figure 24–15. *Severe deformities of the knee can be corrected with modern knee replacement techniques.*

A *Preoperative radiograph of a patient with severe arthritis (probably osteoarthritis) and varus deformities of both knees. On the right there is lateral subluxation of the tibia as well as marked loss of proximal tibial bone. On the left side similar, but less severe, changes are seen.*

B *Postoperative radiograph following total knee arthroplasty. The deformities have been corrected and the joint surfaces have been replaced by metal and plastic components, providing nearly normal motion and relief of pain.*

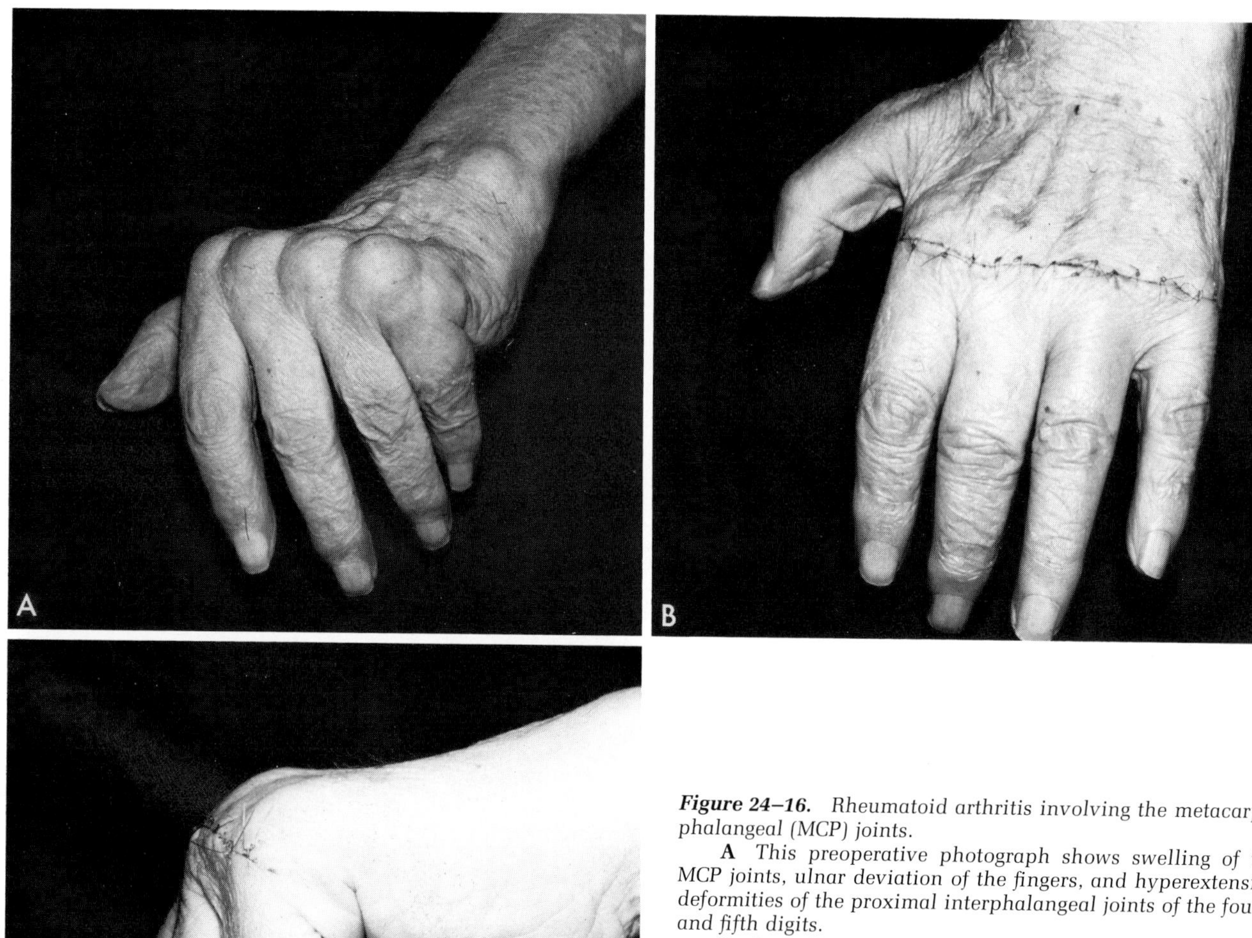

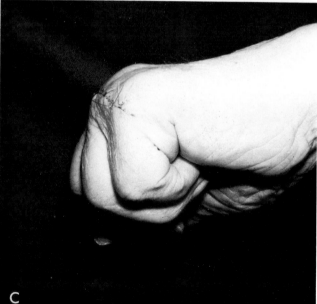

Figure 24–16. *Rheumatoid arthritis involving the metacarpophalangeal (MCP) joints.*

A *This preoperative photograph shows swelling of the MCP joints, ulnar deviation of the fingers, and hyperextension deformities of the proximal interphalangeal joints of the fourth and fifth digits.*

B *Immediate postoperative photograph showing correction of the ulnar drift with implantation of silicone rubber spacers replacing the metacarpophalangeal joints of the second, third, fourth, and fifth fingers.*

C *Restoration of biomechanical function of the hand enables the patient to flex the fingers normally, allowing fine pinch and grasp.*

(Courtesy of Lewis H. Millender, M.D.)

siderations dictate that the polyethylene acetabular component must be very thin. Whether or not this thin polyethylene cup will stand up for long periods of time is problematic.

Substitution arthroplasty recognizes the difficulty of anatomic duplication and substitutes simpler motions for the complex motions found in normal joints. The knee is an excellent example; one of the most complex joints in the body, it normally performs gliding, sliding, and rotating motions during each gait cycle. During its motion, the functional "axis" through which the knee moves changes constantly. To duplicate this complex function in a prosthetic knee has been difficult. Early devices, therefore, substituted a uniaxial artificial joint such as a hinge. Numerous series have now demonstrated quite clearly that this is an inappropriate choice of prosthesis and that the incidence of late loosening in such uniaxial hinges is unacceptably high (Fig. 24–14). In addition, most of the hinges involved a metal-to-metal articulation, which, for unknown reasons, carried a 10 to 15 per cent incidence of late infection.[62] More recent efforts, therefore, have been to provide anatomic replacements for the knee (Fig. 24–15), duplicating the multiaxial function of the normal knee and transferring stresses away from the weak bone-cement interface into the ligaments and other surrounding soft tissues, where these forces may be safely dissipated.[63] In the upper extremity, substitution arthroplasties have been somewhat more successful. Here, silicone spacers ("flexible hinges") have been used in the elbow, wrist, and metacarpophalangeal and interphalangeal joints. In the metacarpophalangeal joint, in which surgical experience is great, the results have been quite good[64] (Fig. 24–16). Breakage of early prostheses was common, but newer, improved materials promise to have greater longevity.[65] In the wrist and elbow, however, silicone hinges have been less satisfactory. Experience with hinge replacement of the knee joint suggests that simple hinges will not suffice in either the elbow[66] or the wrist, and current efforts are being directed toward the development of semiconstrained, nonlinked replacements for both these joints.[39, 67]

POSTOPERATIVE MANAGEMENT

The role of physical therapy in the postoperative management of patients undergoing joint replacement surgery has not been clearly defined. Controlled prospective studies are notably lacking. The nearly universal acceptance of the importance of postoperative physical therapy is based on personal experience. The requirements for such therapy appear to vary from one joint to another. For example, Charnley does not advocate postoperative physical therapy for patients undergoing hip replacements.[5] His early and late follow-up studies suggest that physical therapy may play a minimal role in the rehabilitation of the patients. At the other extreme is the clear-cut advantage of careful and prolonged therapy following surgery of the hand.[41] Regardless of the lack of scientific evidence essentially all surgeons with experience in the field of joint replacement surgery are convinced that the active participation of both the patient and the physical therapist in a postoperative exercise program will improve muscle strength, increase motion, and educate the patient in proper protection of the joint.

Orthoses are frequently useful following reconstructive surgery of the upper extremity, where they may function either as static devices to maintain position and prevent deformity or as dynamic devices to aid in the restoration of motion and strength.[41] In the lower extremity, the most frequently used orthotic device is the crutch.[40] Its function is to protect weakened muscles until they become strong, prevent falls as the patient learns to function with a new prosthetic joint, and protect the bone-cement interface until healing can occur, minimizing, it is hoped, the complication of late prosthetic loosening.

Radiographic evaluation, critical in the preoperative assessment of the need for surgery and the proper technical approach, is the mainstay of the postoperative evaluation. Parameters to be assessed are the alignment of the prosthetic components, the adequacy of cement fixation, the restoration of joint alignment, and the detection of postoperative loosening as indicated by the development of a radiolucent zone between the barium-impregnated methacrylate cement and the bone. Numerous studies of prosthetic placement in the hip have indicated the undesirability of a varus configuration to the femoral component as well as the increased incidence of prosthetic loosening in patients with incomplete filling of the proximal femur with methacrylate and voids in the methacrylate. Increased rates of dislocation have been noted with retroverted femoral components or excessively abducted acetabular components.[68] In the knee, late loosening has been correlated with faulty alignment of the prosthetic components,[69] and the development of a radiolucent line, particularly at the bone-cement interface on the tibial side, has given early warning that certain prosthetic designs are inappropriate.[70]

Since prosthetic loosening is a time-related complication and infection may be delayed in appearance, indefinite follow-up of patients undergoing joint arthroplasty is necessary. If early signs of prosthetic loosening develop, decrease in joint loading by appropriate use of crutches and avoidance of strenuous activities may prevent or slow the progress of such loosening. Because of evidence that patients with artificial joints continue to be at some increased risk for hematogenous infection,[71] careful attention must be devoted to the prevention of infection anywhere in the body and its prompt recognition and treatment. We recommend that patients utilize prophylactic antibiotics before dental or urologic procedures and that they be aware of the potential danger of untreated infections and seek early medical attention.

SUMMARY

In spite of the dramatic advances in joint replacement surgery in the last two decades, all such procedures must still be considered evolutionary. Continuing changes in design, surgical technique, and materials have led to rapid surgical improvements in some joints and slower improvements in other joints, such as the hip. For this reason, such surgery should be delayed as long as possible in patients who continue to function at a satisfactory level with tolerable discomfort. The old and reliable procedures such as arthrodesis and osteotomy should be utilized when appropriate, especially in younger patients. One clear lesson gained from experience with joint replacements is that the more anatomic the replacement, the greater its long-term success is likely to be. The other clear lesson is that there is a close and obvious relationship between the technical expertise with which an arthroplasty is performed and its immediate and ultimate functional result. New materials for prosthetic replacement and for fixation of prosthetic devices to bone will certainly be developed. Clearer understanding of normal joint anatomy and function will result in improved anatomic designs with greater life expectancy. Functional analysis of large numbers of patients who have undergone arthroplasty will determine the appropriate indications for surgery and the choice of prosthetic designs, but medical judgment in selecting patients for surgery and precise surgical technique during the operation will remain the dominant aspects in the surgical management of arthritis.

REFERENCES

1. Burton KE, Wright V, Richards J: Patients' expectations in relation to outcome of total hip replacement surgery. Ann Rheum Dis *38*:471, 1979.
2. Jergesen HE, Poss R, Sledge CB: Bilateral total hip and knee replacement in adults with rheumatoid arthritis. An evaluation of function. Clin Orthop Rel Res *137*:120, 1978.
3. Taylor DG: The costs of arthritis and the benefits of joint replacement surgery. Proc R Soc Lond *192-B*:145, 1976.
4. Wilcock GK: Benefits of total hip replacement to older patients and the community. Br Med J *2*:37, 1978.
5. Charnley J: Low Friction Arthroplasty of the Hip. Theory and Practice. New York, Springer-Verlag, 1979.
6. Poss R, Ewald FC, Thomas WH, Sledge CB: Complications of total hip replacement arthroplasty in patients with rheumatoid arthritis. J Bone Joint Surg *58A*:1130, 1976.
7. Gristina AG, Rovere GD, Shoji H: Spontaneous septic arthritis complicating rheumatoid arthritis. J Bone Joint Surg *56A*:1180, 1974.
8. Kellgren JH, Ball J, Fairbrother RW, Barnes KL: Suppurative arthritis complicating rheumatoid arthritis. Br Med J *1*:1193, 1958.
9. Poss R, Sledge CB: Total hip replacement in rheumatoid arthritis. *In* I Goldie (Ed): Reconstruction Surgery and Traumatology. Vol 18. Rheumatoid Surgery. New York, S Karger (in press).
10. Garner RW, Mowat AG, Hazelman BL: Wound healing after operations on patients with rheumatoid arthritis. J Bone Joint Surg *55B*:134, 1973.
11. Foker JE, Schwartz R, Smith DC, Matas A: Surgical problems in immunodeficient and immunosuppressed children. Surg Clin North Am *59*:213, 1979.
12. O'Loughlin JM: Infections in the immunosuppressed patient. Med Clin North Am *59*:495, 1975.
13. Burry HC: Penicillamine and wound healing — a potential hazard? Postgrad Med J *50*:75, 1974.
14. Deshmukh K, Nimni ME: A defect in the intramolecular and intermolecular cross-linking of collagen caused by penicillamine. J Biol Chem *244*:1787, 1969.
15. Schorn D, Mowat AG: Penicillamine in rheumatoid arthritis: Wound healing, skin thickness and osteoporosis. Rheumatol Rehabil *16*:223, 1977.
16. Cooke TD, Richer S, Hurd E, Jasin HE: Localization of antigen-antibody complexes in intra-articular collagenous tissues. Ann NY Acad Sci *256*:10, 1975.
17. Ohno O, Cooke TD: Electron microscopic morphology of immunoglobulin aggregates and their interactions in rheumatoid articular collagenous tissues. Arthritis Rheum. *21*:516, 1978.
18. Fell HB, Jubb RW: The effect of synovial tissue on the breakdown of articular cartilage in organ culture. Arthritis Rheum *20*:1359, 1977.
19. Steinberg J, Sledge CB, Noble J, Stirrat CR: A tissue-culture model of cartilage breakdown in rheumatoid arthritis. Biochem J *180*:403, 1979.
20. Robinson DR, Tashjian AH Jr, Levine L: Prostaglandin-stimulated bone resorption by rheumatoid synovia. A possible mechanism for bone destruction in rheumatoid arthritis. J Clin Invest *56*:1181, 1975.
21. Kennedy AC, Allam BF, Boyle IT, Nuki C, Rooney PJ, Buchanan WW: Abnormalities in mineral metabolism suggestive of parathyroid overactivity in rheumatoid arthritis. Curr Med Res Opin *3*:345, 1975.
22. Kennedy AC, Allam BF, Rooney PJ, Watson ME, Fairney A, Buchanan KD, Hillyard CJ: Hypercalcaemia in rheumatoid arthritis: Investigation of its causes and implications. Ann Rheum Dis *38*:401, 1979.
23. Bisla RS, Inglis AE, Ranawat CS: Joint replacement surgery in patients under thirty. J Bone Joint Surg *58A*:1098, 1976.
24. Singsen BH, Isaacson AS, Bernstein BH, Patzakis MJ, Kornreich HK, King KK, Hanson V: Total hip replacement in children with arthritis. Arthritis Rheum *21*:401, 1978.
25. Sledge CB: Joint replacement surgery in juvenile rheumatoid arthritis. Arthritis Rheum *20*:567, 1977.
26. Conway W, Bower G, Barnes M: Hypersomnolence and intermittent upper airway obstruction. Occurrence caused by micrognathia. JAMA *237*:2740, 1977.
27. Bryan RS, Scott WT, Bickel WH: Results of surgical management of the hip in patients with rheumatoid arthritis or rheumatoid spondylitis. *In* RL Cruess, NS Mitchell (Eds.): Surgery of Rheumatoid Arthritis. Philadelphia, JB Lippincott, 1971, p 63.
28. Ritter MA, Vaughan RB: Ectopic ossification after total hip arthroplasty: Predisposing factors, frequency and effect on results. J Bone Joint Surg *59A*:345, 1977.
29. Williams E, Taylor AR, Arden GP, Edwards DH: Arthroplasty of the hip in ankylosing spondylitis. J Bone Joint Surg *59B*:393, 1977.
30. Aly R, Maibach HI, Mandel A: Bacterial flora in psoriasis. Br J Dermatol *95*:603, 1976.
31. Lambert JR, Wright V: Surgery in patients with psoriasis and arthritis. Rheumatol Rehabil *18*:35, 1979.
32. Marples RR, Heaton CL, Kligman AM: *Staphylococcus aureus* in psoriasis. Arch Dermatol *107*:568, 1973.
33. Griffiths ID, Maini RN, Scott JT: Clinical and radiological features of osteonecrosis in systemic lupus erythematosus. Ann Rheum Dis *38*:413, 1979.
34. Nakano KK: Neurologic complications of rheumatoid arthritis. Orthop Clin North Am *6*:861, 1975.
35. Rana NA, Hancock DO, Taylor AR, Hill AGS: Upward translocation of the dens in rheumatoid arthritis. J Bone Joint Surg *55B*:471, 1973.
36. Rana NA, Hancock DO, Taylor AR, Hill AGS: Atlanto-axial subluxation in rheumatoid arthritis. J Bone Joint Surg *55B*:458, 1973.

37. Poss R: Total hip replacement in the patient with rheumatoid arthritis. *In* American Academy of Orthopedic Surgeons: Instructional Course Lectures. Vol 28. St. Louis, CV Mosby Co, 1979, p 298.
38. Millender LH, Nalebuff EA: Arthrodesis of the rheumatoid wrist. An evaluation of sixty patients and a description of a different surgical technique. J Bone Joint Surg *55A*:1026, 1973.
39. Volz RG: Total wrist arthroplasty: A new approach to wrist disability. Clin Orthop Rel Res *128*:180, 1977.
40. Convery FR, Minteer MA: The use of orthoses in the management of rheumatoid arthritis. Clin Orthop Rel Res *102*:118, 1974.
41. Melvin JL: Rheumatic Disease: Occupational Therapy and Rehabilitation. Philadelphia, FA Davis Co, 1977.
42. Benjamin A: Double osteotomy for the painful knee in rheumatoid arthritis and osteoarthritis. J Bone Joint Surg *51B*:694, 1969.
43. Simmons EH: Surgery of the spine in rheumatoid arthritis and ankylosing spondylitis. *In* RL Cruess, NS Mitchell (Eds): Surgery of Rheumatoid Arthritis. Philadelphia, JB Lippincott, 1971, p 93.
44. Coventry MB: Osteotomy about the knee for degenerative and rheumatoid arthritis. J Bone Joint Surg *55A*:23, 1973.
45. MacIntosh DL, Welsh RP: Joint debridement — a complement to high tibial osteotomy in the treatment of degenerative arthritis of the knee. J Bone Joint Surg *59A*:1094, 1977.
46. Muller ME: Intertrochanteric osteotomies in adults: Planning and operating technique. *In* RL Cruess, NS Mitchell (Eds): Surgical Management of Degenerative Arthritis of the Lower Limb. Philadelphia, Lea & Febiger, 1975, p 53.
47. Demottaz JD, Mazur JM, Thomas WH, Sledge CB, Simon SR: Clinical study of total ankle replacement with gait analysis. A preliminary report. J Bone Joint Surg *61A*:976, 1979.
48. Thomas WH: Rheumatoid arthritis of the ankle and foot. *In*: American College of Orthopaedic Surgeons: Instructional Course Lectures. Vol. 28. St Louis, CV Mosby Co, 1979, p 325.
49. Ferlic DC, Clayton ML, Leidholt JD, Gamble WE: Surgical treatment of the symptomatic unstable cervical spine in rheumatoid arthritis. J Bone Joint Surg *57A*:349, 1975.
50. Solomon L, Aufranc OE: Vitallium mold arthroplasty of the hip in rheumatoid arthritis. Arthritis Rheum *5*:37, 1962.
51. Harris WH: The role of cup arthroplasty in contemporary reconstructive surgery of the hip: A reappraisal. *In* RL Cruess, NS Mitchell (Eds): Surgical Management of Degenerative Arthritis of the Lower Limb. Philadelphia, Lea & Febiger, 1975, p 79.
52. Potter TA, Weinfeld MS, Thomas WH: Arthroplasty of the knee in rheumatoid arthritis and osteoarthritis. J Bone Joint Surg *54A*:1, 1972.
53. MacIntosh, DL: Arthroplasty of the knee in rheumatoid arthritis using the hemiarthroplasty prosthesis. *In* RL Cruess, NS Mitchell (Eds): Surgery of Rheumatoid Arthritis. Philadelphia, JB Lippincott, 1971, p 29.
54. Insall J, Scott WN, Ranawat CS: The total condylar knee prosthesis. A report of 220 cases. J Bone Joint Surg *61A*:173, 1979.
55. Shoji H, Insall JN: High-tibial osteotomy for osteoarthritis of the knee with valgus deformity. J Bone Joint Surg *55A*:963, 1973.
56. Marmor L: Marmor modular knee in unicompartmental disease. Minimum 4-year follow up. J Bone Joint Surg *61A*:347, 1979.
57. Insall JN, Ranawat CS, Aglietti P, Shine J: A comparison of 4 models of total knee replacement prostheses. J Bone Joint Surg *58A*:754, 1976.
58. Coventry MB, Beckenbaugh RD, Nolan DR, Ilstrup DM: 2012 total hip arthroplasties: A study of postoperative course and early complications. J Bone Joint Surg *56A*:273, 1974.
59. Freeman MAR: Editorial Comment: Total surface replacement hip arthroplasty. Clin Orthop Rel Res *134*:2, 1978.
60. Wagner H: Surface replacement arthroplasty of the hip. Clin Orthop Rel Res *134*:102, 1978.
61. Freeman MAR, Cameron HU, Brown GC: Cemented double cup arthroplasty of the hip: A 5 year experience with the ICLH prosthesis. Clin Orthop Rel Res *134*:45, 1978.
62. Sledge CB, Thomas WH, Arbuckle RH: Hinge arthroplasty of the knee. *In* CM Evarts (Ed): Symposium on Reconstructive Surgery of the Knee, Rochester, NY, 1976. St. Louis, CV Mosby Co, 1978, p 344.
63. Ewald FC: Surgery of the knee in rheumatoid arthritis. *In* American Academy of Orthopaedic Surgeons: Instructional Course Lectures. Vol. 28. St Louis, CV Mosby Co, 1978, p 285.
64. Swanson AB: Silicone rubber implants for replacement of arthritic or destroyed joints in the hand. Surg Clin North Am *48*:1113, 1968.
65. Ferlic DC, Clayton ML, Holloway M: Complications of silicone implant surgery in the metacarpophalangeal joint. J Bone Joint Surg *57A*:991, 1975.
66. Garrett JC, Ewald FC, Thomas WH, Sledge CB: Loosening associated with GSB hinge total elbow replacement in patients with rheumatoid arthritis. Clin Orthop Rel Res *127*:170, 1977.
67. Ewald FC, Thomas WH, Sledge CB, Poss R: Non-constrained metal-to-plastic elbow arthroplasty in rheumatoid arthritis. *In* Joint Replacement in the Upper Limb. London, Mechanical Engineering Publication Ltd, 1977, p 77.
68. Coventry MB, Beckenbaugh RD, Nolan DR, Ilstrup DM: 2012 Total hip arthroplasties: A study of postoperative course and early complications. J Bone Joint Surg *56A*:273, 1974.
69. Lotke PA, Ecker ML: Influence of positioning of prosthesis in total knee replacement. J Bone Joint Surg *59A*:77, 1977.
70. Cracchiolo A III (Ed): Statistics of total knee replacement. Clin. Orthop *120*:1976 (entire volume).
71. D'Ambrosia RD, Shoji H, Heater R: Secondarily infected total joint replacements by hematogenous spread. J Bone Joint Surg *58A*:450, 1976.
72. Poss R, Sledge CB: Rheumatoid arthritis patients are at increased risk to develop infection following total joint replacement (Abstr). Arthritis Rheum *23*:733, 1980.
73. Goldie IF, Bunketorp O, Gunterberg B, Hansson T, Myrhage R: Resurfacing arthroplasty of the hip. Arch Orthop Traumat Surg *95*:149, 1979.

RADIOGRAPHIC EVALUATION OF THE POSTOPERATIVE PATIENT

by Thomas Goergen, M.D.

25

A large variety of surgical procedures are available to the orthopedic surgeon for treatment of pain, joint instability, or decreased range of motion. Extra-articular procedures (e.g., osteotomy) or intra-articular procedures (e.g., arthrodesis and replacement arthroplasty) may be performed. It is important for the radiologist to understand the treatment goals of the various procedures, as well as the normal postoperative appearance and the long-term implications. Without this fundamental appreciation, the radiologist may encounter difficulty distinguishing normal appearances from complications, and will be unable to recognize such complications at an early stage.

A description of every available articular and periarticular procedure is beyond the scope of this chapter; newer techniques are appearing at a rapid rate and, in many instances, are superseding older procedures. However, from a study of some of the available procedures, one can appreciate certain principles that can then be utilized to evaluate newer operations as they appear.

MATERIAL TECHNOLOGY

Metal Arthroplasty Components

Metal implants used in orthopedic surgery most commonly consist of one of the following materials: stainless steel, cobalt-chromium-molybdenum alloy, cobalt-chromium-tungsten alloy, tantalum, or titanium.[1] A total joint arthroplasty may consist of a metal component articulating with either another metal component (metal-metal) or a polyethylene (metal-plastic) component. Friction between various metal-metal and metal-plastic prostheses is greater than that between normal articular cartilage, and ultimately these forces may result in wear of the components and transmission of increased forces across the joint, affecting implant fixation.[2]

Metal-metal prostheses gradually produce large amounts of metallic wear particles in the tissues, whereas fewer metallic fragments are generated by metal-plastic implants.[6, 7] These particles, consisting mainly of cobalt, chromium, and nickel, are released into the periarticular tissues and subsequently pass into the bloodstream.[3] Patch testing has shown an increased incidence of metal sensitivity in patients following placement of metal-metal prostheses.[4, 8, 9, 171] Although less common, allergic reactions may also occur with metal-plastic prostheses.[10, 163] Development of hypersensitivity to metallic wear products has been implicated in some patients who exhibit a severe local tissue reaction with sterile discharge and bone necrosis, which ultimately may result in prosthesis loosening.[3, 5, 8] The issue is clouded by other design defects in these prostheses and by reports of similar local tissue reactions in some patients without demonstrable hypersensitivity.[9, 11] Of interest, cobalt may be carcinogenic in experimental animals, but no cases of sarcomas in humans attributed to cobalt have been reported.[12]

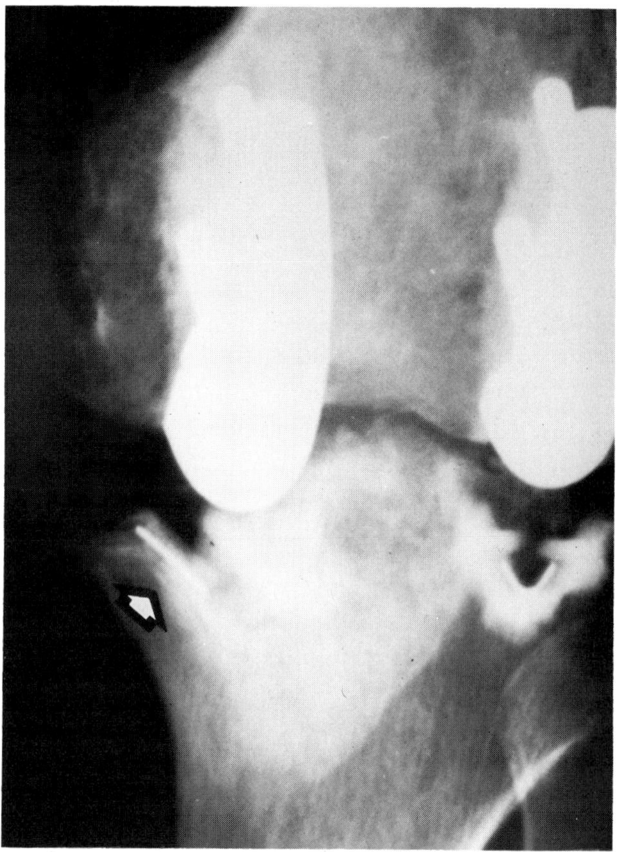

Figure 25–1. Polycentric total knee arthroplasty showing separation of marker wire from medial tibial component (arrow). There was no evidence of component loosening. The wire was subsequently removed via small skin incision.

Ultra High Molecular Weight Polyethylene (UHMWP)

The best combination of currently available materials for joint replacement consists of a metal component articulating with an ultra high molecular weight polyethylene (UHMWP) component. The utilization of a polyethylene-metal interface produces the lowest friction and longest wear properties of currently available implants.[1, 13, 14] UHMWP allows some degree of plastic deformity, which improves congruity between sliding surfaces as the load increases, in turn distributing bearing forces more evenly. Because of the ductility of the plastic, its initial surface finish is less critical than that of the apposing metal surface, whose imperfections may cause a high wear rate of the plastic. When hard and soft materials are used as apposing bearing surfaces, the concave surface is made of the softer material, to take advantage of plastic deformity and to place the softer material in a less stressful situation.

The exterior surfaces of plastic components have grooves or furrows to improve fixation with bone cement. As UHMWP is radiolucent, various metallic wires may be embedded in the external grooves, serving as locator markers for evaluation of alignment, changes in position, and wear.[15] Occasionally a marker wire may detach and migrate from the plastic component (Fig. 25–1). Fixation of plastic hip components to bone is facilitated by drilling holes at various sites in the acetabulum, creating a mechanical anchor. Preshaped fine wire mesh cement retainers may be inserted into these sites, to restrict excessive entry of acrylic bone cement into the pelvis (see Fig. 25–11).

UHMWP components shed wear particles, which may be differentiated histologically from acrylic bone cement.[16, 170] Hypersensitivity or local tissue reaction attributed to UHMWP has not been reported. However, as these prostheses are used in younger patients, debris may accumulate over many years, and the possibility of some reaction to UHMWP cannot be excluded. Although all polymers tested under certain experimental conditions produce tumors in rats, a relationship between plastic implants and malignant change in humans has not been reported.[17]

Polymethylmethacrylate (PMM) Bone Cement

An acrylic bone cement consisting of polymethylmethacrylate (PMM) is used to bond various arthroplasty components.[18-20] It may also be used in fixation of pathologic fractures, often in combination with metallic devices.[21, 22] Acrylic cement does not act as an adhesive or glue; rather, it forms an accurate cast at the interface between the bone and the prosthetic component, facilitating a more perfect mechanical fit, which results in an even distribution of the load over the system, and provides a more gradual transition in elasticity from metal or UHMWP to bone.

PMM cement is prepared at the time of surgery by mixing liquid monomer with powdered polymerized material. Polymerization of the cement results in an exothermic reaction, which causes a temperature increase at the bone-cement interface.[23, 24] Setting of the cement is nearly complete 10 min after mixing, although continued hardening occurs over several hours. Slight contraction (up to 5 per cent) appears with curing.[25]

Currently most bone cement is rendered radiopaque by the addition of 10 per cent barium sulfate during manufacture. Radiopaque PMM bone cement allows evaluation of the prosthesis-cement and bone-cement interfaces as well as radiographic visualization of the distribution of cement and detection of cement fractures or loose fragments. The actual distribution of bone cement around the entire circumference of the prosthetic components has been shown by experimental computed tomography and gross analysis to be less uniform than suspected on routine radiographs.[26] The possibility of allergic reaction to methylmethacrylate has been considered in the etiology of local tissue reaction or loosening of prostheses, but sensitivity to PMM bone cement has not been demonstrated.[27, 28]

Metal-Cement Interface

The interface between a metallic component and bone cement has received less attention than the bone-cement interface. Although the metal-cement interface exhibits fewer problems than the bone-cement interface, alterations at the metal-cement junction may occasionally lead to failure of the system.[29]

Histologic examination of a small series of radiographically normal femoral prostheses disclosed in each case a thin layer of tissue interposed between the metal and the cement.[30] This layer measures 100 micrometers or less in thickness and consists of organizing fibrous tissue containing living fibroblasts. Nourishment of this avascular fibrous layer apparently comes from diffusion of fluid entering at the collar of the prosthesis. Such diffusion implies micromotion of the metal stem within the surrounding cocoon of bone cement. Thermal expansion of the metal stem with subsequent contraction, or contraction of the bone cement itself, has been implicated in the generation of this microscopic space. In some cases, an actual gap may be left if bone cement does not fill the entire space around the metal stem. These phenomena do not adequately explain larger radiolucent areas or progressively increasing lucent regions at the metal-cement interface noted in some cases.

Bone-Cement Interface

Use of barium-impregnated polymethylmethacrylate bone cement allows visualization of the relationship of the cement to the adjacent bone. Ideally, the radiopaque cement should occupy all the spaces between a prosthetic component and adjacent bone; no gaps or spaces should be noted. A thin radiolucent zone may develop along the bone-cement interface in normal patients during the first 6 postoperative months (Fig. 25–9). Since radiolucent zones are also noted in patients with prosthetic loosening or infection, radiographic evaluation must consider the time of appearance, length, width, and progression of such zones to differentiate normal phenomena from complications. Many factors have been implicated in the development of radiolucent zones in normal patients. These phenomena are considered in greater detail later in this chapter.

Elastomers

Polydimethylsiloxane (silicone rubber or Silastic)* or polypropylene prostheses have limited application, with use restricted primarily to the wrist, the hand, and the foot. Medical grade silicones are a combination of quartz, silicone, and oxygen atoms. The product is heat-stable, chemically inert, nonallergenic, and nonadhesive. Silicone joint replacements are generally fabricated as single-piece integral hinge prostheses for replacement of the metacarpophalangeal and proximal interphalangeal joints of the fingers and the carpometacarpal joint of the thumb. The design is simple and relatively inexpensive; a single-piece prosthesis with each stem inserted into the intramedullary cavity allows flexion and extension and provides lateral stability. The Swanson type of prosthesis uses the same grade of silicone rubber throughout, whereas the stems of the Niebauer type are coated with a Dacron mesh that is eventually infiltrated by soft tissue[31, 32] (Figs. 25–2 and 25–3). Most of these prostheses do not require fixation of the stem; the prosthesis is encapsulated and held in place by periarticular fibrous tissue. The lack of need for fixation simplifies insertion and may help distribute stresses over a wide area. The slight

*Silasfic, Dow Corning Corporation, Midland, MI 48640.

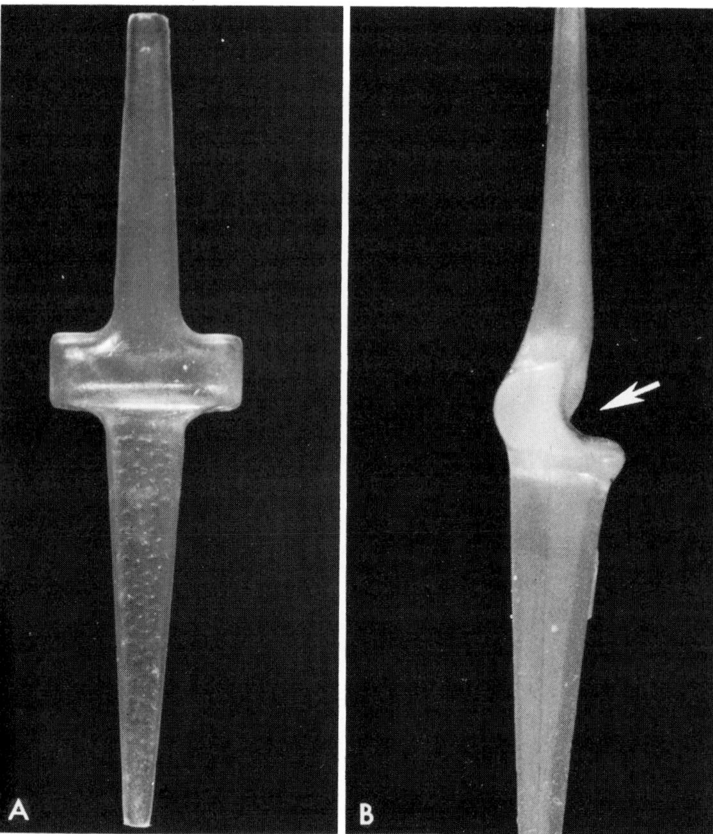

Figure 25–2. Swanson metacarpophalangeal prosthesis. **A**, Dorsal aspect; **B**, lateral aspect. The metacarpal stem is longer. A concavity on the volar aspect allows flexion (arrow).

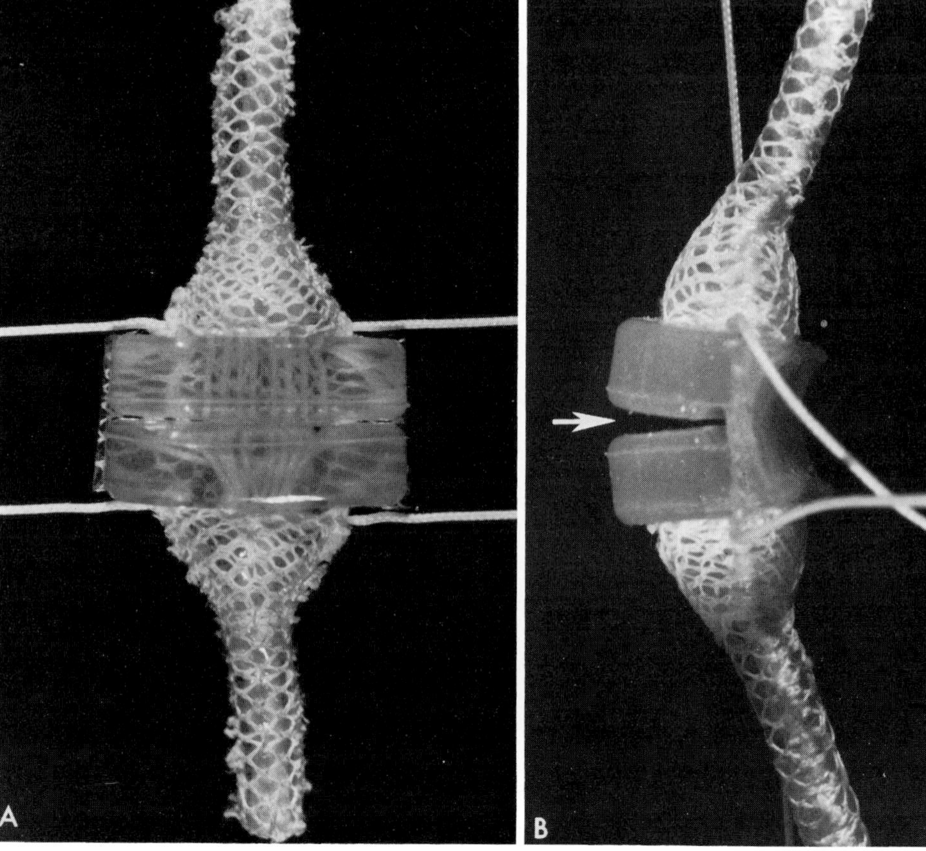

Figure 25–3. Niebauer metacarpophalangeal prosthesis. **A**, Dorsal aspect; **B**, lateral aspect. Both stems covered with Dacron mesh, which is subsequently infiltrated by soft tissue. Sutures are included for fixation. The hinge opens dorsally in flexion (arrow).

motion permitted also allows the implant to find the most functional position. Occasionally, the stems may be fixed in place with suture material or bone cement.

Under laboratory conditions, silicone rubber prostheses are extremely durable, without failure after millions of flexions.[33] Some signs of wear and deterioration have been noted in prostheses that have been removed from humans.[34, 35]

THE HIP

Total Hip Replacement Arthroplasty (THA)

The first successful total hip replacement was performed by McKee and Farrar in 1951, using metal-metal components composed of cobalt-chromium alloy.[36] In recent years, low-friction metal-plastic total hip arthroplasties, which evolved from initial designs and testing by Charnley during the early 1960s have been most commonly employed.[37] Since their initial development, thousands of THA have been performed, representing the most effective therapy for the treatment of advanced arthritic disease of the hip.

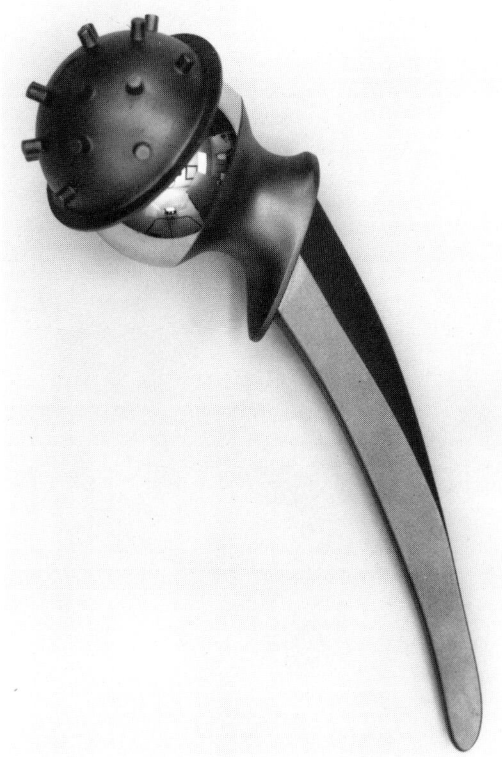

Figure 25–4. *McKee-Farrar total hip arthroplasty (THA). In this type there is metal-metal articulation. The protrusions on the acetabular component aid in fixation.*

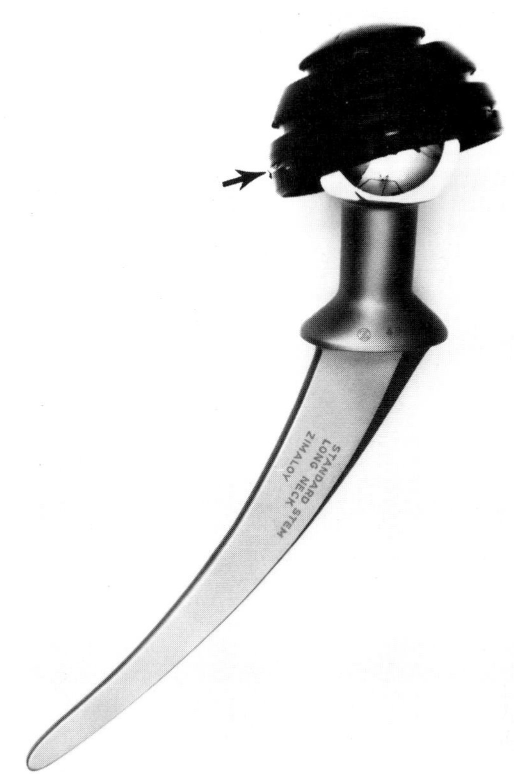

Figure 25–5. *Charnley type THA. The ultra high molecular weight polyethylene (UHMWP) grooved acetabular cup articulates with a metallic femoral component. A locater wire is embedded in the groove (arrow).*

The most common indication for THA is "primary" or secondary osteoarthritis. Rheumatoid arthritis and seronegative spondyloarthropathies constitute additional indications. THA may also be used as a salvage operation for other procedures that have failed or were used as temporary measures prior to a planned THA. Such preexisting procedures include hip fusion, excision arthroplasty of the proximal femur, cup arthroplasty, failed femoral prosthesis, prior THA, and osteotomy. Clinically, the ideal objectives of treatment include relief of pain, increased range of motion, and improved level of function. Relief of pain is expected in all cases, and improved range of motion and function is common. Eight-five to 90 per cent of patients followed for 4 to 5 years have good or excellent results in these clinical parameters.[38]

There are two basic types of THA. A metallic acetabular component articulating with a metallic femoral component is represented both by the McKee-Farrar THA, which is cemented in place, and by the noncemented Ring prosthesis (Fig. 25–4). The other basic type of THA consists of an UHMWP acetabular component articulating with a metallic femoral component; the Charnley and Charnley-Mueller modification are the best known examples (Fig. 25–5). There are many additional modifications of both basic types of THA devices in current use.

Normal Appearance. Routine protocol for evaluation of a THA includes both anteroposterior (AP) and true lateral radiographs. The AP view is obtained with the patient supine and the leg in slight internal rotation to bring the greater trochanter into profile. An 8:1 ratio moving grid is used. The true lateral view is obtained across the table with the opposite leg elevated out of the field. The patient is supine, with the leg in full extension and the patella anterior in position. Either a fixed or a reciprocating grid is employed.

Although the normal radiographic appearance of a THA will vary somewhat depending on the type of prosthesis used, principles of radiographic evaluation are similar. It may be helpful to refer to manufacturers' brochures or available references to identify modifications and suggested alignment of THA units.[29, 39, 40] Radiopaque acrylic bone cement should fill available spaces between the bone and prosthesis components without gaps or trapped air bubbles. Cement entering the pelvis should be noted; excessive intrusion into the pelvis may be associated with complications.[41] No loose cement fragments should be present. Areas of heterotopic bone formation may occasionally be confused with particles of cement. Both components of the prosthesis should be covered with cement, and bone cement should extend at least 2 cm beyond the tip of the femoral stem. Areas of inadequate cement coverage may be subject to increased stresses.

Orientation of the acetabular cup should be approximately 30 degrees (McKee-Farrar type) or 45 degrees (Charnley type) from the horizontal, and in neutral to slight anteversion (10 degrees). Acetabular orientation is easily measured on a nonrotated anteroposterior radiograph of the hip or pelvis by calculating the angle between the base of the metallic acetabular component (McKee-Farrar type) or the orbital wire marker (Charnley type), and the horizontal plane. Anteversion is most easily evaluated on lateral radiographs, but the lateral view is not always available, especially in the immediate postoperative period. An accurate evaluation of anteversion may be determined using anteroposterior radiographs if the central ray is centered over the hip.[42] Acetabular orientation is usually adequately assessed on frontal radiographs by estimation according to the following guides: neutral position (wire appears as a straight line), slight anteversion (wire appears as elongated oval), or increased anteversion (wire assumes a more circular shape). Anteversion may usually be distinguished from retroversion on frontal anteroposterior films (Charnley type prosthesis); on close inspection, the more ventral portion of the wire marker will create a shadow that is slightly larger and less sharp than that of the more dorsal portion of the wire. Formulas are available for more exact calculation of anteversion on anteroposterior radiographs.[43, 159] Excessive deviation from these ideal values predisposes the THA to complications

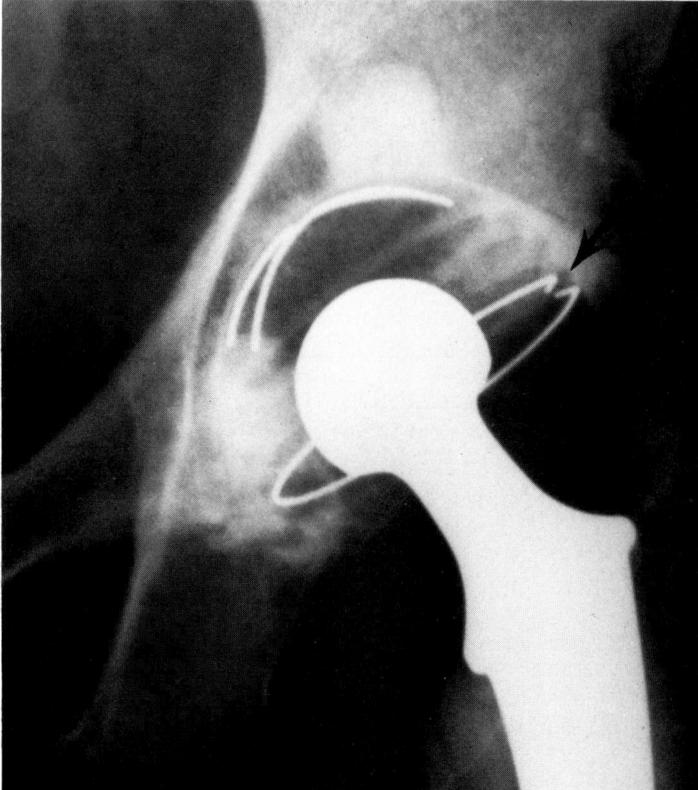

Figure 25–6. *Aufranc-Turner THA. There is an asymmetric acetabular component with thickest portion located laterally. The normal break in the marker wire denotes the thickest portion (arrow).*

of instability, dislocation, or limited range of motion.

The femoral component stem ideally lies in slight valgus position with reference to the femoral shaft or in the central portion of the medullary canal. Slight anteversion, evaluated on the lateral film, is also desirable. The flange at the proximal portion of the metallic stem should rest firmly on the resected femoral neck. The head of the femoral prosthesis should lie centrally within the metal or polyethylene acetabular component, unless an asymmetric acetabular component has been employed[44, 45] (Fig. 25–6).

Osteotomy of the greater trochanter may be performed at the time of THA to facilitate exposure of the hip.[46, 47] The trochanter is often reinserted in a more distal and lateral position for improved stability. Fixation of the trochanter is accomplished with heavy wire suture or a trochanteric bolt[48] (Fig. 25–13). Normal bony union of the trochanteric osteotomy occurs in 6 to 12 weeks.

COMPLICATIONS. In addition to risks associated with any major surgical procedure, patients with THA have a high incidence of thromboembolic disease, which may approach 50 per cent unless prophylaxis is used.[38] There is approximately a 1 per cent risk of deep infection with use of prophylactic antibiotics, although over half of all infections occur as a late complication as long as eight years following surgery.[46, 49, 50] Many potential complications may be evaluated radiographically (Table 25–1).

Table 25–1
COMPLICATIONS OF TOTAL HIP ARTHROPLASTY

Dislocation
Trochanteric avulsion or nonunion
Heterotopic ossification
Fracture
Loosening/infection

Dislocation. Dislocation is an uncommon complication of THA, with most cases appearing in the first few weeks following surgery[50, 51] (Fig. 25–7). Significant deviation from the ideal angles of acetabular orientation and anteversion or trochanteric avulsion predisposes to subluxation or dislocation of the prosthesis. Complete dislocation is obvious when both frontal and lateral radiographs are obtained. Rarely, a complete dislocation may be subtle when only a frontal radiograph is available.[44] Subluxation (eccentric seating) of the metal head within the acetabular component may sometimes be detected in maximum abduction or in internal or external rotation. Persistent subluxation in neutral positions should raise the possibility of interposition of material between the prosthetic components, either soft tissue, osseous, cartilaginous, or cement fragments[52, 53] (Fig. 25–8). Arthrography may be helpful in further evaluation of eccentric seating.

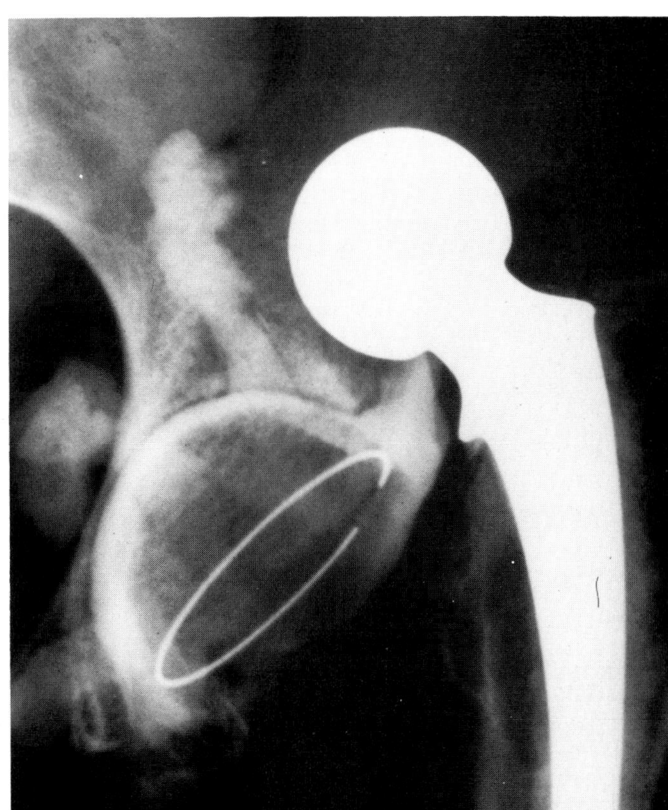

Figure 25–7. Dislocated Charnley type THA. There is slightly increased anteversion of the acetabular component.

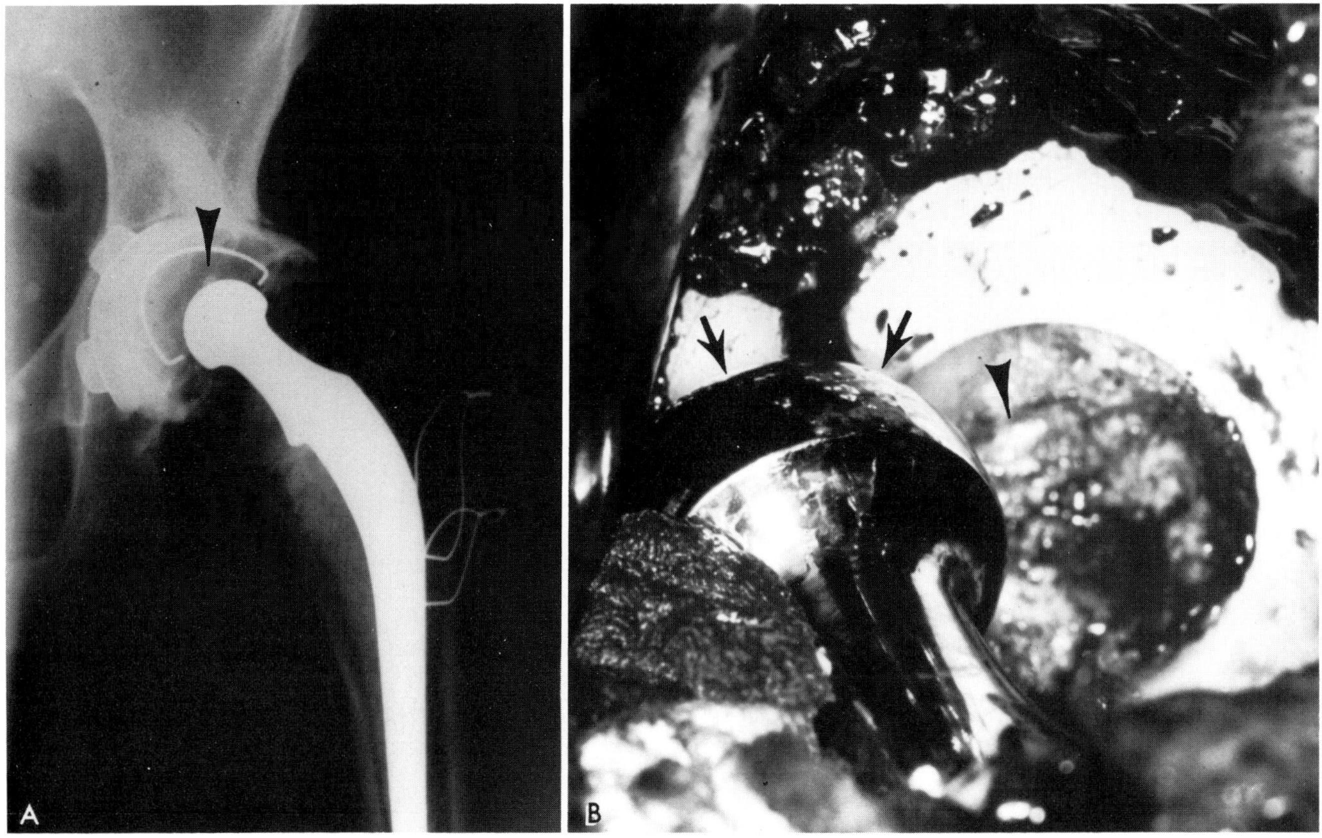

Figure 25–8. **A**, *Slightly eccentric seating of THA related to bone cement fragment trapped between the components (arrowhead).* **B**, *Disarticulated hip at surgery, metallic femoral head at left (arrows). Multiple intra-articular bone cement fragments are noted within the acetabular component (arrowhead). (Courtesy of Dr. R. Convery, University of California, San Diego, California.)*

Trochanteric Avulsion or Nonunion. It is generally agreed that THA performed without trochanteric osteotomy results in less blood loss, a shorter operation, more rapid recovery, and the absence of complications of nonunion, broken or migrating wires, and trochanteric bursitis.[54, 55] However, the majority of patients with radiographic complications related to the osteotomized greater trochanter are asymptomatic. Although bony union between the detached trochanter and the parent bone is usually complete by 6 months, fibrous union occasionally occurs. Fibrous union is inferred radiographically if there is a lack of bony bridging at 6 months and the wires remain intact, without migration of the trochanter. Standing films or films in extreme abduction-adduction may aid in evaluating possible trochanteric nonunion.[29] Breakage of the wire sutures prior to bony or fibrous union may be associated with superolateral migration of the trochanter (Fig. 25–18). Avulsion of the trochanter may also occur without breakage of the wires; in this situation, the wires pull off of the avulsed trochanter, remaining intact and fixed to the femur. Trochanteric avulsion predisposes to chronic recurrent dislocation from lack of abductor muscle support. Fatigue fractures of the wires often occur after bony union or fibrous ankylosis and are generally of no significance. Location of various wire fragments should be noted. Loose wire fragments may cause trochanteric bursitis or may migrate to an intra-articular position.[29, 48, 52, 56]

Heterotopic Ossification. Heterotopic para-articular ossification is a common sequela of THA. The reported incidence of ectopic ossification varies widely.[57, 58] In series specifically evaluating the presence and degree of heterotopic bone formation, the incidence varies from 15 to 50 per cent.[50, 59, 60] Although mild degrees of heterotopic ossification generally cause no clinical disability, 2 to 5 per cent of patients develop extensive ossification, resulting in limitation of motion[60-62] (Fig. 25–9). Para-articular ossification may appear as early as 3 weeks post-THA and, in affected patients, is always evident by 6 months.[61, 63] Early fluffy heterotopic bone is easily overlooked on overexposed radiographs. Maturation of bone is generally achieved by 1 year. Heterotopic bone may show increased uptake on radionuclide bone scanning performed to evaluate possible prosthetic loosening or infection[64] (Fig. 25–10). The para-articular location of the increased uptake with

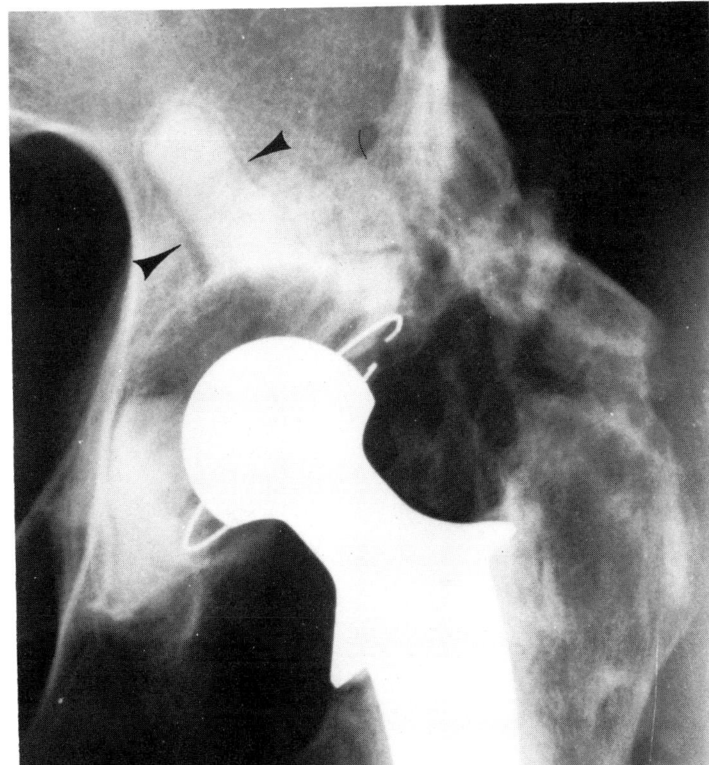

Figure 25–9. *Extensive heterotopic bone formation following THA with limitation of motion clinically. A radiolucent line (1.5 mm) is present along bone-cement interface of acetabular component (arrowheads); there was no clinical evidence of loosening.*

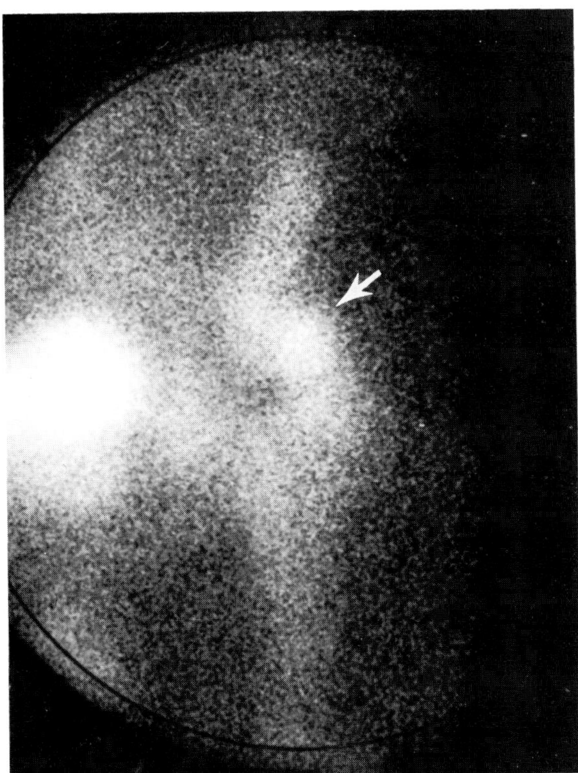

Figure 25–10. *Technetium-99m pyrophosphate scintigram, anterior projection of left hip in patient with heterotopic bone formation following THA. An area of increased activity is noted laterally between the acetabulum and the femur (arrow).*

heterotopic bone formation may occasionally be distinguished from similar changes in the region of the prosthetic components. To avoid misinterpretation of the radionuclide images, it is important to correlate the scan with current radiographs.

The etiology of heterotopic ossification is unknown. Multiple factors have been implicated, including surgical trauma, bone dust, hemorrhage, infection, reoperation, and predisposing systemic illnesses (ankylosing spondylitis, diffuse idiopathic skeletal hyperostosis). Most investigators agree that reoperation results in a higher incidence of this complication.

Fracture. Fractures of the femur and the pelvis may occur during primary THA but are more common at the time of revision or removal of arthroplasty components.[65] Intraoperative fractures of the femoral shaft are more frequent than pelvic fractures and are generally attributed to one or more factors, including severely osteoporotic bone, excessive or misdirected reaming, and rough handling.[164] Placement of a cortical window for removal of bone cement during prosthetic revision may also be a factor. Such fractures are usually recognized at the time of surgery, either from clinical examination (instability) or radiography. Intraoperative films are often obtained in only a single projection, and may not include the entire stem. Frontal films may show only subtle foreshortening in cases of posterior penetration of the femoral cortex. Intraoperative fractures are treated at the time of surgery by several methods: (1) addition of bone cement and encircling bands or compression plates, (2) use of special long-stem implants, and (3) conservative management with bed rest and traction.[65-67] Normal bone healing occurs in the presence of bone cement as long as there is bone apposition.

Postoperative femoral fractures are of two types. Typical fractures of the distal femur occur following major traumatic events, and are treated by standard methods. Fractures of the proximal femoral shaft occur at or just distal to the tip of the femoral stem. These fractures are often spontaneous or follow minor trauma. Factors that predispose to fractures near the tip of the femoral stem include defects in the femoral cortex and inadequate distribution of bone cement. Defects in the femoral cortex may result from placement of a cortical window for removal of old bone cement during revision of a previous arthroplasty. Cortical thinning or unrecognized cortical penetration may occur during reaming of the intramedullary canal. Previous or misdirected screw holes may also cause potential sites of weakening, or weakening may be caused by large bubbles of air trapped in bone cement about the prothesis tip. Recognition of a possible site of femoral weakening prior to or at the time of surgery dictates use of a long-stem prosthesis with additional bone cement. Adequate distribution of bone cement is necessary to prevent concentration of stress forces. Methylmethacrylate should fill the medullary cavity and extend at least 2 cm beyond the tip of the stem.[68] Recognition of faulty bone cement distribution on immediate postoperative films may alert the clinician to protect the hip with crutches.

Fractures of the acetabulum following THA may relate to one or more factors: (1) overrreaming of the acetabulum, (2) severe protrusio acetabuli with thinning of the available acetabular roof, (3) chronic loosening or infection with increased stresses, (4) perforation of the medial wall of the acetabulum during placement of bone cement anchoring holes, (5) metastatic disease, and (6) large acetabular cysts[68-71, 172] (Fig. 25–11). Acetabular reconstruction

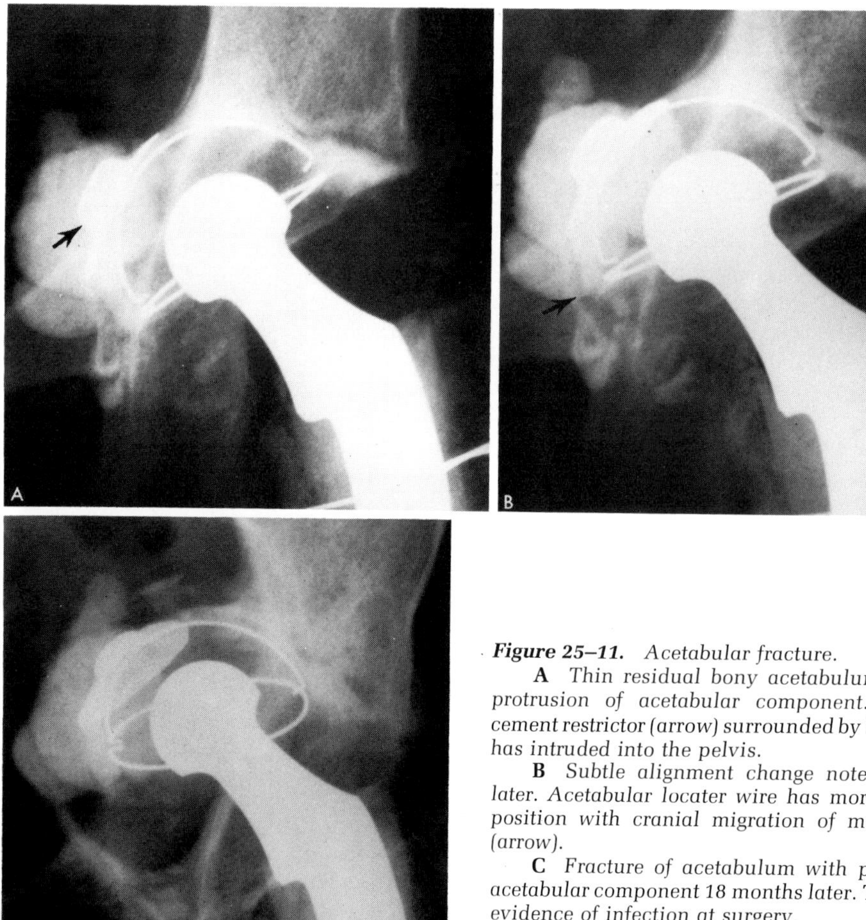

Figure 25–11. *Acetabular fracture.*

A *Thin residual bony acetabulum with mild protrusion of acetabular component. The mesh cement restrictor (arrow) surrounded by bone cement has intruded into the pelvis.*

B *Subtle alignment change noted 6 months later. Acetabular locater wire has more horizontal position with cranial migration of medial aspect (arrow).*

C *Fracture of acetabulum with protrusion of acetabular component 18 months later. There was no evidence of infection at surgery.*

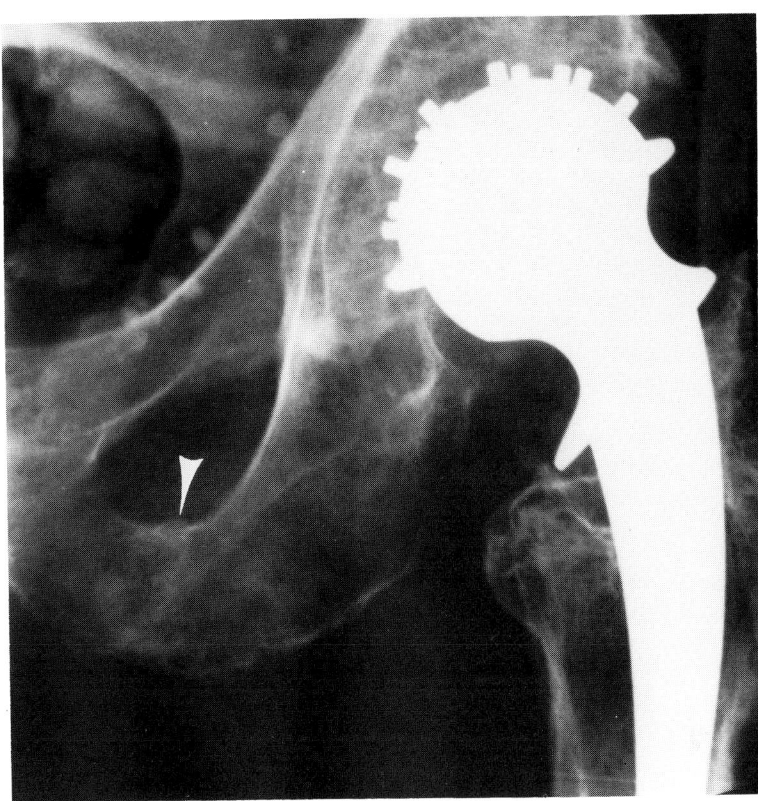

Figure 25–12. *Stress fracture of inferior pubic ramus (arrowhead) following THA (McKee-Farrar type; radiolucent bone cement).*

with heavy wire mesh and bone cement in hips with protrusio acetabuli may decrease the incidence of acetabular component loosening and fracture.

Stress (insufficiency) fractures of the pubic ramus may clinically simulate loosening of a THA.[157] Initial radiographs may be misleading if the stress fracture is not yet visible and a radiolucent line at the bone-cement interface raises the possibility of prosthetic loosening. After several weeks with symptoms, patients with stress fractures generally have positive radiographs (Fig. 25–12). Previously sedentary patients with osteoporotic bone are particularly susceptible to development of insufficiency fractures following increased mobility and stresses in the postoperative period.[68] Radionuclide bone scans may be positive prior to radiographic findings.

Loosening and Infection. The chief long-term complications of THA are infection and loosening. Aside from pulmonary embolism, postoperative infection is the most serious complication and the most frequent indication for reoperation of THA. Loosening of a prosthetic component at the bone-cement interface may occur with or without associated infection. Conversely, deep infection is not always associated with component loosening.

The incidence of deep infection has decreased due to stringent prophylactic measures, including routine administration of antibiotics. The current incidence of deep sepsis is about 1 per cent in large series.[29, 38] A long latent period — up to 8 years in some patients — prior to clinical evidence of infected THA suggests that the actual incidence of infection may be higher. Clinical signs and symptoms of infection may be absent, minimal or indistinguishable from loosening without infection. Predisposing factors associated with the higher incidence of infection following THA include prior hip surgery or revision of THA, rheumatoid arthritis, steroid therapy, and obesity.[72, 166] Although most latent infections are believed to originate from bacteria introduced at the time of surgery, cases of latent THA infections may occasionally be attributed to hematogenous implantation of bacteria from a distant source in the body — e.g., dental, bladder, and respiratory infections.[73-75] Early detection of deep sepsis, usually before the appearance of radiographic changes, may allow successful treatment with antibiotics alone or antibiotics in conjunction with surgical drainage, leaving the prosthesis in place.[76] When infection is more advanced, removal of the prosthesis, bone cement, and necrotic bone (Girdlestone procedure) is required in addition to appropriate antibiotic therapy. A reimplantation may be considered after complete control of the infection (at least 1 year) has been obtained, although there has been some interest in immediate reconstruction after removal of the prosthetic components and necrotic bone.[77] Antibiotic-impregnated methylmethacrylate is currently being utilized outside the United States for revision of THA in patients with pyogenic infections.[78, 79] The antibiotic is slowly and continuously released locally in high concentrations that are not detectable systemically.

Prosthetic loosening is defined as visually evident gross movement observed when the prosthesis is manually stressed at surgery.[80] Loose noninfected components may be primarily revised with likelihood of success, whereas infected components are usually removed. Unfortunately, the distinction between loosening and infection may be difficult even with use of multiple modalities, including (1) plain films, (2) radionuclide scanning, (3) hip aspiration, and (4) subtraction arthrography.

Plain Films. On plain radiographs alone, an infected prosthesis is rarely distinguishable from one that is loosened without infection. Osteomyelitis with bone destruction and irregular periosteal new bone formation is an uncommon manifestation of an infected THA. Development of a radiolucent zone* at the bone-cement interface raises the possibility of loosening. This sign may be detected on plain films only if radiopaque bone cement is utilized.

The presence of a zone is not infallible evidence of loosening; such zones may develop in the normal arthroplasty. Analysis of sequential films aids in distinguishing the normal sequence of events from loosening. Initial postoperative films should show radiopaque bone cement contiguous with the adjacent bone. Occasionally a zone may be noted on immediate postoperative films, limited to the superolateral portion of the acetabular component.[81, 82] Zones of demarcation involving the acetabular component are present in about 70 per cent of patients followed for 10 years.[83] The majority are asymptomatic (Fig. 25–9). Although zones more commonly involve the acetabular component of THA and the tibial component of total knee arthroplasties (TKA), actual loosening is more common in the femoral components of both types of arthroplasties.[38, 83] During the first 6 postoperative months, zones may initially appear and lengthen or widen on sequential films in normal patients. After 6 months, such phenomena may occasionally be noted in normal patients, but changes are less likely to be normal after the first postoperative year. The actual width or appearance of a zone may aid in distinguishing the normal from a loose/infected THA. Zones 2 mm or wider are usually indicative of infection/loosening; zones that extend around the entire bone-cement interface correlate with loosening/infection better than localized zones.[82, 84] Serial widening of a zone that is observed more than 6 months postoperatively also suggests loosening/infection. Although not every zone represents demonstrable prosthetic loosening, essentially every case of loosening is associated with such a zone.

Several theories have been advocated to explain the appearance of radiolucent zones at the bone-cement interface in normal patients: (1) incomplete removal of acetabular articular cartilage, (2) thermal necrosis of bone from the exothermic bone-cement polymerization reaction, (3) surgical trauma, (4) failure to pack the cement tightly or motion of the prosthetic component prior to setting of cement, (5) interposition of soft tissue or blood, (6) chemical damage from the PMM monomer and free radicals in the cement, and (4) micromotion.[81, 85] Internal polymer temperatures may reach 100° C, and some studies have reported temperatures at the bone-cement interface that are of such magnitude as to cause tissue necrosis.[86, 87] More recent investigations report in vivo temperatures below protein denaturation levels.[88, 89] Attempts to isolate chemical effects of bone-cement monomer have shown no increased tissue damage over that of the surgical trauma itself.[90] The remaining factors — surgical trauma, poor packing of cement with interposition of blood or tissue, motion during setting of the bone cement, and micromotion — may all play a role in development of zones.

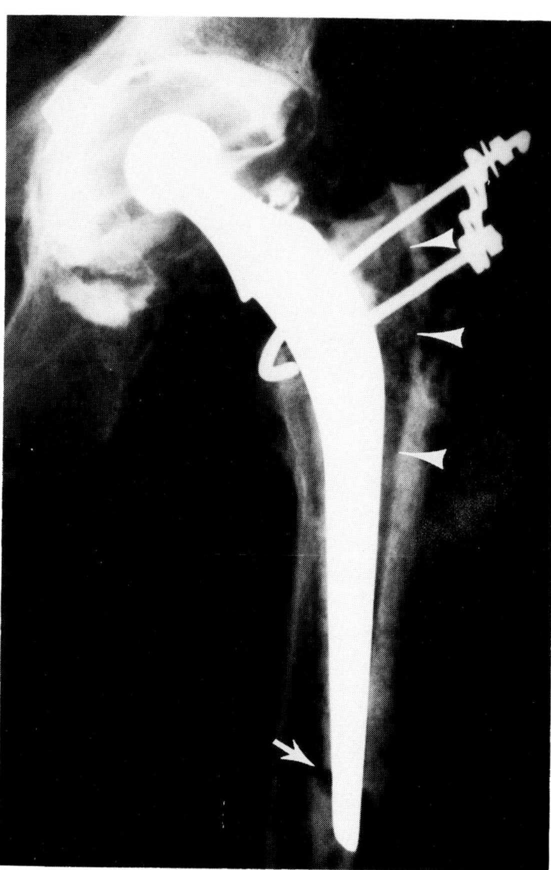

Figure 25–13. *THA with fractured bone cement distally (arrow) and marked subsidence at metal-cement interface along the proximal convex portion of the femoral stem (arrowheads). A special bolt was used for fixation of greater trochanteric osteotomy. (Courtesy of Dr. S. Kleiman, Green Hospital of Scripps Clinic, La Jolla, California.)*

*Hereafter in this chapter "zone" refers to a radiolucent line at the bone-cement interface or metal-cement interface.

The appearance or the interval progression of a radiolucent zone at the metal-cement interface may be noted in some normal patients as well as in patients with loosening of the femoral component.[91] Radiographically detectable lucent areas at the metal-cement interface are most commonly noted along the proximal convex surface of the femoral stem. Fractures of the bone cement near the tip of the stem may precede or be associated with separation of cement at the proximal metal-cement junction (Fig. 25–13). The distal bone-cement fracture often occurs first, resulting from slight movement of the stem within the cement, causing an increased load ("end-bearing") at the distal aspect of the cement.[92] Following cement fracture, the prosthesis may subside to a more distal and varus position in the tapered cavity.[93] In some cases, bending or fatigue fracture of the prosthesis stem may occur as the end result of increased stresses concentrated near the tip of the stem[94-97] (Fig. 25–14).

In patients with stem fatigue fractures, the prosthesis is loose but usually not infected, since rigid fixation distally is a prerequisite for increased stress on the stem. Contributing factors implicated in femoral stem failure include (1) patient weight greater than 91 kg, (2) inadequate valgus positioning of the prosthesis, (3) metallurgical failure, (4) increased patient activity, and (5) bilateral arthroplasty.[96-100] In addition, the complication is more frequent in men.

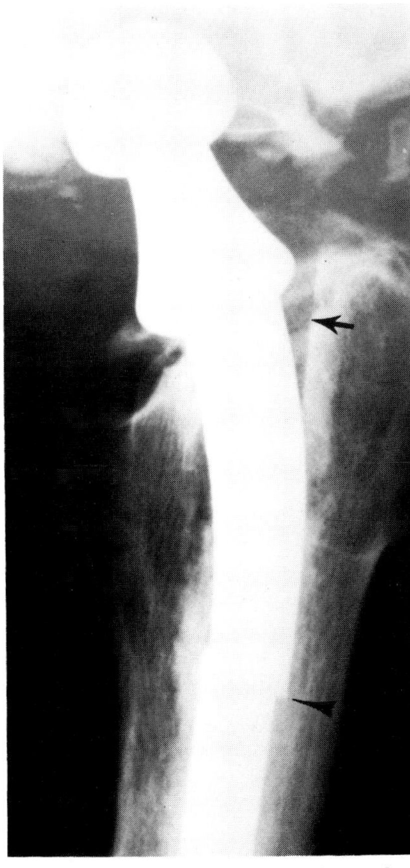

Figure 25–14. Fatigue fracture of metal femoral stem (arrowhead) with separation at the metal-cement interface proximally (arrow).

The development and the progression of radiolucent lines at the bone-cement or the metal-cement interface do not reliably distinguish the normal from the abnormal in many cases. Fracture of the radiopaque cement with subsidence of the femoral stem and migration of the prosthetic component indicates a change in position, but the component may be stable clinically and at surgery. Sequential films should always be carefully analyzed for subtle changes in alignment of prosthesis components. Differences in the centering of the x-ray beam and the positioning of the patient and film must be taken into account. Changes in alignment are not always associated with fractures of bone cement. Stress films (e.g., push-pull or abduction-adduction) may be helpful in evaluation of suspected motion. Fluoroscopic observation and video recording with application of stress may facilitate demonstration of loosening.

In some cases, the Mach effect* is responsible for small (1 to 2 mm) lucent zones at the metal-cement interface that do not progressively widen.[91] Clinical correlation and radionuclide bone scanning will help indicate which patients may benefit from arthrography. Arthrographic demonstration of contrast material tracking into a zone of subsidence along the proximal convex portion of the metal stem or localized to a small portion of the bone-cement interface may indicate only a separation, without actual loosening of the prosthetic component.

Scintigraphy. Radionuclide bone scanning utilizing various radiopharmaceutical agents, such as ^{87m}Sr, ^{18}F, and ^{99m}Tc-phosphate complexes, has recently been employed in the evaluation of patients with painful THA.[156, 167] Anterior and posterior images of the pelvis, including both acetabular regions, are obtained with a diverging collimator. Additional anterior images are obtained with each hip in internal rotation using parallel hole or pinhole collimators for high resolution. Care should be taken to include the full extent of the femoral shaft; radiographs facilitate this optimal positioning. Tape recording and computer processing of data may aid in evaluation of serial studies.[101]

Normally, increased activity with a diffuse distribution is noted in the first postoperative weeks; this gradually decreases over a period of 6 to 9 months.[102, 103] Slightly increased uptake may occasionally be noted in asymptomatic patients, even at 1 year, especially at the superolateral aspect of the acetabulum and region of the calcar.[104] Activity may also persist at the site of a greater trochanteric osteotomy.

*A visual phenomenon caused by the presence of adjacent areas of differing contrast, described by Ernst Mach in 1865 (Radiology *121*:9–17, 1976.)

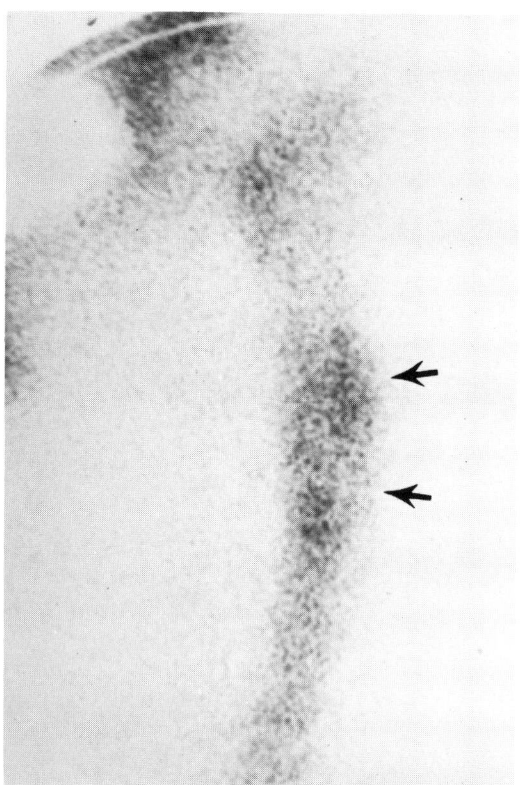

Figure 25–15. Technetium-99m pyrophosphate scintigram, anterior projection of left femur in patient with painful THA. There is a focal area of increased activity near the tip of the femoral stem (arrows). Loosening of the component was confirmed surgically.

A common radionuclide pattern of loosening consists of focal areas of increased uptake, more easily detected on the femoral side, often appearing near the proximal or distal portion of the stem[102, 160, 161] (Fig. 25–15). Another abnormal pattern consists of diffusely increased activity along the prosthesis in patients with either loose or loose and infected components. Increased activity in the region of the femoral neck and para-articular soft tissues may be seen in cases of heterotopic bone formation, even in early stages, when radiographic findings may be subtle.

Radionuclide bone scanning cannot differentiate loosening from infection in THA. However, there has been a recent interest in the use of gallium-67 citrate in an attempt to differentiate these two complications[156, 162] (see Chapter 17). This agent has a normal, weak affinity for bone, and has been widely used to detect abscesses and sites of inflammation. In the absence of infection, gallium activity closely parallels that of the conventional technetium bone scan, although it may not be as prominent. With infection, patchy or diffuse areas of increased gallium uptake may be noted. At this time, the role of gallium scanning in differentiation of infection from loosening remains to be established.

The main deterrents to more routine utilization of the various radionuclide scan modalities in evaluation of the painful THA include the cost of the procedure, the lack of specificity, and the low morbidity and increased specificity of aspiration procedures combined with arthrography.

Table 25–2
UTILITY OF ARTHROGRAPHY IN TOTAL HIP ARTHROPLASTY

Aspiration for culture
Detection of:
- Presence and extent of loosening
- Sinus tracts, communicating abscess cavities
- Intra-articular material in cases of chronic dislocation
- Trochanteric bursitis
- Nonunion of greater trochanter

Arthrography. Arthrography of the painful THA is a valuable preoperative diagnostic modality, which may demonstrate a variety of complications (Table 25–2). Aspiration with culture of intra-articular material is routinely performed at the time of arthrography and is of equal importance to performance of the arthrogram itself. With more routine use of radiopaque bone cement, gross prosthesis loosening is readily detected on plain film radiography, but with this modality, early changes of loosening are difficult to detect. Arthrographic demonstration of opaque contrast material along the bone-cement interface is more difficult to delineate when opaque bone cement has been used; subtraction techniques have been developed to improve the detection of radiopaque contrast material adjacent to the opaque bone cement.

Preliminary internal rotation anteroposterior (AP), true lateral, and frog-leg lateral views are obtained; these views should include the entire prosthesis. Under fluoroscopic control, a marker is placed over the junction of the head and neck of the femoral component, along its medial aspect. The site is marked and confirmed to be below the inguinal ligament and lateral to the femoral vessels by palpation. The marker may be repositioned more distally or laterally if necessary. Following usual skin preparation and local anesthesia, a 20 gauge spinal needle is directed down to the metal of the femoral component near the head-neck junction. The position of the needle tip may be defined by rolling the patient into a posterior oblique position. If no fluid can be aspirated, the needle may be repositioned slightly, sliding along the medial aspect of the neck of the prosthesis. Again, if no fluid is aspirated, the needle position may be confirmed by a small injection of contrast material (0.5 ml Renografin-60). If the needle is in an intraarticular location, the contrast flows away from the needle tip into the intracapsular space. Injection of large amounts of contrast material prior to aspiration of fluid should be avoided to minimize any bacteriostatic effect of the contrast agent.[105, 106, 158] If no fluid is obtained after the intra-articular position is confirmed, normal saline solution (5 to 10 ml, without bacteriostatic agent) is injected and aspirated for smear and anaerobic and aerobic cultures. The lower leg is then stabilized with sand bags and 10 to 15 kg of longitudinal traction is applied utilizing any suitable traction device. A neutral AP film is obtained and corrected for technique and positioning. The patient is instructed not to move the leg and a series of films are obtained: (1) a repeat AP film to be used as a subtraction mask, (2) a series of two to four films following injection of contrast material in 7 to 10 ml increments, using up to 40 ml total volume. The volume is limited by patient discomfort and increasing injection pressure. The needle is removed and the hip is exercised passively and actively if possible, including weight-bearing, for about 5 min followed by a repeat of the initial film series. Subtraction films are prepared from the injection series (Fig. 25–16). Some degree of involuntary flexion of the hip generally occurs as the hip joint is distended. Separate subtraction films of the acetabular and femoral components may alleviate this problem.

Normally, contrast material fills the irregular pseudocapsule, which may vary considerably in volume. No free extravasation should be noted. Lymphatic filling may be observed; some investigators believe that such filling is an ancillary sign of inflammation,[107] although others have noted both antegrade and retrograde filling in patients without demonstrable infection or loosening[84, 106] (Fig. 25–16).

Contrast material penetrating the bone-cement or metal-cement interface clearly indicates a separation or space, although not all areas of communication represent component loosening[108, 109] (Fig. 25–17). The presence of contrast penetration around only a portion of a prosthetic component may merely represent a localized separation of the bone and cement without demonstrable loosening of the component at surgery. The greater the extent of contrast material penetration, the more likely it is that the prosthetic component is loose. Conversely, lack of contrast material penetration at the bone-cement interface does not exclude loosening.[84] Granulation or fibrous tissue may obstruct the opening to a potential space. Demonstration of contrast-filled para-articular cavities or sinus tracts supports a diagnosis of infection.[84, 110] Filling of a single cavity extending over the greater trochanter suggests a trochanteric bursitis, another possible cause of pain following THA[108] (Fig. 25–18).

Imaging Approach in Patients with Painful THA. Evaluation of technical failures and heterotopic bone formation is best accomplished using conventional radiographs. Radionuclide scanning using a ^{99m}Tc pyrophosphate complex aids in localization of symptoms to either the acetabular or the femoral component, the soft tissues (heterotopic

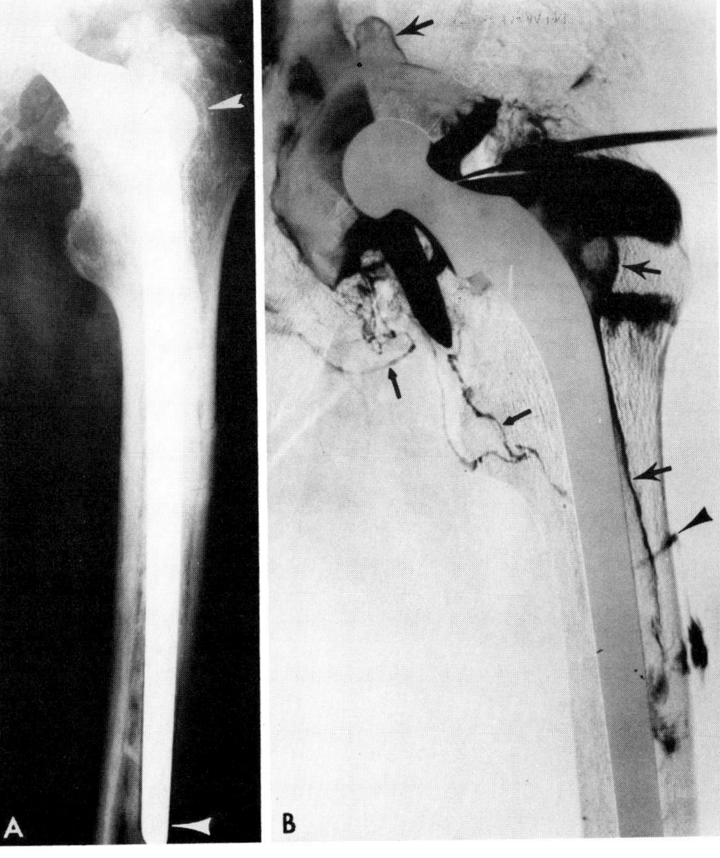

Figure 25–16. *Prosthesis loosening.*

A *Radiograph of revised THA using a long-stem femoral component. There is inadequate bone cement distally with "cutting-out" of distal stem laterally (lower arrowhead). A radiolucent line (1.5 mm) is present at the proximal bone-cement interface (upper arrowhead).*

B *Subtraction arthrogram showing contrast material along bone-cement interface of acetabular and femoral components (large arrows). Contrast material is observed tracking through the site of the cortical window into soft tissues (arrowhead). Lymphatic filling is noted (small arrows). (Courtesy of Dr. S. Kleiman, Green Hospital of Scripps Clinic, La Jolla, California.)*

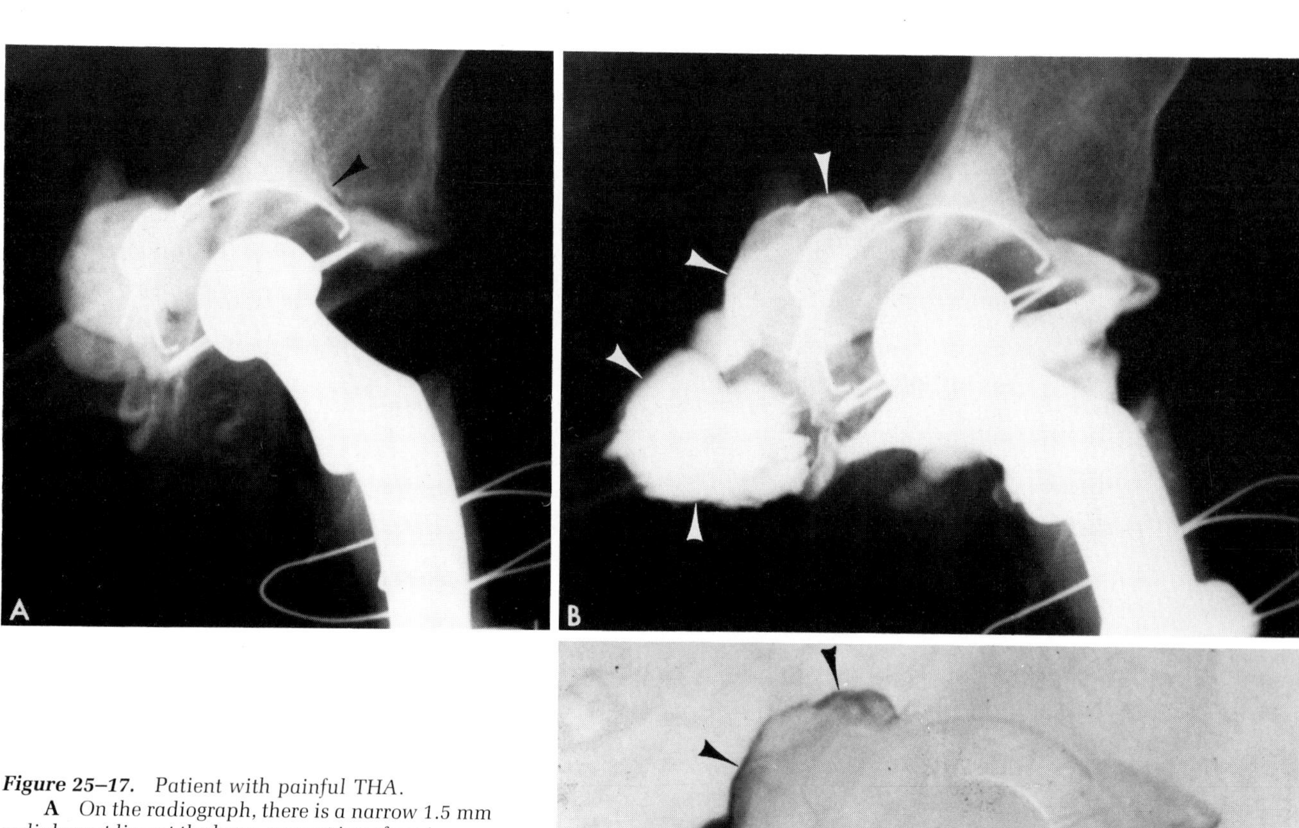

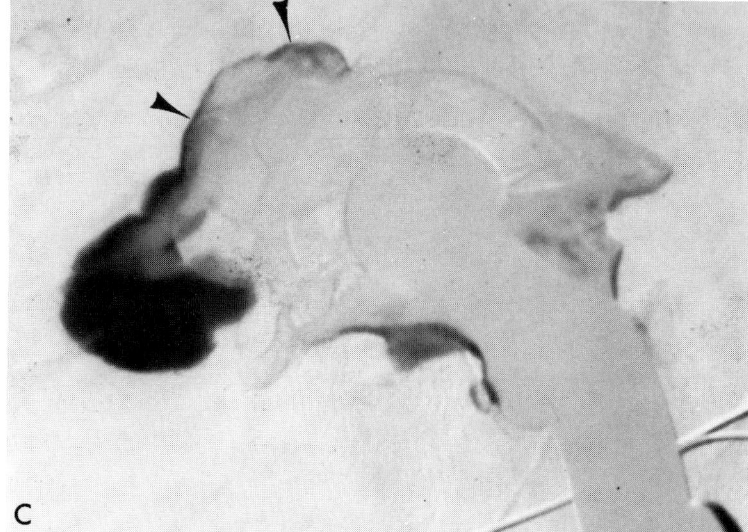

Figure 25–17. *Patient with painful THA.*

A *On the radiograph, there is a narrow 1.5 mm radiolucent line at the bone-cement interface (arrowhead).*

B *Arthrogram demonstrating contrast material around the medial aspect of the acetabular component with extension into the pelvis (arrowheads). There is no contrast filling of radiolucent line superiorly.*

C *Subtraction arthrogram demonstrating contrast material in pelvis (arrowheads).*

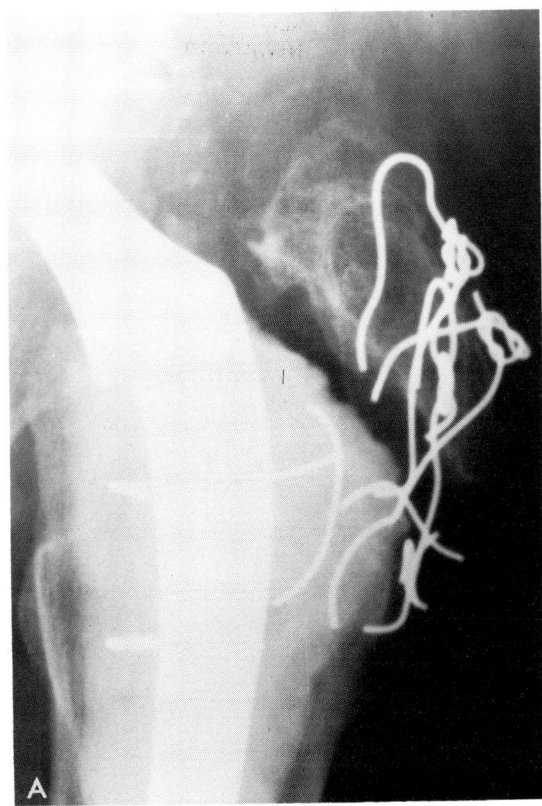

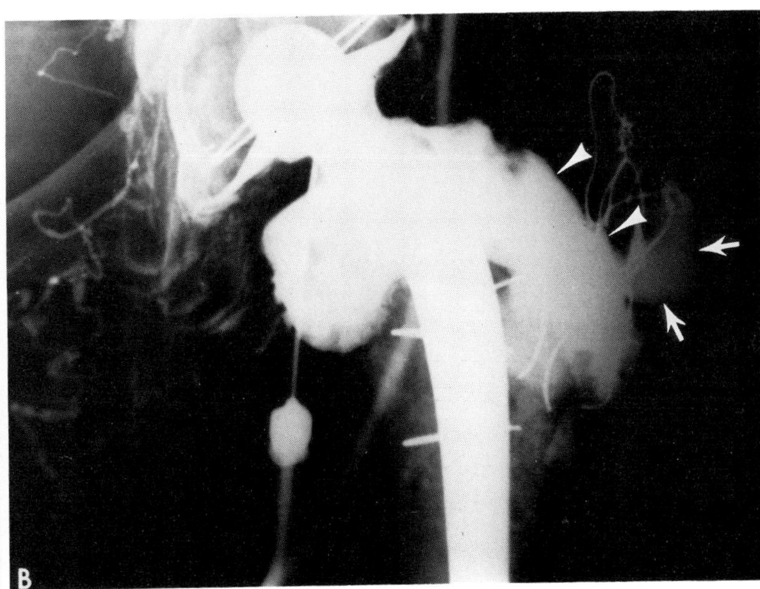

Figure 25–18. Trochanteric abnormalities.
A *Avulsion at trochanteric osteotomy site with fractured wire sutures and separation of trochanteric fragment.*
B *Arthrogram demonstrating contrast material between the femur and separated trochanter (arrowheads) and in a cavity lateral to the trochanter (arrows), representing bursal communication. There is extensive lymphatic filling.*

bone), or the bony pelvis (stress fractures). Patients with abnormal or indeterminate images are referred for aspiration and arthrography. All modalities are complementary and help separate those patients needing surgical intervention from those needing more conservative therapy.

Other Surgical Procedures of the Hip

A variety of surgical procedures preceded and aided development of a successful total hip arthroplasty. The success of THA has changed the indications for use of these earlier procedures, but they continue to be utilized in selected cases, including the salvage of failed hip replacements. These procedures include cup arthroplasty, femoral neck and head replacement, osteotomy, arthrodesis, and the Girdlestone operation.

Cup Arthroplasty. Original indications for cup arthroplasty included pain, loss of motion, instability, and deformity. With advent of the THA, cup arthroplasty has been used in joints complicated by sepsis and in patients who were considered to be too young for THA. Even these indications have been challenged by the current utilization of THA in younger patients and in revision of septic joints.[111, 112]

In the performance of a cup arthroplasty, the affected joint is initially widened by reaming of the acetabulum and the femoral head. A metallic cup is placed over the reamed femoral head, and the hip is reduced. The reparative process following surgery begins with formation of hematoma over the exposed osseous surfaces, which organizes into a fibrous scar. Maturation into fibrocartilage develops over a few months, and some metaplasia to hyaline cartilage may also occur. An extensive rehabilitation program is required, usually lasting 6 months or more, with continued improvement expected over a period of up to 6 years. The prolonged and difficult rehabilitation period is a major disadvantage of cup arthroplasty when compared with THA. Bilateral procedures require even longer rehabilitation. In addition to a long period of rehabilitation, disadvantages of cup arthroplasty include a longer operating time than THA, high revision rates (10 to 22 per cent), and an idiopathic painful cup syndrome in some patients despite an apparently uncomplicated procedure.[113-115] With a successful cup arthroplasty, the hip is strong and stable, permitting activity and loading stresses that are greater than those recommended for THA.

Following the procedure, radiographs outline a metallic cup that obscures the remaining femoral head and much of the acetabulum. The cup should lie in the axis of the femoral neck and rotate with the femur. Sequential films should show no gross alignment changes. Visualization of a joint space is variable. In some cases, progressive diminution of acetabular cartilage may be noted, perhaps related to

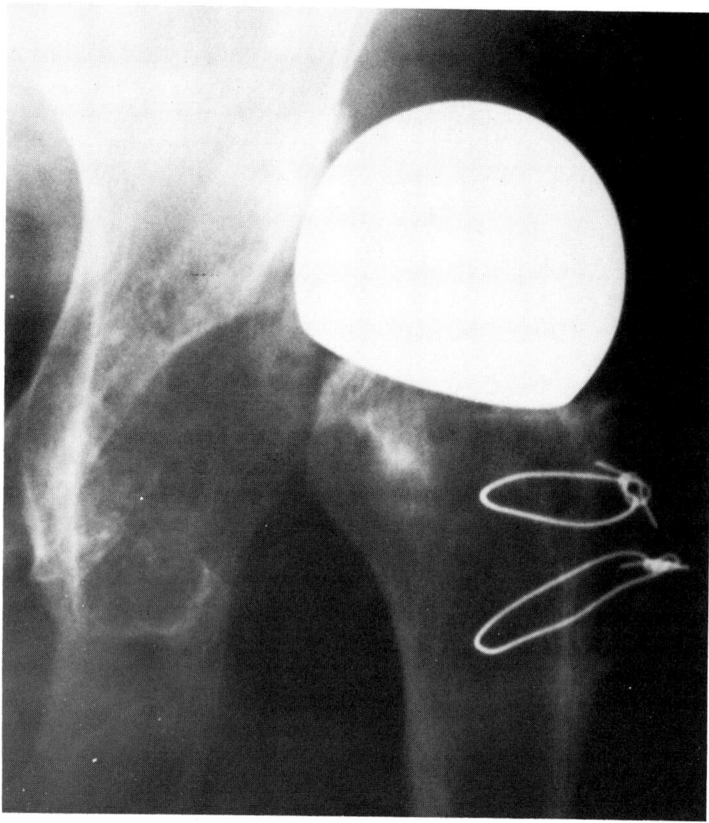

Figure 25–19. *Dislocated cup arthroplasty, in this case related to acetabular dysplasia.*

interference of normal chondral nutrition by the cup.

Several complications of this procedure may be noted. The metallic cup may dislocate or sublux, either along with the remaining femoral head or independently (Figs. 25–19 and 25–20). Poor mobility of the cup within the acetabulum may cause increased stress and ultimate fracture of the femoral neck.[116] An infected cup arthroplasty may show bone destruction and periosteal new bone formation; joint aspiration with culture may aid in diagnosis. Heterotopic bone formation has been reported in as many as 30 per cent of patients, but restriction of motion occurs in only about 3 per cent of patients.[117]

Femoral Hemiarthroplasty. Proximal femoral replacement in patients with arthritic conditions of the hip that affect the acetabular cartilage has been superseded by THA. Femoral head and neck replacement is currently in use for certain types of femoral neck fractures, primarily in older patients. Femoral hemiarthroplasty is occasionally used in children with pathologic fractures and in early stages of osteonecrosis of the femoral head without acetabular involvement. An advantage of this procedure is that the femoral hemiarthroplasty is designed for use without bone cement; thus, the side effects of methylmethacrylate are avoided and revision is facilitated. A new universal proximal femoral hip prosthesis is replacing conventional hemiarthroplasty in some centers.[118] Radiographically, the prosthesis has an appearance similar to that of a cup arthroplasty but with the femoral stem of a total hip arthroplasty (Fig. 25–21). A standard femoral stem and head articulate with a high density polyethylene acetabular cup, enclosed within a metallic cup. The polyethylene and metallic cup may be separate or molded together; the two variations are indistinguishable radiographically. These prostheses function as a double compound bearing, with movement possible at the articulation of the femoral head and polyethylene cup and of the metallic cup and acetabulum. More motion occurs at the metal femoral head–polyethylene articulation than at the cup–acetabular cartilage articulation, sparing articular cartilage from the degree of wear and degeneration that is associated with the conventional hemiarthroplasty. Relative motion of the two articulations may be assessed at fluoroscopy.

Normal Appearance. A variety of metallic femoral head replacements have been utilized. Head size is selected individually for each patient; the metallic head should fit snugly in the acetabulum. Subluxation or dislocation may occur if the head is too large. A small head results in increased wear on acetabular articular cartilage, which may be associated with pain and acetabular sclerosis. Length of the femoral neck must also be properly selected and depends not only on the size of the patient but also on the proposed osteotomy site and the desired degree of anteversion. Special order prostheses are available with extra long stems or necks. These are used in

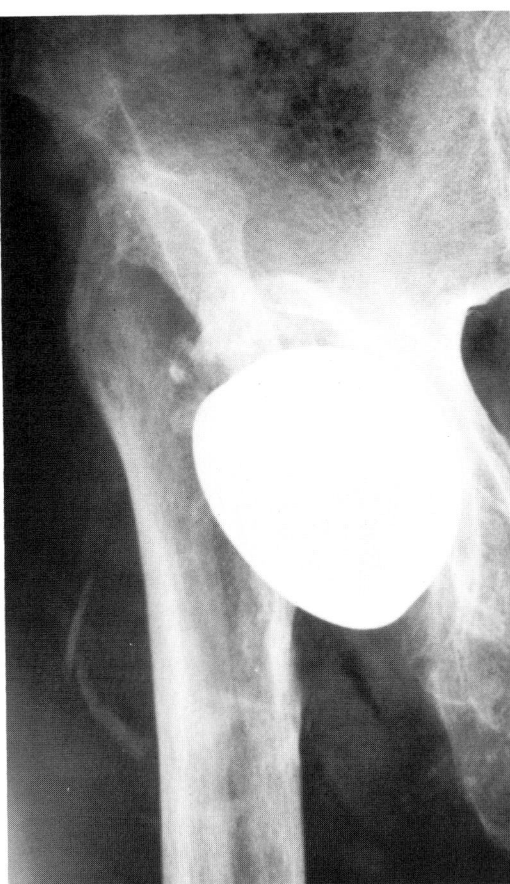

Figure 25–20. Cup arthroplasty with fracture through the femoral neck and superolateral migration of the femur (remaining femoral neck within the cup). The patient was relatively asymptomatic and had some mobility. The fracture may be related to overreaming of the femoral neck or direct trauma.

certain cases of low intertrochanteric fractures or when the proximal femoral shaft is involved with tumor or "bone softening" diseases that might compromise a hemiarthroplasty stem of conventional length. The stem is ideally placed in slight valgus position or centrally in the medullary canal with a modest degree of anteversion. Specific designs utilize varying shapes of the neck, the flange, and the stem. The two most common units are the Austin-Moore and the Thompson prostheses. The flange of the Austin-Moore prosthesis is designed to sit on approximately 1.6 cm (5/8 in) of residual calcar, and until recently, the stem contained fenestrations. Bone bridging through the fenestrations makes removal and revision more difficult. The Thompson prosthesis has a longer neck, and the flange is designed to sit on the base of the resected femoral neck along the intertrochanteric line.

Slight unbroken periosteal reaction along the lateral aspect of the femoral shaft and near the tip of the stem may be seen on follow-up examinations of normal hemiarthroplasties.[119] Localized areas of sclerosis may also be noted at the calcar where the flange contacts bone medially, around the tip of the stem in the intramedullary canal, and over the acetabulum, especially if reaming was performed.[117] A small amount of bone resorption may be noted along the resected margin of the femoral neck, with or without prosthesis settling. A thin radiolucent zone may develop around the stem, demarcated with a sclerotic line of compact bone. This zone usually measures less than 1 mm, and when it exceeds 2 mm, it is often associated with loosening.

Complications. Dislocation is not common and when present is usually related to excessive retroversion or selection of a head size that is too large for the acetabulum. Anchoring the prosthesis with bone cement in some individuals prevents adjustment of excessive retroversion, and such patients are at risk for dislocation.[120] Periarticular heterotopic bone formation has a significance similar to that in THA; symptoms and signs, including decreased range of motion, are more common in patients with extensive deposits. Dynamic studies of the new universal proximal femoral prosthesis are considered abnormal if motion of the outer bearing occurs preferentially to motion at the inner bearing except at the extreme ranges of motion.

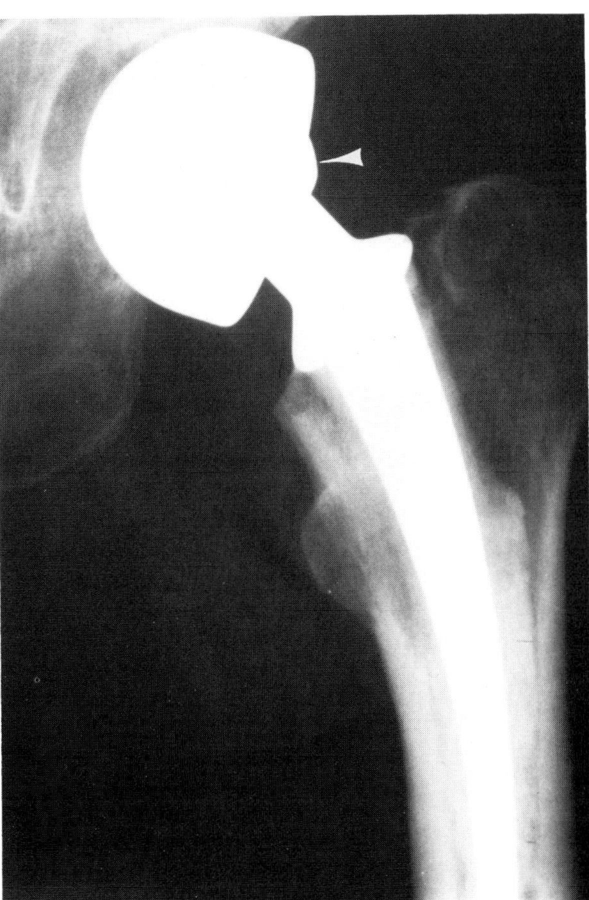

Figure 25–21. Normal universal proximal femoral hip prosthesis, cemented in place. The standard femoral head (arrowhead) articulates with the metal-polyethylene cup.

A radiolucent zone at the stem-bone interface exceeding 2 mm is often associated with loosening or infection. Such zones of less than 2 mm in thickness may be seen in asymptomatic patients as well as in patients with prosthetic loosening and are best evaluated by hip aspiration and arthrography in symptomatic individuals. Differentiation of loosening alone from infection with loosening is generally not possible unless changes of osteomyelitis with permeative bone destruction have occurred. Diagnosis of suspected loosening may sometimes be confirmed with push-pull radiographs which demonstrate gross motion.

Arthrodesis. Arthrodesis has competed with THA as the procedure of choice in the young patient with unilateral hip disease; a successful hip fusion results in a pain-free, stable joint with a high activity tolerance. However, favorable long-term results of THA in younger patients have decreased the use of arthrodesis as a primary method of treatment, although THA does not allow as high an activity level as arthrodesis. In some cases, arthrodesis may be chosen as an interim procedure prior to THA.[121]

The incidence of nonunion with formation of a pseudarthrosis following arthrodesis has decreased with use of bone grafting, internal fixation devices, and prolonged immobilization. Long-term problems include low back and ipsilateral knee pain due to increased stresses on articulations above and below the site of fusion; thus, a preexisting symptomatic ipsilateral knee joint and advanced lumbar disc degeneration are contraindications to hip arthrodesis. Degenerative changes of sacroiliac joints may develop, often on the contralateral side. About 15 per cent of patients with successful hip fusion develop femoral shaft fractures, which may lead to management problems.[122]

Femoral Head and Neck Excision Arthroplasty (Girdlestone Procedure). In the era of THA, resection of the femoral head and neck (Girdlestone procedure) is rarely used as a primary surgical method. In current practice, the Girdlestone procedure is utilized as a salvage operation following the failure of reconstructive procedures or infected THA. The primary advantages of the technique include permanent pain relief, improved range of motion, and correction of deformity.[123] Disadvantages include leg shortening, abnormal gait, and increased fatigability. The degree of instability often requires external support. The addition of a femoral shaft osteotomy has been advocated to improve stability.[124]

The surgical procedure is designed to produce a true pseudarthrosis, without bone-to-bone contact, which would cause recurrent pain. Bony apposition is avoided by interposition of soft tissues, smooth complete resection of the femoral head and neck, and removal of the superolateral portion of the acetabular rim. The resected surfaces of the acetabulum and femoral neck should be parallel (Fig. 25–22).

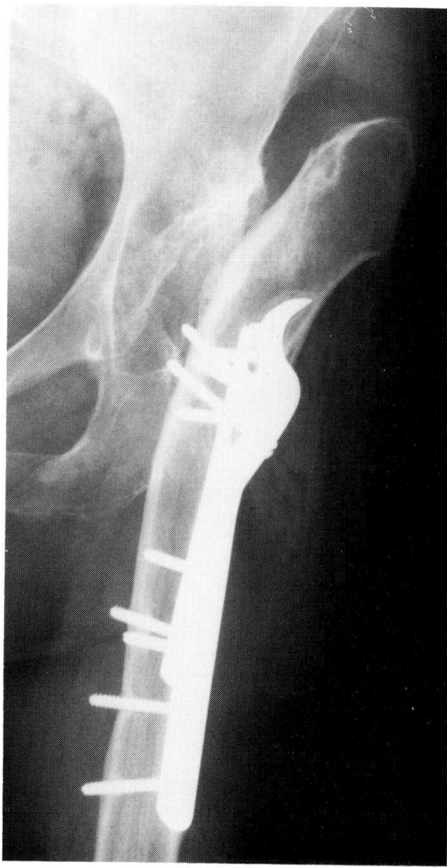

Figure 25–22. Girdlestone procedure with associated femoral osteotomy.

The degree of functional impairment that follows excision arthroplasty is the major contraindication to its utilization as a primary procedure. If used as a salvage procedure, there is the potential for conversion to THA after control of infection.[125]

Femoral Osteotomy. Many types of proximal femoral osteotomy procedures have been described, the common purpose of which is the relief of pain and correction of deformity. Although pain relief is observed in about 80 per cent of patients, the reasons are obscure. Theories used to explain the success of osteotomy implicate several factors, including (1) interruption of blood supply, (2) redistribution of forces across the hip, (3) alteration of joint congruence, and (4) changes of capsular stresses.[126, 127] Arrest or actual reversal of degenerative changes has been noted in some cases, with a measurable increase in joint space and decrease in subchondral sclerosis, osteophytes, and cysts. Such reversal of disease is unpredictable and not well understood.[126, 128, 129]

The radiographs of the proximal femoral osteotomy should be surveyed for changes in position at the osteotomy site and of the fixation device, nonunion, and evidence of progression or arrest of the underlying disease (Fig. 25–23).

Displacement osteotomy has been advocated as

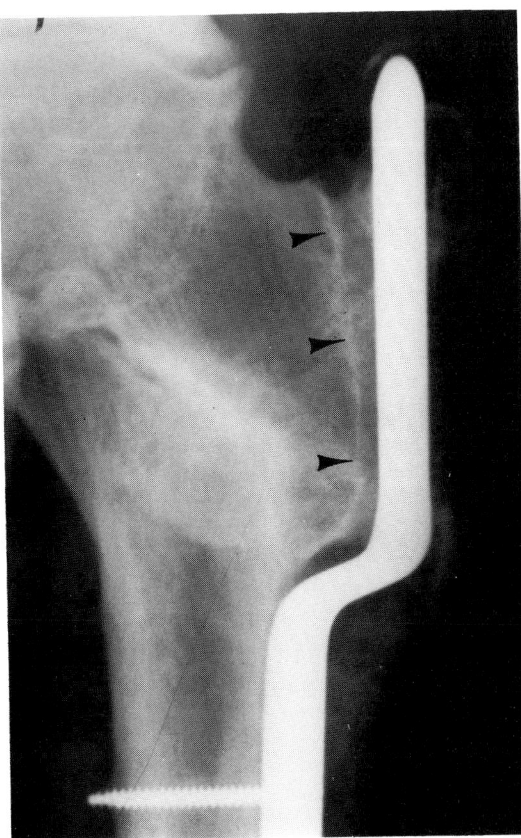

Figure 25–23. Nonunion of femoral osteotomy; gross motion was observed at fluoroscopy. The zone of bone condensation along the fixation device indicates motion (arrowheads).

the procedure of choice in early osteoarthritis, when pain predominates but the radiographs show minimal degenerative changes. The procedure is less extensive than THA and is associated with fewer complications. THA may later be used in those patients in whom residual pain or disease progression is noted.

THE KNEE

Total Knee Arthroplasty (TKA)

The challenge to develop an acceptable total knee arthroplasty (TKA) has logically followed the success of THA. Although the same material technology is utilized, the great variety of available designs and modifications of TKA attests to the greater anatomic and biomechanical complexity of the knee joint. Although attempts to treat arthritic disorders of the knee with resurfacing procedures began in 1861, acceptable knee prostheses required development of metal-polyethylene components and methylmethacrylate bone cement.

The primary indication for TKA is pain; instability, deformity, and decreased range of motion are additional criteria. Rheumatoid arthritis and osteoarthritis are the most common preexisting conditions. With increasing experience and improvements in design, other applications of TKA have included hemophilic arthroplasty, severe posttraumatic problems, and periarticular bone destruction due to benign tumors.

Infection is a major contraindication to the procedure because of the risk of reactivation. Patients with neuroarthropathy are also unacceptable surgical candidates. Although a successful arthrodesis has functional limitations, its conversion to a TKA is not usually recommended because of the possibility of complications, resulting in a worsening clinical situation. Because of the rate of complications in TKA, other acceptable surgical procedures, such as high tibial osteotomy, are usually employed first. TKA places marked limitations on patient activity, including running, jumping, lifting heavy loads, and kneeling. The adverse effects of muscle weakness or paralysis and preexisting hip disease, including arthrodesis, must also be considered in selection of candidates for TKA. Ligamentous instability is not a contraindication but will often dictate the type of prosthesis chosen.

Knee prostheses may be classified by the degree of constraint according to the following scheme: (1) no or minimal constraint; (2) partial constraint; (3) total constraint. For greater degrees of ligament instability, prostheses incorporating design features that impart increasing stability are chosen. Biomechanically, shear forces on the prosthesis increase as constraint increases, resulting in greater stresses on the prosthesis and surrounding bone. Fully constrained prostheses are larger and require more removal of bone, making revision more difficult.

With various modifications, most types of TKA in current use employ metallic femoral components that articulate with polyethylene tibial components, each held in place with radiopaque methylmethacrylate bone cement. The concave polyethylene component(s) are in a dependent position in knee prostheses in contrast with their location in hip arthroplasties. Thus, metallic wear particles and fragments of bone cement are more likely to pool on the concave surface, leading to increased wear.

The polycentric TKA as developed by Gunston is an example of an unconstrained prosthesis.[130, 131] Two stainless steel semicircular runners placed in the distal femur articulate with separate concave polyethylene tracks implanted in the proximal tibia. The shallow grooves of the tibial components provide minimal lateral constraint. Cruciate and collateral ligaments are retained for joint stability.

Partial constraint is provided by the geometric, UCI, and Freeman-Swanson prostheses (Fig. 25–24). The geometric prosthesis consists of a single metal femoral component that articulates with a single polyethylene tibial component[132] (Fig. 25–29*A*). The

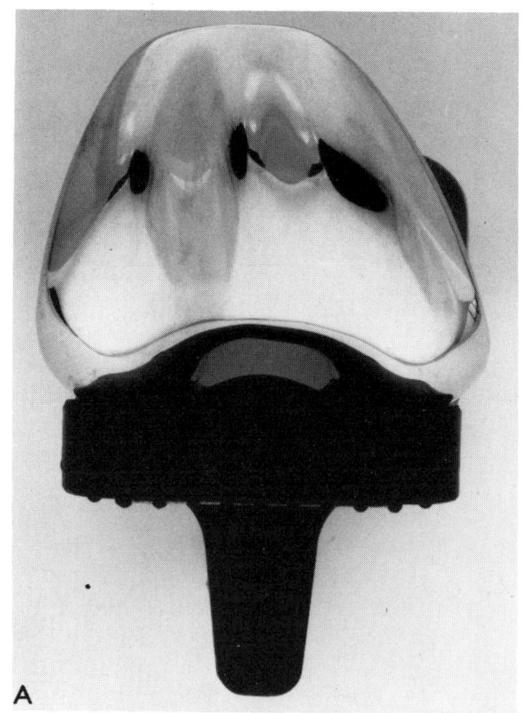

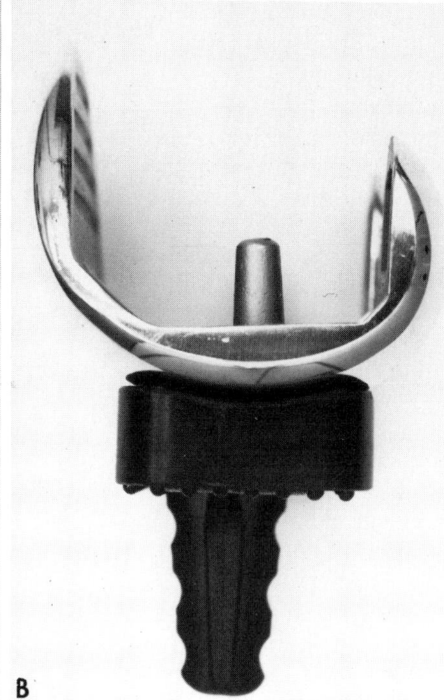

Figure 25–24. *Multiradius (Zimmer, USA) TKA, anterior* **(A)** *and lateral* **(B)** *views. This device is a partially constrained TKA, which allows preservation of posterior cruciate and collateral ligaments. The single metal femoral component articulates with the single polyethylene tibial component.*

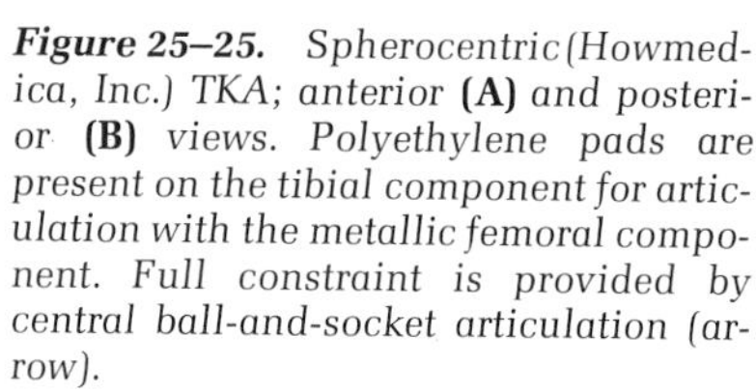

Figure 25–25. *Spherocentric (Howmedica, Inc.) TKA; anterior* **(A)** *and posterior* **(B)** *views. Polyethylene pads are present on the tibial component for articulation with the metallic femoral component. Full constraint is provided by central ball-and-socket articulation (arrow).*

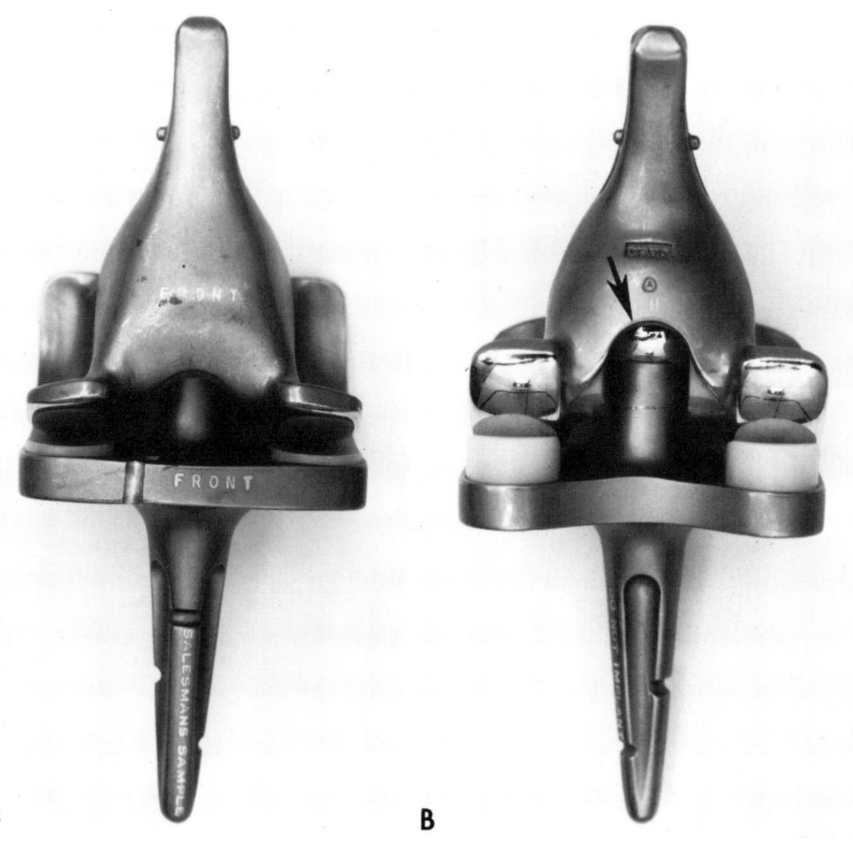

tibial portion is curved in its anteroposterior direction to provide stability in flexion and extension. The cruciate and collateral ligaments are preserved.

Fully constrained knee arthroplasties include the metal-metal Guepar, Walldius, and Shiers hinge arthroplasties and the spherocentric metal-polyethylene arthroplasty.[133-136] The spherocentric replacement is a nonhinged but intrinsically stable prosthesis that allows triaxial rotation (Fig. 25–25). There are three metal-polyethylene articulating surfaces: two runner and track joints between the tibia and femoral condyles and a ball-and-socket joint centrally. This latter joint permits triaxial rotation without the possibility of dislocation.

The knee prostheses discussed previously are not true total knee arthroplasties, since the patellofemoral joint is not replaced. Following TKA, about 15 per cent of patients have severe pain, which may arise from the patellofemoral articulation.[137] Patellofemoral pain is more common in patients with osteoarthritis. To alleviate this situation, various true TKA models have been developed that include patellar resurfacing. The total condylar prosthesis, a typical true TKA, utilizes a polyethylene button that is implanted on the articular surface of the patella and held in place with bone cement[137] (Fig. 25–26).

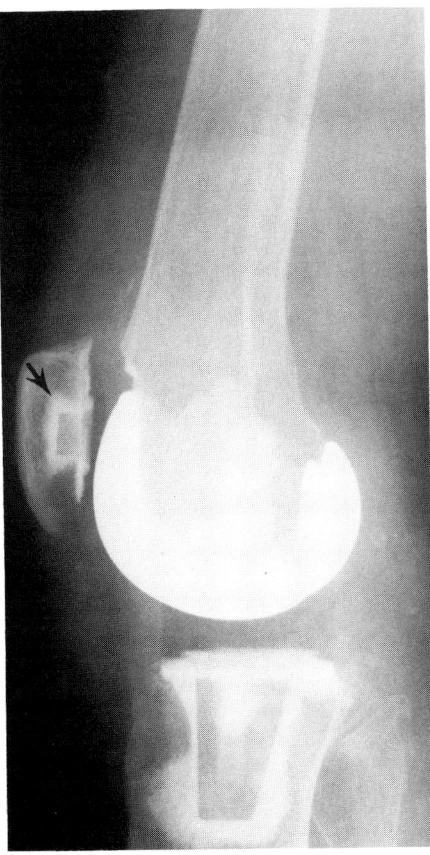

Figure 25–26. *Lateral view of total condylar type TKA. Polyethylene patellar resurfacing implant is cemented in place (arrow).*

Normal Appearance. The alignment and position of the various TKA components must be carefully evaluated on the initial postoperative films. It is helpful to refer to the initial radiographs to detect subtle changes in alignment on follow-up examinations (Fig. 25–27). Ideal alignment and position of the prosthetic components vary with the type of unit that is chosen. Such parameters may be determined by reference to manufacturers' brochures and available literature.[138-140] Alignment of the knee, including residual varus or valgus angulation, should also be noted. Residual angular deformity is usually corrected in the initial plaster cast, but it may become evident on follow-up examinations that are obtained with the patient out of the cast. Intraoperative fractures and intra-articular bone or cement fragments should be noted. Other general guidelines that are derived from experience with hip arthroplasties are applied to the radiographic evaluation of the bone-cement interface of knee prostheses. Normal radiolucent zones at the bone-cement interface appearing during the first 6 months following TKA are much more common about the tibial component than the femoral component of nonhinged TKA with metal femoral and polyethylene tibial components.[141] In metal-metal hinged knee prostheses, normal radiolucent zones are equally frequent about both the femoral and the tibial components. These observations support the role of heat necrosis of bone in the generation of normal radiolucent zones at the bone-cement interface. It is postulated that such zones are less common on the metal side because of its greater heat conductivity.

As in THA, radionuclide scanning and joint aspiration with subtraction arthrography may be used in the evaluation of symptomatic knee prostheses. However, there has been limited experience with radionuclide bone scanning in evaluation of these latter prostheses.[168] In fact, there has not been a comprehensive prospective study of the various imaging modalities that are available for evaluation of the symptomatic TKA. Anecdotal experience with scintigraphy in TKA indicates that focal or unicomponent uptake, especially that which is evidenced 6 months or longer following surgery, suggests loosening or infection, or both. Using lateral images, patellofemoral uptake can be distinguished from activity about the femoral component.[102]

Subtraction arthrography is performed to enhance detection of contrast-tracking within the bone-cement interface. After preliminary AP, lateral, and oblique films are obtained, the joint is punctured in the usual retropatellar fashion. Fluid is aspirated for Gram stain, culture, and sensitivity tests. Nonbacteriostatic saline lavage may be used if no fluid is obtained. If a patellectomy has been performed, the joint may be entered from either an anterior ap-

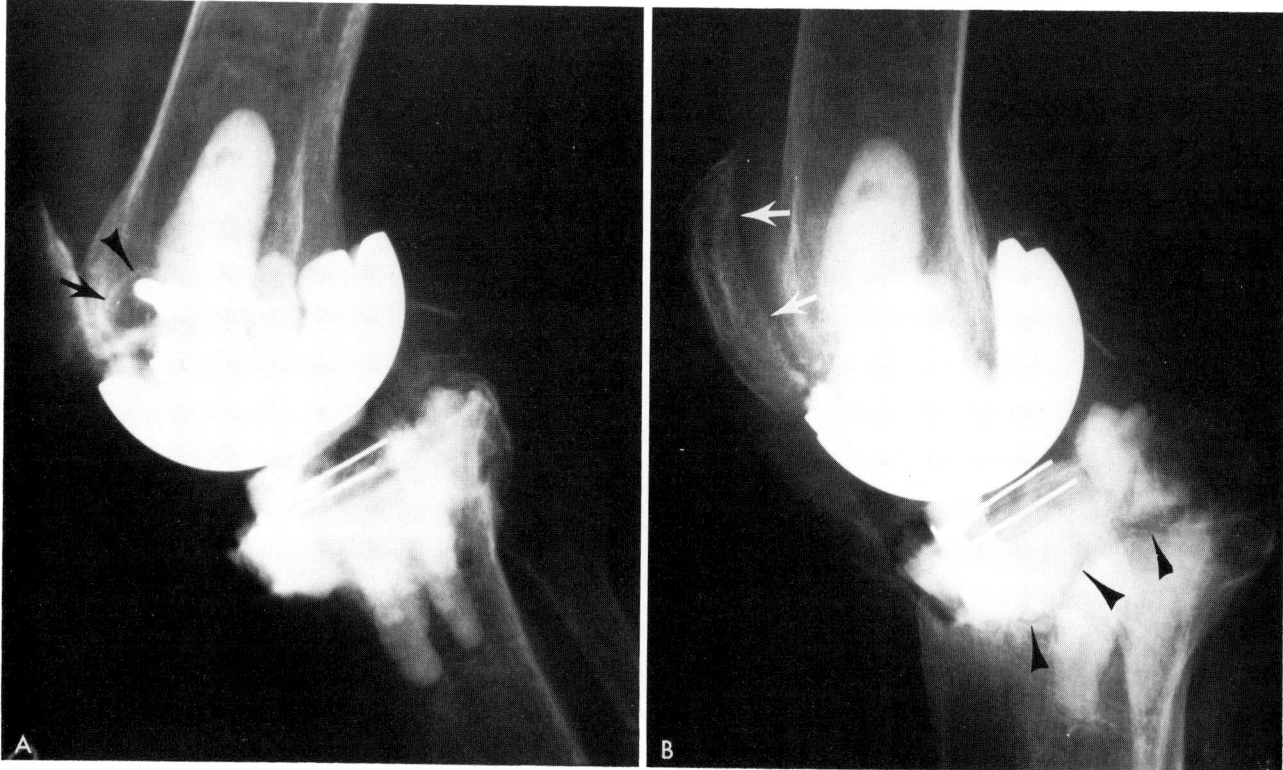

Figure 25–27. *Alignment change in geometric type TKA.*

A *Lateral radiograph. A femoral bone screw is used for stabilization of an intraoperative femoral fracture (arrowhead). The screw was removed subsequently because of adjacent bone resorption suggesting osteomyelitis (arrow).*

B *Follow-up lateral radiograph demonstrating cement fracture (arrowheads) with marked change in alignment of the tibial component. There was interval resorption of the patella in this patient, with an infected prosthesis (arrows).*

proach, directing the needle into the intercondylar region, or a lateral approach, directing the needle in the horizontal plane. In either case, fluoroscopic control is utilized. As always, the intra-articular position is confirmed if a drop of contrast material flows away from the needle tip. The calf is stabilized with sandbags and about 10 kg of traction is applied at the ankle using any convenient device. An AP scout film is obtained with the overhead tube. Without interval motion, three to four additional films are obtained following injection of 16 to 40 ml of contrast medium (methylglucamine — 60 per cent) in 8 to 10 ml increments. The needle is removed and the initial film series is repeated after 2 to 3 min of passive and active exercise. Appropriate subtraction films are made from the initial film series (Fig. 25–28). Resolution may often be improved by positioning the mask separately for the femoral and the tibial components.

Complications. A variety of TKA complications are detectable by radiographic procedures (Table 25–3).

Instability, subluxation, or angulation may be accentuated on weight-bearing or stress views. An asymmetric tibial component that is used to correct varus or valgus angulation should not be misinterpreted as evidence of compartmental widening. As in THA, stress fractures may occur anywhere from the pelvis to the foot owing to increased activity levels following TKA.[165, 169] Migration of wire locator guides has been noted in some of the tibial components[139-142] (Fig. 25–1). "Locking" of the knee in extension may be due to patellar osteophytes that become trapped on an exposed ridge of bone created during the placement of the femoral component.[139]

Distinguishing loosening alone from loosening associated with infection may be difficult. Demonstration of positive cultures, rapid bone resorption or destruction, and draining sinus tracts all support a preoperative diagnosis of infection (Fig. 25–29).

OTHER SITES AND PROCEDURES

Silicone Arthroplasty

Silicone rubber arthroplasties and implants of the hand, the wrist, the elbow, and the foot do not represent true prostheses. They merely act as spacers, separating bone ends and providing a form for periarticular soft tissues. They are most commonly utilized for the replacement of metacarpophalan-

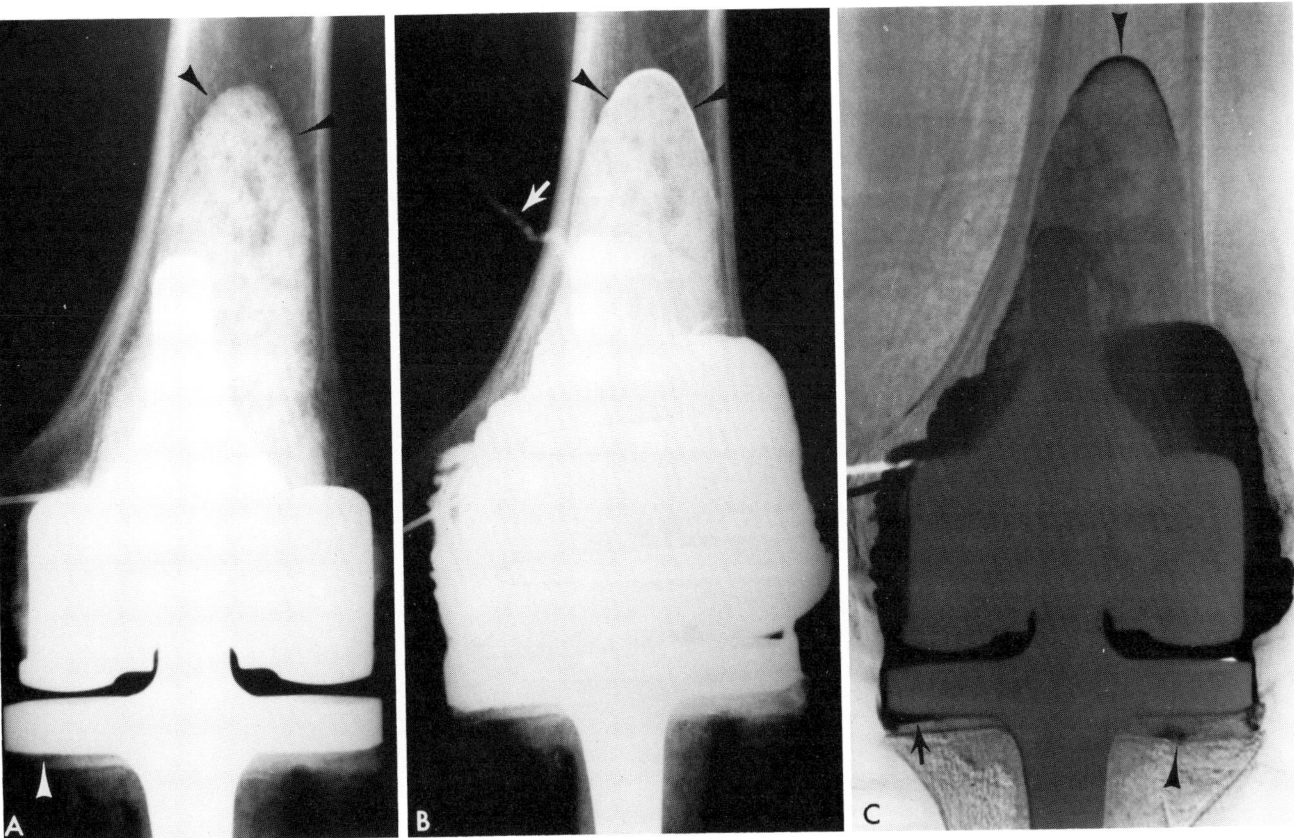

Figure 25–28. Prosthesis loosening.

A *Radiograph of spherocentric TKA. Narrow (1 mm) radiolucent zones are noted at the bone-cement interface of the femoral component and the metal-cement interface of the tibial component (arrowheads).*

B *Arthrogram showing contrast material entering the bone-cement interface of the femoral component (arrowheads) and lymphatic filling (white arrow). Contrast material entering the metal-cement interface along the tibial component is more easily appreciated in the subtraction radiograph* **(C)**.

C *Subtraction arthrogram demonstrating contrast material entering the metal-cement interface of the tibial component (arrow) as well as bone-cement interface of both components (arrowheads).*

Table 25–3
RADIOGRAPHIC COMPLICATIONS OF TOTAL KNEE ARTHROPLASTY

Intraoperative/postoperative fracture
Stress fracture
Patellar dislocation or locking
Instability
Dislocation or subluxation
Migration of wire marker
Loosening/infection

geal (MCP) joints in patients with severe rheumatoid arthritis. Surgical indications include severe pain, joint space loss, osseous destruction due to synovial hypertrophy, and alignment deformity. Carpal, distal ulnar, and radial head implants serve as spacers to restore function in patients with rheumatoid arthritis, osteonecrosis, nonunion, or posttraumatic deformity.

Normal Appearance. Silicone rubber is less dense radiographically than bone, and slightly more dense than the soft tissues (Fig. 25–30). Radiographic examination of MCP joint implants should include posteroanterior (PA), oblique, and true lateral radiographs, supplemented by tomography, especially in the lateral projection. As with any arthroplasty, postoperative films are analyzed for correction and maintenance of desired alignment.

The thicker, hinged portion (midsection) of finger prostheses should abut the adjacent resected margin of the metaphyseal bone. A nonrotated PA radiograph usually shows a symmetrically located rectangular midsection if there is no significant rotation. On the lateral film, the distal palmar aspect of the midsection is concave, allowing flexion but limited hyperextension. It is often difficult to visualize the stem within the medullary canal. In time, a thin sclerotic band of intramedullary bone may form. The tip of the stem may then be noted 1 to 2 mm from the adjacent bone, allowing room for a slight gliding or piston action with flexion-extension. A bone spur may arise from the volar aspect of the metacarpal. Rarely, such a spur may reach the base of the proximal phalanx, resulting in decreased flexion or ankylosis.[143]

Complications. Dislocation of MCP joint implants may occur if a stem slips out of its medullary canal.[144] Radial head, distal ulnar, and carpal bone replacements may sublux or dislocate (Fig. 25–31). Erosion of bone at points of contact between the prosthesis and bone may allow migration of the prosthesis.[143] Although silicone implants withstand millions of machine flexions without breakage, fractures, cracking, and fragmentation have been noted in vivo[143, 144] (Figs. 25–32, and 25–33). Shear forces in vivo may account for this disparity. At the MCP joints, these changes are difficult to detect on the PA

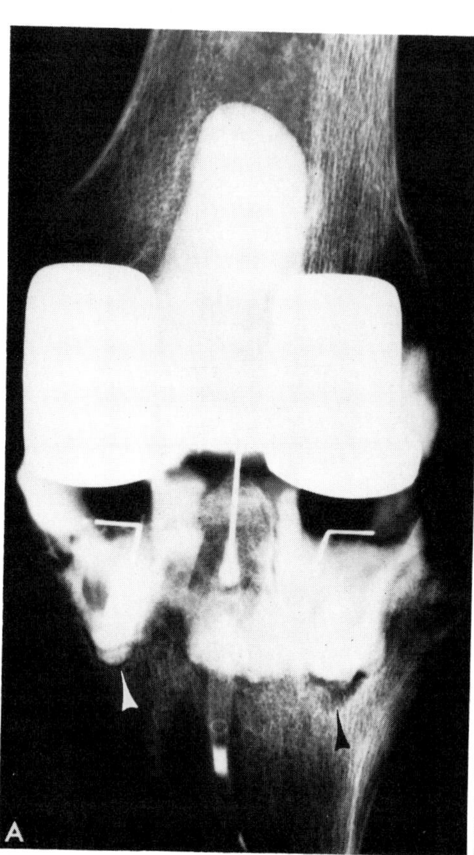

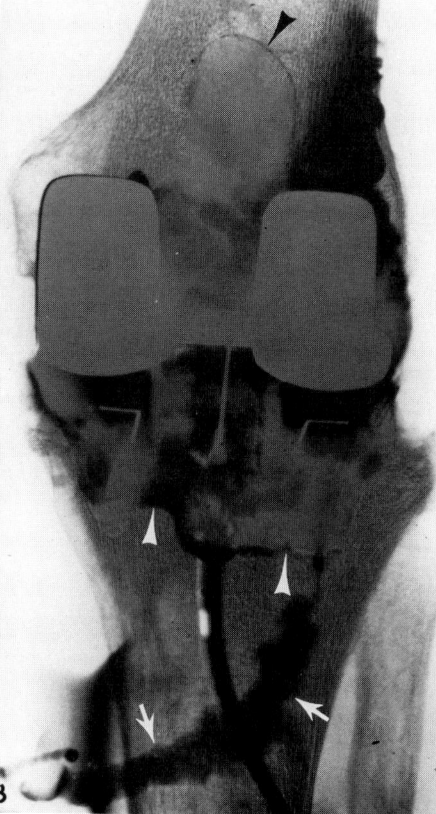

Figure 25–29. *Infection.*
A *Preliminary anteroposterior (AP) radiograph with needle in place (geometric TKA, patella removed). A wide radiolucent zone (2.5 mm) is present around the bone-cement interface of the tibial component (arrowheads).*
B *Anteroposterior subtraction arthrogram showing contrast material tracking along the bone-cement interface of both components (arrowheads). A sinus tract is demonstrated extending from the base of the tibial component to the skin (arrows).*

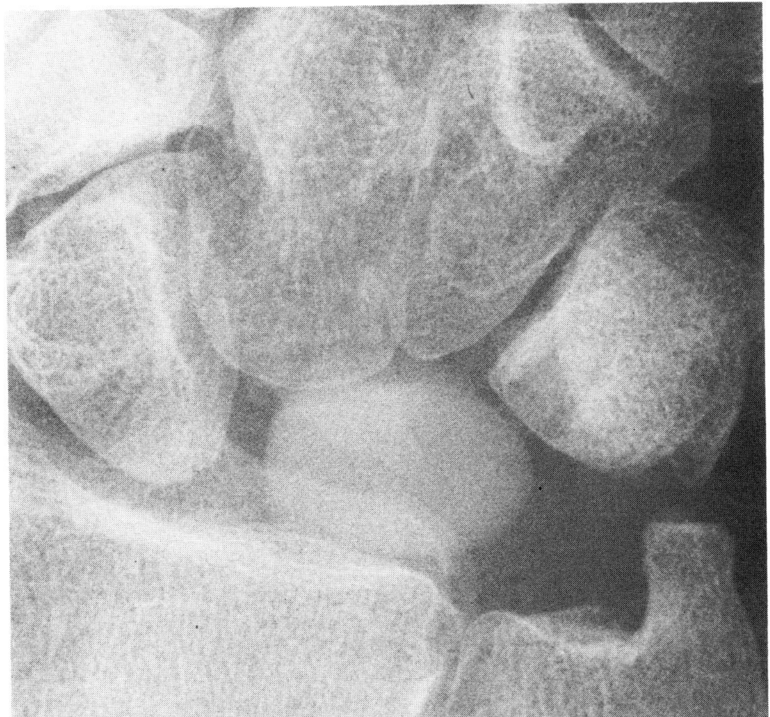

Figure 25–30. *Lunate prosthesis. Posteroanterior (PA) view of wrist following placement of silicone lunate prosthesis, which acts as a spacer between adjacent carpal bones and the radius. There is slight ulnar subluxation of the prosthesis with reference to the capitate.*

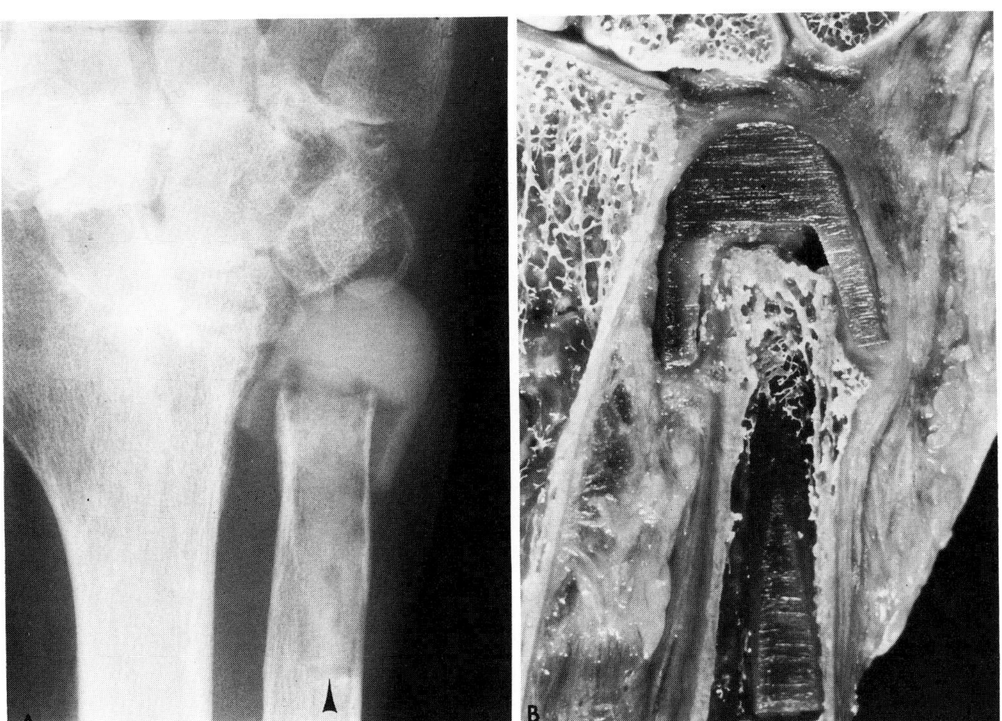

Figure 25–31. *Ulnar head prosthesis.*

A *Silicone ulnar head prosthesis in patient with severe rheumatoid arthritis. There is angulation of the prosthesis from collapse and ulnar subluxation of the carpal bones. A normal space is noted between the tip of the prosthesis stem and the adjacent bone (arrowhead).*

B *Anatomic section of silicone ulnar head prosthesis in a cadaver with rheumatoid arthritis.*

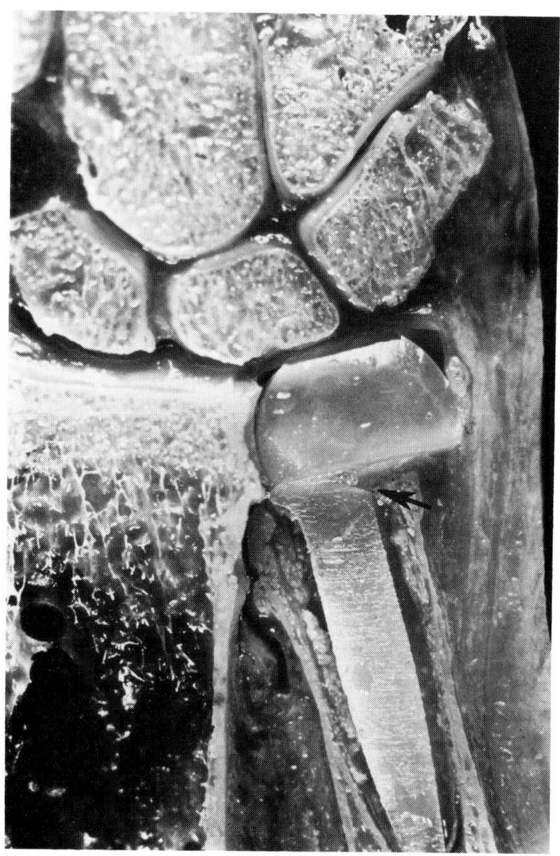

Figure 25–32. Anatomic section of fractured ulnar head prosthesis (arrow).

projections and are best detected on lateral tomograms performed in full flexion or extension.[143] Frank fractures are more easily diagnosed clinically than radiographically. Following fracture of the hinge, the base of the phalanx is usually displaced volarly.[145]

The overall infection rate following MCP joint implants is less than 1 per cent.[146] Increased osteoporosis with soft tissue swelling may be an early sign of infection. Contamination at the time of surgery may be due to implantation of lint or surgical glove powder. More advanced infection may be recognized by periosteal reaction or bone destruction, sometimes with subluxation of the prosthesis.[144]

Osteotomies

Osteotomy, a surgical cutting of bone, is a procedure with widespread application in the pelvis (usually for the hip) and in the long bones.[147] The general goal of treatment is the improvement of function with correction of deformity. This goal may be achieved by a change in angulation, rotation, or bone length.

The need for osteotomy may arise from congenital problems (congenital dislocation of the hip, proximal femoral focal deficiency) or problems acquired during years of growth (slipped capital femoral epiphysis, deformity resulting from epiphyseal in-

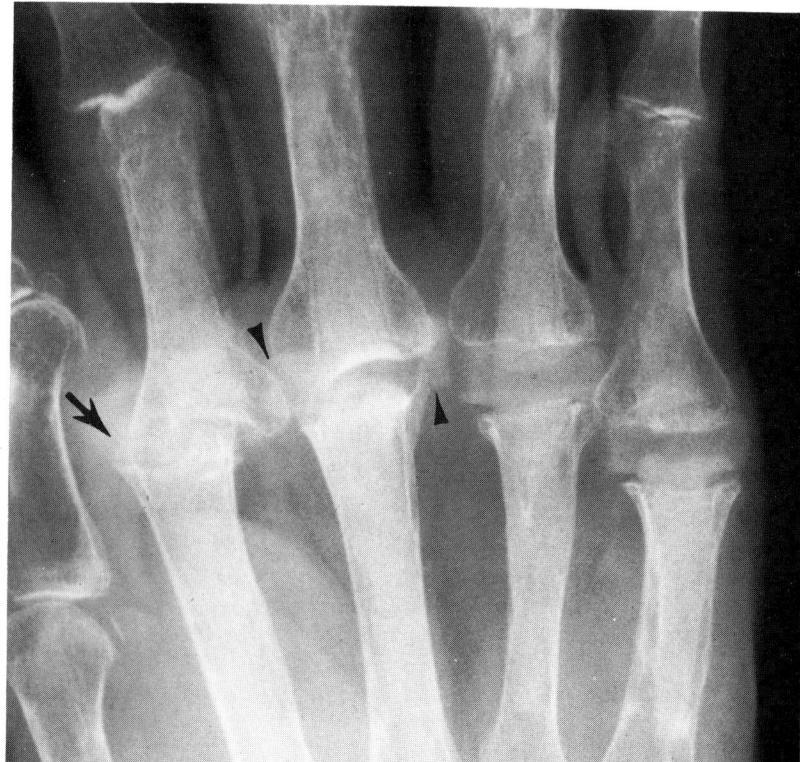

Figure 25–33. Silicone metacarpophalangeal (MCP) joint implants. There is a fracture of the second MCP joint prosthesis manifested by subluxation (arrow). A fracture of the third MCP joint prosthesis shows narrowing of the joint space with extrusion of silicone fragments (arrowheads). The remaining implants appear intact.

jury). More recently, arthritic deformity, especially in weight-bearing joints such as the hip and knee, has been an indication for osteotomy. Osteotomy of the proximal tibia and fibula in the adult is the most commonly performed osteotomy for arthritis.

Tibial Osteotomy. Proximal tibial osteotomy may be performed for degenerative genu varus or valgus. The rationale of tibial osteotomy is the correction of varus or valgus angulation with a shift of the center of weight-bearing forces to the more preserved compartment. Preoperative studies are focused on the evaluation of the "uninvolved" compartment and supporting ligamentous structures in order to determine the best surgical candidates. Preoperative assessment relies heavily on imaging procedures, including plain films, radionuclide bone scanning, and arthrography, in addition to the clinical examination.

Radiographs should include weight-bearing anteroposterior (AP) and lateral films to accurately assess the degree of varus or valgus angulation and subluxation under weight-bearing stress. Deformity may be accentuated if weight-bearing films are obtained while the patient is standing on one leg at a time. Ligamentous instability may be further assessed with stress films. Three-compartment degen-

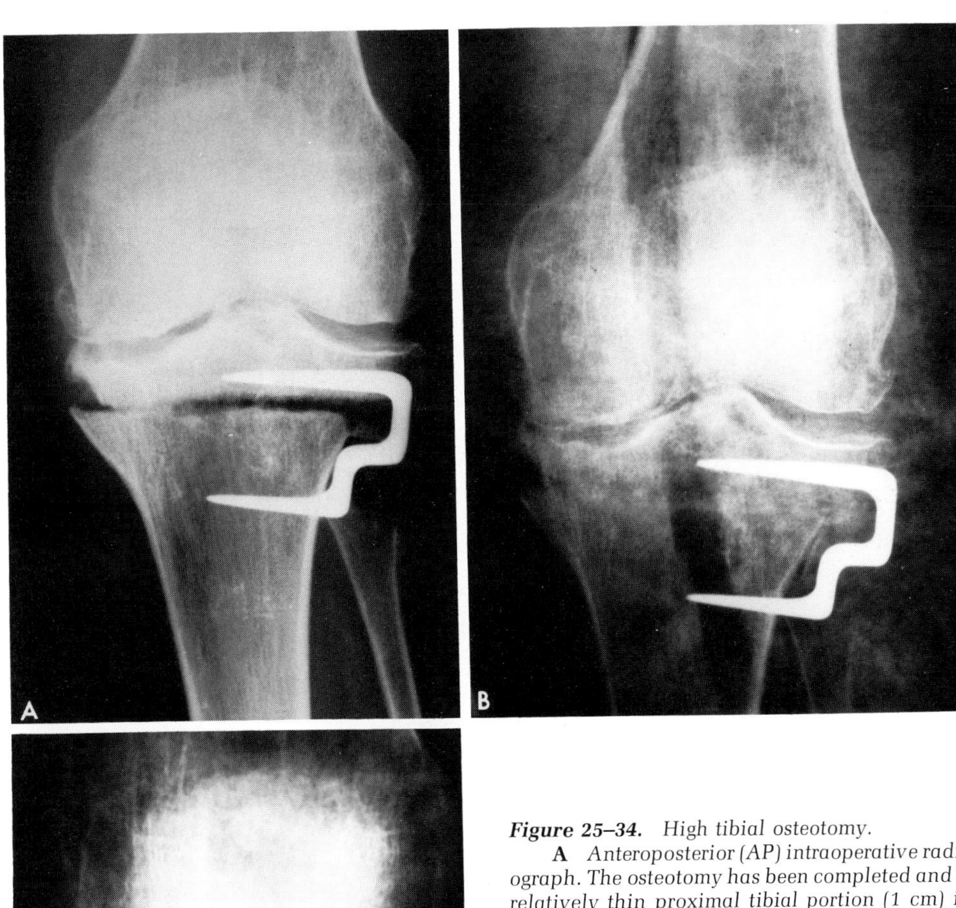

Figure 25–34. *High tibial osteotomy.*

A *Anteroposterior (AP) intraoperative radiograph. The osteotomy has been completed and a relatively thin proximal tibial portion (1 cm) is fixed in place with a stepped staple. A portion of the fibular head has been removed.*

B *Initial AP postoperative radiograph through plaster shows bone apposition across the osteotomy site. Evaluation of postoperative angulation raised the question of whether there was undercorrection, with insufficient valgus angulation for lateral compartment weight-bearing.*

C *AP radiograph 5 weeks later. The narrow proximal tibial fragment has fractured (arrow) and there is lateral subluxation of the fragment, with migration of the staple.*

eration (medial femorotibial, lateral femorotibial, patellofemoral) and severe ligament laxity are among the contraindications to osteotomy. Milder stages of patellofemoral disease rarely present a problem following tibial osteotomy, although advanced disease with large osteophytes may require additional surgical procedures.[148-150]

Patients fulfilling clinical and plain film radiographic criteria for tibial osteotomy may be evaluated further with radionuclide bone scanning, arthrography, and arthroscopy. Radionuclide bone scanning has been shown to be the most sensitive modality in the compartmental evaluation of preoperative patients.[151] Images are obtained in both AP and lateral positions; the lateral position aids in differentiation of patellofemoral from lateral femorotibial compartment involvement. Combined medial and lateral femorotibial compartment involvement is detected more often by bone scanning than by clinical examination and standing radiographs. Double contrast arthrography is useful in detection of meniscal lesions in addition to cartilage erosion or thinning. However, arthrography is more invasive than scintigraphy and has limitations, including (1) difficulty in obtaining a satisfactory examination in patients with advanced osteoarthritis; (2) limited region of articular cartilage that is actually visualized; and (3) difficulty in evaluating the patellar cartilage. Scintigraphy has been shown to be more sensitive than arthrography for the evaluation of the weight-bearing compartments.[151]

High tibial osteotomy (HTO) is performed by removing a wedge of bone above the level of the tibial tubercle. When performed for correction of varus deformity, the tethering effect of the proximal fibula must be considered. This effect is corrected by (1) osteotomy of the fibular shaft; (2) removal of the fibular head; or (3) division of the capsule of the proximal tibiofibular joint. In cases of varus deformity, slight overcorrection to 5 to 10 degrees of valgus angulation is desirable. The width of the wedge may be measured on the preoperative films, allowing for magnification. Use of a long tube-film distance decreases the degree of magnification. It is difficult to appreciate the actual correction at the time of surgery, and intraoperative films are often obtained with marking pins in place prior to removal of bone; immediate postoperative films with the limb in a plaster cast are also obtained. An approximation that the removal of 1 cm of bone at the base of the wedge will correct 10 degrees of angulation can be applied to the "average" tibia, although the actual angle varies with the size of the bone.[152] Following removal of the wedge, the bone fragments are stabilized with a plain or stepped staple and a cylinder cast. Healing is generally rapid, since cancellous bone is involved.

Certain observations are important in the postoperative evaluation of the success of the osteotomy. Alignment in plaster should approximate the desired result. The position of the staple should be noted, since it may enter the intra-articular space or may migrate outward. Fracture or subluxation of a portion of the tibial plateau may also occur; the proximal fragment should be about 2 cm thick[153] (Fig. 25–34). If too large a wedge was removed, the overcorrection will not permit partial weight-bearing on the affected side, which will result in an unstable knee (the "teeter effect").[154] HTO for correction of valgus deformity results in some obliquity of the articular surface with reference to the floor. This obliquity should be limited to about 10 to 15 degrees; excessive obliquity results in medial subluxation of the femur on the tibia.[148, 155] Delayed union is possible with low tibial osteotomy (performed below the tibial tubercle) but is avoidable with HTO. As in any osteotomy, infection is a potential complication.

SUMMARY

In this chapter a limited but representative group of periarticular surgical procedures is considered. Modern arthroplasty techniques have received the most attention; they represent the major thrust in reconstructive joint surgery. Surgical techniques developed prior to arthroplasty are also covered, both as historical elements and as procedures that may still be performed. Radiographic evaluation of such procedures is facilitated by knowledge of material technology, treatment goals, and expected radiographic appearance. Generally, current concepts may be applied in judging the value of newer procedures and prosthetic components as they are developed.

REFERENCES

1. Elloy MA, Wright JTM, Cavendish ME: The basic requirements and design criteria for total joint prostheses. Acta Orthop Scand *47*:193, 1976.
2. Walker PS, Bullough PG: The effects of friction and wear in artificial joints. Orthop Clin North Am *4*:275, 1973.
3. Evans EM, Freeman MAR, Miller AJ, Vernon-Roberts B: Metal sensitivity as a cause of bone necrosis and loosening of the prosthesis in total joint replacement. J Bone Joint Surg *56B*:626, 1974.
4. Benson MKD, Goodwin PG, Brostoff J: Metal sensitivity in patients with joint replacement arthroplasties. Br Med J *4*:374, 1975.
5. Jones DA, Lucas HK, O'Driscoll M, Price CHG, Wibberley B: Cobalt toxicity after McKee hip arthroplasty. J Bone Joint Surg *57B*:289, 1975.
6. Charosky CB, Bullough PG, Wilson P Jr: Total hip replacement failures: A histological evaluation. J Bone Joint Surg *55A*:49, 1973.
7. Swanson SAV, Freeman MAR, Heath JC: Laboratory tests on total joint replacement prostheses. J Bone Joint Surg *55B*:759, 1973.
8. Elves MW, Wilson JN, Scales JT, Kemp HBS: Incidence of metal sensitivity in patients with total joint replacements. Br Med *4*:376, 1975.

9. Webley M, Kates A, Snaith ML: Metal sensitivity in patients with a hinge arthroplasty of the knee. Ann Rheum Dis *37*:373, 1978.
10. Deutman R, Mulder TJ, Brian R, Nater JB: Metal sensitivity before and after total hip arthroplasty. J Bone Joint Surg *59A*:862, 1977.
11. Brown GC, Lockshin MD, Salvati EA, Bullough PG: Sensitivity to metal as a possible cause of sterile loosening after cobalt-chromium total hip replacement arthroplasty. J Bone Joint Surg *59A*:164, 1977.
12. Heath JC, Freeman MAR, Swanson SAV: Carcinogenic properties of wear particles from prostheses made from cobalt-chromium alloys. Lancet *1*:564, 1971.
13. Duff-Barclay I, Spillman DT: Total human hip joint prostheses — a laboratory study of friction and wear. Proc Inst Mech Engineers *181*:90, 1966.
14. Galante JO, Rostoker W: Wear in total hip prostheses. An experimental evaluation of candidate materials. Acta Orthop Scand (Suppl) *145*:1, 1973.
15. Charnley J, Halley DK: Rate of wear in total hip replacement. Clin Orthop Rel Res *112*:170, 1975.
16. Crugnola A, Schiller A, Radin E: Polymeric debris in synovium after total joint replacement: histological identification. J Bone Joint Surg *59A*:860, 1977.
17. Hueper WC, Conway WD: Chemical Carcinogenesis and Cancers. Springfield, Ill, Charles C Thomas, 1964.
18. Wiltse LL, Hall RH, Stenehjem JC: Experimental studies regarding the possible use of self-curing acrylic in orthopaedic surgery. J Bone Joint Surg *39A*:961, 1957.
19. Charnley J: Anchorage of the femoral head prosthesis to the shaft of the femur. J Bone Joint Surg *42B*:28, 1960.
20. Charnley J: The bonding of prostheses to bone by cement. J Bone Joint Surg *46B*:518, 1964.
21. Harrington KD, Johnston JO, Turner RH, et al: Use of methylmethacrylate as an adjunct to the internal fixation of malignant neoplastic fractures. J Bone Joint Surg *54A*:1665, 1972.
22. Carlson DH, Adams R: The use of methylmethacrylate in repair of neoplastic lesions in bone. Radiology *112*:43, 1974.
23. Cameron HU, Pilliar RM, Macnab I: The effect of movement on the bonding of porous metal to bone. J Biomed Mater Res *7*:301, 1973.
24. Charnley J: Acrylic Cement in Orthopedic Surgery. Baltimore, Williams & Wilkins, 1970.
25. Haas SS, Brauer GM, Dickson G: Characterization of polymethylmethacrylate bone cement. J Bone Joint Surg *57A*:380, 1975.
26. Hinderling T, Ruegsegger P, Anliker M, Dietschi C: Computed tomography reconstruction from hollow projections: An application to in vivo evaluation of artificial hip joints. J Comput Assist Tomogr *3*:52, 1979.
27. Charnley J: Sensitivity to acrylic resins. *In* J Charnley: Acrylic Cement in Orthopedic Surgery. Baltimore, Williams & Wilkins, 1970.
28. Charnley J, Follacci FM, Hammond BT: The long-term reaction of bone to self-curing acrylic cement. J Bone Joint Surg *50B*:822, 1968.
29. Beabout JW: Radiology of total hip arthroplasty. Radiol Clin North Am *13*:3, 1975.
30. Fornasier VL, Cameron HU: The femoral stem/cement interface in total hip replacement. Clin Orthop Rel Res *116*:248, 1976.
31. Swanson AB: Silicone rubber implants for replacement of arthritic or destroyed joints in the hand. Surg Clin North Am *48*:1113, 1968.
32. Niebauer JJ, Shaw JL, Doren WW: Silicone-dacron hinge prosthesis: Design, evaluation, and application. Ann Rheum Dis *28* (Suppl):56, 1969.
33. Swanson AB: Flexible implant arthroplasty for arthritic finger joints. J Bone Joint Surg *54A*:435, 1972.
34. Weightman B, Simon S, Rose R, Paul I, Radin E: Environmental fatigue testing of Silastic finger joint prostheses. *In* CA Homsy, CD Armeniades (Eds): Biomaterials for Skeletal and Cardiovascular Applications. New York, Wiley-Interscience, 1972.
35. Swanson AB: Finger joint replacement by silicone rubber implants and the concept of implant fixation by encapsulation. Ann Rheum Dis *28* (Suppl):47, 1969.
36. McKee GK, Watson-Farrar J: Replacement of arthritic hips by McKee-Farrar prosthesis. J Bone Joint Surg *48B*:245, 1966.
37. Charnley J: Total hip replacement by low friction arthroplasty. Clin Orthop Rel Res *72*:7, 1970.
38. Harris WH: Current Concepts: Total joint replacement. N Engl J Med *297*:650, 1977.
39. Gilula LA, Staple TW: A miniature atlas of total hip prostheses. Radiol Clin North Amer *13*:21, 1975.
40. Angell FL, Watts FB: Total hip replacement: Roentgen apperance of current devices. Am J Roentgenol *110*:787, 1970.
41. Switzer PJ, Cooperberg PL, Knickerbocker WJ: Defects in the sigmoid colon caused by placement of a left hip prosthesis. J Can Assoc Radiol *25*:151, 1974.
42. Goergen TG, Resnick D: Evaluation of acetabular anteversion following total hip arthroplasty. Necessity of proper centering. Br J Radiol *48*:259, 1975.
43. McLaren RH: Prosthetic hip angulation. Radiology *107*:705, 1973.
44. Daffner RH, Carden TS, Gehweiler JA: Complication of unrecognized dislocation of Charnley-Müller hip prosthesis. Radiology *108*:323, 1973.
45. Jackson DM: Total hip prosthesis: Real and apparent dislocation. Clin Radiol *26*:63, 1975.
46. Coventry MB, Beckenbaugh RD, Nolan DR, et al: 2012 total hip arthroplasties: A study of postoperative course and early complications. J Bone Joint Surg *56A*:273, 1974.
47. Lazansky MG: Complications in total hip replacement with the Charnley technique. Clin Orthop Rel Res *72*:40, 1970.
48. Volz RG, Brown FW: The painful migrated ununited greater trochanter in total hip replacement. J Bone Joint Surg *59A*:1091, 1977.
49. Müller ME: Total hip prostheses. Clin Orthop Rel Res *72*:46, 1970.
50. Habermann ET, Feinstein PA: Total hip replacement arthroplasty in arthritic conditions of the hip joint. Semin Arthritis Rheum *7*:189, 1978.
51. Campbell RE, Rothman RH: Charnley low-friction total hip replacement. Am J Roentgenol *113*:634, 1971.
52. Campbell RE, Marvel JP: Concomitant dislocation and intra-articular foreign body: A rare complication of the Charnley total hip arthroplasty. Am J Roentgenol *126*:1059, 1976.
53. Tailor CC, Murphy WA, Smith EL: Intra-articular methylmethacrylate: A complication of hip surgery. Am J Roentgenol *131*:1055, 1978.
54. Parker HG, Wiesman HJ, Ewald FC, Thomas WH, Sledge CB: Comparison of immediate and late results of total hip replacement with and without trochanteric osteotomy. *In* Proceedings of the American Orthopedic Association. J Bone Joint Surg *56A*:1537, 1974.
55. Wiesman HJ, Simon SR, Ewald FC, Thomas WH, Sledge CB: Total hip replacement with and without osteotomy of the greater trochanter. J Bone Joint Surg *60A*:203, 1978.
56. Bronson, JL: Articular interposition of trochanteric wires in a failed total hip replacement. Clin Orthop Rel Res *121*:50, 1976.
57. Freeman PA, Lee P, Bryson TW: Total hip joint replacement in osteoarthrosis and polyarthritis. A statistical study of the results. Clin Orthop Rel Res *95*:224, 1973.
58. Bisla RS, Ranawat CS, Inglis AE: Total hip replacement in patients with ankylosing spondylitis with involvement of the hip. J Bone Joint Surg *58A*:233, 1976.
59. DeLee J, Ferrari A, Charnley J: Ectopic bone formation following low friction arthroplasty of the hip. Clin Orthop Rel Res *121*:53, 1976.
60. Riegler HF, Harris CM: Heterotopic bone formation after total hip arthroplasty. Clin Orthop Rel Res *117*:209, 1976.
61. Ritter MA, Vaughan RB: Ectopic ossification after total hip arthroplasty. Predisposing factors, frequency, and effect on results. J Bone Joint Surg *59A*:345, 1977.
62. Brooker AF, Bowerman JW, Robinson RA, Riley LH: Ectopic ossification following total hip replacement. Incidence and a method of classification. J Bone Joint Surg *55A*:1629, 1973.
63. Nollen AJG, Slooff TJJH: Para-articular ossifications after total hip replacement. Acta Orthop Scand *44*:230, 1973.
64. Mall J, Hoffer P, Murray W, Rodrigo J, Anger H, Samuel A: Heterotopic bone, a potential source of error in evaluating hip prostheses by radionuclide techniques (abstract). J Nucl Med *18*:604, 1977.
65. Ali Khan MA, O'Driscoll M: Fractures of the femur during total hip replacement and their management. J Bone Joint Surg *59B*:36, 1977.
66. Rosemeyer B, Jäger M, Witt AN: Femurfrakturen bei Totalendoprosthesen. Arch Orthop Unfall-Chir *76*:40, 1972.
67. Scott RD, Turner RH, Leitzes SM, Aufranc OE: Femoral fractures in conjunction with total hip replacement. J Bone Joint Surg *57A*:494, 1975.
68. McElfresh EC, Coventry MB: Femoral and pelvic fractures after total hip arthroplasty. J Bone Joint Surg *56A*:483, 1974.
69. Miller AJ: Late fracture of the acetabulum after total hip replacement. J Bone Joint Surg *54B*:600, 1972.
70. Salvati EA, Bullough P, Wilson PD: Intrapelvic protrusion of the acetabular component following total hip replacement. Clin Orthop Rel Res *111*:212, 1975.
71. Andersson GBJ, Freeman MAR, Swanson SAW: Loosening of the cemented acetabular cup in total hip replacement. J Bone Joint Surg *54B*:590, 1972.
72. Eftekhar N: Low-friction arthroplasty: Indications, contraindications, and complications. JAMA *218*:705, 1971.
73. Cruess RL, Bickel WS, VonKessler KLC: Infections in total hips secondary to a primary source elsewhere. Clin Orthop Rel Res *106*:99, 1975.
74. D'Ambrosia RD, Shoji H, Heater R: Secondarily infected total hip joint replacements by hematogenous spread. J Bone Joint Surg *58A*:450, 1976.
75. Mallory TH: Sepsis in total hip replacement following pneumococcal pneumonia: A case report. J Bone Joint Surg *55A*:1753, 1973.
76. Coventry MB: Treatment of infections occurring in total hip surgery. Orthop Clin North Amer *6*:991, 1975.

77. Wilson PD, Aglietti P, Salvati EA: Subacute sepsis of the hip treated by antibiotics and cemented prosthesis. J Bone Joint Surg *56A*:879, 1974.
78. Buchholz HW, Engelbrecht H: Über die Depotwirkung einiger Antibiotica bei Vermischung mitt dem Kunstharz Palacos. Chirurg *41*:511, 1970.
79. Elson RA, Jephcott AE, McGechie DB, Verettas D: Antibiotic-loaded acrylic cement. J Bone Joint Surg *59B*:200, 1977.
80. Amstutz HC: Skeletal fixation and loosening of total hip replacements. Instructional Course Lectures AAOS *23*:201, 1974.
81. Reckling FW, Asher MA, Dillon WL: A longitudinal study of the radiolucent line at the bone-cement interface following total joint replacement procedures. J Bone Joint Surg *59A*:355, 1977.
82. Bergström B, Lidgren L, Lindberg L: Radiographic abnormalities caused by postoperative infection following total hip arthroplasty. Clin Orthop Rel Res *99*:95, 1974.
83. DeLee JG, Charnley J: Radiological demarcation of cemented sockets in total hip replacement. Clin Orthop Rel Res. *121*:20, 1976.
84. Dussalt RG, Goldman AB, Ghelman B: Radiologic diagnosis of loosening and infection of hip prostheses. J Can Assoc Radiol *28*:119, 1977.
85. Salvati EA, Im VC, Aglietti P, Wilson PD: Radiology of total hip replacements. Clin Orthop *121*:74, 1976.
86. Schatzker J, Horne JG, Sumner-Smith G, Sanderson R, Murnaghan JP: Methylmethacrylate cement: Its curing temperature and effect on articular cartilage. Can J Surg *18*:172, 1975.
87. Homsy CA, Tullos HS, King JW: Evaluation of rapid-cure acrylic compound for prosthesis stabilization. Clin Orthop Rel Res *67*:169, 1969.
88. Reckling FW, Dillon WL: The bone-cement interface temperature during total joint replacement. J Bone Joint Surg *59A*:80, 1977.
89. Jefferiss CD, Lee AJC, Ling RSM: Thermal aspects of self-curing polymethylmethacrylate. J Bone Surg *57B*:511, 1975.
90. Linder L: Reaction of bone to the acute chemical trauma of bone cement. J Bone Joint Surg *59A*:82, 1977.
91. DeSmet AA, Kramer D, Martel W: The metal-cement interface in total hip prostheses. Am J Roentgenol *129*:279, 1977.
92. Amstutz HC, Markolf KL: Design features in total hip replacements. *In* WH Harris (Ed): The Hip, Proceedings of the Second Open Scientific Meeting of the Hip Society. St. Louis, CV Mosby Co., 1974, p 111.
93. Weber FA, Charnley J: A radiological study of fractures of acrylic cement in relation to the stem of a femoral head prosthesis. J Bone Joint Surg *57B*:297, 1975.
94. Marmor L: Femoral loosening in total hip replacement. Clin Orthop Rel Res *121*:116, 1976.
95. Carlsson AS, Gentz CF, Stenport J: Fracture of the femoral prosthesis in total hip replacement according to Charnley. Acta Orthop Scand *48*:650, 1977.
96. Charnley J: Fracture of femoral prostheses in total hip replacement. Clin Orthop Rel Res *111*:105, 1975.
97. Collis DK: Femoral stem failure in total hip replacement. J Bone Joint Surg *59A*:1033, 1977.
98. Galante JO, Rostoker W, Doyle JM: Failed femoral stems in total hip prostheses. J Bone Joint Surg *57A*:230, 1975.
99. Martens M, Aernoudt E, deMeester P, Ducheyne P, Mulier JC, DeLangh R, Kestelijn P: Factors in the mechanical failure of the femoral component in total hip prosthesis. Acta Orthop Scand *45*:693, 1974.
100. Pellicci PM, Salvati EA, Robinson HJ: Mechanical failures in total hip replacement requiring reoperation. J Bone Joint Surg *61A*:28, 1979.
101. Creutzig H: Bone imaging after total replacement arthroplasty of the hip joint. A follow-up with different radiopharmaceuticals. Eur J Nucl Med *1*:177, 1976.
102. Gelman MI, Coleman RE, Stevens PM, Davey BW: Radiography, radionuclide imaging, and arthrography in the evaluation of total hip and knee replacement. Radiology *128*:677, 1978.
103. Williams ED, Tregonning RJ, Hurley PJ: ^{99m}Tc-diphosphonate scanning as an aid to diagnosis of infection in total hip joint replacements. Br J Radiol *50*:562, 1977.
104. Goergen TG: Unpublished data.
105. Anderson LS, Staple TW: Arthrography of total hip replacement using subtraction technique. Radiology *109*:470, 1973.
106. Melson GL, McDaniel RC, Southern PM, Staple TW: In vitro effects of iodinated arthrographic contrast media on bacterial growth. Radiology *112*:593, 1974.
107. Coren GS, Curtis J, Dalinka M: Lymphatic visualization during hip arthrography. Radiology *115*:621, 1975.
108. Gelman MI: Arthrography in total hip prosthesis complications. Am J Roentgenol *126*:743, 1976.
109. Murray WR, Rodrigo JJ: Arthrography for assessment of pain after total hip replacement. J Bone Joint Surg *57A*:1060, 1975.
110. Brown CS, Knickerbocker WJ: Radiologic studies in the investigation of the causes of total hip replacement failures. J Can Assoc Radiol *24*:245, 1973.
111. Harris WH, Aufranc OE: Mold arthroplasty in the treatment of hip fractures complicated by sepsis. J Bone Joint Surg *47A*:31, 1965.
112. Halley DK, Charnley J: Results of low friction arthroplasty in patients thirty years of age or younger. Clin Orthop Rel Res *112*:180, 1975.
113. Enneking WF, Singsen ET: Pathologic changes in the idiopathic painful cup arthroplasty. Clin Orthop Rel Res *101*:236, 1974.
114. Johnston RC, Larson CB: Results of treatment of hip disorders with cup arthroplasty. J Bone Joint Surg *51A*:1461, 1969.
115. Aufranc OE: Constructive hip surgery with the vitallium mold. J Bone Joint Surg *39A*:237, 1957.
116. Freedman MT: Radiologic aspects of femoral head replacements and cup mold arthroplasties. Radiol Clin North Am *13*:45, 1975.
117. Hamblen DL, Harris WH, Rottger J: Myositis ossificans as a complication of hip arthroplasty. J Bone Joint Surg *53B*:764, 1971.
118. Drinker H, Mall JC: Radiologic aspects of the new universal proximal femoral hip prosthesis. Am J Roentgenol *129*:531, 1977.
119. Thompson FR: Two and one-half years' experience with the vitallium intra-medullary hip prosthesis. J Bone Joint Surg *36A*:489, 1954.
120. D'Ambrosia RD, Chuinard RG, D'Amico DM, Shortley HF, Becker JC: An analysis of dislocation of the cemented femoral hemiarthroplasty. Surg Gynecol Obstet *141*:534, 1975.
121. Brewster RC, Coventry MB, Johnson EW: Conversion of the arthrodesed hip to a total hip arthroplasty. J Bone Joint Surg *57A*:27, 1975.
122. Thompson FR: The role of hip fusion in osteoarthritis. Clin Orthop Rel Res *31*:24, 1963.
123. Nelson CL: Femoral head and neck excision arthroplasty. Orthop Clin North Am *2*:127, 1971.
124. Batchelor JS: Pseudoarthrosis for ankylosis and arthritis of the hip. J Bone Joint Surg *31B*:135, 1949.
125. Ferrari A, Charnley J: Conversion of hip joint pseudoarthrosis to total hip replacement. Clin Orthop Rel Res *121*:12, 1976.
126. Cockin J: Osteotomy of the hip. Orthop Clin North Am *2*:59, 1971.
127. Nissen KI: The arrest of early primary osteoarthritis of the hip by osteotomy. Proc Royal Soc Med *56*:1051, 1963.
128. Adam A, Spence AJ: Intertrochanteric osteotomy for osteoarthritis of the hip. Review of 58 operations. J Bone Joint Surg *40B*:218, 1958.
129. Mensor RC, Scheck M: Review of six years' experience with the hanging hip operation. J Bone Joint Surg *50A*:1250, 1968.
130. Gunston FH: Polycentric knee arthroplasty: Prosthetic simulation of normal knee movement. J Bone Joint Surg *53B*:272, 1971.
131. Bryan RS, Peterson LFA: Polycentric total knee arthroplasty. Orthop Clin North Am *4*:575, 1973.
132. Coventry MB, Upshaw JE, Riley LH, Finerman GAM, Turner RH: Geometric total knee arthroplasty. I. Conception, design, indications, and surgical technique. Clin Orthop Rel Res *94*:171, 1973.
133. Mazas FB: Guepar total knee prosthesis. Clin Orthop Rel Res *94*:211, 1973.
134. Merryweather R, Jones GB: Total knee replacement: The Walldius arthroplasty. Orthop Clin North Am *4*:585, 1973.
135. Shiers LGP: Arthroplasty of the knee. Preliminary report on a new method. J Bone Joint Surg *36B*:553, 1954.
136. Sonstegard DA, Kaufer H, Matthews LS: The spherocentric knee: Biomechanical testing and clinical trial. J Bone Joint Surg *59A*:602, 1977.
137. Insall J, Ranawat CS, Scott WN, Walker P: Total condylar knee replacement: Preliminary report. Clin Orthop Rel Res *120*:149, 1976.
138. Gilula LA, Staple TW: Radiology of recently developed total knee prostheses. Radiol Clin North Am *13*:57, 1975.
139. Goergen TG, Resnick D: Radiology of the total knee replacement. J Can Assoc Radiol *27*:178, 1976.
140. Gelman MI, Dunn HK: Radiology of the knee joint replacement. Am J Roentgenol *127*:447, 1976.
141. Ahlberg A, Linden B: The radiolucent zone in arthroplasty of the knee. Acta Orthop Scand *48*:687, 1977.
142. Mains DB: Marking pin dislocation in total knee arthroplasty. Clin Orthop Rel Res *99*:137, 1974.
143. Hagert CG: Implants designed for finger joints. A roentgenologic study and a study of implant wear and tear. An experimental study. Scand J Plast Reconstr Surg *9*:53, 1975.
144. Calenoff L, Stromberg WB: Silicone rubber arthroplasties of the hand. Radiology *107*:29, 1973.
145. Beckenbaugh RD, Dobyns JH, Linscheid RL, Bryan RS: Review and analysis of silicone-rubber metacarpophalangeal implants. J Bone Joint Surg *58A*:483, 1976.
146. Millender LH, Nalebuff EA, Hawkins RB, Ennis R: Infection after silicone prosthetic arthoplasty in the hand. J Bone Joint Surg *57A*:825, 1975.
147. Ford LT: Osteotomies. Radiol Clin North Am *13*:79, 1975.
148. Coventry MB: Osteotomy about the knee for degenerative and rheumatoid arthritis. Indications, operative technique, and results. J Bone Joint Surg *55A*:23, 1973.
149. Bauer GCH, Insall J, Koshino T: Tibial osteotomy in gonarthrosis (osteoarthritis of the knee). J Bone Joint Surg *51A*:1545, 1969.
150. Torgerson WR: Tibial osteotomy in the treatment of osteoarthritis of the knee. Surg Clin North Am *45*:779, 1965.

151. Thomas RH, Resnick D, Alazraki NP, Daniel D, Greenfield R: Compartmental evaluation of osteoarthritis of the knee. Radiology *116*:585, 1975.
152. Insall J, Shoji H, Mayer V: High tibial osteotomy. A five year evaluation. J Bone Joint Surg *56A*:1397, 1974.
153. Coventry MB: Osteotomy of the upper portion of the tibia for degenerative arthritis of the knee. A preliminary report. J Bone Joint Surg *47A*:984, 1965.
154. Kettelkamp DB, Leach RE, Nasca R: Pitfalls of proximal tibial osteotomy. Clin Orthop Rel Res *106*:232, 1975.
155. Shoji H, Insall J: High tibial osteotomy for osteoarthritis of the knee with valgus deformity. J Bone Joint Surg *55A*:963, 1973.
156. Reing CM, Richin PF, Kenmore PI: Differential bone-scanning in evaluation of a painful total joint replacement. J Bone Joint Surg *61A*:933, 1979.
157. Marmor L: Stress fracture of the pubic ramus simulating a loose total hip replacement. Clin Orthop Rel Res *121*:103, 1976.
158. Kuhns LR, Baublis JV, Gregory J, et al: In vitro effect of cystographic contrast media on urinary tract pathogens. Invest Radiol *7*:112, 1972.
159. Ghelman B: Three methods for determining anteversion and retroversion of a total hip prosthesis. Am J Roentgenol *133*:1127, 1979.
160. Williamson BRJ, McLaughlin RE, Wang G, Miller CW, Teates D, Bray ST: Radionuclide bone imaging as a means of differentiating loosening and infection in patients with a painful total hip prosthesis. Radiology *133*:723, 1979.
161. Weiss PE, Mall JC, Hoffer PB, Murray WR, Rodrigo JJ, Genant HK: ^{99m}Tc-methylene diphosphonate bone imaging in the evaluation of total hip prostheses. Radiology *133*:727, 1979.
162. Rosenthall L, Lisbona R, Hernandez M, Hadjipavlou A: ^{99m}Tc-PP and 67-Ga imaging following insertion of orthopedic devices. Radiology *133*:717, 1979.
163. Carlsson AS, Magnusson B, Moller H: Metal sensitivity in patients with metal-to-plastic total hip arthroplasties. Acta Orthop Scand *51*:57, 1980.
164. Pellicci PM, Inglis AE, Salvati EA: Perforation of the femoral shaft during total hip replacement. Report of twelve cases. J Bone Joint Surg *62A*:234, 1980.
165. Rand JA, Coventry MB: Stress fractures after total knee arthroplasty. J Bone Joint Surg *62A*:226, 1980.
166. Poss R, Sledge CB: Rheumatoid arthritic patients are at increased risk to develop infection following total joint replacement (Abstr). Arthritis Rheum *23*:733, 1980.
167. Pearlman AW: The painful hip prosthesis: Value of nuclear imaging in the diagnosis of late complications. Clin Nucl Med *5*:133, 1980.
168. Hunter JC, Hattner RS, Murray WR, Genant HK: Loosening of the total knee arthroplasty: Detection by radionuclide bone scanning. Am J Roentgenol *135*:131, 1980.
169. Roffman M, Hirsh DM, Mendes DG: Fracture of the resurfaced patella in total knee replacement. Clin Orthop Rel Res *148*:112, 1980.
170. Rose RM, Nusbaum HJ, Schneider H, Ries M, Paul I, Crugnola A, Simon SR, Radin EL: On the true wear rate of ultra high-molecular-weight polyethylene in the total hip prosthesis. J Bone Joint Surg *62A*:537, 1980.
171. Merritt K, Brown SA: Tissue reaction and metal sensitivity. An animal study. Acta Orthop Scand *51*:403, 1980.
172. Baldursson H, Hansson LI, Olsson TH, Selvic G: Migration of the acetabular socket after total hip replacement determined by roentgen stereophotogrammetry. Acta Orthop Scand *51*:535, 1980.

INDEX

Page numbers in *italics* indicate illustrations; (t) indicates tables.